T. Vitale

# Cardiopulmonary Physical Therapy

# *Cardiopulmonary Physical Therapy*

## THIRD EDITION

**Edited by**

**Scot Irwin**, M.S., P.T.

*Regional Director for Physiotherapy Associates*
*Atlanta, Georgia;*
*Instructor in Physical Therapy*
*Emory University*
*Atlanta, Georgia;*
*Adjunct Faculty,*
*Massachusetts General Hospital*

**Jan Stephen Tecklin**, M.S., P.T.

*Associate Professor*
*Department of Physical Therapy*
*Beaver College*
*Glenside, Pennsylvania*

*with 32 contributors*
*with 475 illustrations*

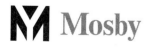 Mosby

St. Louis  Baltimore  Boston  Carlsbad  Chicago  Naples  New York  Philadelphia  Portland
London  Madrid  Mexico City  Singapore  Sydney  Tokyo  Toronto  Wiesbaden

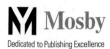
**Mosby**
Dedicated to Publishing Excellence

A Times Mirror
Company

Editor: Martha Sasser
Associate Developmental Editor: Kellie White
Project Manager: Peggy Fagen
Editing and Production: Graphic World Publishing Services
Designer: Jeanne Wolfgeher

**THIRD EDITION**
**Copyright © 1995 by Mosby–Year Book, Inc.**

Printed in the United States of America
Composition by Graphic World, Inc.
Printing/binding by Maple-Vail Book Manufacturing Group

Mosby–Year Book, Inc.
11830 Westline Industrial Drive
St. Louis, MO 63146

**Library of Congress Cataloging-in-Publication Data**

Cardiopulmonary physical therapy / edited by Scot Irwin, Jan Stephen Tecklin.—3rd ed.
        p.      cm.
    Includes bibliographical references and index.
    ISBN 0-8016-7926-5
    1. Cardiopulmonary system—Diseases—Physical therapy.   I. Irwin, Scot.
II. Tecklin, Jan Stephen.
    [DNLM:  1. Cardiovascular Diseases—rehabilitation.   2. Respiration
Disorders—rehabilitation.  3. Physical therapy—methods.   WG 166 C265 1995]
RC702.C37   1995
616.2′00462—dc20
DNLM / DLC
for Library of Congress                                                    95-3210
                                                                            CIP

98  99  /  9  8  7  6  5  4  3  2

# Contributors

**Susan Enriquez Alvarez, B.S., P.T.**
Private Practice
Oxnard, California

**David Arnall, Ph.D., P.T.**
Associate Professor
Department of Physical Therapy
Northern Arizona University
Flagstaff, Arizona

**Raymond L. Blessey, M.A., P.T.**
President
Blessey CV Assessment and Treatment
  Service
Associate Adjunct Professor
School of Physical Therapy
University of Southern California
Los Angeles, California

**Barbara Bernard Butler, M.S., P.T.**
Surgical Chest Clinical Specialist
University Hospital
University of Michigan Medical Center
Ann Arbor, Michigan

**Lawrence P. Cahalin, P.T.**
Staff Development/Clinical Educator and
  Research Coordinator
Physical Therapy Department
St. Luke's Hospital
Cedar Rapids, Iowa

**Frank Cerny, Ph.D.**
Associate Professor and Director of
  Graduate Studies
Department of Physical Therapy and
  Exercise Science
S.U.N.Y. at Buffalo
Buffalo, New York

**Linda D. Crane, M.M.Sc., P.T., C.C.S.**
Instructor
Division of Physical Therapy
Department of Orthopaedics and
  Rehabilitation
University of Miami
School of Medicine
Coral Gables, Florida

**Joan Darbee, M.S., P.T.**
Teaching Assistant
Department of Physical Therapy and
  Exercise Science
S.U.N.Y. at Buffalo
Buffalo, New York

**Jeanne A. DeCesare, M.S., P.T.**
Private Practice
Milton, Massachusetts;
Formerly Research Physical Therapist
Department of Physical Therapy
The Children's Hospital
Boston, Massachusetts

**Barry R. Dix**
Private Practice
Atlanta Cardiopulmonary Associates
Riverdale, Georgia

**Joanne R. Eisenhardt, M.B.A., Ph.D., P.T.**
Associate Professor
Institute for Physical Therapy Education
Widener University
Chester, Pennsylvania

**Ronald Freireich, M.D.**
Private Practice
Atlanta Cardiopulmonary Associates
Riverdale, Georgia

**Joan H. Gault, M.D.**
Associate Professor
Temple University School of Medicine
Department of Physiology
Philadelphia, Pennsylvania

**Anne L. Gould, B.S., P.T.**
Assistant Supervisor of Physical Therapy
Children's Hospital of Boston
Boston, Massachusetts

**Carole A. Graybill-Tucker, P.T.**
Formerly Assistant Supervisor
Cardiopulmonary Rotation
Children's Hospital of Boston
Boston, Massachusetts

**Willy E. Hammon, P.T.**
Director
Rehabilitative Services
Oklahoma Memorial Hospital
Oklahoma Medical Center;
Special Instructor
Department of Physical Therapy
University of Oklahoma Health Science
  Center
Norman, Oklahoma

**Lana Hilling, C.R.T.T., R.C.P.**
Pulmonary Rehabilitation Coordinator
Pulmonary Rehabilitation Program
Mt. Diablo Medical Center
Concord, California

**Thomas R. Holtackers, P.T.**
Hand Clinic
Mayo Clinic
Rochester, Minnesota

**Nancy Humberstone, B.S., M.M.Sc., P.T.**
Roswell, Georgia

**Randolph G. Ice, P.T.**
President
SCOR Physical Therapy
Whittier, California;
President
Lynwood Physical Therapy
Lynwood, California;
President
Laguna Center Physical Therapy
Laguna Niguel, California;
Clinical Instructor
Department of Physical Therapy
Mount St. Mary's College
West Los Angeles, California

**P. Cristina Imle, M.S., P.T.**
Clinical Instructor
Department of Physical Therapy
School of Medicine
University of Maryland
Baltimore, Maryland

**Scot Irwin, P.T.**
Regional Director for Physiotherapy
  Associates
Atlanta, Georgia;
Instructor in Physical Therapy
Emory University
Atlanta, Georgia;
Adjunct Faculty,
Massachusetts General Hospital

**Brenda Rae Lunsford, M.S., P.T.**
Formerly Department of Physical
  Therapy
Rancho Los Amigos Hospital
Downey, California

**Barbara A. Mammen, M.N., R.N.,
C.C.R.N.**
Clinical Nurse Specialist
Clayton General Hospital
Riverdale, Georgia

**Claire Peel, Ph.D., P.T.**
Chairman
Department of Physical Therapy
School of Allied Health Sciences
University of Texas Medical Branch at
  Galveston
Galveston, Texas

**Margery J. Peterson, M.S., P.T.**
Home Health Physical Therapist
Auburn Faith Hospital
Auburn, California

**Thomas H. Shaffer, Ph.D.**
Professor
Department of Physiology and Pediatrics
Temple University School of Medicine
Philadelphia, Pennsylvania

**Z. David Skloven, M.D.**
Associate Medical Director
Arizona Heart Institute, East
Mesa, Arizona

**Jan Smith, M.S., P.T.**
Coordinator of Ergonomic Program
Health and Fitness Institute;
Physical Therapist
Pulmonary Rehabilitation Program
Mt. Diablo Medical Center
Concord, California

**Jan Stephen Tecklin, M.S., P.T.**
Associate Professor
Department of Physical Therapy
Beaver College
Glenside, Pennsylvania

**Jane L. Wetzel, M.S., P.T.**
Academic Coordinator of Clinical
  Education
School of Physical Therapy
Slippery Rock University
Slippery Rock, Pennsylvania

**Marla R. Wolfson, Ph.D., P.T.**
Assistant Professor
Department of Physiology and Pediatrics
Temple University School of Medicine
Philadelphia, Pennsylvania

In Memory of
**Eli Raymond, Jim Thomas, Robert Gauthier,** and **Bill Kennedy**
from whom we learned so much about life and living

*Scot Irwin*


To
**Ashley Joy Tecklin**
and
**Colby David Tecklin—**
each a blessing

*Jan Stephen Tecklin*

# Preface to First Edition

*Cardiopulmonary Physical Therapy* is, first and foremost, a text intended for the entry-level physical therapy student and the practicing therapist inexperienced in either cardiac rehabilitation or respiratory care. We, the editors, believe that since such close interaction exists between the cardiovascular and respiratory systems, a book about one without the other would have been an incomplete effort. Therefore, the first nine chapters of the book describe the essentials of cardiac rehabilitation—structure, assessment, and program planning—and the following twelve chapters discuss assessment and treatment of patients with a wide variety of acute and chronic pulmonary disorders.

Chapter 1 presents the philosophical approach to and the organizational structure of a rehabilitation program for a patient with coronary artery disease. Chapter 2 examines the pathogenesis of atherosclerosis, which accounts for the majority of cases of heart disease among adults in our society. Hemodynamic considerations of the cardiac patient and pharmacological intervention for this patient group are detailed in Chapters 3 and 4, respectively. Although these two topics are not commonly presented in detail in other physical therapy literature, we strongly believe that an understanding of these topics is critical to developing a scientifically sound rationale for the approach to physical rehabilitation of a person with atherosclerotic coronary artery disease. Aberrant physiological responses to exercise that commonly occur in patients who suffer from impaired myocardial circulation and function are delineated in Chapter 5. A comprehensive and systematic evaluation of patients is described in the following chapter. Using information obtained from the evaluation, a treatment approach is offered in Chapter 7 by which a therapist can plan and implement a comprehensive rehabilitation program that is individualized for each patient. Chapter 8 describes the beneficial effects of aerobic exercise for heart patients. This notion is supported by an extensive review of scientific evidence. The final chapter of this portion of the book is a description of the administrative and management strategies necessary for the effective daily operation of a cardiac rehabilitation program.

The second portion of *Cardiopulmonary Physical Therapy* presents basic science and clinical information regarding the pulmonary system. Chapters 10 through 21 are organized differently from the first nine chapters, in that the bulk of the material in the latter chapters is based on specific groups of patients with pulmonary disease or respiratory dysfunction. Chapter 10 describes the normal structure and function of the lungs and chest wall. Chapter 11 discusses the major patterns of acute respiratory failure and the medical management of patients with each type of failure. Chapters 12 and 13 describe the basic knowledge and skills that the physical therapist needs to both assess and treat patients with varying disorders or diseases of the chest.

Each of the remaining eight chapters discusses in depth a major patient group whose members benefit from physical rehabilitation. Chapter 14 reviews the many common types of thoracic and abdominal operative procedures in which physical therapy plays a major role in both preventing and treating pulmonary complications. Chapter 15 examines the acutely ill patient with medical chest disease who is being treated in the intensive care unit. With the enormous increase in the use of mechanical ventilation during the last two decades, a new patient group with a common problem—ventilator dependency—has arisen. Suggestions for physical rehabilitation of patients with ventilator dependency are presented in Chapter 16. Virtually nowhere in patient care has there been a more rapid advance in technology and care than in neonatology. This topic is succinctly described in Chapter 17. Acute and chronic respiratory problems in toddlers and children is the content in Chapter 18. An approach to rehabilitation of patients with chronic obstructive pulmonary disease is suggested in Chapter 19. Respiratory muscle strengthening is a subject that has been discussed at length in the pulmonary literature in recent years. A concise review of the muscular activities that result in improved pulmonary ventilation is found in Chapter 20. The final chapter of the book examines the management of respiratory complications of acute spinal cord injuries.

Since patients with cardiopulmonary disorders frequently require orthopaedic and neurological intervention, we have provided a detailed index to Volume Two, *Orthopaedic and Sports Physical Therapy,* and Volume Three, *Neurological Rehabilitation.*

Each of the patient-problem chapters presents a review of the basic problems associated with the patient group, suggests an approach to patient assessment, describes treatment procedures, and supports the major assertions with a review of the scientific literature on the subject. This last aspect of these chapters—scientific support—is one of the most important aspects of the pulmonary portion of the text. Most other books and monographs about physical therapy for the patient with respiratory problems provide, as this work does, methods of treatment for various problems. Many other textbooks, especially those from Great Britain, provide little if any scientific support for their recommended treatment approaches. One of the major strengths of *Cardiopulmonary Physical Therapy* is the review of published research that supports the assertions of the contributors regarding approaches to treatment; that is, the contributors not only report what to do but also provide, where such information exists, a reasonable scientific rationale for their suggestions.

Although this book is one of a three-volume series, it is particularly important in concept at this time. Cardiac rehabilitation is a relatively new arena in which physical therapists have been working. There is a constant overlapping of perceived responsibility among the several health professions and technical groups that engage in rehabilitation of the patient with coronary artery disease. It is not our intent or that of the contributors to suggest who does what in cardiac care. Rather, the attempt here is to delineate clearly the knowledge and skill necessary for the physical therapist or other professional to provide exemplary care for the patient with heart disease. As physical therapists become more knowledgeable and skillful in providing an optimal level of care, our importance as members of the cardiac rehabilitation effort will become both obvious and unchallengeable.

There exists a similar scenario within respiratory care. Physical therapists in the United States have been involved in acute and chronic respiratory care for more than 50 years. In the last two decades, physical therapists, for many reasons, have often voluntarily disassociated themselves from the patient who had respiratory difficulty. During this period, the development of oxygen technicians to inhalation therapists to respiratory therapists has been remarkable. Is it naïve to believe that there is a cause-and-effect relationship? Regardless, there is a clear need and a clear responsibility for each group. In addition, there is some area of overlap that is dealt with differently from hospital to hospital.

Why discuss this issue here? One of the major purposes of the pulmonary section of *Cardiopulmonary Physical Therapy* is to defuse, at least within physical therapy, the notion that "chest PT" is equivalent to bronchial drainage with manual percussion and vibration. Our skills in assessment and treatment of musculoskeletal disorders, our knowledge of exercise, and our ability to remedy movement dysfunction provide physical therapists a large responsibility for the rehabilitation of the varied groups of patients with pulmonary and respiratory disorders. When these skills are combined with the skills needed for provision of bronchial hygiene and prevention of postoperative pulmonary complications, the physical therapist's major contribution to chest patients should be obvious. To deny this contribution and to ignore our role is, in our opinion, a frivolous abdication of our responsibility to these patients. None of us wants to clap chests for 8 hours each day. Rather, we choose to provide judicious and skillful physical assessment and rehabilitation, combined with appropriate use of bronchial hygiene techniques, to offer wide-ranging therapeutic expertise. This expertise can be appropriately employed in settings that range from the intensive care unit to the home and can include every setting along that recovery route.

This book provides the necessary information for the inexperienced therapist to assume the responsibility to the millions of patients in the United States who suffer from some cardiopulmonary disorder that can be treated with physical rehabilitation methods.

*Scot Irwin*
*Jan Stephen Tecklin*

# Preface to Second Edition

The success enjoyed by the first edition of *Cardiopulmonary Physical Therapy* is gratifying, but it challenges the editors to provide a second edition that is better than the first. We improved this textbook in a number of ways. Almost all authors updated their previous chapters. These updates include an in-depth review of technological advances, such as heart transplantation; an examination of diseases (e.g., AIDS) that have become more prevalent since the first edition was prepared; and an examination of practice trends, such as home care of the ventilator patient.

In addition to the updated material, six new chapters provide a more comprehensive and in-depth discussion of physical therapy for cardiac and pulmonary patients. Barbara Mammen presents the basics of electrocardiography. Ronald Freireich discusses the medical management of the patient admitted with acute myocardial infarction. Joanne Eisenhardt reviews the physiology, pathology, evaluation, and treatment of the peripheral vasculature. Claire Peel bridges the cardiac and pulmonary systems with her excellent presentation of cardiopulmonary changes with aging. Joan Darbee and Frank Cerny offer an approach to a growing area of cardiopulmonary care in their chapter about exercise testing and training for children with chronic lung disease. Finally, Jan Tecklin examines common lung diseases.

We believe this second edition offers educators, students, and clinicians a textbook that is as useful and current as the first edition, and that this edition also provides greater depth and is more comprehensive. *Cardiopulmonary Physical Therapy* should provide the knowledge for physical therapists to continue their 70-year tradition of excellent care for those with heart and lung disease.

*Scot Irwin*
*Jan Stephen Tecklin*

# Preface to Third Edition

The third edition of *Cardiopulmonary Physical Therapy* includes revisions to virtually all chapters and the addition of several new chapters.

Part One: Cardiac Physical Therapy and Rehabilitation includes updated material for each chapter, a complete revision of Chapter 4, "Pharmaceutical Considerations," and major revision and new case studies in Chapter 9, "Program Planning and Implementation." In addition, we moved "Evaluation and Physical Treatment of the Patient with Peripheral Vascular Disorders" into the cardiac section of the book.

Part Two: Pulmonary Physical Therapy and Rehabilitation includes updated chapters and several new chapters. David Arnall presents basic pulmonary pharmacology in Chapter 16. P. Cristina Imle offers a new chapter 20:

"Physical Therapy for Patients with Cardiac, Thoracic, or Abdominal Conditions Following Surgery or Trauma." Chapter 21, "Physical Therapy in Heart and Lung Transplantation," offers a complete perspective in this exciting and difficult new patient group, and is ably described by Barbara Bernard Butler. The final major change is a new Chapter 23: "Pulmonary Rehabilitation," jointly authored by Lana Hilling and Jan Smith. We believe these changes augment and update the third edition of *Cardiopulmonary Physical Therapy* to reflect changes in contemporary practice and technology while maintaining our primary focus of providing an educational tool for entry-level students in physical therapy.

*Scot Irwin*
*Jan Stephen Tecklin*

# Contents

# Cardiopulmonary Physical Therapy

# PART ONE

# *Cardiac Physical Therapy and Rehabilitation*

# CHAPTER 1

# Philosophy and Structure of a Cardiac Rehabilitation Program

*Scot Irwin*

Part One of *Cardiopulmonary Physical Therapy* is devoted to the development, implementation, and potential impact of a program of rehabilitation of patients with coronary artery disease. The approach to cardiac rehabilitation presented in the following pages is derived from a philosophy of patient care that uses available scientific knowledge of coronary artery disease, specific team and patient goals, and specialized clinical skills to create an individualized program. This philosophy has been applied successfully in a variety of hospital settings, from large university-based rehabilitation centers to rural community hospitals.

## PHILOSOPHICAL FOUNDATION

One key to effective cardiac rehabilitation is to thoroughly understand the philosophical principles on which it is based. Our philosophy is based on three essential principles.

The first principle is that coronary artery disease is a progressive, chronic disease process closely aligned with certain epidemiologically documented risk factors. The second is that an exercise program for patients after a heart attack or surgical intervention is beneficial if it is individually designed for each patient and objectively evaluated on an ongoing basis. The final principle is that the process of cardiac rehabilitation requires a team approach. Cardiac rehabilitation requires an enormous amount of patient and family education, covering a multitude of medical specialty areas. No *one* health care professional can adequately provide all the services needed to conduct an effective program of rehabilitation.

## RISK FACTOR MODIFICATION

Patients with coronary artery disease are suffering from a chronic, generally progressive disease process known as atherosclerosis. The exact cause of this disease is not well understood but it is associated with certain well-documented risk factors. These risk factors have been studied extensively and are generally prominent in modern societies where an abundance of high-fat foods and leisure time is available (see Chapter 2).

The program described in this text attempts to reduce those risk factors associated with the atherosclerotic disease process. The goal is to educate all patients about the various risk factors and to give each patient and his or her family a specific list of those risk factors that apply directly to his or her case. It is important to educate patients that reducing their risk factors does not guarantee that the disease will not progress further. Risk factor reduction should not be considered a cure; it is simply a logical approach to a poorly understood disease process. The scientific data to support risk factor modification as a means of reducing coronary mortality and morbidity are extensive (see Chapter 2). Because risk factors increase the chance of developing atherosclerosis, it follows that reducing them will decrease the risk of further disease progression.

Risk factor modification often requires major life-style

changes for the patient with coronary artery disease. Thus one of the principles of our program is to convey to patients that their program of cardiac rehabilitation requires lifelong application. Our educational and exercise programs are directed toward having patients follow through with their program at home.

## OBJECTIVE CONTINUOUS EVALUATION OF EXERCISE RESPONSES

An effective, safe exercise program for patients with coronary artery disease must be based on objective, continuous evaluation of their responses. Exercise responses must be assessed by measuring and interpreting the five available clinical monitoring tools: heart rate, blood pressure, electrocardiogram, heart and lung sounds, and symptoms. Additional elements to be considered when developing an exercise program for cardiac patients include medical history, medications, hemodynamic function, coronary anatomy, extent of and time since infarction, and the patient's goals and psychological condition.

Each change in a patient's exercise program should be based on a thorough objective evaluation. Thus, progression of a patient's activity level throughout the rehabilitation process can be determined using objective measures. If this principle is followed by a therapist with good clinical skills, there is no need for patients to follow arbitrary step-by-step programs to progress their activity levels. Continuous evaluation of patient exercise responses creates an individualized, safe, and effective progression of activity.

## TEAM APPROACH

To achieve a unified approach, the team should be led by a patient care coordinator. The coordinator works with each member of the team to implement team goals and to ensure that all team members advocate the same principles of patient care. The coordinator should have a sound background in electrophysiology, pathophysiology, exercise physiology, and patient care concepts. The coordinator should be responsible for educating the various team members in the principles and philosophy of cardiac rehabilitation. An effective team should include a physician, a nurse, a dietitian, a physical therapist, a psychologist, and a medical social worker. Variables such as space, equipment, and patient population will govern the composition of teams at different institutions.

### Team goals

General team goals should not be equated with the patient treatment goals (discussed later). Team goals should include, but are not limited to, the following:

1. Creation of an educational environment in which patients are given clear, concise, and consistent guidance
2. Agreement that patients should be taught to accept the program goals as part of a lifelong endeavor

3. Delegation of patient problems and questions to the appropriate team member for resolution

### Patient goals

The patient's own goals must be constantly assessed throughout the rehabilitation program and the physical therapist should always keep them in mind. As patients begin to understand and accept the seriousness of their disease and the life-style changes that must be made to improve their chances of survival, these goals may often change dramatically.

Commonly, patients' initial goals are to get home and back to work. They often feel fine, and overtly or covertly deny that they have anything wrong with them. They often believe that their physician has made a mistake. However, as they begin to understand the disease process and accept their condition, their goals begin to change. As the weeks of rehabilitation go by, therapists must continually help patients reassess their goals.

The patient's own goals supersede any other goals that the team members may have determined, because little patient compliance will be achieved unless his or her goals are incorporated into the program.

## CLINICAL KNOWLEDGE AND SKILLS

To participate effectively in a cardiac rehabilitation program, a physical therapist must possess knowledge in cardiopulmonary anatomy and physiology, pathophysiology of arteriosclerosis and coronary artery disease, normal and abnormal cardiac hemodynamics, normal and abnormal exercise physiology, pharmacological effects of cardiac medications, and electrophysiology. The reader is strongly urged to explore these areas in depth by reviewing and studying the selected references listed at the end of each chapter in this book.

## CLINICAL SKILLS DEVELOPMENT

Effective implementation of a cardiac rehabilitation program requires the attainment and use of specialized clinical skills. Therapists with an exceptional level of didactic knowledge may have little success in treating their patients unless their clinical skills are reliable. The clinical data base obtained on every patient must be reproducible and accurate. Without accuracy, physicians will not accept or use the information obtained to modify the patient's medical regimen. Physicians who do not trust the physical therapist's information will be hesitant to refer their patients.

Physical therapists should have the clinical skill and knowledge to rapidly obtain and accurately interpret (1) electrocardiographic changes (ST segments and dysrhythmias), (2) blood pressure responses during exercise, (3) breath sounds and heart sounds, (4) heart rate, and (5) symptoms (especially angina).

Incorporating a philosophical foundation with didactic knowledge and clinical skills helps the physical therapist create a safe, effective, and rewarding program of cardiac rehabilitation.

## BASIC PROGRAM STRUCTURE

The structure of a cardiac rehabilitation program should be directed toward goals common to all patients. The initial goals (phase 1) include (1) screening patients for the appearance of complications, (2) initiating low levels of activity, (3) educating patients and their families, and (4) measuring the effectiveness of medications in controlling patients' cardiovascular status during activity. The emphasis during phase I is on stabilizing the patient's condition and ensuring that general daily activity does not produce undesirable effects. Goals 1 and 4 are not often recognized or listed as goals for an inpatient cardiac rehabilitation program but they are in fact more important to most referring physicians than any other goal.

In general, physicians have a great deal of information about their patients' cardiovascular status in a resting state, but little data about their patients' cardiovascular responses to activity. A physical therapist with the proper knowledge and clinical skills can provide this information. Phase I of a cardiac rehabilitation program should provide the physician with information about patient responses to progressive increases in activity. This information will on occasion cause the physician to make adjustments in patients' medications.

The long-term goals associated with phases II and III of the cardiac rehabilitation program structure echo the philosophy previously discussed. They include (1) reducing risk factors, (2) improving physical work capacity, (3) returning to safe vocational and recreational activity levels, (4) decreasing angina, (5) decreasing fear of the disease, and (6) ensuring frequent objective communication to the physician about patient responses to exercise and medications. The most pronounced impact of phases II and III is achieved when goals 1, 3, 4, and 5 have been attained.

### Postmyocardial infarction

**Phase I: the acute stage.** The acute phase of postmyocardial infarction begins with referral to the cardiac rehabilitation program and ends at discharge from the hospital about 7 to 10 days later. Patients should be referred for cardiac rehabilitation when they are medically stable. This is generally from 3 to 6 days after infarction, depending on whether the patient's condition is complicated or uncomplicated.

As defined by McNeer and others, patients with complications require more time to recover from their acute infarction.* Patients without complications are usually referred to the cardiac rehabilitation program and discharged earlier. Patient rehabilitation programs at this stage consist of a self-care evaluation (see discussions in Chapter

* McNeer JF and others: The course of acute myocardial infarction: feasibility of early discharge of the uncomplicated patient, *Circulation* 51:410, 1975.

7 of patient evaluation, phase I programming, patient and family education, Holter monitoring graduated ambulation, and a predischarge submaximal or low-level treadmill test).

Phase I for patients after bypass surgery is also an inpatient phase, but this usually lasts only 3 to 5 days. The rehabilitation program is often directed more toward preventing the pulmonary complications of the surgery (see Part Two of this text for the pulmonary aspect). Phases II and III are the same for patients after surgery and acute myocardial infarction.

**Phase II: after the acute stage.** Phase II, the subacute phase, begins with completion of the low-level treadmill test and ends when the maximal treadmill test and cardiac catheterization have been completed. This phase may vary from 5 to 12 weeks after infarction or surgery. Six weeks appears to be most common. One may note with some surprise that a cardiac catheterization is included as part of phase II. It has been my experience that proceeding to phase III, high-level exercise training, without catheterization data may be misleading and sometimes unsafe for the patient. The cardiac catheterization gives invaluable and otherwise unobtainable data about heart function and disease severity (see Chapters 2 and 3).

**Phase III: long-term follow-up.** Phase III is the high-level phase, during which the patient continues on an individually designed exercise program based on periodic, formal reevaluations. These reevaluations are in the form of maximal symptom-limited exercise tests conducted 3 months after infarction and annually thereafter. Patients who have appropriate ventricular function and are well controlled medically are encouraged to engage in high levels of aerobic exercise. Phase III ends when the patient's exercise program has achieved a maintenance level. In other words, no further changes in exercise intensity or duration are required.

**Phase IV: lifetime follow through.** When a patient has completed Phase III, he is encouraged to carry out his exercise program independently. This can be completed at a fitness center, health club, hospital, or at home. Patient compliance with lifetime exercise (phase IV) at safe and effective intensities is difficult to achieve. In my experience, most patients will comply best if they remain with a group. Group dynamics and camaraderie help stimulate good compliance. If all phases of cardiac rehabilitation (phases I to IV) are conducted at the same facility, close follow-up and improved compliance may be achieved.

Physical therapy for cardiac patients can be an exciting, rewarding, beneficial experience. Within this text, some key components to developing and conducting a cardiac rehabilitation program are reviewed. Therapists are encouraged to apply the theoretical information and clinical skill descriptions to their individual patient care programs. In this way, the therapist can apply the philosophy, goals, and structure of the cardiac rehabilitation program described herein.

# Atherosclerosis

*An overview of the basic mechanism of atherogenesis, pathophysiology, and natural history*

*Raymond L. Blessey and Scot Irwin*

This chapter is designed to provide essential background information for the chapters that follow. It begins with a review of coronary anatomy and includes discussion of (1) theoretical mechanisms involved with coronary artery and vein graft atherosclerosis, (2) the pathophysiology of the disease process, and (3) the natural history of the disease within the various subsets of patients with coronary artery lesions.

## CORONARY ARTERY ANATOMY

The clinician treating patients with coronary artery disease must have a thorough understanding of coronary anatomy to evaluate and appropriately treat patients. The information that follows is meant to be a review, and one should refer to other texts for a more complete discussion of coronary artery anatomy.[30,36,39,47,95]

There are two major epicardial, or surface coronary, arteries—the right coronary artery and the left main coronary artery. They both originate from the root of the aorta and give off several major epicardial branches and multiple endocardial branches that penetrate the left or right ventricular muscle mass perpendicular to the parent epicardial vessel (Fig. 2-1). The endocardial branches extend to the myocardial wall (referred to as the "subendocardial zone"). It should be emphasized that the exact course of each major epicardial vessel and its branches is variable; therefore, the area of the myocardium each supplies varies as well. Discussions of the most common patterns of coronary artery distribution follow.

### Left coronary artery system

The left main coronary artery is usually 2 to 4 cm long and bifurcates into two major epicardial branches, the left anterior descending artery and the circumflex artery (Fig. 2-2). In some cases, there are one or two additional intermediate epicardial branches that arise at the bifurcation of the left main artery. Such a branch is referred to as a "ramus intermedius."

The left anterior descending artery (LAD) runs along the interventricular groove either up to or around the apex of the heart. In fact, in the majority of cases, the LAD extends beyond the apex and runs up along the posterior interventricular sulcus. The LAD gives off several diagonal branches (epicardial arteries) of varying size. These diagonal branches, along with the parent artery, supply the entire

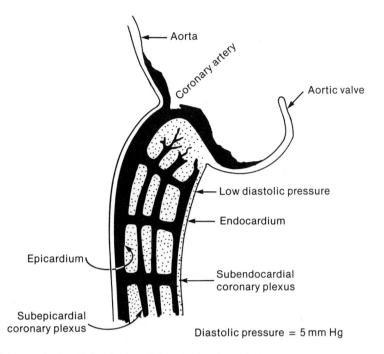

**Fig. 2-1.** Scheme of epicardial, subepicardial, and subendocardial branches. (From Ellestad M: *Stress testing,* Philadelphia, 1976, FA Davis Co.)

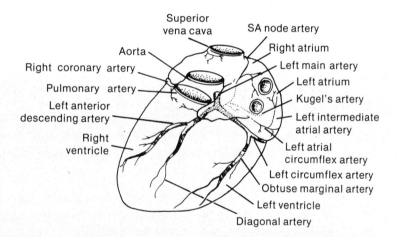

**Fig. 2-2.** Left anterior oblique view of the heart showing the distribution of both the left anterior descending and circumflex arteries and their major epicardial branches. (From Hamby RI, editor: *Clinical-anatomical correlates in coronary artery disease,* Mt Kisco, NY, 1979, Futura Publishing Co, Inc.)

anterior portion of the left ventricle and most of the superior, or lateral, wall of the left ventricle. In addition, the LAD gives off a series of septal perforators (endocardial vessels) that begin at the proximal segment of the parent vessel and run in an anteroposterior plane. These endocardial vessels off the LAD supply two thirds of the upper or superior portion of the interventricular septum and all of the interior aspect of the septum. It is not uncommon for the LAD to supply smaller branches (endocardial vessels) to portions of the right ventricle as well. These branches often anastomose with branches from the right coronary artery (RCA).

The left circumflex artery (LCA) usually arises at a perpendicular angle to the left main artery and runs beneath the left atrial appendage and along the atrioventricular groove (Fig. 2-2). In approximately 12% of the cases, the LCA continues along the atrioventricular groove to the crux (junction between the atrioventricular, interatrial, and interventricular sulci) and gives off a posterior descending artery. In the majority of the cases, the LCA terminates at the obtuse margin (edge between apex of the heart and pulmonary artery root) and gives off a varying number of arteries referred to as obtuse marginal branches. The number of

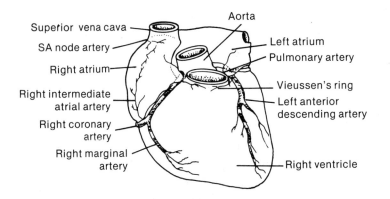

**Fig. 2-3.** Anterior or front view of the heart showing the distribution of the right coronary artery and the left anterior descending artery. (From Hamby RI, editor: *Clinical-anatomical correlates in coronary artery disease,* Mt Kisco, NY, 1979, Futura Publishing Co, Inc.)

branches that the circumflex artery gives off to the posterior wall of the left ventricle is indirectly (and reciprocally) related to the distribution of the RCA and its branches.

In summary, the left coronary artery system supplies up to 70% of the left ventricular muscle mass and at least 54% of the right and left ventricular muscle mass. The LAD and its branches supply the entire anterior wall of the left ventricle, most of the superior wall, the majority of the interventricular septum, the anterior wall of the right ventricle, the anterior papillary muscle, the proximal portion of the right bundle branch, the anterior division of the left bundle branch, and the AV node via an anterior septal perforator. The circumflex artery distribution is variable, but it usually supplies portions of the superior and marginal left ventricular wall, portions of the posterior left ventricular wall, the left atrial muscle mass, and the lateral papillary muscle. Forty percent of the time, the circumflex gives off a sinus node artery, and in approximately 10% of the cases, the posterior descending artery off the circumflex (via a posterior septal branch) supplies the AV node.

### Right coronary artery system

The right coronary artery (RCA) originates from the right, or anterior, sinus of Valsalva and runs directly inferior in the atrioventricular groove beneath the right atrial appendage (Fig. 2-3). The length and number of branches of the RCA, and therefore the amount of myocardial and nerve tissue it supplies, are inversely proportional to the distribution of the circumflex and to a certain degree the LAD. In 86% of the cases, the RCA extends around to the crux of the heart. The RCA and its branches supply most of the right ventricle muscle mass and inferior surface of the left ventricle, portions of the posterior wall, the posteroinferior aspects of the interventricular septum, and the right atrial muscle mass. In 60% of the cases, the RCA supplies the sinus node artery; in 90% of the cases, the posterior descending artery off the RCA supplies the AV node. In addition, the RCA supplies the distal portion of the right bundle branch and the posterior division of the left bundle branch.

As discussed earlier, there is a reciprocal distribution pattern between the RCA and circumflex artery. Autopsy studies have demonstrated that there are three basic patterns of coronary circulation, the particular pattern being determined by which artery is primarily responsible for the blood supply of the posterior wall of the left ventricle. In approximately 86% of the cases, the RCA reaches the crux of the heart and gives off the posterior descending area, supplying the majority of the left ventricular posterior wall area (Fig. 2-4). In 12% of the cases, the circumflex artery reaches the crux and gives off the posterior descending artery (Fig. 2-5), and in 2% of the cases, both the RCA and circumflex arteries reach the crux (Fig. 2-6) and supply an equal portion of the posterior wall (balanced system). The term "dominant" coronary system has been used to designate the coronary artery responsible for the majority of the posterior wall circulation. Based on the above information, 86% of the cases are right dominant, 12% of the cases are left dominant, and 2% of the cases have a balanced coronary system. The term "dominance," however, does not imply that the "dominant" artery system is responsible for the majority of the blood supply, since, as stated previously, the left coronary system always supplies at least 60% to 70% of the left ventricle muscle.

An awareness of the distribution patterns of the coronary arteries as described above and, more thoroughly, in the recommended references is essential to the clinician whose aim is to evaluate and treat each patient as an individual. The remaining sections of this chapter will make the significance of this baseline knowledge even more evident.

## RISK FACTORS AND THE DEVELOPMENT OF CORONARY ARTERY DISEASE
### Framingham study

In 1949 a prospective epidemiological study of 5209 men and women 30 to 62 years of age was initiated in Framingham, Massachusetts, to determine the relationship between life style and antecedent personal attributes to the development of cardiovascular diseases (atherosclerosis).[18]

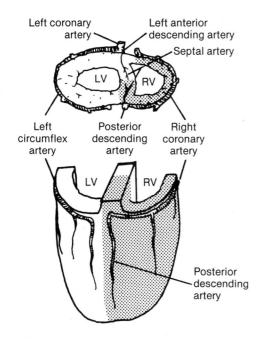

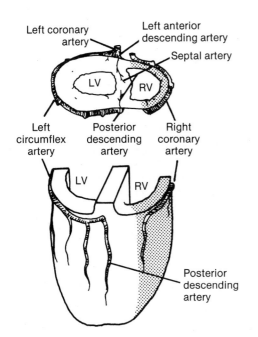

Fig. 2-4. Scheme of a right dominant vascular pattern of the posterior aspect of the heart. In the upper portion of the diagram the heart is viewed from above with the atria removed. *Stippled area.* Portion of the heart supplied by the right coronary artery (RCA). Notice the posterior septal perforator off the RCA supplying the septum and AV node. The clear area of the diagram is supplied by the left coronary artery (left anterior descending and circumflex arteries). (From Hamby RI, editor: *Clinical-anatomical correlates in coronary artery disease,* Mt Kisco, NY, 1979, Futura Publishing Co, Inc.)

Fig. 2-5. Left dominant vascular pattern of the posterior myocardium. Clear area represents portion of the heart supplied by the left coronary artery. See Fig. 2-4 for further explanation. (From Hamby RI, editor: *Clinical-anatomical correlates in coronary artery disease,* Mt Kisco, NY, 1979, Futura Publishing Co, Inc.)

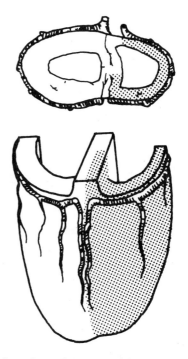

Fig. 2-6. A balanced vascular pattern of the posterior myocardium. Note that both the circumflex and the right coronary artery supply equal portions of the posterior myocardium and the posterior aspect of the septum. See Fig. 2-4 for further explanation. (From Hamby RI, editor: *Clinical-anatomical correlates in coronary artery disease,* Mt Kisco, NY, 1979, Futura Publishing Co, Inc.)

After the initial evaluation, these men and women were followed with biennial examinations including (1) questionnaires dealing with activity level and smoking history, (2) blood chemistry studies, (3) blood pressure evaluation, and (4) resting 12-lead electrocardiogram. The specific design and methods of the study were published in detail in 1963.[18] The study population has been very cooperative, with only 2% of the total population being lost to followup and 80% of the subjects having missed none of the biennial examinations. Because Framingham is a relatively small city with only one general hospital, the investigators have been able to monitor accurately cardiac events in their subjects.

Gordon[33] and Kannel[49] have published papers that update the findings of the Framingham Study and more precisely identify the risk factors for the development of atherosclerosis. Hypertension,[26] smoking, elevated serum cholesterol[26,56] or triglycerides, abnormal glucose tolerance (diabetes), sedentary life-style, family history of coronary disease, age, and male gender are all factors that individually or in combination increase the likelihood or risk of developing coronary artery disease and hence are referred to as risk factors.[31] The studies of Rosenman[81] and Jenkins[48] indicate that personality type (type A versus type B) may be associated with risk of coronary disease. Statistically, the strongest or most predictive risk factors are smoking, elevated cholesterol, and hypertension. The role of genetics and its influence on the individual's resistance to the atherogenic precursors of smoking, hypertension, and so on are not clearly understood. Many experts in the field, most notably Kannel, believe that an adverse family history increases the risk for coronary disease primarily because families share risk factors such as smoking habit, poor diet, sedentary life-style, and tendency to develop hypertension.

Some common misconceptions about these risk factors exist because of the confusion between the so-called normal values, which merely represent the average value for a given population, or because of belief in outdated information. The Framingham statistics indicate that elevation of the systolic blood pressure is as strong a predictor for future coronary disease as elevated diastolic blood pressure for both men and women. Furthermore, the presumably innocuous rise in systolic blood pressure with age is associated with increased risk of future coronary events. The typical "normal" laboratory values for serum cholesterol of 150 to 300 mg/dl that were used as normal values during the 1980s have given way to a new standard. Total cholesterol levels should be 200 mg/dl or less and the total cholesterol to high-density lipoprotein (HDL) ratio should be 5 or less. The Framingham studies indicate that the risk of developing coronary disease varies with the degree of elevation in the serum cholesterol, with a significant increase in risk when the value exceeds 220 mg/dl. Men who smoke as little as 1 to 9 cigarettes per day have 1.6 times the risk of developing atherosclerosis compared with that of the nonsmoker. The statistics for female light smokers are not much different. On the brighter side, quitting smoking can decrease the future risk of a coronary event as much as 50%.

The presence of other coexisting risk factors alters the likelihood of developing coronary artery disease dramatically. For example, a 35-year-old man with elevated systolic blood pressure and serum cholesterol who smokes, can have up to 38 times the risk of a coronary event within 6 years when compared with an age-matched man without risk factors. Table 2-1 illustrates more completely the probability relationship between multiple risk factors at varying levels of severity.[49]

## Cholesterol

As mentioned previously, although total serum cholesterol is a predictor of future coronary events, the studies of Gordon[34] and others[1,14,19,50,70] indicate that it is important to know more about the various components of the serum cholesterol. Cholesterol does not circulate freely in the plasma because it is insoluble in an aqueous solution. Various plasma proteins bind with cholesterol and therefore facilitate transport from the liver to the target organs. These combinations of protein and cholesterol (or triglycerides) are referred to as "lipoproteins." A review article by Grundy[38] provides a more detailed discussion of cholesterol metabolism and transport.

Two major classes of lipoproteins are responsible for the transport of endogenous cholesterol, low-density lipoprotein (LDL) and high-density lipoprotein (HDL).[107] Approximately 70% to 80% of the total serum cholesterol is bound to LDL, the chief transporter of cholesterol to the body cells. HDL functions to transport cholesterol from the body's cholesterol pools (red blood cells, spleen, muscle, adipose tissue) to the liver for excretion. The work of Gordon,[34] and Solymoss,[97] and Miller[70] indicates that elevated serum levels of LDL or low serum levels of HDL or both increase the risk for the development of coronary artery disease. Gordon also reported that the ratio of total cholesterol to the HDL (cholesterol value divided by HDL value) is related to the probability of developing coronary atherosclerosis. A high total cholesterol-to-HDL ratio, such as 10, indicates that only a small portion of the total cholesterol is HDL and places the person at approximately 2 times the normal risk of experiencing a future coronary event.

## Risk factor interrelationships

Finally, in considering the risk factors, it is important to keep in mind that there is a considerable amount of association or interrelationship among them. For example, low HDL values are associated with cigarette smoking,[78] sedentary life-style,[11,61,108] and diabetes.[35] Diabetes is also associated with abnormally elevated serum triglycerides.[57] Thus the risk of developing coronary artery disease is related to multiple factors that are often associated with one another, and the greater the number of risk factors that exist, the greater the likelihood of developing angina, having a myocardial infarction, or dying suddenly from coronary artery disease.

## Venous atherosclerosis

Atherosclerotic changes can and do occur in saphenous vein grafts,[65] and the likelihood of this occurrence relates to the presence or absence of some of the major risk factors. Lie and others[58] reported that 79% of the vein grafts in nine patients with hyperlipidemia who survived for 13 to 75 months after surgery had arteriosclerotic changes. On the other hand, atherosclerosis was found in only 12% of the vein grafts in the patient with normal lipids. Barboriak[8] and Meadows[68] also reported evidence of atherosclerosis in vein grafts of hyperlipidemic patients. The effects of continued smoking, hypertension, and diabetes on vein graft atherosclerosis will require further study.

## Mechanisms of atherogenesis: the relationship to risk factors

Atherosclerosis is a disease process that potentially can affect the majority of the medium and large arteries throughout the body, including the vertebral, basilar, carotid, coronary, femoral, and popliteal arteries, as well as the thoracic and abdominal aortas. Its effects are varied: atherosclerotic changes in the aorta include thinning of the

**Table 2-1.** Probability (per 1000) of having cardiovascular disease within 8 years according to specified characteristics in a 45-year-old man. Framingham Study: 18-year follow-up

| Glucose tolerance | Cholesterol | Does not smoke cigarettes Systolic blood pressure (mm Hg) | | | | | | | Smokes cigarettes Systolic blood pressure (mm Hg) | | | | | | |
|---|---|---|---|---|---|---|---|---|---|---|---|---|---|---|---|
| | | 105 | 120 | 135 | 150 | 165 | 180 | 195 | 105 | 120 | 135 | 150 | 165 | 180 | 195 |
| **No left ventricular hypertrophy by electrocardiogram** | | | | | | | | | | | | | | | |
| Absent | 185 | 22 | 27 | 35 | 43 | 54 | 68 | 84 | 38 | 47 | 59 | 73 | 91 | 112 | 138 |
| | 210 | 28 | 35 | 43 | 54 | 68 | 84 | 104 | 47 | 59 | 73 | 91 | 113 | 138 | 169 |
| | 235 | 35 | 44 | 54 | 68 | 84 | 104 | 129 | 59 | 74 | 91 | 113 | 139 | 169 | 205 |
| | 260 | 44 | 55 | 68 | 85 | 105 | 129 | 158 | 74 | 92 | 113 | 139 | 170 | 206 | 247 |
| | 285 | 55 | 68 | 85 | 105 | 129 | 158 | 192 | 92 | 113 | 139 | 170 | 206 | 247 | 293 |
| | 310 | 68 | 85 | 105 | 130 | 158 | 192 | 232 | 114 | 140 | 170 | 206 | 248 | 294 | 345 |
| | 335 | 85 | 105 | 130 | 159 | 193 | 232 | 277 | 140 | 171 | 207 | 248 | 295 | 346 | 401 |
| Present | 185 | 39 | 49 | 61 | 76 | 95 | 117 | 143 | 67 | 83 | 102 | 126 | 154 | 188 | 226 |
| | 210 | 49 | 61 | 76 | 95 | 117 | 144 | 175 | 83 | 103 | 126 | 155 | 188 | 227 | 271 |
| | 235 | 62 | 77 | 95 | 117 | 144 | 176 | 212 | 103 | 127 | 155 | 189 | 227 | 271 | 320 |
| | 260 | 77 | 95 | 118 | 144 | 176 | 213 | 255 | 127 | 156 | 189 | 228 | 272 | 321 | 374 |
| | 285 | 96 | 118 | 145 | 176 | 213 | 255 | 303 | 156 | 189 | 228 | 272 | 321 | 375 | 431 |
| | 310 | 118 | 145 | 177 | 214 | 256 | 303 | 355 | 190 | 229 | 273 | 322 | 375 | 432 | 490 |
| | 335 | 145 | 177 | 214 | 256 | 304 | 356 | 411 | 229 | 273 | 323 | 376 | 433 | 491 | 550 |
| **Left ventricular hypertrophy by electrocardiogram** | | | | | | | | | | | | | | | |
| Absent | 185 | 60 | 75 | 93 | 115 | 141 | 172 | 208 | 101 | 124 | 152 | 185 | 223 | 266 | 315 |
| | 210 | 75 | 93 | 115 | 141 | 172 | 209 | 250 | 124 | 152 | 185 | 223 | 267 | 315 | 363 |
| | 235 | 93 | 115 | 142 | 173 | 209 | 251 | 297 | 153 | 186 | 224 | 267 | 316 | 369 | 425 |
| | 260 | 116 | 142 | 173 | 209 | 251 | 298 | 349 | 186 | 224 | 268 | 316 | 369 | 426 | 484 |
| | 285 | 142 | 173 | 210 | 252 | 298 | 350 | 405 | 225 | 268 | 317 | 370 | 426 | 485 | 543 |
| | 310 | 174 | 210 | 252 | 299 | 351 | 406 | 464 | 269 | 318 | 371 | 427 | 485 | 544 | 602 |
| | 335 | 211 | 253 | 300 | 351 | 406 | 464 | 523 | 318 | 371 | 428 | 486 | 545 | 602 | 657 |
| Present | 185 | 105 | 129 | 158 | 191 | 231 | 275 | 324 | 170 | 205 | 246 | 293 | 344 | 399 | 456 |
| | 210 | 129 | 158 | 192 | 231 | 275 | 325 | 378 | 206 | 247 | 293 | 344 | 399 | 457 | 516 |
| | 235 | 158 | 192 | 232 | 276 | 325 | 379 | 436 | 247 | 294 | 345 | 400 | 457 | 516 | 574 |
| | 260 | 193 | 232 | 277 | 326 | 380 | 436 | 495 | 294 | 346 | 400 | 458 | 517 | 575 | 631 |
| | 285 | 232 | 277 | 327 | 380 | 437 | 496 | 554 | 346 | 401 | 459 | 518 | 576 | 632 | 635 |
| | 310 | 278 | 327 | 381 | 438 | 496 | 555 | 612 | 402 | 459 | 518 | 576 | 633 | 685 | 734 |
| | 335 | 328 | 382 | 438 | 497 | 556 | 613 | 667 | 460 | 519 | 577 | 633 | 686 | 734 | 773 |

From Kannel WB: Some lessons in cardiovascular epidemiology from Framingham, *Am J Cardiol* 37:269, 1976.

media, weakening of the vessel wall, aneurysm, and rupture, whereas the major change in the coronary artery is a stenotic, occlusive lesion. The focus of the following information is on the atherosclerotic process that leads to the occlusive lesions that typically form in the coronary arteries.

It is clear from the previous discussion that there are certain factors that increase the likelihood of developing coronary artery disease or vein-graft atherosclerosis.[87] However, a cause-and-effect relationship between the risk factors and atherosclerosis cannot be assumed on the basis of the epidemiological studies alone. Salel and others[86] investigated the relationship between a risk factor index (score derived from total number of risk factors) and the presence or absence of coronary disease found at the time of angiography. In this study a significant relationship was found between the risk factor index and coronary disease. In addition, the study results indicated that patients with multivessel disease had significantly higher risk factor indexes than patients with single vessel disease. The specific relationship between the risk factors and atherogenesis is still undetermined.

A brief review of arterial and venous structure and function is warranted before discussion of the theoretical mechanisms involved with the genesis of the atherosclerotic process (atherogenesis). Arteries consist of three distinct layers (tunicae): intima, media, and adventitia (Fig. 2-7). The intima (inner layer) is lined with endothelial cells and supported by connective tissue. The middle layer, or media, consists mainly of smooth muscle cells, and the outer layer, or adventitia, consists of collagenous elastic fibers and small blood vessels (vasa vasorum). Veins, like arteries, have three layers, but the amount of smooth muscle tissue and elastic tissue is considerably less, most likely because veins function in a low-pressure system.

Studies have shown that arteries, in addition to their function as conduits or tubes through which blood is transported from point to point, transport selected plasma proteins through their inner layer, or intima, to the adventitia, and eventually to the lymphatic vessels.[63,89] The disturbance of this selective transport is postulated to be one of the key mechanisms involved in the process of atherogenesis.[6] Further discussion of this point follows.

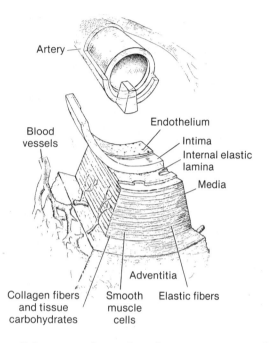

**Fig. 2-7.** Enlargement of a section of a coronary artery and its structural components, namely, the endothelium, the media (consisting primarily of smooth muscle cells), and the adventitia. (From Benditt EP: *Sci Am* 263(2):74, 1977.)

Although not all the mechanisms and processes involved with the formation of atherosclerotic lesions are totally understood, there is enough evidence from animal and human studies to construct a reasonable theoretical model of the process of atherogenesis.[53,102] Two explanations for atherogenesis, the Lipid Infiltration Theory (Insudation Theory) and the Endothelial Injury Theory, have recently been combined into a Unified Hypothesis as a result of the overwhelming scientific evidence in support of each of these two theories. This Unified Hypothesis proposes that there are two primary components of atherosclerosis, endothelial cell injury or damage and lipid infiltration (insudation). Fig. 2-8 summarizes the various steps involved in the Unified Hypothesis of atherogenesis.

There is evidence that the major component of the atherosclerotic plaque is LDL cholesterol and that when LDL cholesterol is allowed to seep into (insudate) the intima, it results in smooth muscle cell proliferation, increased collagen formation, and other reactions that are involved with the pathogenesis of atherosclerosis.* In addition, several identified factors are responsible for alteration of the permeability of the arterial endothelial layer. Table 2-2 summarizes the various factors that have been shown to alter endothelial permeability to lipoproteins and macrophages.

This injury or damage to the arterial endothelial layer[69] allows insudation of several macromolecules, such as LDL and fibrinogen, both of which are believed to be key factors in the atherogenic process. Huper[44-46] and others[7,52,74,105] have shown that hypoxia and elevated levels of serum carbon monoxide alter arterial permeability. These data suggest one

* References 41, 43, 51, 101, 103, 104, 106

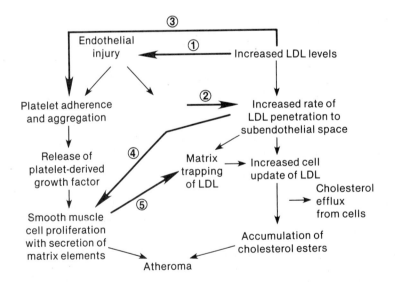

**Fig. 2-8.** A summary of the various steps involved with the Unified Hypothesis of atherogenesis. (From Steinberg D and Olefsky JM, editors: *Hypercholesterolemia and atherosclerosis: pathogenesis and prevention,* New York, 1987, Churchill Livingstone.)

**Table 2-2.** Summary of various factors that have been shown to alter endothelial permeability to lipoproteins and macrophages

| Substance or physical condition | Mechanism involved | Clinical condition |
|---|---|---|
| Hemodynamic forces; tension, stretching, shearing, eddy currents | Separation or damage to endothelial cells, increased permeability, platelet sticking, stimulation of smooth muscle cell proliferation | Hypertension |
| Angiotensin II | "Trap-door" effect | Hypertension |
| Carbon monoxide or decreased $O_2$ saturation | Destruction of endothelial cells | Cigarette smoking |
| Catecholamines (epinephrine, norepinephrine, serotonin, bradykinin) | Hypercontraction, swelling and loss of endothelial cells, platelet agglutination | Stress, cigarette smoking |
| Metabolic products | Endothelial cell damage | Homocystinemia, uremia |
| Endotoxins and other similar bacterial products | Endothelial cell destruction, platelet sticking | Acute bacterial infections |
| Ag-Ab complexes, immunological defects | Platelet agglutination | Serum sickness, transplant rejection, immune complex diseases, lupus erythematosus |
| Virus diseases | Endothelial cell infection and necrosis | Viremias |
| Mechanical trauma to endothelium | Platelet sticking, increased local permeability | Catheter injury |
| Hyperlipidemia with increase in circulating lipoproteins (cholesterol, triglycerides, phospholipids) and free fatty acids | Platelet agglutination in areas of usually hemodynamic damage, over "fatty streaks" | Chronic nutritional imbalance (high-fat and high-cholesterol diets), familial hypercholesterolemia, diabetes, nephrosis, hypothyroidism |

From Braunwald E, editor: *Heart disease: a textbook of cardiovascular medicine,* Philadelphia, 1984, WB Saunders Co.

way in which the risk factor of cigarette smoking plays a direct role in atherogenesis. Hypertension (probably as a result of direct trauma) and angiotensin II also have been shown to damage the endothelial cells and therefore alter permeability of the endothelial layer.[16,87] Catecholamines (epinephrine, norepinephrine, serotonin, bradykinin), which can be elevated by stress or cigarette smoking, also cause endothelial damage.[91,92]

There is also evidence that certain blood components, such as platelets and monocytes, play a role in the pathogenesis of atherosclerosis.[29,55] Mustard's studies[72,73] demonstrated that platelets tend to adhere to the damaged or injured arterial intimal surfaces, and he and his co-workers speculated that this platelet aggregation contributed to the progression of the atherosclerotic process. The work of Ross[82-85] has confirmed that platelet aggregation and eventually degeneration does occur at the site of intimal injury and that a platelet-derived growth factor (PDGF) is released at these sites. Furthermore, this PDGF has been shown to stimulate increased cholesterol synthesis in the smooth muscle cells, to increase the tendency for LDL cholesterol to bind to the smooth muscle cells, and to stimulate proliferation of smooth muscle cells. All the above processes, including the smooth muscle cell proliferation stimulated by the PDGF, are believed to be important to the overall pathogenesis of atherosclerosis (Fig. 2-9).[83] The process of platelet aggregation is not totally unrelated to the known risk factors for coronary artery disease.[55] In fact,

hyperlipidemia, cigarette smoking, and glucose intolerance have been shown to increase the tendency for platelet aggregation.[17,25,72,100]

A study by Faggiotto and others[23] of diet-induced atherosclerosis in nonhuman primates identified the exact sequence of events that occurred over a period of 12 days to 13 months in monkeys whose serum cholesterol was elevated to 500 to 1000 mg/dl. There was evidence, within 12 days after elevated serum cholesterol, of monocytes attached to the arterial endothelium at random sites along the artery. Monocytes were also found subendothelially with accumulated lipids, assuming the appearance of "fatty streaks." After approximately 5 months there was evidence of proliferation of smooth muscle cells with accumulated lipids and separation of endothelial cell junctions primarily at bifurcations and branches of arteries. The separation exposed macrophages and underlying cells and tissue to the circulation, which in turn gave rise to platelet aggregation and mural thrombi. Within the following 2 months, there was evidence of advanced smooth muscle cell proliferation at the sites of platelet aggregation. This work by Faggiotto and others[24] was extremely important in developing a further understanding of atherosclerosis and was supported by numerous studies cited previously. For a more detailed discussion of the pathobiology of atherosclerosis, the reader is referred to texts by Braunwald[12] and Steinberg.[98]

The role of high-density lipoproteins should be considered when one is examining risk factors in the pathogenesis

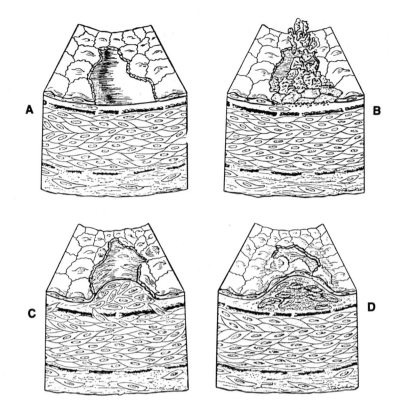

**Fig. 2-9. A,** Diagram of area of endothelial damage or injury, the major initial phase of atherogenesis. **B,** Secondary phase of atherogenesis involving platelet aggregation, a phase that probably precedes smooth muscle cell proliferation. **C,** Diagram of smooth muscle cell proliferation and migration from the media to the intima. **D,** Insudation of low-density lipoprotein cholesterol within the inner layers of the arterial wall. (From Ross R and Glosmet JA: The pathogenesis of atherosclerosis, *N Engl J Med* 295:420, 1976.)

of atherosclerosis.[19] There is evidence that HDL cholesterol protects against the formation of atherosclerotic plaques by (1) removing cholesterol and cholesterol esters from smooth muscle cells in the arterial wall[15,71,96] and (2) blocking the atherogenic action of LDL on the smooth muscle cells of the intima.[110] Further study is currently underway to investigate the protective mechanisms of HDL cholesterol. Based on what is currently known, we can begin to understand why the epidemiological studies referred to earlier have consistently shown low levels of serum HDL to be a strong risk factor for coronary artery disease.

In summary, there is growing scientific evidence relating the major risk factors directly to the pathogenesis of atherosclerosis. These data underscore the importance of therapeutic modalities aimed at risk factor reduction that are used in both primary and secondary prevention programs.

## HEMODYNAMICS OF CORONARY ARTERY FLOW IN NORMAL AND DISEASED STATES

It is important to understand the normal determinants of myocardial oxygen supply and demand before attempting to appreciate the consequences of hemodynamically significant atherosclerotic occlusions in the coronary arteries.

The average resting coronary blood flow in humans is 75

ml of blood per minute per 100 grams of myocardium; this can increase to as high as 350 ml of blood per minute per 100 grams at maximal exercise. Coronary blood flow or supply depends on (1) the driving pressure and (2) the resistance to flow along the coronary vascular bed. During systole, because of the relatively high left ventricular subendocardial pressures (in relation to the distending pressures of the coronary arteries) and because of intramyocardial pressure in general, there is virtually no coronary flow to the subendocardial zones and minimal flow to the subepicardial regions.[59] Therefore the driving pressure is essentially the systemic diastolic blood pressure, since effective coronary filling takes place only during diastole. In the normal person the left ventricular end-diastolic pressure is low (5 to 10 mm Hg) and therefore has little or no adverse effect on the net driving pressure (systemic diastolic blood pressure minus LV end-diastolic pressure). The vascular resistance to flow depends on the tone of the smooth muscle of the arteries and the length of the arteries. A third factor in determining coronary flow is length of filling time. Since the coronary arteries fill during diastole and since diastole comprises two thirds of the entire cardiac cycle at rest, filling time is not a limiting factor. During exercise, as the heart rate increases, the time of systole remains fairly constant and the diastolic filling time can decrease as much as 35% to 40%. Once again, in the normal person filling time, even during maximal exercise, is not a limiting factor. The determinants of myocardial oxygen demand are (1) heart rate, (2) systemic systolic blood pressure, (3) myocardial wall tension, and (4) rate pressure generation in the left ventricle. At rest the average myocardial oxygen demand ($M\dot{V}o_2$) is 10 ml of $O_2$/min/100 gm of myocardium, and with exercise the $M\dot{V}o_2$ can exceed 50 ml of $O_2$/min/100 gm. In the normal person, since the myocardium extracts 75% of the oxygen (a-$\tilde{V}o_2$, or arterial and central venous oxygen difference) from the coronary blood supply both at rest and with exercise, any increase in myocardial oxygen demand is matched by an increase in coronary blood supply. The coronary blood is autoregulated as a result of both neural and metabolic influences. The most potent metabolic coronary vasodilator is hypoxia. In fact it is assumed that the vasodilatory influence of hypoxia overrides the vasoconstricting influence of the alpha-adrenergic fibers that innervate the coronary vessels during exercise. The coronaries are also innervated by beta$_1$- and beta$_2$-adrenergic fibers, which vasodilate the vessels but play a relatively minor role in the regulation of coronary blood flow.

In summary, the coronary blood flow is determined by (1) mechanical factors such as the driving pressure, extravascular pressure and diastolic filling time, (2) metabolic factors such as hypoxia, and to a lesser degree (3) neural influences resulting from innervation of both alpha-and beta-adrenergic fibers.

Since the driving pressure decreases beyond the site of the lesion, the problem that fixed coronary atherosclerotic lesions presents is that they may reduce coronary flow capacity below demand levels. What degree of stenosis is hemodynamically significant? Logan[60] demonstrated that at low flow rates (10 to 30 ml/min) resistance to flow was minimal; however, at flow rates of 30 to 100 ml/min, resistance increased twofold to threefold. More important, he demonstrated that lesions involving less than 70% to 80% stenosis had fairly constant curves of flow versus percent stenosis, but that with lesions greater than a range of 70% to 80% stenosis, minimal increases in luminal narrowing resulted in pronounced increases in resistance to flow and decrease in flow beyond the stenosis. The length of a lesion also is a factor in determining its hemodynamic effect.[37] A diffuse 50% lesion could impair coronary flow as much as, or more than, a discrete 70% lesion. Sequential lesions can also have more of a bearing on flow capacity than a single discrete lesion, depending on the percent stenosis.

The idea that all atherosclerotic lesions are fixed and rigid is somewhat misleading; in fact there is evidence that coronary lesions are dynamic and variable, depending on the degree of vasomotor tone at the lesion site. There is clear evidence that coronary plaque fissures create opportunities for intermittent episodes of platelet aggregation which may result in ischemia and thrombus formation. Sharp increases in vasomotor tone leading to a localized or diffuse spasm of a coronary artery (with or without a fixed lesion) have been shown to reduce coronary flow significantly, resulting in one of several clinical manifestations including resting angina, myocardial infarction, or sudden death.[109] Recent evidence suggests that coronary spasm often occurs in persons with atherosclerotic lesions, and the degree of spasm is more severe at the site of the atherosclerotic lesion than it is at adjacent uninvolved areas of the same artery in the same person.[28] Maseri's work[64] indicates that there is a definite interrelationship between the vasomotor tone of an artery and the integrity of the endothelium, the presence of vasoactive substances, and certain components in the blood. The vasoactive substances that can potentially lead to coronary spasm include catecholamines thromboxane $A_2$ (a substance derived from phospholipids of agglutinated platelets), serotonin, and histamine. Insufficient secretion of the prostaglandin prostacyclin ($PGI_2$) a vasodilator, can also allow for either localized or diffuse vasospasm, especially with higher than normal concentrations of the various vasoactive substances. Persons with periodic coronary spasm that results in myocardial ischemia often exhibit certain characteristic signs or symptoms that include, but are not limited to, (1) a variant angina pattern often involving discomfort at rest and a variable threshold for exertional discomfort, (2) cyclic symptom patterns such as recurrent nocturnal or early morning discomfort, and (3) ST-segment elevation with or without symptoms. The definitive diagnostic procedure for coronary spasm is coronary angiography in conjunction with ergonovine (potent vasoconstrictor) administration. Medical therapy for patients with coronary spasm is discussed in Chapter 4.

In summary, the hemodynamic consequences of a coronary lesion depend on the degree of luminal narrowing, the severity and frequency of plaque fissures ulcerations, the degree of calcification or soft plaque formation, the length of the stenosis, the coronary blood flow rate, and the degree of vasomotor tone of the affected artery. Significant perfusion or driving pressure losses beyond the site of the lesion occur because of these factors and lead to inadequate perfusion to the subendocardium, an area that is most sensitive to decreased driving pressures because of its direct contact with the left ventricular cavity. In the resting state the perfusion pressure beyond the stenosis must exceed a certain threshold (50 to 60 mm Hg). In the person with a hemodynamically significant lesion exercise (with the associated increases in the heart rate and systolic blood pressure) results in (1) increased extravascular pressure, (2) insufficient coronary flow, and (3) increased left ventricular filling pressures, all of which result in decreased coronary perfusion pressures and eventually myocardial ischemia. In addition, as the myocardium becomes ischemic, there is a series of events that is believed to occur that further reduce the capacity for coronary flow.[20] Specifically, the ischemic myocardium does not relax completely, a condition that leads to (1) prolonged period of systole and thus shorter diastolic filling time, (2) decreased compliance of the left ventricle, and (3) increased left ventricular end diastolic pressure and consequently further decreases in the driving pressure, all of which lead to more severe ischemia.

Aortocoronary venous bypass grafts placed in the patient with advanced coronary lesions are subject to perfusion or driving pressures similar to those in the native coronary arteries, since the proximal origin of the grafts is located just distal to the ostium of the native coronary artery. There is recent evidence that blood flow through the grafts in the postoperative state is not determined by the luminal diameter of the graft, provided that it is greater than 3 mm.[93] There is still considerable controversy over the influence of the ratio of the diameter of the graft vessel to the host vessel on graft flow. A more important consideration, however, is the influence of the bypass graft on blood flow beyond the lesion site in the coronary vessel.

Smith and others studied the hemodynamic effects of coronary artery bypass grafts in 24 patients with 29 grafts. In general, the bypass grafts improved coronary blood flow by a mean of 268%. The authors also noted that in native coronary arteries with less than 80% obstruction there were minimal pressure gradients (difference in pressure before and beyond obstruction) and high postobstruction flow (mean of 75 ml/min/100 gm). When these lesions were bypassed, there was no significant increase in flow rates. In coronary lesions of 80% or greater, postobstruction flow was greatly reduced, and after bypass surgery, flow rates improved significantly. Although this study demonstrates that there appears to be a percent stenosis "threshold" above which bypass grafts increase flow, the results (in terms of absolute values) should be interpreted cautiously since the flow studies were done at rest and therefore at low demands for coronary perfusion. It is likely that the degree of improvement in coronary blood flow during exercise after aortocoronary bypass graft surgery is dependent on the severity of the bypassed lesion.

The effects of medications on both myocardial oxygen demand and coronary flow are discussed in Chapter 4.

## ACUTE MYOCARDIAL INFARCTION

Prolonged ischemia as a result of complete occlusion of a coronary artery or a severe occlusion coupled with increased vasomotor tone will result in myocardial cell death or infarction. The exact pathophysiology of the coronary arteries that leads to infarction is not really known; in fact, there are at least four possible mechanisms: (1) progression of the atherosclerotic lesion to complete occlusion, (2) near total obstruction coupled with a thrombosis resulting in total obstruction of the vessel, (3) near total obstruction coupled with coronary spasm, or (4) near total obstruction coupled with prolonged relatively high myocardial oxygen demands. The actual process of infarction appears to involve either a single biological event or, in some cases, a wave of biological functions through which the infarction gradually progresses. Changes in the myocardial tissue (mitochondria, sarcomeres, and so on) begin to occur within 15 minutes after the tissue becomes hypoxic. The necrotic changes are followed by cell absorption and eventually scar formation.

The exact site and extent of necrosis depend on the anatomic distribution of the artery, the adequacy of collateral circulation, presence and extent of previous infarction, and various factors that could influence the myocardial oxygen demand such as catecholamine-release rates, activity of the autonomic nervous system, the systolic blood pressure, and the left ventricular end-diastolic volume and pressure. There are generally two types of myocardial infarctions: (1) transmural infarction, which extends through the subendocardial tissue to the epicardial layer of the myocardium, and (2) subendocardial infarction, which involves only the innermost layer of the myocardium and perhaps, in some cases, portions of the middle layer of tissue but does not extend to include the epicardial region of the myocardium.

The diagnosis of acute myocardial infarction is made from the combination of several findings including clinical history of symptoms, elevation of specific enzyme levels in the blood, presence of acute injury pattern on the 12-lead electrocardiogram, and, most recently, positive findings of special radioisotope studies. It is important to recognize that all the above-mentioned findings are not necessarily evident in every acute myocardial infarction and that, in most cases, the changes in enzyme levels and the 12-lead electrocardiogram are relied on most heavily (see Chapter 6).

The classic symptoms of an acute myocardial infarction involve severe central chest or retrosternal discomfort. The nature of the discomfort varies but most commonly is described as either pain or a pressure or heaviness that the patient states is "like a heavy weight on my chest." The discomfort often will radiate to several areas including the neck or jaw, one or both upper extremities, and the midscapular region. Infarction symptoms usually persist for prolonged periods of time but may wax and wane and are not relieved by nitroglycerin. Associated signs and symptoms commonly include dyspnea, diaphoresis, light-headedness, nausea, apprehension, weakness, vomiting, and hypotension. The clinician must be aware, however, that the so-called classic symptoms described above do not always accompany the infarction and that the nature, location, and intensity of discomfort, along with the associated signs and symptoms, can vary. Finally, myocardial infarctions can occur without symptoms; in fact, based on postmortem and epidemiological studies, 20% to 25% of all infarctions are "silent" or asymptomatic.

The use of serum enzyme levels to diagnose an acute myocardial infarction is based on several assumptions that are still somewhat controversial. First, it is assumed that elevation of the enzyme level occurs only with cell death and not in instances of prolonged ischemia; second, that the enzyme level rise is not attributable to damage in other major organs; finally, that there is a direct relationship between the amount of rise in the enzyme levels and the size of the infarction.

The three enzymes that are characteristically utilized in the diagnosis of acute myocardial infarction include creatine phosphokinase (CPK), aspartate aminotransferase (AST, formerly called serum glutamic oxaloacetic transaminase, SGOT), and lactate dehydrogenase (LDH). The serum levels of all three enzymes will generally increase within the first 36 hours of an infarction. The CPK levels usually elevate within 6 hours of myocardial cell death, followed by rises in the AST and LDH levels 6 to 12 hours later. The CPK values gradually return to normal over a period of 3 or 4 days, whereas the AST and LDH levels resolve by 7 to 9 days after the event. Although all three enzymes are relatively sensitive indicators of myocardial damage, the specificity of serum changes is poor because there are similar enzyme pools in other major organs such as the brain, liver, and skeletal muscle. Recently, isoenzymes (different molecular forms of the same enzyme) of LDH and CPK have been found to be more specific to myocardial cell death.[8] The most specific isoenzyme is the CPK-II, or what is also referred to as the MB-CPK fraction. It usually becomes elevated in the blood serum within 4 hours after infarction and peaks by 36 hours. False positive rises in the CPK-II can occur in patients with myositis, muscular dystrophies, and pericarditis.

The acute changes in the 12-lead ECG that occur as a result of a myocardial infarction depend on (1) the type of infarction, that is, transmural versus subendocardial, and (2) the area of infarction. By definition, subendocardial infarctions result in new T-wave inversion or ST-segment depression or both that persist for 48 hours with no new Q-wave changes or R-wave losses.[62] Transmural infarctions usually result in convex ST-segment elevation associated with T-wave inversion in leads specific to the area of infarction (Table 2-3). In addition, evolutionary changes in the ECG pattern of a patient with a transmural infarction induce a significant Q wave (greater than 0.04 second in duration and greater than 25% of the amplitude of the R wave) and in some cases decreased R-wave voltage. Reciprocal ST-segment depression often occurs in undamaged areas opposite the area of infarction. Studies indicate that ECG changes

establish the correct diagnosis 85% of the time. Postmortem studies indicate that the sensitivity of acute ECG changes in infarction patients is 60% and the false positive rate is 42%. The most common causes of "false positive" 12-lead ECG changes include cardiomyopathies, cerebrovascular accidents, pulmonary emboli, hyperkalemia, idiopathic hypertrophic subaortic stenosis, and 12-lead conduction abnormalities such as left bundle branch block and Wolff-Parkinson-White (WPW) syndrome. It is often 24 or more hours before the acute ECG changes described above appear.

## NATURAL HISTORY OF CORONARY ARTERY DISEASE

An understanding of the natural history of coronary artery disease is important to the clinician who desires to identify the various subsets of patients and the prognostic significance of each subset. Ideally, the awareness of these subsets, along with the data base accumulated from clinical monitoring, exercise testing, results from special studies, patient history, and physical examination, will provide the basis for an individually designed serial evaluation plan and treatment program (see Chapters 8 and 9).

Atherosclerotic coronary artery disease is generally considered to be a progressive disease that can develop as early as the second decade of life.[22,66] The natural history of the disease is a bit difficult to document because of the variables of medical and surgical therapy, risk factor reduction, and the presence or absence of other coexisting illnesses. Yet it is important to have some indication whether certain factors, relative to the severity of the disease at the time of initial evaluation, predict the likelihood of future coronary events such as progression of symptoms, recurrent myocardial infarction, or cardiac death. Unfortunately, most of the studies in the literature are limited by relatively short follow-up periods, except for the work of Bruschke[13,14] and Proudfit[79] from the Cleveland Clinic. The Proudfit study involved a 10-year follow-up period of 601 nonsurgical patients. All these patients had evidence of at least 50% narrowing of one coronary artery at the time of entry into the study and were less than 65 years of age. The study used the end point of sudden death (terminal illness that began 1 hour before death) and did not attempt to examine carefully the likelihood of progression of symptoms or recurrent infarction. The number of arteries involved was an important prognostic factor, with 10-year survival rates for patient with single-vessel, double-vessel, and triple-vessel disease being 63%, 45%, and 23% respectively. The presence of a 50% or greater lesion in the left main coronary artery was also an important prognostic factor with 10-year survival rates of 22%. Survival rates also related to ventricular function. Patients with large myocardial infarctions and therefore poor left ventricular function and low ejection fractions (less than 35%) had lower survival rates than those with small areas of damage and normal ventricular function. Patients with a definite ventricular aneurysm or with ejection fractions less

| Area of infarction | ECG changes |
|---|---|
| Anteroseptal | Q or QS in $V_1$-$V_3$ |
| Anterior (localized) | Q or QS in $V_2$-$V_4$; $V_1$-$V_6$ |
| Anterolateral | Q or QS in I, $aV_L$; $V_4$-$V_6$ |
| Lateral | Q or QS in I, $aV_L$ |
| Inferior | Q or QS in II, III $aV_F$ |
| Posterior | Increased R waves $V_1$-$V_3$ |

**Table 2-3.** Twelve-lead ECG changes and areas of infarction

$V_1$ to $V_6$ are chest leads; I to III and $aV_R$, $aV_L$, and $aV_F$ are extremity leads.

than 40% had 10-year survival rates of 10% to 18%. This finding is supported by the work of Nelson[64] and Hammermeister.[40] Finally, there were other factors that were prognostically influential and were independent of the number of coronary vessels diseased and ventricular function. These factors included the severity of functional impairment imposed by angina pectoris, ECG evidence of left ventricular hypertrophy or conduction defects, and persistence of risk factors such as cigarette smoking, diabetes, and hypertension. Most recently, functional performance or time on the treadmill test has been shown to be an important predictor of survival as well.[56] Further discussion of this point appears in Chapter 8.

## REVERSAL AND RETARDATION OF PROGRESSION OF ATHEROSCLEROSIS

The concept that the normal progression of atherosclerosis can be altered and, in some cases, reversed is no longer theoretical, based on the scientific evidence that has accumulated in the last 5 to 10 years. A thorough review of this literature was recently published by Blankenhorn.[9] There is direct evidence that risk factor reduction has a major impact on the disease process both for those with known coronary disease and for those at high risk of developing hemodynamically significant coronary atherosclerosis. In fact, Blankenhorn[9] states that there is ample evidence indicating that the sclerotic and the atherotic components of arterial lesions can be favorably altered by a reduction in hypertension, hypercholesterolemia, and hyperglycemia.

The Helsinki Heart Study[27] has provided the most impressive clinical evidence thus far, indicating that lipid lowering is an effective primary prevention intervention. This 5-year randomized study of 4081 men demonstrated a 34% lower incidence of coronary heart disease in those men with lower LDL and total cholesterol values and higher HDL values as a result of treatment. In the early 1970s there was definite evidence of coronary lesion size reduction accompanied by decreased arterial lipid content in rhesus and cynomolgus monkeys after hypercholesterolemic diets were withdrawn.[2-4] There have also been several human studies involving coronary angiography that have demonstrated that lipid lowering through diet or medical therapy results in a decreased incidence of coronary lesion progression and an improved clinical course.[5,75,77] Blankenhorn and others recently demonstrated not only that aggressive lipid lowering and elevation of HDL led to a decreased incidence of lesion progression, but that the treated group of post-CABG patients also demonstrated a significantly higher incidence of lesion regression.[10] The exact mechanism through which lipid lowering prevents coronary progression or induces coronary lesion regression is not known, although Harrison and others[42] produced morphological evidence of lesion improvement associated with restored endothelial-dependent relaxation as a result of dietary treatment.

The angiographic evidence of the beneficial effects of aerobic exercise on coronary progression is by no means as extensive (see Chapter 10). However, Kramsch and others[54] have published evidence that moderate exercise carried out over a period of 3 or more years and associated with improvements in HDL, LDL, and triglyceride levels resulted in (1) decreased degree of atherosclerosis, (2) decreased lesion size and collagen accumulation, and (3) increased heart rate and vessel lumen. These authors concluded that regular aerobic exercise may prevent or retard the development of coronary atherosclerosis especially if it is initiated before an atherogenic diet.

## SUMMARY

There are two major epicardial or surface coronary arteries, the right coronary artery and the left main coronary artery. The left coronary system is the major source of blood supply to the left ventricle (LV), perfusing up to 60% to 70% of the LV muscle mass. The precise perfusion distribution patterns of the coronary arteries vary among persons. The exact etiology of atherosclerosis is not fully understood; however, there are certain factors that have been shown to increase the likelihood of the disease process occurring in a given person. The major risk factors include cigarette smoking, increased serum levels of LDL cholesterol and triglycerides, decreased serum levels of HDL cholesterol, hypertension, diabetes, and sedentary life-style. There is evidence that the above factors play a role in the exact mechanisms of atherosclerosis.

The adequacy of coronary blood flow to the myocardium depends on the balance between supply and demand. Atherosclerotic changes in the coronary arteries can significantly decrease coronary supply because of luminal narrowing. Supply can be further compromised by increased vasomotor tone in the coronary arteries leading to acute spasm of the artery. The possible consequences of an imbalance between supply and demand include myocardial ischemia with or without symptoms, myocardial infarction, or sudden death. The diagnosis of an acute myocardial infarction is based on a combination of findings. Clinical symptoms, serum enzyme levels, and changes in the 12-lead ECG are all used to determine the diagnosis of myocardial infarction.

Coronary artery disease is a progressive process. The prognosis of a patient with coronary disease depends primarily on the number of vessels diseased and the degree of left ventricular dysfunction as a result of infarction or ischemia.

Angiographic evidence exists demonstrating that risk factor reduction, including improvement of lipid levels and regular aerobic exercise, does alter the progression of coronary atherosclerosis and, in some cases, leads to regression of the disease process. Further study is needed to uncover the various ways in which risk factor reduction alters the normally progressive course of atherosclerosis.

## REFERENCES

1. Albrink MJ and others: Serum lipids, hypertension, and coronary artery disease, *Am J Med* 31:4, 1961.
2. Armstrong ML and Megan MB: Arterial fibrosis proteins in cynomolgus monkeys after atherogenic and regression diets, *Circ Res* 36:256, 1975.
3. Armstrong ML and others: Lipid depletion in atheromatous coronary arteries in rhesus monkeys after regression diets, *Circ Res* 30:675, 1972.
4. Armstrong ML and others: Regression of coronary atherosclerosis in rhesus monkeys, *Circ Res* 27:59, 1970.
5. Arntzenius AC and others: Diet, lipoproteins and the progression of coronary atherosclerosis, *N Engl J Med* 312:805, 1985.
6. Aschoff L: *Lectures in pathology,* New York, 1929, Paul B Hoeber.
7. Astrup P and others: Enhancing influence of carbon monoxide on the development of atheromatosis in cholesterol fed rabbits, *J Atheroscler Res* 7:343, 1967.
8. Barboriak JJ and others: Atherosclerosis in aortocoronary vein grafts, *Lancet* 2:621, 1974.
9. Blankenhorn DH and Kramsch DM: Reversal of atherosis and sclerosis: the two components of atherosclerosis, *Circulation* 79:1, 1989.
10. Blankenhorn DH and others: Beneficial effects of combined colestipol-niacin therapy on coronary atherosclerosis and coronary venous bypass grafts, *JAMA* 257:3233, 1987.
11. Bovens AM and others: Physical activity, fitness, and selected risk factors for CHD in active men and women, *Med Sci Sports Exer* 25:572, 1993.
12. Braunwald E: *Heart disease: a textbook of cardiovascular medicine,* Philadelphia, 1984, WB Saunders Co.
13. Bruschke AVG and others: Progress study of 590 consecutive nonsurgical cases of coronary disease followed 5-9 years. I. Arteriographic correlations, *Circulation* 47:1147, 1973.
14. Bruschke AVG and others: Progress study of 590 consecutive nonsurgical cases of coronary disease followed 5-9 years. II. Ventriculographic and other correlations, *Circulation* 47:1154, 1973.
15. Carew TE and others: A mechanism by which high density lipoproteins may slow the atherogenic process, *Lancet* 1:1315, 1976.
16. Constantinides P and Robinson M: Ultrastructural injury of arterial endothelium. II. Effects of vasoactive amines, *Arch Pathol* 88:106, 1969.
17. Carvalho AC and others: Platelet function in hyperlipoproteinemia, *N Engl J Med* 290:434M, 1974.
18. Dawber TR and others: An approach to longitudinal studies in a community: the Framingham Study, *Ann NY Acad Sci* 107:539, 1963.
19. Drexel H and others: Relation of the level of high-density lipoprotein subfractions to the presence and extent of coronary artery disease, *Am J Cardiol* 70:436, 1992.
20. Ellestad MH: Ischemic ST segment depression: hemodynamic, electrophysiologic, and metabolic factors in its genesis. In Ellestad MH: *Stress testing: principles and practice,* Philadelphia, 1976, FA Davis Co.
21. Egan B and others: Comparative effects of overweight on cardiovascular risk in younger versus older men, *Am J Cardiol* 67:248, 1991.
22. Enos WF and others: Coronary disease among United States soldiers killed in action in Korea, *JAMA* 152:1090, 1953.
23. Faggiotto A and others: Studies of hypercholesterolemia in the nonhuman primate. I. Changes that lead to fatty streak formation, *Arteriosclerosis* 4:323, 1984.
24. Faggiotto A and Ross R: Studies of hypercholesterolemia in the nonhuman primate. II. Fatty streak endothelium, *Arteriosclerosis* 4:341, 1984.
25. Forbiszewski R and Worowski K: Enhancement of platelet aggregation and adhesiveness by beta lipoproteins, *J Atheroscler Res* 8:988, 1968.
26. French JK and others: Association of angiographically detected coronary artery disease with low levels of high-density lipoprotein, cholesterol, and systemic hypertension, *Am J Cardiol* 71:505, 1993.
27. Frick MH and others: Helsinki Heart Study: primary prevention trial with gemfibrozil in middle-aged men with dyslipidemia. Safety of treatment, changes in risk factors and incidence of coronary heart disease, *N Engl J Med:* 1237, 1987.
28. Friedman B and others: Pathophysiology of coronary artery spasm, *Circulation* 67:705, 1982.
29. Fuchs J and others: Circulating aggregated platelets in coronary artery disease, *Am J Cardiol* 60:534, 1987.
30. Gensini G: *Coronary arteriography,* New York, 1975, Futura Publishing Co, Inc.
31. Genest JJ and others: Prevalence of risk factors in men with premature coronary artery disease, *Am J Cardiol* 67:1185, 1991.
32. Gofman JW and others: Ischemic heart disease, atherosclerosis, and longevity, *Circulation* 34:679, 1966.
33. Gordon T and Kannel WB: Predisposition to atherosclerosis in the head, heart, and legs: the Framingham Study, *JAMA* 221:661, 1972.
34. Gordon T and others: High density lipoproteins as a protective factor against CHD, *Am J Med* 62:707, 1977.
35. Gordon T and others: Diabetes, blood lipids, and the role of obesity in coronary heart disease risk for women: the Framingham Study, *Ann Intern Med* 87:393, 1977.
36. Gorlin R: Coronary anatomy. In Gorlin R: *Coronary artery disease, vol 11, Major problems in internal medicine series,* Philadelphia, 1976, WB Saunders Co.
37. Gorlin R: Physiology of myocardial blood flow and metabolism. In Gorlin R: *Coronary artery disease, vol 11, Major problems in internal medicine series,* Philadelphia, 1976, WB Saunders Co.
38. Grundy SM: Cholesterol metabolism in man, *West J Med* 128:13, 1978.
39. Hamby RI: *Clinical-anatomical correlates in coronary artery disease,* New York, 1979, Futura Publishing Co, Inc.
40. Hammermeister KE and others: Variables predictive of survival in patients with coronary disease: selection by univariate and multivariate analyses from the clinical, electrocardiographic, exercise, arteriographic and quantitative angiographic evaluations, *Circulation* 59:421, 1979.
41. Hanig M and others: Flotational lipoproteins extracted from human atherosclerotic aortas, *Science* 124:176, 1956.
42. Harrison DG and others: Restoration of endothelium-dependent relaxation by dietary treatment of atherosclerosis, *J Clin Invest* 80:1808, 1987.
43. Henry PD: Hypercholesterolemia and angiogenesis, *Am J Cardiol* 72:61, 1993.
44. Huper WC: Arteriosclerosis, *Arch Pathol* 38:162, 1944.
45. Huper WC: Arteriosclerosis, *Arch Pathol* 39:57, 1945.
46. Huper WC: Pathogenesis of atherosclerosis, *Am J Clin Pathol* 26:559, 1956.
47. James TN: *Anatomy of the coronary arteries,* New York, 1961, Harper & Row, Publishers, Inc.
48. Jenkins CD and others: Prediction of clinical coronary heart disease by a test for the coronary-prone behavior pattern, *N Engl J Med* 290:1271, 1974.
49. Kannel WB: Some lessons in cardiovascular epidemiology from Framingham, *Am J Cardiol* 37:269, 1976.
50. Kannel WB and others: Serum cholesterol, lipoproteins, and the risk of coronary heart disease: the Framingham Study, *Ann Intern Med* 24:1, 1971.
51. Kao VCY and Wissler RW: A study of the immunohistochemical localization of serum lipoproteins and other plasma proteins in human atherosclerotic lesions, *Exp Mol Pathol* 4:465, 1965.
52. Kjeldsen K and others: Ultrastructural intitmial changes in the rabbit aorta after a moderate carbon monoxide exposure, *Atherosclerosis* 16:67, 1972.

53. Kottke BA: Current understanding of the mechanisms of atherogenesis, *Am J Cardiol* 72:48, 1993.

54. Kramsch DM and others: Reduction of coronary atherosclerosis by moderate conditioning exercise in monkeys on an atherogenic diet, *N Engl J Med* 305:1483, 1981.

55. Lam JYT and others: Platelet aggregation, coronary artery disease progression and future coronary events, *Am J Cardiol* 73:333, 1994.

56. LaRosa JC: Cholesterol lowering, low cholesterol, and mortality, *Am J Cardiol* 72:776, 1993.

57. Levy RJ and Glueck CJ: Hypertriglyceridemia, diabetes mellitus and coronary vessel disease, *Arch Intern Med* 123:220, 1969.

58. Lie JT and others: Aortocoronary bypass saphenous vein graft atherosclerosis: anatomic study of vein grafts from normal and hyperlipoproteinemic patient up to 75 months postoperatively, *Am J Cardiol* 40:906, 1977.

59. Little RC: Circulation to special areas. In Little RC, editor: *Physiology of the heart and circulation,* Chicago. 1977, Year Book Medical Publishers, Inc.

60. Logan SE: On the fluid mechanics of human coronary artery stenosis, *IEEE Trans Biomed Eng* 22:327, 1975.

61. Lopez A and others: Effect of exercise and physical fitness on serum lipids and lipoproteins, *Atherosclerosis* 20:1, 1974.

62. Madigan MP and others: The clinical course, early prognosis and coronary anatomy of subendocardial infarction, *Am J Med* 62:634, 1976.

63. Mancini RE and others: Extravascular distribution of fluorescent albumin, globulin and fibrinogen in connective tissue structures, *J Histochem Cytochem* 10:194, 1962.

64. Maseri A: Coronary artery spasm and atherosclerosis. In Santamore WP and Boe A, editors: *Coronary artery disease,* Baltimore, 1982, Urban & Schwarzenberg, Inc.

65. Mautner SL and others: Comparison of composition of atherosclerotic plaques in saphenous veins used as aortocoronary bypass conduits with plaques in native coronary arteries in the same men, *Am J Cardiol* 70:1380, 1992.

66. McNamara JJ and others: Coronary artery disease in combat casualties in Vietnam, *JAMA* 216:1185, 1971.

67. McNeer JF and others: The role of the exercise test in the evaluation of patients for ischemic heart disease, *Circulation* 57:64, 1978.

68. Meadows W and others: Risk factors related to progressive narrowing in aortocoronary vein grafts studied 1 and 5 years (abstract), *Circulation* 64 (suppl 4):292, 1981.

69. Meredith IT and others: Role of endothelium in ischemic coronary syndromes, *Am J Cardiol* 72:27C, 1993.

70. Miller GJ and others: Plasma high-density lipoprotein concentration and development of ischemic heart disease, *Lancet* 1:16, 1975.

71. Miller NW and others: Relationship between plasma lipoprotein cholesterol concentrations and the pool size and metabolism of cholesterol in man, *Atherosclerosis* 23:535, 1976.

72. Mustard JF and Murphy CA: Effect of smoking on blood coagulation and platelet survival in man, *Br Med J* 1:846, 1963.

73. Mustard WP and others: The role of thrombogenic factors in atherosclerosis, *Ann NY Acad Sci* 144:848, 1968.

74. Myaskinov AL: Influence of some factors on the development of experimental cholesterol atherosclerosis, *Circulation* 17:99, 1958.

75. Nash DT and others: Effect of lipid lowering therapy on the progression of coronary atherosclerosis by scheduled repetitive coronary arteriography, *Int J Cardiol* 2:43, 1982.

76. Nelson GR and others: Prognosis in medically treated coronary artery disease: influence of ejection fraction compared to other parameters, *Circulation* 52:408, 1975.

77. Nikkila E and others: Prevention of progression of coronary atherosclerosis by treatment of hyperlipidemia: a seven year prospective angiographic study, *Br Med J* 289:220, 1984.

78. Pozner H and Bellimoria JD: Effect of smoking on blood clotting and lipid and lipoprotein levels, *Lancet* 2:1319, 1970.

79. Proudfit WL: Natural history of obstructive coronary artery disease: ten year study of 601 nonsurgical cases, *Prog Cardiovasc Dis* 21:53, 1978.

80. Roberts WC: Factors linking cholesterol to atherosclerotic plaques, *Am J Cardiol* 62:495, 1988.

81. Rosenman RH and others: Coronary heart disease in the Western Collaborative Group Study: final follow-up experience of 8½ years, *JAMA* 233(8):872, 1975.

82. Ross R: Atherosclerosis and the arterial smooth muscle cell, *Science* 180:1322, 1973.

83. Ross R: The pathogenesis of atherosclerosis. In Santamore WP and Boe A, editors: *Coronary artery disease,* Baltimore, 1982, Urban & Schwarzenberg, Inc.

84. Ross R and Glosmet JA: The pathogenesis of atherosclerosis, *N Engl J Med* 295:420, 1976.

85. Ross R and others: A platelet dependent serum factor stimulates the proliferation of arterial smooth muscle cells in vitro, *Proc Natl Acad Sci (USA)* 71:1207, 1964.

86. Salel A and others: Risk factor profile and severity of coronary artery disease, *N Engl J Med* 296:1447, 1977.

87. Schwartz CJ and others: Pathophysiology of the atherogenic process, *Am J Cardiol* 64:23, 1989.

88. Schwartz SM: Assessment of angiotensin endothelial injury by incident light microscopy, *Fed Proc* 35:208, 1976.

89. Scott PJ and Hurley PJ: The distribution of radio-iodinated serum albumin and low-density lipoprotein in tissues and the arterial wall, *Atherosclerosis* 11:77, 1970.

90. Shell W: Specificity of cardiac enzymes in clinical strategies. In Swan G and Corday E, editors: *Ischemic heart disease: new concepts and current controversies,* Baltimore, 1979, The Williams & Wilkins Co.

91. Shimamoto T: The relationship of edematous reaction in arteries to atherosclerosis and thrombosis, *J Atheroscler Res* 3:87, 1963.

92. Shimamoto T: Contraction of endothelial cells as a key mechanism in atherogenesis. In Weigel A, editor: *Atherosclerosis III: proceedings of the third international symposium,* Berlin, 1974, Springer-Verlag.

93. Simon R and others: Blood velocity and dimensions of aortocoronary venous bypass graft in the postoperative state, *Circulation* 66 (suppl I):34, 1982.

94. Smith SC and others: Myocardial blood flow in man: effects of coronary collateral circulation and coronary artery bypass surgery, *J Clin Invest* 51:2556, 1972.

95. Skolow M and McIllroy MB: *Clinical cardiology,* Philadelphia, 1979, Lange Medical Publications.

96. Stein Y and others: The removal of cholesterol from aortic smooth muscle cells in culture and Landschutz ascites cells by fractions of human high-density lipoproteins, *Biochem Biophys Acta* 390:106, 1975.

97. Solymoss BC and others: Relation of coronary artery disease in women <60 years of age to the combined elevation of serum lipoprotein (a) and total cholesterol to high-density cholesterol ratio, *Am J Cardiol* 72:1215, 1993.

98. Steinberg D: Lipoproteins and atherosclerosis: a look back and a look ahead, *Arteriosclerosis* 3:283, 1983.

99. Steinberg D and Olefsky JM: *Hypercholesterolemia and atherosclerosis: pathogenesis and prevention,* New York, 1987, Churchill Livingstone.

100. Sullivan JM and others: Studies of platelet adhesiveness, glucose tolerance, and serum lipoprotein patterns in patients with coronary artery disease, *Am J Med Sci* 264:475, 1972.

101. Tracy RE and others: On the antigenetic identity of human serum beta and alpha-2 lipoproteins, and their identification in aortic intima, *Circ Res* 9:472, 1961.

102. Walton KW: Pathogenetic mechanism in atherosclerosis, *Am J Cardiol* 35:542, 1975.

103. Walton KW and Burkerley DJ: Studies on the pathogenesis of corneal

2222

2222

arcus formation. II. Immunofluorescent studies on lipid deposition in the eye of the lipid-fed rabbit, *J Pathol* 111:97, 1975.

104. Walton KW and others: The pathogenesis of xanthoma, *J Pathol* 109:271, 1973.

105. Wanstrup J and others: Acceleration of spontaneous intimal-subintimal changes in rabbit aorta by prolonged moderate carbon monoxide exposure, *Acta Pathol Microbiol Scand* 75:353, 1969.

106. Wissler RW: Principles of the pathogenesis of atherosclerosis. In Braunwald P, editor: *Heart disease: a textbook of cardiovascular medicine,* Philadelphia, 1980, WB Saunders Co.

107. Wilson PWF: High-Density Lipoprotein, Low-Density Lipoprotein and Coronary Artery Disease, *Am J Cardiol* 66:7A, 1990.

108. Wood PD and others: Plasma lipoprotein distributions in male and female runners, *Ann NY Acad Sci* 301:748, 1977.

109. Yasue H: Pathophysiology and treatment of coronary arterial spasm, *Chest* 78:216, 1980.

110. Yoshida Y and others: Effects of normolipemic HDL on proliferation of aortic smooth muscle cells induced by hyperlipemic LDL, *Circulation* 56 (suppl 3):100, 1977.

# Hemodynamics

*Z. David Skloven*

peptides (Fig. 3-1). The crossbridge formation process occurs during an "active state," when an influx of calcium across sarcomere membranes triggers the troponin-tropomyosin interaction that initiates the contraction process. The energy used by these active state processes is derived ultimately from the oxidative splitting of ATP to ADP with its attendant energy release. The rate of onset and the intensity (rate of cross-bridge formation) of active state are modulated by the activity of various enzyme systems and by sarcolemmal membrane conditions that ultimately govern calcium ion flux and ATP kinetics within the sarcomere. The so-called "contractile state" of the intact heart reflects the rate and intensity the active state processes.

This chapter develops basic concepts of cardiac function in terms of classic muscle mechanics. The hemodynamic principles derived from these concepts are then viewed within the framework of an integrated cardiovascular exercise response. Using the well-known "muscle strip" model, the chapter next reviews fundamental properties of cardiac muscle. These properties will then be studied, with "pressure/volume loops" being used to describe the pump characteristics of the intact heart. Finally, the response of the heart and peripheral circulation to exercise will be described in terms of the muscle mechanics and pump properties that have been defined.

## THE MOLECULAR BASIS OF CONTRACTION

The contractile unit of the heart, the sarcomere, functionally consists of filaments of the contractile proteins *actin* and *myosin* so arranged as to slide parallel to each other in a pattern that causes the sarcomere to shorten and lengthen (Fig. 3-1). Shortening occurs as myosin polypeptide cross-bridge segments alternately attach to and release from active sites on the medially sliding actin poly-

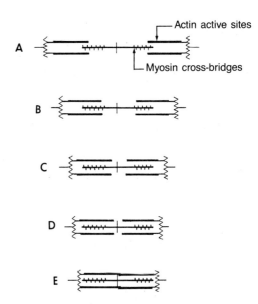

**Fig. 3-1.** Optimal sarcomere length (preload), **C,** results in maximal interaction between actin and myosin cross bridges. Over stretching, **A** and **B,** or understretching, **D** or **E,** of the sarcomere results in submaximal crossbridge linkage.

## Preload

At the start of cardiac contraction, the relative position of the actin and myosin filaments determines the maximum number of cross bridges that can form and thus the maximum shortening force that can be generated. If the sarcomere is overstretched or understretched before contraction, fewer cross bridges can be formed, resulting in suboptimal sliding force generation. At an optimal degree of filament overlap (corresponding to a sarcomere length of about 2.2 μm, maximal crossbridge formation takes place, generating maximal force for shortening. Preload defines the stretch applied to the sarcomere that determines the extent of actin-myosin overlap before the onset of active state. It is important to understand that preload reflects contractile protein geometry only, and that changes during preload occur independent of changes during the contractile state and vice versa.

## Afterload

A thick-walled spherical model of the left ventricle is useful in developing the concept of afterload (Fig. 3-2). To open the aortic valve and eject blood from the ventricle into the aorta, pressure in excess of central aortic pressure must rise in the ventricular chamber. The ventricular pressure results from force generated in the ventricular myocardium. In the thick-walled spherical model, myocardial wall force is depicted as circumferential wall tension throughout the thickness of the myocardium. Idealized mean wall tension at each instant during contraction is determined by the formula for mean midwall tension

$$T = PR/h \qquad (1)$$

where $P$, $R$, and $h$ are, respectively, instantaneous intraventricular pressure, chamber radius, and wall thickness (Fig. 3-2). At the level of the sarcomere, afterload is the force required per sarcomere to generate the midwall tension needed to open the aortic valve and eject blood. Afterload is thus a function of ventricular size and wall thickness and of those factors that determine central aortic blood pressure (e.g., aortic elastic properties, peripheral vascular resistance, and stroke volume).

## Muscle strip model

Study of the interrelation of preload, afterload, and contractile state is facilitated by the papillary muscle strip preparation (Fig. 3-3). Here, one end of a papillary muscle strip is affixed to a strain gauge so that the force produced can be measured. The other end is attached to a lever that can be allowed to move freely on its fulcrum or be kept locked and immobile. With the lever locked, the papillary muscle can develop force when stimulated, but shortening is prevented (isometric contraction). With the lever unlocked, isotonic contraction occurs when the muscle contracts and shortens, lifting a load attached to the other end of the lever. The length of the muscle before stimulation (preload) can be varied by attaching different weights to the opposite end of the lever. Once the resting length (preload) is set, a stop allows additional weight to be added to the lever (afterload). To shorten, the muscle strip must generate force equal to the added afterload.

With the lever locked (isometric contraction), stimulating the muscle strip from various resting lengths (preloads) and plotting the force generated by the stimulus along with the resting length force yields a force-length relation (Fig. 3-4), where developed force equals total force minus resting force (preload). Maximum force occurs at a muscle length, $L_o$, that corresponds to a sarcomere length of 2.2 μm, at which optimal contractile protein filament overlap is obtained. Preloads less than or greater than $L_o$ yield submaximal force generation.

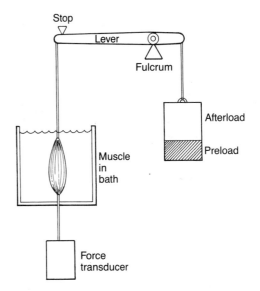

**Fig. 3-3.** The classic muscle strip model. The movable lever can be locked to prevent shortening (isometric) or move freely to allow isotonic contraction. Preload and afterload can be varied to simulate varying hemodynamic loading conditions.

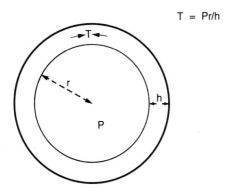

$$T = Pr/h$$

**Fig. 3-2.** Ventricular thickness *(h)*, chamber radius *(r)*, and pressure *(P)* determine circumferential wall tension, according to the equation for a thick-walled sphere.

With the lever free to move, force rises in the stimulated muscle and shortening begins when the force developed equals the afterload. Once shortening starts, force remains constant (equal to afterload) until relaxation occurs, hence the term *isotonic contraction* (Fig. 3-5). Velocity, dl/dt (change in length/change in time), at the onset of shortening and the total extent of shortening (dl) are plotted versus increasing afterloads (Fig. 3-5). Both initial velocity of shortening and the extent of shortening decline with increasing afterloads. At afterload $P_o$, equal to the maximum force the muscle can generate, shortening ceases and the model behaves as an isometric contraction. A velocity-force relation is obtained by plotting initial shortening velocity for increasing afterload (Fig. 3-6). Extrapolation to zero afterload yields a theoretical maximum velocity, $V_{max}$, that has been shown to reflect the intrinsic rate and intensity of force development (i.e., *contractile state*). The force intercept at zero velocity defines $P_o$. At a higher preload the velocity of

shortening is greater for any given afterload. Extrapolated $V_{max}$, however, is not affected by preload, in keeping with the concept that preload alters muscle function by mechanisms independent of contractile state. Adding an inotropic agent, such as digitalis, to the preparation (which increases contractile state) shifts the entire curve upward and to the right. Thus, at a given preload, raising the contractile state yields greater force-generating capacity or, conversely, a higher velocity of shortening at any given afterload. The important result in terms of muscle function is greater shortening at a given preload with higher contractile states.

### Intact heart

In the intact heart, the effects of changes in preload, afterload, and contractility can be described within the context of the ventricular pressure-volume loop, where intraventricular pressure is plotted during diastole and systole against ventricular volume. During diastole venous blood returning to the heart distends the ventricle, and both diastolic volume and pressure rise passively. The elastic properties of the ventricle during diastolic filling determine the relation between diastolic volume and pressure—that is, the compliance characteristics of the ventricle (Fig. 3-7). Thus, from the compliance curve preload can be defined as a function of ventricular diastolic pressure or volume. With the onset of systole, ventricular pressure rises without any net change in ventricular volume (isovolumically) until it equals aortic pressure, at which time the aortic valve opens and ejection begins. The myocardial wall force or tension needed at any instant during systole to generate the required ventricular chamber pressure represents afterload and, in the

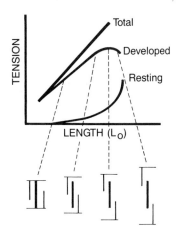

**Fig. 3-4.** Total tension minus initial resting tension gives developed tension. Maximal developed tension occurs at length ($L_o$) corresponding to optimal sarcomeric stretch.

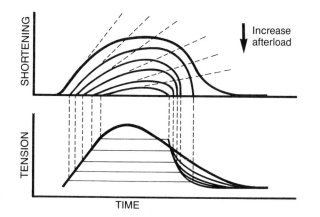

**Fig. 3-5.** Shortening is measured at increasing afterloads. The initial slope of shortening per unit time *(dashes)* can be used to define $V_{max}$ (see text).

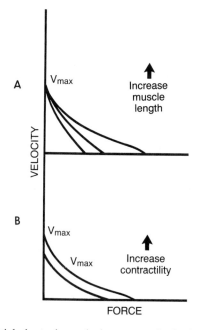

**Fig. 3-6.** Initial shortening velocity versus afterload. **A,** Varying preload; $V_{max}$ is independant of preload. **B,** Varying contractile state.

thick-walled sphere model, is determined by equation 1. If we assume little relative change in $R$ and $h$ over short periods of time, afterload becomes primarily a function of central aortic pressure and those factors affecting it. From equation 2 average systolic pressure, and thus afterload, is a function of cardiac output (CO) and total peripheral resistance (TPR):

$$P \simeq CO \times TPR \qquad (2)$$

Using the ventricular pressure-volume loop (Fig. 3-8), preload is represented by end-diastolic points along the

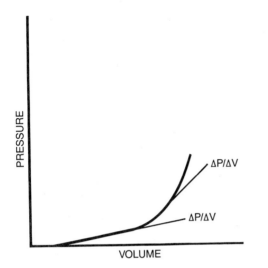

**Fig. 3-7.** Passive diastolic pressure-volume curve defines ventricular compliance. The ventricle stiffens (increased slope) as diastolic volume increases.

passive diastolic filling curve (A-C). Afterload at any instant is depicted as developed ventricular pressure. In the intact ventricular preparation with the aorta cross-clamped, ejection is prevented and the ventricle can thus only develop force without shortening, analogous to the isometric muscle strip contraction. From a given end-diastolic volume (A), pressure rises to a peak (B), which represents the maximum pressure that can be generated from preload A. Repeating the contraction from increasing preloads (end-diastolic volumes) defines an isovolumic pressure curve (B-D) that is the intact heart analog of the force-length relation defined for the muscle strip. Curve B-D represents the maximum force that the ventricle can generate from a given preload. An inotropic intervention that raises contractile state is depicted by line $B_1 - D_1$, where greater peak force is generated from any given preload. This is the intact heart analog of the increase in $P_o$ resulting from increased inotropy in the muscle strip model.

A normal contraction with the ventricle free to eject blood (cross clamp removed) is illustrated in Fig. 3-9. At the onset of systole pressure rises isovolumically until aortic pressure is reached and the aortic valve opens (A-B). Ejection then begins along line B-C until the isovolumic line is reached. Any further decrease in ventricular volume would occur along the isovolumic pressure line thus reducing intraventricular pressure below aortic pressure and causing the aortic valve to close. From C the ventricle at first relaxes

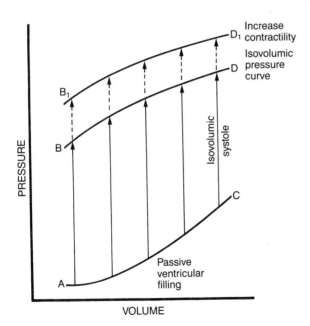

**Fig. 3-8.** Isovolemic contraction from increasing preloads (diastolic volumes) yields isovolemic peak pressure line, *B* to *D,* which represents the maximal pressure attained from a given preload. Increasing contractile state raises the isovolemic pressure line, *B₁* to *D₁.*

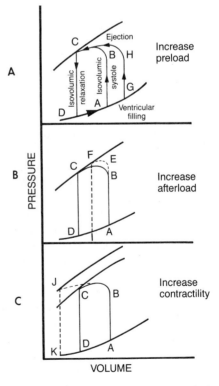

**Fig. 3-9.** Normally ejecting heart (isotonic contraction). *A-B-C-D,* normal control cycle. **A,** *G-H-C-D,* increased preload. **B,** *A-E-F-I,* increased afterload. **C,** *A-B-J-K,* increased contractile state.

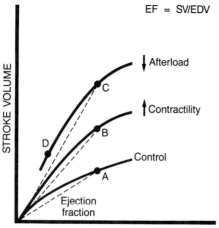

EF = SV/EDV

**Fig. 3-10.** Ventricular function curves. Control SV, A, rises to B with increased contractile astate. SV is augmented further to C with afterload reduction. Failure of venous return to rise in concert with increasing CO to maintain EDV (preload) would limit the increase in SV, D. The dashed lines represent ejection fraction at various points on the function curves, EF = SV/EDV.

isovolumically to D and then fills during diastole along its passive compliance curve (D-A).

B-C, the volume change during ejection, is the stroke volume (end-diastolic minus end-systolic volume). Ejection from a higher preload is illustrated by loop G-H-C-D. Here the ventricle ejecting from a higher end-diastolic volume ejects a larger stroke volume. Ejection ceases at the same point, C, on the isovolumic pressure curve since instantaneous developed ventricular pressure is a function of instantaneous ventricular volume and is not affected by the volume at which ejection began. Loop A-E-F-I illustrates the effect of raising afterload (aortic pressure) on stroke volume. Intraventricular pressure must now rise to the higher aortic pressure, E, in order to open the aortic valve. Ejection then occurs along path E-F to a higher point on the isovolumic pressure curve at which ejection ceases. The net result is a decrease in stroke volume concomitant with an elevation in aortic pressure or afterload. The converse holds true; that is, stroke volume rises as afterload falls (E-F versus B-C). The effect of an increase in contractility is shown by loop A-B-J-K. Here, adding an inotrope to the intact heart preparation shifts the isovolumic pressure curve up and to the left so that from any ventricular volume a greater pressure is generated.

The data from the ventricular pressure-volume loop can be replotted as stroke volume versus preload to obtain the classic ventricular function curve (Fig. 3-10). Here an increase or decrease in preload is reflected by movement to the right or left along the function curve. An increase in contractile state or a reduction in afterload shifts the entire ventricular function curve to a higher level and vice versa. It is apparent from these curves that, from the standpoint of stroke volume, an increase in contractility is equivalent to a

reduction in afterload. During exercise stroke volume is augmented both by increasing contractility and by afterload reduction (A → B → C). Although preload also may rise slightly during upright exercise, the more important point is that it be maintained by increased venous return that matches forward cardiac output; if preload falls, the effects of increased contractile state and afterload reduction are severely limited (Fig. 3-10, D).

## EXERCISE PHYSIOLOGY

At the time of the industrial revolution, human labor supplied about 30% of the energy used in the workplace or on the farm in America. Today this figure has fallen to about 1% and recreational exercise represents a displacement of this physical activity from the workplace. Exercise has become an important element of contemporary life as evidenced by the popularity of running. Other expressions of this trend include bicycling, swimming, and racquet sports, as well as the phenomenal growth of health clubs throughout the country that provide exercise possibilities ranging from weight training to aerobics. Humans have been accustomed to strenuous physical exercise throughout history; it is the sedentary way of life of modern society that is new.

Exercise can be somewhat arbitrarily subdivided into isometric and isotonic work, depending on the type of muscular activity that is performed. Isometric exercise involves an increase in muscle tension without significant muscle shortening. Examples of isometric exercise include handgrip, pushing or pulling against a fixed resistance, or holding a heavy weight. Although no external work is performed (no shortening), high levels of energy may be expended. Isotonic exercise involves shortening of muscle fibers with relatively little tension development. Examples of predominantly isotonic (dynamic) exercise include running, swimming, and bicycling. Most forms of exercise include elements of isometric and isotonic muscle activity. In this chapter we will discuss the physiology of primarily isotonic forms of exercise.

The immediate source of energy for muscular work comes from the breakdown of ATP to ADP and inorganic phosphate. The total available pool of ATP can support exercise such as running for about 1 second but a few more seconds of work are obtained by replenishment of ATP from creatine phosphate stores. After these are expended, high-energy phosphate bonds must be recreated either by aerobic mitochondrial oxidative phosphorylation, in which glycogen, glucose, or fatty acids are used as fuels, or anaerobically by glycogenolysis or glycolysis with lactate formation. The aerobic pathways of oxidative phosphorylation are the main energy source for work of more than 1 or 2 minutes duration (isotonic exercise) and thus systemic oxygen transport is a rate-limiting function. The process of oxygen transfer from the atmosphere to the tissue could be limited at any of several levels (pulmonary, cardiovascular, or peripheral). Pulmonary oxygen transport involves ventilation, diffusion across the alveolar-capillary barrier, and chemical reaction with hemoglobin. The cardiovascular transport is a function of cardiac output and arterial oxygen content. The peripheral elements include distribution of the cardiac output and diffusion of oxygen to metabolizing tissues. The healthy sedentary subject uses about two thirds of his or her pulmonary capacity with maximal exercise, and oxygen transport is limited by cardiovascular and peripheral factors. In the highly trained athlete there is a closer match between pulmonary and cardiovascular oxygen transport capacity, and pulmonary, rather than cardiovascular, function may become the limiting factor in some individuals at sea level when maximal oxygen consumption exceeds 6 $L/min^{-1}$.

The principal characteristic of the normal response to dynamic exercise is a one-to-one match between changes in peripheral oxygen demand and cardiovascular oxygen transport. Thus there is a linear relationship between the intensity of aerobic work and total body oxygen consumption, $\dot{V}O_2$, that characterizes dynamic (isotonic) exercise. From the Fick equation 3 below, minute oxygen consumption, or $\dot{V}O_2$, is the product of cardiac output (oxygen delivery) and a $-\tilde{v}O_2$ difference (oxygen extraction):

$$\dot{V}O_2 = CO \times a - \tilde{v}O_2 \text{ diff} \qquad (3)$$

Since $CO = SV \times HR$, equation (3) can be rewritten as

$$\dot{V}O_2 = HR \times SV \times a - \tilde{v}O_2 \text{ diff} \qquad (4)$$

As exercise intensity increases, a level will be reached where HR and SV can increase no further, because to do so will result in oxygen deficit and increasing use of anaerobic energy pathways with net lactate formation and rapid onset of exhaustion. This plateau level of $\dot{V}O_2$ is termed $\dot{V}O_{2max}$, and it is a reproducible measure of a subject's total aerobic work capacity. Aerobic work at submaximal levels can be quantified as a percent of $\dot{V}O_{2max}$, which is known as relative work intensity and whose formula is given in equation 5:

$$\dot{V}O_{2rel} = \dot{V}O_{2actual}/\dot{V}O_{2max} \qquad (5)$$

The cardiovascular response to dynamic exercise can be described from the standpoint of the central (HR and SV) and peripheral (a $-\tilde{v}O_2$ diff) adaptations that occur with increasing levels of work intensity.

## Cardiac response

Cardiac output during dynamic exercise is a linear function of oxygen consumption ($\dot{V}O_2$). Bruce[1] has studied normal healthy men during treadmill exercise and has found $CO = 4.1 + 5.6$ ($\dot{V}O_2$). The central cardiac response to augment CO reflects the increased sympathetic nervous system activity that accompanies exercise. A linear relationship exists between sympathetic nervous system impulse level and the relative intensity of aerobic work $\dot{V}O_2;\dot{V}O_{2max}$) and thus also between HR, contractile state, and relative

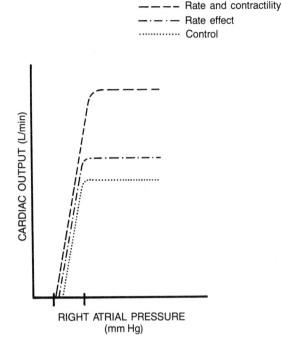

Rate and contractility
Rate effect
Control

**Fig. 3-11.** At a given right atrial pressure (RAP), increases in heart rate and contractile state can augment the cardiac output, CO, up to fourfold. The importance of maintaining venous return (preload) is apparent from the steep drop in cardiac output with a slight reduction in RAP.

work intensity. As exercise intensity increases, the heart rate rises linearly until somewhere between 170 and 190 beats per minute (bpm); any further increment encroaches on diastolic filling time and results in reduced preload, thus limiting SV. The heart rate response alone can increase cardiac output up to 2.5 times resting levels. The inotropic effects of increased sympathetic tone also augment contractility linearly with rising relative work intensity. Thus the characteristic pattern of cardiac response to dynamic exercise is a linear rise in heart rate and contractile strength with increasing work intensity. The combined effects of heart rate and contractile state are additive in augmenting CO (Fig. 3-11).

The contribution of preload to augmented SV during upright exercise remains controversial. End-diastolic volume and filling pressure increase on transition from rest to exercise in both the upright and supine positions, and there is a further rise in end-diastolic volume with increasing workloads. From Fig. 3-11 the critical importance of maintaining right atrial pressure at or above 0 mm Hg relative to atmospheric pressure (the importance of venous return and maintenance of preload) is evident. End-systolic volume decreases during upright exercise. This is consistent with an increased contractile state, since systolic blood pressure (afterload) may increase by as much as 100 mm Hg with maximal exercise even though ventricular ejection has also increased.

## Peripheral response

The peripheral vascular system consists of organ-associated arterio-capillary-venous circuits in a parallel arrangement (Fig. 3-12). Total peripheral resistance, TPR (the pressure gradient between the aorta and the right atrium), is shown in equation 6:

$$1/R_t = 1/R_i + \ldots + 1/R_n \qquad (6)$$

where $R_t$ is TPR, $R_i$ is resistance in each circuit, and $n$ is the total number of circuits. During exercise equation 6 can be rewritten as:

$$1/TPR = 1/R_w + 1/R_{nw} \qquad (7)$$

where $R_w$ is net vascular resistance in the working muscle groups and $R_{nw}$ is net resistance in all other nonworking vascular circuits (Fig. 3-13). At the onset of exercise (actually beginning even before exercise starts), the resistance (arteriolar) and capacitance (venous) components of the working muscle beds dilate, resulting in a large reduction in resistance to blood flow through the working muscle. At the same time, exercise induces a global increase in

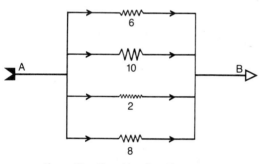

$$1/R_{A-B} = 1/6 + 1/10 + 1/2 + 1/8 = 1/.89 = 1.12$$

**Fig. 3-12.** Resistance in specific vascular beds $R_1$, $R_2$, $R_3$, $R_4$. Total resistance across parallel beds $R_{A-B}$ is given by $1/R_{A-B} = 1/R_1 + 1/R_2 + 1/R_3 + 1/R_4$.

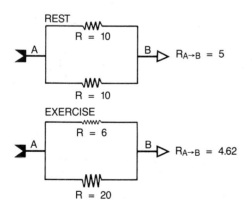

**Fig. 3-13.** During exercise resistance can be partitioned between working and nonworking vascular beds. Total resistance can drop despite substantial nonworking compartment vasoconstriction because of vasodilation in the working compartment.

sympathetic nervous system impulse traffic to all vascular beds, both working and nonworking. Until the higher stages of exercise, when heat loss becomes a major factor, the target organ response to the SNS outflow in all nonworking vascular beds is vasoconstrictive, and vascular tone increases in both resistive and capacitance elements. In the working muscle bed, the local vasodilator response overrides the vasoconstrictor influence. The net result of these two opposing vascular phenomena is a characteristic feature of the behavior of total resistance across parallel circuits: despite a widespread rise in resistance in many beds, a significant drop in resistance in one area can effect a net lowering of resistance across the entire circuit. Table 3-1 illustrates how because of the behavior of resistance across a parallel circuit, even a doubling of nonworking resistance during exercise can be offset by a modest (30% to 40%) reduction in resistance in the working muscular bed to yield a net reduction in TPR.

The entire mechanism underlying the local vasodilator response has not been completely defined, but current thinking supports the role of muscle activity itself as an important mediator of the local response. The possibility that potassium is a principal metabolic vasodilator agent is also intriguing. There is strong evidence that potassium release from working muscle during exercise causes local vasodilation and also activates muscle afferents and mediates the reflex-induced increases in heart rate, cardiac output, contractile state, and arterial pressure. Thus the same agent may serve as a vasodilator (local effects) and a vasoconstrictor (reflex-induced alpha-adrenergic stimulation). Whatever the mechanism, it has been shown that the magnitude of the local vasodilatation response in working muscle is directly proportional to the relative intensity of workload, that is $\dot{V}o_2;\dot{V}o_{2max}$.

The dual pattern of vascular changes that occurs is unique to dynamic exercise involving large muscle groups, and it forms the basis for the integrated functional circulatory exercise response. Local vasodilation, by reducing TPR and thus afterload, can augment the cardiac output independently of any change in heart rate or contractile state. Thus, part of

**Table 3-1.** Net reduction in total peripheral resistance (TPR)

| TPR | Working resistance ($R_w$) | Nonworking resistance ($R_a$) |
|---|---|---|
| At rest, 5 | 10 | 10 |
| 6.7 | 10 | 20 |
| 6.2 | 9 | 20 |
| 5.7 | 8 | 20 |
| 5.2 | 7 | 20 |
| 4.6 | 6 | 20 |
| 4 | 5 | 20 |
| 3.3 | 4 | 20 |

the rise in CO with exercise is directly proportional to the magnitude of the local vasodilatory reaction, which, in turn, is a function of relative workload. The enhanced flow through the dilated working muscle bed serves to augment venous return thus maintaining preload—a prerequisite for augmented stroke volume. In the absence of this increased venous return, preload would fall displacing cardiac function leftward along the ventricular function curve and thus curtailing the rise in stroke volume that results from increases in contractility and afterload reduction (Fig. 3-10, point D). Also, were it not for the vasoconstriction in nonworking organs, the otherwise unopposed local vasodilation would produce, right at the start of exercise, a sudden and profound fall in blood pressure. In general, the balance between vasoconstriction and vasodilation results in a graded fall in the total peripheral resistance (TPR) described by equation 7 and shown in Table 3-1.

Like the local vasodilator response, the SNS response to exercise is also linearly related to relative workload, and thus any parameter modulated by the SNS would be expected to behave similarly. This has been shown to be true for the vasoconstrictive response in nonworking areas. TPR, which reflects a balance between vasodilation and vasoconstriction (both of which are proportional to relative workload), has also been shown to be a linear function of $\dot{V}_{O_2};\dot{V}_{O_{2max}}$. Venoconstriction of capacitance vessels in nonworking beds causes up to 40% of the blood contained in them to be translocated centrally and ultimately to working muscle.

The net result of the circulatory changes accompanying exercise is an augmentation and redistribution of CO, so that the working musculature receives a greatly enhanced blood flow proportional to the relative intensity of exercise whereas nonworking areas maintain sufficient flow for normal homeostatic function during even prolonged exercise. In dynamic exercise involving large muscle groups (e.g., swimming or running), the circulatory response results from the combined effects of central (cardiac) and peripheral circulatory changes. Because the circulatory system is closed, except for beat-to-beat imbalances, venous return to the heart must equal cardiac output. Thus for cardiac output to rise with exercise, venous return also must rise to the same extent. In Fig. 3-14 the points of equilibrium between cardiac output and venous return are represented by the points where these curves intersect. Point A represents normal resting control with RAP near 0 and cardiac output/venous return about 5 L/min. With an increase in central (cardiac) function (increased HR and contractile state), cardiac output rises to point $A_1$, but in the absence of any peripheral effects, a further rise is prevented by the plateau in venous return, which would cause a fall in RAP and ultimately ventricular preload and thus shift the ventricle leftward and down its function curve (Fig. 3-10) curtailing SV. Point B is reached when maximal peripheral venoconstriction occurs, augmenting venous return and cardiac output about twofold. Thus the five- to sixfold rise in CO seen with strenuous dynamic

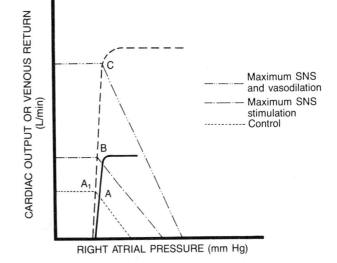

**Fig. 3-14.** The intersection of the cardiac output and venous return curves *(A, A₁, B, C)* determines the maximum cardiac output attainable under the conditions defined for each set of curves.

exercise is largely mediated by the drop in TPR caused by the local vasodilator response in working muscle. As a corollary, when dynamic exercise is performed with smaller muscle groups (i.e., two- legs → one leg → arms → . . . → hands), the relative contribution of the working muscle vasodilator effect diminishes and the circulatory pattern approaches point B (see Fig. 3-14), which is more characteristic of the circulatory response to isometric exercise.

## PHASES OF THE CARDIOVASCULAR RESPONSE TO EXERCISE

The dynamic pattern of circulatory adjustments to exercise can be divided into four fairly distinct phases: (1) the anticipatory phase in which neurological, humoral, and perhaps mechanical factors prepare the cardiovascular system for exercise; (2) an initial phase encompassing the first few minutes of exercise in which large changes in cardiovascular parameters occur as the system rapidly adapts to the requirements of exercise; (3) a period of relative "steady state," during which equilibrium is maintained through minor cardiovascular adjustments; and (4) the stage of "cardiovascular drift," characterized by progressively less efficient delivery of oxygen and metabolic needs and increasing demands on the cardiovascular system to dispose of body heat.

### Anticipatory phase

The earliest changes in response to exercise begin before the onset of actual muscular work. In anticipation of exercise there is frequently a mild increase in the heart rate and in cardiac output along with a modest elevation in systolic blood pressure. Venous tone throughout the body increases slightly, raising peripheral venous pressure, and thus blood volume shifts to the center from the periphery. These changes are all consistent with an anticipatory increase in sympathetic nervous system outflow. The intensity and extent of the changes, however, are highly variable, suggesting a major element of higher cortical modulation of this early response. Thus the physiological changes preceding a routine jog in the park are, not surprisingly, of much lesser magnitude than those preceding the start of an important race.

### Initial phase

The period, usually lasting from 2 to 4 minutes after the onset of exercise until the attainment of a relatively steady state, is termed the "initiation phase." Throughout this stage major alterations in circulatory function occur that, in effect, bring about the integrated circulatory response. The principal effector mechanism is the rapid and intense rise in sympathetic nervous system stimulation that modulates both the central and the peripheral circulatory activity and also the locally mediated muscular vasodilator response.

Although by no means completely delineated, a mechanism appears to be in operation that links the intensity of the sympathetic nervous system stimulation to the level of aerobic exercise defined in terms of percentage of maximum work capacity ($\dot{V}_{O_{2max}}$). In turn, all variables that are affected by sympathetic nervous system activity, that is, heart rate, contractile state, and vasoconstriction, have also been shown to be linearly related to the fraction $\dot{V}_{O_2}/\dot{V}_{O_{2max}}$. In the working muscle as well, the extent of vasodilation is directly proportional to local metabolic needs, which in turn correspond in a linear manner to $\dot{V}_{O_2}/\dot{V}_{O_{2max}}$. The possible role of potassium as mediator of local and ultimately the SNS response has been noted earlier. The total peripheral resistance (TPR) is the net result of opposing vasoconstriction and vasodilation, and because the intensity of the latter two phenomena is proportional to relative workload, TPR too varies in an inverse linear relation to $\dot{V}_{O_2}/\dot{V}_{O_{2max}}$.

Within seconds of onset of exercise, the heart rate begins to rise and may double within 15 seconds. Because it is easily measured, the heart rate response to exercise has been extensively studied and has been found consistently to bear a linear relationship to the relative workload. In fact, measurement of the heart rate alone provides a reliable, reproducible measure of exercise intensity in a given subject.

Blood pressure is not a directly controlled parameter, but rather reflects the net interaction of rising cardiac output and falling TPR ($BP = CO \times TPR$).

Typically, systolic blood pressure at first increases rapidly and then more gradually until a plateau is reached. The final "set" point of systolic blood pressure is, not surprisingly, a direct function of the relative workload intensity (see Chapter 5). Diastolic blood pressure is unchanged or falls slightly, and mean BP increases only slightly, typically by less than 20 mm Hg.

The rise in cardiac stroke volume results from changes in multiple variables rather than from any single direct alteration of cardiac function. Thus stroke volume depends on the level of venous return (preload), the blood pressure and/or TPR (afterload), the contractile state, and the heart rate. In general, in mild to moderate exercise, the stroke volume increases by about 50%, the increase ultimately being proportional to relative work intensity. At more strenuous levels of exercise, further increases in the stroke volume up to about twofold over resting values may occur in trained athletes.

Although all the parameters that determine the cardiac output are seen to be functions of relative workload, the cardiac output itself is a function not of the relative but of the absolute level of aerobic work or oxygen consumption. This reflects the requirement that as absolute $\dot{V}_{O_2}$ rises, the $O_2$ supply or cardiac output must keep pace. In fact, the limiting factor in exercise capacity ($\dot{V}_{O_{2max}}$) is, in most cases, specifically the ability to elevate oxygen delivery. Thus the circulatory pattern that emerges during the initial phase is a rise in the cardiac output directly proportional to $\dot{V}_{O_2}$ and brought about by rapid alterations in multiple hemodynamic parameters that are proportional to the relative level of work, that is, $\dot{V}_{O_2}/\dot{V}_{O_{2max}}$.

At rest the rate of oxygen transport greatly exceeds metabolic demand, and less than one third of the oxygen available in arterial blood is used. During exercise the combined effects of increased systemic oxygen demand and redistribution of increased CO to working muscle are an increase in extraction to about three fourths of the oxygen available in arterial blood.

### Steady state

After the initial rapid adjustment phase, if the level of exercise is submaximal, a stage is reached where the major hemodynamic parameters plateau and, except for minor variations, remain relatively constant for up to several hours. The duration of the steady state largely depends on the intensity of exercise, such that work levels of 50% to 70% of $\dot{V}_{O_{2max}}$ can be sustained for hours, whereas near-maximal exertion leads rapidly to exhaustion within minutes. During the steady state, the needs of the exercising muscle are being adequately met by the cardiovascular system, and any major change in circulatory variables will occur only in response to a change in exercise level itself—homeostasis has been achieved. The unifying factor with which all the cardiovascular variables measured correlate is oxygen uptake as a fraction of $\dot{V}_{O_{2max}}$. Adjustments for minor variations in metabolic need are through two mechanisms—one local and one central. Locally, if flow becomes inadequate for metabolic needs, local vasodilation increases, reducing resistance and directing larger flow to the working muscle bed. Venous return, further enhanced by the additional fall in resistance, augments the cardiac output. Thus a finely tuned system emerges in which minute-to-minute changes in working muscle vascular tone, probably a result of highly sensitive muscle afferent reflexes modulated by the metabolic milieu, can quickly alter the magnitude and distribution of the cardiac output. At the same time, processing of these signals in sympathetic nervous system centers modulates sympathetic nervous system tone, producing a synergism between the locally mediated effects of vasodilation and factors of the heart rate, contractile state, and peripheral vasoconstriction related to the sympathetic nervous system.

### Cardiovascular drift

As exercise continues, at some variable point in time a progressive change begins in the cardiovascular functional pattern just described. This final phase is characterized by a progressive fall in venous return, stroke volume, and blood pressure. Cardiac output, a function of the "absolute" exercise level, remains unchanged, but a progressive redistribution of flow, the result of an increasing need to dissipate body heat, is seen in the final stage of exercise. Before this stage, sympathetic nervous system peripheral influence is vasoconstrictive, but now vasodilation in the skin (mediated by the sympathetic nervous system) begins and becomes a progressively more important factor. As increased blood volume and flow is directed to the skin, splanchnic and nonworking blood flow approaches a minimum. Underlying these changes is a progressive rise in sympathetic nervous system tone, accompanied by a rising heart rate and intense vasoconstriction (except in skin and working muscle) in an effort to meet increasing circulatory demands. At some point, no further effective rise in the heart rate, venous return, or contractile state can occur and now, as further skin vasodilation occurs, less flow is available to working muscles. The metabolic and hemodynamic counterparts of exhaustion soon ensue.

At rest, fats and carbohydrates supply equal amounts of energy. With increasing workloads, carbohydrate use becomes increasingly more important and at maximum workloads energy is obtained exclusively through carbohydrate metabolism. This dependence on carbohydrates during heavy exercise is what limits endurance at work levels that approach but do not reach the capacity of the cardiovascular system to deliver oxygen. Under these conditions glycogen becomes the main source of fuel, and exhaustion sets in at the time of muscle glycogen depletion.

## EXERCISE AND HEART DISEASE

In general the physiological response to exercise in the normal subject and the subject with heart disease is qualitatively the same. There are, however, certain quantitative differences in exercise parameters that characterize the subject with heart disease. Different groups of patients with various forms of heart disease have, as a common denominator, a reduced maximal oxygen uptake. Patients with rheumatic heart disease have, on average, two thirds the normal $\dot{V}_{O_2}$. Patients with angina pectoris or recent myocardial infarction generally develop symptoms (angina, dyspnea) at exercise levels corresponding to 50% to 60% of the normal maximal age and sex specific $\dot{V}_{O_2}$. In the subject with heart disease, as in the normal subject, maximal oxygen consumption depends on cardiac output (delivery) and a-$\tilde{v}_{O_2}$ diff (extraction). It appears that patients with coronary disease, with or without varying degrees of congestive heart failure, retain a normal ability to extract oxygen at the tissue level. Thus the basis for the quantitative reduction in $\dot{V}_{O_{2max}}$ in coronary disease resides in the impairment of left ventricular function, which limits augmentation of stroke volume and cardiac output. Patients with mild left ventricular failure are able to compensate for reduced SV by relative tachycardia with exercise. In this case cardiac output is preserved at submaximal levels of exercise; however, maximal CO and $\dot{V}_{O_{2max}}$ are depressed in proportion to the decrease in maximal SV. As heart failure worsens there is a progressive attenuation of heart rate response, as well as SV, resulting in a subnormal cardiac output at all levels of exercise. Thus the characteristic finding in the coronary subject during exercise is a greater reliance on peripheral oxygen extraction than oncentral delivery mechanisms to sustain $\dot{V}_{O_2}$. Since $HR_{max}$, $SV_{max}$, and thus $\dot{V}_{O_{2max}}$ are lower in the subject with heart disease, it follows that for any level of submaximal exercise and its corresponding $\dot{V}_{O_{2actual}}$ the relative work intensity—defined as $\dot{V}_{O_{2actual}}/\dot{V}_{O_{2max}}$—is greater in the coronary subject. Moreover, all of the cardiovascular parameters that vary as a function of relative work intensity will achieve higher plateau values during steady state in the subject with heart disease. Thus at the same level of exercise, the SNS-mediated vasoconstrictor activity and consequently heart rate and blood pressure responses are more intense in the subject with heart disease than in the normal subject.

Myocardial work (the pumping of blood) is an aerobic process in which myocardial contractile energy requirements are met by oxidative metabolic pathways only (see Chapter 4). At basal conditions, myocardial oxygen extraction is much higher than in resting skeletal muscle, and there is no effective myocardial extractive reserve. Thus increased myocardial oxygen supply depends entirely on augmented coronary blood flow. In the subject with coronary disease and angina pectoris, exercise capacity is limited not by impaired $\dot{V}_{O_2}$ augmentation but, well before this, by the development of chest pain. Angina develops when myocardial oxygen demand outstrips a supply that is limited by obstructive coronary stenoses. Myocardial oxygen consumption, in turn, is a linear function of heart rate, afterload, and contractile state and empirically has been shown to be accurately approximated by the heart rate-blood pressure product, equation 8.

$$M\dot{V}_{O_2} = HR \times BP_{syst} \qquad (8)$$

Since heart rate and BP are both functions of relative workload during exercise, $M\dot{V}_{O_2}$ also correlates closely with exercise intensity. Angina, in a given coronary subject, can be elicited at a constant rate-pressure product that reflects the point where myocardial oxygen demand outstrips supply. This linkage between exercise intensity (relative $\dot{V}O_2$) and $M\dot{V}O_2$ forms the basis for clinical exercise testing (treadmill, bicycle) for diagnostic purposes or for determining exercise capacity in the coronary subject.

## MEASUREMENT OF HEMODYNAMIC PARAMETERS

Clinical measurement of cardiovascular function can be divided generally into two categories of testing, noninvasive and invasive. Widely used noninvasive techniques include radionuclide cardiac imaging (radionuclide ventriculography) and echocardiography (with or without treadmill or bicycle exercise testing). In both techniques end-diastolic and end-systolic left ventricular volumes can be measured and the percentage of blood filling the ventricle that is ejected with each beat (i.e., the ejection fraction) can be calculated at rest and during exercise.

$$\text{ejection fraction} = (EDV - ESV)/EDV \text{ or } SV/EDV \quad \text{(9)}$$

In the normal subject the rise in myocardial contractility and the drop in TPR and attendant augmentation of venous return and preload during exercise result in a characteristic increase in ejection fraction despite increased afterload. In the subject with severe left ventricular dysfunction, there is an apparent absence of exercise-induced changes in ventricular function, and characteristically ejection fraction either remains constant or falls with increasing workload. Because exercise capacity is strongly related to cardiac output (the product of heart rate and stroke volume), it is not surprising that the magnitude of the heart rate response becomes the principal determinant of exercise capacity in the subject with severe left ventricular failure.

In the patient with coronary atherosclerosis, exercise capacity is often symptom-limited by the onset of angina well before the maximal augmentation of total body oxygen consumption is reached. Treadmill or bicycle exercise testing has been the mainstay of clinical noninvasive evaluation in the coronary subject. Here, at a reproducible rate-pressure product reflecting a maximal $M\dot{V}O_2$ in a given subject, electrocardiographic (ST-segment) changes indicating ischemia occur. Clinical exercise testing provides both qualitative and semiquantitative information about the cardiovascular response to exercise in both the normal subject and the subject with heart disease. In the past decade, various myocardial imaging modalities (thallium, Technitium, and positron emission radionuclide techniques, echocardiography, and nuclear magnetic resonance) have been used both with and without exercise testing to obtain information about the distribution and adequacy of blood flow to the myocardium and also to assess myocardial cellular function.

Cardiac catheterization provides invasive data on central (cardiac) and peripheral (vascular) hemodynamics. Pressures can be measured in all of the cardiac chambers during the cardiac cycle, and blood flow (cardiac output) can be quantified. Peripheral vascular parameters such as TPR, pulmonary vascular resistance, and arteriovenous oxygen extraction can be directly assessed. Ventricular volumes, ejection fraction, and the pattern of ventricular contraction can be studied by cineangiographic ventriculography. The extent and severity of coronary atherosclerotic lesions can be determined by selective coronary arteriography. Although typically measured at rest, hemodynamic variables can be assessed during supine leg or arm exercise during cardiac catheterization. Ambulatory hemodynamic monitoring using a Swan-Ganz catheter has also been used to study the circulation.

Cardiac catheterization provides accurate and sophisticated data on cardiac function; however, prediction of exercise capacity or potential for improvement in cardiovascular function through exercise training from these results is not very accurate. In general, there is a striking lack of correlation between exercise capacity and results of measurement of ventricular performance both at rest and during exercise. This divergence stems in part from errors inherent in extrapolation of resting supine data to the upright exercise state. Moreover, exercise performance reflects the interplay of various cardiovascular, muscular, central nervous system, and other system variables as well as compensatory mechanisms that partially mitigate functional impairment in other areas. Despite its shortcomings, catheterization does provide useful data in formulating reasonable therapeutic goals and demonstrates as well the hemodynamic and anatomical substrate with which the patient must function. In general, it can be shown that the extent and severity of the coronary atheromatous process and the degree of left ventricular dysfunction correlates roughly with exercise capacity or potential for improvement. Thus a semiquantitative estimate of coronary stenoses in terms of the number of vessels involved and the severity of individual stenoses can provide some indication of what the possible exercise capacity and symptom level will be. Currently the most widely used measure of total left ventricular pump function is the ejection fraction, and here too a general relation exists between extent of reduction in ejection fraction and exercise performance. Thus the subgroup with normal left ventricular function, in terms of ejection fraction, and single vessel coronary involvement, will, as a whole, be better able to exercise more strenuously and derive greater benefit from it than the subgroup with advanced three-vessel disease and severely impaired ejection fraction. Unfortunately, the degree of overlap within these subgroups, in terms of symptoms and catheterization findings, significantly reduces the sensitivity and specificity of catheterization data. Moreover, in the largest subset of subjects (i.e., those with "moderate" disease), failure to establish the statistical validation for most measures derived from catheterization data is most apparent.

## REFERENCES

1. Bruce RA: Progress in exercise cardiology. In Yu PN and Goodwin JR, editors: *Progress in cardiology,* Philadelphia, 1974, Lea & Febiger.

## SUGGESTED READINGS

Astrand PO and Rodahl K: *Textbook of work physiology,* ed 3, Newark, 1986, McGraw-Hill Book Co.

Blomqvist CG and Saltin B: Cardiovascular adaptations to physical training, *Ann Rev Physiol* 45:169, 1983.

Braunwald E, Ross J, and Sonnenblick EH: *Mechanisms of contraction of the normal and failing heart.* Boston, 1967, Little, Brown & Co. Inc.

Brutsaert DL and Paulus WJ: Loading and performance of the heart as a muscle and pump, *Cardiovasc Res* 11:1, 1977.

Brutsaert DL and Sonnenblick EH: Cardiac muscle mechanics in the evaluation of myocardial contractility and pump function: problems, concepts and directions, *Prog Cardiovasc Dis* 16:337, 1973.

Chapman RA: Control of cardiac contractility at the cellular level, *Am J Physiol* 14:H535, 1983.

Clausen JP: Circulatory adjustments to dynamic exercise and effect of physical training in normal subjects and in patients with coronary artery disease, *Prog Cardiovasc Dis* 18:459, 1976.

Davies KJ, Packer L, and Brooks GA: Biochemical adaptations of mitochondria, muscle, and whole-animal respiration to endurance training, *Arch Biochem Biophys* 209:539, 1981.

Ehsani AA and others: Cardiac effects of prolonged and intense exercise training in patients with coronary artery disease. *Am J Cardiol* 50:246, 1982.

Gobel FL and others: The rate pressure product as an index of myocardial oxygen consumption during exercise in patients with angina pectoris. *Circulation* 57:549, 1978.

Lewis SF and others: Cardiovascular responses to exercise as functions of absolute and relative workloads, *J Appl Physiol* 54:1314, 1983.

Mitchell JH: Cardiovascular control during exercise: central and reflex neural mechanisms, *Am J Cardiol* 55:34D, 1985.

Opie Lionel H: Role of cyclic nucleotides in heart metabolism. *Cardiovasc Res* 16:483, 1982.

Saltin B: Hemodynamic adaptations to exercise, *Am J Cardiol* 55:42D, 1985.

Schaible TF and Scheuer J: Cardiac adaptations to chronic exercise, *Prog Cardiovasc Dis* 27:297, 1985.

# CHAPTER 4

# Drug Therapy of Common Cardiac Disorders

*Barry R. Dix*

The purpose of this chapter is to discuss the clinical pharmacology of medications used in the treatment of cardiac disorders frequently encountered by the cardiovascular physical therapist. These topics are quite extensive, and by necessity, discussion of them will be brief. The reader is encouraged to consult the extensive bibliography at the end of this chapter for additional information.

This chapter will review the following five clinical conditions:

1. Chronic ischemic heart disease
2. Congestive heart failure
3. Hypertension
4. Dyslipidemia
5. Cardiac dysrhythmia

## DRUG THERAPY: CHRONIC ISCHEMIC HEART DISEASE

Chronic ischemic heart disease is usually caused by occlusive disease of the coronary arteries. This most commonly results from atherosclerosis (see Chapter 2) and is typically manifest as angina pectoris. Angina pectoris is discomfort in the chest or adjacent areas, caused by myocardial ischemia. The discomfort is frequently described as a pressure or as being vise-like, crushing, squeezing, heavy, or constricting in quality. In some patients the discomfort is described as a vague sensation of numbness, burning, or shortness of breath. Electrocardiographically, ischemia is manifest as displacement of the ST-segment (depression when ischemia is subendocardial, and elevation if it is transmural or epicardial), with or without T-wave changes (usually inversion). Functionally, segmental left ventricular wall motion disturbances accompany ischemia and may produce an $S_4$ gallop (decreased compliance) or an $S_3$ gallop (left ventricular dysfunction).

Anginal pain is produced when myocardial oxygen *requirements* ($M\dot{V}O_2$) exceed oxygen *delivery*. Myocardial oxygen requirements are directly related to heart rate, myocardial contractility, and myocardial wall stress, which increases as chamber dimension and intracavitary systolic pressure rise. This function is approximated by the familiar double product—heart rate (HR) times systolic blood pressure (SBP) (HR × SBP). In typical angina, increased $M\dot{V}O_2$ is commonly brought about by physical activity. Other factors that increase metabolic demands, such as fever, anemia, hyperthyroidism, tachycardia, emotional stress, and eating may also provoke angina, but usually only if an anatomic coronary artery occlusion is present.

Angina may also be caused by transient reductions of oxygen *supply* as a consequence of coronary vasoconstriction with or without a concomitant increase in myocardial oxygen *demand*. This condition is commonly referred to as coronary artery spasm. Coronary spasm may occur in the presence or absence of anatomical obstruction. It is frequently responsible for symptoms of angina at rest. Delivery of sufficient oxygen may also be limited by severe diastolic hypotension (since most coronary blood flow occurs during diastole) and severe left ventricular hypertrophy.

Typical angina may also occur in severe aortic stenosis, severe pulmonary hypertension (right ventricular angina), and hypertrophic cardiomyopathy even in the absence of significant coronary disease.

Clinically, it is important for the therapist to recognize that not all chest pain is cardiac in origin. Important conditions that may produce chest discomfort, at times resembling angina include: esophageal motility disorders, peptic ulcer disease, cholelithiasis, gastroesophageal reflux, costochondritis, cervical spine disease, pleuritis, pericarditis, pulmonary embolism, aortic dissection, and musculoskeletal chest pain.

### Therapeutic goals

The therapeutic goals in the management of chronic ischemic heart disease include terminating the acute attack of angina, preventing recurrences, and reducing the risk of subsequent myocardial infarction. The medications commonly used are the nitrates, beta blockers, and calcium channel antagonists. These agents are effective principally by restoring the balance between myocardial oxygen supply and demand.

### Classification of agents

**Nitrates.** Organic nitrates (nitroglycerine, isosorbide, and others) are the most frequently used agents in the treatment of angina. Their primary mode of action is to relax vascular smooth muscle. These vasodilating effects are present in both the arterial and venous circulation, but the latter appears to be more critical in patients with ischemic heart disease. The nitrates decrease venous tone that results in a reduction in the return of blood to the heart; this in turn diminishes preload and ventricular dimensions, resulting in lowered wall tension and hence, decreased $M\dot{V}o_2$. The nitrates also lower ventricular afterload, which contributes in part to their antiischemic effect. The arterial vasodilating action of the nitrates on coronary circulation results in improved oxygen delivery. The nitrates, therefore, are excellent agents in that they reduce myocardial oxygen *demand* (principal effect) and increase oxygen *supply,* thereby relieving or preventing myocardial ischemia.

**Types of nitrates and routes of administration.** Nitroglycerin administered sublingually remains the drug of choice for treatment of acute anginal episodes. It is also used prophylactically by patients prior to activity that is likely to provoke chest pain. Nitroglycerin is rapidly absorbed; its onset of action is approximately 1 minute, peaking at 3 to 5 minutes. Its effects are brief, rarely lasting more than 20 to 30 minutes. The typical dose is 0.3 to 0.6 mg sublingually every 5 minutes but no more than 1.2 mg should be used in a 15 to 20 minute interval. Nitroglycerin tablets tend to lose their effect, especially if exposed to light, and therefore should be kept in dark containers. The patient characteristically experiences a burning or tingling under the tongue when taking sublingual nitroglycerin, a useful indicator of its potency.

Other nitrate preparations are available in buccal, oral, spray, topical, and ointment form. Long-acting agents such as the transcutaneous patches and oral isosorbide derivatives are useful in anginal prophylaxis. They should not be employed to abort an acute attack.

Oral long-acting nitrates are effectively absorbed but extensively metabolized by the liver. Therefore, the agents need to be administered in relatively large doses and at frequent intervals. The transdermal varieties offer an advantage in terms of patient compliance, having to be applied only once per day. Although around the clock protection was initially considered desirable, tolerance (loss of efficacy) may develop. Consequently, 10- to 12-hour nitrate-free intervals are currently recommended.

Recently, isosorbide mononitrate (Ismo, Monoket) was released for clinical use. These agents have greater bioavailability than isosorbide dinitrate, and therefore may be used in lower doses and at less frequent intervals. Ismo and Monoket are administered twice per day; Imdur, recently released, is effective once daily.

*Side effects.* As a group the nitrates produce a number of side effects that largely stem from their vasodilating properties. These are common and include headache, flushing, and hypotension. Headache and flushing tend to diminish in severity with continued use of the drugs but frequently are persistent. Hypotension, if severe, can have profound consequences, including loss of consciousness and precipitation of myocardial ischemia. Parodoxically, nitrate-induced hypotension is occasionally accompanied by bradycardia, rather than the expected reflex increase in heart rate. The transcutaneous nitrates share in the group effects but may also cause skin irritation at the administration site, a problem that often limits their use.

In addition to the effect of nitrate tolerance mentioned briefly above, some patients develop nitrate dependence. For this reason, as is often the case with many cardiac medications, discontinuation of the drug, when clinically indicated, should be done gradually to avoid precipitating a rebound ischemic event.

**Beta-adrenoceptor blocking agents.** Beta blockers are instrumental in the treatment of ischemic heart disease. They are generally well tolerated, reduce the frequency of angina, and raise the anginal threshold. Beta blockers work by competitively inhibiting the interaction between catecholamines and beta adrenergic receptors. These receptors are of two types: $beta_1$ receptors are located principally in the heart; their stimulation increases heart rate and myocardial contractility. $beta_2$ receptors are found in the lung and in the peripheral vasculature. Stimulation of $beta_2$ receptors produces bronchodilitation and peripheral vasodilitation. Beta blockers attenuate the cardiac response to adrenergic stimulation (increases in heart rate and contractility), thereby reducing myocardial oxygen *demand* primarily when surges in sympathomimetic activity take place. The beta blockers also reduce blood pressure, which also lowers myocardial oxygen demand. Several beta blockers are currently available for clinical use in the treatment of angina. These include, among others, propanolol (Inderal), atenolol (Tenormin), metoprolol (Lopressor), nadalol (Corgard), and acebutolol (Sectral).

Beta blockers are often classified according to three major properties (see the box below): cardioselectivity, lipid solubility, and intrinsic sympathomimetic activity (ISA). Cardioselective agents preferentially interact with the beta$_1$ receptors located in the heart and not with the beta$_2$ receptors in the lungs and peripheral vasculature. As a result, cardioselective agents may be associated with a reduced incidence of bronchospasm and peripheral vascular insufficiency, two potential important side effects of beta blockade. Cardioselectivity, however, is only apparent at low doses of these drugs; at high doses, even the cardioselective agents will inhibit both types of receptors.

These drugs also differ in their lipid solublity. Lipid soluble medications are more likely to cross the blood brain barrier and enter the central nervous system. Lipid soluble beta blockers, therefore, may produce more central nervous system side effects, such as insomnia, nightmares, and depression.

Some agents also have ISA, that is, *mild* beta-receptor stimulation. This may reduce side effects related to unopposed catecholamine mediated alpha-receptor vasoconstriction that may accompany beta blockade in the peripheral vasculature. Some beta blockers may have an adverse effect on lipid metabolism. Triglyceride levels may be increased and levels of high density lipoprotein cholesterol (HDL) may be reduced. These effects on lipids, which may not be clinically significant, do not appear to occur with agents possessing ISA.

*Side effects.* The side effects of the beta blockers are generally a consequence of the pharmacological blockade of the beta receptor and hence are shared to a greater or lesser extent by all of the agents. These include severe bradycardia, sinus arrest, heart block, reduced left ventricular systolic function, and bronchospasm. Other reported side effects include fatigue, depression, nightmares, sexual dysfunction, peripheral vascular insufficiency, and aggravation of coronary artery spasm. Miscellaneous side effects include alopecia, fever, short-term memory loss, and emotional lability.

---

### Summary of commonly used agents by classification

atenolol: cardioselective, water soluble, -ISA
metoprolol: cardioselective, lipid soluble, -ISA
propranolol: nonselective, lipid soluble, -ISA
nadolol: nonselective, water soluble, -ISA
acebutolol: selective, lipid soluble, +ISA

---

*Contraindications.* The contraindications to the use of beta blockers are also related to the consequences of beta-adrenergic antagonism. These drugs should be avoided in patients with severe sinus bradycardia or second- or third-degree heart block, unless the patient is protected by an electronic ventricular pacemaker. The drugs should also be avoided in patients with bronchial asthma, pulmonary hypertension, overt congestive heart failure, and cardiogenic shock. Patients with peripheral vascular disease may experience circulatory insufficiency if blockage of vascular beta$_2$ receptors leaves adrenergic alpha vasoconstrictor receptors unopposed; using a cardioselective agent or one with intrinsic sympathomimetic properties may minimize this side effect.

Beta blockers may also effect carbohydrate metabolism. Catecholamine stimulation of beta receptors (particularly in response to low blood sugar) leads to increased glucose production by the liver (hepatic glycogenolysis). This is an important defense mechanism against hypoglycemia. Noncardioselective agents may blunt the glucose elevating effect of circulating catecholamines. This could be clinically important, particularly in insulin-dependent diabetics, should they become hypoglycemic for any reason.

As with many cardiac drugs, if discontinuation of beta blockers becomes necessary, it is best to do so gradually. Abrupt withdrawal of a beta blocker from a patient with stable angina could trigger an acute ischemic event.

**Calcium antagonists.** The calcium antagonists are another useful addition to the therapeutic arsenal against cardiovascular disease. These agents are indicated in the treatment of myocardial ischemia (angina, coronary artery spasm), idiopathic hypertrophic subaortic stenosis, hypertension, and certain supraventricular tachydysrhythmias. Their principal mechanism of action is to block calcium receptors that are located in the heart and in vascular smooth muscle. In so doing, these agents promote arterial and venous dilitation. Certain agents may also retard electrical impulse conduction through the atrioventricular node and depress myocardial contractility. The calcium antagonists are also attractive antiangina agents since they favorably affect both aspects of the myocardial oxygen supply-demand balance. As arterial vasodilators they enhance oxygen delivery, and they reduce myocardial oxygen demand by lowering afterload and decreasing myocardial contractility.

Examples of calcium channel blockers include, among others, nifedipine (Procardia), verapamil (Calan, Isoptin), and diltiazem (Cardizem). These drugs are generally considered equally efficacious when used for angina or hypertension. The heart rate-slowing properties of verapamil and diltiazem make these agents particularly useful when there is need to control rapid heart rates. Verapamil and diltiazem are more likely to have a myocardial depressant effect. Nifedipine is therefore preferred when left ventricular dysfunction is present. In addition to being available in oral form, diltiazem and verapamil may be administered intravenously for rapid control of supraventricular tachydys-rhythmias, and nifedipine may be used sublingually when urgent antihypertensive action is needed.

*Side effects.* The principal side effects of the calcium antagonists relate to their pharmacological properties of vasodilation and include headache, flushing, hypotension, syncope, and dizziness. Peripheral edema and reflex tachycardia are more common with nifedipine, whereas bradycardia, heart block, and aggravation of left ventricular dysfunction are more likely to be seen with verapamil and diltiazem. Constipation also occurs, especially with verapamil.

## DRUG THERAPY: CONGESTIVE HEART FAILURE

Congestive heart failure is broadly defined as the condition in which the pumping performance of the heart is inadequate to meet the metabolic requirements of the peripheral tissues. It is usually, but not always, the result of myocardial failure. Myocardial failure, in turn, may have several causes, including severe valvular disease, hypertension, ischemic heart disease, or intrinsic muscle disease (cardiomyopathy). When the myocardium fails, several adaptive mechanisms are recruited in an effort to maintain the heart's pumping performance. Unfortunately, these adaptations often produce the signs and symptoms of congestive heart failure.

Principal among these compensatory responses is an increase in preload, primarily brought about by the salt and water retention that occurs when decreased blood flow to the kidneys activates the renin-angiotensin-aldosterone system. This dilates the ventricle and orients the heart muscle cells to contract more efficiently. The increased ventricular end diastolic pressure, however, may lead to pulmonary and sytemic venous congestion. As a consequence, dyspnea, paroxysmal nocturnal dyspnea, orthopnea, cough, hemoptysis, peripheral edema, jugulo-venous distension, and hepatomegaly may occur.

Cardiac output is improved by the increase in heart rate and contractility that occurs as a result of activating the sympathomimetic adrenergic system. The heart muscle may also hypertrophy in order to increase the mass of contractile tissue. However, both of these adaptations may increase myocardial oxygen consumption, which could be counter-productive by causing ischemia.

### Therapeutic strategy

The pharmacologic therapy of congestive heart failure addresses three areas:

1. Preload-reducing agents (control excess salt and water retention)
   a. Nitrates
   b. Diuretics
2. Inotropic agents (improve cardiac pumping performance)
   a. Cardiac glycosides (digitalis)
   b. Catecholamines (dobutamine, dopamine)

3. Afterload-reducing agents (reduce cardiac workload)
   a. Vasodilators
      1. ACE inhibitors
      2. Hydralazine
      3. Alpha$_1$ adrenergic blocking agents (prazocin, terazocin, doxazocin)
      4. Sodium nitroprusside

### Classification of agents

**Preload-reducing agents.** Preload-reducing agents act by reducing venous return to the heart. This in turn decreases intraventricular volume, which results in reduced intracavitary pressure. As this pressure is lowered, pulmonary and sytemic venous congestion are diminished. The nitrates, discussed earlier, do this by dilating the venous capacitance vessels. The diuretics perform this function by promoting enhanced salt and water loss via increased urine flow. This reduces intravascular volume that in turn lowers ventricular filling pressures. Fortunately, patients with congestive heart failure function can tolerate fairly significant reductions in filling pressure before cardiac output is compromised.

Numerous diuretic agents are currently available. They differ in potency, duration of action, metabolic effects, and in their site of action in the kidney. They all may cause excess volume depletion, hypotension, and electrolyte disturbances. Hypokalemia is always an important concern and may occur even when "potassium-sparing" agents are used. A summary of the most commonly observed side effects of diuretics is found in the box below.

The loop diuretics, furosemide and bumetenide, are the most potent. They inhibit sodium reabsorption in the ascending limb of the Loop of Henle in the renal nephron; they are almost always required when significant impairment of renal function exists (creatinine, level in excess of 2.5 mg/100 ml). The thiazides act on the distal tubule. Potassium-sparing agents, spironolactone, amiloride, and triampterine, act at the level of the collecting duct. Simultaneous use of agents acting at different sites in the renal nephron may enhance the diuretic effect, particularly in refractory cases.

---

### Side effects of diuretics

1. Hypokalemia (decreased potassium)
2. Hypochloremia (decreased chloride)
3. Hypomagnesemia (decreased magnesium)
4. Metabolic alkalosis
5. Hypercalcemia (increased calcium)—thiazide diuretics
6. Hypocalcemia (loop diuretics)
7. Hyperuricemia (which may precipitate an acute attack of gout)
8. Insulin resistance (which can lead to hyperglycemia, especially in diabetics)
9. Volume depletion, dehydration, and pre-renal azotemia
10. Hypotension
11. Hypercholesterolemia (increased cholesterol levels)

**Inotropic agents.** Currently, the cardiac glycosides are the only inotropic drugs available for chronic oral use. Several parenteral catecholamines, such as epinephrine, norepinephrine, dopamine, and dobutamine, may be used for short-term treatment of severe heart failure, but all attempts to create effective and safe oral derivatives have thus far proved unsuccessful.

Many different digitalis preparations exist, but digoxin, available both orally and parenterally, is by far the most frequently prescribed. Digoxin has a half life of 36 hours, is 60% to 85% absorbed by the gastrointestinal tract, and has a duration of action of approximately 3 to 6 days. It is eliminated primarily by the kidney. Digitalis exerts its inotropic action by binding to and inhibiting the function of a cell membrane enzymatic receptor, $Na^+/K^+$-ATPase (the $Na^+/K^+$ "pump"). The function of this enzyme is to move sodium out of the cell and potassium into the cell. When deactivated, the intracellular concentration of sodium increases. This in turn stimulates another transport system that exchanges the intracellular sodium for extracellular calcium. As a result, more calcium is available intracellularly to interact with the myocardial contractile proteins; hence, it augments contractility.

Digitalis also has significant electrophysiological effects that are mediated by its inhibition of the $Na^+/K^+$ pump. Clinically, its most important action is to retard conduction through the atrial-ventricular node, slowing the ventricular response to atrial fibrillation, atrial flutter, and certain types of supraventricular tachycardia.

Although clinically effective, digitalis preparations must be used cautiously, and patients need to be carefully monitored since the therapeutic to toxic ratio of these drugs is relatively narrow. Digitalis intoxication is a common and occasionally fatal problem. The combination of hypokalemia and digitalis toxicity is particularly dangerous as it frequently provokes ventricular dysrhythmia. A summary of commonly seen side effects of digitalis is found in the accompanying box.

**Afterload-reducing agents.** Afterload is broadly defined as impedance to ventricular emptying. Its components are complex and consist of the interaction among the aortic valve, elasticity of the arterial circulation, peripheral vascular resistance, and left ventricular wall stress. In the nonfailing heart, an increase in afterload results in a compensatory augmentation of myocardial contractility so that cardiac output is maintained. In heart failure, however, similar increases in afterload are not accompanied by this appropriate positive inotropic response. Cardiac output drops, ventricular end diastolic volume and pressure increase, and venous congestion occurs.

Afterload-reducing agents improve cardiac performance by lowering the resistance against which the ventricle ejects blood, thereby augmenting cardiac output. Myocardial contractility is not increased. Currently, the afterload-reducing agents clinically available consist of the vasodilators, which function as vascular smooth muscle relaxants. These drugs are classified as arterial, venous, or balanced (arterial and venous) vasodilators.

Hemodynamically, arterial vasodilation lowers peripheral vasculature resistance. Ordinarily, this would produce a drop in blood pressure. However, in patients with congestive heart failure, cardiac output (CO) is sufficiently increased so that mean arterial pressure (MAP) is maintained or only mildly diminished (MAP = CO × TPR*). Similarly, heart rate tends to remain the same or increases only slightly (CO = SV† × HR).

The venodilators work primarily by reducing preload; hence, they improve cardiac performance by lowering ventricular end diastolic pressure and volume. The nitrates, discussed earlier, are examples of these agents.

**Arterial vasodilators.** Hydralazine is a direct-acting, arterial vasodilator. It has no significant effect on venous circulation. Hemodynamically, cardiac output is improved with little or no change in ventricular filling pressures.

*Side effects.* Flushing and vascular headaches are frequent side effects. Hypotension and reflex tachycardia occur more often when the drug is used as an antihypertensive agent in the absence of heart failure. Secondary salt and water retention and tolerance (diminished efficacy) may follow long-term use. Hydralazine may produce a peripheral neuropathy that is related to drug induced pyridoxine (B-complex vitamin) deficiency. Chronic high-dose administration (300 to 400 mg per day) may also lead to a lupus-like syndrome (rash, joint swelling, pericarditis). This occurs more often in patients who metabolize the drug slowly (slow acetylators), but it is usually reversible upon its discontinuation. More effective results are seen when hydralazine is combined with isosorbide to achieve balanced arterial and venous relaxation. This combination recently has been shown to prolong survival in patients with chronic congestive heart failure.

**Balanced vasodilators (preload-afterload reducing agents).** The balanced arterial-venous vasodilators include

---

| Side effects of digitalis |
| --- |
| 1. Bradydysrhythmia: sinus bradycardia, sinus arrest, sinus node exit block, first-degree heart block, second-degree heart block (usually Wenckebach), complete heart block, asystole. |
| 2. Tachydysrhythmia: atrial tachycardia with AV block, nonparoxysmal junctional tachycardia, premature ventricular beats, ventricular tachycardia, ventricular fibrillation. |
| 3. Anorexia, nausea, vomiting, abdominal pain |
| 4. Disturbed color vision (especially yellow-green), halos, scotoma, fatigue, malaise, headache, delerium, psychosis |
| 5. Worsening congestive heart failure |

* TPR: total peripheral resistance
† SV: stroke volume

sodium nitroprusside, the alpha$_1$ receptor blockers (prazocin, terazocin), and the angiotensin converting enzyme inhibitors (captopril, enalapril, and others).

Nitroprusside is a rapid-acting, short-duration agent available only intravenously for the treatment of severe congestive heart failure. It is designed primarily for short-term therapy. Prazocin and terazocin inhibit the postsynaptic vascular alpha$_1$ receptors, thereby producing arterial and venous dilitation. Reduced ventricular filling pressures and improved cardiac output with little change in heart rate and mean arterial pressure are the predominant hemodynamic effects following short-term use. These responses, may become attenuated, however, with long-term use.

*Side effects.* Prolonged administration of nitroprusside may lead to the accumulation of thiocyanate (a byproduct of nitroprusside metabolism), especially in the presence of renal insufficiency. Thiocyanate toxicity may cause hypothyroidism, neuromuscular irritability (twitching, seizures), abdominal pain, and psychosis. Hypotension, particularly orthostatic, an important side effect when prazocin and terazocin are used as antihypertensive drugs, is less common in the heart-failure patient. A major limitation is that these agents have not been shown to improve long-term survival.

**ACE inhibitors.** The ACE inhibitors have become a valuable addition to the therapeutic arsenal for the treatment of congestive heart failure. These agents have balanced arterial and venous effects and therefore improve cardiac output and relieve venous congestion. They improve quality of life, increase exercise tolerance, and prolong survival (recently demonstrated for enalapril and captopril), even more so than the isosorbide-hydralazine combination.

Several ace inhibitors are available. They differ in their frequency of administration and duration of action. They all inhibit converting enzyme leading to reduced levels of angiotensin, a potent vasoconstrictor. Until recently this effect was believed to be their principal mode of action. It is now felt that other actions, such as reduced breakdown of bradykinin (a potent vasodilator), reduced levels of catecholamines, and direct effects at the cellular level may be equally important.

*Side effects.* The ACE inhibitors also share similar side effects. These include chronic dry cough (usually reversible and not dose related), angioneurotic edema, hyperkalemia, hypotension, and renal insufficiency (especially in the presence of renal artery stenosis). Taste disturbances, agranulocytosis, and proteinuria have been reported. In general, the ACE inhibitors are effective agents for long term use. Tolerance does not seem to occur. Quality of life and long-term prognosis are both improved.

## DRUG THERAPY: HYPERTENSION

Hypertension is the most common cardiovascular disease. It is a major risk factor for the development of coronary artery disease, cerebral vascular disease, peripheral vascular disease, and congestive heart failure.

---

### Criteria for hypertension

**Diastolic blood pressure**

1. Less than 85 mm Hg normal
2. 85 to 89 mm Hg high normal
3. 90 to 104 mm Hg mild hypertension
4. 105 to 114 mm Hg moderate hypertension
5. Greater than 114 mm Hg severe hypertension

**Systolic blood pressure**

1. Less than 140 mm Hg normal
2. 140 to 159 mm Hg borderline
3. Greater than 159 mm Hg elevated

---

Hypertension is usually defined as an elevated systolic and/or diastolic blood pressure based on the average of two or more readings taken on two or more occasions using proper technique and an appropriately sized blood pressure cuff. The criteria listed in the accompanying box are generally accepted.

Hypertension is generally classified into two main groups. The first group, essential or idiopathic hypertension, constitutes 90% to 95% of cases. The second classification, secondary hypertension, although relatively infrequent, must be recognized since therapy for the underlying cause is often the definitive treatment for the associated elevated blood pressure. Secondary causes of hypertension include the following diagnoses:

1. Pheochromocytoma (characterized by increased blood levels of catecholamines)
2. Cushing's syndrome (characterized by increased levels of cortisol and its metabolites)
3. Primary aldosteronism (characterized by increased levels of mineralocorticoids such as aldosterone)
4. Hyperthyroidism
5. Hyperparathyroidism (characterized by hypercalcemia)
6. Renal parenchymal disease (glomerulonephritis, chronic pyelonephritis, polycystic kidney disease, and others)
7. Renal vascular disease (renal artery stenosis—atherosclerotic, fibromuscular dysplasia)
8. Coarctation of the aorta
9. Oral contraceptive use

Specific tests are available to establish these diagnoses and should be ordered when appropriate. Clinically, secondary hypertension should be suspected in the following instances:

1. Development of hypertension in patients less than 20 or older than 50
2. Evidence of symptoms of paroxysmal hypertension, tachycardia, and sweating (pheochromocytoma)
3. Evidence of unprovoked hypokalemia or unexplained hyperglycemia (aldosteronism, Cushing's syndrome)

4. The presence of a flank or abdominal bruit (renal vascular disease)
5. Elevated serum creatinine [greater than 1.5 mg/100 ml (renal parenchymal disease)]

Family history of hypertension or renal disease, use of oral contraceptives, use of proprietary pharmaceuticals containing catecholamines (cold remedies), and use of laxatives (mineralocorticoids), should also be pursued.

### Essential hypertension

The pathogenesis of essential hypertension is not definitively understood. A primary disorder of renal sodium handling leading to salt and water retention is thought to play an early role. A defect in cellular calcium metabolism leading to increased intracellular calcium levels (causing arterial vasoconstriction) may also be a contributing factor. Hormonal factors are also important and include the renin-angiotensin-aldosterone system, growth hormone, insulin, and atrial natriuretic hormone. Angiotensin is a potent vasoconstrictor and may also promote vascular growth; aldosterone contributes to salt and water retention. Growth hormone may play a role in vascular hypertrophy, and natriuretic hormone is important in fluid balance. Insulin has been shown to promote vascular hypertrophy, sodium retention, and to increase sympathomimetic activity. Insulin resistance and hyperinsulinemia are common in hypertensives, particularly those who are obese.

Hemodynamically, blood pressure is defined by the equation $MAP = CO \times TPR$ (mean arterial pressure is a function of cardiac output and peripheral vascular resistance). No matter how hypertension is initiated, the final common denominator is a sustained increase in peripheral vascular resistance. Once the diagnosis is established, therapy is crucial. Although a conclusive reduction in the incidence of acute myocardial infarction has not been demonstrated, treatment of hypertension leads to reduced morbidity and mortality from stroke, renal failure, and congestive heart failure.

Although pharmacologic treatment is the cornerstone of medical management, dietary sodium restriction (at least a no-added-salt diet), weight reduction (to ideal body weight), relaxation techniques, and regular isotonic exercise, are important adjunctive factors.

### Classification of agents

Antihypertensive drugs can be divided into the following main categories:

1. Diuretics: thiazides, loop, potassium-sparing
2. Beta blockers
3. Peripheral alpha$_1$ adrenergic blockers
4. Central alpha$_2$ adrenergic agonists
5. Vasodilators
6. Calcium channel blockers
7. Angiotensin converting enzyme (ACE) inhibitors

**Diuretics.** Diuretics were discussed previously in the section on congestive heart failure. In general, diuretics are effective antihypertensive agents leading to a reduction in diastolic blood pressure to below 90 mm Hg in approximately half of all patients. Thiazide diuretics are the most frequently prescribed. They are effective when used alone and particularly when combined with additional agents, such as potassium-sparing agents (spironolactone, triampterine, amiloride) to limit hypokalemia. The loop diuretics are needed, however, when renal insufficiency is present and serum creatinine exceeds 1.5 to 2.5 mg/100 ml, or when refractory edema is present.

The antihypertensive mechanism of diuretics is poorly understood. Initially, there is a reduction in plasma volume brought about by enhanced renal salt and water excretion. This is accompanied by a small drop in cardiac output. After several weeks, cardiac output and plasma volume return to normal (probably secondary to compensatory activation of the renin-angiotensin-aldosterone system). The antihypertensive effect is maintained by a reduction in peripheral vascular resistance. This may be achieved by a direct vasodilating effect, increased vascular compliance (less sodium in the vascular wall), or altered vasoreceptor sensitivity.

The side effects of diuretics are listed in the box on p. 37. Principally, these include hypokalemia, hyponatriemia, hypomagnesemia, hypochloremia, hyperuricemia, hypercalcemia, hypercholesterolemia, volume depletion, and orthostatic hypotension.

**Beta blockers.** The beta blockers were discussed previously in the section on ischemic heart disease. Their antihypertensive effect is not thoroughly understood. Beta blockade with resultant decrease in heart rate, cardiac output, and hence blood pressure has only a minor role. It is thought that suppression of renin (and therefore decreased angiotensin production) is a more important mechanism.

**Peripheral alpha$_1$ blockers.** Peripheral alpha$_1$ blockers, which include prasocin (Minipress), terazocin (Hytrin), and doxazosin (Cardura), competitively block the vascular alpha$_1$ receptors in both arteriolar resistance vessels and venous capacitance vessels. Presynaptic alpha receptors are unaffected (stimulation of these receptors leads to inhibition of norepinephrine release). These agents, therefore, lower blood pressure without significant reflex tachycardia or an increase in plasma-renin activity. The most frequent side effects are postural dizziness, and occasionally, syncope due to orthostatic hypotension (often following the first dose). Other less frequent side effects include nausea, vomiting, diarrhea, constipation, male impotence, urinary frequency, weakness, fatigue, and headache.

**Direct vasodilators.** Hydralazine (Apresoline) is a direct-acting arterial vasodilator. Its blood pressure lowering effect is accompanied by reflex tachycardia, renin release, and salt and water retention. Use in conjunction with beta blockers and diuretics blunts these secondary effects. Further discussion of hydralazine may be found in the section on congestive heart failure (CHF).

Minoxidil (Loniten) is similar to apresoline but considerably more potent. Concomitant use of beta blockers and diuretics is almost always required. The drug is usually reserved for patients with refractory severe hypertension and renal failure. Hirsutism and pericardial effusion may complicate its use.

**Central alpha$_2$ agonists.** Central alpha$_2$ agonists act by stimulating central alpha$_2$ receptors, causing a decrease in sympathomimetic outflow from the central nervous system (CNS). Blood pressure is lowered by a drop in peripheral vascular resistance. Cardiac output is usually maintained; renal blood flow is preserved; and significant postural hypotension is uncommon. Sedation, dry mouth, sexual dysfunction, galactorrhea, and mild orthostatic hypotension are side effects common to this class of drug. Bradycardia and worsening of CHF are rare, but they may occur in patients with severely compromised cardiac function.

Methyldopa (Aldomet) has been accompanied by unique side effects that include an autoimmune Coombs positive hemolytic anemia, fever, and a syndrome resembling viral hepatitis.

Clonidine is available in a transdermal preparation that may be applied once per week. It may also be used hourly in 0.1 to 0.2 mg doses to lower urgently severe hypertension. A withdrawal syndrome characterized by tachycardia, sweating, and overshoot severe hypertension has been described following abrupt discontinuation of clonidine, but these symptoms have been seen with other agents as well.

Guanabenz (Wytensin) and guanfacine (Tenex) are recent additions to this group of drugs. Guanabenz may cause less secondary fluid retention; guanfacine has a long duration of action and is often used once daily.

**Calcium channel blockers and ACE inhibitors.** Calcium channel blockers and ACE inhibitors have been discussed in some detail in earlier sections of this chapter. Suffice it to say, that these agents are effective antihypertensives that are well tolerated. They are frequently used alone as initial therapy, but they can be used in combinations with other antihypertensive agents as well. These drugs are currently among the most commonly prescribed medicines in the treatment of hypertension.

# DRUG THERAPY: DYSLIPIDEMIA

A detailed discussion of dyslipidemia is beyond the scope of this chapter. Treatment consists of nonpharmacologic (diet, exercise) and pharmacologic measures. Drug therapy is generally reserved for those patients who fail to achieve satisfactory results from nonpharmacologic measures or in whom lipid levels are so high that diet and exercise alone are unlikely to be effective. Secondary causes of dyslipidemia need to be recognized and treated. These include hypothyroidism, uncontrolled diabetes mellitus, dysglobulinemia, nephrosis, ethanol abuse, and estrogen administration.

## Classification of lipid-lowering drugs

The drugs commonly used in the treatment of lipid disorders include:

1. Bile acid resins
2. Nicotinic acid
3. Fibric acid derivatives
4. Probucol
5. HMG CoA reductase inhibitors

In general, the goal of therapy is to reduce total cholesterol levels to less than or equal to 200 mg/100 ml, LDL cholesterol to less than 130 mg/100 ml, and triglycerides to below 150 mg/100 ml. Pharmacologic measures to elevate HDL cholesterol are of limited effect. Achieving these therapeutic endpoints has been demonstrated to significantly reduce the incidence of ischemic heart disease.

The bile acid resins (cholestyramine, colestipol) sequester cholesterol laden bile salts in the bowel thereby leading to their excretion and limiting their reabsorption (enterohepatic circulation). This lowers total serum cholesterol levels and leads to a secondary increase in hepatic receptors (LDL receptors) that causes an increased clearance of LDL from the blood. Thus, these agents are effective in lowering both total cholesterol and LDL cholesterol. If properly taken, a 20% to 25% reduction in cholesterol and LDL may be expected. These agents are difficult to use, however, because of frequent unpleasant gastrointestinal side effects, especially nausea, bloating, abdominal pain, constipation, and unpleasant taste. They may also interfere with the absorption of other medications such as Coumadin or digitalis.

Nicotinic acid (niacin, a B-vitamin), when used in large doses, lowers total cholesterol, LDL cholesterol, and triglycerides. HDL levels are increased. Its mechanism of action is largely unknown. Side effects are frequent and include a prostaglandin mediated flushing reaction (which may be blunted by aspirin), pruritus, gastritis (which could lead to peptic ulcer), liver function abnormalities, glucose intolerance (caution when used in diabetics), and hyperuricemia (especially in patients with gout).

The fibric acid derivatives reduce both cholesterol (through increased cholesterol secretion in the bile) and triglycerides (through increased lipoprotein lipase activity, resulting in increased triglyceride clearance from the blood). HDL levels are mildly increased. Side effects include an increased incidence of gall stones, a possible increased incidence of GI malignancy, liver function test abnormalities, myositis, diarrhea, and nausea. The effects of warfarin anticoagulants (coumadin) are potentiated.

Probucol lowers LDL via a scavenger-mediated pathway. It also lowers HDL level (uncertain clinical significance), and may prolong the $QT_C$ interval of the electrocardiogram (potential arrhythmic effect). The drug also causes diarrhea, nausea, and flatulence.

The HMG CoA Reductase inhibitors act by competitively blocking the rate limiting step in hepatic cholesterol synthesis. A secondary rise in hepatic LDL receptors ensues. These agents are quite effective in lowering total and LDL cholesterol levels. A mild increase in HDL also occurs. Liver function test abnormalities may occur. Myositis may occur, particularly when these drugs are combined with nicotinic acid, gemfibrozil, or the antibiotic erythromycin. An initial concern over the development of cataracts has not materialized.

## DRUG THERAPY: DYSRHYTHMIAS
### Review of electrophysiology

Cardiac cells are electrically excitable; that is, they are capable of generating an action potential in response to an appropriate stimulus. Once initiated, the excitatory wave propagates along the cell membrane as a regenerative response. The heart is a functional syncytium of cells. The excitatory stimulus generated by the pacemaker cells within the SA node spreads to adjacent atrial myocardium and then, sequentially, to the AV node, His bundle, right and left bundle branches, distal Purkinje system, and ventricular myocardium (see Chapter 5). The envelopment of the heart by this excitatory process and the subsequent restoration of the resting equilibrium are responsible for the familiar characteristics of the surface electrocardiogram (ECG). The propagated electrical impulse causes changes in myocardial cell membrane permeability and produces the action potential. Calcium and sodium ions enter the cells, triggering an interaction between the myofibrillar proteins that results in myocardial contraction.

There are two types of action potentials in the heart, termed "fast" and "slow." The fast action potentials occur in normal atrial and ventricular myocardium and in the specialized conduction tissue of the His-Purkinje system. The fast response action potential has five phases. Phase 0 is the upstroke in which membrane potential moves from a resting level of about −90 to about +30 mV. This represents depolarization of the cell and is mediated by a rapid inward movement of sodium (Na$^+$) ions. After the upstroke, a brief outward flow of potassium (K$^+$) ions (or an influx of chlorine [Cl]) causes a slight drop in membrane potential toward baseline (phase 1). This is followed by phase 2, the plateau phase, during which membrane potential remains relatively constant. Phase 3 is repolarization and is primarily due to a net outward movement of K$^+$ ions. Phase 4 represents electrical diastole and remains flat except in those cells that exhibit automaticity, such as the SA and AV nodes, His-Purkinje system, and specialized atrial cells. During phase 4 a net inward current of positive ions gradually moves the resting membrane potential back toward its activation threshhold. Automaticity is a characteristic of pacemaker cells, but it may occur in nonpacemaker tissue under abnormal conditions.

The second type of action potential is the slow response action potential found primarily in the SA and AV nodes. These action potentials are principally mediated by the slow inward movement of calcium ions.

The surface ECG is correlated to the action potential. Atrial depolarization is responsible for the P wave. Activation of the AV node and His-Purkinje system produces the PR interval. The QRS interval occurs during ventricular depolarization; the ST-T segment represents ventricular repolarization. Atrial repolarization occurs during the QRS complex and usually is not depicted on the surface ECG. Repolarization of the His-Purkinje system is thought to produce U waves when they are present. (See Fig. 4-1.)

In summary, in the resting state myocardial cells are polarized: that is, the inner aspect of the cell membrane is negatively charged with respect to the outside. The resting potential is the result of electrochemical gradients established by the selective permeability of the cardiac cell membrane. Stimulation of the cell provokes specific changes in membrane permeability and ion conductance, alterations in transmembrane voltage, and changes in the internal ionic composition of the cell. These changes in cellular electrical activity are responsible for the monophasic action potential (MAP).

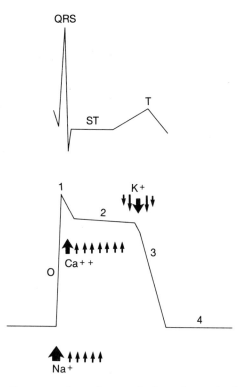

**Fig. 4-1.** Representation of monophasic action potential in a nonpacemaker cell and relationship to surface ECG. Depolarization, phase 0, is carried by the fast sodium current, which continues at reduced levels throughout the plateau. The slow calcium current is maximum towards the end of phase 0 and phase 1, and continues at a low level throughout the plateau. Repolarization is carried by a potassium current which is maximal during the latter portions of phase 2 and phase 3. (Modified from Lassara R and Scherlag BJ: Generation of arrhythmias in myocardial ischemia and infarction, *Am J Cardiol* Symposium Arrhythmia Therapy 61(20A-26A):2, 1988.)

## Mechanisms of dysrhythmia

Cardiac dysrhythmias reflect disordered electrical activation of the heart. The following three phenomena observed during microelectrode studies of myocardial cell preparations may be operative in the genesis of clinical dysrhythmias:

1. Abnormal automaticity
2. Reentry
3. Afterpotentials

Ordinarily, the pacemaker cells of the SA node exhibit the fastest intrinsic rate. Pacemaker cells situated elsewhere are suppressed by the depolarization wave originating from the SA node (overdrive suppression). Disease, metabolic derangement, hypoxia, drugs, mechanical stresses, and altered autonomic nervous activity may permit normally dormant pacemakers to assume dominance. This may become manifest as single or multiple extrasystoles or as sustained ectopic tachycardia. The specific type of dysrhythmia will depend on the location of the ectopic pacemaker and its frequency and regularity.

Reentry refers to the propagation of an electrical impulse in a circuit or loop. In order for reentry to occur the different "limbs" of the circuit must display *slowed conduction* and *unidirectional block.* When an electrical impulse arrives at the circuit it is propagated slowly down one limb, but its passage down the other limb is blocked. At some other point the impulse engages the other limb of the circuit and is propagated in the opposite direction since the block is unidirectional. When conditions are appropriate, this process becomes self-perpetuating, producing tachydysrhythmia.

Two types of reentry phenomena have been described. The first type, macroreentry (circus-movement reentry), involves pathways that may be found in the SA node, the AV node, bypass tracts [preexcitation syndromes such as Wolff-Parkinson-White (WPW)], and possibly within the atria. Circus-movement reentry may underlie atrial flutter, AV nodal reentrant tachycardia, supraventricular tachycardia, and some instances of ventricular tachycardia. The second type, microreentry, is the result of focal reexcitation between myocardial cells in close proximity. Ischemia, drugs, and other injury may alter the action potential durations and refractory periods of adjacent cardiac cells, resulting in microscopic regions of slowed conduction and block, thereby creating the conditions favorable for microreentry circuits. Ventricular tachycardia complicating chronic ischemic heart disease is probably related to this mechanism.

Afterpotentials are fluctuations in transmembrane potential observed during the plateau or at the end of the monophasic action potentials. The precise mechanism responsible for their appearance is unknown. Afterpotentials may be provoked or exaggerated by certain toxins and drugs, including the cardiac glycosides (digitalis, digitalis derivatives), and may play a role in the genesis of the dysrhythmias associated with these agents.

## Classification of agents

The antidysrhythmic drugs may be categorized according to their dominant electrophysiological effects. The following outline lists four major classes of antidysrhythmic drugs and (where appropriate) subgroups within these classes:

1. Class 1: Membrane depressants/local anesthetics
   a. Quinidine, procainamide, disopyramide
   b. Lidocaine, tocainide, mexiletine, phenytoin
   c. Flecainide, propafenone
2. Class II: Beta adrenergic blocking drugs (beta blockers)
3. Class III
   a. Bretylium, amiodarone, sotalol
4. Miscellaneous agents: Calcium-channel blockers

**Class Ia agents.** Quinidine (Quinaglute, Quinidex), procainamide (Pronestyl, Procan SR), and disopyramide (Norpace) produce moderate slowing of phase 0 (rapid $Na^+$ channel) of the MAP. On the surface ECG this is manifested as an increase in QRS duration. Repolarization, phase 3, is prolonged. $QT_c$ interval increases in duration, and changes in the ST segment and T waves are observed. Diastolic depolarization is normal and ectopic pacemaker cells are suppressed. Rhythm disturbances related to abnormal pacemaker activity may be responsive to these agents. They are useful in the management of a variety of supraventricular and ventricular dysrhythmias. Quinidine in particular and, to a lesser degree, procainamide and disopyramide, may convert atrial fibrillation and flutter to normal sinus rhythm. Class Ia agents effectively suppress atrial and ventricular premature complexes and may prevent the recurrence of atrial and ventricular tachycardias. The direct effect of these drugs is to slow AV nodal conduction. Quinidine and disopyramide, however, may indirectly accelerate AV conduction through vagolytic anticholinergic mechanisms. In the case of atrial flutter or fibrillation, a dangerous acceleration in ventricular response may be observed, necessitating the simultaneous administration of digitalis, a beta blocker, or a calcium-channel blocker. Combined therapy with quinidine and digoxin may result in serum glycoside levels higher than observed when the same dosage of digoxin is given alone. Thus the dosage of digoxin must be diminished when quinidine is added to the therapeutic regimen.

Because of their extensive electrophysiological activity, quinidine, procainamide, and disopyramide are potentially dysrhythmogenic. Suppression of normal automaticity may result in sinus arrest or asystole. Preexisting atrioventricular and intraventricular conduction disturbances may be aggravated when large dosages of these drugs are given. Particular caution is demanded in patients with evidence of impaired sinus node function (i.e., "sick sinus syndrome"). Quinidine, disopyramide, and, less frequently, procainamide have been associated with a paradoxical increase in ventricular ectopic complexes, recurrent ventricular tachycardia, and recurrent ventricular fibrillation ("quinidine syncope"). This reaction is usually observed in patients who demonstrate pronounced QT-interval prolongation.

Although quinidine is a versatile antidysrhythmic agent, its use is often limited by unacceptable gastrointestinal side effects, particularly nausea, abdominal cramping, and diarrhea. Abnormal bleeding may be observed as a result of drug-induced thrombocytopenia ("quinidine purpura"). Quinidine is an optical isomer of the antimalarial drug quinine, first isolated from the bark of the cinchona tree. Symptoms of "cinchonism," including tinnitus, headache, nausea, and visual disturbances, may complicate quinidine therapy.

Procainamide may also cause gastrointestinal symptoms, including anorexia, nausea, and vomiting. Potentially more serious, however, is the appearance of abnormal immunoglobins or antinuclear antibodies. Accompanying the serological perturbations, in approximately 15% of patients, are signs and symptoms resembling systemic lupus erythematosus, including fever, rash, arthralgias, and pleural and pericardial effusions.

The most troublesome side effects observed in patients receiving disopyramide relate to this agent's marked anticholinergic activity, which may result in blurred vision, dry mouth, urinary retention, constipation, and impotence. The concomitant administration of an acetylcholinesterase inhibitor such as physostigmine may minimize these side effects. Disopyramide interferes with myocardial calcium transport, and may exert significant negative inotropic effects. Congestive heart failure may be aggravated or precipitated, particularly in patients with preexisting left ventricular dysfunction. It may also provoke marked hypotension or circulatory collapse in patients with limited cardiac reserve.

**Class Ib agents.** Both mexiletine (Mexitil) and tocainide (Tonocard) are chemically related to lidocaine, and are classified as group Ib local anesthetic agents. These drugs cause a minimal slowing of phase 0 and suppress phase 4 of the MAP. Phase 3 is accelerated and repolarization is shortened. Few changes are noted on the surface ECG when they are administered in therapeutic dosages. Their usefulness is limited to treatment of ventricular dysrhythmias, including premature ventricular complexes, ventricular tachycardia, and ventricular fibrillation.

Lidocaine (Xylocaine) has been employed in the coronary care unit setting for over 2 decades. It remains the drug of choice for the control of ventricular dysrhythmia complicating acute myocardial infarction. Some have recommended its use prophylactically in all patients presenting with infarction to reduce the risk of primary ventricular fibrillation. Others reserve administering it until warning dysrhythmias appear. It is routinely employed after successful resuscitation from ventricular fibrillation to prevent recurrence. Lidocaine is available only for parenteral use. Extensive hepatic degradation precludes oral administration. Prominent side effects resulting from central nervous system toxicity include paresthesias, apprehension, tinnitus, drowsiness, respiratory depression, somnolence, coma, and convulsions. Hypotension, circulatory collapse, marked bradycardia, and asystole have also been observed. Toxicity is directly related to the speed of administration and total dosage. Patients with marked right heart failure or preexisting hepatic disease may rapidly accumulate toxic blood levels because of impaired degradation of the drug.

Tocainide (Tonocard) is a chemical congener of lidocaine. Therapeutic blood levels can be maintained with oral dosing making this agent suitable for chronic treatment. Frequent side effects include paresthesias, tremor, nausea, vomiting, and rash. Pulmonary fibrosis and agranulocytosis are two less common but more serious side effects requiring careful drug monitoring and immediate termination of therapy. Because a significant fraction of the administered dose is excreted unchanged by the kidneys, dosages must be adjusted in patients with impaired renal function or diminished renal perfusion. The hemotologic side effects of this drug, however, have severely limited its use.

Mexiletine (Mexitil) is another lidocaine analog. Similar to both lidocaine and tocainide, its usefulness is limited to the treatment of ventricular dysrhythmia. Frequent side effects include heartburn, nausea, and vomiting, which sometimes can be avoided by administering the drug with antacids or food. Central nervous system toxicity including nervousness, insomnia, tremor, dizziness, and lightheadedness are also common. The drug is extensively metabolized by the liver, and dosage must be adjusted in patients with impaired hepatic function.

Phenytoin (Dilantin) is used primarily for control of epileptic seizures. Electrophysiologically it resembles lidocaine, and it is included as a Class Ib drug. Phenytoin's antidysrhythmic activity is quite modest. It is useful in the management of supraventricular and ventricular dysrhythmia secondary to digitalis intoxication. Phenytoin suppresses pacemaker activity in the SA node and may produce marked sinus slowing or sinus arrest.

**Class Ic agents.** Drugs in this category principally affect the rapid sodium channel. Phase 0 of the MAP is markedly slowed, resulting in QRS widening on the surface ECG. The ST segment and T wave exhibit only minimal alteration, reflecting the minor effects exerted by these drugs on the repolarization process. Cardiac conduction is slowed in all areas of the heart, with the most pronounced effects being observed in the cells of the specialized conduction system (His-Purkinje fibers).

Two drugs are currently available for clinical use in this class: flecainide (Tambocor) and propafenone (Rhythmol). Indications for their use, contraindications, and toxicity profiles are quite similar. These drugs are clinically effective in a wide variety of both supraventricular and ventricular tachydysrhythmias including atrial fibrillation, atrial flutter, supraventricular tachycardia, the supraventricular dysrhythmias associated with the Wolff-Parkinson-White (WPW) syndrome, premature ventricular contractions (PVCS), and ventricular tachycardia. Prodysrhythmic effects (i.e., a propensity to increase the frequency and severity of dysrhythmia) are particularly troublesome with this class of drugs. New and potentially life-threatening ventricular dysrhythmias, including ventricular tachycardia may be observed in up to 10% to 15% of patients receiving these agents. Prodysrhythmia is most likely to appear in patients with marked left ventricular dysfunction and in those presenting with sustained monomorphic ventricular tachycardia. Such patients must be carefully monitored during initiation of therapy.

Sinus node depression may result in severe bradycardia or asystole. This is a particular risk in patients who exhibit evidence of sinus node dysfunction (i.e., "sick sinus syndrome"). These agents probably should not be used in the presence of second degree heart block without the protection of a permanent pacemaker and should be used cautiously in patients with preexisting intraventricular conduction disorders. Propafenone possesses beta-blocking properties approximately 5% the potency of propranolol. This needs to be taken into consideration when prescribing this agent.

Drugs in this category exhibit negative inotropic activity and their use may therefore lead to worsening congestive heart failure. This is particularly true of flecainide. They should thus be used cautiously, if at all, in patients exhibiting evidence of severe left ventricular dysfunction.

Recently, the empiric treatment of ventricular dysrhythmias, other than life-threatening ventricular tachycardia, with type I agents has been seriously questioned. Not only is there no definite proof of efficacy in preventing sudden cardiac death, but also these agents may actually increase mortality in certain patients [The Cardiac Arrhythmia Suppression Trial (CAST)]. Asymptomatic ventricular ectopy may require no treatment at all, even in the presence of heart disease. When therapy for symptomatic ventricular ectopy is deemed necessary (troublesome palpitations, angina, hypotension), beta blockers, provided no serious contraindications exist, are useful agents. Treatment of life-threatening sustained ventricular tachycardia (documented survival of sudden cardiac death, syncope) may require type III drugs, electrophysiologic guided therapy, or the implantation of an automatic implantable cardiac defibrillator (AICD).

**Class II agents (beta blockers).** The antidysrhythmic potential of the beta blockers may be attributed to one or more of their pharmacological effects:

1. Direct membrane depressant ("quinidine-like") activity
2. Prevention or reduction of myocardial ischemia
3. Inhibition of dysrhythmogenic effects of catecholamines

Commercially available propranolol is a mixture of both D and L isomers. The D isomer does not provide beta-blocking activity but does produce membrane depressant effects. Propranolol reverses catecholamine-induced acceleration of diastolic depolarization (suppresses automaticity). Sinus node slowing and prolongation of AV-nodal conduction are observed at low dosages and are a function of beta blockade. These effects explain the drug's usefulness in controlling ventricular response during atrial fibrillation and flutter and in slowing the sinus rate in patients with excessive adrenergic drive (e.g., hyperkinetic heart syndrome). Excessive adrenergic activity or increased sensitivity to circulating catecholamines may also contribute to dysrhythmias associated with thyrotoxicosis, general anesthesia, digitalis intoxication, and myocardial infarction.

Higher concentrations of propranolol produce alterations in the MAP of Purkinje cells, suppression of spontaneous diastolic depolarization, and decreased membrane responsiveness. The importance of these direct membrane effects has been questioned, since the plasma concentrations achieved with the customary dosages employed are considerably smaller than the concentrations required to alter MAP properties in microelectrode preparation.

Recently, several large-scale, multicenter studies have demonstrated a reduced risk of sudden death following acute myocardial infarction in patients maintained on certain beta-blocking drugs. It is not known whether the observed effect is a direct result of the antidysrhythmic activity (membrane effects) of this class of drugs, is secondary to their ability to favorably influence the balance between $M\dot{V}o_2$ and myocardial $O_2$ supply, or is the result of a change in the natural history of the underlying atherosclerosis.

**Class III agents.** Bretylium (Bretylol) is available for parenteral use only. Bretylium has no effect upon the action potential of atrial muscle. Accordingly, it is ineffective in controlling supraventricular dysrhythmias. Bretylium does not suppress and may actually accelerate the slope of phase 4 depolarization in Purkinje fibers. Its predominant effect appears to be on the repolarization phase of the action potential in Purkinje and ventricular myocardial fibers. Bretylium may indirectly hyperpolarize cells by eliciting a transient release of catecholamines, resulting in enhanced membrane responsiveness in abnormally depressed fibers. It also exhibits some adrenergic blocking activity, which may contribute to the hypotension observed during rapid intravenous administration. Bretylium's clinical usefulness is confined to control of recurrent or refractory ventricular tachycardia and fibrillation, particularly in the case of acute myocardial infarction. It is contraindicated in the presence of digitalis intoxication.

Amiodarone (Cordarone) is an iodinated benzofuran derivative with unique and novel electrophysiological properties. It was developed originally as an antianginal agent and possesses coronary vasodilatory activity. Subsequent investigation demonstrated its potent antidysrhythmic potential. Its mechanism of action is unknown. Amiodarone markedly prolongs repolarization and refractory period duration in all cardiac fibers. Striking increases in QT-interval duration are observed on the surface ECG. Phase 4 depolarization is suppressed in pacemaker cells located in the SA and AV nodes and in the His-Purkinje system. The drug also noncompetitively blocks alpha and beta adrenergic receptors. Amiodarone inhibits the binding of thyroid hormone to its receptors.

Amiodarone exhibits an extraordinary spectrum of antidysrhythmic activity, although at present it has been approved only for management of malignant ventricular dysrhythmias (ventricular fibrillation, ventricular tachycardia). In particular, amiodarone has proven effective in treating a significant proportion of patients presenting with recurrent ventricular fibrillation unresponsive to all other antidysrhythmic agents. It favors the reestablishment of normal sinus rhythm or may facilitate electrical cardioversion in patients with persistent atrial fibrillation and flutter. It is effective in controlling persistent atrial ectopic activity, including recurrent supraventricular and AV-nodal tachycardia and reentrant tachycardia related to the WPW syndrome.

Despite its proven effectiveness and versatility, amiodarone is not considered a first-line antidysrhythmic drug. It has been associated with serious and potentially life-threatening side effects, and therefore its use is reserved for serious dysrhythmia that has proven unresponsive to more conventional agents. Progressive and sometimes fatal pulmonary fibrosis may occur in a small minority of patients. Thyroid dysfunction, including both hyperthyroidism and hypothyroidism, is relatively common. Corneal microdeposits and abnormal skin pigmentation are commonly observed. The very long half life allows for infrequent dosing. It also presents particular problems when evidence of toxicity has appeared. Amiodarone interacts with many other drugs commonly administered to cardiac patients, including warfarin (intensifies anticoagulant effect) and digoxin (increases serum concentration). Therapy with amiodarone demands careful monitoring.

Sotalol is a type III agent that has been available in Europe for several years. Like amiodarone, it is effective against a wide variety of supraventricular and ventricular dysrhythmias. However, it has been approved in this country only for the treatment of life-threatening ventricular tachycardia. It shares the potential prodyshythmic effect of other agents. As its name implies, sotalol is also a beta blocker and therefore the precautions associated with beta blockers apply to sotalol as well.

**Class IV: calcium-channel blockers.** Cardiac fibers may be classified as fast or slow, depending on the speed at which they conduct electrical impulses. Fast fibers are characterized by rapid conduction velocity, high resting potential, high threshold potential, rapid rate of depolarization, and large spike amplitude. Fast fiber depolarization (phase 0) is dependent on activation of a "fast" membrane sodium channel. Cell types in this group include ordinary atrial and ventricular myocardium and Purkinje fibers. Slow cardiac fibers are characterized by their slow conduction velocity, low resting potential, slow rate of depolarization, and small spike amplitude. Depolarization (phase 0) of slow fibers is carried by an inward calcium current. Myocardial cells with these characteristics are located in the sinoatrial and atrioventricular nodes.

The calcium antagonist drugs retard depolarization in slow fibers, resulting in sinus bradycardia and AV conduction delays. These drugs also interfere with the calcium current responsible for the plateau phase (phase 2) of the MAP.

Nifedipine is devoid of important antidysrhythmic activity. Indirectly, it may reduce dysrhythmia by alleviating myocardial ischemia.

Parenteral verapamil is considered by some to be the drug of choice for termination of paroxysmal supraventricular tachycardia. It is useful both parenterally and orally in slowing ventricular response in atrial fibrillation and flutter and suppressing recurrent atrial tachycardia. Its usefulness with respect to ventricular dysrhythmia is controversial. Verapamil is contraindicated in patients with the WPW syndrome who present with atrial fibrillation and antegrade conduction through the bypass (accessory) tract. In this situation, verapamil may accelerate ventricular response and precipitate ventricular fibrillation.

Diltiazem is also useful in the control of the ventricular response to supraventricular tachydysrhythmia. It is now available for intravenous administration and is quite effective for this purpose.

Adenosine is an endogenous nucleoside that has recently been approved for the treatment of supraventricular tachycardia. It functions primarily by blocking the AV node. It is administered by rapid IV bolus; its effect dissipates within 6 to 12 seconds. Adenosine is now competing with verapamil as the drug of choice to pharmacologically acutely terminate AV-nodal reentrant SVT.

## SUMMARY

This concludes the discussion of pharmacological therapy used in the treatment of ischemic heart disease, congestive heart failure, hypertension, dyslipidemia, and cardiac arrhythmia. Although brief out of necessity, effort was made to provide the cardiovascular therapist with clinically useful and appropriate information. As is apparent from the preceding discussion, there is considerable overlap in the indications for the usage of several of these agents. The reader is encouraged to consult the bibliography for more details regarding specific topics.

## SUGGESTED READINGS

Abrams J: Tolerance to organic nitrates, *Circulation* 74(6):1181, 1986.

Braunwald E: Control of myocardial oxygen consumption, *Am J Cardiol* 27:416, 1971.

Braunwald E: *A textbook of cardiovascular medicine,* Philadelphia, 1992, W.B. Saunders Company.

Calcium-entry blockade: basic concepts and clinical implications, *Circulation Monograph* No. 5 75(6) June 1987.

The Cardiac Arrhythmia Suppression Trial (CAST) Investigators: Effect of encainide and flecainide on mortality in a randomized trial of arrhythmia suppression after myocardial infarction, *N Engl J Med* 321:406, 1989.

The Cardiac Arrhythmia Suppression Trial (CAST II) Investigators: *N Engl J Med* 327:227, 1992.

Chatterjee K and Parmley WW: The role of vasodilator therapy in heart failure, *Prog Cardiovasc Dis* 19:301, 1977.

Cohn JN and others: Effect of vasodilator therapy on mortality in chronic congestive heart failure: results of a Veterans Administration cooperative study, *N Engl J Med* 314:1547, 1986.

Cohn JN and others: A comparison of enalapril with hydralazine-isosorbide dinitrate in the treatment of chronic congestive heart failure, *N Engl J Med* 325:303, 1991.

The CONSENSUS Trial Group: Effect of enalapril on mortality in severe congestive heart failure: results of the Cooperative North Scandinavian Enalapril Survival Study, *N Engl J Med* 316:1429, 1987.

The CONSENSUS Trial Study Group: Effects of enalapril and neuroendocrine activation on prognosis in severe congestive heart failure. *Am J Cardiol* 66:400, 1990.

Doherty JE and others: Clinical pharmacokinetics of digitalis glycosides, *Prog Cardiovasc Dis* 21(2):141, 1978.

Epstein S and others: Angina pectoris: pathophysiology, evaluation, and treatment, *Ann Intern Med* 75(2):263, 1971.

Goodman LS and Gilman A, editors: *The pharmacological basics of therapeutics,* New York, 1985, Macmillan, Inc.

Gorlin R: Regulation of coronary blood flow, *Br Heart J* 33(suppl):9, 1971.

James TN: The delivery and distribution of the coronary collateral circulation, *Chest* 58(3):183, 1970.

Lucchesi BR and Leighton WS: The pharmacology of the beta adrenergic blocking agents, *Prog Cardiovasc Dis* 11(5):410, 1969.

Mason DT: Digitalis pharmacology and therapeutics: recent advances, *Ann Intern Med* 80(4):520, 1974.

*The Medical Letter On Drugs and Therapeutics:* Choice of cholesterol lowering drugs, vol 35 (891):19-22, March 5, 1993.

*The Medical Letter On Drugs and Therapeutics:* Sotalol for cardiac arrhythmias, vol 35 (893):27, April 2, 1993.

*The Medical Letter On Drugs and Therapeutics:* Drugs for chronic heart failure, vol 35 (896):40, May 14, 1993.

The 1988 Report of the Joint National Committee on Detection, Evaluation, And Treatment of High Blood Pressure. US Department of Health and Human Services *Arch Intern Med* 148(5):1023, 1988.

Packer M: Therapeutic options in the management of chronic heart failure, *Circulation* 79(1):198, 1989.

Proceedings of the workshop on implications of recent beta-blocker trials for post-myocardial infarction patients, *Circulation Monograph,* No. 96, 67(6), June 1983.

Rosen MR and Gelband H: Antiarrhythmic drugs, *Am Heart J* 81(3):428, 1971.

Singer DJ and others: Cellular electrophysiology of ventricular and other dysrhythmias, *Prog Cardiovasc Dis* 24(2):97, 1981.

Singer I and Kupersmith J: *Clinical manual of electrophysiology,* Baltimore, 1993, Williams & Wilkins.

Singh BN and others: New perspectives in the pharmacologic therapy of cardiac arrhythmias, *Prog Cardiovasc Dis* 22(4):243, 1980.

Smith TW and Haber E: Digitalis, *N Engl J Med* 289(18):945, 1973.

Smith TW and Haber E: Digitalis, part 2, *N Engl J Med* 289(19):1010, 1973.

Smith JW and Haber E: Digitalis, part 3, *N Engl J Med* 289(20):1063, 1973.

Smith TW and Haber E: Digitalis, part 4, *N Engl J Med* 289(21):1125, 1973.

The SOLVD investigators: Effect of enalapril on mortality and the development of heart failure in asymptomatic patients with reduced left ventricular ejection fractions, *N Engl J Med* 327:685-691, 1992.

The SOLVD investigators: Effect of the antiarrhythmic agent Moricizine on survival after myocardial infarction. The Cardiac Arrhythmia Suppression Trial (Cast II) Investigators, *N Engl J Med* 327:227-233, 1992.

A symposium: antiarrhythmia therapy—controversies, directions and challenges, *Am J Cardio* 61(2):(entire issue) 1988.

A Symposium: Clinical evaluation of response to antiarrhythmic therapy, *Am J Cardiol* 62(12):1988.

Zipes DP and Troup PJ: New antiarrhythmic agents: amiodarone, aprindine, disopyramide, ethmozin, mexiletine, tocainide, verapamil, *Am J Cardiol* 41(6):1005, 1978.

## CHAPTER 5

# Basic Electrocardiography

*Barbara A. Mammen*

This chapter describes basic principles of electrocardiography with a primary focus on single-lead strip analysis relating to common and benign, as well as life-threatening, dysrhythmias. When the electrical conduction system and the electrocardiogram (ECG) are understood, it becomes relatively simple to interpret cardiac waveforms.

## ELECTROPHYSIOLOGY OF THE HEART

The cardiac muscle is comprised of two basic cell types: *electrical* conductive cells that initiate the electrical activity and conduct it through the heart and *mechanical* cells that

☐ NOTE: Rhythm strips included in this chapter are, for the most part, sample strips obtained at Southern Regional Medical Center in Riverdale, Georgia. The two monitoring systems currently in use at this facility are Nihon-Kohden and Care Monitoring Systems.

respond to the electrical stimulus and contract to pump blood. There cannot be a mechanical response without an electrical stimulus first.

The processes of contraction and relaxation in the myocardium are referred to as *depolarization* and *repolarization,* respectively. During depolarization the cells are stimulated and the myocardium contracts; during repolarization it relaxes.

During the resting phase, the cells of the myocardium are said to be *polarized.* This means that they have positive charges on the outside of each cell and an equal number of negative charges on the inside. In other words, in a polarized or resting state the charges are balanced and no electricity flows. Electrical stimulation makes the cell membrane permeable to the flow of ions. The primary ions involved in this

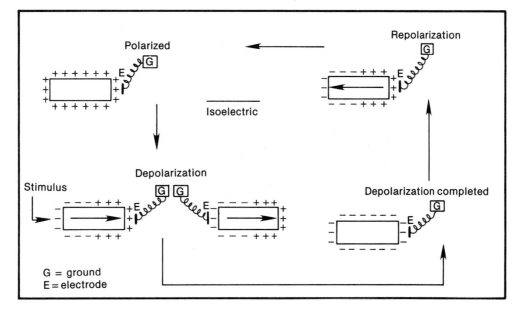

**Fig. 5-1.** Depolarization-repolarization process.

electrical activity are sodium and potassium. In the resting cell, potassium is mostly on the inside of the cell while sodium is mostly on the outside. During *depolarization,* the current flow consists of sodium ($Na^+$) ions moving from the outside to the inside of the cell, until the outside of the cell becomes negatively charged and the membrane is fully depolarized. The pathway allowing for this ion exchange is referred to as the fast channel. The flow of potassium ($K^+$) ions from the inside to the outside of the cells begins shortly after the $Na^+$ ions start to move in. When the $K^+$ ions flow exceeds that of the $Na^+$ ions, *repolarization* begins and the outer surface of the membrane again becomes positively charged. This depolarization process is illustrated in Fig. 5-1. It is important to note that other mechanisms are involved in current flow.

## THE CONDUCTION SYSTEM

The electrical cells in the heart are arranged in a pathway called the conduction system. This conduction system is designed to allow for the spread of electrical activity throughout all four heart chambers. Fig. 5-2 illustrates the conduction system.

The primary pacemaker of the heart is the sinoatrial (SA) node. It is located in the right atrium near the orifice of the superior vena cava. The normal cardiac impulse originates in the SA node and then travels through the intraatrial pathways, also located in the right atrium; simultaneously, the impulse moves across Bachman's bundle and the left atrium is depolarized. The impulse arrives next at the atrioventricular (AV) node, also known as the junctional node, located near the intraventricular septum in the inferior wall of the right atrium close to the tricuspid valve. Conduction is slowed through the AV node. The depolarization wave then spreads to and through the bundle of His.

Ventricular depolarization now proceeds by way of the bundle branches that follow along the intraventricular septum. The right bundle branch is responsible for right ventricular depolarization, and the left bundle branch is responsible for left ventricular depolarization. Because the left ventricle is physically larger than the right ventricle, there are two divisions of the left bundle branch. The main pathway is called the anterior fascicle: the smaller second division is called the posterior fascicle. At the terminal ends of the bundle branches are thousands of smaller fibers called Purkinje fibers that penetrate the myocardium and distribute electrical impulses to the muscle cells. Mechanical contraction is then completed (see Fig. 5-2).

The three major "pacemakers" of the heart are the SA node, which is the primary pacemaker, and the AV node and ventricles (Purkinje fibers), the latent or secondary pacemakers. In the event of a default of the SA node, the latent pacemakers, if functional and intact, should initiate conduction and stimulate contraction. Each of the three pacemakers has an inherent rate or expected rate of firing at which impulses are usually produced. A site can exceed or fall below its inherent rate under certain conditions. The inherent rates of the SA node, AV node, and ventricles are as follows:

SA node 60 to 100 times or beats per minute
AV node 40 to 60 times or beats per minute
Ventricles 20 to 40 times or beats per minute

Ideally, the SA node maintains control and initiates the impulse of a sinus rhythm, the normal expected cardiac rhythm. Should the SA node fail as a pacemaker, the AV node or ventricles should assume control and act as a secondary pacemaker.

The concept of refractoriness is important to the understanding of the completion of depolarization. There are two

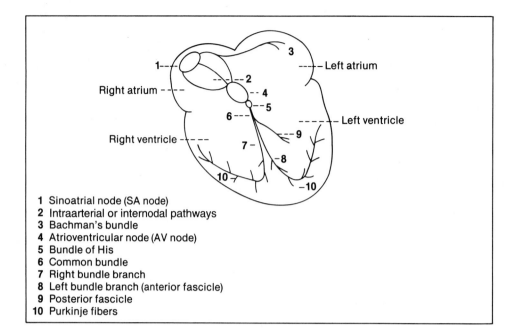

**Fig. 5-2.** The conduction system.

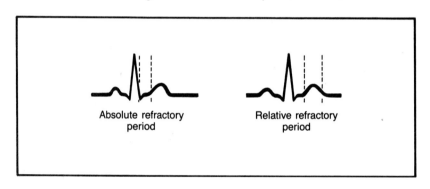

**Fig. 5-3.** Periods of refractoriness.

refractory periods: (1) the absolute refractory period and (2) the relative refractory period. During the absolute refractory period, no matter how much stimulation is applied to the cells, depolarization cannot occur because repolarization is not complete. In the relative refractory period some cells are ready to be depolarized and others have not completed repolarization. During the relative refractory period, abnormal depolarization may result since some cells can be stimulated and others cannot. Potentially lethal dysrhythmias may occur. Fig. 5-3 illustrates these periods.

There are two electrophysiological properties of a cardiac cell that should be mentioned. They are *automaticity* and *conductivity*. Automaticity refers to the ability of cardiac cells to discharge an electrical current without stimulation from the nervous system. The highest degree of automaticity is found in the SA node, but the entire conduction system possesses some degree of automaticity. Disturbances in automaticity can produce a speeding up or slowing down of the sinus node (sinus tachycardia or sinus bradycardia) or a premature beat from the atria, junction, or ventricles.

Conductivity enables the cardiac cells to transfer impulses to successive cells very rapidly. Conduction velocity or speed varies in cardiac tissue but ranges from 200 to 4000 mm/sec. Alterations in conductivity can produce very rapid rhythms such as supraventricular tachycardias or slow rhythms such as heart blocks.

Innervation of the heart is also influenced by the autonomic nervous system and its two branches—the sympathetic and the parasympathetic nervous systems. The sympathetic branch influences the SA node, the AV node and the ventricles and, when stimulated, increases the heart rate, increases conduction through the AV node, and increases irritability. The parasympathetic system, primarily through the vagus nerve, creates the opposite responses. There is a decrease in heart rate, slowed conduction through the AV node, and a decrease in irritability.

## WAVEFORMS AND RECORDED ACTIVITY

The waveforms that are recorded on the ECG tracing are representative of the electrical stimulation that precedes the mechanical contraction and relaxation of the heart. The

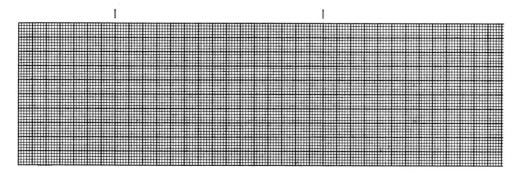

**Fig. 5-4.** ECG graph paper.

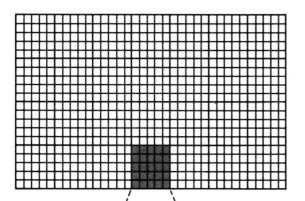

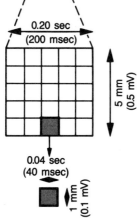

**Fig. 5-5.** Graph paper and time in seconds.

electrical patterns of the heart are recorded by the application of electrodes to the skin and connection to a monitor or ECG machine, which inscribes the patterns on graph paper.

Standard ECG paper for a single-lead system is shown in Fig. 5-4. The graph paper provides a determination of time. The standard speed that ECG paper advances past the stylus is 25 mm/sec. At this rate, each very small square represents 0.04 seconds so that 5 small squares are equivalent to 0.20 seconds. Voltage is measured by the vertical lines on the graph paper, and each very small square equals 1 mm. Voltage criteria are generally not used in basic ECG interpretation. Fig. 5-5 shows the relationship between time intervals and the graph paper.

## LEAD CONFIGURATIONS

The application of electrodes to the skin's surface provides the picture that will enable interpretation of the cardiac rhythm. The selection of a particular lead is determined by the health care professional who will be monitoring the patient. The three most common lead configurations are shown in Fig. 5-6.

Selection of a lead configuration is based upon which lead will provide the clearest picture. Lead II is the most common monitoring lead. Modified chest lead 1 (MCL 1) is also a popular choice for monitoring. Each of these leads has certain advantages; however, waveform clarity will help to determine which lead will be selected. Lead I may be used when monitoring on a single lead system; however, it provides the least information. All of these leads are bipolar, meaning that there is a *positive* electrode, a *negative* electrode, and a ground. The positioning of these electrodes on the chest determines the lead configuration that is being used. It is important to remember that a single-lead system has as its primary purpose rhythm identification. Time and voltage plus 12-lead views of the electrical activity of the heart enable the interpreter to make more advanced assessments of cardiac status. A 12-lead ECG provides information about ischemic processes, chamber size, axis determination, drug effects, and bundle branch blocks in addition to rhythm identification.

## WAVEFORMS

The primary purpose of the conduction system is to depolarize the four cardiac chambers—the right atrium, left atrium, right ventricle and left ventricle. The waveforms that represent the mechanical contractions have been arbitrarily labeled the P, QRS, T, and U waves. Each P, QRS, and T wave represents one cardiac cycle or heart beat. Refer to Fig. 5-7 for an illustration of these waveforms.

The P wave, which is generally rounded and upright in lead II, represents atrial (right and left) depolarization. The QRS complex represents ventricular (right and left) depolarization. It has multiple deflections and is recorded with numerous variations. Fig. 5-8 shows examples of typical QRS morphologies. The T wave represents ventricular repolarization and may be upright, inverted, elevated, or depressed. Occasionally a U wave may follow the T wave.

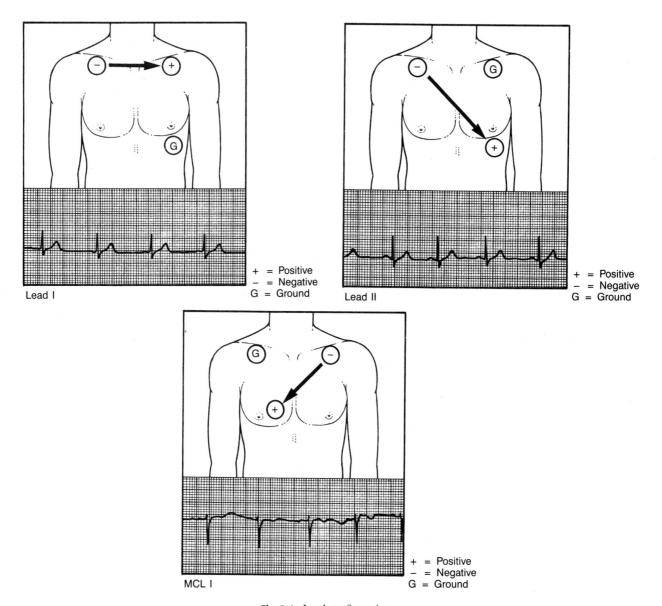

**Fig. 5-6.** Lead configurations.

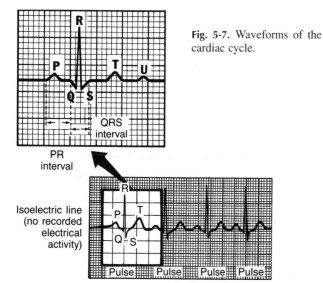

**Fig. 5-7.** Waveforms of the cardiac cycle.

The exact cause of the U wave is unknown, but clinically it provides little information.

The period between each cardiac cycle is referred to as the baseline or isoelectric line. No electrical activity occurs during the isoelectric period. When a waveform is *positive* it is deflected above the baseline; when a waveform is *negative* it is deflected below the baseline. In Fig. 5-9 the P wave, R wave, and T wave are positive; the Q wave and the S wave are negative.

## CALCULATIONS AND INTERVALS

To interpret dysrhythmias it is important to calculate rate, as well as, intervals. Rate is most easily calculated by noting 3-second intervals that are marked on ECG paper. By selecting a 6-second period, counting the number of cardiac cycles during that 6-second period, and then multiplying by 10, an approximate 1-minute heart rate is obtained. Most

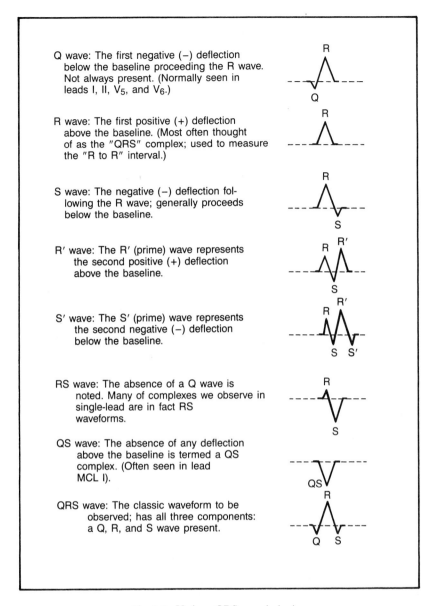

Q wave: The first negative (−) deflection below the baseline proceeding the R wave. Not always present. (Normally seen in leads I, II, $V_5$, and $V_6$.)

R wave: The first positive (+) deflection above the baseline. (Most often thought of as the "QRS" complex; used to measure the "R to R" interval.)

S wave: The negative (−) deflection following the R wave; generally proceeds below the baseline.

R′ wave: The R′ (prime) wave represents the second positive (+) deflection above the baseline.

S′ wave: The S′ (prime) wave represents the second negative (−) deflection below the baseline.

RS wave: The absence of a Q wave is noted. Many of complexes we observe in single-lead are in fact RS waveforms.

QS wave: The absence of any deflection above the baseline is termed a QS complex. (Often seen in lead MCL I).

QRS wave: The classic waveform to be observed; has all three components: a Q, R, and S wave present.

**Fig. 5-8.** Various QRS morphologies.

monitors also feature a digital readout that measures each R to R interval or cardiac cycle; the heart rate is displayed on the screen. Fig. 5-10 shows a sample rhythm strip.

Two intervals are measured in basic ECG. These are called the *PR interval* and the *QRS duration.* The PR interval represents atrial depolarization by measuring conduction time from the SA node to the AV node. The PR interval is normally 0.12 to 0.20 seconds. The PR interval is measured from the onset of the P wave to the onset of the QRS wave. The QRS duration reflects the time it takes the ventricles to depolarize and conduction to proceed from the AV node to the Purkinje fibers. Normal QRS duration is 0.04 to 0.11 seconds. The QRS duration begins at the end of the PR interval, noted by a change in waveform deflection (either positive or negative) and ends generally with the return to baseline. The interval that occurs between the end of the QRS complex and the beginning of the T wave is called the

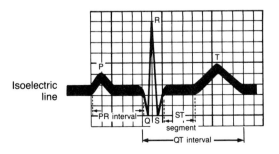

**Fig. 5-9.** Waveform deflections and intervals.

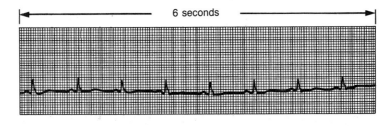

6 seconds

Heart rate is approximately 80; digital readout
would show 78

**Fig. 5-10.** Rate calculation.

*ST segment.* It represents the time during which the ventricles have completed depolarization and when repolarization begins. This is not a measured interval; instead ST-segment depression or elevation is noted. The 12-lead ECG is used to detect abnormalities of the ST segment (see Chapter 7 for more about ST segments). The *QT interval* (see Fig. 5-9), which represents electrical systole, is measured from the beginning of the Q wave (or the R wave if no Q is present) to the end of the T wave. The normal QT interval is 0.32 to 0.40 seconds if the heart rate is 65 to 95 (bpm). The QT interval should be noted when using single-lead interpretation since a gradually prolonged QT interval may be caused by drug toxicities.

## ARTIFACT AND INTERFERENCE

The single-lead tracing can be affected by artifact or interference. Common causes of artifact are: (1) muscle tremors, (2) patient movement, (3) loose electrodes, and (4) 60-cycle electrical interference. Fig. 5-11 shows several examples of artifact and interference. Dysrhythmia interpretation requires understanding of some basic principles. It also requires practice and a knowledge of the physiology behind the normal process and the disturbance. There are certain patterns noted in rhythm disturbances. Fig. 5-12 illustrates these patterns.

Each rhythm strip should be analyzed in a systematic fashion. The following questions should be asked and answered with each strip that is interpreted.

- Is the rate fast or slow? (tachycardia or bradycardia)
- Is the rhythm regular or irregular? (Are there early, late, or absent beats?)

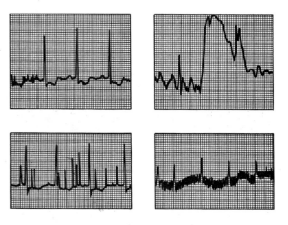

**Fig. 5-11.** Artifact and interference.

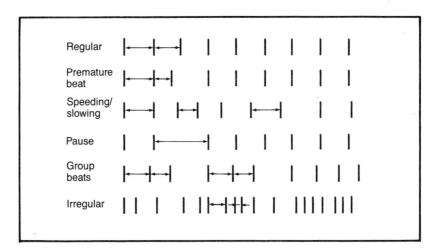

**Fig. 5-12.** Rhythm patterns.

- Are a P wave and QRS wave present with each cycle?
- Do the P waves always look alike?
- Do the QRS waves all look alike?
- Is there a P wave preceding every QRS?
- Is the PR interval within normal limits?
- Is the QRS duration within normal limits?
- Does the rhythm come from the SA node, atria, AV node, or the ventricles?

- Does the atrial rate equal the ventricular rate?
- When correlated with clinical observation of the patient, what is the significance of the rhythm?

The remainder of this chapter will focus on rhythm identification using this criteria-based approach.

*Text continued on p. 74.*

## Cardiac rhythm

| ECG characteristics | Etiology | Treatment |
|---|---|---|
| **Normal sinus rhythm (NSR, RSR, SR)*** | | |
| P waves present and regular | Impulse originates in the SA node and follows the normal conduction pathways for depolarization | None |
| QRS constant and regular | | Significance: optimal cardiac output |
| Each P wave is followed by a QRS | | |
| PR interval is 0.12 to 0.20 | The SA node readily responds to autonomic stimuli; *parasympathetic* (cholinergic) slows while *sympathetic* (adrenergic) speeds the rate of discharge | |
| QRS duration is 0.04 to 0.11 | | |
| Ventricular rate is 60 to 100 | | |

---

*Illustration from Beare PG and Myers JL: *Principles and practice of adult health nursing,* St Louis, 1990, The CV Mosby Co.     *Continued.*

## Cardiac rhythm—cont'd

| ECG characteristics | Etiology | Treatment |
| --- | --- | --- |

### Sinus tachycardia (S-tach, ST)*

P waves present, regular and of constant configuration
P waves may encroach on the T waves
PR interval is 0.12 to 0.20
QRS is constant and regular
QRS duration is 0.04 to 0.11
Each QRS is preceded by a P wave
Ventricular rate is greater than 100

Impulse originates in the SA node and follows the normal conduction pathways
Conditions in which SA node automaticity is increased:
Response to pain, emotion, exertion
Increased demands for $O_2$, fever, CHF, MI, infection, hemorrhage, anemia, hyperthyroidism
Caffeine, nicotine, atropine, adrenalin, amyl nitrate

Treat the underlying cause
Occasionally beta blockers may be used to slow an ST
Significance: under normal circumstances, no compromise of cardiac output

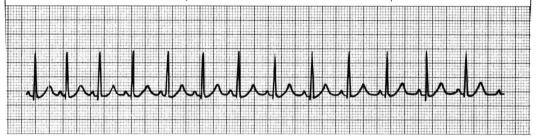

### Sinus bradycardia (S Brady, SB)*

P waves present, regular and of constant configuration
PR interval is 0.12 to 0.20
QRS is constant and regular
QRS duration is 0.04 to 0.11
Each P wave is followed by a QRS
Ventricular rate is 40 to 59
When sinus bradycardia (by criteria) is less than 40 beats per minute, it is referred to as "marked" sinus bradycardia

Impulse originates in the SA node and follows the normal conduction pathways
Occurs in conditions when automaticity of the SA node is decreased
Vagal response (parasympathetic stimulation sleep, fear, suctioning, vomiting)
SA node hypoxia (MI)
Well-trained athletes
Glaucoma
Increased ICP, brain tumors
Drugs—digoxin, morphine, beta blockers
Hypothyroidism, hypercalcemia

Usually none
Remove source of vagal stimulation
If symptomatic (BP, syncope, angina pale, diaphoretic, ventricular ectopy), may use: atropine, isuprel, temporary pacemaker (rare)
Use morphine with caution
Use beta blockers, digoxin, quinidine with caution—confer with physician
Significance: generally no compromise of cardiac output

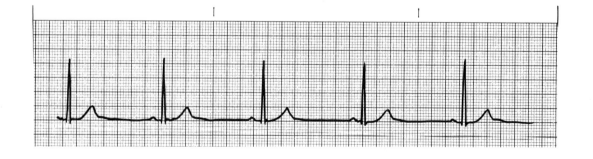

## Cardiac rhythm—cont'd

| ECG characteristics | Etiology | Treatment |
|---|---|---|

### Sinus dysrhythmia*

Ventricular rate is usually 40 to 100
Overall rhythm is irregular
P wave precedes each QRS
P wave morphology remains the same
QRS morphology remains the same
PR interval is 0.12 to 0.20
QRS duration is 0.04 to 0.11

Impulse is initiated by the SA node;
  irregularity is caused by variation in
  vagal stimulation
Types:
  Respiratory (common)
    Rate increases with inspiration
      and decreases with expiration
    Cycles are short (3 to 4 beats)
    Occurs commonly in the young
      or elderly
    Is easily simulated
  Nonrespiratory
    Cycles are longer and are not
      associated with respiration
    Can occur with atelectasis, rheu-
      matic fever, infection, digoxin,
      and morphine administration

Respiratory type is benign
  Nonrespiratory type—treat underly-
    ing cause
  Give morphine and digoxin with
    caution
  Increasing the heart rate abolishes
    the respiratory type
Significance: no compromise of car-
  diac output

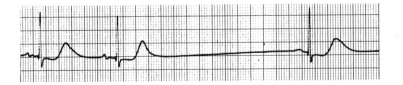

### Sinus pause†

Underlying rhythm is sinus
Occasional pause is noted
Usually 1½ to 2½ missing beats are
  noted
PR interval of underlying rhythm is
  0.12 to 0.20
P waves are always followed by QRS
QRS duration is 0.04 to 0.11

Momentary failure of SA node to ini-
  tiate an impulse caused by:
  Sudden surge of parasympathetic
    activity
    Carotid sinus pressure
    Fear or emotional upset
    Pharyngeal stimulation
  Acute infection (rare)
  Organic disease of the SA node
    Infarct
    Inflammation
    Rheumatic disease
    Sick sinus syndrome
  Digoxin

Infrequent episodes do not require in-
  tervention
Treat underlying cause
Remove source of vagal stimulation
  (i.e., tight clothing)
Stop digoxin
Give atropine, isuprel (rare)
Consider permanent pacemaker (rare)
Significance: rare episodes do not
  compromise cardiac output

†Illustration from Vinsant MO and Spence MI: *Commonsense approach to coronary care: a program,* ed 5, St Louis. 1989, The CV Mosby Co.

*Continued.*

## Cardiac rhythm—cont'd

| ECG characteristics | Etiology | Treatment |
|---|---|---|

**Sinus arrest‡**

Underlying rhythm is sinus

Long "pauses" with no cardiac rhythm are noted

Three or more beats must be missing

PR interval of underlying rhythm is 0.12 to 0.20

P waves are followed by a QRS complex

QRS duration is 0.04 to 0.11

Failure of SA node to initiate an impulse

Back-up pacemakers also fail to respond

Causes:

    Sudden surge of parasympathetic activity

        Fear (rare)

        Carotid sinus pressure

        Pharyngeal stimulation

    Organic disease of the SA node and latent pacemaker

        Infarct

        Sick sinus syndrome

        Inflammation

        Rheumatic process

Treat as emergency

Assess patient status

Remove source of vagal stimulus if applicable

Give atropine

If organic disease, patient will be a candidate for permanent pacemaker

Significance: *no* cardiac output during periods of arrest

**SA exit block (SA block)‡**

Underlying rhythm is sinus

Occasional "pause" is noted

One whole complex is missing—*P, QRS, T*

Should map out to exactly one missing cycle

PR interval of underlying rhythm is 0.12 to 0.20

P waves are always followed by QRS

QRS duration is 0.04 to 0.11

Lack of emergence of an impulse from the SA node

Lasts for just one cycle or beat

Causes:

    Increased vagal tone

    Carotid sinus sensitivity

    Acute infection (rare)

    Increased levels of digoxin (common), quinidine, salicylates

    Coronary artery disease

Potassium intoxication

Treat underlying cause if possible

Is a rare phenomenon

Remove source of vagal stimulation (i.e., tight clothing around the neck)

Hold digoxin or other drugs

May treat with atropine (rare)

May consider permanent pacemaker (rare)

Significance: rarely any compromise to cardiac output

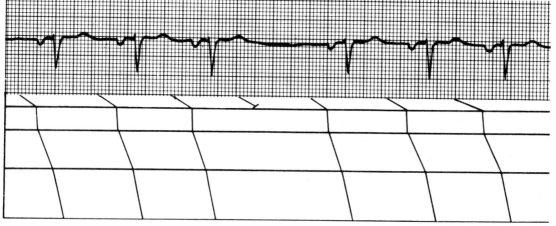

‡Illustration from Conover MB: *Understanding electrocardiography: arrhythmias and the 12-lead ECG,* ed 4, St Louis, 1984, The CV Mosby Co.

## Cardiac rhythm—cont'd

| ECG characteristics | Etiology | Treatment |
| --- | --- | --- |

**Wandering atrial pacemaker (WAPM)§**

Rhythm is not sinus in origin

P waves are present, but vary in configuration

QRS will follow each P wave

PR intervals may vary; R to R will vary

Most often appear in groups of one P wave configurations followed by three to four beats with a different P wave (type 1)

Each P wave may look different (type 2)

QRS duration is 0.04 to 0.11

Ventricular rate is less than 100

Irritable foci initiate impulse in the atria, but at a normal rate of discharge and control wanders; may be caused by increased vagal tone

Control may also pass from the atria to the AV node

Occurs in:
  Advanced age
  Adolescence

May be abolished by increasing the heart rate

Generally requires no treatment

Significance: does not compromise cardiac output

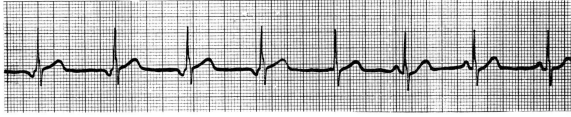

**Sinus with premature atrial contractions (PACs)\***

Underlying rhythm is sinus

Normal complexes have one P wave configuration and one QRS configuration

Sinus PR intervals are 0.12 to 0.20

QRS duration is 0.04 to 0.11

*Early beat occurs*
  P wave will be present but with different configuration (PR interval of the early beat will differ from the sinus beats)

May be multifocal PACs with variable P wave morphologies

P wave of the early beat may be "buried" in the T wave

Often compensatory pause will follow a PAC

Ectopic or irritable focus in the atria (either right or left) cause atrial firing

Causes:
  Emotional stress
  Caffeine, nicotine
  Myocardial ischemia
  CAD
  Renal disease
  Rheumatic disease
  Hypoxemia
  Infection
  Hyperthyroidism

If infrequent, no intervention is required

May give quinidine

May give small dose beta blockers

If organic disease may give digoxin

Frequent PACs may lead to SVT or A-fib

Significance: rarely compromises cardiac output

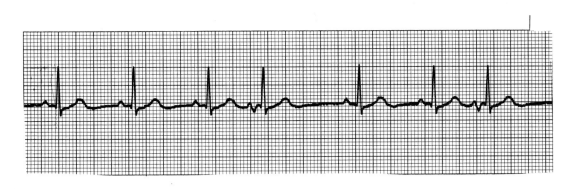

§Illustration from Phibbs B: *The cardiac arrhythmias*, ed 3, St Louis, 1978, The CV Mosby Co.

*Continued.*

## Cardiac rhythm—cont'd

| ECG characteristics | Etiology | Treatment |
|---|---|---|

### Nonconducted PACs (blocked PACs)‡

Underlying rhythm is sinus
Normal complexes have one P wave configuration and one QRS configuration
Sinus PR intervals are 0.12 to 0.20
QRS duration is 0.04 to 0.11
*Early beat occurs*
   P wave will be present but with different configuration
*There will be no QRS!*
P may be buried in the T wave
There will be a compensatory pause

Premature beat originates in the atria, but the impulse arrives when the ventricles are still refractory so the atria contract but not the ventricles (absolute refractory period)
Occurs in patients:
   With renal disease
   With ischemic heart disease
   As a benign process

Intervention is not required
Rhythm occurs rarely
Significance: generally no compromise to cardiac output

### Atrial flutter (A. flutter)‡

Rhythm is not of sinus origin
P waves are present as "F" waves or flutter waves that have a characteristic "sawtooth" pattern
There is AV block and conduction ratios are recorded as 2 : 1, 3 : 1, up to 8 : 1
Atrial firing rate is 250 to 350
The T wave is often dominated by the atrial wave
QRS duration is 0.04 to 0.11

Ectopic focus in the atria gains control and the depolarization impulse originates there
Rate of discharge is rapid
Causes:
   Advanced age
   CAD
   Rheumatic heart disease
   Hyperthyroidism
   Constrictive pericarditis
   Cor pulmonale
   Infection
   Hypoxemia
   Exercise; stress
   Myocardial infarct
   Drugs (digoxin, epinephrine, quinidine)
   Renal failure

Medications:
   Digoxin
   Quinidine
   Beta blockers
   Calcium-channel blockers
Cardioversion: 10 to 50 WS
Temporary atrial pacing-used to override the irritable focus
May lead to atrial fibrillation
Occurs commonly
Significance: usually no compromise to cardiac output except when too rapid or too slow

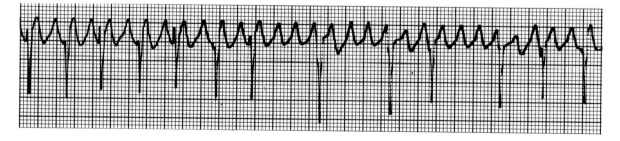

## Cardiac rhythm—cont'd

| ECG characteristics | Etiology | Treatment |
| --- | --- | --- |

### Atrial fibrillation (A. fib)*

Rhythm is not of sinus origin
P waves are absent, "F" waves are absent and are replaced by a "wavy" or flat baseline
Atrial rate is 350 or more
Hallmark of this rhythm: *irregular*
QRS duration is 0.04 to 0.11

Ectopic focus in the atria gains control and the depolarization impulse originates there
Rate of discharge is extremely rapid
Atria no longer contract
Causes:
  Rheumatic heart disease
  Hypertension
  Thyrotoxicosis
  Stress, pain
  CAD
  Renal failure
  Infection
  Hypoglycemia
  CHF
  Pericarditis
  Cardiomyopathy
  Illegal drug use
  Digoxin toxicity

Medications:
  Digoxin
  Verapamil
  Quinidine
Cardioversion (occasionally)
Treat underlying cause
*Mural thrombi may develop and lead to emboli; anticoagulants may be needed
Thirty percent of all patients with A fib develop emboli—pulmonary or systemic
Common rhythm
Significance: cardiac output generally intact; compromise occurs if rate is too fast or too slow

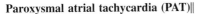

### Paroxysmal atrial tachycardia (PAT)‖

Rhythm is not of sinus origin
Rapid rate rhythm; most often 160 to 250
P waves may be present but are often buried in the T wave and not visible
QRS duration is 0.04 to 0.11 unless there is aberration
Rhythm starts and stops abruptly; lasts less than 24 hours
ST elevation or depression is frequently noted
Is one of two forms of supraventricular tachycardia (SVT)

Result of repetitive firing of a single atrial focus or circus reentry
Causes:
  Pulmonary emboli
  Emotional factors
  Overexertion
  Hypokalemia
  Caffeine, nicotine
  Aspirin sensitivity
  Rheumatic heart disease
  Hyperventilation
  Hypertension
If PAT last longer than 24 hours, it is called sustained atrial tachycardia
Frequent PACs may induce PAT

Treat underlying cause
If digoxin toxic, stop digoxin
Carotid sinus massage
Valsalva maneuver
Gagging, coughing
Atrial pacing (rare)
Cardioversion (rare)
Medications:
  Digoxin
  Verapamil
  Quinidine
  Pronestyl
  Beta blocker
Short bursts fairly common
Significance: if prolonged will compromise cardiac output even of a healthy heart

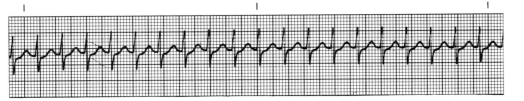

‖Illustration from Goldberger AL and Goldberger E: *Chemical electrocardiography: a simplified approach,* ed 3, St Louis, 1986, The CV Mosby Co.

*Continued.*

## Cardiac rhythm—cont'd

| ECG characteristics | Etiology | Treatment |
| --- | --- | --- |

### Atrial tachycardia with AV block (PAT with block)‖

Rhythm is not of sinus origin

P waves present; rhythm may or may not be regular

P wave morphology is abnormal (focus is atrial)

AV block exists; QRS may not follow a P wave

Ventricular rate is 75 to 200

*There are isoelectric intervals between the P waves*

Ventricular response may be regular or irregular

QRS duration is 0.04 to 0.11

Ectopic atrial focus with slower discharge rate; block created when ventricles are unable to respond

Causes:

Digoxin toxicity (50% to 70% of the patients with this rhythm)

Significant organic disease (cor pulmonale)

Discontinue digoxin, if toxic

If not on digoxin, start the drug

After digitalization, may require quinidine or pronestyl

Rapid rates—may cardiovert or use verapamil

Inderal may be used up to a total of 3 mg

Occurs rarely

Significance: with block, rate is generally within a normal range so cardiac output is maintained

III

### Multifocal atrial tachycardia (MAT)‡

Rhythm is not of sinus origin

P waves have variable morphology

P waves may or may not be followed by a QRS

PR interval will vary

P to P interval will vary

Atrial rate is 100 to 250

QRS duration is generally 0.04 to 0.11

R to R interval will vary

Multiple irritable foci in the atria at a moderate to rapid rate discharge; ventricles will respond whenever possible, hence irregularity

Cause: severe pulmonary disease with coexisting hypoxemia, hypokalemia, pulmonary hypertension, altered pH

Usually none

May require the same treatment as for PAT if very rapid rate

Commonly occurs in COPD patients

Significance: if too rapid may compromise cardiac output

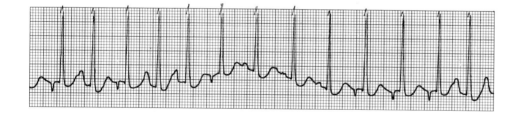

## Cardiac rhythm—cont'd

| ECG characteristics | Etiology | Treatment |
|---|---|---|

### Sinus rhythm with premature junctional contractions (PJCs)*

Underlying rhythm is sinus in origin

Normal complexes have one P wave configuration and one QRS configuration

Sinus PR intervals are 0.12 to 0.20

QRS duration is 0.04 to 0.11

*Early beat occurs*

The early beat may have three presentations:

Short PR interval (less than 0.12) (inverted)

Absent P wave

Retrograde P wave

AV node becomes irritated and initiates an impulse, thus causing an early beat

Causes:

Carotid sinus pressure

Digoxin on board

CAD

Rheumatic heart disease

Generally requires no treatment

Can give quinidine and pronestyl

Common with cardiac disease

Significance: cardiac output generally intact

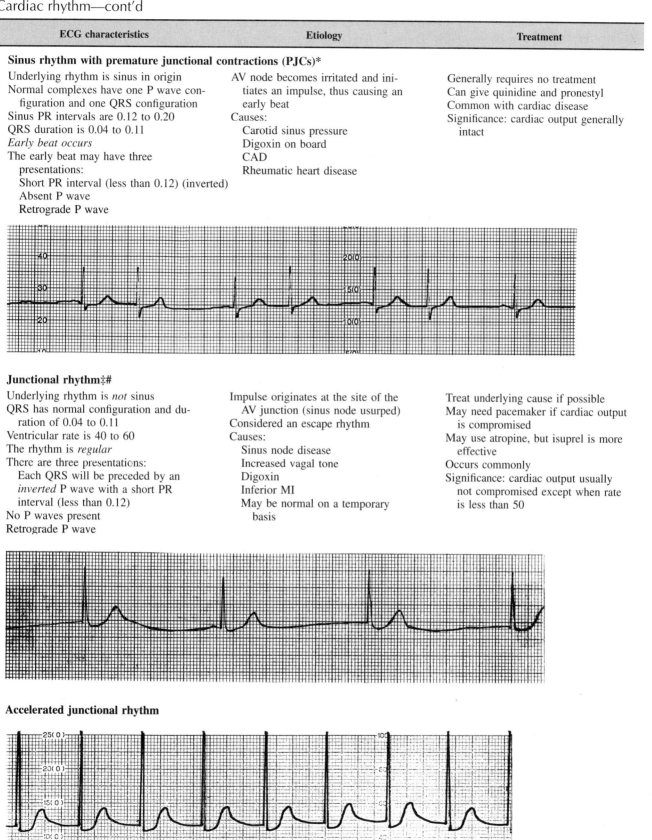

### Junctional rhythm‡#

Underlying rhythm is *not* sinus

QRS has normal configuration and duration of 0.04 to 0.11

Ventricular rate is 40 to 60

The rhythm is *regular*

There are three presentations:

Each QRS will be preceded by an *inverted* P wave with a short PR interval (less than 0.12)

No P waves present

Retrograde P wave

Impulse originates at the site of the AV junction (sinus node usurped)

Considered an escape rhythm

Causes:

Sinus node disease

Increased vagal tone

Digoxin

Inferior MI

May be normal on a temporary basis

Treat underlying cause if possible

May need pacemaker if cardiac output is compromised

May use atropine, but isuprel is more effective

Occurs commonly

Significance: cardiac output usually not compromised except when rate is less than 50

### Accelerated junctional rhythm

---

¶Junctional rhythms with rates of 60 to 100 should be referred to as accelerated junctional rhythms.

#Form of supraventricular tachycardia (SVT).

*Continued.*

## Cardiac rhythm—cont'd

| ECG characteristics | Etiology | Treatment |
|---|---|---|

### Junctional tachycardia‡#

Underlying rhythm is *not* sinus
QRS has normal configuration and duration of 0.04 to 0.11
Ventricular rate is 100 to 180
The rhythm is usually regular
There are three presentations:
   Each QRS will be preceded by a P wave with a short PR interval (less than 0.12) that is *usually* inverted
No P waves present
Retrograde P wave present

Impulse arises in the AV junctional tissue with an accelerated rate of discharge
May be paroxysmal or nonparoxysmal
Causes:
   *Paroxysmal*: hyperventilation, myocardial infarction, pulmonary emboli, rheumatic heart disease, hypertension, emotional factors, overexertion, caffeine, nicotine
   *Nonparoxysmal*: digoxin toxicity, after heart surgery, acute myocarditis

Treat underlying cause
Digitalize if not digoxin toxic
Vagal stimulation
   (cough, gag, ice water)
Cardioversion (if patient compromised)
Verapamil, inderal

Significance: cardiac output is compromised when rate is rapid

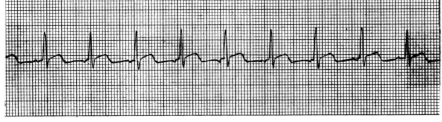

### Sinus rhythm with premature ventricular contractions (PVCs)*

The underlying rhythm is sinus (occasionally junctional or atrial)
The PR interval is 0.12 to 0.20 for the sinus rhythm
The QRS duration is 0.04 to 0.11 for the sinus rhythm
*An early beat occurs*
The early beat is wide and bizarre
QRS duration of the early beat is greater than 0.11
The P wave is absent
The ST segment often slopes in the opposite direction of the normal complexes
PVCs are generally followed by a compensatory pause
If every other beat is a PVC, the rhythm is termed *bigeminy*
If every third beat is a PVC, the rhythm is termed *trigeminy*
If every fourth beat is a PVC, the rhythm is termed *quadrigeminal*
If PVC complexes differ in appearance, they are called *multifocal* or *multiformed*
If each PVC looks alike, the term is *unifocal* or *uniformed*
If three or more consecutive PVCs appear in a row at a rate above 100, they are called V-tach, a salvo, or a triplet
If two PVCs appear in a row, they are called couplets
If a PVC occurs at the same place in each cycle it is called "fixed"

Impulses arise from single or multiple foci in the ventricles or Purkinje fibers
Causes:
   *Ischemia*
   Cardiac disease
   Electrolyte imbalance (hypo- or hyperkalemia)
   Digoxin toxicity
   Quinidine or pronestyl toxicity
   Caffeine, nicotine
   Stress, overexertion
   Acute MI
   Irritation from insertion of a pacer or hemodynamic catheter
   Overdistention of ventricular tissue (CHF, cardiomyopathy)
   Chronic lung disease

Know patient—if chronic PVCs, observe
Administer $O_2$
Treat underlying cause if possible (give potassium supplements, hold digoxin)
Lidocaine IV bolus and drip
Pronestyl IV bolus and drip
Oral antidysrhythmics—quinidine, pronestyl, mexitil, enkaid, tambocor, tonocard, calan, amiodarone
PVCs may be benign
Significance: increase in number of PVCs and positive cardiac history require close monitoring; cardiac functioning may decrease

## Cardiac rhythm—cont'd

| ECG characteristics | Etiology | Treatment |
| --- | --- | --- |

If a PVC migrates in the cycle it is called nonfixed

If a PVC falls between two sinus beats that are separated by a normal R to R interval, the PVC is described as *interpolated*

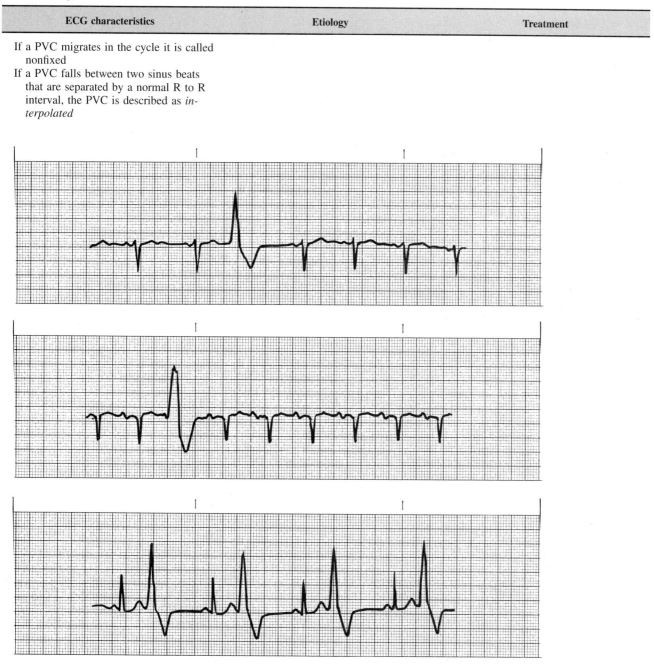

**Ventricular tachycardia (V-tach)\***

Underlying rhythm is not sinus
Ventricular rate is 100 to 250
P wave is absent
QRS is wide and bizarre

Rapid firing by a single ventricular focus with enhanced automaticity
Causes:
    Ischemia
    Fresh (acute) MI
    Electrolyte imbalance (hypo- or hyperkalemia)

Lidocaine IV and bolus
Pronestyl IV and bolus
$O_2$
Cardioversion/defibrillation
Oral drugs (quinidine, Pronestyl, mexitil, enkaid, tambocor, tonocard, amiodarone)

*Continued.*

## Cardiac rhythm—cont'd

| ECG characteristics | Etiology | Treatment |
|---|---|---|
| | Cardiac disease<br>CHF, cardiomyopathy<br>Irritation from intracardiac catheters<br>Toxicities digoxin, pronestyl, quinidine, enkaid<br>Idiopathic | Significance: V-tach with rate less than 140 may allow for adequate cardiac output; higher rates compromise cardiac output and cause loss of consciousness |

**V-tach: torsade de pointes***

| | | |
|---|---|---|
| Underlying rhythm is not sinus<br>Ventricular origin<br>Ventricular rate 100 to 250 | Called "twisting of the points"<br>Polarity pattern swings from positive to negative<br>Often converts to v-fib | Class I antidysrhythmics may be dangerous (lidocaine, pronestyl)<br>May see Isuprel ordered; cardiovert<br>Significance: inadequate cardiac output; may lead to no cardiac output |

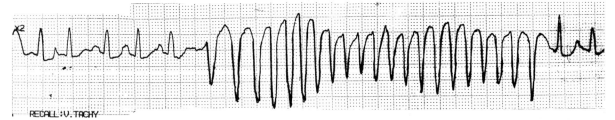

## Cardiac rhythm—cont'd

| ECG characteristics | Etiology | Treatment |
| --- | --- | --- |

**Bidirectional v-tach‡**

Underlying rhythm is not sinus
Ventricular origin
Ventricular rate 100 to 250

Ventricular complexes alternate in polarity, positive to negative
Etiology may also be two ectopic foci in the ventricles
Sometimes associated with digoxin toxicity—prognosis poor

Conventional for v-tach (lidocaine, pronestyl)
Cardiovert
Significance: inadequate cardiac output; may herald impending loss of function

**Ventricular fibrillation (v-fib)‡**

Underlying rhythm is not sinus
Essentially no QRS complexes noted
Bizarre, erratic electrical activity noted
Usually either "fine" v-fib or "coarse" v-fib

Random, asynchronous ventricular electrical activity
Results in the ventricular muscle merely quivering
There is no cardiac output!
Causes:
  Digoxin and quinidine toxicity
  Cardiac disease
  Acute MI
  Electrocution
  Hyperkalemia
  Hypothermia

Medical emergency
CPR
Most important—defibrillate as quickly as possible
Epinephrine
Lidocaine, bretylol, or pronestyl
Oxygenate
Significance: *no* cardiac output; no tissue perfusion

*Continued.*

## Cardiac rhythm—cont'd

| ECG characteristics | Etiology | Treatment |
| --- | --- | --- |

**Idioventricular rhythm or "dying heart"‡**

Underlying rhythm is not sinus
Ventricular origin; QRS is wide and bizarre
Ventricular rate is 20 to 40
Complexes may be multifocal

Impulse originates in the ventricles because of loss of other (primary) pacers
Last-ditch effort to provide cardiac output

CPR—emergency
Epinephrine
May attempt temporary pacemaker
Significance: compromise cardiac output with a highly unfavorable prognosis

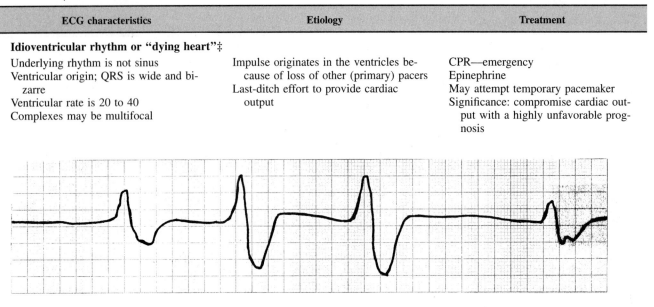

**Accelerated idioventricular rhythm (AIR)‡**

Underlying rhythm is not sinus
Ventricular origin, QRS duration is greater than 0.12
Is generally is regular rhythm
Rate is 50 to 100

Impulse originates in the ventricles; rate more controlled and therefore adequate cardiac output occurs
Often a reperfusion phenomenon
Considered benign; generally does not lead to more lethal dysrhythmias

Generally none; observe for v-tach
If rate too slow and patient symptomatic, stimulate the SA node with atropine
Significance: generally provides adequate cardiac output

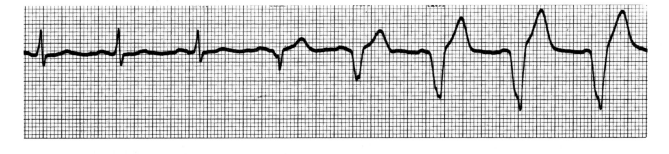

## Cardiac rhythm—cont'd

| ECG characteristics | Etiology | Treatment |
|---|---|---|

**Ventricular standstill‖**

| | | |
|---|---|---|
| Rhythm is initially sinus<br>Sudden cessation of QRS wave<br>P waves will be present and regular | Failure of the lower pacemakers and conductile tissue; SA node intact; impulse does not reach the ventricles<br>Essentially no cardiac output<br>Causes:<br>　Acute MI<br>　Ventricular rupture<br>　Can occur with CHB | Medical emergency<br>CPR<br>Epinephrine<br>Isuprel<br>Pacemaker insertion<br>Significance: atrial contraction with no ventricular contraction, hence no cardiac output |

**Asystole‖**

| | | |
|---|---|---|
| No underlying rhythm<br>Absence of P, QRS, and T waves<br>May occur abruptly | Failure of all pacers to initiate an impulse<br>No cardiac output<br>Causes:<br>　Conduction system failure<br>　Acute MI<br>　Ventricular rupture | Medical emergency<br>CPR<br>Epinephrine<br>Isuprel<br>Pacemaker insertion<br>Significance: no cardiac output |

**Cardiac phenomenon: electromechanical dissociation (EMD)‖, also called PEA (pulseless electrical activity)**

| | | |
|---|---|---|
| Underlying rhythm may appear to be junctional or sinus<br>Criteria will be met for these rhythms (i.e., rate and intervals as would be expected)<br>No palpable pulses or BP may be measured or recorded | Conduction system remains intact<br>Cardiac muscle is badly damaged and is unable to respond to the impulse<br>There is no cardiac output<br>Causes:<br>　Acute MI<br>　Ventricular rupture<br>　Hypothermia<br>　Hypoxemia<br>　Acidosis<br>　Pulmonary emboli<br>　Cardiac tamponade<br>　Tension pneumothorax<br>　Sepsis | Medical emergency<br>CPR<br>Epinephrine<br>Occasionally isuprel<br>Pacemaker-aid (transcutaneous pacemaker)<br>*Must know the patient and practice sound assessment skills<br>Significance: nonviable rhythm<br>*Generally irreversible |

*Continued.*

## Cardiac rhythm—cont'd

| ECG characteristics | Etiology | Treatment |
| --- | --- | --- |

### Ventricular fusion (summation beats)‡

Underlying rhythm is often sinus
PR interval is 0.12 to 0.20; QRS duration is 0.04 to 0.11
There will be PVCs
There is a "fusion"; the beat takes on the appearance of both the PVC and the normal beat

Ventricles are partly activated by a descending atrial impulse and partly by an ascending ectopic ventricular focus
Seen most often when PVCs occur late in a cycle
Common with:
  Accelerated idioventricular rhythm
  Pacemakers: permanent and temporary

None
Benign
Significance: cardiac output intact

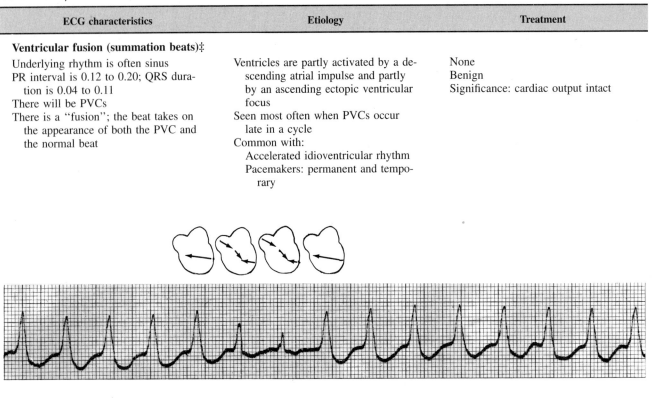

### Sinus rhythm with first-degree heart block (first-degree AVB)*

Underlying rhythm is sinus
QRS duration is 0.04 to 0.11
P wave is present and with normal configuration
There is a P wave preceding every QRS
PR interval is *lengthened* and is greater than 0.20 (generally does not exceed 0.40)

Impulse from the SA node is delayed on the way to the AV tissue or in the AV tissue and the AV conduction time is prolonged
Causes:
  CAD
  Rheumatic heart disease
  Myocardial infarct
  Digoxin
  Beta blockers

Usually none
Hold digoxin or beta blockers if indicated
May lead to higher degree of block
Significance: cardiac output intact

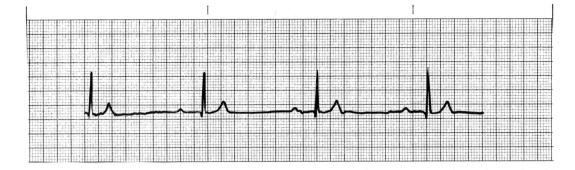

## Cardiac rhythm—cont'd

| ECG characteristics | Etiology | Treatment |
|---|---|---|

### Second-degree heart block, type I (Mobitz I; Wenckebach)*

Underlying rhythm is sinus, but there is intermittent AV block

Initially a P wave precedes each QRS

QRS is normal in configuration and duration is 0.04 to 0.11

PR interval begins to *lengthen*

As the PR interval increases a *QRS will be dropped* (P wave occurs, but no QRS)

This occurs in a repetitive cyclic manner

Cycles vary (i.e., 2 Ps, 1 QRS drop, or 3 Ps, 1 QRS drop)

Pattern is characteristic and is referred to as "footprints of Wenckebach"

The block occurs high in the AV junction

It is a benign, transient disturbance

Rarely progresses to higher forms of block

Causes:
Inferior MI
Rheumatic heart disease
Digoxin toxicity
Beta blockers
CAD

No intervention necessary if cardiac output is uncompromised

Could give atropine or isuprel

Rarely pacemaker

Significance: transient rhythm; cardiac output most often intact

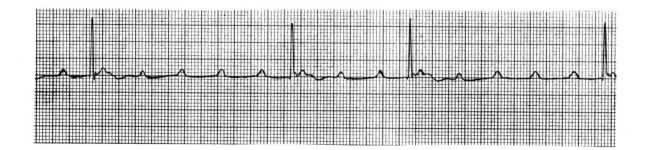

### Second-degree heart block, type II (Mobitz II)*

Intermittent underlying sinus rhythm

Ratio of P waves to QRS is altered; there may be 2, 3, or 4 P waves to every one QRS

Atrial rate is regular and P to P interval can be measured

QRS rate is usually regular and R to R intervals can be measured

QRS duration is 0.04 to 0.11

Every time a P wave precedes a QRS, the PR interval will remain the same

The site of the block is usually below the bundle of His and is a periodic bilateral bundle branch block

Occurs with:
MIs, especially those involving the LAD
CAD
Rheumatic heart disease
Digoxin toxicity

With MI can do prophylactic pacemaker

If patient symptomatic, give atropine

May progress to CHB

Significance: adequate cardiac output if 2 : 1 ratio; potential for compromise if ratio is 4 : 1 and rhythm is continuous

*Continued.*

## Cardiac rhythm—cont'd

| ECG characteristics | Etiology | Treatment |
| --- | --- | --- |

### Complete heart block (CHB); third-degree heart block*

Underlying rhythm is not sinus

P waves are present, regular, and of uniform configuration, but have *no relationship with regard to the QRS*

QRS complexes are regular and R to R can be measured

Rate will depend on the site of the latent pacemaker

*Junctional*-QRS will be normal in appearance and duration will be 0.04 to 0.11 (rate 40 to 60)

*Ventricular*-QRS will be wide, occasionally bizarre QRS duration will be greater than 0.12 (rate 20 to 40)

Complete block in conduction system in which no supraventricular impulses are conducted to the ventricles

Latent pacemakers respond; either the AV node or the ventricles

Each system is independent (atria and ventricles)

Causes:
 CAD
 Rheumatic heart disease
 Acute MI
 Degenerative disease of the conduction system

Determine the site of the block (junctional or ventricular)

Assess the patient's status

Can use atropine or isuprel

Pacemaker

If patient is unconscious, initiate CPR

Significance: CHB with junctional escape is not usually compromised; CHB with ventricular escape may be medical emergency

### Aberrant ventricular conduction (aberrancy)‡

Underlying rhythm is usually sinus

Usually the presence of a P wave

If a P wave, it will be followed by a wide QRS (greater than 0.12)

Initial QRS deflection will be the same as for the normal beat

Many have an RSR[1] pattern

Three forms exist

Temporary abnormal intraventricular conduction of supraventricular impulses

The impulse arrives early so that some portions of the bundle branches remain refractory; conduction is aberrant or through an abnormal pathway, or down the opposite branch

Not dependent on refractoriness; caused by anomalous conduction down the ventricles (Mahaim tract)

Late aberrancy: spontaneous depolarization of one fascicle

None

Do not treat as PVCs

Common, benign

Significance: generally no compromise of cardiac output

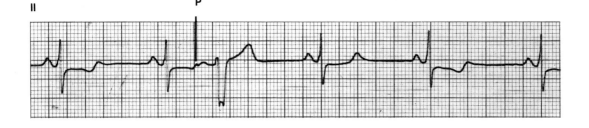

## Cardiac rhythm—cont'd

| ECG characteristics | Etiology | Treatment |
| --- | --- | --- |

**Sinus rhythm with IVCD (intraventricular conduction delay)∥**

Underlying rhythm is sinus
PR interval is 0.12 to 0.20
QRS duration is greater than 0.11
Rhythm is regular

Bundle branch block exists
Unable on single-lead system to determine if right or left
12-lead ECG will confirm origin of block
Causes:
  CAD
  Post-MI
  Benign

None; document only
Common
Significance: no compromise to cardiac output

**Left bundle branch block on 12 lead**

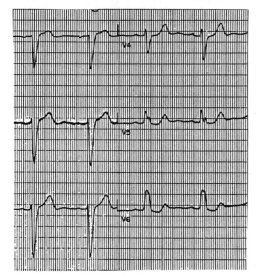

**Right bundle branch block on 12 lead**

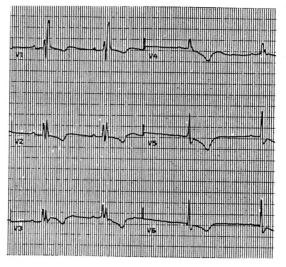

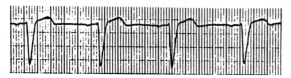

**Left bundle branch block on single lead**

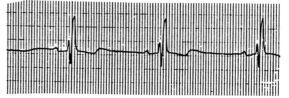

**Right bundle branch block on single lead**

## SUMMARY

- The heart has two cell types: electrical and mechanical.
- In a polarized state, the electrical charges are balanced.
- Depolarization is the discharge of energy that accompanies the transfer of ions across the cell membrane.
- Repolarization is the return of the electrical charges to their original state. Sodium and potassium are the primary ions responsible for changes in the electrical current.
- Depolarization is an electrical phenomenon; contraction is mechanical and is expected to follow depolarization.
- The conduction system is composed of electrical cells arranged in a pathway that allows the two atrial and two ventricular chambers to be depolarized.
- The conduction system begins with the SA node, continues through the intraatrial pathways and Bachman's bundle, to the AV node, the bundle of His, along the common bundle, which divides into the left and right bundle branches and terminates in the Purkinje fibers.
- Because the left ventricle is thicker than the right, the left bundle has two divisions, the anterior fascicle (left bundle) and the smaller posterior fascicle.
- The primary pacemaker of the heart is the SA node: its normal firing range is 60 to 100 times per minute.
- The secondary pacemakers or latent pacemakers are the AV node and the ventricles (Purkinje fibers). The normal firing rates are as follows: AV node = 40 to 60 times per minute and ventricles = 20 to 40 times per minute. Should the primary pacemaker fail, the latent pacemakers, if intact, will initiate the impulse.
- The electrical cells possess automaticity, meaning that they can discharge an electrical current without an external stimulus.
- There are two periods of refractoriness—the absolute and the relative refractory periods. During the absolute refractory period, no amount of stimulation can cause the cells to fire; during the relative refractory period, some cells can be depolarized and others cannot.
- The autonomic nervous system with its two branches influences heart rate, conduction, and irritability. The sympathetic speeds and the parasympathetic slows.
- Basic ECG uses a single-lead system to interpret dysrhythmias.
- Each very small square on ECG paper equals 0.04 seconds; five small squares equal 0.20 seconds.
- Voltage is measured in millimeters; each very small square equals 1 mm. Voltage criteria are not routinely used in basic ECG.
- A lead is a single view of the electrical activity of the heart produced by the application of electrodes.
- Electrodes are gel-coated conductors that, when applied to the skin, detect electrical activity and convey it to an ECG machine for display.
- Three common lead configurations are lead I, lead II, and MCL 1. They each have a positive electrode, a negative electrode, and a ground.
- Movement toward an electrode creates a positive waveform; movement away from an electrode creates a negative waveform.
- The waveform corresponding to mechanical depolarization of the four heart chambers are called arbitrarily the P, QRS, T, and U waves.
- The P wave equals atrial (left and right) depolarization. It is generally rounded and upright in lead II.
- The QRS wave represents ventricular (left and right) depolarization. It is a complex waveform with multiple morphologies.
- One cardiac cycle or heart beat is equivalent to one P, QRS, T, and occasionally a U wave.
- Several intervals and durations are important in basic ECG. They are the PR interval and the QRS duration.
- The PR interval represents the onset of atrial depolarization to the onset of ventricular depolarization. A normal PR interval is 0.12 to 0.20 seconds.
- The QRS duration represents ventricular depolarization, onset to completion. A normal QRS duration is 0.04 to 0.11 seconds.
- The T wave represents ventricular repolarization and follows the QRS waveform. The U wave occasionally follows the T wave: its significance is relatively unknown.
- The ST segment represents the termination of ventricular depolarization and the onset of ventricular repolarization. It is of little significance in basic ECG.
- The QT interval begins with the onset of ventricular depolarization and ends with the completion of ventricular repolarization. It generally lasts from 0.32 to 0.40 seconds.
- Artifact and interference are also recorded on the ECG tracing. Common forms of artifact include muscle tremors, loose electrodes, patient movement, and 60-cycle electrical interference.
- Rhythms may be regular, irregular, or in group patterns. There may be premature beats, pauses, and late beats.
- It is important to analyze rhythms in a systematic fashion.
- Rhythms that were discussed were those that originated in the sinus node (sinus rhythms), atria (atrial rhythms), AV node (junctional rhythms), ventricles (ventricular rhythms), and the heart blocks.
- Rhythms were presented with basic treatment and also identified as normal, benign, or potentially lethal.

This chapter has focused on basic concepts of single-lead ECG interpretation. Principles of depolarization and repolarization were discussed and related to the major waveforms associated with the mechanical contraction of the four heart chambers. Common lead configurations were illustrated to show how a cardiac cycle presents when electrodes are applied to the skin and an ECG device is used. The conduction system was presented in an effort to provide an understanding of how normal and abnormal rhythm patterns are initiated. Recognition of the normal waveforms (P, QRS, and T) and normal intervals and durations (PR and QRS) was stressed. Criteria for normal, common, and abnormal rhythms were presented. Use of a criteria-based, systematic approach enables the interpreter to correctly identify cardiac rhythms.

## SUGGESTED READINGS

Andreoli KG and others: *Comprehensive cardiac care,* ed 6, St Louis, 1987, Mosby.

Jaffe AS and others: *Textbook of advanced cardiac life support,* Dallas, 1987, American Heart Association.

Meter MV and Lavine PG: *Reading EKGs correctly,* Jenkintown, Pa, 1977, Intermed Communications.

Walraven G: *Basic arrhythmias,* Bowie, Md, 1980, Prentice Hall, Inc.

# CHAPTER 6

# Medical Management of Acute Myocardial Infarction

*Ronald Freireich*

Acute myocardial infarction is the most dramatic presentation of coronary atherosclerosis. In most instances, infarction is the first clinical manifestation of the presence of atherosclerosis.

Acute myocardial infarction strikes almost 1.5 million persons each year, although that number has been progressively declining over the past 10 to 20 years. Over 50% of the deaths attributable to acute myocardial infarction (AMI) occur within the first hour, and most are related to dysrhythmias, chiefly ventricular fibrillation. Approximately one-half (500,000 persons) are hospitalized annually with acute infarction. Over the past 10 to 20 years, a definite decrease in both incidence and mortality from myocardial infarction has been noted. The exact causes of this reduction are still open to some debate. Among the reasons cited are increased awareness, better attention to diet, increased interest by the public in exercise and limiting other risk factors, and improvements in emergency transport and treatment. A decrease in mortality of as much as 43% since 1950 has been documented recently. Data from life insurance companies show that the mortality rate for women decreased

from 240/100,000 population, to about 120; and for men, from about 385/100,000 population to 210.

Among the important new treatment modalities of infarction recently adopted for widespread use are thrombolytic therapy and early use of pharmacological agents such as beta-blocking agents. The full impact of these changes in treatment has yet to be completely realized, and new drugs and treatment regimens continue to be implemented as the results of various medical trials, both here and abroad, are announced.

Recent dramatic improvements in the modes of treatment available for acute infarction are only partially responsible for the improvement in survival statistics. In addition, there has been a slow but progressive decrease in the incidence of infarction as well.

The majority of patients identified as candidates for cardiac rehabilitation programs will have suffered at least one myocardial infarction at some point before their rehabilitation. The aim of this chapter is to introduce the therapist to this acute, dramatic presentation of cardiac disease, with consideration of diagnosis, initial care, and features of the hospitalization period.

## DIAGNOSIS

In its classic presentation, AMI presents little difficulty in diagnosis. However, in many patients, initial manifestations of infarction may be extremely variable and a straightforward means of definite, early diagnosis remains elusive. The present climate of cost containment, preadmission screening, and attempts to limit unnecessary hospitalization is counterbalanced by the potentially grave consequences of misdiagnosis. These and the availability of new, definitive treatment modalities, such as reperfusion, which may allow significant reduction in mortality and morbidity of infarction, all place an added emphasis on diagnostic accuracy and, even more important, speed of diagnosis.

In the traditional sense, diagnosis proceeds from the

history, the physical examination, and finally, from assistance provided by laboratory determinations. This approach remains unaltered, though the time course may be compressed.

## History

Acute myocardial infarction usually begins with a feeling of pressure or discomfort in the midsternal region. This gradually worsens over a period of 5 to 15 minutes or longer, becoming progressively more disagreeable. The discomfort is felt as a deep, heavy, and diffuse pressure, and is not usually identified by the patient as "pain." This has been a frequent cause of unnecessary delay in the patient's recognition of the seriousness of the condition. There is a widespread misconception among the general public that the pain of AMI is sudden and severe in onset, sharp in nature, and localized to the left side of the chest (where most people think the heart is located).

As the severity of discomfort increases, there is usually some radiation or a feeling that the discomfort is spreading in a specific direction. Frequent sites of radiation include the shoulders, inner aspects of the arms and elbows (in the distribution of the ulnar nerve to the fourth and fifth fingers of the hand) especially on the left side, and the neck and jaw. At times radiation will occur toward the epigastric region or to the interscapular region, suggesting severe indigestion or peptic ulcer disease.

Additional variations in presentation commonly occur. Discomfort may occasionally begin at one of the locations of radiation and remain dominant there, suggesting, for example "toothache" or "elbow ache." The epigastric pain presenting as possible "ulcer attack" has already been mentioned. Less commonly, the discomfort may occur solely in a nonthoracic location.

The reason for the type of discomfort of AMI and its peculiar radiation pattern is the embryologic derivation of the heart as a midline structure. The innervation of the embryonic heart arises from the lower two cervical and upper four thoracic nerves, and is thus shared by other midline structures in the chest; it is represented in the cortical pain center in proximity to other structures in the upper extremities, the left mandibular area, the left ulnar area and the upper abdomen. In contrast to the precise "map" of the body surface in the cortical pain center, cortical representation of internal organs is imprecise, allowing for misinterpretation of afferent impulses. This is particularly apt to occur when the appropriate area has been "conditioned" (as, for example, with a patient who has previously suffered peptic ulcer disease and then months or years later develops myocardial ischemia or infarction).

Other symptoms invariably occur in the presence of AMI. Among these additional symptoms are nausea and vomiting; diaphoresis (usually profound and associated with cutaneous vasoconstriction, presenting as cold, ashen skin); occasional sudden urge for a bowel movement; profound weakness; and

a sense of impending doom. These generally reflect reflexes mediated through the vagus nerve and serve as an important indication of a potentially serious or life-threatening event. In some cases, such as "silent infarction," *only* these vagal reflexes may occur and chest discomfort may be completely lacking. This is also commonly seen in diabetic patients because of diabetic neuropathy.

## Differential diagnosis

The diagnosis of AMI presents little difficulty in most cases, and almost all alternative diagnostic possibilities would require equally prompt hospitalization. Among these are acute pulmonary embolus, aortic aneurysm, or aortic dissection. Less critical, though possibly confusing, diagnoses would include acute pericarditis, pleuritis, pneumothorax, or gastrointestinal conditions, including peptic ulcer disease, esophagitis, or Mallory-Weiss syndrome. Less serious medical conditions that may be confused with the diagnosis of AMI include various musculoskeletal disorders that present with chest pain, including acute muscular strain, costochondritis, various disorders of the bones and joints of the thoracic spine, shoulder girdle, and ribs, and their associated musculature.

A careful history will usually suggest the correct diagnosis. In cases where the patient is obviously seriously ill, the history may be abbreviated, and attention given to differentiating life-threatening conditions that require rapid admission to a critical care unit where additional diagnostic and therapeutic measures may be undertaken.

In the hemodynamically stable patient, historical features useful in the differential diagnosis would include the type of pain (recognizing again that the sensation may not be interpreted as pain, but rather pressure or discomfort), its severity, the time from development to maximum intensity, the activity being performed when the discomfort began, and a history of previous similar symptoms with their frequency, severity, and any provocative factors. A prior history of heart disease or myocardial infarction is an important historical feature. The perceived depth of the discomfort and its boundaries provide useful information, as do factors that aggravate or relieve the discomfort. Among these factors would be respiratory motion, body position (lying versus sitting or standing), relationship to any particular activity or emotional stress, relationship to meals, or to anatomical motion of the upper extremities, head and neck, or chest.

Note should be taken of the known risk factors for coronary atherosclerosis, including a smoking history, presence of hypertension, diabetes mellitus, or known lipid abnormalities, and a family history of atherosclerosis.

A very important part of the history is the prior presence of angina pectoris. Although AMI will frequently develop in the absence of a clear-cut provocation, and, in fact, frequently occurs at rest, or awakens victims from sleep, the presence of angina pectoris provides an important clue to the prior presence of coronary atherosclerosis, the substrate for occurrence of AMI. Angina pectoris is a clinical syndrome of chest discomfort, *less intense, though similar to that of AMI*. It is frequently initiated by physical or emotional exertion or stress, and is thought of as representing a "supply-demand imbalance" in the myocardium, frequently caused by the underlying presence of coronary atherosclerosis with its consequent narrowing of one or more coronary arteries. It usually is relieved promptly after cessation of the offending activity or stress, and is not associated with any myocardial damage. Its importance in the history is that it is an important marker for the process of coronary atherosclerosis, which is the general precursor to AMI. In patients who suffer angina pectoris, a pattern of instability, referred to as "unstable angina" or "preinfarction angina" is a frequent precursor to AMI. This unstable pattern is characterized by a worsening in any one or more of several features of the angina pattern, such as frequency and/or severity of episodes, a decrease in provocation needed to precipitate an episode, a delay in resolution or a decrease in response to sublingual nitroglycerine, or a recurrence of discomfort after relief.

### Physical examination

The initial examination is usually dominated by the patient's pain, hemodynamic abnormality, cardiac rhythm, or vagal response. The patient will appear apprehensive, in obvious discomfort, and may be restless and moving about in an attempt to find relief. The patient may hold or clutch the chest. The skin color will be ashen or gray, and diaphoresis is common, and is often profuse.

Initial vital signs are quite variable and may depend on the extent and location of infarction. Blood pressure is frequently elevated as a result of sympathetic response to pain, and, if low, is a cause for concern. Respiration is commonly rapid but shallow. The heart rate may be rapid, but it is usually normal or slow. If extremely slow, the presence of acute heart block should be considered.

Physical findings of the neck, chest, and heart vary, depending on the degree of left ventricular dysfunction associated with the infarction. Patients can be categorized according to a scheme proposed in 1967 by Killip,[1] who grouped patients into four classes of increasing severity of infarction, based on the presence of pulmonary rales, a third heart sound gallop, and shock (Table 6-1). A moderate percentage of patients (30% to 45%) present with no striking cardiac abnormalities that is, there is no jugular venous distension, the chest is clear or has only a few basal rales, and the cardiac examination is unremarkable (although a fourth heart sound gallop is present in almost all cases). A similar percentage will present with mild abnormalities, including more pronounced rales or a third heart sound gallop. Severe infarcts fall into classes three and four, with clinical evidence of left ventricular failure and/or shock, and may demonstrate neck vein distention, pulmonary rales with cough and possible hemoptysis, an $S_3$ gallop rhythm, and possibly a

**Table 6-1.** Killip classification of patients with acute myocardial infarction

| | Percent of patients in this category admitted to CCU | Approximate mortality rates |
|---|---|---|
| Class I (no dysfunction; no $S_3$ gallop) | 30-40 | <10% |
| Class II (rales ≤ ½ way or $S_3$) | 30-50 | ~30% |
| Class III (rales ≥ ½ way or pulmonary edema) | 5-10 | ~45% |
| Class IV (shock) | 5-10 | 80%-100% |

murmur of mitral regurgitation, suggesting papillary muscle dysfunction.

### Laboratory data

The laboratory evaluation of the patient with AMI includes electrocardiogram, serum enzyme analysis, and chest radiograph studies, as well as other nonspecific and specific studies.

**The electrocardiogram (ECG).** In the typical or classic presentation of AMI, specific changes are noted in the electrocardiogram. These begin subtly, within as early as 5 to 15 minutes after onset of infarction, and progress through a series of alterations, frequently called "evolutionary changes," that reflect electrophysiological alterations resulting from the pathological process.

In addition to confirming the history, the electrocardiogram is probably the most useful laboratory modality to confirm the diagnosis of AMI, and it often shows changes early enough to be of significant diagnostic value in the emergency room. On the other hand, the changes described may occur in an extremely variable fashion, and some features may be missed or may not occur at all. Under observation, electrocardiographic changes tend to "flow" into one another over a period of several days, with a slowing in subsequent changes that may then occur for months or longer after the acute event. With the advent of thrombolytic therapy (see below), the sequence of electrocardiographic changes may be accelerated and/or blunted.

The earliest change usually seen in the electrocardiogram is the development of tall, peaked T waves. The next change is a progressive elevation in the ST segment in those ECG leads "facing" the area of infarction. This may progress until the magnitude of the ST elevation is equal to or higher than the R-wave amplitude, and it blends with the T wave in a pattern sometimes referred to as "tombstone ST segments." In areas electrocardiographically opposite to the site of injury there will be ST-segment depression. This is referred to as "reciprocal depression," and its cause and significance are open to some debate. The appearance of this ST depression, however, provides important additional support to the acute nature of the ST-segment elevation occurring in other leads, since ST elevations may occasionally occur on a chronic basis (such as in the case of ventricular aneurysm), and, therefore, they may not connote acute injury. In addition, it lends diagnostic clarity by highlighting the regional nature of infarction, a process involving only one area of myocardium. In contrast, conditions such as acute pericarditis can result in widespread ST elevation involving almost all recorded leads. In some cases, physiologic variants of normal (so called "physiologic early repolarization") may be associated with ST-segment elevations. In these cases, the "reciprocal" ST-segment depressions in ECG leads "opposite" to the area of infarction are almost never seen. These variant changes, however, can sometimes lead to diagnostic errors in anxious patients who have (noncardiac) chest pain.

As ST elevation progresses, changes begin to occur in the QRS complex, consisting chiefly of the development of progressively deeper (and wider) Q waves—commonly considered the electrocardiographic hallmark of transmural myocardial injury. In association with this increase in Q-wave magnitude, there is a reduction in R-wave amplitude. It is sometimes normal for small Q waves to be present, and the usual criterion for a pathological Q wave is one having a duration of 0.04 seconds or more, or one exceeding 50% of the magnitude of the R wave.

As the Q wave develops over the course of the first several hours to days, the T wave also develops progressive changes, usually beginning as an inversion of the terminal portion of the T wave, progressing to symmetrical, deep T-wave inversion. The ST segments during this time gradually return toward baseline, though at times prolonged ST deviation may persist. If ST segments have returned to baseline, a subsequent change, particularly an elevation, is an important suggestion of recurrent myocardial ischemia or injury.

Table 6-2 lists ECG leads in which changes of acute injury are seen, corresponding to the anatomic area infarcted. In addition, the leads demonstrating reciprocal ST-segment depression are listed. In the case of direct posterior infarction, no electrocardiographic lead records this area. Therefore, changes seen in direct posterior infarction are represented by the inverse changes seen on the anterior wall, indicated by deep ST-segment depression (rather than elevation) and development of tall R waves (rather than Q waves).

The typical pattern of development of electrocardiographic change is illustrated in Fig. 6-1.

The changes mentioned are highly variable, and the earliest change, that of peaked T wave, is frequently missed because of delay in presentation to the hospital or in ordering the electrocardiogram. ST-segment changes are labile though they may persist for months. When present for longer

**Table 6-2.** ECG leads and their approximate anatomical correlation

| Location of infarction | Leads showing "injury current" (ST elevation) | Leads showing "reciprocal changes" (ST depression) |
|---|---|---|
| Anteroseptal | $V_1$-$V_3$ or $V_4$ | II, III, AVF, I, AVL |
| Anterior | $V_2$-$V_4$ or $V_5$ | II, III, AVF, I, AVL |
| Anterolateral | $V_2$ or $V_3$-$V_6$ I, AVL | II, III, AVL |
| Inferior | II, III, AVF | I, AVL, $V_1$-$V_2$ or $V_3$ |
| Inferoaprial | II, III, AVF, $V_4$ or $V_5$-$V_6$ | I, AVL, $V_1$-$V_2$ |
| "True" posterior | ST *depression* $V_1$-$V_3$ and tall $R$ $V_1$ | |

than 6 months, ST-segment elevation usually suggests the development of ventricular aneurysm. Echocardiography has been very valuable in confirming this diagnosis noninvasively. T-wave inversion will frequently return to normal, although this takes several months or years. Pathological Q waves are usually permanent, though infrequently, these too, may return toward normal (small magnitude or short duration) or disappear completely.

**Non–Q-wave infarctions.** Distinct from the pattern described above is that seen in about 20% to 30% of cases, previously called "subendocardial infarction." In these cases, Q waves do not occur, but the pattern of ST elevations and T wave changes, leading to symmetrical deep T-wave inversions, is seen. Non–Q-wave infarction can be as severe as the typical Q-wave infarction, and there is some controversy as to the specific meaning of this pattern. It is seen more commonly in cases where an incomplete occlusion or no occlusion of a coronary artery can be found pathologically. This pattern may also be seen in cases of severe aortic stenosis or severe hypertension, where an increase in myocardial oxygen demand can actually lead to infarction in the absence of coronary artery occlusion. In addition, the advent of reperfusion therapy (see pp. 85-86) with reestablishment of coronary blood flow after occlusion has led to an increased frequency of this electrocardiographic variant.

Clinical experience has demonstrated that non–Q-wave infarctions are associated with a high incidence of recurrent ischemic episodes and occurrence of reinfarction of a more typical Q-wave type. For this reason, more careful evaluation and follow-up of patients with this type of infarction have been recommended during the postinfarction period. In addition, the specific usefulness of a calcium-channel antagonist, diltiazem, has been demonstrated in a number of

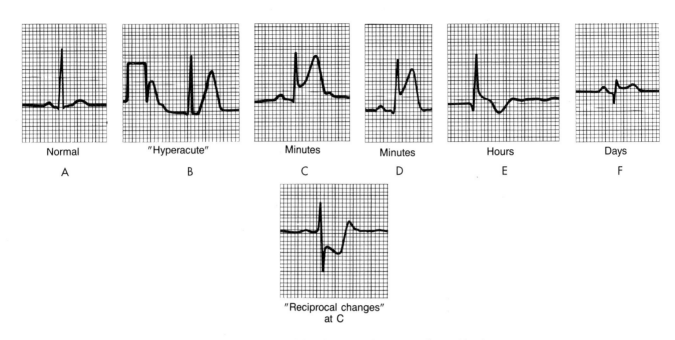

**Fig. 6-1.** Typical pattern of development of electrocardiographic change.

clinical studies, except in cases of severe left ventricular dysfunction.

**Serum enzymes.** Enzyme analysis has been a mainstay in the diagnostic evaluation of acute myocardial infarction. Enzymes are best used to confirm the diagnosis and in some cases to aid in assessing the degree of myocardial damage or the effectiveness of reperfusion attempts.

It has been shown that irreversibly damaged myocardial tissue, in distinct contrast to ischemic (but not dead) cardiac muscle, loses its cellular integrity and releases a variety of intracellular components into the bloodstream. These components are released at a variable rate and are likewise cleared by the kidney and other organs at a variable rate. By assessing the level of these substances, some of which may be unique to or predominantly present in myocardial tissue, the diagnosis of myocardial infarction may be established.

Because of the variable delay that can occur in enzyme release, the absence of any of these components cannot be taken as excluding the diagnosis.

The most frequently used tests are those that measure the level of specific enzymes in the blood, particularly creatine phosphokinase (CPK), glutamic-oxaloacetic transferase (SGOT) and lactic dehydrogenase (LDH). SGOT has more recently been referred to as AST, or aspartate aminotransferase.

Each of these enzymes has a typical temporal course of appearance, peak level, and decline in the serum after acute infarction. CPK demonstrates the most rapid release and peak reaching abnormal levels within 3 to 6 hours after the onset of infarction, peaking at 1 to 2 days, and lasting 3 to 4 days. SGOT is released more slowly, commonly peaking at 18 to 36 hours. LDH is the slowest to peak, at 3 to 6 days, and lasts longest in the circulation, frequently remaining in

an abnormal range for up to 5 to 7 days after infarction (Fig. 6-2). None of these enzymes appears rapidly enough to be reliable in the emergency room assessment of the patient. Additionally, they are nonspecific, and each occurs in a wide variety of tissues. Abnormal elevations may appear under a variety of different conditions. Although the absence of an enzyme rise cannot be used to exclude the diagnosis of infarction, the presence of elevated enzymes in the circulation at the time of presentation can be used as additional data to support a clinical diagnosis of acute infarction.

The enzymes CPK and LDH demonstrate some variation specific to different tissues containing these enzymes. These variations in enzymes are called "isoenzymes," and measuring the specific isoenzyme patterns present in cardiac tissue can provide additional diagnostic accuracy. CPK has three major isoenzyme forms, MM, MB, and BB, of which the MB type is the most specific for myocardial origin. LDH has five isoenzymes, differentiated by specialized laboratory techniques. The cardiac fraction is high in isoenzymes $LDH_1$ and $LDH_2$. A ratio of $LDH_1/LDH_2$ greater than 1.0 is strongly suggestive of infarction.

Among the disadvantages in using isoenzyme studies are the delay in obtaining the specialized test results, the special equipment required to perform these assays, and the lack of definite specificity.

In attempting to find faster and more accurate diagnostic markers for acute infarction, various other cell constituents have been examined. Among these myoglobin may be the most promising. Myoglobin is a protein released from injured myocardial cells that peaks in the circulation within 4 hours after infarction. Myoglobin is highly sensitive but less specific than CK-MB and thus may have an extremely useful negative predictive value in the emergency room

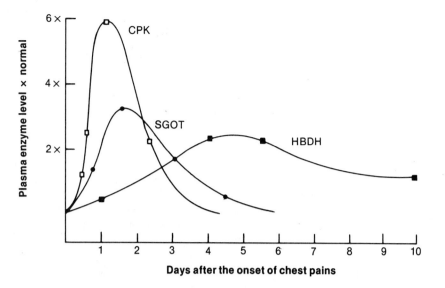

**Fig. 6-2.** Typical plasma profiles for creatine kinase (CPK), glutamate oxalocetate transaminase (SGOT), and hydroxybutyrate dehydrogenase (HBDH, LDH) activities following the onset of acute myocardial infarction. (From Hearse DJ: Myocardial enzyme leakage, *J Molec Med* 2:185, 1977.)

**Table 6-3.** Hemodynamic subsets in acute myocardial infarction

| Clinical subset | Cardiac index (L/min/m²) | Pulmonary capillary wedge pressure (mm Hg) | Mortality (%) |
|---|---|---|---|
| I. No pulmonary congestion or peripheral hypoperfusion | 2.7 ± 0.5 | 12 ± 7 | 2.2 |
| II. Isolated pulmonary congestion | 2.3 ± 0.4 | 23 ± 5 | 10.1 |
| III. Isolated peripheral hypoperfusion | 1.9 ± 0.4 | 12 ± 5 | 22.4 |
| IV. Both pulmonary congestion and hypoperfusion | 1.6 ± 0.6 | 27 ± 8 | 55.5 |

From Forrester JS and others: Medical therapy of AMI by application of hemodynamic subsets, *N Engl J Med* 295:1404, 1976.

setting. If the myoglobin level is not elevated by 3 to 4 hours after the onset of symptoms, then the likelihood of infarction is extremely small.

Confounding factors such as muscle trauma, skeletal injury, or cardiopulmonary resuscitation attempts will result in the release of similar enzymes in the circulation, limiting the utility of all enzyme studies. In these situations, however, isoenzyme assays may still have some diagnostic value.

In the setting of acute infarction treated with thrombolytic therapy (see below), frequent determinations of CK-MB have been used to assess the occurrence of reperfusion. In this setting, an early or a secondary peak followed by a more rapid decline in CK-MB levels after thrombolytic therapy is suggestive of successful reperfusion.

**Other tests.** Additional laboratory tests performed on patients presenting with acute onset of chest pain have value in the overall assessment of the patient, in excluding alternative diagnoses of chest pain, and in providing data useful in the subsequent management of the patient. Among these tests are complete blood count (CBC), chest radiography, amylase level, and coagulation profile.

***Complete blood count (CBC).*** The complete blood count is usually normal. Significant anemia, if present, may represent an unrecognized stress factor in the cause of infarction and may need to be corrected to increase myocardial oxygen supply. The white blood count is almost always normal on initial determination, but over the course of the first several days after infarction, leukocytosis may appear, reflecting the response to necrotic myocardium.

***Chest radiography.*** Chest radiography is useful in assessing several parameters. Cardiac size is usually normal, and enlargement may be an indication of preexisting heart disease. Specific chamber enlargement may be suggested by the appearance of the cardiac contour. Examination of the aortic shadow may provide clues regarding atherosclerotic calcifications or widening, which may suggest dissection.

Careful attention is paid to the status of the pulmonary vascular bed. Pulmonary congestion, if present, is an extremely important finding and suggests extensive infarction or impending or actual congestive heart failure. It thus has important therapeutic and prognostic implications (Table 6-3).

*Amylase.* The amylase level is sometimes obtained to exclude pancreatitis in cases presenting with severe epigastric pain, nausea and vomiting.

*Coagulation profile.* A coagulation profile is frequently obtained in preparation for thrombolytic therapy and before routine anticoagulation.

## MANAGEMENT

The management of the patient with acute infarction depends on careful attention to the patient's clinical status, constant reassessment of the ongoing effects of the pathological process, initiation of therapy, and assessment of the intended effects of therapy, and whether therapy should continue or be changed. For the purpose of discussion only, these can be separated somewhat, though in the actual event no clear separation points are evident.

In most cases the patient will be transferred from the emergency room setting to the coronary care unit (CCU) as soon as the diagnosis is made and the patient's condition is stabilized. Most therapeutic interventions take place therefore in the setting of the CCU. Specially trained nursing and ancillary personnel, as well as specific monitoring, diagnostic, and therapeutic equipment are available in the CCU.

If the patient's condition is unstable or if a suitable CCU bed is not immediately available, much of the early intervention and therapy may take place while the patient is in the emergency room. The importance of transferring the patient to the CCU once the diagnosis is established cannot be overstressed.

### General measures

Even before the initial diagnosis is established by history and physical examination and the important early decision regarding thrombolytic or other therapy is made, certain general measures are initiated. These include use of analgesics to alleviate severe discomfort and associated anxiety. Potent narcotic analgesics are commonly used, usually morphine or meperidine (Demerol).

Oxygen is almost always provided to ensure maximal hemoglobin saturation. Intravenous access routes (usually several) are established while blood samples are obtained for laboratory testing. Rhythm monitoring is initiated with appropriate intervention, if necessary. Depending on the clarity of presentation, some initial pharmacological measures may be undertaken. Among these are administration of nitroglycerin by the sublingual or transdermal routes and administration of lidocaine, an antidysrhythmic medication which may be given prophylactically, especially if ventricular ectopy is noted. In addition, it has become standard practice to initiate salicylate therapy immediately on presentation, usually with chewable aspirin (to achieve rapid blood levels), if no contraindication exists. This is done in recognition of the effect of aspirin on reducing platelet adhesion.

### Abnormalities of blood pressure, rhythm, and cardiac output

As part of the initial assessment, careful attention must be given to the presence of specific hemodynamic derangements. Significant abnormalities of blood pressure (particularly hypotension), the presence of congestive heart failure, and significant dysrhythmias must be addressed. Both hypotension and congestive heart failure have a significant negative prognostic implication in the setting of acute infarction, especially if present in combination. Malignant dysrhythmias, although not of specific prognostic influence, can lead to sudden clinical deterioration or death and must therefore be dealt with promptly.

Some of the potential interventions undertaken with the aim of reducing infarct size may have a significant effect on blood pressure, congestive heart failure, and dysrhythmias.

**Hypotension.** Although increased sympathetic tone related to anxiety and pain may be responsible for the initial elevation of blood pressure readings seen on presentation, greater importance is attached to hypotensive blood pressures. Systolic blood pressure readings of less than 90 to 100 mm Hg suggest significant impairment in the contractile function of the left ventricle. At least in part, hypotension commonly may be the result of fluid losses associated with the onset of infarction, including those caused by emesis and by profuse diaphoresis. In addition, administration of morphine analgesics and nitrates could produce venodilation, compounding the effect of fluid losses and creating a further relative hypovolemia. In some cases, profound bradycardia, particularly in the setting of inferior infarction or right ventricular infarction, may account for hypotension.

Profound hypotension results in diminished perfusion, particularly that of the coronary arteries, that occurs primarily during diastole (when pressures are even lower). In addition, cerebral perfusion and renal blood flow are reduced. It is considered of utmost importance in the management of acute infarction to maintain coronary perfusion pressure.

Initial measures used in correcting hypotension usually include a fluid challenge. Bolus infusion of saline solution or similarly osmotically active fluid in volumes of 250 to 500 ml/hr may be undertaken while carefully observing the patient for the development of pulmonary congestion and heart failure. If the fluid challenge is unsuccessful, vasopressor agents may be required, being titrated to achieve a systolic blood pressure of 100 mm Hg or greater (see Chapter 4).

**Congestive heart failure.** In the setting of acute infarction, congestive heart failure indicates more profound ventricular impairment and is associated with a worse prognosis. Congestive heart failure usually implies a significant degree of infarction of the left ventricle, usually considered at least 30% to 40% of left ventricular mass. In these cases, impairment of left ventricular systolic function is usually associated with similar impairment in left ventricular diastolic function (ventricular relaxation), and recent treatment modalities have attempted to address both of these aspects of left ventricular dysfunction.

The mainstay of treatment of congestive heart failure in the setting of acute infarction has been the use of potent parenteral diuretics such as furosemide (Lasix). The therapeutic value of furosemide lies in its ability to reduce pulmonary capillary pressure and preload.

Vasodilators are used to reduce left ventricular afterload. Among these agents are parenteral nitroglycerin, sodium nitropresside, and nifedipine, a calcium-channel antagonist that can be administered sublingually. Nitroglycerin has an additional use as a venodilator and is effective in reduction of preload, or left ventricular filling pressure, when appropriate.

Digitalis has been used less frequently during recent years as an inotropic agent, though it still plays a valuable role in selected cases, particularly in the setting of ventricular dilation. In addition, digitalis may be useful in situations in which its other effects may prove advantageous, such as in the presence of supraventricular ectopy.

Of less clear benefit is the use of parenteral inotropic agents (beta$_1$ agonists) such as dopamine, dobutamine, and nonadrenergic inotropes including the phosphodiesterase inhibitors, such as amrinone, which may operate physiologically in an additive manner with adrenergic agents. This area is currently the subject of intense scrutiny, and several new agents are on the verge of introduction.

A more detailed description of the effects and uses of the various pharmacological agents has been provided in Chapter 4 and will not be repeated here.

The most ominous hemodynamic impairment seen with acute myocardial infarction is the combination of hypotension (or cardiogenic shock) and congestive heart failure. In the clinical setting, combination therapy consisting of vasopressors with vasodilators and diuretics is used. To enable continuous accurate assessment of ventricular function in this condition, as well as to monitor hemodynamic changes from moment to moment in response to therapy, the technique of hemodynamic monitoring has proved invaluable.

Hemodynamic monitoring depends on the placement of a balloon-tipped (flow-directed) monitoring catheter in the pulmonary artery, using a percutaneous approach at the bedside. Blood pressure measurements obtained from this catheter reflect the pressure at its tip. When the balloon is deflated, this pressure reflects pulmonary arterial pressure, but when inflated, the pressure records "pulmonary capillary wedge pressure," a reasonably accurate reflection of left atrial pressure and, therefore, of left ventricular filling pressure. In practice, the balloon is inflated periodically when actual measurements approximating left ventricular filling pressure are required; then it is deflated. This catheter and technique for introduction was developed by Drs. Swan and Ganz, and their names have become synonymous with this pressure-measuring device.

At the same time, careful blood pressure measurements reflecting systemic arterial pressures are recorded by using typical blood pressure cuffs or, even more accurately, by peripheral arterial cannulation and direct pressure measurement.

By providing the pulmonary artery, or Swan-Ganz catheter, with a temperature-sensitive probe at its tip and providing an additional lumen that communicates with the right atrium, repeated measurements of cardiac output can be made using thermodilution techniques.

In critically ill patients hemodynamic monitoring as described above is employed to enable use of pharmacological agents in such a way that the ventricular function curve is optimized for each patient.

A traditional left ventricular function curve (see Chapter 3) is constructed by plotting left ventricular stroke work against left ventricular filling pressure. This defines a region in which the "muscle stretch" of the ventricular sarcomere is optimal. In the setting described above, a close approximation of left ventricular stroke work can be derived from the stroke volume (the cardiac output divided by the heart rate). Left ventricular filling pressure is closely approximated by the pulmonary capillary wedge pressure. With such a monitoring system a personal ventricular function curve can be plotted for each patient by measuring the change in stroke volume and pulmonary capillary wedge pressure after various interventions. In practice it has been found that when pulmonary capillary wedge pressure begins to exceed 20 mm Hg, left ventricular systolic performance deteriorates.

The relationship between the presence or absence of pulmonary congestion and hypoperfusion as reflected in measurements of cardiac index and pulmonary capillary wedge pressure, and subsequent mortality was outlined by Forrester and others and is reproduced in Fig. 6-3. Please note that these statistics are based on work performed in 1976 and mortality figures would be expected to be lower today.

**Dysrhythmias.** Both supraventricular and ventricular dysrhythmias, as well as a variety of conduction abnormalities, occur in the setting of acute infarction.

*Premature ventricular contractions.* Premature ventricular contractions (PVCs) with bursts of ventricular tachycardia and ventricular fibrillation occur commonly during the initial phase of myocardial infarction and account for the high mortality rate during the prehospital phase of AMI (see Chapter 5).

Occurrence of PVCs is almost universal in AMI, and deterioration to the more lethal dysrhythmias, ventricular tachycardia (VT), and/or ventricular fibrillation (VF) may be sudden and unpredictable. Spontaneous VT or VF without prior recording of PVCs has been described. This occurs as a result of stimulation, usually by an isolated PVC, during the so-called "vulnerable phase" (the region electrically represented by the interval from the end of the QRS wave and the peak, or midportion, of the T wave.) The likelihood that such a PVC or other stray electrical signal will initiate

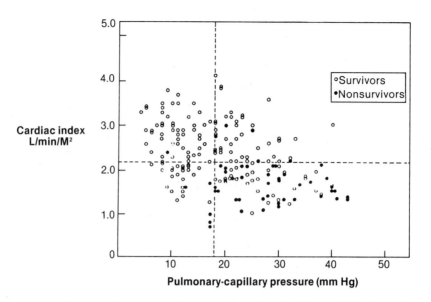

**Fig. 6-3.** Relation between pulmonary-capillary pressure and cardiac index in 200 patients with acute myocardial infarction. The dotted lines are placed at the levels of 18 mm Hg for pulmonary-capillary pressure and 2.1 L/min/m² for cardiac index. There is a wide degree of variability in left ventricular performance in patients with acute myocardial infarction, and mortality rate increases as cardiac performance deteriorates. (From Forrester JS and others: Medical therapy of acute myocardial infarction by application of hemodynamic subsets, *N Engl J Med* 295:1356, 1976.)

an episode of VT or VF depends on the "fibrillation threshold" of the ventricular muscle. This threshold is significantly lowered during periods of ischemia and infarction. This is why PVCs rarely cause problems in a setting of chronic irritability, but are a cause for concern in the setting of acute infarction.

Preventing these malignant forms of dysrhythmias is, therefore, particularly important during the acute phase of infarction. Important steps include prevention and correction of electrolyte abnormalities (especially hypokalemia), correction of hypoxemia and acidosis, and use of antidysrhythmic agents (particularly lidocaine). In addition, beta blockers decrease the incidence of malignant ventricular dysrhythmias. Other antidysrhythmic agents may be required (see Chapter 4).

The chief benefits of the CCU in reducing early mortality and morbidity associated with AMI are the continuous monitoring of cardiac rhythm and the detection and treatment of ventricular dysrhythmias as soon as they occur.

*Supraventricular tachycardia.* Supraventricular tachycardia—including sinus tachycardia, paroxysmal atrial fibrillation or atrial flutter, or paroxysmal atrial tachycardia (PAT)—is often a manifestation of left ventricular failure and bears significant prognostic importance. Initially, sinus tachycardia may simply be a response to pain and anxiety and its associated increase in adrenergic tone. Other causes may include fever, pericarditis, hypovolemia, or anemia. Rapid heart rates exert a detrimental effect through various mechanisms. Myocardial oxygen demand is increased as a direct result of increased heart rate. Cardiac output is reduced at rapid heart rates as a result of decreased diastolic filling

time. Diastolic time per minute is decreased at rapid heart rates, resulting in less time for myocardial perfusion, further exacerbating ischemia. In the case of atrial fibrillation, the loss of the atrial contribution to left ventricular filling can have a significantly detrimental effect on cardiac output. This atrial contribution has been found to be of increased importance during AMI. Increased ventricular stiffness as a result of infarction leads to impaired diastolic filling. Atrial contraction in this situation significantly augments diastolic filling and increases sarcomere stretch, thereby increasing contractility (by Starling's Law).

Initial therapy usually includes the use of analgesics and sedatives. Other pharmacological agents may be required, including digitalis, beta blockers, and some of the calcium-channel antagonists (see Chapter 4). Treatments specific to some of the causes of tachycardia, such as congestive heart failure, fever, pain, or anxiety, may be indicated.

*Bradydysrhythmias.* Bradydysrhythmias are extremely common in AMI particularly during the acute phase, usually because of vagal stimulation. This is particularly true of inferior or posterior infarctions. The normal heart adapts to bradycardia by increasing stroke volume, and cardiac output is usually not affected until the heart rate drops below 40 or even less. In AMI, however, even rates in the range of 50 beats per minute may be associated with a decrease in stroke volume and cardiac output and result in hypotension.

Asymptomatic bradycardia is usually not treated. Mildly symptomatic bradycardia may be treated with parenteral atropine, and placement of a temporary pacemaker may be required if bradycardia is severe or prolonged or associated with significant hypotension.

***Atrioventricular block.*** Atrioventricular (AV) block may occur, again usually in cases of inferior infarction, and may be well tolerated, though pharmacological treatment or pacemaker implantation may be required. When AV block occurs in anterior infarction, it usually indicates extensive myocardial injury and is associated with progression to sudden, complete AV block or cardiac standstill. Pacemaker implantation is almost always required in these cases. Cases of anterior infarction complicated by AV block (because of the associated extensive myocardial injury) have an extremely high mortality rate independent of the treatment applied, often resulting from cardiogenic shock or "pump failure."

## Limitation of infarct size

**Thrombolysis.** The management of patients with acute myocardial infarction has undergone significant change within just the past few years. This is the result of the increasingly widespread availability and use of thrombolytic therapy in an attempt to achieve reperfusion of the infarcted segment. This has made it possible, for the first time, to attempt to reduce the degree of myocardial infarction with a corresponding improvement in morbidity and mortality, and to achieve a superior functional recovery with less residual disability. Until recently, a patient with acute infarction underwent stabilization and treatment of known or possible complications, with little ability to reverse the pathophysiological injury. Potential complications could be anticipated and prevention attempted. Hemodynamic derangements could be measured and correction attempted. With the advent of clinical availability of thrombolytic agents, therapy can be directed at an actual reversal of the disease process; it offers the hope of recovery with some degree of reduction, even possibly prevention or reversal, of permanent myocardial damage.

It is now generally recognized and accepted that acute myocardial infarction is the result of a thrombotic occlusion of a major coronary artery—usually one that has had its lumen narrowed to a variable extent by the process of atherosclerosis. It is thought that fracture, fissuring, or disruption of the plaque surface results in a break in the endothelial lining, exposing plaque material to the flowing blood. This initiates the process of clotting, resulting in complete occlusion of the affected artery, where the actual atheromatous narrowing may not even have been severe.

If the thrombotic occlusion could be dissolved or lysed and reperfusion of the myocardium effected, the process of myocardial necrosis might be aborted. It is clear that the more rapidly this can be achieved, the greater the potential benefit. Although some improvement in ventricular function has been described after reperfusion times as long as 12 or more hours following onset of infarction, it is generally agreed that a maximum of 6 hours should be the limit beyond which the risks of reperfusion therapy probably outweigh any potential advantages to be gained (though this is still being evaluated in clinical trials). Best results can be anticipated if reperfusion therapy is instituted within 4 hours of onset of infarction, but the current maxim appears to be, "the sooner the better." Studies are currently underway of possible medications or electrolyte solutions that might be infused to stabilize the ischemic or anoxic myocardium, increasing the "therapeutic window" in which reperfusion therapy might be expected to be of benefit.

The precise technique of reperfusion therapy is currently under intense investigation, with several large-scale multinational trials underway (see Suggested Readings), and it is clear that changes in the details of treatment will occur frequently as new information is acquired and new thrombolytic agents or combinations of agents become available, or demonstrate efficacy.

Initially, it was proposed that reperfusion therapy would require an intracoronary route of administration, in order to maximize the therapeutic agent at its intended site of action and to minimize bleeding complications, but this proved to have several major disadvantages when compared with the intravenous route of administration. Chief among these disadvantages is the additional time required to perform the necessary cardiac catheterization for placement of the perfusion catheter and the need for a catheterization laboratory and personnel available on 24-hour call in all community hospitals. In addition, catheterization generally requires arterial cannulation, posing a significant risk of complications related to bleeding. The intravenous route is now almost universally used, allowing rapid initiation of therapy in all hospitals, even those not equipped with catheterization laboratory capabilities. Although overcoming the major disadvantages of the intracoronary route, intravenous thrombolytic therapy poses the disadvantage of creating a "systemic lytic state" in the patient. The risk of serious, perhaps fatal, bleeding as a result of thrombolytic therapy has limited its universal applicability and has therefore demanded careful patient selection. This has also led to a judicious balancing of the dosage of thrombolytic agents used, in an attempt to maximize the percentage of successful clot lysis while minimizing the risk of major bleeding complications.

A variety of agents have been used for thrombolytic therapy and several others are currently under investigation. Streptokinase and urokinase were widely used initially. More recently tissue-type plasminogen activator (t-PA) has become clinically available through techniques using recombinant DNA technology. By this technique, plasminogen activator, a normal human enzyme present in minute quantities in tissue, is manufactured in therapeutic doses by genetically altered bacteria.

Studies currently underway are attempting to identify the ideal agent or combination of agents, appropriate doses and schedules of administration. Streptokinase appears to be highly efficacious, but because it is a bacterial (streptococcal) enzyme, it is potentially antigenic in humans. There have been occasional allergic reactions reported with its use, some of them serious. In addition, streptokinase has the theoretical disadvantage of producing a systemic lytic state because it nonselectively produces widespread plasmin activation. Episodes of hypotension, sometimes profound, have been associated with streptokinase therapy.

In contrast, the newer agent, t-PA, is nonallergenic and is theoretically clot specific. Its chief disadvantage currently is its extremely high cost when compared with streptokinase. There is also some clinical evidence that there may be an increased incidence of reocclusion following t-PA compared with streptokinase. The relative efficacy of streptokinase and t-PA continues to be studied. The most recent large scale trial (GUSTO) suggests a definite advantage to the use of t-PA, though the benefit is surprisingly small.

It is currently estimated that more than 60% of patients diagnosed as suffering AMI are denied thrombolytic therapy because of delay in presentation, advanced age, potential bleeding risks, and an over-cautious approach by the treating physician. Other contraindicating factors include recent major surgery, severe hypertension, ulcer disease, and a prolonged or traumatic resuscitation attempt.

Use of any of the currently available thrombolytic agents demands careful patient selection and close attention to technique and potential complications. This has limited their use during the very earliest phase of myocardial infarction (i.e., use in the field or in the ambulance en route to the hospital, where very early administration of a thrombolytic agent might be expected to provide maximum benefit).

All currently used forms of thrombolytic therapy involve a single dose infusion, though this may progress over the course of several hours. To prevent subsequent reocclusion, all agents are currently followed by continuous therapeutic anticoagulation, using heparin intravenously by continuous infusion and maintaining the partial thromboplastin time at between 2 and 2½ times control value. In addition, it has been demonstrated that initiation of salicylate therapy at the time of thrombolytic therapy has been of additional benefit in preventing reocclusion. The agent used is aspirin, at a dose of 1¼ to 5 grains orally per day. Anticoagulation is expected to continue during the subacute phase.

The increasing attention to use of thrombolytic therapy and the recognition that time is critically important in maximizing the benefit of such therapy, has had the effect of increasing the need for rapid assessment and diagnosis of patients presenting with chest pain, and has led, therefore, to an abbreviation of the traditional diagnostic pathway previously outlined. Patients presenting with a strong clinical history are now subjected to emergent ECG, and, if suggestive, the history is abbreviated to one of ascertainment of contraindications to thrombolytic therapy, which often may be initiated while the more traditional examination procedure is resumed.

Some controversy exists over whether patients who have been successfully reperfused should be routinely subjected to coronary angiography before discharge from the hospital, or whether patients may be safely selected for this procedure by appearance of ischemic symptoms before discharge or by ischemia elicited by stress testing before discharge. Further studies should provide an answer to these questions (see Suggested Readings). This has led to an intense effort at "risk stratification."

**Direct angioplasty.** Over the past several years, the technique of percutaneous transluminal coronary angioplasty (PTCA) has been developed and has become increasingly widely used. Initially, this technique was employed as an alternative to coronary artery bypass grafting. In this role, PTCA was considered in patients who were stable, and in the recovery phase of their infarct, or, more commonly, were identified as a result of clinical evaluation of angina pectoris; as such, they would not have a place in discussion of AMI and its treatment.

PTCA recently has undergone an expansion of its indication to include the treatment of acute infarction. The possible use of PTCA in this setting was investigated as a means of treating patients who, for one reason or another, were unsuitable for thrombolytic therapy; later, investigations included patients who had undergone thrombolytic therapy, but were clinically suspected to have been "treatment failures" (i.e., they demonstrated no evidence of reperfusion, and, often, were suspected to be at high risk as a result of continuing infarction and clinical instability). This technique is highly "technology intensive" and requires the availability of suitable, trained staff and a catheterization laboratory facility on a 24-hour basis. This has significantly limited its clinical usefulness to date. Studies comparing efficacy, risk, and relative benefits of this technique versus immediate thrombolytic therapy are ongoing. Practical difficulties imposed by this approach will continue to limit its application, though in the clinical subsets described, direct PTCA would seem to offer a definite advantage.

**Other measures.** Although thrombolytic therapy offers the patient the benefit of substantial reversal of the disease process, significant advances in other modalities have occurred in the treatment of patients with AMI. These modalities are generally widely applicable and have had a definite impact on reducing the morbidity and mortality of infarction independent of, and possibly in addition to, the improvement offered by thrombolysis.

As a result of a series of sophisticated studies dating to the late 1960s, a method was established to experimentally assess the degree of infarction, thereby allowing careful analysis of the improvement or harm afforded by various interventions and therapeutic approaches. Extrapolations from these studies were applied to humans and ushered in a new era of therapy aimed at limiting infarct size, not by affecting the basic disease process but by optimizing factors affecting heart work, metabolic demand, and energy supply.

Despite the subsequent development of thrombolytic therapy to achieve reperfusion (a modality that has become the premier method of limiting infarct size), lessons learned from this earlier phase of infarct management still play an extremely important role in the current treatment of patients with infarction. This remains an area of intense research interest.

***Adjusting filling pressure and oxygen demand.*** General measures are aimed at optimizing coronary filling pressure, while minimizing myocardial oxygen demand ($M\dot{V}O_2$.) Systolic blood pressure is maintained between 90 and 120 mm Hg, oxygen is administered, sedatives are provided to allay anxiety, analgesics are given to relieve pain, and the patient is kept at bed rest in a quiet environment.

***Beta blockers.*** Beta-adrenergic blockade has been found to be of significant benefit in a number of recent large-scale trials. Beta blockers exert a beneficial effect on a number of parameters influencing $M\dot{V}O_2$ (see Chapter 4). In the uncomplicated infarction, beta blockers are now routinely used at the time of admission or in the emergency room setting, beginning with parenteral therapy and continuing with oral therapy through the hospital phase and for years following discharge. Relative contraindications to their use have included hypotension, bradycardia, the presence of significant AV block, or history of severe bronchospastic lung disease. Use of beta blockers has been associated with a significant reduction in pain duration, ectopy, in-hospital mortality, and late mortality. Enzyme analysis and various functional studies have confirmed a reduction in infarct size coincident with the use of beta blockers. The beta-blocking agents used in the setting of acute infarction are those without intrinsic sympathomimetic activity and include metoprolol, propranolol, and atenolol. Although these agents have been thought of as contraindicated in the presence of hypotension and congestive heart failure, cautious use has been found to offer a definite survival advantage (see ISIS trials, Suggested Readings). In fact, it has been shown that patients who are considered most critically ill, usually because of severe impairment of left ventricular function, are the ones who demonstrate the greatest degree of benefit from this form of therapy.

***Nitrates.*** Nitroglycerin has been shown to reduce infarct size, particularly if used early in the course of acute infarction. Nitrates are commonly given sublingually before or shortly after the patient arrives at the emergency room. Subsequently, nitroglycerin may be given by continuous intravenous infusion, with careful regulation of the dosage to avoid hypotension.

***Other agents.*** A number of other potential approaches to treatment of acute infarction are currently under study, and over the next several years at least some of these will be proved useful in limiting infarct size by preserving ischemic myocardium. Among the more promising of these interventions under study are the following:

*Angiotensin converting enzyme (ACE) therapy.* Recent studies have demonstrated that the use of ACE inhibitors, including captopril, enalapril, and others, has conferred a definite survival advantage, especially in patients with moderately severely impaired left ventricular function (i.e., those with left ventricular ejection fraction 40% or less). It is now recommended that these agents be cautiously instituted as early as possible, certainly during the acute hospitalization, and continued indefinitely. The exact mechanism by which survival advantage is conferred is unknown; however, it may relate to amelioration of factors resulting in increased wall stress, and, thereby, $M\dot{V}O_2$, and also to the process of left ventricular remodeling that occurs following infarction. The direct action of these agents is inhibition of conversion of angiotensinogen, a precursor peptide, to angiotensin, a potent vasoconstrictor and mediator of several important pathways of inflammation and clotting. Work is currently underway in development of direct angiotensin inhibitors, but none are clinically available as yet.

*Calcium-channel antagonists.* Calcium-channel antagonists affect the slow calcium membrane channel in a variety of cells, particularly cardiac and vascular smooth muscle cells. There appears to be a pronounced variability in the specific effects on the heart and peripheral vascular system of each individual drug in this category. Cardiac effects include alterations in contractility and effects on the intracardiac conduction system, particularly on AV-node conduction. Vascular smooth muscle effects usually mediate vasodilation, particularly affecting small arteries, thereby reducing afterload and peripheral resistance. There are currently numerous drugs in this pharmacological category, with several others poised for release.

Particular agents in this drug class offer specific benefits for individual problems and complications encountered in cases of acute infarction. Verapamil demonstrates a moderate degree of inotropic inhibition and has potent effects on AV node conduction. Its use is considered in the setting of supraventricular tachycardia or dysrhythmias. Diltiazem is beneficial in cases of acute infarction, particularly in non-Q wave infarction, in which it has been shown to reduce the incidence of in-hospital reinfarction, though its use may be hazardous in patients with marked ventricular dysfunction. Nifedipine is a potent vasodilator and may result in reflex tachycardia and hypotension. Its use may be indicated in cases of hypertension and/or bradycardia if additional afterload reduction is desirable. Some evidence that nifedipine may increase infarct size has led to reluctance to use it in this setting. Nicardipine is an agent very similar to nifedipine in action. Further details on these agents may be found in Chapter 4. There is a fair amount of controversy over the routine use of calcium-channel agents in the setting of acute infarction. This has resulted from disappointing results of various studies, in which these agents have failed to result in improvement, and in many instances, may have had an adverse effect on recovery.

*Free radical scavengers.* Much attention has been paid recently to so-called "oxygen derived free radicals," particularly in the setting of reperfusion, where hypoxic tissue is suddenly reperfused with oxygen-rich blood. These agents have been found to cause additional injury and to blunt the beneficial effects of reperfusion. A new area of drug research involving free radical scavenging agents has therefore arisen and is showing some early promise. Among these agents is superoxide dismutase (SOD), and it is expected that use of this or an analogous agent will be routine in association with reperfusion therapy in the future. The role of nitric oxide has been the most recently studied intermediary.

*Prostaglandin modifying agents.* Aspirin and other so-called nonsteroidal antiinflammatory agents are under careful scrutiny as modifiers of various stages of myocardial injury, as well as in platelet activity and the coagulation cascade. Aspirin has been beneficial in cases of acute infarction and may have a role as a primary prevention agent. Numerous other drugs in this group are currently available. Their efficacy in the cases of acute infarction has yet to be determined. As with the calcium-channel antagonists, an overall similarity in the mode of action of these drugs should not obscure the widespread subtle differences that may exist, making one agent perhaps more effective for specific indications than others.

*Magnesium.* Recent tentative data suggesting that use of magnesium, as one of several salts, in the acute setting, is associated with significant improvement in survival, led to great excitement in the medical community. Magnesium is intimately associated with muscle and conduction system physiology, is inexpensive, generally available and convenient to use. Additional data has been somewhat disappointing, and the exact role of magnesium therapy in the setting of AMI is currently unclear.

Other approaches are currently underway, spurred by increasing understanding of the basic process of ischemic injury and by advances recently made in the field of cardiac surgery.

During cardiac surgery, marked disturbances of cardiac metabolism for periods as long as 12 hours have been managed successfully, allowing recovery of contractile function. It is obvious that some techniques possible in the operating room, such as hypothermia, cannot be duplicated in the patient with acute infarction, but important advances have been made regarding other factors that may prove of significant benefit. These may involve infusion of altered electrolyte solutions or other agents to stabilize ischemic myocardium.

Mechanical approaches, including intraaortic balloon pump and coronary sinus reperfusion, are beyond the scope of this chapter.

### The coronary care unit

Much of the decrease in mortality due to AMI in recent years has been attributed to the advent of the coronary care unit (CCU). Although the chief incidence of significant ventricular ectopy (VT and VF) occurs during the first 6 hours following infarction, over the ensuing 36 to 48 hours an appreciable number of patients will continue to experience life-threatening dysrhythmias. The CCU places the patient in an environment of continuous electrocardiographic monitoring and is staffed by nurses trained in recognizing potentially serious rhythm disturbances and other complications of early infarction. CCU nurses are trained to immediately initiate appropriate therapy, including electrical defibrillation, external cardiac pacing, and use of the pharmacological armamentarium available under specific guidelines established for this type of unit and trained personnel.

In addition, much of the physician-directed early intervention already discussed will occur in the setting of a CCU. The trend over the past 10 years has been to transport the patient with acute infarction to the CCU setting as rapidly as possible, with most of the initial therapy frequently administered in the CCU rather than in the emergency department. The CCU has been particularly valuable for those patients requiring hemodynamic monitoring, frequent assessment of vital signs, and continual adjustment of the variety of pharmacological agents that often are administered simultaneously, including thrombolytic agents, antidysrhythmics, nitrates, vasopressors and anticoagulants.

For patients without complications a stay of probably 2 or 3 days in the CCU is sufficient. Patients who develop complications may require a significantly longer period of close observation and therapy. These patients should remain in a CCU until they no longer need close nursing supervision are no longer dependent on parenteral vasoactive agents, or no longer require hemodynamic monitoring. Patients who remain unstable, with evidence of recurrent ischemia or significant dysrhythmia, should continue under close scrutiny in the CCU.

### The stepdown unit

Once the patient has been stable for at least 24 hours (with stable blood pressure and heart rate and no significant rhythm disturbance) and has been weaned of most, if not all, vasoactive parenteral medications, transfer may be made to an "intermediate CCU" or "stepdown unit."

This type of facility is usually characterized by a lower nurse/patient ratio, although still allowing for more careful supervision than on a regular medical floor. This includes the capability of continuous rhythm monitoring, usually with some form of telemetric monitoring system, which allows the patient greater physical mobility.

The purpose of the intermediate CCU is to allow initial ambulation of the patient to proceed in a monitored environment. This consists of self-help tasks, such as in-bed hygiene, sitting at bedside to eat, and use of a bedside commode, then allowing ambulation to a sink for facial and oral hygiene, and progressing to ambulation outside the room in the hallway, which is usually equipped for telemetric monitoring.

Relatively frequent vital signs assessment, although not as frequent as in the acute CCU, allows identification of abnormal blood pressure and heart rate responses to early progressive ambulation, and monitoring detects unexpected rhythm abnormalities. These may occur as a result of increased myocardial workload, and as a function of myocardial injury resulting from the infarction. Patients at higher risk at this stage of recovery are those with extensive myocardial injury as evidenced by persistent sinus tachycardia and supraventricular dysrhythmias, intraventricular conduction delays of new onset, persistent ST-segment elevation, and recurrent pain. Patients with anteroseptal infarction are more prone to complications than those with inferior or posterior wall infarction.

## Convalescence

After 2 to 3 days in an intermediate CCU setting the patient may be transferred to a regular hospital room for further convalescence, with plans to gradually increase ambulation.

Development of complications in the intermediate CCU, such as ambulation-associated ischemic pain or significant ectopy, would be considered an indication to prolong observation or to transfer the patient back to the acute CCU. In addition, this may be considered an indication for predischarge coronary angiography.

In the patient without complications, onset of ambulation has gradually been initiated earlier. This has been the result of an increased appreciation of actual workloads associated with specific activities, as well as the tolerance of the acutely infarcted heart to limited activity. A complicating feature in this regard has been the trend to initiate complex intervention strategies early during the hospitalization, a practice that progresses rapidly in many cases to invasive diagnostic techniques in an attempt to detect those who are candidates for further intervention (either balloon angioplasty or bypass surgery). This has led to delay, or alteration of the traditional ambulation process until the patient has been completely treated, studied, and "corrected."

Recent studies, such as the TIMI trials, (see Suggested Readings) have suggested that, following thrombolytic therapy, patients should undergo more routine hospitalization, with selection of patients for further invasive diagnostic studies based on symptoms of recurrent angina during convalescence or in the course of predischarge noninvasive testing (so-called risk stratification). On the basis of these and other studies, it seems likely that the trend to earlier angiography followed by balloon angioplasty or surgical correction will be slowed and applied selectively to patients demonstrating post infarction instability.

Patients with uncomplicated AMI usually begin early ambulation activities by the second day of infarction with mild in-bed activity while in the CCU. Initial ambulation involves assuming a sitting posture usually with feet suspended from the bed ("dangling"), and progresses to sitting in a chair at bedside for periods of 10 to 15 minutes, with gradual lengthening of the out-of-bed time and increased frequency. These early ambulation maneuvers balance the increased workload of the activity with the harmful effects associated with prolonged bed rest. Immobilization is associated with the pooling of blood in the legs and pelvis, loss of muscular and vascular tone, and mobilization of calcium out of bone. A relative contraction of intravascular volume may occur in response to the diuresis induced by these shifts. In addition, bed rest is known to predispose to development of thrombophlebitis and its risk of pulmonary embolization.

Careful evaluation of the cardiac response to early activity, such as sitting in a chair while the bed linen is being changed rather than rolling from side to side in bed, and using a bedside commode rather than a bedpan, has shown no significant additional stress and these mild forms of activity are much preferred by patients. Although it is advisable for a nurse or attendant to perform the bed bath during the first 2 to 3 days, the energy requirements for a basin, shower, or tub bath have been found to be similar.

Gradual progressive walking ambulation may be generally undertaken by the third to fifth day, using parameters of heart rate, blood pressure, and ectopic activity as guidelines. In addition, symptoms such as fatigue, breathlessness or shortness of breath, dizziness, and chest discomfort are carefully monitored. In the absence of a "stepdown unit," portable telemetry monitors may be used for this purpose allowing periodic rhythm strips to be obtained. These are analyzed for heart rate, cardiac rhythm or development of conduction defects (which may be rate related), and ST-segment shifts.

Discharge of the patient without complications from the hospital has reflected the trend toward earlier ambulation, and, partially in response to cost-containment pressures, has been reduced to between 7 and 10 days, occasionally even earlier. Some studies have suggested that in the absence of specific risk factors identified at the outset of AMI, some patients may do as well at home as in the hospital, though it is highly unlikely that acute infarction will be managed with less than 1 week of hospitalization. An exception might be in cases where early successful reperfusion is followed by symptomatic ischemic pain, early angiograph, and balloon angioplasty. In this setting, it is conceivable that a patient may be discharged within 5 to 6 days of admission. In the case of direct angioplasty, discharge may occur even sooner, perhaps in 3 days.

Before the patient is discharged from the hospital, and as part of the risk-stratification strategy, it is customary to have the patient undergo "low-level" exercise testing. This procedure helps identify high-risk patients and provides some assurance that the activities engaged in during the postdischarge convalescence period can be done safely. End points to the low-level test include: achievement of submaximal heart rate, usually 120 to 130 bpm; development of

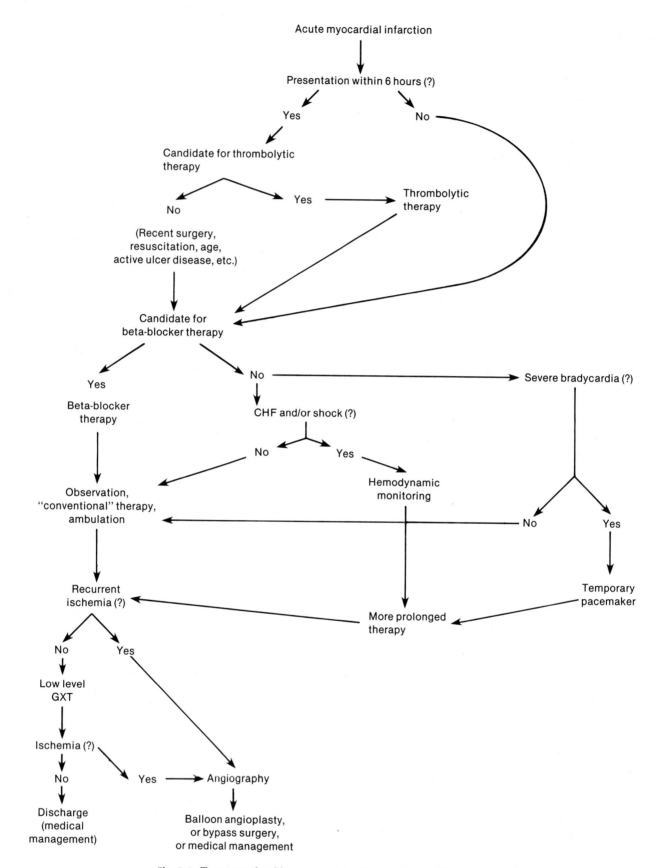

**Fig. 6-4.** Treatment algorithm summarizing the decision-making processes.

ischemic pain; ischemic ST-segment depression; hypotension, or a drop in systolic blood pressure of 20 mm Hg or more; or development of increasingly frequent ventricular ectopy. The protocol is completed in 9 minutes (consisting of three 3-minute segments—0%, 5%, and 10% grades—all at 1.7 mph) (see Chapter 8).

Other testing done before discharge may include 24-hour Holter electrocardiography to assess the patient's rhythm response to ambulation on a general medical floor at a time just before discharge. In some cases this can be delayed to the postdischarge period, offering demonstration of the representative rhythm and ST-segment shifts occurring in the outpatient setting.

## SUMMARY

This chapter has attempted to present a brief summary of the current treatment of a patient with acute myocardial infarction. It is hoped that the sense of urgency in completing a large number of tasks, including initiation of an increasing array of pharmacological therapies, has been transmitted to the reader. An attempt has also been made to convey a sense of the rapidity of change in treatment of this serious manifestation of coronary atherosclerosis, the leading cause of death in the United States and the cause of 750,000 annual hospital admissions. Despite changes that may occur as a result of increased knowledge of the pathophysiology of myocardial injury and introduction of new medications and techniques, the principles described above will remain generally valid. In review, a treatment algorithm is presented below to summarize the decision-making processes in schematic form (Fig. 6-4).

## REFERENCES

1. Killip T and others: Treatment of myocardial infarction in a coronary care unit, *Am J Cardiol* 20:457, 1967.

## SUGGESTED READINGS

Braunwald E, editor: *Heart disease: a textbook of cardiovascular medicine,* ed 3, Philadelphia, 1988, WB Saunders Co.

Comparison of invasive and conservative strategies after treatment with intravenous tissue plasminogen activator in acute myocardial infarction (TIMI II), *N Engl J Med* 320:618, 1989.

Gersh, BJ and Rahimtoola, S, editors: *Acute myocardial infarction,* New York, 1991, Elsevier Science Publishing Co. Inc.

Gruppo Italiano per lo Studio della Streptochinasi nell'Infarcto Miocardico (GISSI), *Lancet* I:397, 1986.

Gruppo Italiano per lo Studio della Streptochinasi nell'Infarcto Miocardico (GISSI-2), *Lancet* 336:61, 1990.

GUSTO (Global Utilization of Streptokinase and t-PA for Occluded Coronary Arteries Trial), *N Engl J Med* 329:1127, 1993.

ISIS-4 Collaborative Group. Fourth International Study of Infarct Survival; *Am J Cardiol Suppl* 68:87D, 1991.

*Prog Cardiovasc D* 29:165-468 (1986-87), 30:1-306 (1987-88).

# CHAPTER 7

# Abnormal Exercise Physiology

*Scot Irwin*

## OUTLINE

This chapter's purpose is to expand the knowledge base of physical therapists conducting cardiac or pulmonary rehabilitation programs. To understand the clinical observations discussed, one must have a sound understanding of *normal* human responses.[1]

To the purist the term "abnormal" is a misnomer, because a clear-cut definition of "normal" has not been established. Normal values may range from those less than average to those above average. This makes it difficult to distinguish normal variations from true aberrations. However, to describe some peculiar exertional responses found in patients with cardiac or pulmonary disease, the term "abnormal" will be used.

There are several established physiological responses to exercise. For example, heart rate and systolic blood pressure rise as the workload is increased, and cardiac output limits the increase in oxygen consumption and determines the maximal physical work capacity. Furthermore, numerous articles describe the angina threshold (the point at which a patient first perceives angina) as a fixed phenomenon based on myocardial oxygen demand, which is strongly correlated

to the product of heart rate and systolic blood pressure.[24] Each of these well-established norms has an abnormal counterpart. Various pathological conditions and treatments (including medications) can create demonstrable changes in normal heart rate, blood pressure, and anginal responses during exercise. These abnormal responses and the occurrence of respiratory limitations to maximum oxygen consumption are discussed in the following format. First the abnormal response is defined, then the supporting literature is cited, clinical examples that illustrate the abnormality are presented, followed by a brief theoretical discussion of the possible causes, and finally the clinical implications of the abnormal phenomenon are summarized.

## HEART RATE RESPONSE
### Normal

At normal and submaximum levels of exercise, cardiac output and heart rate response increase linearly as the workload and oxygen consumption demands increase[39] (Fig. 7-1). At near-maximum and maximum levels of exertion, however, the heart rate response becomes less linear and increases disproportionately to the workload imposed (Fig. 7-2).

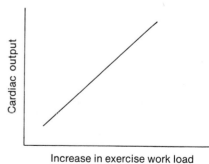

**Fig. 7-1.** Cardiac output is linearly related to workload. When the workload is progressively increased, cardiac output matches the demand until maximum cardiac output is achieved. (Normal.)

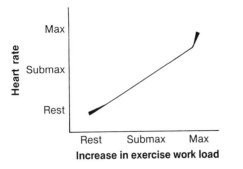

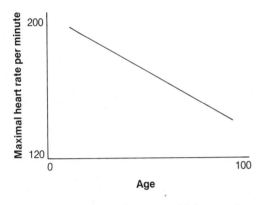

**Fig. 7-2.** Heart rate response to increases in workload. Submaximum effort is closely related to heart rate response, but at the extremes of exertion the relationship is generally less linear.

**Fig. 7-3.** Maximum heart rate decreases with increase in age.

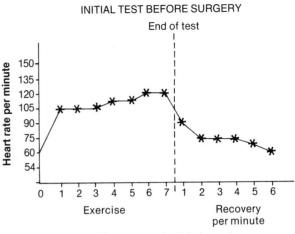

**Fig. 7-4.** Heart rate response to Bruce Protocol Treadmill Test in patient A, a 45-year-old man, before surgery. Patient completed 6 minutes and 6 seconds of the Bruce Protocol. He was limited by angina. Resting heart rate was 54, and maximum heart rate was 118. Resting blood pressure was 164/98, and maximum blood pressure was 244/126. He demonstrated moderate systolic and severe progressive diastolic hypertension with exercise. No ST-segment changes were found in any of the six leads: $V_1$, $V_5$, $V_6$, X, $CM_4$, Y. There were no dysrhythmias. His medications were nitroglycerin as needed and Dyazide (triamterene and hydrochlorothiazide). A fourth heart sound was auscultated.

In addition, a person's maximum attainable heart rate decreases with age. A useful but limited formula for predicting a maximum heart rate is to subtract the patient's age from 220 (Fig. 7-3). The accuracy of this formula is limited because of the effects of medications (see Chapter 4), abnormal heart rate responses, and the wide range of individual variations in maximum heart rate response (± 10%). It is preferable to obtain a patient's true maximum heart rate by performing a maximum symptom-limited exercise test (see Chapter 8).

## Abnormal

In the clinical setting, a small subset of patients with coronary artery disease demonstrates a clearly abnormal heart rate response to exercise. This phenomenon has been described by Ellestad,[15] Miller,[28] and Blessey and others.[3] Although each describes slightly different criteria for the response, and thus a slightly different population of patients, they do agree that this response is a sign of an advanced pathological condition. Generally the following criteria are observed:

1. Low resting heart rate (50 to 70 bpm)
2. Poor physical condition (untrained)
3. Advanced coronary artery disease
4. Maximum symptom-limited heart rate achieved during exercise testing is well below the person's predicted maximal heart rate (PMHR), obtained by subtracting the individual's age from 220
5. Men between the ages of 40 and 60
6. Nonuse of chronotropic-inhibiting medications (chronotropic means "influencing the rate of the heart beat")
7. Poor, slow heart rate increase in response to incremental increases in exercise workload
8. Poor exercise tolerance

A classic example of this phenomenon in the same patient tested before and after bypass surgery is presented in Figs. 7-4 and 7-5. A summary interpretation of each of these tests follows the graph. Each exercise test was performed in the same manner according to the protocol described in Appendix A in Chapter 11.

It is extraordinary that patient A's exercise tolerance was unchanged despite a 42-beat-per-minute increase in his maximum heart rate between the first test before surgery and the second test 8 weeks after surgery. In effect, this patient had a 36% increase in his heart rate reserve but essentially no change in his physical work capacity.

The following findings were recorded on patient A's catheterization: (1) 25% narrowing of the left main coronary artery; (2) less than 50% narrowing at the junction of the proximal and middle thirds of the left anterior descending artery, plus a somewhat narrowed appearance throughout its length; (3) about 75% stenosis at the origin of the second

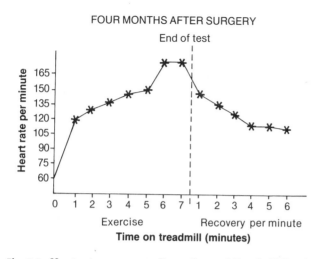

**Fig. 7-5.** Heart rate response to Bruce Protocol Treadmill Test in patient A ( 7-4) 8 weeks after bypass surgery. Patient completed 6 minutes and 7 seconds of the Bruce Protocol. He was limited by leg pain. Resting heart rate was 62, and maximum heart rate was 160. Resting blood pressure 176/110 and maximum blood pressure was 292/120. He demonstrated severe systolic and diastolic blood pressure response throughout the test. He had no angina or ST-segment changes. There was one premature ventricular contraction during exercise. He was not using medications. Fourth heart sound was auscultated.

posterolateral branch of the circumflex and mildly irregular throughout; (4) right coronary artery 75% stenotic at the ostium and midpoint; (5) hemodynamically, the right ventricle and atrium had greatly elevated end-diastolic and systolic pressures; (6) left ventricular end-diastolic pressure was greatly elevated; (7) ejection faction was normal; and (8) the left ventricular contractile pattern was normal. An abnormal heart rate response to exercise testing using the criteria listed may be the only abnormality found on the exercise test. Yet this finding often signifies advanced coronary artery disease and a poor prognosis.

**Mechanisms.** There appears to be a close relationship between patient A's heart rate response and ischemia. (Note that there were no ST-segment changes on either test.) The first test, which vividly demonstrates chronotropic incompetence, illustrates the need to watch all the factors involved in exercise testing, not just ST segments.

Neither Ellestad nor Blessey has presented a consistent explanation for this abnormal heart rate response. Hinkle, Carver, and Plakum[19] believe that it is attributable to ischemia of the sinoatrial node. On the other hand the work of Jose[22] indicates that as myocardial contractility decreases, as occurs with increasing levels of ischemia, the intrinsic heart rate response decreases. Ellestad has found that this decreased response is an ominous sign of advanced coronary artery disease associated with accelerated rates of mortality and morbidity (Figs. 7-6 and 7-7), especially when compared with patients with normal heart rate responses.[15]

The exact cause of this response is unknown; however, one may speculate that patients who exhibit it have a neurological, vascular, or humoral reflex that works through the autonomic nervous system to keep their heart rates down. Another possibility is that the ischemia causes a reflex inhibition of the electrical activation in the sinoatrial node, thus decreasing the rate at which the sinoatrial node can fire.

If ischemia is the cause of this decreased heart rate response, the body's defense mechanism is appropriate because a lower heart rate certainly facilitates improved coronary blood flow and decreases myocardial oxygen demand. A lower heart rate lengthens the diastolic period, and thus the coronary artery filling time is lengthened so that an improved perfusion can be achieved. A lower heart rate also decreases myocardial oxygen requirements. Alternatively, an increased diastolic filling time may, especially during exercise, cause large increases in end-diastolic volume. Volume increases are well tolerated by a normal, well-perfused myocardium, but in the ischemic myocardium volume changes are associated with increased pressures and thus decreased subendocardial perfusion (see Chapter 2). As the reader may note from the patient example, his end-diastolic pressure was greatly elevated, 20 mm Hg, at rest (0 to 12 mm Hg is normal). One could speculate that the rising end-diastolic pressures that undoubtedly occur with increased venous return during exercise may somehow be the impetus to a reflex inhibition in heart rate.[22]

Further speculation and research into the probable causes of abnormal heart rate responses to exercise should focus on all the factors that normally control heart rate. This would be an exhaustive review and not within the purview of this text. Perhaps future clinicians and researchers will determine the exact cause of this abnormal response.

The normal heart rate response in a well-trained athlete to increasing levels of exercise is to have a slow resting heart and a gradual but linear rise to a normal maximum rate. The pathological chronotropic incompetence exhibited by the nonathlete should not be taken lightly by therapists, but instead interpreted as a highly abnormal response to exercise.

### Summary of clinical significance

1. Failure to perform symptom-limited, maximum-exercise tests may mask the patient with abnormal heart rate responses.

2. A slow heart rate at rest and a slow heart rate response to exercise does not always signify a good state of fitness.

3. Abnormal heart rate response to exercise may be an ominous sign, predictive of severe coronary artery disease and all its manifestations.

4. Patients who exhibit an abnormal heart rate response to exercise should be monitored carefully and medically supervised closely if they are enrolled in a cardiac rehabilitation program.

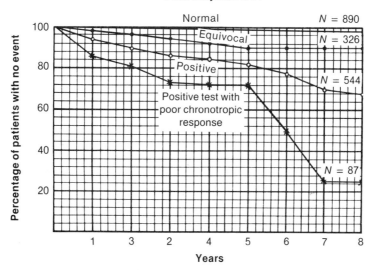

**Fig. 7-6.** Abnormal rate response. Life table display of incidence of myocardial infarctions. Notice the higher incidence of infarction in those with poor chronotropic response to exercise. (Redrawn from Ellestad MH: *Stress testing,* ed 2, Philadelphia, 1981, FA Davis Co.)

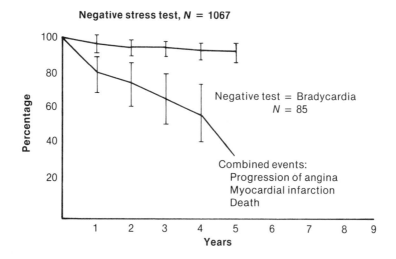

**Fig. 7-7.** Combined-events bradycardia. Those with bradycardia (pulse fell below 95% confidence limits for age and sex) and normal ST segments have a high incidence of combined events (similar to those with ST-segment depression). (Redrawn from Ellestad MH: *Stress testing,* ed 2, Philadelphia, 1981, FA Davis Co.)

## BLOOD PRESSURE RESPONSE
### Normal

In normal adult men, blood pressure response to increasing levels of exertion is not nearly so clearly described as a heart rate response. Systolic pressure rises with increasing levels of workload, and diastolic pressure either rises slightly (less than 10 mm Hg), remains the same, or drops slightly (less than 10 mm Hg) (Fig. 7-8). In healthy individuals who can achieve or exceed their predicted maximum heart rates, the systolic pressure may rise steadily during the submaximum workloads and then flatten off or even fall at peak exercise. This is not an abnormal finding. Generally, the systolic blood pressure response to exercise is flatter in adult women than that found in men.

The primary reason that blood pressure responses are difficult to categorize is that the auscultatory method of obtaining blood pressure during exercise may be highly inaccurate. It requires good clinical skill to obtain any blood pressure readings when someone is exercising on a treadmill, but reliable readings are difficult to obtain because of the excessive extraneous noise of the treadmill and the arm movement that occurs during an exercise test. At low levels of exercise it is possible to get fairly reliable and reproducible data, but at high levels of exercise they are not at all

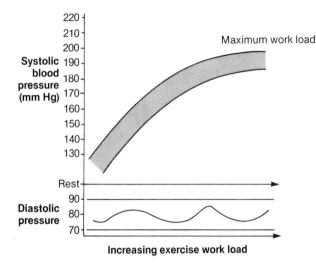

**Fig. 7-8.** Normal systolic and diastolic blood responses to exertion.

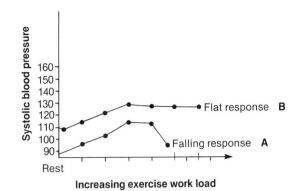

**Fig. 7-9. A,** Abnormal systolic blood response to exertion. *Top graph,* Flat response. *Bottom graph,* Poor response with an abnormal fall at peak exercise, **B.**

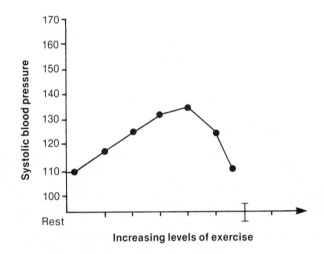

**Fig. 7-10.** Abnormal systolic blood pressure response to exertion. Striking fall in systolic pressure with exercise despite a normal response at submaximum levels of exertion.

accurate.[25] This limitation of obtaining accurate blood pressure measurements has a direct bearing on the discussion in the following section of the abnormal blood pressure response, where only major changes in blood pressure are considered significant. An arterial indwelling pressure sensor in the arm would be the most accurate means of obtaining blood pressures, but it is highly impractical.

Systolic blood pressure rises during exercise because the increase in cardiac output is greater than the decrease in peripheral vascular resistance (see Chapter 3 for specifics). In well-conditioned athletes and in younger persons, the diastolic blood pressure may fall precipitously during exercise creating a wide pulse pressure. This phenomenon is rarely seen in patients or older persons (40 or more years of age).

### Abnormal

Significant abnormalities in blood pressure responses to increasing levels of exertion occur both in systolic and in diastolic blood pressure. Both abnormalities often represent the existence of significant pathological conditions and should be recognized, interpreted, and incorporated into each patient's data base.

**Systolic abnormality.** There are three abnormal systolic blood pressure responses that occur during increasing levels of exertion. The first is the flat response, in which the pressure may rise slightly but fails to continue to rise and remains generally below 140 mm Hg (Fig. 7-9, *A*). The second is a response in which the systolic pressure is low to begin with (less than 110 mm Hg), rises slightly, and then begins to fall despite increases in workload (Fig. 7-9, *B*). The third and clinically most common response, especially in patients following an infarction, is a normal submaximum response with a precipitous fall in systolic pressure at higher workloads (Fig. 7-10). This response is often associated with pronounced ST-T depression or elevation changes in the patient's electrocardiogram.

Bruce[6] and Irving and others[20] have found that this response is highly indicative of serious pathological conditions. They found that patients not on medications, with poor systolic blood pressure responses, and peak systolic pressures less than 140 mm Hg had a much higher incidence of sudden death. In addition, they found that this response was most commonly found in three patient groups: those with severe obstructive coronary artery disease, which caused pronounced ischemia with exertion but with normal ventricular function; those with cardiomegaly or gross myocardial damage and poor ventricular function; and those with a combination of these two conditions. Fig. 7-11 presents graphs and data for two patients who exhibited the abnormal blood pressure response during exercise testing.

The abnormal systolic blood pressure response should not remove a patient for consideration in a cardiac rehabilitation program, but the exercise prescription must be adjusted to accommodate this abnormality. Patients with these responses must be monitored closely.[12]

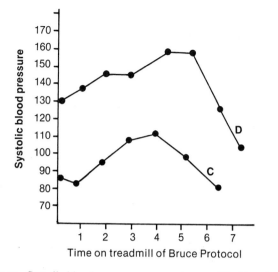

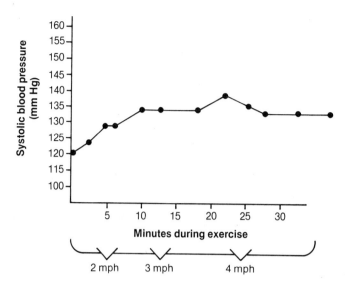

**Fig. 7-11.** Systolic blood pressure response to a modified low-level Bruce Protocol Treadmill Test in patient *C,* a 67-year-old man, 2 weeks after anteroseptal myocardial infarction. Initial pressure was taken standing. Resting heart rate was 63; maximum heart rate 82. Test stopped because of blood pressure response and shortness of breath. Patient developed a third heart sound. He had frequent ventricular dysrhythmias after exercise. His medications were Inderal (propranolol), Procardia (nifedipine), and nitroglycerin, and they may have played a role in his abnormal blood pressure response. ST elevation throughout showed no change. *D,* Abnormal systolic blood pressure to a Bruce protocol symptom-limited maximal-exercise test. Patient D was a 50-year-old man taking no medications and having no previous history of infarction. Maximum heart rate was 155 bpm, no dysrhythmias, positive ST-segment depression of 2.0 mm horizontal change during and after exercise, and positive for angina. $S_4$ after exercise. Resting pressure was 132/84 mm Hg; maximum pressure was 162/90 mm Hg.

*Mechanisms.* When we look at the normal systolic blood pressure response, it is common to see a person's blood pressure flatten or fall at peak exercise. Theoretically, as heart rate exceeds 190 bpm, the filling time for the ventricle decreases to a point at which stroke volume actually falls. As stroke volume falls, cardiac output levels off, but peripheral vascular resistance normally should continue to fall so that a decrease in systolic pressure results. This normal response gives us a clear, logical sequence to explain the mechanism of abnormal responses.

The documentation and descriptions given to us by Bruce,[6] Irving,[20] Benz,[2] and their associates reveal what the cause of this response may be. An ischemic ventricle or a ventricle with a large scar will quickly achieve a maximum stroke volume. Normally, during progressive incremental increases in exercise workloads, venous return rises, causing elevation in the end-diastolic volume. In the normal heart, this elevation in volume is met by increased contractility with a resultant increase in ejection fraction (see Chapter 3). On the other hand, patients with severe pathological conditions (ischemia, large infarcts) are not able to increase contractility. Stroke volume does not increase and in fact may fall. A decreasing stroke volume places severe restric-

**Fig. 7-12.** Normal flattening of systolic blood pressure due to prolonged exercise at the same workload.

tions on increases in cardiac output. Because systolic pressure is a result of the relationship between cardiac output and peripheral vascular resistance, an abnormal cardiac output response with a normal fall in peripheral vascular resistance during exercise may be the cause of a falling systolic blood pressure.[26]

As with all of the responses described in this text, a single abnormality, such as a fall in systolic blood pressure, should not be acted upon unless additional abnormalities are noted. A fall in systolic pressure is often associated with shortness of breath, deep ST-T–segment depression or elevation, angina, and pallor. After exercise, patients frequently will exhibit a third heart sound. The clinician should look for these additional signs and symptoms to confirm the significance of a fall in systolic pressure (Fig. 7-11). Care should be taken not to overinterpret a flat or falling systolic response in middle-aged women or in any patient on antihypertensive or beta-blocking medications. These patients may exhibit this response, but unless there are additional signs or symptoms, it may not be significant.

The clinician should be sure that the blood pressure fall occurs with an increase in workload. In Fig. 7-11 the workloads were increased at minutes 3 and 6. Systolic pressure fell 20 mm Hg or more with an increase in workload. Patient C also became dyspneic, had some angina, and became palloric during the test. Patient D exhibited angina and 2.0 mm of horizontal ST-segment depression.

It is common and normal for systolic pressure to flatten and fall with prolonged (30 to 45 minutes) bouts of exercise at the same workload (Fig. 7-12). This should not be considered an abnormal response. For example, a patient exercising at a continuous workload of 3.8 mph at 2% grade for 40 minutes may typically exhibit the following pressures: at rest, 138/86; after 3 to 5 minutes of exercise, 166/90; after 15 minutes or more exercise, 144/84. This is not an abnormal

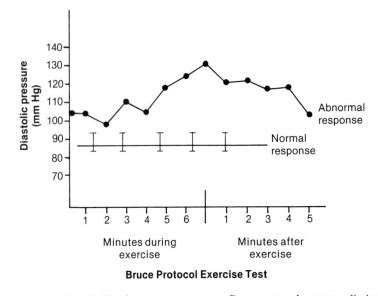

**Fig. 7-13.** Abnormal diastolic blood pressure response to Bruce protocol symptom-limited exercise test. Patient E was a 47-year-old man who completed 7 minutes and was limited by leg fatigue and shortness of breath. Resting blood pressure (BP) standing was 176/104 mm Hg, and maximum BP was 246/126 mm Hg. He exhibited 2.0 mm of ST-segment depression in four leads and mild angina 4 minutes after exercise. He had frequent multifocal premature ventricular contractions throughout the test and an $S_4$ after exercise.

response. The patient's peripheral resistance has decreased as a result of an increase in body temperature, or a redistribution of blood has caused a decrease in cardiac output. Either will result in a fall or flattening of the systolic pressure response, and this should be considered normal unless concomitant symptoms arise.

### Summary of clinical significance

1. Abnormal systolic blood pressure responses are exhibited by patients with severe ischemia, poor ventricular function, or a combination of these pathological conditions.
2. This abnormality is commonly associated with other significant signs and symptoms.
3. Patients who demonstrate falling systolic blood pressure have higher annual morbidity and mortality.
4. These patients can still undergo exercise conditioning, but must be closely monitored for signs of ventricular dysfunction and the advent of serious dysrhythmias.

**Diastolic abnormality.** The second, less commonly cited, abnormal blood pressure response is a persistent rise in diastolic pressure with increases in exercise workloads. There are numerous articles in the literature that describe normal diastolic blood pressure responses.[25] Many of these contradict one another, but generally the normal response to exercise is to have diastolic blood pressure fall slightly (10 to 20 mm Hg) in younger persons and to rise slightly, fall slightly, or remain the same in older persons.

A common sequel to a progressive rise in diastolic pressure with exercise is for the diastolic pressure to remain elevated several minutes after exercise. There is no literature that describes the significance of this finding, but in the author's clinical experience it is an abnormal finding.

For the purposes of this discussion, an abnormal diastolic blood pressure response occurs when the pressure rises 15 to 20 mm Hg or more above 90 mm Hg with exercise. A patient's actual abnormal response and the generally accepted normal response are depicted in Fig. 7-13. Patients who exhibit this response may have coronary artery disease even in the absence of ST-segment changes.[36] Patient E (Fig. 7-13) exhibited the following findings upon cardiac catheterization: all atrial and ventricular pressures were mildly to moderately elevated; the left ventricular end-diastolic pressure was 22 mm Hg at rest (0 to 12 mm Hg is normal); ejection fraction contractile pattern was normal; right coronary was irregular throughout its course but without severe stenosis; the left main and circumflex were normal; the left anterior descending artery (LAD) was normal to its midpoint, where a 95% to 100% lesion appeared to end the LAD, but a large diagonal branch took off at this same point; this branch and the remnants of the LAD continued to be irregular throughout the rest of their course, but without significant stenosis.

*Mechanisms.* The cause or causes for progressive diastolic response to exercise are open to speculation. Once again, any of the humeral, neurological, or hemodynamic factors could be the cause. It is of interest, though, to speculate that patients exhibiting the progressive diastolic response to exercise may have a reflex mechanism that senses a need for increased coronary blood flow. This as yet unidentified mechanism may exert an influence on the peripheral vascular tree to increase diastolic pressures and thereby cause an increase in coronary artery driving pressure. The cause or causes may also be simple coincidence. Patients with severe coronary disease generally have some additional peripheral vascular disease, which can dramatically affect systolic and diastolic pressures.

Again, a rise in progressive diastolic pressure with exercise is a clinical sign that adds to each patient's data base and should be recognized and incorporated into exercise test interpretations and individualized exercise training programs.

### Summary of clinical significance

1. A progressive rise in diastolic blood pressure with exercise may indicate severe coronary artery disease.
2. The rise should be at least 20 mm Hg or more above 90 mm Hg and persist after exercise testing.

## ANGINAL RESPONSES

Angina is classically described as a discomfort caused by an impaired blood supply to cardiac muscle. This impairment results in an imbalance between myocardial oxygen supply and demand (see Chapter 2). It is a well-documented finding that a patient's threshold for angina is roughly equivalent to a fixed, clinically recordable product of heart rate multiplied by the systolic blood pressure. This multiple is referred to as the "rate-pressure product" and is linearly correlated with myocardial oxygen demand.[24] Numerous texts, articles, and scientific papers have been written to describe the reproducibility of a patient's angina at the same rate-pressure product.[9,33,38,39] The purpose of this section is to discuss how patients can increase their angina threshold and even eliminate their angina completely.

### Angina threshold

Most current practitioners and authors will state that patients with stable angina can improve their exercise tolerance and maximum preangina working capacity, but patients with angina are unable to exceed their anginal rate-pressure product.[8,33] An example of this is given below.

*Preexercise training* (HR, heart rate; SBP, systolic blood pressure)

| | | |
|---|---|---|
| Workload | 2.5 mph | 12% grade |
| Angina threshold | HR 120 | SBP 150 |
| | angina | |
| Rate-pressure product | $1.8 \times 10^3$ | |

*Postexercise training*

| | | |
|---|---|---|
| Workload | 2.5 mph | 12% grade |
| | HR 110 | SBP 150 |
| | no angina | |
| Rate-pressure product | $1.65 \times 10^3$ | |
| Workload | 3.0 mph | 12% grade |
| Angina threshold | HR 120 | SBP 150 |
| | angina | |
| Rate-pressure product | $1.8 \times 10^3$ | |

The patient in this example has increased his maximum preangina workload, but his angina threshold and rate-pressure product are unchanged since his pretraining status.

One of the most rewarding clinical improvements is when a patient exceeds the angina threshold by raising the rate-pressure product he or she can attain before experiencing angina. There is even a small percentage of patients who actually eliminate their angina completely. Those who are capable of increasing or eliminating their angina threshold commonly have the following characteristics:

1. Inoperable coronary artery disease or patients who refuse surgery
2. Highly motivated to exercise
3. Chronic, stable angina
4. Capable of walking through their angina within the first 3 months of their training program

Walk-through angina is angina that occurs during a training session at a specific workload but gradually diminishes and finally goes away despite the fact that the workload is the same or even slightly higher. It is common for patients to get angina when they initiate an exercise session, but with a prolonged warm-up this can be avoided. When they do get angina, walk-through angina occurs when the patient's workload is maintained and the angina abates.

Increasing or eliminating angina thresholds in patients with coronary artery disease is not a quick process. It often takes 12 to 24 months of training (see Chapter 9).

The actual patient example on p. 100 (Case 1) dramatically demonstrates the phenomenon of increasing a patient's angina threshold and then eliminating the discomfort completely.

**Mechanisms.** As with the other abnormal findings, it is difficult to explain how a person's angina threshold can be increased or eliminated. These patients still exhibit ST-segment depression at the same rate-pressure product as they did before their exercise training program, and the depth of the depression is unchanged. This indicates that ischemia may still be present, but the discomfort that previously accompanied it is gone.

There are numerous potential explanations for the occurrence of this phenomenon, but none of them has been scientifically proven in humans. Following is a list of possible explanations:

1. Increased oxidative enzymes in the heart muscle
2. Improved coronary blood flow through the development of collateral arteries
3. Accommodation of the pain stimulus created by the ischemia via the central nervous system

Any argument that proposes methods to improve coronary blood flow or decrease myocardial oxygen demands should be considered. For the three arguments listed above, neither the first nor second adequately explains why ST changes still occur at the same rate-pressure product.[39]

## CASE 1    Patient E

*Brief medical history*

Inferior myocardial infarction, July 1986
Subsequent stable but frequent exertional angina
Two-year documented history of hypertension
Family history of atherosclerosis and diabetes
Thirty-year 2-pack-a-day smoker who quit July 1986
Entered outpatient program, 4/17/88
Age 55, 5'7", 155 lb
Newspaper publisher
Medications: propranolol (Inderal) 160 mg/day, furosemide (Lasix), nitroglycerin (see Chapter 4)

*Initial exercise test results* (R resting; M, maximum)

Exercise tolerance 30% below predicted for a sedentary man
Limited by level 2 angina
RHR 52 bpm, MHR 96 bpm, RBP 140/100 mm Hg, MBP 150/100 mm Hg
Angina began at HR 90 bpm, BP 140/100 mm Hg
No ST-segment depression

Exercise training began at 2.5 mph 0% grade for 30 minutes. The patient experienced level 1 angina at a heart rate of 90 bpm early in the exercise period, but this gradually abated during the exercise training session without a decrease in workload. Over the next 6 months, the patient progressed to a workload of 4.0 mph with the same angina threshold, but he experienced frequent episodes of the walk-through phenomenon. At this point the patient's physician began to reduce his Inderal gradually (see Chapter 4). The patient's maximum heart rate before the onset of angina rose steadily over the next 6 months. He began a walk-jog program of 3 miles in 45 minutes 5 times a week. His revised exercise training heart rate was now 126 bpm. A repeat treadmill test was performed 13 months after beginning the program, and the patient was off all medications.

Completed 9 minutes of Bruce Protocol
MHR 145 bpm, MBP 158/86 mm Hg
Limited by leg fatigue
No angina ST-segment depression 2.5 to 3.0 mm
Initial ST shift occurred at HR of 120 bpm
Exercise tolerance is 8% below predicted for a sedentary man

Fig. 7-14 graphically depicts the change in this patient's angina threshold.

This patient was well-motivated and continued to exercise four or five times a week jogging 45 to 60 minutes (4 to 5 miles) per session. The reader should realize that this patient is an extraordinary case; his unusual success would not be reproduced easily in other patients. This example does, however, demonstrate that angina thresholds are not fixed at immovable rate-pressure products.

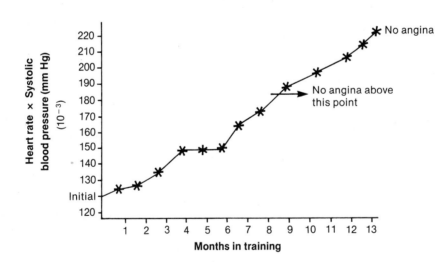

**Fig. 7-14.** Patient E. Improvement of anginal threshold (by increasing rate pressure product) in a patient over a 13-month period of exercise training.

Regardless of the cause for increasing or eliminating angina thresholds, the therapist conducting a cardiac rehabilitation program for patients with reproducible angina thresholds should consider this threshold as a symptom that can be successfully treated and, in some cases, eliminated completely.

**Summary of clinical significance**

1. Angina may be successfully treated by exercise training.
2. Angina threshold measured by multiplication of the heart rate and systolic blood pressure is not a fixed value.
3. Extensive research into the mechanisms of elimination of angina in humans through exercise training is necessary.

# RESPIRATORY LIMITATIONS TO MAXIMUM OXYGEN CONSUMPTION

## Normal oxygen consumption limitations

The basis of exercise physiology is derived from the formula for oxygen consumption, $\dot{V}O_2 = CO \times (aO_2 - \tilde{v}O_2)$, or the volume of oxygen consumed per minute ($VO_2$) is equal to the cardiac output (CO) multiplied by the difference in arterial ($a$) and central venous ($\tilde{v}$) oxygen content. When the components of this formula are analyzed, a wealth of clinically useful information becomes available. Oxygen consumption is one of the foundations of human life. Exertion is dependent on oxygen transport, either during the activity (aerobic) or after the activity as a means of repayment of oxygen deficits created during anaerobic activities. Oxygen is essential for normal cell function, and the primary function of our cardiopulmonary system is to maintain a continuous adequate supply.

Cardiac output has been discussed in this chapter and in previous chapters. For our purposes, those discussions will suffice. The discussion will now turn to the second part of the formula, the a-$\tilde{v}O_2$ difference.

Arterial oxygen content, $a$, is normally equal to 20.1 vol%. This number is obtained by multiplication of hemoglobin concentration (in grams per 100 ml of blood) by 1.34 ml of $O_2$, per gram of hemoglobin and then multiplication of that by the percent saturation of the hemoglobin. For example, 15 grams of hemoglobin per 100 ml of blood, (a normal value for males) times 1.34 ml of $O_2$ per gram of hemoglobin equals 20.1 ml of $O_2$ per 100 ml of blood, or 20.1 vol% (15 gm of Hb × 1.34 ml of $O_2$ = 20.1 vol%). This would be true if the hemoglobin was 100% saturated. Normal percent saturation ranges from 95% to 100%.[29]

Changes in arterial oxygen content are dependent on many variables, including but not limited to percent saturation, oxygen content of the atmosphere, pH of the blood, temperature of the blood, minute ventilation, carbon monoxide concentration in the atmosphere, and the pulmonary ventilation/perfusion ratio. To appreciate some abnormal responses found in pulmonary patients, a sound understanding of the effects of these variables is essential. For the purpose of this text, only the variables of ventilation and ventilation perfusion ratio are discussed.[35]

The normal, accepted limitation to maximum oxygen delivery is considered to be attainment of a maximum cardiac output. Patients with chronic obstructive pulmonary disease do not appear to be limited by achieving their maximum cardiac output. Instead, they are limited by chest wall and pulmonary mechanics that appear to be intimately associated with ventilation, respiratory muscle oxygen cost, and oxygen saturation.

## Ventilation responses

**Normal.** Ventilation, specifically alveolar ventilation, is one of the keys to the determination of the percent saturation and oxygen content of arterial blood. Alveolar ventilation,

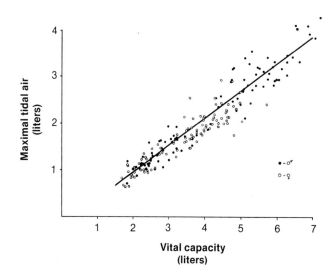

**Fig. 7-15.** Highest tidal volume measured during running at submaximum and maximum speed (work time about 5 minutes) related to the person's vital capacity measured in the standing position. (From Åstrand, P-O and Kaare R: *Textbook of work physiology,* ed 2, New York, 1977, McGraw-Hill Book Co.)

$V_A$, is determined by the total tidal volume, $V_T$, which is equal to the alveolar ventilation plus the deadspace ventilation, $V_D$: $V_T = V_A + V_D$. Thus alveolar ventilation is $V_A = V_T - V_D$. For the patient with chronic obstructive pulmonary disease, dead-space ventilation inflicts major restrictions on alveolar ventilation capacity and thus oxygen content of arterial blood. Patients with obstructive pulmonary disease have severely limited tidal volume reserves. In other words, they are unable to increase their tidal volume appreciably. Åstrand states that normal persons can rarely achieve tidal volumes in excess of 50% of their vital capacities during maximum exercise[1] (Fig. 7-15). All patients do not have the same capacity. In fact, many have tidal volumes that are relatively fixed. For example a patient with a fixed or nearly fixed tidal volume is totally dependent on the frequency of respiration to increase pulmonary ventilation ($V_E$). In healthy people, the tidal volume ($V_T$) accounts for a majority of the increase in ventilation at low levels of exertion. It is not until they reach higher levels of exertion that healthy people require increases in the frequency of respiration (see Fig. 7-16).

**Abnormal.** Because patients with obstructive pulmonary disease depend on frequency to improve their ventilation, they also ventilate a greater amount of dead space. For example if we assume that dead space is the same amount and fixed in both cases, it is apparent that the net alveolar ventilation is decreased in obstructive disease. Thus a normal person who has a ventilation of 10 liters per minute, a dead space of 0.20 liter, and a respiratory frequency of 10 has an alveolar ventilation that is $10 - (0.20 \times 10) = 8$ liters per minute. The same level of ventilation, 10 liters per minute, achieved by a patient with pulmonary disease through a higher respiratory rate (20) has an alveolar ventilation that is

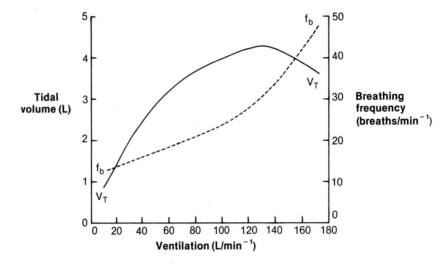

**Fig. 7-16.** Changes in tidal volume and breathing frequency with increasing levels of ventilation in exercise. (Data from Jensen JI and others. The relationship between maximal ventilation, breathing pattern, and mechanical limit of ventilation, *J Physiol (Lond)*, 309:521, 1980. In Pardy RL and others: The ventilatory pump in exercise, *Clinics in chest medicine.* 5 (1):35, 1984.)

$10 - (0.20 \times 20) = 6$ liters per minute. The alveolar ventilation is where gaseous exchange takes place and thus is one of the key components in determining arterial oxygen saturation.

Another key to oxygen saturation is the ventilation/perfusion ratio. This is the ratio that matches the lung ventilation to the perfusion of blood from the right side of the heart. Briefly, when one is at rest sitting, the apex of the lung is well ventilated but poorly perfused, the midportions of the lungs have nearly equal ventilation to perfusion and the lower lobes have high perfusion and moderate ventilation. The net effect is very close to an equal match between ventilation and perfusion.

The person with obstructive pulmonary disease not only is ventilated poorly but also often has a very poor ventilation/perfusion ratio. Areas that are poorly ventilated are matched with good perfusion and well-ventilated areas may be underperfused. The result of this mismatching is that venous blood may pass through the lungs without coming into contact with fresh air. This blood is then mixed with oxygenated arterial blood in the left atrium and ventricle. As the venous blood and arterial blood gases attain equilibrium, the $O_2$ concentration decreases. $CO_2$ concentrations increase, and the pH decreases (see Chapter 12).

### Normal oxygen consumption response to exercise

During maximal levels of exertion a normal person progressively matches cardiac output (to the lungs) to the ventilation of the alveoli. This remains true up to near-maximal levels of exertion, when alveolar oxygen tension may continue to increase but arterial $P_{O_2}$ may diminish slightly. Arterial $CO_2$ pressure tends to fall gradually as maximal levels of exertion are achieved (Fig. 7-17). Thus normal arterial oxygen content is essentially unchanged at

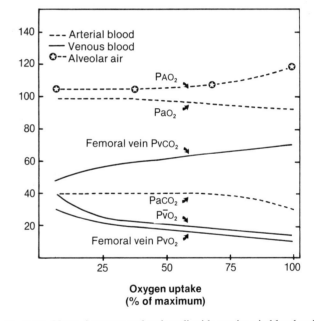

**Fig. 7-17.** Normal oxygen and carbon dioxide tensions in blood and alveolar air at rest and various levels of work up to and exceeding the load necessary to achieve maximum oxygen uptake. (From Åstrand P-O and Kaare R: *Textbook of work physiology*, ed 2, New York, 1977, McGraw-Hill Book Co.)

maximal levels. This argument strongly supports the theory that maximum cardiac output, not respiration, is the limiting factor to maximal oxygen uptake. It is apparent from the work of Åstrand that increases in pulmonary ventilation at maximum oxygen uptake do not increase oxygen uptake in normal persons.[1]

In healthy persons, the respiratory muscles use from 0.5 to 1.0 ml of $O_2$ per liter of ventilation. It is estimated that this unit of oxygen cost per liter of ventilation increases linearly

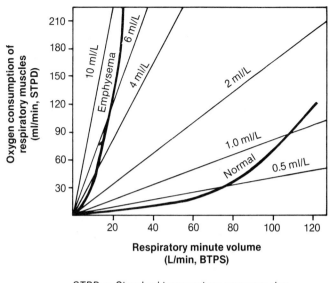

STPD = Standard temperature pressure, dry
BTPS = Barometric temperature pressure, saturated

**Fig. 7-18.** Oxygen cost of breathing in normal subject and in subject with emphysema, measured as increase in whole-body oxygen consumption during respiratory response to added dead space. Cost of breathing in normal men over usual range of activity is less than 0.5 ml of $O_2$ per liter of air breathed. (Adapted from Mountcastle VB editor: *Medical physiology*, ed 14, St Louis, 1980, Mosby.)

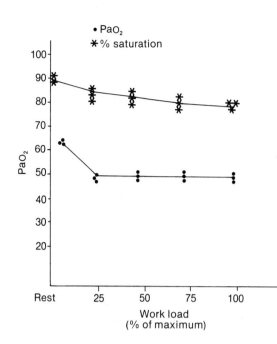

**Fig. 7-19.** $Pao_2$ tension and arterial oxygen saturation falling with exercise in three patients with obstructive pulmonary disease. Tests were limited by dyspnea.

with heavy workloads. The respiratory muscles may use as much as 10% of the total oxygen uptake in normal persons at maximum levels of work.[1] Recently, there has been an increased debate and review of the significance of ventilation as a limit to maximum exercise tolerance. In effect, many authors are now questioning whether the ventilatory system, and not maximum cardiac output, is the limiting factor to maximum exercise tolerance, especially in well-trained athletes. The reader is encouraged to review these discussions in depth by reading Dempsey's article,[11] "Is the lung built for exercise?" A thorough understanding of this article will more clearly illustrate how abnormal pulmonary mechanics can severely impair exercise tolerance in spite of normal heart function.

### Abnormal oxygen cost of ventilation

There are only estimates of respiratory muscle costs for the patient with chronic obstructive disease. The mechanical patterns that develop with the various disease processes limit the reliability of any absolute measures. Fig. 7-18 does demonstrate the extreme difference in oxygen cost of respiration between a healthy subject and a subject with emphysema. This high cost of breathing is directly related to the patient's (1) high dead-space ventilation, (2) frequency-dependent breathing, and (3) hyperexpanded chest wall, which decreases diaphragmatic function and demands that accessory muscles of respiration be aggressively employed.

**Mechanisms.** When cardiac output rises but ventilation does not improve, the ventilation/perfusion mismatch wors-

ens. The result is a fall in arterial oxygen pressure and saturation. Arterial oxygen tension drops precipitously (Fig. 7-19) with exertion, with the resultant decrease in oxygen saturation and thus oxygen content of the blood. This puts great limitations on the oxygen extraction reserve, (a-$\bar{v}o_2$ differences), which should cause a strong increase in cardiac output as a compensatory mechanism for improving oxygen consumption. At rest, many pulmonary patients have greatly elevated heart rates. But it is clear from the exercise arterial graph (Fig. 7-20) that maximum heart rates are not attained before termination of exercise. If we surmise that less than maximum cardiac outputs are achieved and that these patients exercised to their maximum symptom limits (which they all did), then cardiac output was not their limiting factor. In fact, dyspnea appears to be the limiting factor in all these tests. The patients were all limited by their abnormal ventilation and not by achievement of maximal cardiac output as in the normal state.

### Summary of clinical significance

1. Poor respiratory mechanics combined with limited tidal volume reserves may lead, with exertion, to hypoxia and desaturation.
   a. Pronounced hypoxia as seen in each case is a significant finding. Hypoxia causes the pulmonary vasculature to constrict. The exact neurochemical cause can be examined in Åstrand.[1] The ultimate effect is an increase in pulmonary artery pressure. In turn, constant elevation in pulmonary artery pressures (pulmonary hypertension) leads to right-sided hypertrophy. Chronic hypertension often leads to right-sided

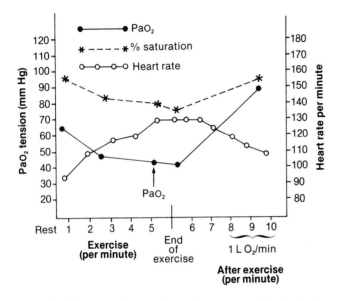

**Fig. 7-20.** Oxygen tension and saturation compared to heart rate response to maximal exercise in patient F, a 46-year-old woman. Note heart rate levels off at 130 at the same time oxygen tension and saturation fall to their lowest levels.

heart failure, also called cor pulmonale, a common complication of obstructive pulmonary disease.

b. The implication to the clinician involved in pulmonary rehabilitation is to identify those patients who become hypoxic during even submaximum levels of exertion. A progressive exercise program with a pulmonary patient suffering from exercise-induced hypoxia may quickly be to the patient's detriment.

2. Respiration can be the limiting factor to maximum exertion, specifically in patients with obstructive pulmonary disease.

3. Clinicians should be working to devise treatment techniques that result in improved respiratory mechanics and thus decreased costs of breathing.

4. Controlled research of the exercise responses of pulmonary patients is needed.

## SUMMARY

This chapter contains a clinician's view of some abnormal responses to exercise. One should not accept these simple examples as scientific proof of the cause and effect of certain pathological conditions on human exercise response. On the other hand, physical therapists should understand that these phenomena—abnormal heart rate response, bradycardia, abnormal blood pressure responses, hypotension, increased or unlimited angina threshold through exercise training, and oxygen desaturation during exercise—do occur. They are indications in some cases of severe pathological conditions and often of a poor prognosis for the patient. With this in mind, physical therapists working with cardiac and pulmonary patients should carefully assess their conditions and interpret the findings against the predicted normal responses

that have been scientifically delineated by Åstrand, Mountcastle, and others.[2,6,25,29]

## REFERENCES

1. Astrand P-O and Kaare R: *Textbook of work physiology,* ed 2, New York, 1977, McGraw Hill Book Co.
2. Benz H and Sambrano J: *The significance of a hypoadaptive blood pressure response during maximal stress testing in patients with coronary artery disease,* master's thesis, Los Angeles, 1977, University of Southern California.
3. Blessey R and others: Aerobic capacity and cardiac catheterization results in 13 patients with exercise bradycardia, (abstract), *Med Sci Sports Exer* 8:50, 1976.
4. Brouha L and Harrington ME: Heart rate and blood pressure reactions of men and women during and after muscular exercise, *Lancet* 77:79, 1957.
5. Bruce RA and others: Maximal oxygen intake and nomographic assessment of functional aerobic impairment in cardiovascular disease, *Am Heart J* 85:546, 1973.
6. Bruce RA and others: Noninvasive predictors of sudden death in men with coronary heart disease, *Am J Cardiol* 39:833, 1977.
7. Campbell EJM and others: Simple methods of estimating oxygen and efficiency of muscles of breathing, *J Appl Physiol* 11:303, 1957.
8. Clausen JP and others: Heart rate and arterial blood pressure during exercise in patients with angina pectoris: effects of training and of nitroglycerin, *Circulation* 43:436, 1976.
9. Cokkinos DV and Voridis EM: Constancy of pressure-rate product in packing-induced angina pectoris, *Br Heart J* 38:39, 1976.
10. Conn EH and others: Exercise responses before and after physical conditioning in patients with severely depressed left ventricular function, *Am J Cardiol* 49:296, 1982.
11. Dempsey J: Is the lung built for exercise?, *Med Sci Sports Exer* 18:143, 1986.
12. Efraim Ben-Ari AE and others: Significance of exertional hypotension in apparently healthy men: an 8.9-year follow-up, *J Cardiopulm Rehab* 10:92, 1990.
13. Ehsani AA and others: Effects of 12 months of intense exercise training on ischemic ST-segment depression in patients with coronary artery disease, *Circulation* 64(6):1116, 1981.
14. Ehsani AA and others: Cardiac effects of prolonged and intense exercise training in patients with coronary artery disease, *Am J Cardiol* 50:246, 1982.
15. Ellestad MH: *Stress testing,* ed 2, Philadelphia, 1981, FA Davis Co.
16. Ferguson RJ and others: Effect of physical training on treadmill exercise capacity collateral circulation and progression of coronary artery disease, *Am J Cardiol* 34:764, 1974.
17. Fraser RS and Chapman CB: Studies on the effect of exercise on cardiovascular function: blood pressure and pulse rate, *Circulation* 9:193, 1954.
18. Henschel A and others: Simultaneous direct and indirect blood pressure measurements in a man at rest and work, *J Appl Physiol* 6:506, 1954.
19. Hinkle LE and others: Slow heart rates and increased risk for cardiac death in middle-aged men, *Arch Intern Med* 129:732, 1972.
20. Irving JB and others: Variations in and significance of systolic pressure during exercise (treadmill) testing *Am J Cardiol* 39:841, 1977.
21. Iskandrian AS and others: Mechanism of exercise-induced hypotension in coronary artery disease, *Am J Cardiol* 69:1517, 1992.
22. Josc AD and Taylor RR: Autonomic blockade by propranolol and tropine to study the intrinsic muscle function in man, *J Clin Invest* 48:2019, 1969.
23. Kariv I and Kellermann JJ: Effects of exercise on blood pressure, *Malattie Cardiovasc* 10:247, 1969.
24. Kitamura K and others: Hemodynamic correlates of myocardial oxygen consumption during upright exercise, *J Appl Physiol* 32:516, 1972.
25. Loskutoff DW: *Study of the relationship of arterial blood pressure*

*response to Bruce Protocol Exercise Tolerance testing,* master's thesis, Atlanta, 1981, Emory University.

26. Mazzotta G and others: Significance of abnormal blood pressure response during exercise-induced myocardial dysfunction after recent acute myocardial infarction, *Am J Cardiol* 59:1256, 1987.
27. Metheny E and others: Some physiological responses of women and men to moderate and strenuous exercise: a comparative study, *Am J Physiol* 137:318, 1942.
28. Miller, Todd and others: Sinus node deceleration during exercise as a marker of significant narrowing of the right coronary artery, *Am J Cardiol* 71:371, 1993.
29. Mountcastle VB, editor: *Medical physiology,* ed 14, St Louis, 1980, Mosby.
30. Nagle FJ and others: Comparison of direct and indirect blood pressure with pressure-flow dynamics during exercise, *J Appl Physiol* 21:317, 1966.
31. Neill WA and others: Respiratory alkalemia during exercise reduces angina threshold, *Chest* 80(2):149, 1981.
32. Ricci B: *Physiological basis for human performance,* Philadelphia, 1967, Lea & Febiger.
33. Robinson BF: Relation of heart rate and systolic blood pressure to the onset of pain in angina pectoris, *Circulation* 35:1073, 1967.
34. Schwarz F and others: Coronary collateral vessels: their significance for left ventricular histologic structure, *Am J Cardiol* 49:291, 1982.
35. Shapiro BA and others: *Clinical application of blood gases,* ed 2, Chicago, 1977, Year Book Medical Publishers, Inc.
36. Sheps DS and others: Exercise-induced increase in diastolic pressure: indicator of severe coronary artery disease, *Am J Cardiol* 43:708, 1979.
37. Sim DN and others: Investigation of the physiological basis for increased exercise threshold for angina pectoris after physical conditioning, *J Clin Invest* 54:763, 1974.
38. Wahren J and Bygdeman S: Onset of angina pectoris in relation to circulatory adaptation during arm and leg exercise, *Circulation* 44:432, 1971.
39. Wilmore JH: Acute and chronic physiologic responses to exercise. In Amsterdam EA and others, editors: *Exercise in cardiovascular health and disease,* New York, 1977, Yorke Medical Books.

# CHAPTER 8

# Patient Evaluation

*Scot Irwin and Raymond L. Blessey*

This chapter describes the evaluation of a patient with coronary heart disease in terms of the significant data available in the medical record, the information that can be obtained from an initial evaluation process, and the methods for obtaining useful clinical data from a patient's response to exercise. It should be noted that relevant clinical findings are usually found in combinations. Each informational item relates to the others, and the incorporation of all findings completes the patient assessment.

There are two precepts to our evaluation process:

1. The therapist should understand the scientific prin-ciples underlying the clinical data being observed and recorded.
2. The data obtained should be accurate and inter-pretable.

Selection of appropriate evaluation techniques depends on an understanding and application of the sciences, and the validity of the assessment depends on the accuracy of the data collected.

Objective patient information is obtained from the medical record, including historical data, diagnostic tests performed, laboratory values recorded, and patient interview findings.

The initial evaluation of the coronary patient should begin with a review of the medical record followed by the patient interview and examination. The general purpose of these three preliminary tasks is to allow the therapist to formulate an accurate assessment of the clinical status of the patient, including the severity of the disease, the stability of the symptoms, and the presence of significant medical problems other than the primary diagnosis. Once these tasks have been completed, an informed decision can be made to proceed or not to proceed with definitive evaluation procedures. These procedures include assessment of the patient's responses to activities of daily living, ambulation, aerobic exercise, and low-level exercise testing. The following is a suggested evaluation and program-planning sequence for patients with coronary artery disease beginning with the acute stage of the hospital course:

1. Review of medical records and extraction of perti-nent data
2. Interview and examination of patient
3. Preliminary assessment of clinical status
4. Determination of candidacy for further evaluation
5. Evaluation of functional activities (if indicated)
6. Evaluation of activities of daily living
7. Monitored ambulation
8. Low-level exercise test
9. Definitive assessment regarding candidacy for exer-cise therapy

INITIAL EVALUATION AND PLAN

Name _____ Hospital no. _____

Age _____ Sex _____ Height _____ Weight _____

   Referring physician _____ Date _____

   Patient address (home) _____ Phone no. _____

   Patient address (work) _____ Phone no. _____

I. MEDICAL HISTORY

II. RISK FACTORS     Family history _____

     Cholesterol _____ Triglycerides _____ HDL ____ LDL _____

      Smoking _____ Hypertension _____ Diabetes _____
     (packs/year)

     Sedentary _____ Obesity _____ Type A _____

     Uric acid level _____ PFTs

III. MEDICATIONS (dosage and frequency) _____

_____

_____

IV. CARDIAC CATHETERIZATION:   Date _____ LVEDP ____ Ejection fraction _____

    Ventricular function _____

    Vessels involved/degree of occlusion _____

    _____

    _____

V. CORONARY ARTERY BYPASS SURGERY   Date _____ Hospital _____

    Grafts _____

    Surgeon _____ Complications (if any) _____

VI. MUSCULOSKELETAL EXAMINATION _____

    Orthopedic or foot problems _____

    Strength and range of motion _____

    Chest wall examination _____

VII. EXERCISE TEST RESULTS   Date _____ Duration _____

    Limiting factors _____ MHR _____ MBP _____

    Blood pressure response _____ Angina _____

    ST change _____ Dysrhythmia _____

    Physical work capacity _____ Heart sounds

VIII. PATIENT'S GOALS

_____

_____

**Fig. 8-1.** An example of an initial evaluation form designed with major points of interest in mind.

IX. ECG   Date _____   Interpretation _____

X. INITIAL PHYSICAL FITNESS STAGE _____

XI. SOCIAL HISTORY   Marital status _____

Occupation _____

Leisure time activity _____

XII. ASSESSMENT

_____

_____

_____

XIII. PLAN

_____

_____

_____

_____

_____ Date _____
Registered physical therapist

© Copyright Blessey, Huhn, Ice, Irwin, Oschrin, Physical Therapy, Inc., 1982.

**Fig. 8-1, cont'd.** For legend see the preceding page.

10. Individually monitored aerobic exercise and strengthening program (phase II)
11. Maximal exercise test
12. Additional invasive and noninvasive testing as indicated
13. Group aerobic and strengthening program (phase III)
14. Evaluation of monitored job simulation as indicated
15. Serial follow-up testing
16. Additional noninvasive testing as indicated
17. Serum lipid profile
18. Maximal exercise test

## MEDICAL RECORD REVIEW

The therapist can use clinical information from the medical record to formulate a basis for the development of both the definitive evaluation sequence and the treatment plan. The therapist should focus his or her attention on at least the following major areas of interest when reviewing the medical record:

1. Primary diagnosis
2. Additional significant medical problems
3. Medical therapy

4. Clinical subset of the patients, based on the number of diseased coronary arteries and left ventricular function
5. Contraindications for proceeding with the self-care evaluation
6. Priorities for cardiovascular monitoring with activity
7. Risk factors for coronary disease
8. Classification of the postevent hospital course into either complicated or uncomplicated, according to the criteria of McNeer and others[43]

The recommended points of interest or concerns in both the preliminary and the definitive aspects of the evaluation, along with the specific evaluation tasks, are listed in Table 8-1. An initial evaluation form designed with the above considerations in mind (Fig. 8-1) can help the therapist extract key information from the medical record.

It is not within the scope of this chapter to discuss in detail how the clinician would use the medical record review to obtain data and insight related to all the major points of interest listed in Table 8-1. The selected case examples and discussions that follow illustrate both the methods of obtaining the pertinent data base and the way in which the information taken from the medical record can be used to develop the subsequent evaluation and treatment plan.

**Table 8-1.** Points of interest and specific evaluation tasks involved with the preliminary and definitive assessment of the patient

| Major concerns and points of interest | Evaluation tasks |
|---|---|
| **Preliminary assessment** | |
| Primary diagnosis | Medical record review |
| Additional significant medical problems | Physical examination |
| Clinical subset | Patient interview |
| Hospital course (complicated versus uncomplicated) | |
| Etiology and stability of symptoms | |
| Medical therapy | |
| Psychosocial status | |
| Mobilization (indications versus contraindications) | |
| Monitoring needs and protocol | |
| | |
| **Definitive assessment** | |
| Signs and symptoms of myocardial ischemia | Functional ability to perform activities of daily living |
| Ventricular function (good or poor) | Monitored ambulation |
| Appropriateness of cardiovascular response to activity | Exercise test |
| Candidacy for exercise therapy | Individually monitored exercise therapy |

## Primary diagnosis

### CASE 1 ▼ Case Example A

A 57-year-old man was documented as having a myocardial infarction 10 years ago. A cardiac catheterization at that time revealed multiple vessel disease and that the patient was not a candidate for bypass surgery because of the diffuse nature of his disease. The patient had been asymptomatic until 2 months ago, when he noted onset of retrosternal pain associated with neck and jaw discomfort precipitated by vigorous activity, such as running to catch the bus or rapidly climbing numerous flights of stairs. In the last few weeks the patient noted onset of similar symptoms with mild activity, such as casual walking or carrying packages for short distances. The evening before admission to the hospital, the patient had 3 hours of moderate-to-severe retrosternal discomfort while at rest. These symptoms were not relieved by one nitroglycerin tablet.

*Reason for referral to cardiac rehabilitation.* To evaluate effectiveness of antianginal medications during functional activities.

*Time of entry to program.* Four days after hospital admission.

*Discussion.* The medical history shows that the patient has documented coronary artery disease by angiography and he has had a prior myocardial infarction. The key question after reviewing the medical history of case A is, has this patient suffered a second infarction or is the current primary diagnosis unstable angina (also referred to as coronary insufficiency or coronary intermediate syndrome)? To answer this question, the clinician must review the results of at least two other tests contained in the medical record. First, the serum enzyme (CPK, LDH, SGOT) results should be examined to see if there has been a significant rise above the normal level in these values since the patient has been admitted. If, in fact, there has been a rise in the enzymes, a review of the more precise isoenzyme results should be obtained. Additionally, a review of the serial ECG interpretations made from studies taken since

the patient has been admitted should be completed. Only then will the therapist know whether a myocardial infarction has been ruled out or documented. Presuming that the primary diagnosis in this case is coronary insufficiency, a careful review of the ECG and enzyme values just before mobilization of the patient should be completed to ensure that his clinical status has not changed since the order for rehabilitation was issued.

In addition to the above, the medical record should be reviewed in an attempt to uncover the presence of other medical problems that may have precipitated the unstable angina. Based on the admitting note and the nurse's notes, is there evidence that the patient has recent onset of poorly controlled hypertension?

Based on the complete blood count (CBC) results, does the patient have significant anemia? Based on review of the echocardiogram, is there evidence of a valve lesion that may contribute to the unstable pattern of symptoms? Based on chest radiograph findings and results of the physician's physical examination and interview, has the patient recently demonstrated findings consistent with congestive heart failure?

Having a clear understanding of the patient's primary diagnosis is essential in formulating both the evaluation and the treatment plan. In this case the primary diagnosis of coronary insufficiency should encourage the clinician to build into his or her evaluation protocol careful questioning regarding the stability of the patient's symptoms and regular review of pertinent lab and ECG results when available. In terms of program planning, the diagnosis in this case should influence the therapist to schedule the patient for relatively frequent outpatient visits (e.g., 3 times per week) and to educate him regarding a method for quantifying the intensity of his angina, documenting his anginal symptoms, and taking action in the event his symptoms become unstable again.

## CASE 2 ▼ Case Example B

A 42-year-old woman has had several hospital admissions secondary to chest pain and frequent premature ventricular contractions. Approximately 1 week ago, the patient was readmitted to the hospital because of crushing chest pain that had started while she was doing housework. ECG studies and enzyme levels were negative, and therefore a myocardial infarction was ruled out. An echocardiogram done at the time of this most recent admission suggested mitral valve prolapse. The patient continued to have chest discomfort, and so she was sent for a cardiac catheterization, which revealed normal coronary arteries and moderate mitral regurgitation.

*Reasons for referral to cardiac rehabilitation*
1. To improve exercise tolerance
2. To evaluate rhythm response to exercise

*Time of entry to program.* Two weeks after hospital admission.

*Discussion.* Based on the medical history, this is a patient with organic heart disease and chest discomfort; however, the chest discomfort is not related to myocardial ischemia, but, instead, it is attributable to a valvular lesion.

Awareness of the primary diagnosis of mitral valve prolapse (with significant mitral regurgitation) should encourage the clinician to examine the echocardiogram and catheterization results to determine whether there is evidence of the following:
1. Additional valve dysfunction
2. Ventricular or atrial enlargement
3. Compromised resting left ventricular function

In addition, one should review the rhythm strips and results of the 24-hour Holter monitor to become aware of the frequency and complexity of dysrhythmias and the association of the rhythm disturbance to activities. Finally, the clinician should be aware of the medical therapy for rhythm control so that responses to exercise can be interpreted appropriately, an adequate data base can be accumulated documenting the degree of effectiveness of the medication, and potential side effects of the medications can be recognized and reported to the patient's physician.

The primary diagnosis in this case should influence the therapist's approach to the patient's educational requirements. In this case, it would be important to point out the cause of the chest discomfort and its benign nature to the patient. In addition, in terms of further evaluation procedures for this patient, it would be important not to "overmonitor" and thereby encourage her to exercise only in a supervised environment.

In summary, the primary diagnosis of the patient obtained from the medical chart should alert the therapist to the additional priority areas of the medical record review that must be completed and should help the therapist begin to formulate the subsequent evaluation plan and treatment plan.

## Additional medical problems

## CASE 3 ▼ Case Example C

A 68-year-old man was documented as having a myocardial infarction 2 years ago. Patient has had onset of exertional chest pressure and shortness of breath in the last 3 months and reports that his exercise tolerance has diminished. A recent treadmill test was done with these major findings: very poor exercise capacity [with functional aerobic impairment (FAI) at 45%] with 2.0 mm ST depression at the maximum heart rate. The major limiting factor on the test was dyspnea. The patient has a 120-pack-per-year smoking history and has been diagnosed as having bronchitis. Other medical problems include adult-onset diabetes mellitus and peptic ulcer disease. The patient has had two previous admissions because of bleeding ulcers.

*Reason for referral to cardiac rehabilitation.* Patient was referred to the cardiac rehabilitation program as an outpatient for the purpose of improving his exercise tolerance and reducing his risk factors.

*Discussion.* From the medical history, it is clear that the patient has coronary artery disease and appears to be experiencing exertional symptoms consistent with angina. The key points, though, are to begin considering:
1. What other medical problems are identified in the history

that may have an impact on the patient's acute and chronic response to exercise?
2. Which other portions of the medical record may contain additional information documenting the severity of these problems?

Chronic obstructive pulmonary disease (chronic bronchitis) may be at least partly responsible for the patient's poor exercise capacity. Review of the results from the chest radiograph, pulmonary function test, arterial blood gas analysis at rest and with exercise (if available), and 12-lead ECG should give the clinician a better idea of this patient's pulmonary dysfunction.

The history of peptic ulcer disease with recurrent bleeding ulcers should encourage the therapist to review the results of the complete blood count (hemoglobin and hematocrit levels) to rule out anemia, which, if severe enough, could have a profound effect on this patient's exercise tolerance.

Finally, the history of adult-onset diabetes mellitus should lead to a review of serum glucose levels and the urinalysis to determine how well controlled the patient's glucose levels are. In addition, there should be periodic repeat values to be sure the patient's glucose levels remain normal.

## Medical therapy

### CASE 4  Case Example D

A 48-year-old man had "flu-like" symptoms for approximately 2 weeks. His primary complaint was weakness and shortness of breath. The patient reported that it was not uncommon to wake up feeling short of breath. Patient finally sought medical attention and was found to have evidence of an anterior myocardial infarction on the 12-lead ECG.

*Physical findings*
Lungs: rales at both bases
Heart: $S_3$, $S_4$, no murmur
Extremities: 1 +/4 + pretibial edema
*Medications*
Digoxin, 0.25 mg/day
Furosemide (Lasix), 40 mg/day
Procainamide (Procan), 200 mg a day

*Discussion.* The combination of digoxin and furosemide should be a "red flag" to the clinician that the patient has probably had evidence of congestive heart failure at one time. The clinician needs to review the medical chart to see if there is or has been evidence of congestive failure. The physical findings in case D of $S_3$ and pedal and pulmonary edema, along with the medical history, are compatible with heart failure. In addition, the clinician should be alerted to the fact that the patient has had significant dysrhythmias (even though there is no mention of it in the history) since the medical therapy includes Procan. Further review of the medical record and discussion with the physician is indicated to identify the exact nature of the rhythm disturbance.

### CASE 5  Case Example E

A 57-year-old male has a long history of hypertension and premature ventricular contractions. Patient had onset of exertional chest discomfort and was referred for exercise testing. The exercise test was positive for ischemia and angina and the patient was referred for coronary angiography. Just before the cardiac catheterization, the patient suffered a myocardial infarction. The patient became stabilized and eventually had coronary angiography and subsequent bypass surgery. After surgery, the patient had recurrent pericarditis and frequent premature ventricular contractions that did not respond to class I antidysrhythmics [quinidine, procainamide, disopyramidephosphate (Norpace); refer to Chapter 4]. During a maximal exercise test done postoperatively, the patient had a sustained run of ventricular tachycardia. As a result he was started on a combination of propranalol and quinidine therapy, which was found to be reasonably effective in controlling the ventricular ectopy. After a 6-month trial on propranolol, however, the patient continued to complain

about lethargy and depression. Therefore the decision was made to change medications and evaluate the patient's cardiovascular responses to exercise during an individually monitored exercise session.

*Current medications*
Atenolol (Tenormin), 50 mg/day
Quinidine, 300 mg 4 times a day
*Discussion.* Both propranolol and atenolol are beta-blocking drugs that act to significantly lower resting and exercise heart rate and blood pressure. Therefore it is essential that the therapist be aware of the use of medications and follow adjustments in the dosage given to interpret exercise responses and to design exercise programs appropriately. Awareness of the relative strength of the various beta blockers is important as well. We have found atenolol to be a potent beta blocker that in some patients results in significant exercise hypotension, even at mild levels of activity.

### Summary

These cases demonstrate the importance of carefully reviewing the medical record and identifying the patient's current medical therapy. The medications listed often will give an indication of the cardiovascular abnormalities a patient has had, such as dysrhythmias, hypertension, congestive heart failure, or angina. Familiarity with the action, purpose, and side effects of the numerous cardiac drugs will help the therapist provide the most pertinent information to the physician. Finally, many cardiac drugs will alter the cardiovascular responses to exercise, and therefore their effects must be taken into consideration when one is evaluating and designing a treatment plan (see Chapter 4).

### CLINICAL SUBSETS OF CORONARY ARTERY DISEASE

One of the major reasons to thoroughly review the medical record is to determine which clinical subset the patient is in because of its implications for evaluations and program planning. As has been mentioned in Chapter 2, the prognosis of the coronary patient is strongly influenced by the degree of left ventricular dysfunction and number of arteries diseased. There are several items in the medical record that should give the therapist some insight regarding the patient's clinical course.

In the acute patient who has had a myocardial infarction, the description contained in the admitting note of the hospital course during the first 4 days after the myocardial infarction is of great value. Patients with a complicated early hospital course, as defined by the criteria in the box at right, commonly have either poor left ventricular (LV) function as a result of a large infarction or multiple vessel disease. One should keep in mind that the absence of these complications does not rule out poor LV function or multivessel disease.

The 12-lead ECG may also be of some value in predicting poor LV function if it contains evidence of a large myocardial infarction or a ventricular aneurysm, or both. The degree of rise in the enzyme levels during the infarction also correlates with the amount of myocardial damage. Currently, there are several noninvasive methods available to evaluate LV function at rest, of which two-dimensional echocardiography and radioisotope studies seem to be of the greatest value. The results of these studies should be reviewed carefully whenever they are available. The most definitive study is, of course, the cardiac catheterization, since it identifies the degree of disease in the coronary arteries and documents resting LV function. One should keep in mind that to appreciate the hemodynamics and functional consequences of the patient's disease, one should take the patient through a series of activities that are graduated in terms of physiological demand. This series of activities should include procedures such as the activities of daily-living (ADL) evaluation, monitored ambulation, low-level exercise testing, and eventually maximal exercise testing.[36] Noninvasive evaluation of LV function during either the low-level exercise test or the maximal test, especially in suspected cases of poor LV function, can be most helpful.

## CONTRAINDICATIONS FOR PROCEEDING WITH A SELF-CARE EVALUATION

On occasion an inpatient may be quite stable at the time of referral to cardiac rehabilitation. Then, before being seen by the therapist, he or she becomes unstable. Not all patients are candidates for self-care evaluation, even if a referral for cardiac rehabilitation has been made. The following pieces of data from the medical record may preclude proceeding with the self-care evaluation: (1) a sudden rise in cardiac enzyme profile (see Chapter 2); (2) nursing notes and communication indicating a new onset of resting angina; (3) chest radiograph evidence of overt congestive heart failure; (4) overt ECG changes indicating a new infarction; (5) any other data that may correspond with an unstable cardiac or metabolic status (e.g. anemia, uncontrolled

| Criteria for a complicated post—myocardial infarction hospital course* |
| --- |
| Ventricular tachycardia or fibrillation<br>Rapid supraventricular dysrhythmia<br>Second- or third-degree atrioventricular block<br>Persistent sinus tachycardia (≥100 bpm)<br>Persistent hypotension (systolic blood pressure, 90 mm Hg)<br>Pulmonary edema<br>Cardiogenic shock<br>Persistent angina or extension of infarction |

*McNeer JF and others: *Circulation* 51:410, 1975.

diabetes, severe hypoxia or hypercarbia). These pieces of data do not necessarily represent absolute contraindications to self-care evaluation, but a therapist should give serious consideration to proceeding with an exercise evaluation of a patient who exhibits any resting cardiopulmonary instability, especially early after an infarction or bypass surgery. Each patient's case history requires a thorough review, and if there is any doubt about the patient's status, further consultation with the medical staff (physicians and nurses) is recommended.

## PRIORITIES FOR CARDIOVASCULAR MONITORING WITH ACTIVITY

During the medical chart review and accumulation of patient data, the therapist should begin to formulate monitoring priorities. For example, the patient's history may indicate recurrent serious dysrhythmias. The dysrhythmia history will key the monitoring activities to focus on ECG monitoring and identification of dysrhythmia-created symptoms. The following questions should be formulated. Will the dysrhythmia cause hypotension, shortness of breath, or the onset of angina? Will the dysrhythmia worsen with increasing levels of exercise or higher rate-pressure products? Are the current medications controlling the dysrhythmia during activity?

Although each monitored parameter, heart rate, blood pressure, ECG, symptom, or heart sound change requires continuous assessment during exercise, the medical record review may create monitoring priorities that will cause a therapist to focus on specific areas. On the other hand, because of the patient's medications, especially beta-blocking medications (see Chapter 4), some monitored parameters, specifically heart rate and blood pressure, may be much less useful. These medications may blunt the patient's heart rate and blood pressure to such a degree that minimal, if any, changes occur even with increasing levels of activity. This makes the patient's symptoms, ECG, and heart sound changes higher monitoring properties.

# INITIAL PHYSICAL THERAPY EVALUATION

The foundation for patient assessment and treatment is established through the initial evaluation process. At any stage of cardiac disease and treatment (acute, subacute, chronic, postmyocardial infarction, pre- and post-bypass, angioplasty, or valvular surgery) the patient's treatment program will be based on the evaluation findings. The evaluation process includes both the patient interview and a physical examination.

## Patient interview

The patient interview is a dynamic interchange of information between the therapist and the patient. An interview session introduces the concept of cardiac rehabilitation to patients and their families. It is also the mechanism to establish the therapist-patient relationship. Conversations centered around the subjects listed in the box above right provide insight for the therapist regarding the patient's knowledge about his or her own disease, perspective on how it affects his or her life, and what support mechanisms are available.

**Understanding of the disease.** The patient's understanding of cardiac disease is essential before participation in the rehabilitation process. Each person approaches the program with his or her personal biases regarding cardiac disease and the degree and progress of the disability. The patient's level of knowledge then affects the willingness and ability to participate. Additionally, assessment of the patient's educational level provides the therapist with the information needed to accurately educate and motivate the patient at the appropriate level.

**Patient description of symptoms.** The patient's description of symptoms specifies familiar terminology for use in future communications. The terms each patient uses to describe his or her cardiac symptoms (e.g., chest tightness shortness of breath, discomfort, pain, burning, shoulder ache, or dizziness) are highly variable. For example, when a patient describes his or her symptoms as a fullness, the therapist should use this description when asking about the patient's symptoms. Personal descriptions will aid the therapist during reassessment. An established base line allows judgment regarding the severity of symptoms if they reoccur.

**Family.** Family participation is integral to the success of the rehabilitation program. Family members are needed both to support the patient and to participate in the educational experience. Educating the family helps them understand both the disease process and the need for life-style modification. Inpatient programming should be directed at the patient's family. Most of the information presented in an inpatient education program is not well retained and must be repeated in phases II and III. Often a spouse can contribute to or detract from the patient's ability to cope with the disease. Children also benefit from involvement because education can inform them and provide incentives for the prevention of coronary disease.

---

> ## Topics for discussion in a patient interview
>
> Understanding of the disease
> Patient symptoms
> Family
> Vocation
> Psychological profile
> Risk-factor profile
> Leisure activities and exercise history
> Patient's goals

---

**Vocation.** Discussion concerning the specifics of the patient's vocational history aids in the assessment of his or her functional capabilities. Important aspects to consider include both physical activity on the job and level of responsibility and stress. This information is valuable for setting goals and planning the patient's return to work.

**Psychological profile.** Consultation with the team member responsible for psychological care before or after the patient's interview helps to place the assessment of the patient in the proper perspective. The recommendations from the psychological assessment often indicate appropriate ways to approach the patient and to make suggestions for program modifications. Both the patient's ability to participate in the rehabilitation program and his or her attitude toward education are closely linked to his or her psychological status, that is, denial, fear, depression. The majority of inpatients deny their infarctions and disease. Repeated, direct, and truthful responses to their denial by all team members have proven most effective in moving them through this phase. Once they are out of the denial phase, they will often become depressed. Again, a team approach, with appropriate psychological support, can move them through this phase.

**Risk factor profile.** While interviewing the patient and discussing his or her history, one can obtain specifics such as the family history of cardiac disease, smoking history, or social eating and drinking habits. This information is recorded and a personal "risk factor profile" is formed. Identifying individual problem areas is the key to focusing the patient's education and accomplishing modification of risk factors.

The importance of risk factor identification and analysis has been presented in Chapter 2. The importance of identifying each patient's risk factors from his or her medical record relates directly to future educational priorities with that patient. A patient with a smoking history, diabetes, and obesity needs specific educational programming in those areas. Other patients will have different risk factors and, thus, different educational priorities.

The clinician should be careful not to accept the risk factor review found in the patient's medical record. During the interview process, a more useful and thorough profile can be obtained. Also, cholesterol values recorded early after an infarction may not be representative of the patient's normal values. A reassessment of the lipid profile 6 weeks after the infarction or surgery should be used to determine the importance of this risk factor in each patient.

**Leisure activities and exercise history.** A list of the patient's leisure activities provides information necessary for individual program planning. Specific activities patients enjoy can be used to achieve increased function and performance. Early discussion of the potential to return to vigorous leisure activities often has a positive effect on the patient's psychological status.

**Patient's goals.** Recognition of the patient's goals throughout the rehabilitative process is essential. When the program goals and patient goals are not synchronized, there will be less chance for the patient's compliance.

### Physical examination

Physical examination of a cardiac patient by the physical therapist requires the skills of observation, palpation, and auscultation. Observation includes the analysis of musculoskeletal deficits such as posture, gait, muscle strength and tone, skin color and tone, and facial expression. Notation of the musculoskeletal deficits is necessary because these patients may require program adaptation and modifications based on their disability. Traditional walking, or jogging programs may not be a possibility for a patient with a cerebrovascular accident or lower-extremity amputation. Skin color, tone, and facial expression changes can be significant indications of abnormal circulatory responses to exercise or indicative of the patient's attitude and degree of discomfort or weariness.

When observation has been completed, palpation is performed to collect further information. Palpation of the thorax, chest wall, head, neck, shoulder girdle, arms, and upper thoracic spine provides feedback on specifics about complaints of chest wall pain. During the period after myocardial infarction, many patients experience residual chest wall pain or musculoskeletal soreness. It is essential to determine the origin of that pain and distinguish it from angina. Palpation also focuses on circulation to the extremities. Many patients with coronary artery disease have accompanying peripheral vascular disease. It is therefore necessary to include palpation of femoral and peripheral pulses during the examination. Although the point of maximal impulse and some heart sounds can be palpated, heart sounds are primarily evaluated through auscultation.

Auscultation of heart sounds is an art and a science (see Goldberger).[31] The additional information obtained from establishment of a base line and then detection of a change or continued stability of a patient's heart sounds may be critical to his or her program planning. The therapist should be able to identify normal heart sounds, rubs, murmurs, third heart sounds (gallops), and fourth heart sounds. Auscultation of breathsounds is discussed in Chapter 18.

The findings of the gross physical examination are continuously used as referrence points for future evaluation and assessment of the patient and are essential to program development and revision throughout the rehabilitation process.

### Dynamic evaluation

After completion of the chart review, patient interview, and gross evaluation, there is a sufficient data base to initiate further evaluation, including response to activity. The patient's inpatient (phase 1) exercise program is based on the results of (1) a self-care evaluation and (2) monitored ambulation. A third exercise activity, low-level treadmill testing, is done before discharge. The exercise test results are the foundation for program planning and progression in phase II. The common objective for all evaluation procedures is the identification and interpretation of any abnormal or unsafe responses in heart rate, blood pressure, ECG symptoms, or heart sounds that the patient exhibits during progressively increasing levels of activity.

**Self-care evaluation.** The self-care evaluation is performed for evaluation of the cardiac patient's response to activities of daily living. The evaluation is usually initiated 3 to 6 days after infarction and is optimally completed before transfer out of the coronary care unit. (Resting values are obtained in the supine, sitting, and standing positions.)

Patients are asked to perform several activities including: tooth brushing, hair combing, dressing, ambulation, and a Valsalva maneuver. Heart rate, blood pressure, ECG changes, symptoms, and heart sound responses are recorded for each activity. This information is documented on a self-care evaluation form and subsequently placed in the patient's chart (Fig 8-2).

*Collection procedures.* To perform a self-care evaluation, two trained persons are required. One person continuously observes the patient's ECG response, obtains sample ECG strips during each activity, and records the responses on the evaluation form. The other person takes the patient's blood pressure and monitors clinical signs and symptoms during the activity and continuously through observation and questioning. Heart sounds are auscultated supine, at rest, and immediately after ambulation.

The activities included in the self-care evaluation are known to cause mild increases in heart rate and blood pressure in various body positions. A study by Butler and others[9] demonstrated that the heart rate, blood pressure, and ECG changes that occur with self-care are strongly correlated to the responses of the patient during monitored ambulation activities later in the inpatient stay.

**Monitoring clinical responses to exercise.**

*Heart rate.* Heart rate is a simply obtained, yet extremely useful indicator of patient response to activity. It can be counted from the pulse or read from the ECG tracing. The heart rate is dependent on many factors, including medication levels, ventricular function, and level of patient activity.

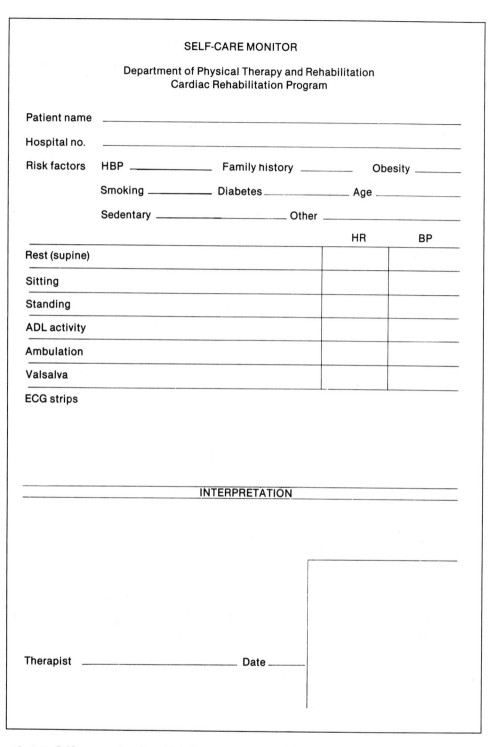

**SELF-CARE MONITOR**

Department of Physical Therapy and Rehabilitation
Cardiac Rehabilitation Program

Patient name _____

Hospital no. _____

Risk factors    HBP _____ Family history _____ Obesity _____

Smoking _____ Diabetes _____ Age _____

Sedentary _____ Other _____

|  | HR | BP |
|---|---|---|
| Rest (supine) |  |  |
| Sitting |  |  |
| Standing |  |  |
| ADL activity |  |  |
| Ambulation |  |  |
| Valsalva |  |  |

ECG strips

INTERPRETATION

Therapist _____ Date _____

**Fig. 8-2.** Self-care monitor form. This form serves to record data and can be used as an initial progress note.

The highest heart rates achieved clinically occur during upper-extremity activities, such as hair combing and tooth brushing. However, these activities rarely cause heart rates in excess of 100 bpm. Most self-care activities require a minimal increase in oxygen consumption. Thus there should be a minimal change in the patient's heart rate with the activities listed.

Patients with large infarctions, continuing ischemia, or borderline heart failure may exhibit a sharp increase in the heart rate (20 to 40 bpm) over resting. Poor ventricular function dictates that the heart rate must rise rapidly to meet the demand for increased cardiac output. If a rapid heart rate is documented (greater than 100 bpm), the therapist immediately determines the significance of this response by noting blood pressure, symptoms, and heart sounds. A patient with poor ventricular function may also exhibit a flat, low blood pressure response (systolic less than 100 bpm), shortness of breath, and a third heart sound. A rapid heart rate response alone may have minimal significance except to indicate anemia or deconditioning. The combination of a heart rate greater than 100 bpm with low blood pressure, shortness of breath, and a third heart sound indicates a severely limited cardiac reserve. Thus, careful monitoring and a slower progression of the patient's activities are necessary. Discussion of the evaluation findings with the referring physician is mandatory.

**Blood pressure.** A major key to the clinical usefulness of the blood pressure response is to record accurate and interpretable blood pressures.[34] Blood pressure recordings are most useful if obtained during an activity and recorded as such. Therapists can then use base-line or resting pressures and compare them to those taken during an activity and those recorded as the patient completes an activity. For example, a single resting blood pressure obtained sitting cannot be used as a base line for interpretation of upright activities. A blood pressure obtained only 15 seconds after a patient has stopped walking may have already fallen significantly and thus is of little value. Therefore, because of the dynamic nature of blood pressure, it should be taken during an activity to measure the real blood pressure response.

In addition to recording blood pressures during an activity, it is most accurate to record pressures using a mercury manometer and an appropriately sized cuff. Mercury manometers are the standard for blood pressure measurement and therefore, if at all possible, should be used in patient evaluation. Cuff size is also very important. Leg or thigh cuffs may be required for patients with very large arms; pediatric cuffs should be used for patients with small arms. Failure to use the appropriate cuff size can give extremely erroneous measures of blood pressure.

The blood pressure response to self-care activities and ambulation is generally unremarkable. Low levels of self-care activity should not evoke even moderate elevations in systolic or diastolic pressure. A 30 mm Hg rise in systolic pressure is uncommon. A fall in systolic pressure with an increase in heart rate or the development of symptoms of shortness of breath may be quite ominous (see Chapter 7). Again, an isolated finding of a flat or falling systolic pressure may be of little significance. However, when found in combination with angina or shortness of breath, a fall in systolic pressure may indicate significant ischemia or abnormal ventricular function.

**ECG changes.** Physical therapists require knowledge of and the ability to interpret the full spectrum of electrocardiogram changes. An excellent reference for learning basic ECG interpretation is *Rapid Interpretation of EKG's* by Dubins.[15] Although dysrhythmias and conduction defects can be identified and recorded using telemetry monitoring (see Chapter 5), ST-segment changes cannot be quantified. Telemetry units cannot be calibrated; therefore, any ST-segment interpretation is at best subjective and limited.

The significance of ECG interpretation lies in its relation to the patient's clinical picture. Three factors of major importance to the ECG are (1) the patient's pharmacological regimen, (2) the severity and, therefore, the potential danger of the dysrhythmia or conduction defect, and (3) the symptoms associated with a dysrhythmia or conduction defect.

*Antidysrhythmic medications.* A description of the effects and side effects of antidysrhythmic medications is found in Chapter 4. Because some of these medications can cause dysrhythmias or conduction defects, a clear identification and understanding of the type and effects of the medication the patient is taking are required (see Chapter 4). It is not unusual to find that patients well controlled on their antidysrhythmic medications at rest do not have the same control with activity.

*Severity and potential danger of dysrhythmias or conduction defects.*

DYSRHYTHMIA. A therapist involved in a cardiac rehabilitation program should be clinically competent in defining, recognizing and determining the significance of all dysrhythmias (see Chapter 5).

Categorization of dysrhythmias from least dangerous to most dangerous is difficult because their severity is relative to the symptoms evoked and the frequency of the dysrhythmia. Asymptomatic patients who exhibit dysrhythmias are generally categorized as less serious, but this is not always true. Patients can be asymptomatic while in ventricular tachycardia, but this dysrhythmia frequently deteriorates into fibrillation, which is lethal.

Ventricular dysrhythmias may be ranked from least serious to most serious in the following order:

Unifocal premature ventricular contraction (PVC)
Multifocal PVCs
Coupled PVCs (R-on-T PVCs)
Ventricular tachycardia
Ventricular fibrillation

Atrial dysrhythmias without conduction block are generally less dangerous (lethal) than ventricular dysrhythmias. Their primary effect is to reduce cardiac output by decreasing preload (see Chapter 3). Thus a true ranking is really not related to the dysrhythmia as much as to the ventricular impairment produced.

1. Premature atrial contractions (PACs)
   a. Premature nodal contractions (PNCs)
2. Atrial fibrillation
3. Paroxysmal atrial tachycardia (PAT)
4. Atrial flutter (is a block)

CONDUCTION DEFECTS. There are two categories of conduction defects. One category results in an interruption of the electrical transmission of an impulse from the atrioventricular node to the ventricular bundle branches. These are called "AV blocks." The other category involves the bundle of His and its branches. These are called "bundle-branch blocks" (see Chapter 5).

*Symptoms.* The most difficult patient responses to interpret are symptoms. The symptoms are as varied and widespread as are the patients in the program. The primary symptom, which the therapist learns to recognize, is angina.

The classic description of angina is a dull, substernal ache or pain that is brought on by eating, exercise, or emotional upset. In the clinical experience of Scot Irwin, the best description of angina is as follows: "Angina is any discomfort that occurs above the waist and is reproduced by exertional activities." Angina *must be differentiated* from other musculoskeletal or neurological discomforts. The therapist should understand and recognize the significance of the difference to educate and reassure patients and to inform the patient's physician. Differentiation of nonanginal discomforts from angina is not easy. Some guidelines and suggestions are listed in Table 8-2.

Angina can be described by patients as a burning, tightness, pressure, indigestion, shortness of breath aching, fullness, jaw pain, backache, toothache, shoulder pain, or arm pain.

Each patient will use his or her own term(s) to describe the anginal discomfort. A therapist should record carefully the patient's description of angina and consistently use his or her term(s). Failure to use the patient's terminology can result in serious miscommunication. For example, if a patient describes his or her angina as a *tightness* or a *fullness* and a therapist asks if he or she has any chest *pain,* the patient may respond negatively and in fact be experiencing angina. The appropriate question would have used the patient's term(s), "fullness" or "tightness," not chest "pain."

The content of Table 8-2 may suggest that distinguishing angina from nonanginal discomforts should be fairly easy. This is not true. The differentiation of angina from nonanginal chest discomfort is made difficult by the existence of two other types of angina: unstable angina and Prinzmetal's angina. Unstable, preinfarction angina can occur at any time, even at rest, may last longer than stable anginal episodes, and may be associated with chest wall soreness or a frozen shoulder. Prinzmetal's angina, caused by coronary vasospasm, has characteristics similar to unstable angina. It also can occur at anytime and is improved only slightly by administration of nitroglycerin.

In addition, chest pain that is caused by pericarditis can create some confusion and misinterpretation. Pericarditis can occur following bypass surgery. Thus, a patient population is created that has chest wall soreness from surgery, a previous history of angina, and pericarditic pain. Differentiating among these discomforts is critical to the therapist's evaluation process and the patient's prognosis. Pericarditis is a contraindication to exercise and requires medical attention. Pericarditic pain is characterized by (1) sharp, stabbing substernal pain and (2) nonexertional occurrence. This pain may also be associated with fever and malaise.

The therapist should also recognize and appropriately interpret symptoms of shortness of breath, dizziness, pallor, and general fatigue.

Shortness of breath has numerous causes, but for the purposes of this discussion there are four major causes that require differentiation by a therapist. First, shortness of breath can be a description of angina. This is referred to as an angina equivalent. A patient may not describe any chest discomfort; he or she simply has a reproducible shortness of breath with exercise and concomitant ST-segment changes. This angina equivalent description for shortness of breath is rare, and it is difficult to ascertain because exercise-induced shortness of breath is a normal response to increased blood lactate levels during moderate to severe exercise. Clinically, however, the differences are striking. Angina equivalent shortness of breath generally occurs at low heart rates and low levels of exercise and may be associated with a flattened systolic blood pressure and ST-segment depression.

A second cause of shortness of breath may be pulmonary pathology. Abnormal pulmonary function test results may indicate quickly the cause of the shortness of breath to be pulmonary in origin. Thus, it is important that a therapist review the results of these tests before evaluating a patient's response to exercise.

**Table 8-2.** Differentiation of nonanginal discomforts from angina

| Stable angina | Nonanginal discomfort (chest wall pain) |
| --- | --- |
| 1. Relieved by nitroglycerin (30 seconds to 1 minute) | 1. Nitroglycerin generally has no effect |
| 2. Comes on at the same heart rate and blood pressure and is relieved by rest (lasts only a few minutes) | 2. Occurs any time; lasts for hours |
| 3. Not palpable | 3. Muscle soreness, joint soreness, evoked by palpation or deep breaths |
| 4. Associated with feelings of doom, cold sweats, shortness of breath | 4. Minimal additional symptoms |
| 5. Often seen with ST-segment depression | 5. No ST-segment depression |

A third cause of shortness of breath is limited cardiovascular reserve. Patients with borderline congestive heart failure, cardiomegaly, or right ventricular failure may suffer from shortness of breath at very low levels of activity. The pathological cause of the shortness of breath is abnormal ventricular function. A patient's data base—including an enlarged heart on chest radiograph; low ejection fraction at rest; need for inotropic medications (digitalis derivatives); age, number, and size of infarctions; or a combination of these findings—points towards a cardiogenic cause for the symptom of shortness of breath.

A fourth cause of shortness of breath is the normal exercise-induced shortness of breath as described previously.

The differentiation of the cause of the shortness of breath is a key part of the therapist's evaluation process. A patient's exercise program prescription and progression will have to be adjusted according to the reason for his or her shortness of breath.

Dizziness and pallor are also associated with signs of failure and ischemia. Hypotension will cause dizziness and pallor. Although these symptoms are not as common as shortness of breath and angina in cardiac patients, they can be more ominous. Pallor that occurs during exercise testing can be a significant sign of impending cardiovascular collapse. These signs and symptoms should be added to all the other pieces of information in a patient's data base and interpreted appropriately.

*Auscultation.* The final clinical tool to be discussed is auscultation of heart sounds. Effective auscultation requires clinical experience under the tutelage of a knowledgeable clinician. A physical evaluation starts with auscultation of the patient's heart sounds. Recognition of different heart sounds is essential. The ability to auscultate does not need to be at a diagnostic level. A level of expertise that affords the therapist clinical recognition of heart sound changes is sufficient. A change in heart sounds can indicate a change in heart function because of infarction, ischemia, failure, or inflammation. A complete review of heart sounds will not be discussed here, but some common clinical examples are worth review.

Early after bypass surgery (less than 6 weeks) some patients will develop pericarditis. Pericarditis can cause a heart sound change. The patient may develop an abnormal heart sound called a pericardial rub. Some patients will have audible rubs, and some will only develop an audible rub after exercise. Patients with pericarditis or those who develop pericardial rubs during exercise training should be referred back to their physician. Another example of a significant heart sound change is when a patient develops a third heart sound after exercise. Although a third heart sound may be auscultated in children and athletes, it is generally pathological when found in patients over 40 years of age. Third heart sounds correspond strongly with a decrease in ventricular compliance. Loss of compliance results from either a distended ventricle or large areas of ischemia or

infarction. A combination of these changes produces the same loss. Patients who exhibit normal heart sounds at rest and develop a third heart sound perhaps are being exercised too strenuously. Their heart is literally being distended to its limits to compensate for the increased demand for cardiac output. Again, the presence of a third heart sound alone may have minimal significance. When this heart sound change occurs in conjunction with shortness of breath, falling systolic blood pressure, or pronounced ST-segment depression, the patient's exercise should be terminated and a lower level of activity should be assumed during any future exercise sessions.

**Summary.** Dynamic cardiac patient evaluation requires incorporation of good clinical skill (to obtain data) and rapid, accurate interpretation of the data obtained. Self-care evaluation and monitored ambulation are performed to obtain guidelines for exercise programming and progression. The five dynamic clinical monitoring skills available to assist the therapist in evaluation and treatment are heart rate, blood pressure responses, ECG and heart sound changes, and symptoms.

### Low-level exercise testing

Low-level exercise testing is usually the final procedure of the definitive evaluation in phase I. As discussed earlier, it provides the data base from which the hemodynamics and functional consequences of the patient's disease can be assessed. Furthermore, it provides the additional information needed to decide whether the patient is a candidate for exercise therapy (phase II) and, if so, what intensity of exercise appears to be indicated.

The low-level exercise test is a multistage procedure progressing from a workload equivalent of 2 to 3 metabolic equivalents (METs) up to a workload equivalent of no greater than 6 to 7 METs. There are numerous protocols for low-level testing in the literature. The key is to correlate the protocol with the purpose of the test and with the patient population to be evaluated. With any evaluation of exercise responses on a treadmill, the evaluator should allow minimal or no handrail support. Handrail support cannot be measured, but the effect can increase workloads and decrease myocardial oxygen demand per a given workload.[34] Table 8-3 defines the various stages and corresponding estimated MET levels for the protocol employed with our postmyocardial infarction and, when indicated, postbypass surgery patient population. Two additional treadmill protocols for low-level testing are listed in Table 8-4.

It has become standard medical practice to perform a low-level exercise test before hospital discharge for the postmyocardial infarction patient. The realization that the patient is likely to perform activities soon after discharge that are equivalent to the work loads performed on a low-level test has definitely influenced the physician's thinking regarding the timing of the test. The precise timing of the test will depend on the hospital course of the patient; generally,

**Table 8-3.** Low-level treadmill test protocol and estimated metabolic equivalent (MET) for each workload

| Stage | Speed (mph) | % grade | Duration (min) | Estimated MET level |
|---|---|---|---|---|
| I | 1.7 | 0 | 3 | 2.3 |
| II | 1.7 | 5 | 3 | 3.5 |
| III | 1.7 | 10 | 3 | 4.6 |
| IV | 2.5 | 12 | 3 | 6.8 |

From Schwartz KM and others: Limited exercise testing soon after myocardial infarction: correlation with early coronary and left ventricular angiography, *Ann Intern Med* 94:727, 1981.
NOTE: For a more debilitated, deconditioned patient we sometimes precede stage I with a stage A of 1.3 mph, 0% grade for 3 minutes.

**Table 8-4.** Additional commonly utilized low-level treadmill test protocols

| Stage | Speed (mph) | % grade | Time (min) | Metabolic equivalent |
|---|---|---|---|---|
| Lerman-Bruce protocol | | | | |
| I | 1.2 | 0 | 3 | 2.1 |
| II | 1.2 | 3 | 3 | 2.3 |
| III | 1.2 | 6 | 3 | 3.0 |
| IV | 1.7 | 6 | 3 | 3.3 |
| Modified Naughton protocol | | | | |
| I | 2 | 3.5 | 3 | 3 |
| II | 2 | 7.0 | 3 | 4 |
| III | 2 | 10.5 | 3 | 5 |
| IV | 2 | 14.0 | 3 | 6 |
| V | 2 | 17.0 | 3 | 7 |
| VI | 3 | 12.5 | 3 | 8 |
| VII | 3 | 15.0 | 3 | 9 |
| VIII | 3 | 17.5 | 3 | 10 |

From Hassack RF and Bruce RA: *Primary Cardiol*, pp. 106-112, Feb 1980, and from Starling MR and others: Exercise testing early after myocardial infarction: predictive value for subsequent unstable angina and death, *Am J Cardiol* 46:909, 1980.

the uncomplicated postmyocardial infarction patient is tested as early as 7 to 10 days after the event. The interval for testing in the complicated patient will depend on the length of time required for stabilization, but generally these patients are tested within 2 to 3 weeks after the event. The safety of the procedure when performed within 1 to 3 weeks after the myocardial infarction has been borne out by numerous reports in the literature. According to an editorial published in the June 1981 issue of the *Annals of Internal Medicine* there have been only two deaths related to low-level testing and "the concern about safety need not arise," provided that the test is designed to reproduce the physiological demands of the activities that the patient is likely to perform early after discharge.[53]

**Purpose.** The low-level exercise test has at least three major purposes:

**Table 8-5.** Prevalence of ischemic findings during low-level testing in 134 postmyocardial infarction patients

| | N | % |
|---|---|---|
| Angina pectoris | 29 | 22 |
| ST-segment depression | 23 | 17 |
| Drop in systolic blood pressure of 10 mm Hg | 13 | 10 |
| Complex dysrhythmias | 1 | 1 |

1. To help identify the higher-risk patient (i.e., the patient who demonstrates signs or symptoms of myocardial ischemia or poor left ventricular function at low workloads)
2. To evaluate the effectiveness of medical therapy designed to control hypertension, dysrhythmias, and angina
3. To provide the basis from which to make recommendations for activity and exercise therapy (phase II)

The ability to identify the high-risk patient by low-level testing is essential to the process of determining the candidacy of a given patient for early exercise therapy. Starling and others[54,55] reported that uncomplicated postmyocardial infarction patients, with the combination of exercise-induced ST-segment depression and inadequate blood pressure response (peak systolic blood pressure less than 140mm Hg, or a 20 mm Hg or more drop from peak systolic pressure during exercise) on low-level testing, had a significantly greater incidence of cardiac death within 11 months than patients without ischemic treadmill abnormalities. Schwartz and others[51] found that 90% of patients with ischemic ECG changes or angina had multiple vessel disease compared with 55% of patients with no ischemic treadmill abnormalities. In addition, his group reported that exercise-induced ST-segment elevation predicted poor left ventricular function. The work of both Schwartz and Starling has been supported by Théroux[57] and Fuller[29] with others.

A review of the data of 134 postmyocardial infarction patients tested in our laboratory within 7 to 10 days after the event revealed that the most prevalent ischemic treadmill abnormality was angina pectoris (Table 8-5). However, our data suggest that ST-segment depression of 2 mm or a hypoadaptive systolic blood pressure response (drop from peak exercise pressure of 10 or more mm Hg) is highly predictive of the high-risk subset of patients with triple vessel or left main coronary disease. The sensitivity, specificity, and predictive value of these two markers for severe coronary disease is summarized in Table 8-6. In essence, our findings possibly indicate that if the patient has less than 2 mm of ST-segment depression and an adequate blood pressure response, he or she has an 88% chance of not having severe coronary disease, whereas two thirds of the

**Table 8-6.** Significant ST-segment depression and exercise hypotension as predictors of severe coronary artery disease

| | |
|---|---|
| Positive test | 2 mm ST-segment depression or decrease in peak exercise systolic blood pressure of 10 mm Hg |
| "Significant" coronary disease | Triple vessel or left main disease |
| Sensitivity | 62% |
| Specificity | 90% |
| Predictive value of a negative test | 88% |
| Predictive value of a positive test | 67% |

**Table 8-7.** Contraindications to low-level exercise testing

Patient less than 5 days after myocardial infarction or after coronary artery bypass graft surgery
Incomplete pretest data base
Acute congestive heart failure
Severe aortic stenosis
Recent episodes of chest pain suggestive of unstable angina
Hypotension (BP, 80/50 mm Hg)
Hypertension (BP, 170/100 mm Hg) at rest
Uncontrolled dysrhythmias before exercise, such as atrial fibrillation, frequent, or complex premature ventricular contractions

**Table 8-8.** End points for low-level treadmill tests

Achievement of heart rate equivalent to 75% to 80% of the age-predicted maximum value (unless the patient is taking beta blockers)
Hypoadaptive systolic blood pressure response
Onset of symptoms consistent with mild angina pectoris
Two or more millimeters of ST-segment depression
Frequent multifocal premature ventricular contractions (PVC), paired PVCs, ventricular tachycardia
Sustained supraventricular tachycardia
Fatigue
Patient request

**Table 8-9.** Low-level test end points (N = 134)

| | N | % |
|---|---|---|
| Reached target heart rate | 57 | 43 |
| Fatigue | 36 | 27 |
| Angina | 22 | 16 |
| Hypotension | 8 | 6 |
| Hypertension | 4 | 3 |
| Leg pain, claudication | 3 | 2 |
| Dyspnea | 3 | 2 |
| Dysrhythmias | 1 | 1 |

time if a patient has either or both of the ischemic treadmill abnormalities discussed above, he or she will demonstrate triple vessel or left main disease by angiography. (See Case 6 and Case 7 on p. 121.)

**Contraindications and termination points.** As mentioned earlier, low-level testing is a safe procedure. This is especially true when specific contraindications for testing are observed, and appropriate end points for testing are enforced. Table 8-7 lists the contraindications for testing we use at our facilities. The end points for testing, like the test protocols, should be determined with the test objectives and patient population in mind. The criteria for terminating a low-level test are listed in Table 8-8. Our data (Table 8-9) indicate that 60% of the patients tested have their test terminated because they achieve their target heart rate or fatigue. Ischemic abnormalities (angina and hypotension) account for 22% of tests being terminated, and only 1% of the tests are stopped because of serious dysrhythmias.

**Summary.** In summary, the low-level exercise test is a safe and extremely useful procedure, especially as part of the definitive evaluation of the postmyocardial infarction patient. For this procedure to be as useful as possible, the therapist should consider all the available data, including the total test time and maximum workload completed, the heart rate and blood pressure response, ECG changes, rhythm, exertional symptoms, reasons for terminating the test, and heart sounds before and after exercise. The therapist should carefully examine the test results (even if he or she is not directly involved in the procedure) to finalize the assessment of the patient and if indicated, begin designing the treatment program.

## MAXIMAL EXERCISE TESTING

In general, physical therapists who are involved with cardiac rehabilitation are not often directly involved with maximal exercise testing although they should be involved because this test is perhaps the most definitive evaluation for a patient prior to entering a cardiac rehabilitation program. Just as therapists evaluate strength and range of motion (ROM) before treating a musculoskeletal problem they should consider an exercise test as a definitive evaluation tool before treating a cardiac patient.

As the emphasis shifts from inpatient rehabilitation to outpatient rehabilitation, the importance of the data base provided by the maximal exercise test will become more evident. The objectives of the next section in this chapter are to provide an overview of the purposes of maximal exercise testing, to illustrate how the test results influence treatment program planning, to provide examples of protocols used in testing, and to provide references that include a more detailed discussion of the various subjects addressed.

## CASE 6 ▼ Mr. E. B.

Consider the case of Mr. E. B., who had a documented myocardial infarction and a hospital course complicated by congestive heart failure, persistent chest pain, sinus tachycardia, and complex ventricular dysrhythmias. The complicated postmyocardial infarction hospital course suggests either a large myocardial infarction or severe coronary artery disease. After Mr. E.B.'s course in the hospital became stabilized, he underwent activities of daily living evaluation and monitored ambulation without demonstrating any major cardiovascular abnormalities. Fourteen days after the myocardial infarction, Mr. E.B. was referred for exercise testing before being referred for exercise therapy. His 12-lead ECG appears in Fig. 8-3. There is evidence of an anteroseptal myocardial infarction on the cardiogram but no suggestion of extensive myocardial damage. The heart rate and systolic and diastolic blood pressure responses to exercise are summarized on the graph in Fig. 8-4. Note the sharp drop in systolic blood pressure occurring after 2 minutes of exercise at 1.7 mph, 0% grade at a heart rate of 104 bpm. Figs. 8-5 and 8-6 show the base line ST-segment changes (preexercise standing) and the pronounced ST-segment changes occurring in multiple-exercise leads at maximal exercise. Based on the prior discussion, the findings on Mr. E.B.'s exercise test suggest that he has severe coronary disease and that he was not a candidate for rehabilitation until the degree of his coronary disease had been documented by angiography. In fact, the patient was found to have 80% occlusion of the left main coronary artery and significant occlusions in the right coronary, the left anterior descending, and the circumflex arteries. After bypass surgery, Mr. E.B. was referred to the cardiac rehabilitation program.

On the other hand, the absence of significant ischemic treadmill abnormalities usually clears the way for hospital discharge and referral for early outpatient rehabilitation.

Figures 8-3 to 8-6 for this case are on pages 122-124.

## CASE 7 ▼ Ms. J. T.

Ms. J.T. was a 44-year-old woman with a documented myocardial infarction and an uncomplicated course. The activities of daily living evaluation and monitored ambulation were unremarkable, and thus the patient was referred for low-level exercise testing 6 days after the myocardial infarction. The 12-lead ECG shown in Fig. 8-7 indicates that this patient had an anterior myocardial infarction and that there were the corresponding T-wave abnormalities. The graph of Ms. J.T.'s blood pressure response (Fig. 8-8) and the preexercise and maximal exercise testing ECG strips (Figs. 8-9 and 8-10) demonstrate appropriate cardiovascular responses to exercise. Because of the age of this patient, she did undergo coronary angiography, which documented single-vessel coronary disease (left anterior descending) and good left ventricular function, as would be predicted from the postmyocardial infarction hospital course and the exercise test results. This patient was discharged from the hospital 7 days after the infarction and returned on day 9 after the infarction to begin outpatient cardiac rehabilitation.

The value of low-level exercise testing in providing the database from which to design an individualized exercise prescription is discussed in Chapter 9. Case examples are included to illustrate the exact method in which exercise prescriptions are formulated with these data at hand.

Figures 8-7 to 8-10 for this case are on pages 125-128.

It is most common to perform maximal exercise tests on the post myocardial infarction patient and the postcoronary artery bypass surgery patient as early as 3 to 6 weeks after the event. In fact, the maximal test is usually done at the completion of the early outpatient phase (phase II) of the exercise rehabilitation program and it precedes the point in time at which the patient is cleared to return to work. The maximal exercise test, by definition, involves exercising a patient to a symptom-limited end point, which is most commonly severe leg fatigue or dyspnea. Heart rate, magnitude of exercise-induced ST-segment depression, and mild angina, unlike those produced by the low-level exercise test, are not used as test end points (see Appendix A).

### Purposes of maximal exercise testing

**Diagnosing coronary artery disease.** The fact that the majority of patients who arc referred to exercise rehabilitation programs have known coronary artery disease does not diminish the importance of being knowledgable of the diagnostic parameters of maximal exercise testing. Not only do the electrocardiographic and physiological ischemic indicators seen on exercise testing identify those patients who are likely to have coronary artery disease, but also these indicators are useful in predicting the severity of the disease. Furthermore, when exercise testing is done serially, as it is on most patients involved with long-term rehabilitation, changes in the ischemic indicators correlate with changes in the hemodynamics of the native coronary vessels or the bypass grafts.

**ECG changes and ischemia.** There are a number of changes in the electrocardiogram induced by exercise that are predictive of myocardial ischemia; hence, coronary artery disease. ST-segment changes are the most commonly referred to electrocardiographic indicators of exercise-induced ischemia.[5] The various types of alterations in the ST-segment that can occur during or after exercise as a result of myocardial ischemia are illustrated in Fig 8-11 on page 129 and include a normal ST-segment, a slowly upsloping

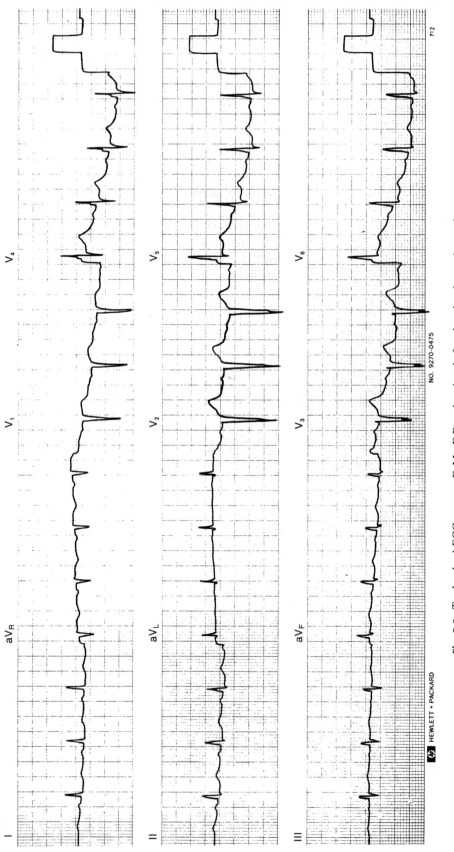

**Fig. 8-3.** Twelve-lead ECG on case F, Mr. E.B., taken just before low-level exercise testing.

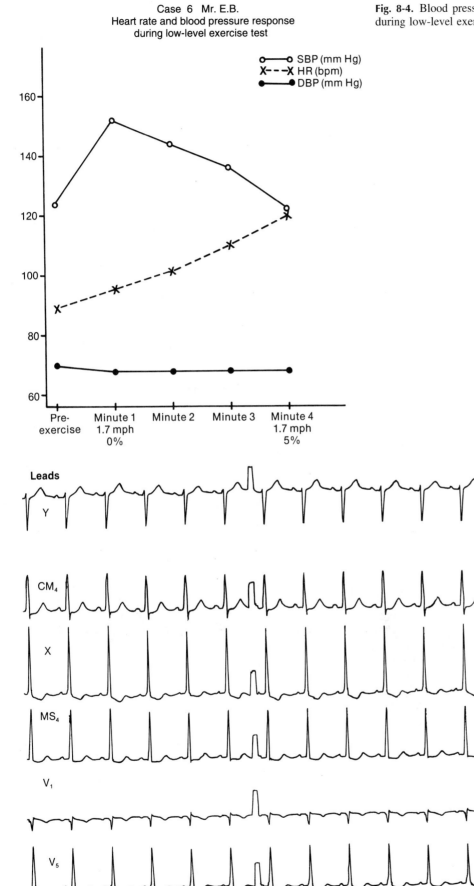

Case 6 Mr. E.B.
Heart rate and blood pressure response
during low-level exercise test

**Fig. 8-4.** Blood pressure and heart rate response of Mr. E.B. during low-level exercise testing.

**Fig. 8-5.** Preexercise multiple-lead ECG tracing demonstrating ST depression in the X, MS$_4$, and V$_5$ leads.

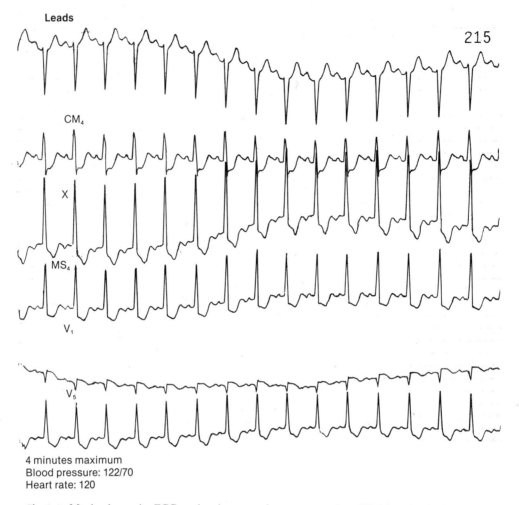

**Fig. 8-6.** Maximal exercise ECG tracing demonstrating pronounced net ST depression in four of the six leads and ST elevation in $V_1$.

ST-segment depression, a horizontal ST depression, a downsloping ST depression, and a horizontal ST elevation. The precise causes of the shift in the ST-segments that are associated with ischemia are not clearly understood. Ellestad[20] has proposed that the ischemic electrophysiological changes result from both hemodynamic and metabolic factors, including elevated left ventricular end-diastolic pressures, incomplete relaxation of the myocardium, and potassium leak from the myocardial cells.

Research has provided the clinician with some guidelines for understanding the value and limitations of exercise-induced ST-segment changes or shifts. In most exercise laboratories, the electrocardiographic criteria for ischemia involve a net change (when compared with the base-line preexercise tracing) of 1 mm or more of either horizontal or downsloping ST-segment depression or horizontal ST-segment or 1.5 to 2 mm of slow upsloping ST-segment depression when measured 0.08 seconds from the J point.[20] However, the predictive accuracy of the above criteria for myocardial ischemia is not 100% and, in fact, is related directly to the prevalence of the disease in the population of

patients being tested (Table 8-10, p. 129). In other words, the predictive value of exercise-induced ST-segment changes is poor in a population of patients with low prevalence of coronary disease such as asymptomatic males less than 35 years of age[33] or premenopausal females.[13] On the other hand, in a population of older males or females with multiple risk factors or typical angina pectoris, or both, the predictive value of ST changes occurring with exercise for ischemia is very high. Furthermore, in a population of patients who previously had normal exercise electrocardiograms and who develop ST changes with exercise on subsequent tests, there is a very high likelihood of progression of disease either in the native coronary arteries or in the bypass grafts.

Finally, it has recently been shown that the sensitivity, specificity, and the predictive value of ST changes can be enhanced when examining the degree of ST displacement in relation to the change in heart rate from rest to maximal exercise.[35,39,46] An index of 1.6 $\mu$V ST-segment depression/beat/minute resulted in a sensitivity and specificity in excess of 90% according to Kligfield and others.[39]

One should keep in mind that exercise-induced ST-

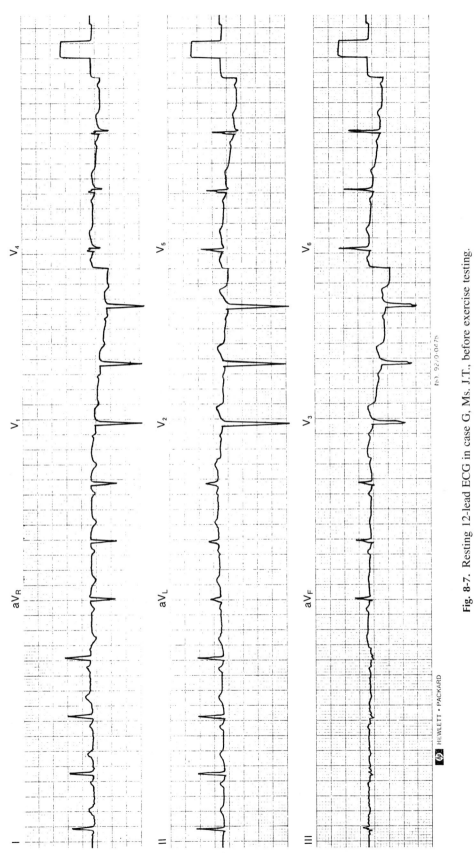

**Fig. 8-7.** Resting 12-lead ECG in case G, Ms. J.T., before exercise testing.

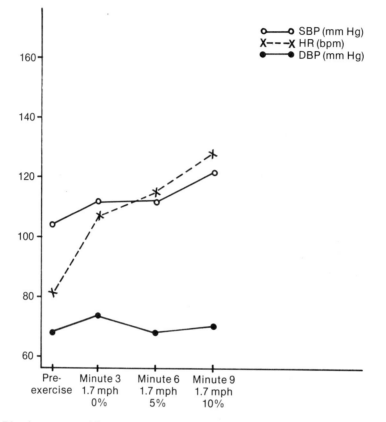

**Fig. 8-8.** Blood pressure and heart rate response of Ms. J.T. during low-level exercise testing.

segment changes can result from a number of factors other than ischemia including (1) conduction abnormalities such as Wolff-Parkinson-White syndrome, left ventricular hypertrophy, and left and right bundle-branch block, (2) medications such as digitalis and diuretics, (3) valvular disorders such as mitral valve prolapse and aortic stenosis, (4) extreme base-line ST-segment abnormalities, and (5) electrolyte disturbances such as hypokalemia. Therefore when any of the above conditions exist, the ST-segment changes must be interpreted cautiously.

On the other hand, the absence of ST-segment changes does not by itself rule out myocardial ischemia, especially in a population of patients with either a high prevalence of coronary disease or known ischemic heart disease. The predictive accuracy of a negative test (absence of electrocardiographic changes) depends on a number of factors such as (1) absence of physiological indicators for ischemia (i.e., hypotension, dysrhythmias, angina), (2) achievement of a maximum heart rate that is equivalent to at least 85% of the age-predicted maximum, (3) the use of multiple exercise electrocardiographic leads, and (4) the clarity and stability of the exercise and postexercise electrocardiographic tracing.

In addition to exercise-induced ST-segment changes, studies have indicated that there are a number of other electrocardiographic indicators of myocardial ischemia. Recently, R-wave amplitude changes with exercise have been reported to be a useful indicator of myocardial ischemia and left ventricular function, though there is some controversy in the literature. Theoretically, R-wave amplitude is directly related to left ventricular end-diastolic volume.[7] In the normal subject, R-wave amplitude decreases when the preexercise standing voltage is compared with the immediate postexercise value. It is assumed that this decrease in R-wave amplitude is attributable to the decrease in the left ventricular end-diastolic volume that occurs in the person with normal coronaries and normal left ventricular function. In the patient with coronary disease who becomes ischemic with exercise and whose left ventricular function deteriorates resulting in increased end-diastolic volumes, one would expect the R-wave amplitude to increase. In fact, there are studies indicating that R-wave amplitude changes increase the diagnostic value of exercise testing.[3,29] The problem with R-wave changes is that they can occur in patients with poor ventricular function without ischemia and in a small

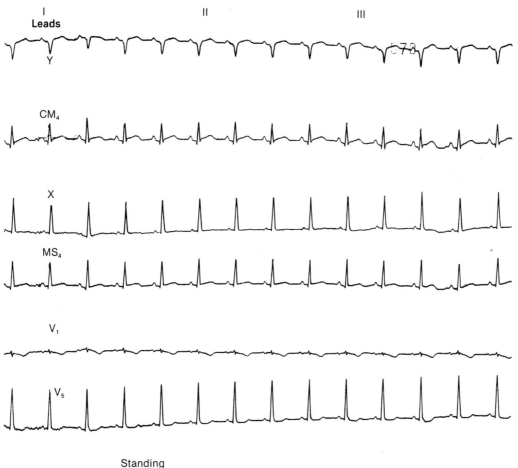

Leads I II III

Y

CM₄

X

MS₄

V₁

V₅

Standing
blood pressure: 108/70
Heart rate: 94

**Fig. 8-9.** Preexercise multiple-lead ECG tracings demonstrating essentially isoelectric ST segment.

percentage of "normal" subjects, and therefore there are studies questioning their usefulness.[60] It seems that the most reasonable approach for use of R-wave changes is to combine ST-segment changes with R-wave changes as done by Ellestad[24] (Fig. 8-12). According to Ellestad, if the net ST-segment changes are a "positive" 1 mm or more, once the R-wave changes have been taken into consideration, there is a stronger likelihood of coronary disease.

Exercise-induced septal Q-wave changes have been studied, and the results indicate that decreases in the amplitude of the Q wave (in lead $CM_5$) are highly predictive of disease in the left anterior descending artery.[45] Finally, although it is a rare finding, postexercise inversion of the U wave is highly predictive of coronary disease even in the absence of ST-segment depression according to Gerson and others.[30] There appears to be some question as to the usefulness of exercise testing in the detection of ischemia in patients. An article by Ehrman and others concluded that exercise electrocardiograms have a very low sensitivity for ischemia in 36 post-heart transplant patients.[19]

**Physiological changes and ischemia.** As mentioned earlier, there are a number of physiological indicators of myocardial ischemia that can develop during exercise testing in conjunction with the various electrocardiographic changes or despite the absence of electrocardiographic changes such as ST-depression or R-wave amplitude changes. Blood pressure response to exercise is one physiologic parameter that must be evaluated carefully throughout the test (see Chapter 7). Another hemodynamic indicator of compromised left ventricular function, usually associated with myocardial ischemia, is exercise bradycardia, also referred to as "chronotropic incompetence" (see Chapter 7). When the exercise bradycardia accompanies other electrocardiographic and hemodynamic indicators of ischemia, the patients are more likely to have severe coronary disease.[4]

Exercise-induced ventricular dysrhythmias by themselves (in absence of electrocardiographic changes and other signs of myocardial ischemia) are not predictive of coronary disease. The combination of ST changes and exercise-

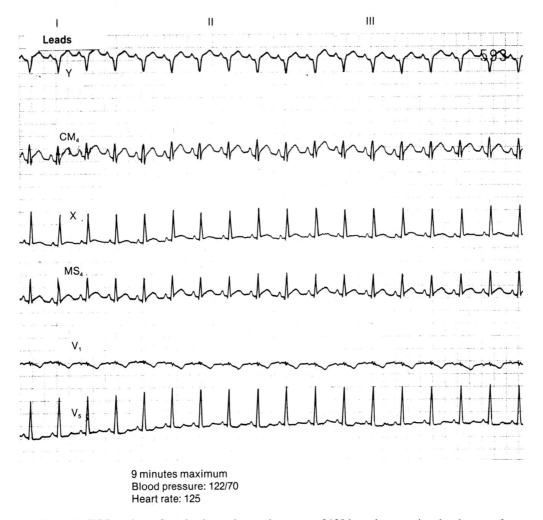

I    II    III

Leads

Y

CM₄

X

MS₄

V₁

V₅

9 minutes maximum
Blood pressure: 122/70
Heart rate: 125

**Fig. 8-10.** ECG tracings of maximal exercise at a heart rate of 128 bpm documenting the absence of ischemic ST changes.

induced dysrhythmias is, however, predictive of more severe coronary disease.

The presence of anginal discomfort during exercise testing without electrocardiographic changes has been shown to be as predictive as electrocardiographic changes alone.[61] The nature of the anginal discomfort can be quite variable, involving burning, pressure, tightness, tiredness in the chest, upper extremities, neck, jaw, or midscapular region. The common denominator, however, is that the discomfort becomes more intense with increased heart rate and systolic blood pressure, and it is usually relieved within 5 minutes after exercise or after nitroglycerin administration.

It should be clear at this point that exercise-induced myocardial ischemia can be detected during and after testing by a variety of electrocardiographic and physiological indicators. It is obviously inappropriate to use the "tunnel-vision" approach of equating ischemia with ST changes alone.

## Prognostic implications from exercise testing

Exercise testing provides a great deal of information regarding the prognosis of patients with known coronary disease. It is the most important functional assessment of the consequences of the degree of coronary disease and left ventricular dysfunction seen at the time of cardiac catheterization. For therapists involved with phase III cardiac rehabilitation candidates, the prognostic implication of exercise testing is important because it (1) identifies the priority for involvement in an ongoing program based on the likelihood of a future cardiac event (i.e., myocardial infarction, progression of angina, or sudden death), (2) provides part of the data base from which decisions can be made regarding the frequency of phase III visits, and (3) provides part of the data base from which decisions about the specific exercise program can be made.

As mentioned in Chapter 2, the two major determinants of prognosis for the patient with coronary disease are the

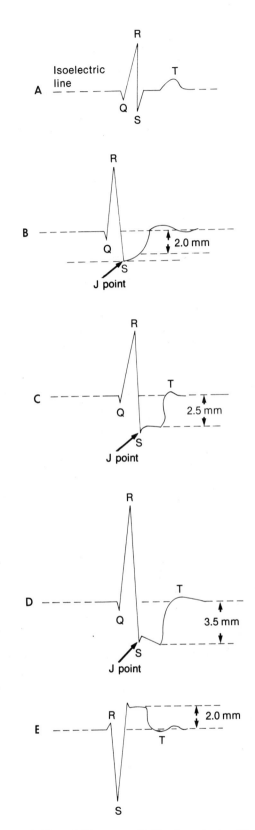

**Fig. 8-11. A,** Normal ST segment. **B,** Slowly upsloping ST-segment depression. **C,** Horizontal ST-segment depression. **D,** Downsloping ST-segment depression. **E,** Horizontal ST-segment depression.

**Table 8-10.** Predictive accuracy of ST-segment changes related to prevalence of disease in the population being tested

| Disease prevalence (%) | Predictive accuracy of ST depression | Predictive accuracy of no ST depression |
|---|---|---|
| 5 | 50 | 99.7 |
| 10 | 68 | 99.4 |
| 20 | 83 | 98.7 |
| 30 | 90 | 97.5 |
| 50 | 95 | 95.0 |

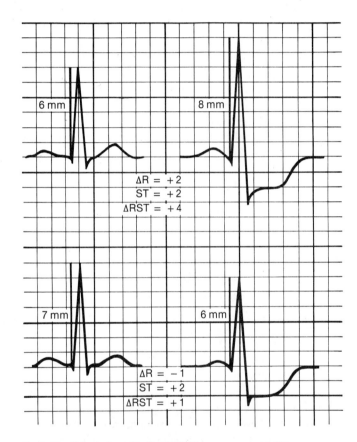

**Fig. 8-12.** Calculation of index (RST) in two cases with ST-segment depression and R wave increased and decreased. (From Bonoris PE and others: Evaluation of R wave amplitude changes versus ST segment depression in stress testing, *Circulation* 57(5):904, 1978.)

number of diseased arteries and the degree of left ventricular dysfunction. There are several electrocardiographic and physiological indicators obtained from exercise testing that predict the likelihood of a future coronary event since they relate directly to the degree of coronary disease and left ventricular impairment. A discussion of these prognostic variables follows.

The slope, magnitude, time of onset, and persistence of ST-segment abnormalities after exercise have been shown to be related to the severity of coronary disease and therefore the likelihood of future coronary events. Goldschlager and others[32] found downsloping ST depression (versus horizontal or slow, upsloping ST depression) to be more commonly associated with multivessel or left main coronary disease. Patients who demonstrate significant ST-segment depression within the first 3 minutes of the test are at a much higher risk of a future coronary event.[21] In addition, the magnitude (number of millimeters of depression) of the ST change is predictive of future coronary events, especially when one compares ST changes occurring within the first 6 minutes of a Bruce or treadmill test. For example, according to Ellestad's data, a patient with 3 mm of ST-segment depression has an 82% chance of a future event compared with 50% likelihood of a future event for the patient with 1 mm at the same point on the test. However, those with 1 to 2 mm ST depression at 5 minutes of the test have approximately a 35% likelihood of a future coronary event compared with a 42% likelihood in patients with 4 mm of ST depression at the same point on the test. From these data it appears that the time of onset is the more powerful prognostic variable. The onset of angina early in the test (within the first 3 minutes), in combination with early onset of ST depression, worsens the prognosis for the patient as well.[18] The persistence of the ST-segment depression after exercise appears to be a predictor of more severe coronary disease provided that 1 to 2 mm of horizontal or downsloping ST depression are used as end points for testing. Goldschlager[32] found that over 40% of patients whose ischemic ST depression resolved within 1 minute after exercise had normal coronary arteries or single-vessel disease. Ninety percent of those whose ischemic ST depression persisted for 9 or more minutes had multivessel disease, however. One should note that the predictive value for postexercise persistence of ST-segment changes might differ in patients who are taken to a symptom-limited end point despite the magnitude of ST-segment depression.

McNeer and others[43] demonstrated that patients (not on beta adrenergic receptor-blocking agents) with impaired chronotropic reserve (low maximum heart rate) had a poor prognosis with clear distinctions among those with a maximum heart rate (1) equal to or greater than 160 bpm, (2) between 120 to 159 bpm, and (3) less than 120 bpm. Forty percent of patients with a maximum heart rate below 120 had died within 4 years of follow-up. Likewise, Irving and others[35] found patients with a limited inotropic reserve to have a poor prognosis. The annual rate of sudden death was 97.9 per 1000 men if the maximum systolic pressure was less than 140 mm Hg, 25.3 if the response was between 140 and 155, and 6.6 if the systolic pressure was equal to or greater than 200 mm Hg.

The exercise capacity of the patient has also been shown to be an important prognostic indicator. McNeer and others[42] showed that patients able to perform through the third stage or longer on the Bruce test have a significantly better prognosis than those able to complete only stage I or II. In fact, patients able to complete only stage I had a 2-year survival rate less than 60%. Podrid[48] and Danegais[14] both found that even in patients with 2 or more millimeters of ST depression, the survival was closely correlated with exercise duration, and those able to enter the third or fourth stage of the Bruce test had an excellent prognosis.

Udall and Ellestad[59] have shown in the past that exercise-induced premature ventricular contractions have prognostic value in a population of patients with known coronary artery disease. Their results indicate that the annual incidence of a new coronary event (progression of angina, myocardial infarction, or death) was 1.7% in patients without premature ventricular contractions or ischemic ST changes, 6.4% in those with premature ventricular contractions alone, 9.5% in those with only ischemic ST changes, and 11.4% in those exhibiting both premature ventricular contractions and ischemic ST changes. A thorough review and analysis of the use of exercise testing as a diagnostic, prognostic and clinical tool can be found in a 1991 article by Dubach and Froelicher.[17]

## Exercise prescription and activity recommendations based on maximal exercise test results

Exercise testing to a true symptom-limited end point (versus terminating a test at a predetermined end point such as 85% of the predicted maximum heart rate) allows for an objective measurement of the patient's physical work capacity. Each workload on a test, whether it be a treadmill or bicycle ergometer, has an oxygen requirement equivalent, and there are tables or nomograms from which the predicted values can be obtained (Fig. 8-13). Therefore by taking a patient to a symptom-limited end point, one can predict his or her maximal oxygen-uptake capacity and compare the results to age- and sex-matched norms to assess the patient's degree of impairment. For clinical purposes, predicting the maximal oxygen-uptake capacity may be useful. However, one must keep in mind that the majority of tables and nomograms that exist for oxygen-uptake workload equivalent are based on normal data and therefore, there is a tendency to over estimate the cardiac patient's values by as much as 10% to 15%. As Adams and others[1,36] suggest, the prediction error is probably directly related to the severity of the patient's disease and the degree of ventricular dysfunction during exercise.[36] Bruce[8] has published a nomogram for male cardiac patients from which the degree of impairment in maximal oxygen uptake can be calculated based on the treadmill test duration and the age of the patient. Once again, Bruce's nomogram is a useful clinical tool; however, the nomogram was developed from an undefined group of cardiac patients in terms of their ventricular function and the severity of their disease.

Another point to keep in mind when assessing maximal oxygen uptake from symptom-limited exercise testing is that

| Functional class | Clinical status | O₂ requirements (ml O₂/kg/min) | Treadmill tests — Bruce* 3-min stages | Treadmill tests — Kattus+ 3-min stages | Treadmill tests — Balke# % grade at 3.4 mph | Bicycle ergometer |
|---|---|---|---|---|---|---|
| | | | mph %gr | mph %gr | | For 70 kg body weight |
| | Physically active subject | 56.0 | | | 26 | kg/min |
| | | 52.5 | | mph %gr | 24 | |
| Normal and I | | 49.0 | | 4   22 | 22 | |
| | | 45.5 | 4.2   16 | | 20 | 1500 |
| | | 42.0 | | 4   18 | 18 | 1350 |
| | Sedentary healthy | 38.5 | | | 16 | 1200 |
| | | 35.0 | | 4   14 | 14 | 1050 |
| | | 31.5 | 3.4   14 | | 12 | 900 |
| | | 28.0 | | 4   10 | 10 | |
| | Diseased, recovered / Symptomatic patients | 24.5 | 2.5   12 | 3   10 | 8 | 750 |
| II | | 21.0 | | | 6 | 600 |
| | | 17.5 | 1.7   10 | 2   10 | 4 | 450 |
| | | 14.0 | | | 2 | 300 |
| III | | 10.5 | | | | 150 |
| | | 7.0 | | | | |
| IV | | 3.5 | | | | |

**Fig. 8-13.** Classification and oxygen requirements for various workloads on treadmill and bicycle ergometers. *gr* = Grade. (From Fortuin N and Weiss JL: Exercise stress testing, *Circulation* 56(5):699, 1977.)

both the protocol and the mode of exercise can be important variables. Studies have shown that normal sedentary subjects achieve a 10% to 15% higher value for maximum oxygen uptake on a treadmill protocol compared with bicycle ergometry testing.[33,44] Our unpublished results on cardiac patients indicate that a similar disparity in the actual measured maximal oxygen uptake obtained during treadmill and bicycle testing is evident in both the sedentary and the active patient using jogging as the primary mode of training. However, in the active cardiac patient using cycling as the primary mode of training, we found no significant difference in the measured maximal oxygen uptake obtained from the two testing modes. Based on a review of the literature and our results, it appears that part of the reason for the difference in maximal oxygen uptake values obtained on treadmill and bicycle testing is attributable to the local muscle fatigue (quadriceps) that prevents a true maximal cardiovascular effort during bicycle testing of the untrained or noncyclist subject. Froelicher and others[27] compared maximal oxygen-uptake obtained on three treadmill protocols in 15 normal subjects. Their results indicate that the highest oxygen-uptake values were obtained on the Taylor protocol (com-

pared with the Bruce and Balke protocols) and the smallest coefficient of variation (a measure of reliability) was seen on the Taylor and Bruce tests.

In light of the above discussion, it would appear that ideally it is better to measure directly the cardiac patient's physical work capacity or maximum oxygen-uptake capacity by expired-gas collection and analysis. Our results indicate that the reliability of measured oxygen uptake in cardiac patients is equal to that of sex-matched inactive and active normals.[34]

The value of objective assessment of the patient's physical work capacity is at least threefold. First, the decision to allow a patient to return to work (especially a job involving relatively high levels of energy expenditures) cannot be appropriately made without knowing the patient's maximal capacity. As a guideline, the Committee on Exercise of the American Heart Association suggests that the vocational-setting work intensity during an 8-hour shift should fall within 25% to 40% range of the difference between the resting oxygen uptake and the maximal oxygen uptake. Similarly the decision to clear the patient to perform activities of daily living and recreational activities should be based in part on the relationship between the energy demand of a given activity and the patient's maximal capacity. Finally, objective evaluation of the patient's work capacity will allow for evaluation of the effectiveness of exercise therapy, medications, and surgery when the results of future tests are compared.

The results of the maximal exercise test also provide the basis on which the intensity of the therapeutic aerobic exercise program is initially formulated. Studies indicate that the minimum aerobic training needed to stimulate improvement in the oxygen-consumption capacity of patients with coronary-disease is a workload equivalent to 60% of the person's maximum oxygen consumption (which corresponds to 70% of his maximum heart rate). The desired training threshold for each patient in terms of the workload and heart rate range, can be calculated from the results of the maximal exercise test. In addition, the exercise test results provide guidelines for the therapist to determine whether it is appropriate to exercise the patient at the desired training threshold, that is, heart rates equivalent to 70% or greater of the maximum heart rate achieved on the exercise test. In other words, does the patient develop significant hypotension or hypertension, dysrhythmias, angina, and dyspnea at heart rates below 70% of maximum? Obviously, the current clinical status and medical history have a bearing as well on the establishment of the patient's recommended therapeutic intensity of exercise. Once the exercise prescription has been formulated, it is the responsibility of the therapist to evaluate the patient at the established therapeutic heart rate range, using the same skills needed for exercise testing, to determine the appropriateness of the initial exercise treatment plan (see Chapter 9).

### Interpretation of maximal exercise test results

The following is a guideline for obtaining the key results from the maximal exercise test, whether it be from the standpoint of extracting the data from a test administered by the physician or by the therapist. Refer to Appendix B for an example of a test result work sheet.

1. Demographic data
   a. Age, sex, activity level of patient (i.e. sedentary, mildly active, training)
   b. Current medication list including dose, frequency, and time of last dose taken before test
   c. Time of test
2. Protocol used (Appendix C)
   a. Sheffield, Bruce, Ellestad, Balke
   b. Intermittent versus continuous, bicycle ergometer, arm ergometer
3. Minutes or maximum workload completed
4. Resting heart rate and blood pressure
   a. Note if significant changes occur in heart rate or blood pressure with position change (i.e. supine to sitting to standing)

5. Base-line ST-segment depression or elevation and slope
   a. Note if changes occur with position changes or breathing maneuvers (10-second breathholding and 30 seconds of hyperventilation)
6. R-wave amplitude in standing position
7. Maximum heart rate and percentage of age-predicted rate achieved
8. Maximum blood pressure achieved and pressure at peak workload if different
9. Interpretation of resting and exercise systolic and diastolic blood pressures
10. Major limiting factors of test or reason test was terminated (Appendix D)
11. Statement regarding presence or absence of anginal symptoms
    a. If symptoms noted, description of the location and nature of symptoms, time and heart rate at onset and postexercise persistence should be given
12. Summary of ST-segment changes
    a. To include time and heart rate at onset, maximum magnitude of ST changes, ST-segment slope, and time required for resolution of ST changes
13. Description of significant pre- and postexercise auscultatory findings
    a. Including heart sounds, lung sounds and carotid or femoral bruits
14. Description of dysrhythmias
    a. Including the type(s) and frequency (range in terms of numbers per minute)
15. Assessment of physical work capacity
    a. To include predicted maximum oxygen consumption value and a comparison to age- and sex-matched norms

**Table 8-11.** Specific diagnoses of patients tested at Cigna 4 health plans: 1980 to 1985

| N | Diagnoses |
|---|---|
| 10,577* | |
| 5356 (51%) | Diagnostic to rule out CAD; 590 inpatients |
| 4393 (41%) | Patients with known CAD (angiographic evidence, S/P MI, or S/P CABG) |
| | 280 low-level tests on patients with recent MIs (5-21 days postevent) |
| 828 (8%) | Other (hypertension evaluations, dysrhythmia evaluations, IHSS, cardiomyopathies, valvular heart disease, COPD, or previously positive exercise test—asymptomatic) |

From Cahalin LP and others: The safety exercise testing performed independently by physical therapists, *J Cardiopulm Rehab* 7(6):269, 1987. CAD = coronary artery disease; S/P = status post; MI = myocardial infarction; CABG = coronary artery bypass graft surgery; IHSS = idiopathic hypertrophic subaortic stenosis; COPD = chronic obstructive pulmonary disease.
*Total number of exercise tests.

**Table 8-12.** A summary of the complication rates of exercise testing: 1969 to 1985

| Investigator | Number of tests | Morbidity rate (per 10,000) | Mortality rate (per 10,000) | Total complications (per 10,000) |
|---|---|---|---|---|
| Rochmis and Blackburn[49] | 170,000 | 2.4 | 1.0 | 3.4 |
| Stuart and Ellestad[56] | 514,448 | 8.3 | 0.5 | 8.8 |
| Scherer and Kaltenback[50] | 353,638* | 0 | 0 | |
| | 712,285† | 1.4 | 0.2 | 1.6 |
| Atterhog and others[2] | 50,000 | 5.2 | 0.4 | 5.6 |
| CIGNA, Cahalin[10] | 10,577 | 3.8 | 0.9 | 4.7 |

*Athletes.
†Coronary patients.

## Safety of maximal exercise testing by physicians and health care professionals

The rationale for performing maximal symptom-limited exercise tests has been discussed earlier and is summarized in Appendix A. How safe is it to perform maximal exercise tests? In 1970 Rochmis and Blackburn,[49] based on a survey of 170,000 exercise tests performed by physicians, reported a mortality rate of 1 in 10,000 and a morbidity rate (prolonged chestpain or dysrhythmia requiring hospitalization) of 2.4 per 10,000. A more recent survey by Stuart and Ellestad[56] involving over 500,000 tests, revealed a mortality rate of 0.5 per 10,000 and a morbidity rate of 9 per 10,000.[56]

Independent exercise testing by nonphysician health care professionals has been carried out in a number of laboratories for at least the last 20 years. Despite this, it was not until 1980 that the American Heart Association Committee on Stress Testing, chaired by Dr. Myrvin Ellestad, endorsed the idea of delegating exercise testing to "experienced paramedical personnel."[22,23] In a 1988 article Robert DeBusk, cardiologist and professor of medicine at Stanford, strongly advocated the use of properly trained health care professionals for exercise testing. He bases his opinion on 10 years experience at Stanford University Hospital.[15] In his opinion this practice is preferable to the use of physicians because it is more cost effective and time efficient and because physicians rarely receive formal training in exercise testing.

Because there had not been any documentation of the safety of exercise testing by health care professionals, in 1980 we began to systematically track the complications that occurred during testing performed independently by physical therapists with advanced clinical competencies. For every test, we recorded the primary diagnosis, the reason for the evaluation, and any complication during or within 24 hours after the test. At the time of our 1987 publication, our staff had performed a total of 10,577 tests.[10] A summary of the patient population tested is given in Table 8-11. A review of Table 8-12 reveals that our overall complication rate, and our morbidity and mortality rates, compare favorably with those reported previously during physician-supervised tests.

Since the 1987 article we have completed an additional 8500 tests, bringing our total to over 19,000 tests with no additional mortalities and a similar morbidity rate.

The safety and quality of patient care is obviously a reflection of the competencies of the staff performing the tests. It has been our practice to identify the advanced clinical skills necessary for the thorough evaluation of the cardiopulmonary patient first,[11,12] and then to apply these competencies to the exercise testing laboratory setting. Using this approach, we have identified specific evaluation skills that enable our staff to function safely and independently in the testing laboratory. An abbreviated form of an evaluation instrument we use to systematically determine our staff's readiness for independent exercise testing is shown in the box on p. 134.

Based on our statistics and the experience of other physical therapists performing exercise testing (including Scot Irwin's staff at Southern Regional Medical Center in Riverdale, Georgia and the nursing staff at Stanford University Hospital), it is clear that health care professionals can safely and independently perform exercise tests. Equally as important, these individuals with advanced clinical skills and knowledge are also capable of completing an accurate and thorough exercise assessment of patients with known cardiopulmonary disease. In the future it is likely that the use of qualified physical therapists and other health care professionals for testing will increase as a result of the increased demand for testing, the ongoing need for cost containment and physician time constraints.

## SUMMARY

Patient evaluation is performed systematically throughout the cardiac rehabilitation program. To effectively evaluate a patient with coronary artery disease, the therapist should be able to obtain useful clinical data and understand the relationships of that data to the basic sciences of exercise physiology, pathology, hemodynamics, and pathophysiology. As the patient moves through his or her program (phase I) to hospital discharge (phase II) to independent exercise

## Performance evaluation for independent exercise testing

| | Points | Score | | Points | Score |
|---|---|---|---|---|---|
| **I. Pretest preparation and assessment of patient** | 5 | — | F. Adequate supervision and instruction of electrocardiograph technician during the test | 5 | — |
| A. Adequate preparation in terms of having necessary materials and information (knowledge of testing protocols/guidelines) | | | | | |
| B. Consistently obtains *all* necessary information from patient's medical record | 5 | — | **III. Test interpretation** | | |
| C. Seeks additional information directly from referring physician when necessary | 5 | — | A. Demonstrates consistent accuracy in interpretation, assessment of physical work capacity/functional aerobic impairment, and summary remarks/recommendations | 55 | — |
| D. Consistently completes a thorough patient interview and physical examination | 5 | — | | | |
| E. Accurately assesses the medical data base and results from the patient interview and physical examination | 21 | — | B. Completes test interpretation within allotted time and adequately supervises electrocardiograph technicians to ensure compliance with testing schedule | 5 | — |
| F. Checks for proper calibration of testing instrumentation and correct functioning of emergency equipment | 5 | — | | | |

TOTAL    176

| | Points | Score |
|---|---|---|
| **II. Test performance** | | |
| A. Consistently makes correct judgments regarding the conducting of the test | 10 | — |
| B. Consistently obtains accurate data before, during, and after the test | 30 | — |
| C. Accurately uses above information to determine test end points | 10 | — |
| D. Accurately uses above information to determine point at which postexercise monitoring can be discontinued | 5 | — |
| E. Makes correct decision regarding need for patient follow-up of patient | 10 | — |

**IV. Ability to respond to life-threatening situations**

To test independently the therapist must have:

A. Clearance from the medical director of the exercise testing laboratory to take definitive action in event of an emergency    —

B. Current American Heart Association certification in Advanced Cardiac Life Support    —

(phase III), a matching exercise evaluation is performed. Using the clinical monitoring tools of heart rate, blood pressure, ECG changes, symptoms, and heart sounds, as well as the patient's demographic information and medical status, the therapist can make useful assessments of the patient's activity tolerance. Phase I begins with the self-care evaluation. Phase II begins with a low level exercise test, and phase III can be initiated after maximal exercise testing and cardiac catheterization.

Each assessment will afford the therapist the clinical information necessary to develop a safe, yet effective, program of exercise and education.

We recommend that each exercise-testing laboratory develop specific policies and procedures that take into consideration the patient population to be tested, the expertise of the staff involved with performance of the tests, and the equipment utilized.

**REFERENCES**

1. Adams GE and others: Oxygen uptake in cardiac patients during treadmill testing, *Cardiovasc Pulm Tech* 2:11, 1980.
2. Atterhog JH and others: Exercise testing: a prospective study of complication rates, *Am Heart J* 98:572, 1979.
3. Berman JL and others: Multiple-lead QRS changes with exercise testing, *Circulation* 63:53, 1980.
4. Blessey RL and others: Aerobic capacity and cardiac catheterization results in 13 patients with exercise bradycardia (abstract), *Med Sci Sports Exer* 8:50, 1976.
5. Bobbio M and others: How the exercise electrocardiogram is used in

clinical practice in patients with suspected coronary artery disease, *Am J Cardiol* 72:763, 1993.

6. Bonoris PE and others: Evaluation of R-wave amplitude changes versus ST-segment depression in stress testing, *Circulation* 57:904, 1978.

7. Brody DA: A theoretical analysis of the intercavity blood mass influence on the heart lead relationship, *Circ Res* 4:731, 1956.

8. Bruce RA and others: Maximal oxygen uptake and nomographic assessment of functional aerobic impairment in cardiovascular disease, *Am Heart J* 85:846, 1973.

9. Butler SM: *Phase one cardiac rehabilitation: the role of functional evaluation in patient progression,* master's thesis, Atlanta, 1983, Emory University.

10. Cahalin LP and others: The safety of exercise testing performed independently by physical therapists, *J Cardiopulm Rehab* 7(6):269, 1987.

11. Cardiopulmonary Specialty Council: *Physical Therapy Advanced Clinical Competencies,* Washington, DC, 1983.

12. Cardiopulmonary Specialty Council: *Cardiopulmonary Patient Care Competencies,* Washington, DC, ed rev, 1987.

13. Cumming GR and others: Exercise electrocardiography in normal women, *Br Heart J* 35:1055, 1973.

14. Danegais GR and others: Survival of patients with a strongly positive exercise electrocardiogram, *Circulation* 65:452, 1982.

15. DeBusk RF: Exercise test supervision: time for a reassessment, *The Exercise Standards and Malpractice Reporter* 2(5):65, 1988.

16. Deedwania PC and others: Role of myocardial oxygen demand in the pathogenesis of silent ischemia during daily life, *Am J Cardiol* 70:19F, 1992.

17. Dubach P and Froelicher VF: Recent advances in exercise testing, *J Cardiopulm Rehab* 11:29, 1991.

18. Dubin D: *Rapid interpretation of EKG's,* ed 3, Tampa, 1971, Cover Publishing Co.

19. Ehrman JK and others: Exercise stress tests after cardiac transplantation, *Am J Cardiol* 71:1372, 1993.

20. Ellestad MH: *Stress testing: principles and practice,* ed 2, Philadelphia, 1980, FA Davis Co.

21. Ellestad MH and Wan MKC: Predictive implications of stress testing, *Circulation* 51:363, 1975.

22. Ellestad MH and others: Stress testing: clinical application and predictive capacity, *Prog Cardiovasc Dis* 21:431, 1970.

23. Ellestad MH and others: Standards for adult exercise testing laboratories. In *The exercise standard book,* Dallas, 1979, The American Heart Association, Communication Division.

24. Ellestad MH and others: Changes noted in report "Adult Exercise Testing," *Circulation* 61:49, 1980.

25. Fairbarn MS and others: Prediction of heart rate and oxygen uptake during incremental and maximal exercise in healthy adults, *Chest* 105:1365, 1994.

26. Fortuin N and Weiss JL: Exercise stress testing, *Circulation* 56(5):699, 1977.

27. Froelicher VF and others: The correlation of coronary angiography and the electrocardiographic response to maximal testing in 76 asymptomatic men, *Circulation* 48:597, 1973.

28. Froelicher VF and others: A comparison of three maximal treadmill exercise protocols, *J Appl Physiol* 38:720, 1974.

29. Fuller CM and others: Early post-myocardial infarction treadmill stress testing: an accurate predictor of multivessel coronary disease and subsequent cardiac events, *Ann Intern Med* 94:734, 1981.

30. Gerson MC and others: Exercise-induced U-wave inversion as a marker of stenosis of the left anterior descending coronary artery, *Circulation* 60:1014, 1979.

31. Goldberger E: *Textbook of clinical cardiology,* St. Louis, 1981, Mosby.

32. Goldschlager N and others: Treadmill stress test indicators of presence and severity of coronary artery disease, *Ann Intern Med* 85:277, 1976.

33. Hermansen H and Salten B: Oxygen uptake during maximal treadmill and bicycle exercise, *J Appl Physiol* 26:31, 1969.

34. Ice R and others: The reliability of maximal oxygen uptake in trained and untrained normal and cardiac patients (abstract), *Med Sci Sports Exer* 14:168, 1982.

35. Irving TB and others: Variations in and significance of systolic blood pressure during maximal exercise testing, *Am J Cardiol* 39:841, 1977.

36. Iyriboz Y and Hearon CM: Blood pressure measurement at rest and during exercise, *J Cardiopulm Rehab* 12:277, 1992.

37. Kelsey MA, Kirby TE and Leier CV: Exercise response to a high incremental and low incremental treadmill protocol in patients with left ventricular dysfunction, *J Cardiopulm Rehab* 11:248, 1991.

38. Kligfield P and others: Relation of the exercise ST/HR slope to simple heart rate adjustment of ST-segment depression, *J Electrocardiol* 20:135, 1987.

39. Kligfield P and others: Heart rate adjustment of ST-segment depression for improved detection of coronary artery disease, *Circulation* 79:245, 1989.

40. Linhart SW and others: Maximum treadmill exercise electrocardiography in female patients, *Circulation* 50:1173, 1974.

41. McConnell TR and others: Prediction of functional capacity during treadmill testing: effect of handrail support, *J Cardiopulm Rehab* 11:255, 1991.

42. McNeer JF and others: The course of acute myocardial infarction: feasibility of early discharge of the uncomplicated patient, *Circulation* 51:410, 1975.

43. McNeer JF and others: The role of the exercise test in the evaluation of patients for ischemic heart disease, *Circulation* 57:64, 1978.

44. Miyamura M and Honda Y: Oxygen intake and cardiac output during maximal treadmill and bicycle exercise, *J Appl Physiol* 32:185, 1972.

45. Morales-Ballejo H and others: Septal Q wave in exercise testing: angiographic correlation, *Am J Cardiol* 48:247, 1981.

46. Morris SN and others: Incidence and significance of decreases in systolic blood pressure during graded treadmill exercise testing, *Am J Cardiol* 41:221, 1978.

47. Okin RM and others: Identification of anatomically extensive coronary disease by the exercise ECG ST segment/heart rate slope, *Am Heart J* 115:1002, 1988.

48. Podrid PJ and others: Prognosis of medically treated patients with coronary artery disease with profound ST-segment depression during exercise testing, *N Engl J Med* 306:111, 1981.

49. Rochmis P and Blackburn H: Exercise tests: a survey of procedures, safety, and litigation experience in approximately 170,000 tests, *JAMA* 217:1061, 1971.

50. Scherer D and Kaltenback M: Frequency of life-threatening complications associated with stress testing, *Dtsch Med Wochenschr* 104:1161, 1979.

51. Schwartz KM and others: Limited exercise testing soon after myocardial infarction: correlation with early coronary and left ventricular angiography, *Ann Intern Med* 94:727, 1981.

52. Sheps DS and others: Exercise-induced increase in diastolic pressure: indicator of severe coronary artery disease, *Am J Cardiol* 45:708, 1979.

53. Stange JM and Lewis RP: Early exercise test after MI, *Ann Intern Med* 94:814, 1981.

54. Starling MR and others: Exercise testing early after myocardial infarction: predictive value for subsequent unstable angina and death, *Am J Cardiol* 46:909, 1980.

55. Starling MR and others: Treadmill exercise tests pre-discharge and six weeks post-myocardial infarction to detect abnormalities of known prognostic value, *Ann Intern Med* 94:721, 1981.

56. Stuart RJ and Ellestad MH: National survey of exercise stress testing and facilities, *Chest* 77:94, 1980.

57. Theroux P and others: Prognostic value of exercise testing soon after myocardial infarction, *N Engl J Med* 301:341, 1979.

58. Thompson PD and Deleman MH: Hypotension accompanying the onset of exertional angina: a sign of severe compromise of left ventricular blood supply, *Circulation* 52:28, 1975.

59. Udall JA and Ellestad MH: Predictive implications of ventricular premature complexes associated with treadmill stress testing, *Circulation* 56:985, 1977.

60. Wagner S and others: Unreliability of exercise-induced R-wave change as indexes of coronary artery disease, *Am J Cardiol* 44:1241, 1979.

61. Werner DA and others: The predictive value of chest pain as an indicator of coronary disease during exercise testing, *Circulation* 54(suppl 2):10, 1976 (abstract).

# APPENDIX A     *GUIDELINES FOR MAXIMAL EXERCISE TESTING*

*Definition*

A maximal symptom-limited exercise test is an electrocardiographically monitored evaluation of a person's maximum oxygen consumption during dynamic work (exercise) using large muscle groups. It begins with submaximal exertion, allows time for physiological adaptations, and has progressive increments in workloads until individually determined end points of fatigue are reached or limiting symptoms or signs occur.

*Purpose*

1. To establish the diagnosis and severity of coronary artery disease through exercise-induced ECG changes. This may occur as confirmation of clinically suspected coronary artery disease or detection of latent coronary artery disease in an asymptomatic individual.
2. Evaluate the functional cardiovascular capacity and reserve in response to exercise in patients with coronary artery disease for assessment of return to work or leisure activities and candidacy for exercise-training programs.
3. To evaluate prescribed therapy as an objective measure of medical or surgical intervention. This is particularly important in the assessment of the effect of a person's participation in an ongoing aerobic exercise program.

4. To serve as motivation and as stimulus to make needed changes in behavior or life-style (e.g., to stop smoking, alter diet, or adhere to an exercise program).

*Indications for procedure*

1. After myocardial infarction or coronary artery bypass graft surgery, 4 or more weeks after either event in uncomplicated patients, greater than 4 weeks in complicated patients.
2. Outpatient referral for admission to a cardiac rehabilitation program in a patient suspected of having coronary artery disease.
3. To distinguish angina from noncardiac chest pain.
4. Development of a change in the patient's medical status that requires reevaluation of cardiovascular status (onset of hypertension, inability to maintain habitual exercise program because of onset of dyspnea, excessive fatigue, or angina), or evaluation of a change in medications.
5. Ongoing periodic reevaluation of the patient's cardiac status and physical work capacity as part of a treatment program (i.e., exercise conditioning, surgery).
6. To assist in determining whether a coronary patient can return to a particular type of vocational or recreational activity.

# APPENDIX B

## TREADMILL TEST WORKSHEET

INSTITUTION: _____

Name _____ Patient No. _____ Date _____ Age _____

Sex _____ Weight _____ Height _____ Diagnosis _____

Reason for test _____ Protocol _____

12-Lead ECG interp. _____

Time _____ Medications _____

Time last dose _____ Time last cigarette _____ Time last meal _____

Physician: _____ Activity status: _____

## TEST RESULTS

Minutes completed _____ Limiting factors _____

Resting heart rate _____ Max. heart rate _____ Resting BP _____ / _____

Max. BP _____ / _____ BP response _____

Chest pain _____

Summary ST segment changes _____

Heart sounds _____ Dysrhythmias _____

Physical work capacity _____

_____ Remarks/recommendations _____

Interpreted by _____ M.D. _____

*Continued.*

| Stage | Workload | Time | HR | BP | Angina | Dysrhy. | Y | ML | X | |
|---|---|---|---|---|---|---|---|---|---|---|
| Supine pre-exercise | | 1 | | | | | | | | |
| Supine pre-exercise | | 2 | | | | | | | | |
| Breath-holding | | 3 | | | | | | | | |
| Hyperventilation | | 3 | | | | | | | | |
| Sitting pre-exercise | | 4 | | | | | | | | |
| Standing pre-exercise | | 5 | | | | | | | | |
| | | 1 | | | | | | | | |
| | | 2 | | | | | | | | |
| | | 3 | | | | | | | | |
| | | 4 | | | | | | | | |
| | | 5 | | | | | | | | |
| | | 6 | | | | | | | | |
| | | 7 | | | | | | | | |
| | | 8 | | | | | | | | |
| | | 9 | | | | | | | | |
| | | 10 | | | | | | | | |
| | | 11 | | | | | | | | |
| | | 12 | | | | | | | | |
| | | 13 | | | | | | | | |
| | | 14 | | | | | | | | |
| | | 15 | | | | | | | | |
| Immed. post-exercise | | 0 | | | | | | | | |
| | | 1 | | | | | | | | |
| | | 2 | | | | | | | | |
| | | 3 | | | | | | | | |
| | | 4 | | | | | | | | |
| | | 5 | | | | | | | | |
| | | 6 | | | | | | | | |
| | | 7 | | | | | | | | |
| | | 8 | | | | | | | | |
| | | 9 | | | | | | | | |

| ST changes | | | V L/min | Vo$_2$ L/min | Vo$_2$ ml/kg/m | O$_2$ Pulse | RQ |
| MS 4 | V$_1$ | V$_5$ | | | | | |
|---|---|---|---|---|---|---|---|
| | | | | | | | |
| | | | | | | | |
| | | | | | | | |
| | | | | | | | |
| | | | | | | | |
| | | | | | | | |
| | | | | | | | |
| | | | | | | | |
| | | | | | | | |
| | | | | | | | |
| | | | | | | | |
| | | | | | | | |
| | | | | | | | |
| | | | | | | | |
| | | | | | | | |
| | | | | | | | |
| | | | | | | | |
| | | | | | | | |
| | | | | | | | |
| | | | | | | | |
| | | | | | | | |
| | | | | | | | |
| | | | | | | | |
| | | | | | | | |
| | | | | | | | |
| | | | | | | | |
| | | | | | | | |
| | | | | | | | |
| | | | | | | | |
| | | | | | | | |
| | | | | | | | |
| | | | | | | | |
| | | | | | | | |
| | | | | | | | |
| | | | | | | | |
| | | | | | | | |
| | | | | | | | |

## APPENDIX C  *EXERCISE TEST PROTOCOLS*

*Bruce Multistage Continuous Procotol*

| Stage | Speed (mph) | Grade (%) | Time (minutes) | Metabolic equivalents (workloads) |
|-------|-------------|-----------|----------------|-----------------------------------|
| 1 | 1.7 | 10 | 3 | 4-5 |
| 2 | 2.5 | 12 | 3 | 6-7 |
| 3 | 3.4 | 14 | 3 | 8-9 |
| 4 | 4.2 | 16 | 3 | 10-12 |
| 5 | 5.0 | 18 | 3 | Greater than 14 |

*Arm ergometry tests*
1. Continuous protocol
   a. Initial workload not less than 150 kg
   b. A total of 4 or 5 workloads, each with a duration of 2 minutes
   c. Workload increments not less than 50 kg
   d. Crank speed 50 to 60 rpm

2. Intermittent protocol
   a. Initial workload not less than 150 kg
   b. A total of 4 or 5 workloads each 3 minutes in duration followed by 3-minute recovery periods
   c. Workload increments not less than 50 kg
   d. Crank speed 50 to 60 rpm

*Bicycle ergometry tests—intermittent protocol*
1. Initial workload not less than 150 kg
2. A total of 4 or 5 workloads, each 4 minutes long, followed by 4-minute recovery periods
3. Seat height adjusted so that there is no more than 5 to 10 degrees of flexion in the knee at the lowest point in the pedal revolutions
4. Workload increments should be 20% to 25% of the difference between the initial workload and the estimated maximum workload
5. Crank speed should be maintained at 50 to 60 rpm

## APPENDIX D  *CRITERIA FOR TERMINATION OF TEST*

1. Patient's report of fatigue, which would make continued exertion uncomfortable
2. Patient's report of dizziness
3. Increasing premature ventricular contractions becoming multifocal
4. Recurrent coupled premature ventricular contractions or ventricular tachycardia (three PVCs in a row)
5. Development of rapid atrial dysrhythmias
6. Level III angina (scale of I to IV)
7. A progressive fall in systolic blood pressure of 20 mm Hg or more in the presence of increased heart rate and workload, confirmed by second blood pressure taken within 20 seconds
8. Extreme hypertensive response (systolic 250/diastolic 130)
9. Severe musculoskeletal pain as in leg claudication
10. Uninterpretable electrocardiographic tracing
11. Patient signs such as cold and clammy skin, ataxic gait, or other signs of vascular insufficiency

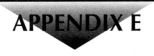

# APPENDIX E   *CONTRAINDICATIONS AND PRECAUTIONS TO EXERCISE TESTING*

1. Contraindications
   a. Overt congestive heart failure
   b. Rapid intensifying or unstable angina
   c. Recent acute myocardial infarction (less than 3 weeks)
   d. Dissecting aneurysm
   e. Second- or third-degree heart block
   f. Recurrent ventricular tachycardia
   g. Rapid atrial dysrhythmias
   h. Acute myocarditis or pericarditis
   i. Severe aortic stenosis
   j. Recent pulmonary embolus
   k. Acute infections or other active disease process

2. Precautions (attending physician to be consulted before beginning of test)
   a. Repetitive or frequent ventricular ectopic activity at rest (more than 10 premature ventricular contractions per minute)
   b. Resting hypertension (systolic 180/diastolic 110)
   c. Severe cardiomegaly
   d. Resting tachycardia of greater than 110 bpm or a recent change in cardiac symptoms

# CHAPTER 9

# Program Planning and Implementation

*Lawrence P. Cahalin, Randolph G. Ice, and Scot Irwin*

In 1978 Jan Kellerman, one of the early pioneers in the field, gave the following definition of cardiac rehabilitation: "Rehabilitation of cardiac patients is the sum of activities required to insure the best possible physical, mental and social conditions so they may, on their own efforts, regain an active and productive life."[74] The key phrase in this definition is "on their own efforts," which implies that for a cardiac patient to be rehabilitated, he or she must assume control and direction of the program. In this chapter, the rationale, design, and sequence for planning and implement-

ing such a program in a team-oriented fashion will be presented for the inpatient (phase I), subacute patient (phase II), and stable long-term patient (phase III). A brief review of primary prevention programs will also be included, as well as a review of the goals of each of the three phases, several case studies and supportive literature.

## RATIONALE AND PROGRAM DESIGN FOR CARDIAC REHABILITATION

Since the original writing of this chapter, numerous advances in technology and medical therapy have changed not only patient prognosis, but also the planning and implementation of cardiac rehabilitation programs. Percutaneous transluminal coronary angioplasty (PTCA), tissue plasminogen activator (t-PA), streptokinase, and urokinase have decreased the incidence of myocardial infarction (MI) and the amount of myocardial damage during an MI.[48] During PTCA, atherosclerotic plaques are decreased by a balloon attached to the tip of a catheter. The diameter of the balloon increases and compresses the plaque as pressure is directed into the balloon through the catheter. Streptokinase, urokinase, and t-PA are anticlotting agents that, when administered during the evolution of an MI, can lessen myocardial damage if the MI is in part the result of a thrombus.[76,80,126,161] Streptokinase and urokinase are exogenous activators that activate circulating plasminogen to plasmin, dissolving thrombi. Finally, t-PAs are natural products that attach to fibrin and only activate plasminogen already attached to fibrin, thus dissolving the fibrin clot.[24] These thrombolytic agents can be administered intravenously or directly to the coronary artery (intracoronary) (see Chapter 5). The goal of the above therapies is to preserve left ventricular function and promote a quicker recovery, after which the quality and expectancy of life may be improved.

Will these recent advances and the improved prognosis of cardiac patients lessen the need for cardiac rehabilitation in the future? This question was addressed at a conference in Mainz, West Germany, entitled "Expected Developments in Cardiology 1986-2000: Scientific, Clinical, and Economic Aspects," and resulted in the following statements: (1) aggressive therapy for coronary artery disease (CAD) increases the need for cardiac rehabilitation programs, because more patients are detected and treated earlier; (2) coping with the experience of an acute MI, bypass surgery, or acute PTCA and coping with the detection of a chronic lifelong disease needs time, help, and knowledge that can be best given in the form of organized rehabilitation programs; and (3) "The problem of coronary heart disease will not be solved with better curative therapy and comprehensive rehabilitation programs, but only with better success in starting and performing primary prevention programs."[46]

Cardiac rehabilitation programs and primary prevention programs appear to be necessary adjuncts for the treatment and continued decline of CAD, but sound scientific data supporting such a relationship have been sparse.[19,28,30,88,124,129,136,153,160] Scientific data supporting the effects of cardiac rehabilitation upon improved functional capacity,[30] psychosocial function,[39,144] health education,[18,114,118,119] morbidity and mortality,[12,99,124,129,136,153,160] and risk factor modification[19,88,102,153,160] have been inconclusive. However, a study by Kallio[70] did show substantial changes in risk factors as well as a reduction in cardiac mortality in the intervention group receiving cardiac rehabilitation. In addition, a recent meta-analysis of 10 previous studies of cardiac rehabilitation after MI estimated that cardiovascular mortality and death from all causes were reduced 25% and 24%, respectively, in patients undergoing cardiac rehabilitation.[111] Many of the studies reviewed were planned and implemented in a way similar to that advocated by the American College of Physicians.

In the October 1988 *Annals of Internal Medicine,* two articles were developed by the American College of Physicians. One reviewed the efficacy of cardiac rehabilitation services with an emphasis on patients after myocardial infarction. The other was a position paper on cardiac rehabilitation services. The review article[49] was based on patients with CAD and a history of MI, since most reports on cardiac rehabilitation are about such patients. Articles on cardiac rehabilitation published from 1976 to 1986 were reviewed for quality of data, study design, sample size, pertinence of endpoints, and clarity of presentation of the intervention procedures. Each study was then evaluated for the effects cardiac rehabilitation had on functional (work) capacity, psychosocial functioning, health-related knowledge, risk factor modification, morbidity and mortality, and cardiac function. The position papers[50] resulted from the above review and provided rationale and recommendations for cardiac rehabilitation services.

It is interesting and worth mentioning that the paper ended with a summary of costs and charges for cardiac rehabilitation services. It was estimated that a minimum of

$108 million is spent each year for medically supervised cardiac rehabilitation. The concluding sentence stated that "It is clear that on a national basis, judicious selection of candidates, combined with discharge at the earliest appropriate time, could reduce the costs substantially without jeopardizing care to properly selected patients."[50] This sentence reflects what we believe to be the beginning of a new era in cardiac rehabilitation. It is not a new thought (see the APTA position paper on cardiac rehabilitation services developed for the National Center for Health Services, October 1985) or a new practice.[116,154] At the CIGNA Healthplans of California (Los Angeles and Pomona), cardiac rehabilitation services are provided in a manner similar to that implied in the position paper of the American College of Physicians. In fact, our delivery of cardiac rehabilitation services has resulted in the formation of a new model for the design of a cardiac rehabilitation program. This model is based on individual patient need, but generally consists of one *cardiovascular assessment* per week until patient status progresses to the level necessary for maximal exercise testing. Subsequent assessments depend on the results of the maximal exercise test. Usually the reassessments are performed 1 to 2 times per month for approximately 3 to 6 months, depending on patient need. The once-a-week cardiac rehabilitation schedule can be referred to as phase II cardiac rehabilitation and the 1 to 2 times per month schedule as phase III.

In no way does this model depart from what cardiac rehabilitation is defined to provide. In contrast, it may provide more. Such assessments are *individually* designed, which improves the quality of patient care and cost effectiveness and possibly increases patient compliance with routine physical exercise. Compliance to home exercise training was studied in a random sampling of patients undergoing phase II cardiac rehabilitation once a week versus those undergoing rehabilitation three times per week. Home exercise diaries of patients in each group were compared, and the results showed significantly greater short-term and long-term compliance to home exercise in the one-time-per-week group. Although the patients were treated in two different health care delivery systems (HMO and private hospital), other studies of patients provided with less frequent cardiac rehabilitation also observed high levels of compliance to exercise training.[116,154] It is important to note that neither we nor others[95] have observed increased morbidity or mortality rates with such a reduction in medically supervised exercise.

The American College of Physicians recommends that certain high-risk patients be assessed more frequently in phase II until stabilized.[50] These include patients with the following:

1. Severely depressed left ventricular function (ejection fraction <30%)
2. Resting complex ventricular dysrhythmias (Lown type IV or V)

3. Ventricular dysrhythmias appearing or increasing with exercise
4. A decrease in systolic blood pressure of 15 mm Hg or more with exercise
5. Recent myocardial infarction (less than 6 months) complicated by serious ventricular dysrhythmias
6. Marked, exercise-induced ischemia, as indicated by either anginal pain or 2 mm (or more) ST depression by ECG
7. Survival of sudden cardiac arrest.

The allocation of cardiac rehabilitation services to patients with specific risk has been recognized and advocated by the American Association of Cardiovascular and Pulmonary Rehabilitation (AACVPR). The practice of "risk stratification" has evolved to the point of assigning a certain number of cardiac rehabilitation treatments for specific disease processes. For example, a patient with an uncomplicated inferior myocardial infarction may be assigned a specific number of treatments. However, this varies from state to state and has not been organized from a national standard of practice. The AACVPR has recently awarded a million-dollar grant to assess and define cardiac rehabilitation that should provide a national standard of practice to assist with risk stratification and legislative/reimbursement issues.

Recent advances in technology and medical therapy have demonstrated other indications for routine cardiovascular assessments, including, but not limited to, the prevalence of silent ischemia in patients with CAD,[2,4,40,146] potential need for PTCA soon after an acute MI,[61] continued evidence supporting atherosclerotic regression,[5,7,12] evaluating and reprogramming pacemakers, mild to moderate congestive heart failure,[148] poor left ventricular function,[25,59,148] and heart transplantation. Such treatment provides primary physicians with information necessary for the management of their patients, increasing the role and responsibilities of the physical therapist, and ensures quality patient care. The long-range effects of such individualized cardiac rehabilitation appear to promote patient independence and self-care. In this way, patients "regain an active and productive life" as a result of their own efforts.[74]

## PHASE 1: INPATIENT CARDIAC REHABILITATION

Phase I cardiac rehabilitation is undergoing rapid change because of a remarkable evolution in the overall care of patients with CAD.[75] Treatments for acute MI (streptokinase, t-PA), coronary insufficiency (PTCA, bypass surgery), congestive heart failure, as well as dysrhythmias (electrophysiologic study followed by dysrhythmia assessments to evaluate effectiveness of drug therapy),[75] and heart transplantation have required changes to be made in the planning and implementation of cardiac rehabilitation programs. These changes have created a noticeable reduction in the number of hospital days for patients. Data now available for post-myocardial infarction patients classify them into complicated or uncomplicated categories within the first 4 days of hospital admission (see Chapter 8). Research studies have found that patients without complications during the first 4 days after infarction can be discharged from the hospital at 7 days without increasing their mortality during the next 6 months.[93] This population usually does very well in phase I and is quickly progressed to phases II and III. Patients with complications are often not referred to cardiac rehabilitation for fear that increased activity may provoke a catastrophic event (e.g., repeat infarction, cardiac arrest).

Work by our group with this type of patient at the CIGNA Healthplans of California in Los Angeles and Pomona, the Presbyterian Intercommunity Hospital in Whittier, California, and at other sites[141] has indicated that the safety of progressive ambulation in patients with complications is as good as that in those without complications, provided that an individualized program is formulated and good communication with the referring physician is maintained. Quite often, day-to-day adjustments in antidysrhythmic, antihypertensive, or antianginal medications will help stabilize the patient much more rapidly, and facilitate progress and an earlier hospital discharge.

The rationale for many inpatient phase I programs has previously centered around the need to prevent the detrimental effects of bed rest.[157] Although that is still a goal, it is clear that most patients do not require extended periods of bed rest. Early mobilization and discharge have required phase I programs to assume an alternate emphasis and rationale. With careful activity assessment (see Chapter 8), patients without complications may be out of bed performing self-care activities and ward ambulation as early as the second or third day after an infarction. Patients with complications may be up as early as the fourth or fifth day after an infarction. Thus the goals and rationale for phase I are:

1. Assessment of hemodynamic responses to self-care and progressive ambulation activities
2. Determination of the effectiveness of the patient's medications in controlling abnormal physiological or electrocardiographic responses to activity
3. Establishment of clinical data that contribute to the patient's prognosis and thus to optimal medical management
4. Early behavior modification and risk factor reduction
5. Family education

These goals, along with the approach to patient evaluation discussed in detail in Chapter 8, encompass the treatment program for phase I. In other words, the purpose of phase I treatment for all patients (status: post-MI, CABG, PTCA, t-PA infusion, heart transplantation) is simply to evaluate progress through ever-increasing levels of activity. In addition, emphasis is placed on educating the patient's family. The patient is included in these educational activities, but in the acute setting, denial, anxiety, and medications make cognitive learning difficult.[26]

**Table 9-1.** Protocol for phase I cardiac rehabilitation program

| Day | Protocol | Team member responsible |
|---|---|---|
| 1<br>2<br>3 | Coronary care unit<br>(stabilization)<br>↓ | Physician |
| 4 | Self-care evaluation | Physical therapist, nurse, or occupational therapist |
| 5<br>6 | Monitored ambulation<br>↓ | Physical therapist |
| 7 | Low-level exercise test | Physical therapist or physician |
| 8 | Discharge | Physician |

To facilitate the cardiac rehabilitation team's effectiveness, an overall protocol for patient progression in phase I was developed. Table 9-1 illustrates the protocol for progressing a patient through phase I cardiac rehabilitation. This protocol is based on literature indicating the safety and efficacy of early ambulation programs[14,30,42,56] and on the prognostic value of early exercise testing before hospital discharge.[1,45,143,151] The protocol permits individualized treatment programs to be formulated based on objective findings during evaluation. Nonindividualized programs based on predetermined activity levels should be discouraged because such a structured system would be overly optimistic for some patients and not progressive enough for others.

### Phase I protocol

Phase I calls for a self-care evaluation as the first activity after a cardiac event (see Chapter 8). If no serious abnormalities are observed during the self-care evaluation, this level of activity is determined to be safe. The patient is then instructed to perform the self-care activities as part of the daily routine. (See the boxed material for a list of activity levels.) The program is based on the physical assessment and the evaluation and treatment procedures performed by the cardiac rehabilitation team. If the patient completes the self-care evaluation (levels 1 through 3) without significant cardiovascular problems, the patient progresses to activity level 4, which consists, in part, of monitored ambulation.

**Monitored ambulation.** Monitored ambulation refers to an individualized form of treatment in which the patient participates in a walking program while being monitored one-on-one by a physical therapist. Initially, supine, sitting, and standing heart rates and blood pressures are obtained, and a resting, single-lead electrocardiographic tracing is recorded. Heart and breath sounds may also be auscultated in selected patients (see Chapter 8). The patient is then ambulated under supervision by the therapist.

The initial distance walked is individualized for each patient. The total walk may vary from 10 to 20 feet for those in severely poor condition, to unlimited distances in those patients whose responses remain normal. During the course

## Activity levels

1.  a. Complete bed rest
    b. Independent morning care; wash hands, face, brush teeth with arms supported
    c. Feed self, with arms supported
    d. Complete bed bath; male shaved by nurse
    e. Bedside commode
2.  a. Complete bed bath; male patient may shave self; patient does own genital area
    b. Teaching materials given to patient
    c. Bedside commode
    d. Up in chair, at bedside with feet elevated, 20 to 30 minutes twice a day
    e. Flat, sitting, and standing blood pressure and apical pulse before moving to the chair on the first day
    f. Monitored self-care evaluation
3.  a. In bed, patient bathes arms, chest, and genitals; nurse bathes back, legs, and feet.
    b. May walk to bathroom with help. Flat, sitting, and standing blood pressure and pulse before ambulation on the first day.
    c. Walk to chair and sit for 30 to 60 minutes three times a day
4.  a. Same as level 3
    b. Up to bathroom as desired
    c. Up in room and chair three times a day for 30 to 60 minutes
    d. Monitored ambulation
5.  a. Sponge-bathe self, sitting in bathroom (nurse bathes back)
    b. Up in room and chair as desired
    c. Continue progressive monitored ambulation
6.  a. Sit down shower
    b. Walk in hall three times a day
7.  Walk up and down one flight of stairs
8.  Low-level treadmill test before discharge.

of ambulation, the physical therapist obtains ambulating blood pressure readings while a telemetry electrocardiogram is continuously observed and occasionally recorded (Fig. 9-1). When ambulation is completed, the therapist reevaluates the patient's hemodynamic and cardiovascular responses to determine whether activity progression is warranted (see Chapter 8).

One method of further evaluating the effectiveness of therapeutic intervention in the phase I patient population with end-stage heart disease is to assess the cardiopulmonary response and total distance ambulated during the six-minute walk test. Multivariate analysis of a number of patient characteristics before and during the six-minute walk test (age, height, weight, distance ambulated, cardiopulmonary response to exercise, cardiac output, cardiac index, and pulmonary artery pressure) identified the total distance ambulated to be the best single predictor of maximal oxygen consumption ($r = 0.74$; $p < 0.0001$). In view of this, an equation was developed to predict maximal oxygen consumption ($\dot{V}o_{2max} = 0.012 \times$ distance (feet) $- 0.735$).

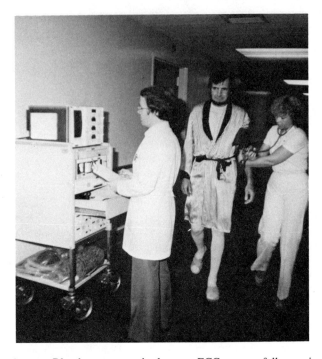

**Fig. 9-1.** Blood pressure and telemetry ECG are carefully monitored during ambulation. Blood pressures should be taken *while* walking, not afterwards.

**Monitored bicycle ergometry.** For patients unable to ambulate or in need of variety, bicycle ergometry or restorator bicycling are effective modes of increasing strength and endurance and assessing cardiopulmonary performance. Patients may begin with restorator bicycling while seated in a surgical or other supportive chair, and progress to upright bicycle ergometry when strength and endurance or mental status have improved. Unfortunately, workload is very difficult to assess with restorator bicycling, and for this reason, bicycle ergometry with workload settings is preferable.

During phase I, most patients begin with 2 to 5 minutes of continuous monitored ambulation or bicycling, and often progress to 15 to 30 minutes of treadmill or bicycle ergometry exercise. The goal is to increase endurance at a relatively mild level of energy expenditure while continuously evaluating the patient's stability and effects of medical therapy.

In most patients, this level of activity will provoke heart rates in the range of 80 to 125 beats per minute and systolic blood pressures of 120 to 150 mm Hg. If the patient is on drug therapy that alters heart rate or blood pressure, values will be significantly lower. The overall rate-pressure product during phase I will usually not exceed $20 \times 10^3$ and is usually in the range of 7 to $15 \times 10^3$. Thus, activities that progress at low rate-pressure products should not induce ischemic or other detrimental cardiovascular responses and thus should allow the patient to progress to higher levels of independent self-care and endurance. Abnormal responses at low rate-pressure products are a signal that further medical interven-

tion is necessary. The following are criteria for modifying or terminating monitored ambulation or the self-care evaluation during phase I:

1. Hypertensive blood pressure response (systolic >180 mm Hg, diastolic >110 mm Hg)
2. Hypotensive systolic blood pressure response (>10 to 15 mm Hg fall) (see Chapters 7 and 8)
3. Narrowing of the pulse pressure to <20 mm Hg between systolic and diastolic pressures
4. Development of coupled premature ventricular contractions (PVCs) or a salvo of three or more PVCs in a row (ventricular tachycardia)
5. PVCs with R-on-T phenomenon during exercise
6. Level I/IV angina pectoris
7. Onset of severe fatigue or dizziness
8. 2+/4+ dyspnea with ambulation

When any of these signs or symptoms occur, the patient's physician must be notified and appropriate documentation made in the medical chart.

In keeping with McNeer's definition of patient complications,[92] the following criteria are proposed as contraindications to the initiation of phase I therapy:

1. Overt congestive heart failure
2. MI or extension of infarction within the previous 2 days
3. Second- or third-degree heart block, coupled with PVCs or ventricular tachycardia at rest
4. Hypertensive resting blood pressure (systolic >160 mm Hg, diastolic >105 mm Hg)
5. Hypotensive resting blood pressure (systolic <80 mm Hg)
6. More than 10 to 15 PVCs per minute at rest, particularly if there is a variable coupling interval
7. Severe aortic stenosis (gradient of ≥80 mm Hg)
8. Unstable angina pectoris with recent changes in symptoms (<24 hours)
9. Dissecting aortic aneurysm
10. Uncontrolled metabolic diseases
11. Psychosis or other unstable psychological condition

Further medical management should precede phase I cardiac rehabilitation in these instances. Although phase I therapy is contraindicated in overt congestive heart failure, recent animal and human studies suggest that exercise therapy may be beneficial for patients with mild to moderate congestive heart failure.[100,101,121,140,148] Although we do not routinely train patients with significantly decompensated congestive heart failure, we do occasionally perform self-care evaluations or monitored ambulation with patients in mild to moderate congestive heart failure. Such evaluations provide the primary physician with important information to better direct medical therapy[91] and make discharge planning decisions.

The deconditioning effects of bed rest are often cited as

```
10-60    18-108
11-66    19-114
12-72    20-120         Name_____ Dr._____
13-78    21-126
14-84    22-132
15-90    23-138         INPATIENT EXERCISE LOG
16-96    24-144
17-102   25-150         TARGET HEART RATE _____
```

SPECIAL INSTRUCTION/PRECAUTIONS _____

_____

_____

| Date | Rest. HR | Distance | Time | Peak HR | Symptoms or comments |
|------|----------|----------|------|---------|----------------------|
|      |          |          |      |         |                      |
|      |          |          |      |         |                      |
|      |          |          |      |         |                      |
|      |          |          |      |         |                      |
|      |          |          |      |         |                      |
|      |          |          |      |         |                      |
|      |          |          |      |         |                      |
|      |          |          |      |         |                      |
|      |          |          |      |         |                      |
|      |          |          |      |         |                      |
|      |          |          |      |         |                      |
|      |          |          |      |         |                      |
|      |          |          |      |         |                      |
|      |          |          |      |         |                      |
|      |          |          |      |         |                      |
|      |          |          |      |         |                      |

**Fig. 9-2.** During the last few days of hospitalization, inpatients may ambulate independently using this inpatient exercise log to record results.

an indication that patients should receive inpatient cardiac rehabilitation.[157] However, with the shorter length of stay in coronary care units and earlier out-of-bed activities, the complications of excessive bed rest are rarely seen. Therefore, passive movement of the patient's extremities while in bed should be discouraged and patients should be encouraged to independently perform self-care activities (after evaluation by appropriate personnel) in and out of bed, which provides more effective and appropriate range of motion.

Quite frequently, patients without complications perform their individualized ambulation services on the ward several times each day. Instructions are given to capable patients to keep a record of their ambulation distance, time, and heart rate response as illustrated in Figs. 9-2 and 9-14. When the ambulation prescription is progressed, electrocardiographic monitoring should be employed to further assess the status of the cardiopulmonary system (i.e., ischemia, dysrhythmias). If the patient's exercise prescription update is performed safely without ischemia, ectopy, or adverse blood pressure response, subsequent similar ambulation can be performed independently with the ward clerk monitoring the telemetry electrocardiogram. This monitoring method is most cost-effective, because the patient requires only one or two formal supervised ambulation sessions per day. The patient can then exercise an additional two or three times per day on his or her own. This independent ambulation improves self-confidence and helps to prepare the patient both physiologically and psychologically for subsequent predischarge exercise testing.

**Low-to-moderate-level exercise testing.** Exercise testing soon after a cardiac event provides important information pertaining to a patient's stability and prognosis, as well as medical therapy.[79] Several studies have documented the significance of this prognostic information and the safety of such testing.[1,45,143,151] In fact, since January 1980, we have performed 400 low-level tests 5 to 21 days after MI. Twenty-five of these were begun as low-level tests, but progressed to moderate or maximal levels. No complications occurred during these tests.

Such testing is important because there are subsets of patients admitted with an MI or unstable angina who are at high risk of repeat infarction or of sudden death, particularly in the first few months after discharge. An exercise test performed to a heart rate of 120 to 140 beats per minute is the best physiological evaluation tool currently available to uncover patients at higher risk (see Chapter 8). During predischarge exercise testing, high-risk persons may demonstrate a hypoadaptive blood pressure response,[132,152] 2 mm or more of ST-segment depression,[47,155,156] angina pectoris,[152] or complex ventricular dysrhythmias[155] (see Chapters 7 and 8). For example, Stein[143] elicited angina in 29% of his post-MI patients during early exercise testing, 55% of whom were not expected to have angina. Severe dysrhythmias were also seen in 31% of his patients, 60% of whom then required the addition of antidysrhythmic therapy. As a result of the testing, 47% of the population had their post-MI medical therapy altered. It is, therefore, evident that with these test results, the physician can accurately provide appropriate therapy to improve abnormal cardiovascular responses and patient prognosis. In addition, the physical therapist can more appropriately prescribe proper exercise training and recommend a return to normal activities or prescribe a lower functional level of activity.

Therefore, the low-level exercise test provides the rehabilitation team with important information regarding the safety of home activities of daily living requiring from 4 to 6 metabolic equivalents of exertion (e.g., driving, housework, sexual activity) and base-line information required to develop an initial exercise training program. For example, if a patient exhibits a poor work capacity, angina, and pronounced ST-segment changes (>2 mm), this suggests that other vessels are at risk or a zone of ischemia exists around an infarcted area. Low-level exercise with additional drug therapy, such as beta-blocking agents and long-acting nitrates, may be needed for these patients to exercise comfortably and safely. These drugs should optimally be used after discharge in a phase II program where close monitoring is available.

Very little has been written on the value of this type of test for the postbypass patient; however, we believe it to be an essential part of the overall patient evaluation before discharge. It helps determine readiness for discharge and establish activity guidelines. Some centers have progressed to the use of symptom-limited maximal exercise testing for their post-bypass patients before discharge.[128] The rationale is that with successful myocardial revascularization, it is unlikely that the patient will demonstrate abnormal responses to testing such as ST-segment depression or angina. However, it is expected that these patients will have blunted or hypoadaptive blood pressure responses because of anemia or temporary postoperative ventricular dysfunction. They will usually be very tachycardic with exertion, fatigue easily, and quite often demonstrate atrial irritability (e.g., premature atrial contractions, shorts runs of supraventricular tachycardia) during exercise.[128]

Four of the six case studies included at the end of this chapter illustrate individualized program planning and its effective use in phase I cardiac rehabilitation. Among them is a typical postbypass patient without complications, a severely impaired patient with multiple complications after infarction, and a complicated patient who underwent many of the more recent medical interventions.

## PHASE II: OUTPATIENT CARDIAC REHABILITATION

The term "phase II" refers to that part of the cardiac rehabilitation program conducted on an outpatient basis immediately after hospitalization. It involves a closely supervised and carefully monitored exercise program with a structured basic education series. This program may include patients who have been recently discharged from the hospital after myocardial infarction, coronary bypass surgery, or PTCA. Others who may be included in a phase II program are those with stable angina pectoris, hypertension, dysrhythmias, compensated congestive heart failure, mitral valve prolapse with ventricular dysrhythmias, or asymptomatic patients with latent coronary disease.

The following are purposes of phase II programs:

1. Increase exercise capacity and endurance in a safe and progressive manner
2. Ensure the continuity of the exercise program with a transition to the home environment
3. Assess the cardiovascular responses of mild to moderate external workloads and give feedback to the referring physician
4. Teach the patient to apply techniques of self-monitoring to home activities
5. Obtain monitored objective information on medication effectiveness in such areas as angina, blood pressure regulation, and dysrhythmia control
6. Relieve anxiety and depression
7. Increase the patient's knowledge of the atherosclerotic disease process and how personal health habits affect it

It is advantageous for patients to be referred to phase II immediately after hospital discharge. In addition to the medical reasons previously discussed, coronary patients are more easily influenced and educated at this time because of fear and anxiety about their health and longevity. As many studies have documented, coronary patients go through an adjustment period after an MI consisting of initial denial or anger, followed by depression.[26,144] Cardiac rehabilitation is the process that directs and supports physical, emotional, and psychological recovery. We believe it is a process that should begin in the hospital and continue without interruption.

## Training program

Physical training of patients in phase II requires consideration of many variables, including exercise intensity, duration, frequency, and mode; age, sex, general musculoskeletal status of the patient; time since MI, PTCA, or coronary bypass surgery; size of the infarction; subsequent complications such as development of angina pectoris or other signs of myocardial ischemia; medications; and the patient's own goals. In addition, specific skills in assessment are needed to assist in individualizing the training programs. The five key areas to assess include (1) heart rate, (2) blood pressure, (3) electrocardiogram, (4) heart sounds, and (5) signs and symptoms. An individualized approach to each patient must use these variables (see Chapter 8).

Identifying spinal or lower-extremity problems before initiating cardiovascular training may prevent the development of orthopedic problems. These kinds of problems are common in middle-aged and older people who embark on exercise programs. A musculoskeletal evaluation is necessary to identify lower-extremity problems such as arthritis, old orthopedic injuries, and unusual biomechanical abnormalities (excess pronation of the foot, genu valgum). Although in many cases these biomechanical abnormalities are of no consequence in a patient's everyday routine, under specific lower-extremity training they may develop into symptomatic orthopedic problems that interfere with the normal cardiovascular conditioning program.

The current literature supports a phase II training program that is varied in nature and includes a combination of upper- and lower-extremity training.[44,159] Training of the lower extremities is specific to the lower extremities, and there is little cardiovascular carry-over to upper-extremity work and vice versa.[21] Therefore, since a goal of physical conditioning is to reduce myocardial oxygen demand with arm or leg activities at any given level of submaximal work, it is essential to train both arms and legs (Fig. 9-3). Lower-extremity aerobic exercise is accomplished with stationary equipment such as treadmills and bicycle ergometers (Fig. 9-4). Upper-extremity training is done with arm ergometer units and rowing machines. Programs that employ these types of equipment can improve both endurance and physical work capacity of all patients involved in phase II cardiac rehabilitation. A variety of programs that include

oxygen-demanding cardiovascular exercises can be planned with such equipment; however, upper-extremity training is not started until 3 to 4 weeks after surgery in postbypass or valve replacement patients. Chest soreness and bone healing precludes aggressive arm work for several weeks after bypass surgery.

## Intensity of exercise

Before entering phase II, patients undergo a low- to moderate-level or maximal exercise test. A low-to-moderate-level test with a predetermined end point is appropriate for the early post-MI and postbypass patient. The training intensity of exercise during phase II should be a percentage of the maximum heart rate achieved on this exercise test. One goal of phase II is to improve aerobic endurance; therefore, training levels are set at an intensity of work that will not interfere with the healing process or produce cardiovascular complications.

In our experience training post-MI, post-PTCA, and post bypass patients, we noted that patients are able to tolerate training at 80% to 100% of the heart rate achieved during the low-level test. Training at this level is not associated with any increased risk of reinfarction, congestive heart failure, or other morbidity or mortality.[11] Occasionally we have found that patients who demonstrate no dysrhythmias or symptoms on a low- to moderate-level exercise test may exhibit one or more of these abnormalities during the initial sessions in phase II. Again, close communication with the physician and medical director is required to ensure medical stabilization of these patients.

Early post-MI and postbypass patients can usually only

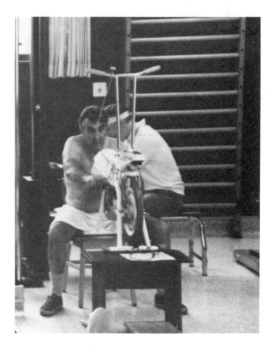

**Fig. 9-3.** Upper extremity ergometry may be done when a stationary bicycle is placed on a chair and stool.

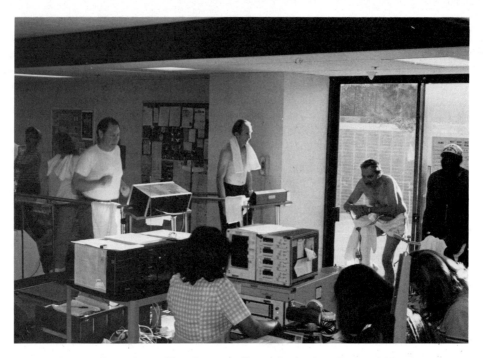

**Fig. 9-4.** Many cardiac patients will prefer treadmill exercise in phase II, though bicycle ergometers are necessary for those with lower extremity orthopedic problems.

tolerate 10 to 15 minutes of continuous low-intensity training. Patients who have undergone PTCA without previous or subsequent myocardial bypass generally exercise continuously for 20 to 30 minutes during the initial assessment. The emphasis during this initial 2 to 4 weeks is on increasing the peak exercise interval time to 30 to 45 minutes of continuous exercise.

After the first 2 to 3 weeks of phase II, patients with good blood pressure responses, no ECG abnormalities, and no angina are progressed to higher levels of work by increasing the target heart rate by 10 beats per minute. For patients without complications, the target heart rate during exercise may be raised 10 beats every 1 to 2 weeks. Patients with complications may have their target heart rate increased, or they may stay at the same level until the maximum exercise test is done. Increases in the intensity of training (target heart rate increases) are determined by careful review of the patient's monitored responses. If the patient exhibits angina, serious dysrhythmias, poor blood pressure responses, symptoms of *poor* ventricular function, or musculoskeletal difficulties, the intensity of exercise should remain unchanged or even be decreased. As these abnormalities resolve or decrease in severity, closely supervised workload increases can be applied. Each time the peak exercise heart rate is raised to a higher level, close monitoring of symptoms and physiologic adaptations is required. Patients with complications who require close monitoring are those who (1) are limited by angina, (2) have excessively hypertensive or hypotensive (≥15 mm Hg) blood pressure responses, (3) develop rapid supraventricular dysrhythmias, (4) develop

ventricular dysrhythmias, or (5) have severely depressed left ventricular function.[50] Oral and written communication regarding these medical problems is maintained with the patient's physician (see Chapter 11). Phase II is similar to phase I in its monitoring methods and examination of the effectiveness of medical management during the early recovery process.

### Supervision and program progression

Progression to an independent exercise program is an important goal during phase II. Promoting the ability to exercise only within the monitored hospital-based sessions fosters an attitude of dependency on the electronic hardware and supervisory personnel who conduct the exercise sessions. Ultimately, a cardiac rehabilitation program should attempt to develop an attitude of self-responsibility for medical care, including the physical exercise program. It has been our experience that patients more rapidly improve psychologically when they reach a state of illness adjustment that acknowledges their contribution to their health status and a willingness to accept the responsibility for performing home exercise. During phase II, the patient usually progresses to 30 to 45 minutes of continuous lower-extremity exercise and is encouraged to perform 10 to 15 minutes of continuous upper-extremity exercise as well. With this combination, the overall peak exercise period is approximately 45 to 60 minutes. A 5-minute warm-up and cool-down period precedes and terminates all training sessions. Supervised, monitored exercise is performed 1 to 3 or more times per week, based on patient status and need.

The patients assume personal responsibility for monitoring and completing additional exercise sessions at home. Home sessions begin in the first 1 to 2 weeks of phase II. The patients exercise for the same period of time and at similar training intensities as they did in the sessions conducted at the hospital. The total number of exercise sessions recommended per week is five or six. Exercise performed at home should be documented in an exercise diary similar to that used in phase I cardiac rehabilitation (Fig. 9-2). However, the home exercise information is better appreciated over a month's duration (Fig. 9-14). The monthly summary of information can be helpful for the assessment and progression of a patient's exercise prescription. With this information, the physical therapist can review problems the patient has during home exercise sessions when the individual comes in for monitored follow-up sessions. Medical intervention and program modifications are made at that time.

Monitoring of patients during phase II exercise employs continuous and intermittent portable radiotelemetry electrocardiographic equipment (see Chapter 11). Continuous ECG monitoring of every exercise session does not last more than 8 to 12 weeks unless serious dysrhythmias are consistently documented. Each patient is "weaned" from the monitor by decreasing use to every other and then every third session. This process continues until "spot" checks are performed with paddle defibrillators. By the end of phase II, most patients rely only on self-monitoring of their heart rate.

In addition, we have found it of value to incorporate some forms of "anaerobic" training into the second half of phase II. An individualized weight training program that emphasizes high repetitions and low weights is a safe and effective adjunct[73] (Fig. 9-5). This type of training has proved valuable in helping patients recover quickly from myocardial infarction or coronary bypass surgery. Weight training improves both peripheral muscle tone and strength. It adds to patients' self-confidence, and they are better able to perform daily activities. Most daily activities, either around the home or at work, are not aerobic in nature and often require some degree of static effort. Examples of anaerobic activities include yard work, grocery shopping, and housework such as vacuuming, mopping, or window washing. Because these activities require muscle strength, incorporating mild strength training into the phase II program is essential.

Selected patients who are candidates for weight training include myocardial infarction patients a minimum of 3 weeks after the event and surgical patients 3 to 4 weeks after the surgery. PTCA patients without MI can begin weight training immediately upon discharge. A multistation apparatus is used for three selected arm and leg exercises. Patients are instructed to avoid the Valsalva maneuver and to coordinate inhalation and exhalation with the concentric and eccentric phases of the exercise movements (Fig. 9-6). Usually two sets of a weight that can be handled easily for 10 to 12 repetitions is the starting point. The emphasis is initially on adding sets the first 2 to 3 weeks, and weight, usually 5 to 10 pounds at a time, is added the next 2 to 3 weeks. Continuous ECG monitoring is done during the initial anaerobic exercise sessions. In our experience, the myocardial oxygen demand is lower during anaerobic training than during the aerobic portion of the training program, as indicated by lower rate-pressure products. We have observed few ventricular dysrhythmias and have had no complications during this type of "isotonic" exercise. As the patient is weaned from telemetry monitoring at the end of phase II, we encourage non–ECG-monitored weight training with therapist supervision. Many patients who graduate from our phase II program continue with weight training at home, in phase III, or at a local health club.

### Safety in phase II

The early post-MI and postbypass patient is at high risk of cardiovascular complications during the first 3 to 6

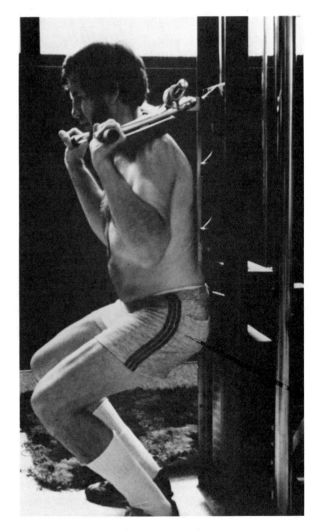

**Fig. 9-5.** This cardiac patient, who had coronary artery bypass surgery (CABG) 8 weeks before, is performing half-squats with 70 pounds.

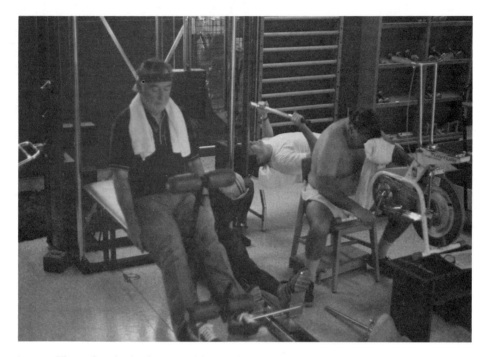

**Fig. 9-6.** The patient in the foreground is exhaling during concentric work with 40 pounds (knee extensions), whereas the other patient is inhaling during eccentric work with 50 pounds (bench press).

months after discharge from the hospital.[99] Statistics show that early exercise conditioning during this period and later is not associated with any higher risk of morbidity or mortality.[10,11,13,150] At the Ross-Loos Medical Center, we studied 85 post-MI patients who were entered into an early exercise training program immediately after hospital discharge.[11] They were classified according to McNeer's criteria (see Chapter 8) into groups of those with complications and those without. During 802 patient hours of early exercise training, there were no adverse effects noted in either subgroup. Since 1979 in the rehabilitation programs at Presbyterian Intercommunity Hospital in Whittier, California, and CIGNA Healthplans in Los Angeles and Pomona, we have accumulated over 30,000 hours of early exercise conditioning in phase II with no cardiovascular mortality and no cardiac arrest.

### Basic patient education lecture series

Our phase II program offers a series of lectures conducted by several team members. These talks are designed to educate the cardiac patient about atherosclerosis, risk factors for heart disease, and the effects of exercise, diet, stress, and medications upon cardiac disease (see the box on p. 153). Often, patients do not retain the educational information provided during phase I because they are not receptive to learning during their acute hospitalization. Learning is enhanced when the patient is out of the hospital and living in a familiar environment. A variety of audiovisual aids (slides, movies, posters) is used to simplify concepts (atherogenesis, role of smoking, and diet in disease progression).

Individual conference sessions are also helpful. For example, fasting serum lipid panels are routinely obtained (cholesterol, triglycerides, HDL, LDL, and VLDL cholesterol, and phenotype) on all patients 4 weeks after a myocardial infarction, surgery, or PTCA (Fig. 9-7). These lipids are reviewed individually with each patient and covered again during the dietitian's lecture, and serve as a baseline for measuring the effects of the intervention program every 6 months thereafter (see Chapter 10). A written, multiple-choice pretest was recently developed by our team to measure the level of knowledge and understanding of outpatients before starting the education series. The same test was given at the end of the 4-week lecture series for assessment of each patient's learning. Analysis of data from the before and after tests over the last few years has been helpful in improving our teaching methods and determining the level of understanding and knowledge obtained by individual patients.

### Termination of phase II

Because phase II is considered a recovery period, as well as a physical conditioning time, the process usually takes a minimum of 6 to 8 weeks. Patients who make initial endurance gains by 6 to 8 weeks after the event are often anxious to pursue higher-intensity exercise and other activities (bowling, dancing, golf, hiking, swimming, running, camping in the mountains). At this point, our protocol calls for a maximal symptom-limited exercise test. The patient is exercise tested through a symptom-limited end point (see Chapter 8). This test serves as a diagnostic procedure to further evaluate the extent of coronary artery

---

## Cardiac rehabilitation program: basic patient education series

*Time:* 4:00 to 5:00 PM                                                          *Place:* Santa Fe Springs Room

| Date | Lecture topic | Instructor |
|---|---|---|
| Jan. 5 | Structure and function of the heart, coronary atherosclerosis, heart attack, angina pectoris, coronary bypass | Larry Cahalin, PT |
| Jan. 7 | The causes of atherosclerosis (risk factors and atherosclerosis) | Diane Tatman, PT |
| Jan. 10 | Cardiac medications: their purposes and side effects | Joyce Knopp, RN |
| Jan. 12 | The therapeutic effects of exercise | Peggy Johnson, PT |
|  | *Film: Quite an Accomplishment* |  |
| Jan. 14 | Managing stress: film and discussion | Barbara Lane, MSW |
| Jan. 17 | Diet, blood fats, and coronary artery disease | Karen Broxson, RD |
| Jan. 19 | Sex and the heart patient* | Barbara Lane, MSW |
| Jan. 21 | Shaking the salt habit: relationship of diet and hypertension | Karen Broxson, RD |
| Jan. 24 | *Film: Coping with Life on the Run* | Dr. George Sheehan |
|  | *Film: The Cardiac TransAmerica Express* | Randy Ice, PT |

* Please bring spouse or significant other to the January nineteenth talk on sex

LIPID PROFILE

| Name: | | Risk | Total Chol/HDL |
|---|---|---|---|
| Date: | Men: | ½ Average | 3.43 |
| Initial ___ F/U ___ | | Average | 4.97 |
| Cholesterol ___ | | 2X Average | 9.55 |
| Triglycerides ___ | | 3X Average | 23.39 |
| HDL ___ | Women: | ½ Average | 3.27 |
| LDL ___ | | Average | 4.44 |
| VLDL ___ | | 2X Average | 7.05 |
| Total Chol/HDL ___ | | 3X Average | 11.04 |

**Fig. 9-7.** This lipid profile form is used to give feedback to each patient on initial and serial lipid results.

disease in post-MI patients, and provides an objective measurement of physical work capacity. A maximal symptom-limited test will also indicate the effectiveness of revascularization procedures or PTCA and document any symptomatic changes with exercise.

If the patient does exceptionally well on the maximal exercise test, the physician may clear the patient to return to either full-time or part-time work and the patient will have completed phase II. At the completion of phase II, the patient is encouraged to continue a physical training program independently at home with further instructions from the physical therapist. Our patients are encouraged to continue the cardiac rehabilitation participation in a phase III program.

### Return to work after phase II

Literature regarding return-to-work statistics for post-MI or postbypass patients participating in phase II cardiac rehabilitation programs has been inconclusive.[62,77,116,135] There are many variables that influence return to work after the onset of coronary artery disease, many of which are completely unrelated to the degree of coronary disease or myocardial damage. Such factors as employment before myocardial infarction or bypass surgery, job satisfaction, employer attitudes, financial incentives, physician attitude, and other socioeconomic factors play a role in determining whether a post-MI or postbypass patient will return to work. Cardiac rehabilitation promotes a positive attitude toward return to work for such patients.

This attitude is instilled early in a phase II training program.

In our experience, 75% to 80% of rehabilitated patients will return to work within 8 to 10 weeks after myocardial infarction.[150] In our rehabilitation program, of the 75% of the total postbypass patients who worked before surgery, 62% went back to work after surgery. In a control group of patients who did not undergo cardiac rehabilitation, the percentages before and after surgery were very similar; however, cardiac rehabilitation patients returned to work an average of almost 40 days sooner than nonrehabilitation patients.[150] Our work supports the concept that a cardiac rehabilitation environment fosters the concept of early return to work and may reduce the length of disability after bypass surgery. This finding is significant in light of the fact that many studies have lamented the clear-cut lack of improvement in return to work after coronary surgery.[6,52,86]

## Results of training

The effect of exercise training on functional capacity has been a topic of investigation for many years. Previous studies have shown that gradual improvement in physical work capacity will occur in patients after an MI even without formal cardiac rehabilitation.[30,164] Therefore, the role of supervised exercise training in cardiac rehabilitation is to expedite the improvement in physical work capacity and evaluate patient status (i.e., blood pressure, rhythm, and symptoms) so that medical therapy can be directed better. A recent review[49] of previous studies that evaluated the improvement in physical work capacity in patients after MI[19,30,64,88,95,117,129,160] indicated that the differences in physical work capacity between training groups and control groups *in all studies* were statistically significant, and suggested that "the magnitudes of the differences reported are relatively small (averaging 20% to 25%)."[49] This may appear to be a relatively small difference, but in patients with CAD, such an improvement or less could be the difference between climbing a flight of stairs with angina or climbing stairs without symptoms.

Blessey and others[13] examined the effects of early exercise training in 85 post-MI patients. Patients were divided into two groups, those with complications and those without, based upon McNeer's criteria. Exercise training was initiated within 7 to 14 days after MI and was performed at 70% of the patient's maximum heart rate obtained from predischarge exercise tests. Exercise testing was repeated after the early exercise training period. The patients without complications had an improved performance on both the predischarge exercise test and the posttraining exercise test when compared to the patients with complications. In addition, both groups demonstrated significantly improved exercise capacity during exercise testing after training when compared with age- and sex-matched controls.[13]

During the phase II follow-up period, 9% of patients in each group demonstrated either resting or exercise hyper-

tension or the new onset of angina. Complex ventricular dysrhythmias were observed in a total of six patients, with five of these being in the group with complications. Follow-up of 802 patient hours of early exercise training revealed no cardiovascular morbidity or mortality in either group.[13] Thus, it was concluded that selected patients, those with complications and those without, could safely participate in and respond favorably to early exercise training. Patients without complications had a tendency to demonstrate a better exercise tolerance initially, as well as after training, and they were less likely to have complex ventricular dysrhythmias.[13]

Is cardiac rehabilitation beneficial for patients with poor left ventricular function? To answer this question, it is important to first define "beneficial." Previous studies evaluating the effects of training in subjects with left ventricular dysfunction have defined beneficial as an increase in physical work capacity or $\dot{V}O_{2max}$[81,83] (see Chapter 10). Such an increase is very important for a patient with poor left ventricular function. Cardiovascular assessments of symptoms, blood pressure, and rhythm responses to varying levels of exercises are also important to determine patient stability and to better direct medical therapy. Such assessments also allow the patient to better understand his or her fitness level, expectations, and prognosis. In our experience, routine cardiovascular assessments appear to improve patient prognosis and quality of life.

A lack of data exists regarding the evaluation of symptoms, blood pressure, and rhythm responses, the effect of exercise training on patient prognosis, and quality of life in patients with poor left ventricular function. However, previous and recent literature has suggested significant improvements in exercise tolerance and ischemia after a program of routine aerobic exercise.[23,25,59,81,83,148] Conn and colleagues[25] discovered a 20% increase in exercise capacity in a small group of patients (n = 10) who had ejection fractions ranging from 13% to 26%. The mean duration of supervised exercise training was 12 months, during which time no morbidity or mortality occurred.

In addition, a larger number of subjects (n = 41) with impaired left ventricular function following an acute MI were recently studied.[59] These individuals demonstrated moderately impaired left ventricular function, determined by the presence of at least two of the following echocardiographic parameters: (1) left atrial diameter ≥35 mm, (2) end-diastolic left ventricular diameter ≥60 mm, or (3) distance between the E-point and the interventricular septum ≥12 mm. The ejection fraction was not estimated. Of the 41 patients, 21 were assigned to a control group, while 20 participated in a 4-month supervised outpatient exercise training program. Initial bicycle ergometry exercise tests revealed no significant difference in exercise tolerance between groups. The exercise training group attended a 50-minute training session three times per week and performed unsupervised training at home. Follow-up testing revealed that the intervention group significantly increased its maximal working capacity, exercise duration, total work, and maximal aerobic power compared with the control group. These effects were achieved without complication.

Other studies evaluating the effects of aerobic exercise training in patients with poor left ventricular function and mild to moderate congestive heart failure also demonstrated the importance of regular aerobic exercise.[23,148] Regular aerobic exercise that is supervised occasionally and performed at levels within an individual's exercise capacity can avoid the deleterious effects of deconditioning and augment peak exercise capacity, which in turn can improve patient comfort during submaximal effort.[23] This was exemplified in two recent studies that evaluated the effects of exercise training in patients with chronic heart failure attributed to left ventricular dysfunction (ejection fraction of 19.6% to 24%).[148] In the study by Sullivan and others, left ventricular dysfunction was the result of either CAD or idiopathic cardiomyopathy. Twelve ambulatory patients with stable symptoms underwent maximal bicycle exercise testing before and after a 4- to 6-month training program consisting of stationary bicycling, walking, jogging, and stairclimbing 4 hours per week at approximately 75% of $\dot{V}o_{2max}$. Central hemodynamic and peripheral metabolic adaptations to heart failure were improved after exercise training. These changes allowed for an increased exercise tolerance, apparently due to increased blood flow to the exercising legs at peak exercise.[148] The second study, performed by Coats and others, demonstrated significantly increased exercise duration, peak oxygen consumption, and submaximal and maximal cardiac output after an 8-week bicycle crossover trial of 17 men with stable, moderate to severe congestive heart failure. They also demonstrated decreased rate-pressure products, patient-related symptom scores, and submaximum heart rates. The reduction in submaximum heart rates during exercise testing was highly correlated to improved maximal oxygen consumption. The physiologic basis for this improvement was suggested to be due to either an improvement in myocardial contractile performance or diastolic compliance. The above studies, which were performed without significant complications, demonstrate the importance of proper exercise training in patients with chronic congestive heart failure.

Despite these recommendations, two other important studies have suggested that specific criteria must be present for training effects to occur in subjects with poor left ventricular function.[3,69] Arvan[3] evaluated the results of a 12-week cardiac rehabilitation program in high-risk patients after an acute MI.

He observed that patients who had both significant left ventricular dysfunction and myocardial ischemia did not demonstrate training effects, but that those with left ventricular dysfunction without myocardial ischemia demonstrated significant improvement in exercise performance and peak oxygen consumption. The relatively short duration of the study (12 weeks) may have prevented training effects from occurring in the group with left ventricular dysfunction and myocardial ischemia. A longer period of exercise training may have produced training effects while also reducing risk factors.

Another study by Jugdutt and others[69] evaluated the importance of regional left ventricular function during exercise training, and discovered that exercise training in patients with a large acute transmural anterior MI may cause more left ventricular dysfunction, resulting in a decreased ejection fraction and functional capacity. These changes were evaluated via two-dimensional echocardiography and allowed the investigators to determine optimal left ventricular performance necessary to prevent the above effects. A level of <18% regional left ventricular asynergy (an index of contractile dysfunction) was associated with no further functional or topographic deterioration during exercise training. Cardiac catheterization and echocardiographic findings of significant akinesis or dyskinesis should alert clinicians to closely observe such patients during exercise training. These patients may also benefit from serial echocardiographic studies to assess left ventricular function. This information and occasional cardiovascular assessments can better direct the medical treatment of these complicated patients.

In conclusion, several studies have shown substantial increases in exercise tolerance in patients with impaired left ventricular function and an initial poor physical work capacity. These findings are supported by the American College of Physicians position statement on cardiac rehabilitation, which states that "Patients with cardiac disease with significant limitation of maximal work capacity, for example, less than 7 METS soon after infarction, may expect to achieve meaningful improvement in work capacity by participating in an exercise training program. The 15% to 25% greater improvement in work capacity that may be expected to occur in an exercise program is likely to be of greatest clinical benefit in such patients."[49]

The case studies at the end of this chapter illustrate examples of post-MI and postbypass patients who have progressed through a phase II training program and responded very favorably.

## PHASE III: OUTPATIENT CARDIAC REHABILITATION

A phase III cardiac rehabilitation program (also known as phase IV or "maintenance" in some facilities) is an ongoing, supervised exercise conditioning program. It provides the coronary artery disease patient the opportunity to achieve a higher level of physical, mental, and sociological function. Typically, a phase III program provides incentives for the patient to continue a lifelong habit of exercise, risk factor reduction, and ongoing education. These programs should also provide a mechanism for serial evaluation to assess progress and disease stability.

Typically, patients are referred to phase III rehabilitation programs at least 4 to 6 weeks post-MI, postbypass surgery, or PTCA. Patients with stable angina pectoris, abnormal exercise tests, or who are asymptomatic and have a high risk for the development of symptomatic coronary disease are also referred to phase III. Ambitious patients who are 1 to 4 weeks post-PTCA, who have been educated and assessed in phase II, and who do well during maximal exercise testing are quickly progressed into phase III. Many phase III programs are open-ended without discharge criteria. The patient also assumes a greater financial burden in a phase III program after the initial 6 months to 1 year since phase III cardiac rehabilitation is frequently not a reimbursed service.

Although several nonrandomized studies have suggested a decreased morbidity and mortality for patients who participate in long-term cardiac rehabilitation,[57,58,72] randomized trials have not been as supportive.[122,136,160] Compliance with the prescribed program is a major problem in both types of study. This difficulty exists because of the nature of the life-style changes involved. Typically, the noncompliant cardiac rehabilitation patient is a habitual smoker, a blue-collar worker, spends leisure time in sedentary activities, and works at a job that requires little energy expenditure.[109] Frequently with long-term rehabilitation programs, the participant rate may drop to as little as 30% to 40% after the first year and decrease at a rate of 10% per year thereafter (see Chapter 10). The reasons for this high drop-out rate may relate to psychological changes the patient is experiencing. Fear will motivate most patients for only a short period of time, and compliance with exercise, diet, and nonsmoking directives will lessen as fear abates. Over the long run, compliance will come only with external and internal rewards for behavior modification. If the patient perceives the life-style changes to mean deprivation and giving up enjoyable habits, and if these needs are not replaced with habits that are equally or more rewarding, it will be only a matter of time before the patient returns to the premorbid life-style with previous level of risk factors for coronary artery disease. The phase III program should, therefore, provide ongoing rewards, feedback, and encouragement to help the patient adjust to this kind of problem and successfully adhere to the cardiac rehabilitation program.

## Location of phase III program

To establish a phase III program, one has to examine the personnel available to staff it, the geographical location, and the medical support systems available. The minimum equipment requirement for phase III includes a radiotelemetry system with the capability to monitor patients exercising on a track, and outdoor exercise area (preferably with lights), locker rooms with shower facilities, and an educational room with facilities for audiovisual aids such as slides, movie projectors, or videocassette systems (see Chapter 11).

Because the patient has achieved a higher level of fitness by phase III and requires less supervision and monitoring, a greater variety of exercise modalities and procedures can be carried out. For this reason, phase III programs can be established at either a hospital facility or a community facility such as a YMCA, health club, or college. Hospital-based facilities have the advantage of maintaining greater continuity for patients progressing from phase I through phase III. They also provide complete medical support systems for any emergencies that occur. Unfortunately, however, many hospitals lack both space and varied exercise equipment. Another disadvantage is that hospitals are often considered a place for "sick people." On the other hand, community-based facilities have the advantage of often being closer to patients' homes and usually have adequate equipment and space. Their disadvantages are that they offer less medical support and they break up the continuity from phase to phase. In addition, a competitive environment, which may cause patients to exceed safe exercise limits, sometimes exists in these facilities.

## Purpose of phase III

The designated purposes of the phase III program are to improve the physical fitness and endurance level in coronary patients and to produce long-term reductions in coronary risk factors (see Chapter 10). In addition, the program should improve the patient's knowledge of his or her disease process and role in health maintenance. Because most patients referred to phase III programs are working, the program is usually conducted in the early morning between 6:00 and 8:00 AM or in the evening between the hours of 6:00 and 8:00 PM. This scheduling encourages the patient to continue working as a productive, contributing member of society while participating in an ongoing individualized training program that allows for evaluation of his or her progress and disease stability. Coronary artery disease is a progressive disease process. Despite maximal medical therapy, the disease may jeopardize the patients' lives and may produce unstable symptoms from time to time. By being seen on a regular basis in a phase III program, patients have an ongoing weekly to monthly evaluation that may detect changes in the course of the disease.

Phase III programs can also incorporate an advanced educational series that continues to build on the knowledge from previous patient education series. Such a series provides continued information about new therapeutic or diagnostic techniques for coronary disease, ongoing dietary management, cooking workshops, psychological intervention to reduce stress and adjust to illness, and motivational talks from inspirational speakers (see the box on p. 157).

A major objective of cardiac rehabilitation is to enhance the patient's quality of life. Indeed, phase III programs—through group interaction, peer support, and camaraderie—help contribute to this improved quality of life. We have also found that if the program can be oriented toward the production of research, patients are more likely to comply because they feel as though they are contributing to a body of knowledge that will benefit others, including their family members and children.

---

### Cardiac rehabilitation program advanced lecture series: January and February 1983

*Time:* 6:00 PM                                                                                    *Location:* Hacienda Heights Room
*Date*           *Lecture topic*                                                                   *Speaker*
Jan. 3           Cardiopulmonary "Heartsaver" course (open to all)                                 Rehab. faculty
                 *note:* On this night we will have "Dance For Your Heart." All
                 rehab. members and spouses will participate in an aerobic
                 dance session led by Sarah Shea. I will personally sponsor all
                 participants for 1¢ per minute of dancing.
Jan. 10          *Videocassette and discussion:* "Treatment of Obesity"                            Karen Broxson, RD
Jan. 17          *Film: Stress and the "Hot Reactor"*                                              John Camp, MD
Jan. 24          *Film: Heart Attacks*                                                             Randy Ice, PT
Jan. 31          *Guest speaker:* The U.S.C. Lipid-Lowering Study                                  Miguel Sanmarco, MD
Feb. 7           *Discussion:* Coping with illness                                                 Barbara Lane, MSW
Feb. 21          *Lecture:* Oh my aching back! Prevention and treatment of low                     Randy Ice, PT
                 back pain
Feb. 28          *Lecture:* A survey of home exercise devices: their cost and effectiveness        Sarah Shea and Randy Ice, PT
                 *AEROBIC DANCING*
For the month of January, we will have aerobic dancing offered *every* Monday as part of the American Heart Association's Dance
    For Heart program. The idea is to get sponsors to pay you for dancing aerobically for 1 to 4 hours (it's your choice). All
    participants will be expected to dance on January 3, while the other dates are optional. Aerobic dancing will be on February 14
    and 28.
*Remember on February 12 the Fourth Annual Walk/Jog/Run/Wheel For your Heart 5 or 10 km.*

---

## Training program

Patients referred into the phase III program must undergo an evaluation procedure not unlike phase II; that is, the patient is interviewed and goals are established. A chart review to obtain the clinical medical history and pertinent laboratory data must be performed (see Chapter 8). We require all of our patients to have a lipoprotein profile—including total serum cholesterol, total serum triglycerides, HDL cholesterol, LDL cholesterol, VLDL cholesterol, and phenotype—before beginning the exercise program. A maximal symptom-limited exercise test is also required. The results of this test are used to determine initial levels of physical fitness and to establish initial training heart rates and monitoring needs. Establishing a training intensity entails developing a target heart rate range. This range of target heart rate training intensity should be high enough to produce peripheral and central "cardiac" improvements. Peripheral effects are attained when prolonged aerobic exercise is performed at a level that is at least 60% of the total chronotropic reserve; that is, the target heart rate should be at least the resting heart rate plus 60% of the difference between resting and maximum heart rate.[159] This formula is referred to as Karvonen's formula. Central improvements are attained at levels of 80% to 90% of the total chronotropic reserve.[36,51]

This is only a rough estimate of proper training intensity, however, because many other clinical variables should be considered. These variables include angina, drop in systolic blood pressure, ST-segment depression of greater than 1 mm, medications, severe dyspnea, fatigue, musculoskeletal limitations, and the patient's goals.

In phase III, emphasizing distance goals rather than speed is of primary importance.[71] It is our impression that, in cardiac rehabilitation, not enough emphasis is placed on encouraging the patient to train for longer periods of time, particularly for those with greater degrees of lipid or carbohydrate metabolism abnormalities. Research we have done on coronary patients who either ran or bicycled more than 5 to 6 hours per week demonstrated consistently higher HDL cholesterol levels as compared to men who exercised only 1 to 2 hours per week. The former subset also demonstrated higher HDL cholesterol than patients who did no training at all (Fig. 9-8).

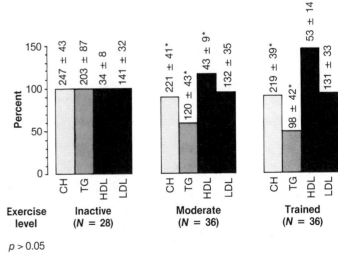

**Fig. 9-8.** *Inactive,* no exercise. *Moderate,* 1 to 2 hours of exercise per week. *Trained,* 5 to 6 hours of exercise per week. Mean follow-up time, 36 months (unpublished data). *HDL,* High-density lipoproteins; *LDL,* low-density lipoproteins; *CH,* carbohydrates; *TG,* triglycerides.

Many patients may not desire to train at high intensities and prefer only the minimum level of training that is required to maintain fitness. This may be achieved with low to moderate levels of exercise training by increasing the duration of exercise. Thus, the mode, intensity, frequency, and duration of each program is individualized to the capabilities and interests of the patient. It is the physical therapist's responsibility to direct patients' progress from week to week. This may include telemetry monitoring, particularly in the first several weeks for new patients or only periodically for those who have graduated from the phase II program. All patients are oriented to proper clothing and, in particular, are given instructions in proper footwear. The patient will often progress from walking to jogging or running, and needs good footwear to prevent orthopedic injuries. Our sessions are conducted on a track either at the hospital or at a local community school site. The therapist works with each patient individually and helps the patient achieve a desired level of training intensity, gradually increasing the duration from 30 minutes to 40 to 60 minutes per session.

### Advanced lecture series

Prior to or immediately after the phase III exercise program, an advanced educational lecture is provided by a cardiac rehabilitation team member. The dietician may discuss weight-loss programs, diets, or the polyunsaturated versus saturated fat controversy. The social worker or psychologist may discuss stress and its management and coping with illness or family adjustments. Current advances in diagnostic or therapeutic cardiology are often presented by an invited speaker. Individual case study presentation of patients who have shown excellent improvement serve to give many patients a pat on the back and motivate newer patients to persevere in their own rehabilitation efforts.

A basic CPR course (usually the heart-saver course) is taught every 6 to 12 months so that all patients and family members are certified in basic life support. This is done not only out of concern over the patient's risk of sudden death, but also because these patients are educated about the causes of coronary artery disease and its risk factors and can, therefore, respond to other emergency situations in an appropriate fashion.

In summary, we have found these advanced patient education lectures to be valuable in maintaining an active and interesting phase III program. To help enhance overall compliance, rewards are given to the patients, and inspirational guest speakers are often invited.

### Phase II and III compliance programming

Compliance to health-promoting behaviors has been a topic of investigation for many years. Compliance with weight reduction and exercise conditioning programs in healthy subjects[90,97,103,138] and with exercise training in cardiac rehabilitation programs[104-106,108,110] has tradition-

ally been low. Reasons for this include behavioral, socioeconomic, and programmatic problems. Early drop-out from cardiac rehabilitation is predictably about 76% if two or more of the following are present: (1) smoking, (2) blue-collar work, or (3) inactive leisure habits.[107] Late drop-out (12 months or greater) from cardiac rehabilitation is apparently a result of changes in the physical environment (job or residence change), social setting (divorce or increased family demand), or medical reasons.[89,104]

An article by Ice suggests that specific strategies be implemented to improve patient compliance.[65] These include (1) early entry into a formal exercise program (no later than 2 to 3 weeks after hospital discharge); (2) coordination of the exercise program with the patient's schedule; (3) frequent, positive reinforcement from the therapist; (4) use of cues and prompts to stimulate desired behavior (e.g., exercise diaries posted on the refrigerator door may control abnormal dietary habits and remind patients to exercise); (5) cognitive strategies (short-term and long-term goal setting); (6) behavioral contracting between patient and therapist (patient signs an agreement to participate in the rehabilitation program); (7) adjunct programs focusing on patient concerns; (8) increased physician presence and interaction with patients; (9) increased feedback on progress (periodic reevaluations); and (10) creation of long-range exercise, diet, or spouse clubs.[65]

Several years ago, we started weekend activity programs (jogging and cycling clubs) as one means of facilitating patient compliance and assisting in the achievement of maximum fitness levels in an environment of social camaraderie and support. The SCOR Cardiac Cyclists Club and SCOR Jogging Club have now been in existence 20 and 18 years, respectively. Cardiac patients, spouses, and family members comprise each club and participate in weekend endurance-building activities.

**SCOR Cardiac Cyclists Club.** The cycling club began in 1974 with a flat 15-mile bike ride on a Saturday morning with four or five selected patients from our phase III program. The club now has over 35 cardiac patients, many of whom complete 100-mile ("century") rides routinely. Several ambitious patients in the cycling club decided to bicycle across the United States. The Cardiac Transamerica Relay Ride was a 24-hour-per-day, nonstop bicycle relay ride that left Los Angeles on June 5, 1982, and set a United States Cycling Federation Relay Ride record of 12 days, 1 hour, and 50 minutes, arriving in Central Park in New York City on June 17, 1982. Fourteen men with coronary artery disease made the trip to demonstrate the benefits of cardiac rehabilitation and the value of an anticoronary life-style. In this ride, each person rode 1 to 2 hours at his own pace each day. There were no cardiovascular complications during the 3000-mile trip, and none were anticipated. The actual physical exercise of 1 to 2 hours of daily bicycling was less than what most of these men do during their own training sessions with the cycling club and at home. Environmental factors of heat, altitude, and hills were the only variables that imposed additional demands on them, but even these factors were well tolerated by all the riders.

Recently, we conducted a retrospective clinical study examining the medical outcome of 68 self-referred cardiac patients who undertook bicycling as an adjunct to standard cardiac rehabilitation procedures.[66] Between October 1974 and September 1985, 68 patients (67 men, 1 woman) with various cardiovascular diagnoses voluntarily began a bicycling exercise program on Saturdays with the SCOR Cardiac Cyclists Club. The majority of these patients became involved after seeing or talking to other club members during phase II or phase III cardiac rehabilitation programs between 1974 and 1985 at Rancho Los Amigos Hospital, Ross-Loos

Medical Center, Presbyterian Intercommunity Hospital, or the Human Performance Center in Whittier. A minority came to the club through word of mouth or press exposure in Southern California.

The average length of participation in the club was 4.4 years, with a range of 2 months to 11 years. At entry, 73% were employed, 15% retired, 6% disabled, and 6% were working and have subsequently retired. The average age of this group was 56.6 years.

For the purpose of this study, long-distance bicycling (LDB) was defined as bicycle rides of 10 miles or more at least once a week. Weekly Saturday morning rides began in November 1974 with initial distances of 10 to 15 miles per session. Distance, not speed, was always emphasized.

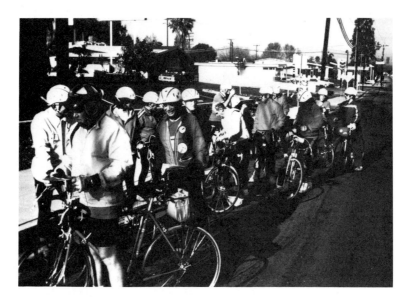

**Fig. 9-9.** All SCOR CCC rides start at 8:00 AM on Saturday mornings and emphasize distance and camaraderie rather than speed.

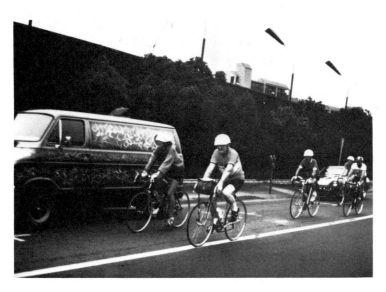

**Fig. 9-10.** SCOR CCC out for a Saturday 40-mile ride.

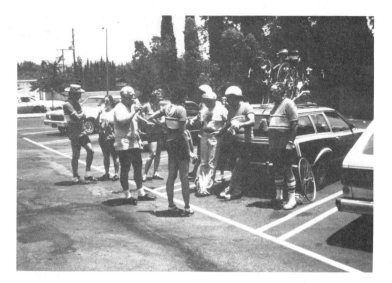

**Fig. 9-11.** SCOR CCC riders relaxing after a Saturday ride. The discussion usually centers around when to eat lunch.

Distances ridden had increased to 25 to 50 miles by early 1976. In late 1976, 5 patients completed their first 100-mile ("century") bike ride from Santa Barbara to Los Angeles. As a group, all 68 patients have averaged 60 miles per week with a range of 10 to 800 miles per week.

From direct observation, home training logs, and self-reports, club members ride at peak heart rates of 120 to 135 bpm (range 90 to 170) an average of 3 to 4 times per week.

Average Saturday rides are now either 15 to 25 (short) or 35 to 50 (long) miles, with 12 to 15 members riding each Saturday (Figs. 9-9 to 9-11). As a group, 948,000 miles, requiring 90,000 hours of bicycling, have been accumulated.

Currently, 40 of the 68 members (59%) have ridden a century in one day, the cycling equivalent of a marathon (Fig. 9-12). A smaller number have completed double or triple centuries, with the furthest distance being 380 miles in 32 hours by a 56-year-old, postbypass patient.

At entry into the club, the following cardiovascular diagnoses were observed (no patient was denied access to participation in the club because of the severity of underlying CAD or left ventricular dysfunction):

Bypass surgery—32 (47%)
Myocardial infarction—one: 22 (32%); two: 2 (3%); three: 1 (1.5%)
Angina pectoris—6 (9%)
Atrial dysrhythmias—2 (3%)
History of congestive heart failure—1 (1.5%)
Heart transplant—1 (1.5%)

Among the 52 patients who had previously undergone coronary angiography, three-vessel CAD was present in 33 (64%), two-vessel CAD in 6 (12%), and single-vessel CAD in 13 (25%).

Ventricular function of the 68 patients was evaluated via cardiac catheterization or echocardiography, or assumed to

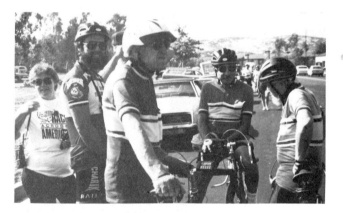

**Fig. 9-12.** Randy Ice, P.T., C.P.S., with SCOR CCC members Henry Torrey (age 83), Leo Charm (age 64), and Guido Orquitapan (age 65). All three ride 400 to 500 miles each month for cardiovascular conditioning and have ridden multiple one-day century rides (100 miles).

be greater than 50% if a normal electrocardiogram was present, yielding the following categories:

Good (EF > 50%)—51 patients (80%)
Fair (EF > 30% but <50%)—7 (11%)
Poor (EF < 29%)—6 (9%)

Currently, of 62 survivors, 35 are active in the club, while 27 have dropped out for a variety of reasons, including moving out of the area, increased vocational demands, retirement, progression of CAD, lack of interest, change in motivation (several became runners), and personality conflicts with other club members. The dropout rate among this self-selected group was 8% a year.

During LDB, two episodes of cardiac arrest occurred (one fatal, one nonfatal), for an incidence rate of 1/45,000 patient-hours of exercise. One myocardial infarction occurred during a Saturday ride in a 57-year-old, postbypass patient, for an incidence rate of 1/90,000 patient-hours of LDB. Two episodes of congestive heart failure occurred in two patients with EF <35%. One was treated with diuretics, the other with rest, and both returned to bicycling without further episodes.

Orthopedically, LDB represents a different risk from that posed by traditional cardiac rehabilitation programs. No overuse syndromes were observed in any patient between 1974 and 1985. Traumatic injuries were observed at a rate of 1/11,250 patient-hours of bicycling. Seven fractures resulted from falls, and one patient sustained a mild concussion when he ran into the back of a parked car while pedaling at a 17-mph pace, shattering the car's rear windshield. A hard-shell helmet prevented certain brain damage, and the patient was discharged after an overnight hospital stay without complications.

Independent of LDB, primary fatal cardiac arrests were observed in two patients who had reduced ejection fractions of 20% and 25%, respectively. The former was 19 years post-MI and the latter was 2 years post-MI at the time of death. Three other patients developed bladder, jaw, and lung cancer and died from advanced carcinoma (4.2%).

Among 62 survivors, 19 nonfatal cardiac events unrelated to bicycling occurred during the 4.4-year follow-up:

Cardiac arrest—3 (4.9%)
New onset angina pectoris—2 (3.2%)
Second bypass surgery—1 (1.6%)
Myocardial infarction—5 (4 patients) (8%)
Bypass surgery—6 (9.8%)
Pacemaker—2 (3.2%)

Of six patients with exertional angina pectoris at the time of starting LDB, four (6.6%) became asymptomatic 1 to 5 years later, requiring no antianginal drugs. The mortality and morbidity rates for the 68 subjects were calculated from natural history studies that have been published in the last 5 years for patients who have equivalent medically or surgically treated CAD. From this data, it was assumed that with good, fair, or poor left ventricular function, a mortality rate of 3% per year and a morbidity rate of 4% per year would be observed among the 64 known CAD patients. The observed death rate was 1.1% per year, or 35% of predicted. Repeated MI rate was 1.7% per year, or 44% of predicted.

In conclusion, the cardiovascular risk of LDB in a group of patients with heart disease is comparable with published risks for supervised and unsupervised exercise programs in known CAD patients. Sudden death not associated with LDB was observed more frequently in patients with reduced ejection fractions (EF < 31%), confirming other reports that ventricular function is a major predictor of subsequent mortality.

From this data, we conclude that the natural history of CAD may be beneficially altered by LDB when done in conjunction with standard risk factor reduction measures.

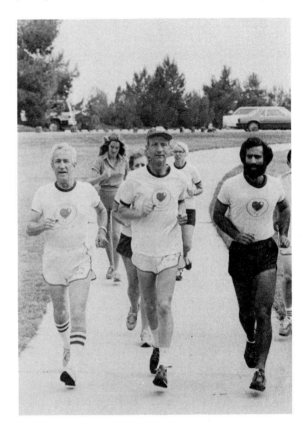

**Fig. 9-13.** Ray Blessey, P.T., runs with several cardiac patients, their spouses, and family members on a typical Saturday morning SCOR Jogging Club meeting.

Although this group of patients reduced their risk factors and altered the progression of their CAD, the complications noted illustrate an important factor to remember in long-term cardiac rehabilitation. Despite the medical and surgical interventions currently available, CAD is an enigma, and episodic recurrent events are sometimes unpredictable. Their temporal relationship to exercise may imply a slightly greater risk of training that is probably offset by the long-term protective effects observed in multiple nonrandomized, uncontrolled rehabilitation studies[58,72,134] (see Chapter 10).

**SCOR Jogging Club.** The SCOR Jogging Club has undergone a metamorphosis similar to that of the cycling club, with over 75 patients now participating in Saturday morning training sessions at various locations around Los Angeles (Fig. 9-13). Thirteen patients have trained to a level of successfully completing a marathon. One man with triple-vessel disease completed over 85 marathons between 1976 and 1981. Many patients routinely participate in weekend 5 and 10 km runs in a noncompetitive fashion. Family participation is strongly encouraged, and spouses, as well as children, often train with patients on weekend outings.

Patient participation in the jogging club usually begins in phase III cardiac rehabilitation by either track walking or

S.C.O.R.
(Specialized Coronary Outpatient Rehabilitation) ——————————
Exercise Diary

Prescription:  Distance_____mile(s)

Time:_____minutes    Physical fitness stage:_____

Target heart rate:_____bpm    Weight (end of month):_____

| Day | Rest. HR | Exercise mode | Distance (peak) | Time (peak) | Work load | W-U HR | Peak HR | C-D HR | Symptoms or remarks |
|---|---|---|---|---|---|---|---|---|---|
| 1 | | | | | | | | | |
| 2 | | | | | | | | | |
| 3 | | | | | | | | | |
| 4 | | | | | | | | | |
| 5 | | | | | | | | | |
| 6 | | | | | | | | | |
| 7 | | | | | | | | | |
| 8 | | | | | | | | | |
| 9 | | | | | | | | | |
| 10 | | | | | | | | | |
| 11 | | | | | | | | | |
| 12 | | | | | | | | | |
| 13 | | | | | | | | | |
| 14 | | | | | | | | | |
| 15 | | | | | | | | | |
| 16 | | | | | | | | | |
| 17 | | | | | | | | | |
| 18 | | | | | | | | | |
| 19 | | | | | | | | | |
| 20 | | | | | | | | | |

**Fig. 9-14.** All exercise sessions, both at the hospital and at home, are logged on this exercise diary form. The physical therapist reviews it at the end of each month, makes comments, and gives a copy back to the patient. Exercise diary.

treadmill walking. Patients then progress to walk-jogging and finally to continuous jogging as tolerated. When the physical therapist observes that the patient is stable, requires infrequent monitoring, and has developed a basic fitness level that is compatible with that necessary for weekend activities, the patient is encouraged to join the jogging club. This occurs usually at least 2 months after starting the phase III program, but is determined by each patient's status.

The overall accomplishments of patients in both of these clubs provide good public relations for the patient's hospital and cardiac rehabilitation program and help motivate new patients. The tremendous life-style changes and fitness improvements that these patients have demonstrated over relatively short periods of time are inspira-

| Day | Rest. HR | Exercise mode | Distance (peak) | Time (peak) | Work load | W-U HR | Peak HR | C-D HR | Symptoms or remarks |
|-----|----------|---------------|-----------------|-------------|-----------|--------|---------|--------|---------------------|
| 21  |          |               |                 |             |           |        |         |        |                     |
| 22  |          |               |                 |             |           |        |         |        |                     |
| 23  |          |               |                 |             |           |        |         |        |                     |
| 24  |          |               |                 |             |           |        |         |        |                     |
| 25  |          |               |                 |             |           |        |         |        |                     |
| 26  |          |               |                 |             |           |        |         |        |                     |
| 27  |          |               |                 |             |           |        |         |        |                     |
| 28  |          |               |                 |             |           |        |         |        |                     |
| 29  |          |               |                 |             |           |        |         |        |                     |
| 30  |          |               |                 |             |           |        |         |        |                     |
| 31  |          |               |                 |             |           |        |         |        |                     |

```
MONTHLY SUMMARY                              DEFINITIONS

Average resting heart rate =                 Level of angina
Average peak heart rate =                       L₁  mild discomfort
Total days exercise =                           L₂  moderately painful
Average peak interval = _____ miles           L₃  severe pain
Average peak duration =                         L₄  intolerable
Total monthly mileage =
                                             SOB—Shortness of breath
                                             PVC—Premature ventricular
                                                   contraction



Recommendations: _____

_____

_____

_____
```

**Fig. 9-14, cont'd.**  Exercise diary

tional and motivational for everyone involved in the program.

**Reevaluation in phase III**

Patients who participate in phase III programs for longer than 6 months need periodic assessment of their disease status. We have developed a protocol that is standardized, yet flexible enough to meet specific patient needs.

The protocol consists of: (1) periodic ECG monitoring during exercise, (2) recording hospital and home exercise sessions in a monthly exercise diary (Fig. 9-14), and (3) maximal symptom-limited exercise tests every 6 months to 1 year, depending upon the patient's status. These exercise logs are returned to the physical therapist at the end of each

month. A review of the exercise log by the physical therapist may uncover subtle changes in performance or the presence of new symptoms. Either finding can indicate disease progression and the need for repeat assessments.

For example, the assessment of lipid changes, particularly HDL cholesterol, requires sufficient training time. A lipid profile is routinely repeated after 3 months in the program and every 6 to 12 months thereafter. These results are always sent to the referring physician and are individually reviewed by the therapist or dietitian with the patient. If the patient's lipid values are worse than they were at the time of admission to the program and the change appears to be the result of an improper diet, individual counseling is done with the team dietitian. If all dietary and training modes of intervention fail to improve lipid values, the referring physician will be contacted and alternative therapy (drugs, medication changes) will be discussed.

We attempt to electrocardiographically monitor all phase III patients at least once every 4 to 8 weeks during an exercise session. Although some patients will tell you when they feel dysrhythmias in their pulse, others will not feel them or perhaps do not regularly take their pulse. Routine monitoring during moderate- to high-intensity exercise, particularly in the cool-down phase, may help detect asymptomatic ventricular dysrhythmias or ST-segment changes. Blood pressure responses to exercise are monitored during each exercise session (see Chapters 7 and 8).

We repeat a maximal symptom-limited exercise test every 6 months to 1 year on patients enrolled in phase III. This is the best noninvasive means of measuring functional improvement (increased time or increased maximal oxygen uptake) and coronary disease stability. A decrease in exercise tolerance, an increase in ST-segment abnormalities, abnormal blood pressure responses, and the appearance of ventricular dysrhythmias or angina may be indicative of worsening coronary disease. Communicating these findings to the patient's referring physician often results in medication changes or further evaluative and therapeutic procedures to prevent any additional cardiac events. Finally, patients who are unstable or in whom new signs or symptoms suggest instability should undergo more frequent exercise testing (every 3 to 6 months). An important point to emphasize is that coronary patients demonstrate training effects that develop more slowly than those in healthy subjects of the same age. Thus, testing may not show improvement if it is done after a short training interval (less than 3 months). Likewise it is not unusual to see compliant, well-motivated patients continue to improve objectively (increased treadmill duration, increased $\dot{V}o_{2max}$) over a 3- to 5-year period from the time of their initial training program.[67,71,72] Such improvement during phase III cardiac rehabilitation is demonstrated in the case studies at the end of this chapter.

## PRIMARY PREVENTION

As previously mentioned, more emphasis must be placed on primary prevention to reduce risk factors and the prevalence of CAD. This emphasis is apparently increasing in view of the growing number of primary prevention (wellness) programs and the recent use of cardiovascular assessments as a part of work hardening evaluations. Individuals at risk for CAD (e.g., those with hypertension, hypercholesterolemia, or a history of cigarette smoking) have benefited significantly from primary prevention programs.[8,29,137]

In 1985, Huhn and Volski[63] published a comprehensive review of primary prevention that included a model for the development of a primary prevention program in business and industry. This model is divided into five phases: history questionnaire, medical screening and evaluation, consultation, exercise performance, and progress assessment. The *history questionnaire* is given to each potential participant and contains questions regarding general health, exercise, physical activity levels, weight, and eating habits, as well as a cardiovascular risk factor analysis. *Medical screening and evaluation* by a physician and physical therapist include testing of cardiovascular endurance, joint screening, body composition, muscle strength, flexibility, job tasks, pulmonary function, and blood chemistry. After testing, each participant *consults* with a physical therapist who provides test results and exercise performance comparisons of others of the same age and sex, as well as individualized exercise programs. The possible types of *exercise performance* programs in which those in a primary prevention program may participate include home programs, company-sponsored programs at in-house facilities, and company-sponsored programs outside of the work place. Each type of program has advantages and disadvantages, but successful fitness programs generally have the following characteristics: executive participation, employee involvement in program planning, promotional planning, convenience, conducive environment, management information systems to provide data for program evaluations, and professional leadership.[63] *Progress assessment* is performed every 1 to 3 months, depending on individual need. Physical therapists with cardiopulmonary and musculoskeletal expertise appear to be best suited for the planning and implementation of such primary prevention programs.

At the CIGNA Healthplans of California (Los Angeles and Pomona), we have implemented a primary prevention program that incorporates many of the above ideas. We have provided this service to approximately 250 individuals who are reevaluated every 3 months after undergoing an initial treadmill stress test and receiving extensive counseling regarding risk factor reduction. A repeat exercise test is performed after approximately 1 year. Significant improvement in treadmill duration and reduction of risk factors have been observed in many of the participants. Individuals enrolled in the CIGNA Healthplans Optifast Program (a medically supervised weight-reduction program for the morbidly obese) are assessed similarly with goals similar to those for the primary prevention participants. Approximately 200 Optifast participants have been assessed and provided with home exercise programs to facilitate weight loss. In addition to offering the above programs, we have extended our primary prevention program to the siblings of patients in our cardiac rehabilitation program. Approximately 60 individuals (ages 5 to 18) have been evaluated and recommendations made to decrease risk factors and the likelihood of CAD. With these primary prevention programs and others like them, the decline of CAD can only continue.

## CASE 1 ▼ Mr. J. M.

This case history demonstrates the use of a one-time-per-week *exercise assessment* in a patient with complications (impaired left ventricular function and history of ventricular ectopy), who underwent t-PA infusion and PTCA with poor results (in view of the extensive left ventricular dysfunction). These exercise assessments were done safely, provided information to the primary physician, and in no way impaired the patient's compliance or safety.

**Patient:** Mr. J.M.

**Age:** 48

**Risk factors**

Strong family history of CAD (father and mother both died of MI at age 53 and 59, respectively)

Smoking 2 ½ to 3 packs a day for many years

Obesity

Increased stress (recent death of his wife and increased job responsibilities)

**Medical history.** At 8:30 AM on October 13, 1988, while preparing for work, he developed severe anterior chest pressure that radiated to the left arm. Because of the severity of the pain, he called paramedics, who arrived within 5 minutes to witness a cardiac arrest. The patient was given lidocaine IV and morphine sulfate, and was defibrillated two times. The patient converted to sinus rhythm, but quickly went into a junctional rhythm at 68 bpm that sufficiently maintained the blood pressure at 130/100 mm Hg and permitted transport to the nearest emergency room.

**Hospital course.** Because of continued chest pain, Mr. J.M. was immediately started on intravenous nitroglycerin and again given morphine sulfate. The ECG confirmed the evolution of an extensive anteroseptal MI. Despite repeat doses of morphine and intravenous nitroglycerin, the chest discomfort persisted. Because of the severity, recent onset, and persistence of the chest pressure, and the ECG signs of an evolving MI, the patient was administered 100 mg of t-PA, followed by a heparin drip. The pain abated considerably after 15 minutes from the initiation of the t-PA. The patient was transferred to the ICU, where he continued to complain of intermittent chest pain, was observed to be in congestive heart failure, and ECG recordings revealed occasional runs of ventricular tachycardia. By October 17, 1988, the patient experienced only rare chest pain and the rhythm was normal sinus. On this date, a cardiac catheterization was performed that revealed 90% occlusion of the left anterior descending (LAD) artery at the second diagonal, 50% occlusion of the mid-right coronary artery, 50% occlusion of a diagonal artery off the circumflex artery, and extensive left ventricular dysfunction. Because of continued chest pain, it was decided that PTCA of the LAD artery occlusion might improve the patient's condition. The PTCA was performed on the evening of October 17, 1988, during which the occlusion was reduced from 90% to 30%. This was considered a successful PTCA, as determined by excellent blood flow to the distal portions of the LAD and a significant decrease in the pressure gradient of the LAD artery (58 mm Hg to 16 mm Hg). After the PTCA, the patient's condition improved significantly. He was asymptomatic and his rhythm was normal during daily activities and increased levels of exertion during phase I cardiac rehabilitation. The patient was discharged home on October 20, 1988 with the following medications: Cardizem 60 mg tid, one aspirin qd, and nitroglycerin sublingual prn.

**Rehabilitation program.** The patient was referred for outpatient cardiac rehabilitation after a maximal symptom-limited treadmill stress test was performed on October 28, 1988, which was limited by dyspnea and fatigue. The patient demonstrated a poor exercise tolerance (3 minutes, 19 seconds of the Bruce protocol) without angina or enhancement of resting ST-segment changes. The patient underwent his initial phase II exercise assessment on October 30, 1988, during which he tolerated 15 minutes of bicycle ergometry at 1.75 to 2.25 KP and was counseled extensively regarding atherosclerotic heart disease, risk factors, and exercise. During this assessment, the patient's diastolic blood pressure was consistently high (96 to 98 mm Hg), both at rest and during exercise. This information was provided to the primary physician, who increased the dose of Cardizem to 90 mg tid. Persantine 75 mg tid was also added for dilation of the coronary arteries and anticoagulation. Repeat exercise assessments were performed weekly, during which workloads were gradually increased to the patient's tolerance. During these reassessments, the patient was asymptomatic and exhibited a normal blood pressure and rhythm at rest and during exercise. He underwent another maximal treadmill stress test on December 23, 1988 and completed 6 minutes, 10 seconds of the Bruce protocol without angina or enhancement of resting ST-segment changes. The patient returned to work on January 3, 1989. He will be followed monthly for 3 to 6 months and will continue his home exercise program, which will be reviewed (via home exercise diary) at each monthly exercise assessment.

## CASE 2    ▼    Mr. F. D.

The following case study illustrates long-term training changes that can occur in a well-motivated man with single-vessel coronary artery disease and angina pectoris. Both peripheral and central training adaptations have accounted for the tremendous improvement in symptoms this man achieved.

**Patient:** Mr. F.D.

**Age:** 48 (at onset of symptoms in early 1977)

**Medical history:** Beginning in January 1977, Mr. F.D. noticed the onset of substernal chest pain while walking uphill to his office in downtown Los Angeles. It was relieved by rest or with nitroglycerin. He saw his family doctor, who referred him to a cardiologist at the Ross-Loos Medical Center for evaluation. His risk factor profile at the time included the following:

**Risk factors**

Pipe smoker for many years, overweight (6 feet tall, 193 pounds), inactive, sedentary life-style, family history of coronary disease with a father who died at age 54 from a myocardial infarction, serum lipids unknown, and no history of hypertension or diabetes. He worked as a construction inspector for the City of Los Angeles, which he considered a very stressful occupation.

He underwent a symptom-limited treadmill exercise test to confirm the diagnosis of angina pectoris and to define noninvasively the extent of coronary artery disease.

**Treadmill test results** (January 24, 1977)
*Time completed:* 6 minutes (Bruce Protocol Test)
*Limiting factor:* moderate angina pectoris (level 2+/4)
*Resting heart rate:* 56 bpm
*Maximum heart rate:* 119 bpm
*Resting blood pressure:* 128/84 mm Hg
*Maximum blood pressure:* 160/80 mm Hg
*Maximum rate-pressure product (RPP):* $19 \times 10^3$
*RPP at onset of angina:* $14 \times 10^3$
*RPP at onset of ST-segment changes:* (not measured)
1.5 mm ST-segment depression at maximum RPP
No dysrhythmias
Fair symptom-limited physical work capacity

The cardiologist subsequently started the patient on Inderal (propranolol) 20 mg qid and Nitrobid (nitroglycerin) 2.5 mg bid. A cardiac catheterization was done on Feb. 14, 1977, revealing:

*Ventriculogram:* Normal left ventricular contractility with an ejection fraction of 70%
*Coronary angiogram:*
    *Left anterior descending artery:* 90% obstruction distal to the first septal perforator and first diagonal
    *Circumflex artery:* intimal irregularities
    *Right coronary artery:* intimal irregularities

Because of continuing angina symptoms, Inderal was increased to 40 mg qid and subsequently to 60 mg qid. The latter dosage caused the patient to feel dizzy and the dosage was decreased to 40 mg qid, and Nitrobid was increased to 5 mg bid. To assess the effectiveness of this medical regimen, his treadmill test was repeated.

**Treadmill test results** (June 1977)
*Time completed:* 5 minutes
*Limiting factor:* severe angina (level 3+/4)
*Resting heart rate:* 45 bpm
*Maximum heart rate:* 90 bpm
*Resting blood pressure:* 100/60 mm Hg
*Maximum blood pressure:* 114/72 mm Hg
*Maximum RPP:* $10.3 \times 10^3$
*RPP at onset of angina:* $7.0 \times 10^3$
*RPP at onset of ST-segment changes:* (not measured)
1.5 mm ST-segment depression at maximal RPP
Decreased symptom-limited performance with increased symptoms at lower RPP's

After this test, Nitrobid was increased to 5 mg tid. The patient was not exercising in any systematic fashion and underwent another exercise test in August 1985 with the same results.

As discussed in Chapter 8, in some patients beta blockade will produce adverse effects by significantly reducing the heart rate and strength of myocardial contraction. This may increase the myocardial oxygen demand as more blood fills the ventricle and increases the right and left end-diastolic volume and pressure. The elevated pressure increases the myocardial oxygen demand. Because of this, the patient's Inderal was reduced to 40 mg qid, and his cardiologist referred him to begin an exercise program with the SCOR Cardiac Cycling Club. The goals of his phase III cardiac rehabilitation program were to (1) improve physical work capacity and endurance, (2) decrease anginal symptoms with exertion, and (3) reduce risk factors through patient education and life-style changes.

He began a home bicycling program with instructions on how to train, the frequency of exercise, at what intensity to train, and how to deal with exertional angina. The emphasis was on increasing the duration of bicycling time at a mild (level 1/4) exertional angina threshold. Within 2 months, Mr. F.D. was cycling outdoors 4 to 15 miles on a 10-speed bicycle. Nitroglycerin was required to relieve his angina about 50% to 60% of the time during these exercise sessions.

Subsequently, the patient's Inderal was reduced from 40 mg qid to 20 mg qid, then to 10 mg qid. A routine follow-up exercise test revealed:

**Treadmill test results** (November 1977):
*Time completed:* 7.5 minutes
*Limiting factor:* severe angina (level 3+/4)
*Resting heart rate:* 58 bpm

## CASE 2 ▾ Mr. F. D. —cont'd

*Maximum heart rate:* 125 bpm
*Resting blood pressure:* 114/72 mm Hg
*Maximum blood pressure:* 154/68, mm Hg, dropping to 148/64 mm Hg the last minute of exercise
*Maximum RPP:* $19.2 \times 10^3$
*RPP at onset of angina:* $15.4 \times 10^3$
*RPP at onset ST-segment changes:* $15.4 \times 10^3$
2.0 mm ST-segment depression at maximal RPP
Improved symptom-limited performance

Over the next 6 months, Mr. F.D. continued cycling, began riding longer distances of 20 to 35 miles on Saturday morning outings with the cycling club, and began a formal phase III hospital-based rehabilitation program for periodic monitoring and educational lectures. He rapidly progressed from 95 to 400 miles per month of bicycling and completed a 100-mile ("century") ride in one day in May 1978. In August 1978, his Inderal was reduced to 5 mg qid, and then discontinued in January 1979. Nitrobid was also discontinued in late 1979. Table 9-2 illustrates the continuing improvement Mr. F.D. has made from May 1978 to June 1982 as a result of his continued excellent compliance to endurance exercise and life-style changes.

As Mr. F.D.'s symptoms have abated over the years, he has expanded his recreational pursuits into other areas. He has become an avid cross-country skier with minimal symptoms in cold weather and at altitudes up to 8000 feet. He continues long-distance cycling and has completed two "double centuries" in one day. In the summer of 1980, he took a 4-week cycling trip through England, Scotland, and Ireland with one of the authors and two cardiac patients from the SCOR Cardiac Cycling Club.

Mr. F.D. had a decrease in angina symptoms at progressively higher rate-pressure products until he became completely asymptomatic during the tests. The ST-segment depression initially became more prominent as he was able to exercise at higher rate-pressure products; however, their magnitude has decreased in the last 2 years. The onset of ST changes has also been occurring at progressively higher rate-pressure products. Concurrently, the patient's medications (beta blockade and vasodilator therapy) were tapered off. It is planned that yearly exercise tests will be continued to assess his stability and freedom from angina symptoms. Certainly, the quality of his life is infinitely better in terms of the many vigorous leisure activities in which he is now capable of participating.

**Table 9-2.** Improvement in cardiac capacities over a 4-year period

|  | May 78 | Nov. 78 | June 79 | Dec. 79 | Sept. 80 | Sept. 81 | June 82 |
|---|---|---|---|---|---|---|---|
| Treadmill time | 9.0 | 10.5 | 10.5 | 10.5 | 10.5 | 10.5 | 10.33 |
| Limiting factor | $L_3AP$ | $L_3AP$ | $L_2$ and fatigue | $L_2$ and fatigue | Fatigue | Fatigue | Fatigue |
| Resting heart rate (bpm) | 51 | 46 | 44 | 53 | 50 | 46 | 53 |
| Maximum heart rate (bpm) | 135 | 141 | 160 | 170 | 170 | 170 | 168 |
| Resting blood pressure (mm Hg) | 108/62 | 112/74 | 112/80 | 104/68 | 106/76 | 124/76 | 122/72 |
| Maximum blood pressure (mm Hg) | 152/62 | 170/70 | 190/90 | 176/70 | 204/74 | 200/92 | 192/78 |
| Maximum rate pressure product ($\times 10^3$) | 20.8 | 22.5 | 30.4 | 28.1 | 34.6 | 34.0 | 32.3 |
| Rate pressure product at angina pectoris ($\times 10^3$) | 20.2 | 21.8 | 23.2 | 22.7 | AP after exercise only | No AP | AP after exercise only |
| Rate pressure product at ST ($\times 10^3$) | 14.2 | 19.5 | 16.8 | N.A. | 23.7 | 26.8 | 24.1 |
| Maximum ST depression (mm) ($CM_4$ lead) | 2.5 | 3.0 | 5.0 | 5.0 | 4.5 | 3.0 | 2.5 |
| Medications | Inderal 5 mg qid Nitrobid 6.5 mg bid | Same | Nitrobid 6.5 mg bid | None | None | None | None |

*L*, Level; *AP*, angina pectoris; *N.A.*, not applicable.

## CASE 3 ▼ Mr. D. D.

The following case study demonstrates an uncomplicated phase I post-coronary artery bypass surgery program. Clear-cut goals, set by the patient, helped to speed his recovery and allow for early hospital discharge.

**Patient:** Mr. D.D.

**Age:** 57

**Medical history:** This 57-year-old man noted the onset of substernal chest pains occurring after running or hiking in the mountains. He had been an active jogger before the onset of these symptoms; however, he had cut back considerably on the amount of running he had done in the last 3 to 4 years. During the time that he was jogging, he would do 2 to 4 miles, 2 to 3 days each week. The patient saw his private physician, who referred him to a cardiologist, who subsequently did a Bruce Treadmill Test (see Chapter 8) This test showed abnormalities of both angina and ischemic ST changes with greater than 1 mm of depression during exercise. The patient subsequently was catheterized on September 20, 1986.

### Results

*Ventriculogram*
    Normal contractility, ejection fraction 60%
*Coronary angiogram*
    *Right coronary artery:* proximal 70% obstruction
    *Left anterior descending artery:* proximal 70% obstruction
    *Circumflex artery:* 30% stenosis midportion

On October 7, 1986, the patient had coronary artery bypass graft surgery with independent grafts to the left anterior descending, right coronary artery, and diagonal. The patient had an uncomplicated postoperative course except for a temporary right bundle branch block.

### Phase I cardiac rehabilitation

The cardiologist referred Mr. D.D. for inpatient cardiac rehabilitation on October 10, 1986, 3 days postoperatively. His medical history was reviewed and it was noted at that time that his hemoglobin was 12.0 and his hematocrit was 40.

After completion of a normal self-care evaluation, the patient began monitored ambulation sessions.

*October 10, 1986:* monitored ambulation 200 yards, 5 minutes, no ectopy, no symptoms, and no ST changes
*Resting heart rate:* 102 bpm
*Peak heart rate:* 114 bpm
*Resting blood pressure:* 112/80 mm Hg
*Peak blood pressure:* 120/62 mm Hg

*October 11, 1986:* monitored ambulation 200 to 300 yards, 10 minutes, no symptoms, no ectopy
*Resting heart rate:* 96 bpm
*Peak heart rate:* 120 bpm
*Resting blood pressure:* 108/76 mm Hg
*Peak blood pressure:* 124/70
*October 12, 1986:* monitored ambulation 300 to 400 yards, 9 minutes, no symptoms
*Resting heart rate:* 96 bpm
*Peak heart rate:* 120 bpm
*Resting blood pressure:* 112/70 mm Hg
*Peak blood pressure:* 120/70 mm Hg
*October 13, 1986:* Mr. D.D. underwent a low-level treadmill test using the modified protocol described in Chapter 8.

### Treadmill test results

*Time completed:* 11 minutes (Sheffield)
*Limiting factor:* reached target heart rate
*Resting heart rate:* 98 bpm
*Peak heart rate:* 155 bpm
*Resting blood pressure:* 142/70 mm Hg
*Peak blood pressure:* 148/70 mm Hg
*Flat systolic blood-pressure response*
No angina
No changes
No dysrhythmias

On October 13, 1986 (6 days after coronary artery bypass graft surgery), the patient was discharged home. His only medication was Fergon (ferrous gluconate), one tablet tid.

### Phase II cardiac rehabilitation

The patient returned on October 16, 1986, for an initial interview with the rehabilitation team. The physical therapy interview identified a 57-year-old man who was strongly motivated to improve his physical condition, only 9 days after bypass surgery with an uncomplicated course. The low-level treadmill test suggested good revascularization results with a flat blood pressure response. The patient's goals upon entering phase II were (1) to return to work by 2 months after the operation, and (2) to build up to 5 miles of continuous jogging as soon as possible.

### Phase II exercise program

On October 18, 1976, the patient began phase II as an outpatient. He began with bicycle ergometry, using 62.5 watts for 15 minutes.

## CASE 3 ▼ Mr. D. D.—cont'd

*Resting heart rate:* 108 bpm
*Peak heart rate:* 132 bpm
*Resting blood pressure:* 92/70 mm Hg
*Peak blood pressure:* 132/60 mm Hg
No ST changes, no ectopy

In addition, the patient was instructed to walk three-fourths of a mile, four times a day.

On October 22, 1986, patient performed 40 minutes of bicycle ergometry with a peak workload of 87.5 watts.

*Resting heart rate:* 102 bpm
*Peak heart rate:* 150 bpm
*Resting blood pressure:* 100/70 mm Hg
*Peak blood pressure:* 138/66 mm Hg

On October 24, 1986, the patient came to phase II. His resting heart rate was 92 bpm, and it was noted that he had frequent premature atrial contractions at rest on the radiotelemetry system. He performed his usual bicycle ergometry workout of 87.5.

At a peak heart rate of 144 bpm, the patient developed multiple premature atrial contractions and a burst of supraventricular tachycardia immediately after exercise at a rate of 160 to 170 bpm. This resolved spontaneously during the postexercise period. Cardiac examination revealed an $S_4$ heart sound with no $S_3$ and no pericardial friction rub, nor any paradoxical pulse. The program cardiologist examined the patient and found again no obvious signs or symptoms of pericarditis, and the cause of the supraventricular tachycardia remained unknown. The physician subsequently used digoxin to slow the heart rate and recommended continuing telemetry exercise sessions.

*October 29, 1986:* 40 minutes at 100 watts, peak heart rate 144 bpm, no ectopy
*November 3, 1986:* 40 minutes at 112 watts, peak heart rate 150 bpm
*November 13, 1986:* 40 minutes at 3.5 mph 7% grade, peak heart rate 144 bpm (resting heart rate 66)
*November 13, 1986:* 40 minutes at 3.5 mph 10% grade; peak heart rate 150 bpm; initiation of arm ergometry at 50 watts for 8 minutes, peak heart rate 126 bpm
*December 12, 1986:* 40 minutes at 3.5 mph, 11% grade, peak heart rate 140; 10 minutes at 62.5 watts for arm ergometry, peak heart rate 120 bpm

*December 19, 1986:* 40 minutes at 3.5 mph, 13% grade, peak heart rate 144 bpm; arm ergometry 10 minutes at 62.5 watts, peak heart rate 120 bpm

### Home program

The patient was now walk-jogging 2 to 4 miles at a peak heart rate of 138 to 144 bpm and progressed from 4 miles in 57 minutes to 4 miles in 45 to 50 minutes by the end of November. On November 13, 1986, the patient returned to work part-time as a worker's compensation adjuster for the state of California, and on December 12, 1986, resumed full-time work.

### Phase III cardiac rehabilitation

*December 22, 1986:* Initial phase III visit with 4-mile peak jog, 38 minutes, peak heart rate 150 bpm, no ectopy
*January 12, 1987:* 4-mile peak jog, 36 minutes, peak heart rate 144 bpm
*January 26, 1987:* 5-mile peak jog, 42 ½ minutes, peak heart rate 150 bpm
*January monthly exercise log summary*
  *Number of workouts:* 27
  *Average resting heart rate:* 66 bpm
  *Average peak heart rate:* 144 bpm
*Total miles:* 155
*Average peak:* 5.1
*Average peak time:* 55 minutes

The patient subsequently joined the SCOR Jogging Club and began training on Saturdays with this group. He continued to gradually increase his distance up to 8 to 12 miles, and in March 1987 was taken off his Lanoxin (digoxin) without recurrence of supraventricular dysrhythmias. Through the course of the next year, Mr. D.D. continued to attend phase III, one or two times per month, while working full-time and running at home. With the help of several other members in the SCOR Jogging Club, Mr. D.D. began to increase his mileage with the idea of training for a full marathon. He did complete the Los Alamitos marathon in March 1988 in 4 hours and 15 minutes and was extremely proud of his accomplishment.

The patient continues with his long-distance running program and maintains an excellent level of risk factor reduction, having improved his cholesterol/high-density lipoprotein ratio to 3.9 and maintaining a nonsmoking status and a normotensive blood pressure.

## CASE 4 ▼ Mr. P. P.

The following case study illustrates the effects of a complicated acute myocardial infarction upon right and left ventricular performance, and how cardiac rehabilitation assisted in the medical management of this patient.

**Patient:** Mr. P.P.

**Age:** 72

**Medical history:** The patient felt well until January 9, 1987, when at work he developed a severe, pressure-like discomfort in the retrosternal area associated with nausea. After going home from work and having the pain persist, the patient called the paramedics to his house and he was transferred to the Presbyterian Intercommunity Hospital emergency room. According to the patient's wife, he lost consciousness for 2 to 3 minutes and was found by the paramedics to have occasional premature ventricular contractions. He was admitted to the coronary care unit and suddenly went into ventricular tachycardia at a rate of 140 bpm, with a stable blood pressure of 120/80 mm Hg. This was treated with intravenous lidocaine. The electrocardiogram revealed an acute inferoposterior myocardial infarction with first-degree atrioventricular block and left atrial enlargement. Myocardial enzyme changes were positive for myocardial damage.

### Risk factors

1. Previous cigarette smoker, one pack per day for 30 years; quit cigarettes in 1974 and subsequently smoked a few pipefuls of tobacco or cigars daily
2. *Hypertension:* 22 year history of high blood pressure
3. *Lipids* on January 14, 1987: *cholesterol* 197; *triglycerides* 100; *HDL* 55; *LDL* 128; *cholesterol/HDL ratio* 3.9
4. *Diabetes:* negative
5. *Sedentary life-style:* positive
6. *Obesity:* negative: height 5'10", weight 155 pounds
7. *Stress:* mild levels of stress associated with part-time work as a salesperson for a hardware store
8. *Diet:* extremely high in saturated fats, cholesterol, and caffeine

### Hospital course

*January 9, 1987:* Potassium 3.1; therefore, it was believed that hypokalemia secondary to diuretic used for hypertension may have contributed to his dysrhythmia.

*January 12, 1987:* The patient was weaned from lidocaine and developed coarse rhonchi and wheezing in both lungs, believed to be acute bronchitis.

*January 13, 1987:* Cardiac rehabilitation ordered. The patient was transferred from the coronary care unit to the telemetry ward.

### Phase I cardiac rehabilitation
### Monitored self-care evaluation

*Chest wall examination:* negative
*Resting heart rate:* 92 bpm
*Resting blood pressure:* 108/62 mm Hg
*Peak heart rate:*
   104 bpm (during dressing and ambulation)
   108 bpm (during hygiene and grooming)

*Peak blood pressure:* 110/60 mm Hg throughout all self-care activities, except for 140/60 mm Hg during Valsalva maneuver. There were no dysrhythmias and no ST changes. An $S_4$ heart sound was auscultated at rest and after ambulation.

### Self-care evaluation summary and recommendations

The patient was asymptomatic without ST-segment changes or dysrhythmias. However, the blood pressure failed to rise with increasing heart rate.

**Plan:** Increase current activity levels; closely monitor HR, BP, ECG, breath and heart sounds, and symptoms.

*January 14, 1987;* initial monitored ambulation session
   *Resting heart rate:* 90 bpm
   *Peak heart rate:* 110 bpm
   *Resting supine blood pressure:* 110/74 mm Hg
   *Resting sitting blood pressure:* 102/66 mm Hg
   *Resting standing blood pressure:* 102/64 mm Hg
   *Peak blood pressure:* 110/70 mm Hg

Patient ambulated 50 yards initially and then 75 yards after a 5-minute rest period, with no ectopic beats.

*January 15, 1987:* monitored ambulation
   *Resting heart rate:* 94 bpm
   *Peak heart rate:* 111 bpm
   *Resting blood pressure:* 114/70 mm Hg
   *Peak blood pressure:* 136/76 mm Hg

Patient ambulated 100 yards with 5 minutes of rest and then 200 yards, with occasional premature arterial and ventricular contractions.

*January 16, 1987*
   *Resting heart rate:* 90 bpm
   *Peak heart rate:* 112 bpm
   *Resting blood pressure:* 116/80 mm Hg
   *Peak blood pressure:* 110/70 mm Hg

Patient ambulated 200 yards, 5 minutes rest, then 300 yards, with occasional premature atrial and ventricular contractions.

*January 17, 1987:* Patient noticed the onset of slight precordial chest pain lasting approximately 30 minutes and subsiding without medications. Repeat electrocardiogram revealed extension of an inferior wall infarction with deeper Q waves in leads 2, 3, and $aV_L$, with hyperacute ST-segment changes in the same leads, as well as reciprocal ST-segment depression in leads 1 and $aV_L$.

The patient was returned to bed rest. He was promptly started on lidocaine because of increased ectopy, and on January 20, 1987, was switched to Pronestyl (procainamide). Inderal (propranolol) and Isordil (isosorbide dinitrate) were also started at this time.

A self-care evaluation was again ordered and completed on January 23, 1987.

### Results

*Resting heart rate:* 84 bpm
*Peak heart rate:* 102 bpm
*Resting blood pressure:* 100/62 mm Hg

*During hygiene and grooming, peak blood pressure:* 82/58 mm Hg

It was noted that the patient had a progressive drop in blood pressure to 82/58 mm Hg while dressing upper extremities and 80/52 mm Hg during Valsalva maneuver, returning to 102/166 mm Hg 1 minute after activity. No ST-segment changes were seen. Occasional premature atrial contractions were noticed.

*January 23, 1987:* monitored ambulation restarted
*Resting heart rate:* 89 bpm
*Peak heart rate:* 105 bpm
*Resting blood pressure:* 112/72 bpm
*Peak blood pressure:* 118/78 mm Hg

Patient ambulated 100 yards without chest discomfort, had one premature atrial contraction with ambulation, and was mildly short of breath.

*January 24, 1987:* monitored ambulation
*Resting heart rate:* 88 bpm
*Peak heart rate:* 96 bpm
*Resting blood pressure:* 114/68 mm Hg
*Peak blood pressure:* 92/60 mm Hg

Patient ambulated 100 yards, with 5 minutes of rest, and then 200 yards. This hypotensive response was slightly greater than that observed during hygiene and grooming on the previous day.

*January 25, 1987:* monitored ambulation
*Resting heart rate:* 89 bpm
*Peak heart rate:* 102 bpm
*Resting blood pressure:* 102/70 mm Hg
*Peak blood pressure:* 90-96/60 mm Hg

Patient ambulated 200 and then 400 yards with no ST changes: however, multiple premature ventricular contractions with short runs of trigeminy and occasional coupled premature ventricular contractions were noticed.

Because of the possibility that the dysrhythmias represented an ischemic response, the patient's beta blocker (propranolol), nitrates, and Pronestyl were increased. Later in the day, the patient had several long runs of ventricular tachycardia that required intravenous lidocaine.

*January 28, 1987:* Because of multiple dysrhythmias and an abnormal blood pressure response, the patient underwent a low-level treadmill test.

**Treadmill test results**
*Time completed:* 8.5 minutes
*Limiting factor:* a 36 mm Hg fall in systolic blood pressure during the last 2 minutes of exercise.
*Resting heart rate:* 80 bpm
*Peak heart rate:* 108 bpm
*Resting blood pressure:* 110/70 mm Hg
*Peak blood pressure:* 84/60 mm Hg

Blood pressure fell to 84/60 mm Hg by minute 8.5. During recovery, the patient again developed ventricular tachycardia at a rate of 140 bpm. This lasted for 3 minutes and required intravenous lidocaine for conversion to sinus rhythm. The patient was symptomatic before, during, and after exercise. No significant ST changes were seen. The test was interpreted as being abnormal with a hypoadaptive blood pressure response and ventricular dysrhythmias suggestive of ischemic left ventricular dysfunction. It was suspected that the patient may have had extensive, severe, three-vessel coronary artery disease.

*January 30, 1987:* cardiac catheterization
*Ventriculogram:*
Akinesis of the inferior wall of the left ventricule because of moderate-sized inferior infarction
Left ventricular end-diastolic pressure 8
Ejection fraction 43%
*Coronary angiogram:*
*Right coronary artery:* proximal 100% obstruction (distal to the first diagonal)
*Left anterior descending artery:* 40% obstruction
*Circumflex artery:* 30% obstruction proximally with an additional 30% obstruction distal to the first marginal artery

*January 31, 1987:* monitored ambulation (reordered)

While walking at a very slow pace, patient again demonstrated a decrease in blood pressure from 120/70 to 94/60 mm Hg with a heart rate rise from 80 to 96. No ventricular ectopic beats were observed.

The patient had a short episode of ventricular tachycardia that occurred while at rest in the afternoon and resolved spontaneously. It was believed that the recurring ventricular tachycardia was caused by a reentry mechanism in peri-infarction tissue. The exertional hypotension in the face of a moderate-sized inferior infarction with apparently good perfusion through the left coronary artery system indicated a myocardial depressant effect of the patient's antidysrhythmics and beta-blocking medications. Subsequently, Isordil (isosorbide dinitrate) and Inderal (propranolol) were decreased; however, Pronestyl (procainamide) was increased to one gram every 6 hours.

*February 1, 1987:* monitored ambulation
The patient continued to show a 15 to 20 mm decrease in blood pressure with a 12 to 20 beat per minute increase in heart rate over resting levels. Occasional premature atrial and ventricular contractions were observed.

*February 4, 1987:*
Because of the persistent dysrhythmias and poor blood pressure response, an exercise radionuclide wall motion study was done. The patient exercised on a supine bicycle ergometer for three stages (200, 300, and 400 KPM) at 3 minutes per stage. The test was terminated by the patient because of leg fatigue.

**Bicycle ergometry test results**
*Resting heart rate:* 72 bpm
*Maximum heart rate:* 90 bpm
(Blunted heart rate because of beta blockade)
*Resting blood pressure:* 112/70 mm Hg
*Peak blood pressure:* 80/50 mm Hg

A fourth heart sound was auscultated before exercise and

## CASE 4 ▼ Mr. P. P.—cont'd

an $S_4$ developed after exercise. There were no dysrhythmias and no significant ST-segment changes.

The right ventricle was dilated with inferior wall akinesis, and the remaining portion of the right ventricle was severely hypokinetic.

An interpretation of this study revealed that left ventricular function was mildly impaired at rest and improved with exercise, while the right ventricle was greatly dilated and demonstrated a very poor ejection fraction at rest and with exercise. It was postulated that this patient's limitation in cardiac reserve was not attributable to left ventricular dysfunction, but rather to right ventricular dysfunction (hypothesis and akinesis with possible aneurysm). Diastolic tamponade of the left ventricle caused by the dilated right ventricle during exercise was also considered as an explanation, in which case filling of the dilated right ventricle during diastole may have compressed the aortic outflow tract and decreased the cardiac output during exercise. Inderal (propranolol) was discontinued, and Dyazide (triamterene and hydrochlorothiazide) was added to decrease the right ventricular preload.

> February 5, 1987: monitored ambulation
> Resting heart rate: 92 bpm
> Peak heart rate: 110 bpm
> Resting blood pressure: 89/70 mm Hg
> Peak blood pressure: 130/70 mm Hg

Occasional premature ventricular contractions were noticed, and an adaptive blood pressure response was observed with ambulation of 100 yards.

> February 6, 1987: monitored ambulation
> Resting heart rate: 88 bpm
> Peak heart rate: 120 to 132 bpm
> Resting blood pressure: 102/70 mm Hg
> Peak blood pressure: 134/70 mm Hg
> One premature ventricular contraction with ambulation of 300 yards

February 7, 1987: Patient discharged home on Pronestyl (procainamide) 1000 mg qid, Isodril Tembids (isosorbide dinitrate) 40 mg bid, and Aldactazide (spironolactone and hydrochlorothiazide), one tablet bid, with K-Lyte for potassium supplementation. With a normal blood-pressure response and no significant dysrhythmias, it was believed that the patient was safe to perform self-care and home activities to a heart rate of 130 bpm.

This case clearly demonstrates three aspects of Phase I cardiac rehabilitation. First, the monitoring activities (self-care and ambulation), when completed accurately and interpreted appropriately, correlated well with the patient's ventricular performance. This patient's hypotension, tachycardia, and heart sounds repeatedly described a person with poor ventricular function. Second, these data were used by the patient's physician to make decisions about further diagnostic tests and medication changes. Finally, the monitored ambulation was used to make appropriate discharge decisions.

### Phase II cardiac rehabilitation

February 9, 1987: The patient was interviewed by the entire cardiac rehabilitation team for entry into the phase II program. The physical therapy assessment determined that this was a 72-year-old man with a very complicated hospital course, with recurrent ventricular dysrhythmias and hypoadaptive blood pressure response to activity because of severe right ventricular failure during exercise. The patient has been quite depressed at times in the hospital because of the multiple complications and setbacks; however, he was very well motivated to improve his physical capacity and to return to work.

### Goals

1. Improve physical work capacity and endurance
2. Reduce risk factors
3. Educate the patient regarding coronary artery disease, risk factors, diet, exercise
4. Return to work as soon as possible

### Plan

1. Begin phase II, three times a week, for outpatient exercise program with arm and leg ergometry; add weight training in 4 weeks
2. Basic education lecture series
3. Schedule for maximal exercise test in 4 weeks

> February 11, 1987: initial phase II session
> Resting heart rate: 90 bpm
> Peak heart rate: 120 bpm
> Resting blood pressure: 92/62 mm Hg
> Peak blood pressure: 100/60 mm Hg

Fifteen minutes of lower-extremity ergometry with 50 watts, 5 minutes of upper-extremity ergometry with 30 watts, no dysrhythmias, moderate dyspnea.

> February 23, 1987:
> Resting heart rate: 84 bpm
> Peak heart rate: 114 bpm
> Resting blood pressure: 106/76 mm Hg
> Peak blood pressure: 120/70 mm Hg

## CASE 4 ▼ Mr. P. P.—cont'd

25 minutes of lower-extremity ergometry at 50 watts, 10 minutes of upper-extremity ergometry at 37 ½ watts, no ectopy.

*March 11, 1987:*
*Resting heart rate:* 84 bpm
*Peak heart rate:* 114 bpm
*Resting blood pressure:* 110/60 mm Hg
*Peak blood pressure:* 120/74 mm Hg
35 minutes of lower-extremity ergometry at 62 ½ watts, 10 minutes of upper-extremity ergometry at 55 watts; only occasional premature atrial contractions were noticed.

*March 25, 1987:*
*Resting heart rate:* 78 bpm
*Peak heart rate:* 114 bpm
*Resting blood pressure:* 104/60 mm Hg
*Peak blood pressure:* 120/62 mm Hg
35 minutes of lower-extremity ergometry at 68 watts, 10 minutes of upper-extremity ergometry at 62 ½ watts, no ectopic beats.

*April 3, 1987:* Maximum treadmill test results
Completed 9.2 minutes of Sheffield Protocol
*Limiting factor:* Dyspnea
*Resting heart rate:* 76 bpm
*Peak heart rate:* 136
*Resting blood pressure:* 146/92 mm Hg
*Peak blood pressure:* 92/70 mm Hg
No angina
$S_4$ before and after exercise
No dysrhythmias, no ST-segment changes
Fair physical work capacity for a 72-year-old man

Upon entering phase II, the patient began a home program of walking, consisting of one-half mile, twice a day, for 15 minutes each time to similar heart rates seen in monitored exercise sessions. By the end of February, he had increased his walking to 2 miles in 43 minutes, and in March through April, he increased this to 3 to 4 miles in 60 to 70 minutes, at a peak heart rate of 120 bpm. The patient elected to retire from work at this point, and in mid-May was transferred to our phase III program.

### Phase III

On May 18, 1987, the patient began the phase III program with a large group exercise class. Because of the absence of dysrhythmias in late April and early May, he had been weaned from the continuous telemetry monitoring, but was monitored the first two sessions in phase III as a routine check.

*May 18, 1987:* initial phase III program
*Resting heart rate:* 78 bpm
*Peak heart rate:* 114 bpm
*Resting blood pressure:* 120/90 mm Hg
*Peak blood pressure:* 130/68 mm Hg

Patient completed 3 miles of a fast walk without dysrhythmias.

The patient continued weekly phase III visits for the next 6 months, while continuing to exercise at home 5 or 6 days a week. During this time, he gradually increased his endurance to 3 miles of walking in 50 minutes with a peak heart rate of 108 to 114 bpm. His resting heart rate had decreased to 72 bpm. At this point, the patient was interested in beginning a walk-jogging program. Since he had been in the program 9 months, it was elected to repeat his maximum treadmill test first.

*November 25, 1987:* maximum treadmill test results
Completed 12.2 minutes of Sheffield Protocol
*Resting heart rate:* 76 bpm
*Peak heart rate:* 136 bpm
*Resting blood pressure:* 146/92 mm Hg
*Peak blood pressure:* 126/80, 104/64 mm Hg
Blunted blood pressure response with 16 mm Hg fall in last 6 minutes
Occasional premature ventricular contractions throughout
No ST-segment changes: R-wave amplitude increased 8 mm
Mildly impaired physical working capacity (PWC) for 72-year-old man
Functional aerobic impairment (FAI): 2%
Three-minute improvement since last test of April 1987

*November 30, 1987:* The patient began short-distance jogging, reducing his 3-mile time from 50 to 45 minutes, while maintaining a peak heart rate of 114 to 120 bpm with an appropriate, albeit blunted, blood pressure response. The patient continues to feel well and participates in all of his premorbid recreational activities, including golfing, bowling, and hiking, and continues to maintain his walk-jogging program. It is planned that yearly treadmill tests will be performed to assess the stability of the patient's disease and to document any further improvement in his physical work capacity.

To summarize, this 72-year-old man demonstrates how a carefully prescribed and supervised cardiac rehabilitation program can significantly improve physical performance and assist in determining the appropriate medical therapy, despite multiple complications and severe ventricular dysfunction.

---

**CASE 5  ▼  Mr. G. F.**

---

The following case study illustrates the difficulties that may be encountered with an extremely complicated myocardial infarction. Although this is clearly a "high-risk" patient, a carefully monitored program allowed this completely bedridden man to become quite vigorous.

**Patient:** Mr. G.F.

**Age:** 63

**Medical history:** This 63-year-old man was well until January 5, 1986. While walking after lunch in Newport Beach, he experienced the onset of retrosternal pain. The pain persisted on and off all afternoon, and he went to a local emergency room at 11 PM. An ECG was normal, and he was given Mylanta and Dalmane (fluorazepam) and sent home. The pain continued and the patient had a more severe episode at 1 AM, associated with pronounced diaphoresis. Early that morning (January 6), his wife drove him to Presbyterian Intercommunity Hospital, where he was admitted.

### Risk factors

1. Negative family history
2. Cigarette smoking: one-third pack per day for 30 years, quit before myocardial infarction
3. *Lipids: cholesterol* 189; *triglycerides* 118; *HDL* 33; *cholesterol/HDL ratio* 5.9 (see Chapter 8)
4. *Obesity:* admission weight 220 pounds, height 6 feet
5. Sedentary
6. Negative for hypertension and diabetes
7. *Stress:* worked as president of local bank

On admission, he had evidence of an acute anterolateral wall myocardial infarction with chest pain. He developed congestive heart failure with cardiomegaly and pulmonary vascular congestion on chest radiography, and auscultation of the lungs revealed inspiratory rales bilaterally. He was medically controlled with morphine and Lasix (furosemide) until January 8, when he developed atrial fibrillation and Lanoxin (digoxin) was added. Nitropaste, Isordil, and Dyazide were also added. Atrial fibrillation continued intermittently through January 11, but his chest radiograph showed signs of improvement. He was allowed by his physician to be up in a chair and walk around in his coronary care unit room by January 12. On January 14, he had increasing premature ventricular contractions requiring intravenous lidocaine, but was transferred from the CCU to a telemetry ward the same day. On January 15, the intravenous lidocaine was removed and the physician ordered "increased activity."

On January 16, the patient had a cardiac arrest requiring defibrillation several times, and he was returned to the CCU, where a Swan-Ganz catheter was inserted, the patient was intubated, and lidocaine was started intravenously with additional diuretic added because of basilar rales. He was weaned from lidocaine on January 20 and started on Norpace (disopyramide phosphate) which proved to be ineffective. The chest radiograph showed an increase in pulmonary congestion, and more Lasix was given. Oral Pronestyl and quinidine were added.

On January 20, it was believed that the patient was in impending cardiogenic shock, and intraaortic balloon coun-

terpulsation was started. A cardiac catheterization was done because of these multiple complications.

*Coronary angiogram*
*Left anterior descending artery:* 99% occluded from first to fourth septal perforators (pattern suggessted recanalization)
*Circumflex artery:* marginal branch irregularity
*Right coronary artery:* normal
*Ventriculogram*
   *Left ventricular end-diastolic pressure:* 12 mm Hg, 24 mm Hg after angiography (normal 0 to 12)
*Pulmonary artery pressure:* 38/20 mm Hg (mean 27, normal 25/10)
*Aortic blood pressure:* 132/68 mm Hg (mean 96)
*Stroke volume:* 107 ml
*Heart rate:* 84
*Cardiac index:* 2.4 L/min $M_2$
*Ejection fraction:* 24%

On January 23, the intraaortic balloon was removed. The patient was encouraged to sit at bedside, but multiple attempts at this and at standing were unsuccessful because of severe hypotension (BP 50/0). Various dysrhythmias continued despite high doses of Pronestyl, quinidine, Norpace, Inderal, and intravenous lidocaine. (Inderal was discontinued January 30.)

In early February, the Pronestyl was increased to 875 mg q4h and Anturane (sulfinpyrazone) 100 mg twice a day was added. Intravenous lidocaine was discontinued on February 6; however, on February 13 an asymptomatic episode of prolonged ventricular tachycardia occurred. Mr. G.F. was transferred to a telemetry bed on February 20, but his congestive heart failure persisted (basilar rales were present) and required more Dyazide. By early March the patient could sit at bedside for only a few minutes because of hypotension and lightheadedness.

### Phase I cardiac rehabilitation

On March 12, cardiac rehabilitation was ordered for Mr. G.F.

After 2 months in the hospital with multiple complications, this patient was totally incapacitated, severely depressed, and dependent on nursing care for all his self-care needs. The goals of phase I cardiac rehabilitation for this patient were as follows:

1. Reduce orthostatic hypotension and increase sitting and standing tolerance
2. Increase self-care capabilities
3. Progress to short-distance ambulation and improve blood pressure response
4. Decrease depression; improve self-confidence
5. Prepare patient for hospital discharge and phase II cardiac rehabilitation immediately after discharge

### Phase I program

Phase I included a self-care evaluation, physical therapy evaluation, and interview.

## CASE 5 ▼ Mr. G. F.—cont'd

1. Sitting out of bed four times a day to tolerance, with blood pressure, heart rate, and telemetry ECG recorded continuously while up
2. Lower-extremity resistive exercise conditioning while seated
3. Monitored ambulation twice a day (10 to 20 feet)
4. Bicycle ergometry twice a day (less than 5 minutes)

### Initial session

*Resting heart rate:* 78 bpm
*Peak heart rate:* 84 bpm
*Resting blood pressure:* 56/38 mm Hg (sitting) after 5 minutes of sitting with active toe raises
*Standing blood pressure:* 50/28 mm Hg
Walking 50 feet, with blood pressure of 48/20 mm Hg while ambulating

*By March 21:*
*Resting heart rate:* 78 bpm
*Peak heart rate:* 88 bpm
*Resting blood pressure:* 90/60, but 82/50 mm Hg with walking 200 feet, repeated four times per day

*By March 23:*
96/60, but 84/50 mm Hg while walking 1000 to 1400 feet; also riding bicycle ergometer at 25 watts for 5 minutes

*By March 31:*
Discharged home
Walking 1700 feet with assistance
*Blood pressure:* 85/50 mm Hg
Infrequent hypotensive episodes
*Discharge medications:* Lanoxin, Pronestyl, quinidine, Norpace, Anturane, Isordil, and Coumadin (warfarin)

A low-level treadmill test was not attempted. The results of the monitored ambulation indicated that further workloads would not be tolerated.

### Phase II goals

Although this patient was able to walk a few hundred feet and perform most self-care activities at the time of discharge, his physician did not believe that a low-level treadmill test was indicated. Based on the knowledge of his ventricular function from catheterization and the physiological detrimental effects of bed rest, the following goals were set for this patient:

1. Decrease exercise-induced hypotension
2. Increase walking distance initially and then speed and intensity, if indicated
3. Increase upper-extremity strength and endurance
4. Increase self-confidence

The limitations were probably the result of a number of pathophysiological mechanisms, including peri-infarction ischemia, the myocardial depressant effects of multiple antidysrhythmic drugs, prolonged bed rest with muscle atrophy and deconditioning (the patient lost 40 pounds in the hospital), and infarcted myocardium.

### Phase II program

Phase II for Mr. G.F. was a three-times-a-week outpatient program.

1. Monitored ambulation, with increases in distance as physiological responses and tolerance warrant
2. Bicycle ergometry, emphasizing low resistance and increasing time and endurance
3. Add arm ergometry when capable

### Program progress

*April 2, 1986:* first phase II session
Walked 2000 feet in 15 minutes; bicycle ergometry at 37 watts for 5 minutes

*Resting heart rate:* 72 bpm
*Peak heart rate:* 90 bpm
*Resting blood pressure:* 84/60 mm Hg
*Peak blood pressure:* 86/50 mm Hg

*May 5, 1986*
Walked 1 mile in 25 minutes
*Resting blood pressure:* 76-84/42 mm Hg
*Peak blood pressure:* 96-106/60 mm Hg
Bicycle eregometry at 50 watts for 20 minutes

*June 9, 1986*
Walked 3 miles in 56 minutes
*Resting blood pressure:* 84/50-60 mm Hg
*Peak blood pressure:* 88-96/40 mm Hg
Started arm ergometry for 10 minutes at 30 watts (discontinued Norpace and Pronestyl was decreased)

*June 20, 1986:* low-level exercise test: 4-minute Sheffield Protocol stopped secondary to a decrease in blood pressure
*Resting heart rate:* 85 bpm
*Maximum heart rate:* 100 bpm
*Resting blood pressure:* 90/50 mm Hg
*Maximum blood pressure:* 90/50 mm Hg, which fell to 80/36 mm Hg during the last minute of exercise
Negative for angina, ST changes or dysrhythmias
$S_4$ before exercise
Pronestyl and quinidine dosages decreased again

*July 2, 1986:* Resting gated blood pool study with first-pass angiogram results: "diffuse hypokinesis of the left ventricle with the apex and interior wall akinesis."

*July 9, 1986*
Walked 3 miles in 46 minutes
*Peak heart rate:* 96 bpm
*Resting blood pressure:* 80/50 mm Hg
*Peak blood pressure:* 102/40 mm Hg, doing 15 minutes of aerobic exercise at 50 watts

*August 9, 1986*
Began walk-jogging 3 miles in 46 minutes, jogged 100 feet, alternated with walking 900 feet
*Peak heart rate:* 102-108 bpm
*Resting blood pressure:* 90/52 mm Hg
*Peak blood pressure:* 102/44 mm Hg

**CASE 5** ▼ **Mr. G. F.—cont'd**

*September 9, 1986*
Walk-jogged 3 miles in 45 minutes, 200-foot jog,
*Peak heart rate:* 102/114 bpm
*Resting blood pressure:* 94/60 mm Hg
*Peak blood pressure:* 110/60 mm Hg

September 29, 1986: started phase III program (one time a week in phase III, two times a week in phase II); arm ergometry increased to 15 minutes at 60 to 65 watts.

Because of the history of multiple cardiac arrests and alternating antidysrhythmic therapy, continuous ECG monitoring in phase II was continued for many months. Only occasional premature ventricular contractions were observed.

In December 1988, the patient's physician cleared Mr. G.F. to return to work. He desired to work part-time and did so on January 5, 1987.

**Phase III program**

With return to work, phase II was completed and Mr. G.F. was seen once a week for continued endurance building and periodic monitoring.

*January 5, 1987*
Walk-jogged for 3 miles in 43 minutes
*Resting heart rate:* 72 bpm
*Peak heart rate:* 72 bpm
*Resting blood pressure:* 102/66 mm Hg
*Peak blood pressure:* 130/68 mm Hg
No dysrhythmias
(See figure 9-15.)

*February 1, 1987:* Mr. G.F. participated in the Presbyterian Intercommunity Hospital 5 and 10 km "Walk-Jog-Run for Your Heart." Exactly one year earlier, he had watched the race from a wheelchair while still an inpatient. He completed the 5 km race in 40 minutes, winning a first-place award for predicting his running time.

Mr. G.F. continues to participate in phase III on a weekly basis, walk-jogging 3 miles in 37 to 39 minutes, and demonstrates appropriate cardiovascular responses. All antidysrhythmics have been eliminated except quinidine. He exercises two to three times a week on his own, continues to work 20 hours a week, fishes at high altitudes, and travels around the country to see relatives from time to time.

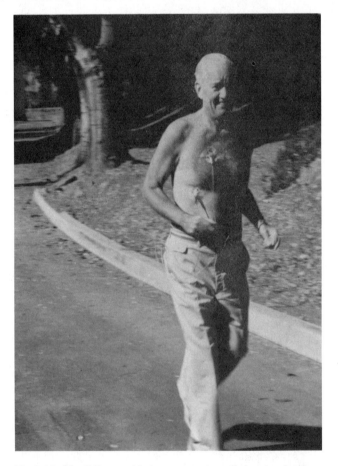

**Fig. 9-15.** Mr. G.F. was able to progress to walk-jogging in phase III despite his poor left ventricular function on angiography. His resting and exercise blood pressures gradually became adaptive over a 12-month period.

## CASE 6 ▼ Mr. E. R.

This case study is another example of the long-term training effects that may be seen in patients who comply with a vigorous aerobic exercise program. Despite severe triple-vessel coronary artery disease and angina, this patient was able to alleviate his symptoms through an exercise conditioning program, improve his physical work capacity by nearly 50% over an 8-year period, and demonstrate some apparent degree of regression of his coronary atheroma.

**Patient:** Mr. E.R.

**Age:** 61 (at time of entry into rehabilitation program)

**Medical history:** This 61-year-old man first began to note the onset of substernal chest pressure in 1965 at 48 years of age. He began a limited walking program on his own, gradually progressing up to 2 miles per day. His angina symptoms improved with this self-prescribed exercise program until 1978, when they became more frequent and more severe. He saw his private physician, who referred the patient for a bicycle ergometry test in July 1978.

**Bicycle ergometry test results:**
*Completed:* 800 kgm (kilogram meters)
*Limiting factor:* fatigue and falling blood pressure
*Resting heart rate:* 62 bpm
*Peak heart rate:* 145 bpm
*Resting blood pressure:* 140/70 mm Hg
*Peak blood pressure:* 160/60 mm Hg (falling to 120/50 mm Hg at peak heart rate)
Patient experienced level 1 angina pectoris during the third and fourth workloads, which was not limiting
No dysrhythmias
4 mm of flat ST-segment depression noted in $V_5$ lead at peak rate
*Physical work capacity:* fair to good in a mildly active 61-year-old man
*Resting electrocardiogram:* normal

The patient was subsequently referred for catheterization because of the hypoadaptive blood pressure response along with pronounced ischemic ST changes and angina symptoms.

**Cardiac catheterization** (July 13, 1978)
*Ventriculogram*
   Normal contractility of the left ventricle
   *Left ventricular end-diastolic pressure:* 12 mm Hg
   *Stroke index:* 65 ml/m$^2$
   *Cardiac index:* 4.7 1/min/m$^2$
   *Ejection fraction:* 78%
*Coronary angiogram*
   Left anterior descending artery: 95% obstruction proximal to first septal perforator with an additional long, narrow segment of 70% to 85% obstruction between the first and second septal perforators with good distal runoff
   *Circumflex artery:* 95% occlusion just proximal to the marginal branch with rapid filling of the marginal and distal circumflex arteries
   *Right coronary artery:* 75% obstruction 2 cm from the origin with excellent distal runoff

**Risk factors**
1. Positive family history of coronary disease: patient's brother died of a myocardial infarction at 55 years of age
2. Negative for smoking
3. Positive for hypertension: systolic blood pressures found to be 140 to 160 mm Hg
4. *Lipids:* only one cholesterol was available in 1978 (215 mg/dl)
5. No history of diabetes
6. *Body weight:* at the onset of the patient's angina in 1965, he weighed 145 pounds, height 5'9"
7. *Stress:* type A personality; patient worked as a shoe salesman for many years under a considerable amount of stress, in the patient's estimation.

**Phase III rehabilitation program**

After the patient's initial catheterization in July 1978, he began exercising on his own and progressed to walking up to 4 miles per day and bicycling a stationary ergometer 6 miles per day. His physician subsequently referred him to a phase III program in April 1979.

Initial evaluation revealed a well-motivated, 61-year-old man who experienced mild to moderate anginal symptoms with walking. He had severe triple-vessel coronary artery disease with normal ventricular function; however, he developed a severely ischemic ventricle at heart rates above 120 bpm with a hypoadaptive blood pressure on objective testing.

**Goals**
1. Reduce angina pectoris symptoms
2. Improve physical work capacity and endurance
3. Reduce risk factors
4. Educate patient on the value of exercise and risk factor reduction in reducing the risk of coronary atherosclerosis progression

Mr. E.R. began phase III and was monitored while performing his usual level of exercise, that is, 4 miles of walking to a peak heart rate of 96. He would experience level 1 angina with an appropriate blood pressure response and no dysrhythmias. During bicycle ergometry, he would train up to a heart rate of 114 to 120 bpm, also with level 1 angina, but with an appropriate blood pressure response (probably secondary to warm-up).

Over the course of the next year, the patient maintained this level of exercise and found his anginal symptoms progressively decreasing to the point where he required very infrequent nitroglycerin use. No other cardiac medications were required.

In September 1979, the patient underwent repeated cardiac catheterization.

**Cardiac catheterization results** (September 1979)
*Ventriculogram*
   Normal contractility
   *Ejection fraction:* 63%

*Left ventricular end-diastolic pressure:* 18 mm H
*Coronary angiogram*

Unchanged except for the circumflex artery, where a new 60% proximal obstruction was observed

Despite the progression of the patient's coronary artery disease, it was elected to continue to treat him medically because of the symptomatic improvement he had experienced in the previous year from his exercise conditioning program. In addition, objective exercise testing revealed an improved physical work capacity (900 kgm) with very mild angina in the fourth and final workload, compared to exercise testing in July of 1978 when angina occurred during the third workload.

Over the next 7 years, as seen in Fig. 9-16, the patient maintained a very high level of compliance to an exercise conditioning program. He consistently averaged between 5 to 7 days per week of training during this time with very infrequent interruption. In 1983, he became virtually asymptomatic and began to jog, and by 1984, he was jogging continuously 5 miles. In addition to his early-morning jogging program, the patient would exercise again in the late afternoon riding a stationary bicycle, progressing up to 10 miles in 45 minutes. Fig. 9-17 reveals that over this 7-year period, the patient was able to train to higher heart rates, ultimately training at pulse rates of 120 to 138 bpm with no angina symptoms. Fig. 9-18 reveals that Mr. E.R. averaged, through a combination of cycling and walk-jogging, between 1 to 2 hours of exercise per day throughout this 7-year period.

Mr. E.R. was seen in phase III on a weekly basis for 7 years and monitored periodically with radiotelemetry ECG and blood-pressure measurements while jogging. With an appropriate warm-up interval, even at higher heart rates, it was found that the patient's blood pressure was almost always adaptive, with only infrequent premature ventricular contractions observed. In 1983, the patient joined the SCOR Jogging Club as a result of his new-found jogging abilities, and did his Saturday morning training sessions with this group. Between 1983 and 1986, he participated in a number of local 10-km runs, enjoying the friendship and camaraderie of doing these physical activities with other cardiac runners.

During this 7-year period of time, bicycle ergometry testing demonstrated rather dramatic physiological changes despite his severe coronary disease and advancing age. His resting pulse rate dropped progressively into the mid-40s, while his maximum chronotropic reserve also increased to 159 bpm by 1985 (Fig. 9-19). Consequently, the patient's maximum rate-pressure product improved dramatically from $174 \times 10^2$ in 1973 to $257 \times 10^2$ by April 1985. From 1980 on, no anginal symptoms were experienced during the patient's yearly exercise tests. Interestingly, the hypoadaptive blood pressure response progressively improved over this time, and by April 1985 the patient experienced a rather small drop of 12 mm Hg (from 180 to 168 at peak exercise) at 1250 kgm. Only occasional premature ventricular contractions were observed during all these tests, and the degree of ST-segment depression

remained stable at 4 to 6 mm in the $V_5$ lead. Thus, this patient demonstrated a 50% improvement in his work capacity over a 7-year period of time with complete resolution of angina symptoms and an ability to exercise at a progressively higher rate-pressure product.

In May 1985, because of the tremendous improvement this patient had experienced with medical management, it was believed that another cardiac catheterization was warranted to examine the stability of the patient's severe coronary obstruction.

**Cardiac catheterization results** (May 1985)
*Ventriculogram*
Normal contractility
*Ejection fraction:* 65%
*Coronary angiogram*
*Left anterior descending artery:* unchanged with a proximal 95% obstruction
*Circumflex artery:* 60% proximal obstruction with apparent regression of the second lesion from 95% to 70%
*Right coronary artery:* apparent regression from 75% in 1973 to 30% to 40% in 1979

Thus, this patient showed regression of coronary atherosclerosis in two of his three major coronary arteries, with symptomatic relief of angina pectoris. Excellent adherence to exercise conditioning and risk factor modifications may have accounted for these findings. The following lipids were observed in 1985:

*Cholesterol:* 151
*Triglycerides:* 54
*HDL:* 51
*LDL:* 109
*Cholesterol/HDL ratio:* 3.0

The patient lost a total of 15 pounds over this 7-year period of time and was 130 pounds in 1985. His percent body fat had decreased from 19% in 1979 to a very lean 13% in 1985. Blood pressure was well controlled with exercise, weight loss, and sodium restriction. The average systolic blood pressure was 120 to 130 mm Hg.

Again, because of these findings, it was elected to continue to treat the patient medically, and he became somewhat of a celebrity in the program because his was the most dramatic example of atherosclerotic regression. (Approximately 5% of middle-aged patients in our long-term phase III program were found to have some degree of regression on repeat coronary angiograms.)

The patient had elected to retire from his job as a shoe salesman in 1972 and often took 2- to 3-week vacations, during which he would continue to exercise either by running around the deck of a ship or running up and down the stairs of a hotel where he was staying.

On January 20, 1986, the patient died during his sleep, apparently suffering a fatal dysrhythmia. A subsequent au-

Figures 9-16 to 9-19 for this case are on pages 179-180.

**CASE 6** ▼   **Mr. E. R.—cont'd**

topsy revealed no evidence of acute myocardial infarction or coronary thrombosis, with stable coronary atherosclerotic lesions, as described at angiography in 1985. Patchy fibrosis of the myocardium was observed, however. The cause of the fatal dysrhythmia during sleep is unknown, but many theories have been advanced in an attempt to explain such occurrences, including myocardial ischemia, low-potassium or low-magnesium levels within the myocardium, inadequate intake of linoleic acid in the diet, and so on.

In any case, we can certainly say that this man experienced a greatly improved quality of life over the 21-year history of his coronary disease, and may well have extended his life as a result of his compliance to the overall cardiac rehabilitation program. His dedication, compliance, and tremendous improvement served as an inspiration for other patients to adhere to life-style changes.

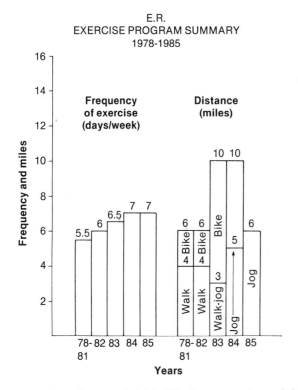

**Fig. 9-16.** Over a 7-year period, Mr. E.R. demonstrated remarkable consistency in his adherence to an aerobic conditioning program. He attended phase III weekly during the entire time.

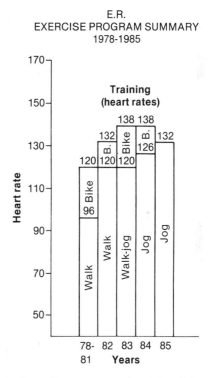

**Fig. 9-17.** As his angina symptoms abated, Mr. E.R. was able to train at higher heart rates, eventually being able to jog continuously at a heart rate of 132 to 138 bpm without symptoms.

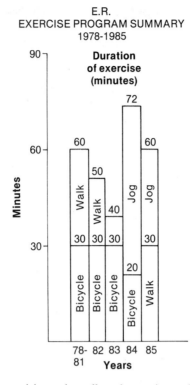

**Fig. 9-18.** Mr. E.R. enjoyed exercising and usually rode a stationary bicycle 20 to 30 minutes in the afternoon after walk-jogging or jogging 40 to 70 minutes in the morning.

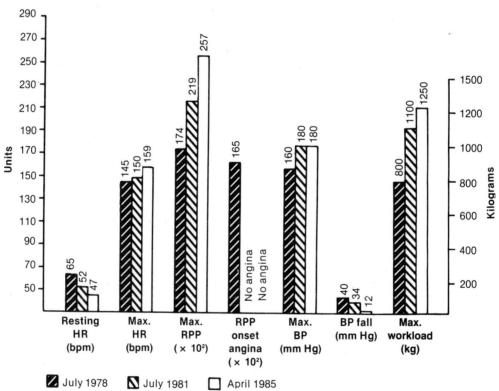

**Fig. 9-19.** This graph demonstrates the tremendous central and peripheral changes Mr. E.R. developed over a 7-year period.

## SUMMARY

These case histories exemplify the importance of proper program planning and implementation for patients involved in phases I, II, and III cardiac rehabilitation programs.

## REFERENCES

1. Akhras F and others: Early exercise testing and coronary angiography after uncomplicated myocardial infarction, *Br Med J* 284: 1293, 1982.
2. Arnim TV: Silent ischaemia in patients with coronary heart disease: prevalence and prognostic implications, *Eur Heart J* 8 (suppl G):115, 1987.
3. Arvan S: Exercise performance of the high risk acute myocardial infarction patients after cardiac rehabilitation, *Am J Cardiol* 62:197, 1988.
4. Assey ME: Prognosis in stable angina pectoris and silent myocardial ischemia, *Am J Cardiol* 61:19F, 1988.
5. Barndt R Jr and others: Regression and progression of early femoral atherosclerosis in treated hyperlipoproteinemia patients, *Ann Intern Med* 86:109, 1977.
6. Barnes GK and others: Changes in working status of patients following coronary bypass surgery, *JAMA* 238:1259, 1977.
7. Bemis CE and others: Progression of coronary artery disease: a clinical arteriographic study, *Circulation* 47:55, 1973.
8. Bjurstrom LA: A program of heart disease, intervention for public employees, *J Occup Med* 20:521, 1978.
9. Blankenhorn DH and others: Beneficial effects of combined colestipol-niacin therapy on coronary atherosclerosis and coronary venous bypass grafts, *JAMA* 257:3233, 1987.
10. Blessey R and others: Therapeutic effects and safety of exercising coronary patients at their angina threshold (abstract), *Med Sci Sports Exer* 11:110, 1979.
11. Blessey R and others: Early exercise training in complicated and uncomplicated post-myocardial infarction patients (abstract), *Med Sci Sports Exer* 12:100, 1980.
12. Blessey R and others: Angiographic, clinical and exercise data in marathoning coronary patients (abstract), *Med Sci Sports Exer* 13:131, 1981.
13. Blessey R and others: Post-myocardial infarction hospital course and response to early exercise training (abstract), *Med Sci Sports Exer* 114:1551, 1982.
14. Bloch A and others: Early mobilization after myocardial infarction: a controlled study, *Am J Cardiol* 34:152, 1974.
15. Block TA and others: Improvement in exercise performance after unsuccessful myocardial revascularization, *Am J Cardiol* 40:673, 1977.
16. Brown CA and others: Prospective study of medical and urgent surgical therapy in randomizable patients with unstable angina pectoris: results of in-hospital and chronic mortality and morbidity, *Am Heart J* 102:959, 1981.
17. Bruce RA and others: Difference in cardiac function with prolonged physical training for cardiac rehabilitation, *Am J Cardiol* 40:597, 1977.
18. Burgess AW and others: A randomized control trial of cardiac rehabilitation, *Soc Sci Med* 24:359, 1987.
19. Carson P and others: Exercise after myocardial infarction: controlled trial, *J R Coll Physicians* (London) 16:147, 1982.
20. Clausen JP: Circulatory adjustments to dynamic exercise and effect of physical training in normal subjects and in patients with coronary artery disease, *Prog Cardiovas Dis* 18:459, 1976.
21. Clausen JP and others: The effects of training on the heart rate during arm and leg exercise, *Scand J Clin Lab Invest* 26:295, 1970.
22. Clement DB and others: A survey of overuse running injuries, *Phys Sports Med* 9:47, 1981.
23. Cohn JN: Current therapy of the failing heart, *Circulation* 78:1099, 1988.
24. Collen D and others: Coronary thrombolysis with recombinant human tissue-type plasminogen activator: a prospective randomized placebo-controlled trial, *Circulation* 70:1012, 1984.
25. Conn EH and others: Exercise responses before and after physical conditioning in patients with severely depressed left ventricular functions, *Am J Cardiol* 49:296, 1982.
26. Cook R: Psychological responses to myocardial infarctions, *Heart Lung* 2:62, 1973.
27. Cookey JD and others: Exercise training and plasma catecholamines in patients with ischemic heart disease, *Am J Cardiol* 42:372, 1978.
28. Cox MH: Fitness and lifestyle programs for business and industry: problems in recruitment and retention, *J Cardiac Rehabil* 4:136, 1985.
29. Cox MH and others: Influence of an employee programme upon fitness, productivity and absenteeism, *Ergonomics* 24:10, 1981.
30. DeBusk RF and others: Exercise training soon after myocardial infarction, *Am J Cardiol* 44:1223, 1979.
31. Detry JM and others: Effects of physical training on exertional ST-segment depression in coronary heart disease, *Circulation* 44:390, 1971.
32. Detry JM and others: Increased arteriovenous oxygen difference after physical training in coronary heart disease, *Circulation* 4:109, 1971.
33. DeWood MA and others: Medical and surgical management of myocardial infarction, *Am J Cardiol* 44:1356, 1979.
34. Dion WF and others: Medical problems and physiologic responses during supervised inpatient cardiac rehabilitation: the patient after coronary bypass grafting, *Heart Lung* 11:248, 1982.
35. Ehsani AA and others: Effects of 12 months of intense exercise training on ischemic ST-segment depression in patients with coronary after disease, *Circulation* 64:1116, 1981.
36. Ehsani AA and others: Improvement of left ventricular contractile function by exercise training in patients with coronary artery disease, *Circulation* 74:350, 1986.
37. Eikelans DW and others: High density lipoprotein-cholesterol in survivors of myocardial infarction, *JAMA* 242:2185, 1979.
38. Erdman RAM: Psychological evaluation of an existing cardiac program: a randomized clinical trial in patients with myocardial infarction. In *II World Congress on Cardiac Rehabilitation: abstracts of free communications,* Jerusalem, 1982.
39. Erdman RA and Duivenvoorden HJ: Psychologic evaluation of a cardiac rehabilitation program: a randomized clinical trial in patients with myocardial infarction, *J Card Rehab* 3:696, 1983.
40. Feldman RL: Ambulatory electrocardiographic monitoring: the test for ischemia in 1988, *Ann Intern Med* 109:608, 1988.
41. Felig P and others: Fuel homeostasis in exercise, *N Engl J Med* 293:1078, 1975.
42. Ferguson RJ and others: Changes in exercise coronary sinus blood with training in patients with angina pectoris, *Circulation* 58:41, 1978.
43. Freedman B and others: Pathophysiology of coronary artery spasm, *Circulation* 66:705, 1982.
44. Froelicher VF: Does exercise conditioning delay progression of myocardial ischemia in coronary atherosclerotic disease? *Cardiovasc Clin* 8:11, 1977.
45. Fuller CM and others: Early post-myocardial infarction treadmill stress testing: an accurate prediction of multivessel coronary disease and subsequent cardiac events, *Ann Intern Med* 94:734, 1981.
46. Gleichmann U: Will there be less need for cardiac rehabilitation programmes when acute treatment is intensified and shortened? *Eur Heart J* 8 (suppl G):29, 1987.
47. Goldman S and others: Marked depth of ST-segment depression during treadmill exercise testing: indicator of severe coronary disease, *Circulation* 71:572, 1980.
48. Greenfield JC Jr: An explosion of technology, *Am J Cardiol* 62:1F, 1988.
49. Greenland P and Chu JS: Efficacy of cardiac rehabilitation services

with emphasis on patients after myocardial infarction, *Ann Intern Med* 109:650, 1988.

50. Greenland P and Chu JS: Cardiac rehabilitation services, *Ann Intern Med* 109:671, 1988.

51. Hagberg JM and others: Effect of 12 months of intense exercise training on stroke volume in patients with coronary artery disease, *Circulation* 67:1194, 1983.

52. Hammermeister KE and others: Effect of surgical vs medical therapy on return to work in patients with coronary disease, *Am J Cardiol* 44:105, 1979.

53. Harri MNE: Physical training under the influence of beta blockade in rats. III. Effects in muscular metabolism, *Eur J Applied Physiol* 45:25, 1980.

54. Hartman CW and others: The safety and value of exercise testing soon after coronary artery bypass surgery, *J Cardiac Rehabil* 1:142, 1981.

55. Haskell JH: Physical activity after myocardial infarction, *Am J Cardiol* 33:776, 1974.

56. Hayes MJ and others: Comparison of mobilization after two and nine days in uncomplicated myocardial infarction, *Br Med J* 3:10, 1974.

57. Hellerstein HK: Effects of an active physical reconditioning intervention program on the clinical course of coronary artery disease, *Med Cardiovasc* 10:461, 1969.

58. Hellerstein HK and others: The influence of active conditioning upon subjects with coronary disease, *Can Med Assoc J* 96:901, 1967.

59. Hoffman A and others: The effect of training on the physical working capacity of MI patients with left ventricular dysfunction, *Eur Heart J* 8 (suppl G): 43, 1987.

60. Hoffman WE: The effect of propranolol on change in HDL level in cardiac patients involved in exercise training (abstract), *Med Sci Sports Exer* 14:124, 1982.

61. Holt GW and others: Results of percutaneous transluminal coronary angioplasty for angina pectoris early after acute myocardial infarction, *Am J Cardiol* 61:1238, 1988.

62. Honegger R: Rehabilitation von Herzinfarktpatienten, *Praxis* 56:752, 1967.

63. Huhn RR and Volski RV: Primary prevention programs for business and industry, *Phys Ther* 65:1840, 1985.

64. Hung J and others: Change in rest and exercise myocardial perfusion and left ventricular function 3 to 26 weeks after clinically uncomplicated acute myocardial infarction: effects of exercise training, *Am J Cardiol* 54:943, 1984.

65. Ice R: Long-term compliance, *Phys Ther* 65:1832, 1985.

66. Ice R and others: Descriptive data on marathon runners with severe coronary artery disease: results from cardiac catheterization, exercise tests and serum lipids (abstract), *Med Sci Sports Exer* 10:35, 1978.

67. Ice R and others: The safety and effectiveness of long distance bicycling in the treatment of coronary artery disease, *Proceedings of the First International Conference on Sports Cardiology,* Rome, 1978, Aulo Gaggi.

68. Ice R and others: The effects of long-distance bicycling on heart disease patients. In Burke ER and Newsom MM, editors: *Medical and scientific aspects of cycling,* Champaign, Ill, 1988, Human Kinetics.

69. Jugdutt BI and others: Exercise training after anterior Q wave myocardial infarction: importance of regional left ventricular function and topography, *J Am Coll Cardiol* 12:362, 1988.

70. Kallio V and others: Reduction in sudden deaths by a multifactorial intervention program after acute myocardial infarction, *Lancet* 2:1091, 1979.

71. Kavanaugh T and others: Characteristics of post-coronary marathon runners, *Ann NY Acad Sci* 301:455, 1978.

72. Kavanaugh T and others: Prognostic indices for patients with ischemic heart disease enrolled in an exercise-centered rehabilitation program, *Am J Cardiol* 44:1230, 1979.

73. Keleman MH and others: Circuit weight training for cardiac rehabilitation: a new direction, *Sports Med* 2:385, 1985.

74. Kellerman J: *Proceedings of the International Conference on Sports Cardiology,* Rome, 1978, Auto Gaggi.

75. Kelly T and others: Exercise training in high risk patients (abstract), *J Cardiopulmonary Rehabil* 10:404, 1988.

76. Kennedy JW and others: Western Washington randomized trial of intracoronary streptokinase in acute myocardial infarction, *N Engl J Med* 309:1477, 1983.

77. Kentala E: Physical fitness and feasibility of physical rehabilitation after myocardial infarction in men of working age, *Ann Clin Res* (suppl) 91, 1972.

78. Kimbiris D and others: Devolutionary pattern of coronary atherosclerosis in patients with angina pectoris, *Am J Cardiol* 33:7, 1974.

79. Krone RJ and others: Low-level exercise testing after myocardial infarction: usefulness in enhancing clinical risk stratification, *Circulation* 71:80, 1985.

80. Laffel GL and Braunwald E: Thrombolytic therapy: a new strategy for the treatment of acute myocardial infarction, *N Engl J Med* 311:710, 1984.

81. Lee A and others: Long-term effects of physical training on coronary patients with impaired ventricular function, *Circulation* 60:1519, 1979.

82. Lehtonen A: The effects of exercise on high density lipoprotein (HDL) apoproteins, Acta Physiol Scand 106:487, 1979.

83. Letac B and others: A study of left ventricular function in coronary patients before and after physical training, *Circulation* 56:375, 1977.

84. Lie JT and others: Aortocoronary bypass saphenous vein graft atherosclerosis: anatomic study of 99 vein grafts from normal and hyperlipoproteinemic patients up to 75 months postoperatively, *Am J Cardiol* 40:906, 1977.

85. Lindberg HA and others: Totally asymptomatic myocardial infarction: an estimate of its incidence in the living population, *Arch Intern Med* 106:628, 1960.

86. Logue B and others: A practical approach to coronary artery disease with special reference to coronary artery bypass surgery, *Curr Probl Cardiol* 1:5, 1976.

87. Lopez SA and others: Effect of exercise and physical fitness on serum lipids and lipoproteins, *Atherosclerosis* 20:1, 1974.

88. Marra S and others: Long-term follow-up after a controlled randomized post-infarction rehabilitation programme: effects of morbidity and mortality, *Eur Heart J* 6:656, 1985.

89. Martin JE and Tubbert PM: Exercise applications and promotion in behavioral medicine: current status and future directions, *J Consult Clin Psychol* 50:1004, 1982.

90. Massie JF and Shephard RJ: Physiological and psychological effects of training—a comparison of individual and gymnasium programs with a characterization of the exercise "dropout," *Med Sci Sports* 3:100, 1971.

91. McElroy PA and others: Cardiopulmonary exercise testing in congestive heart failure, *Am J Cardiol* 62:35A, 1988.

92. McNeer JF and others: The course of acute myocardial infarction: feasibility of early discharge of the uncomplicated patient, *Circulation* 51:410, 1975.

93. McNeer JF and others: Hospital discharge one week after acute myocardial infarction, *N Engl J Med* 298:229, 1978.

94. Miller NE and others: The Tromsø Heart study: high density lipoproteins and coronary artery disease a prospective case control study, *Lancet* 1:965, 1977.

95. Miller NH and others: Home versus group exercise training for increasing functional capacity after myocardial infarction, *Circulation* 70:645, 1984.

96. Mitchell JH: Exercise testing in the treatment of coronary heart disease, *Adv Intern Med* 20:249, 1975.

97. Morgan WP: Involvement in vigorous physical activity with special reference to adherence. In Gulvilas LI and Kneer ME, editors: *National College of Physical Education Proceedings,* Chicago, 1977, Office of Public Service, University of Illinois at Chicago.

98. Morganroth J and others: Echocardiographic detection of coronary artery disease, *Am J Cardiol* 46:1178, 1980.

99. Moss AJ and others: Cardiac deaths in the first six months after myocardial infarction: potential for mortality reduction in the early post-hospital periods, *Am J Cardiol* 39:816, 1977.

100. Musch TI and others: Endurance training in rats with chronic heart failure induced by myocardial infarction, *Circulation* 74:431, 1986.

101. Musch TI and others: Effects of dynamic exercise training on the metabolic and cardiocirculatory responses to exercise in the rat model of myocardial infarction and heart failure, *Am J Cardiol* 62:20E, 1988.

102. Oberman A and others: Changes in risk facotrs among participants in a long-term exercise rehabilitation program, *Adv Cardiol* 31:168, 1982.

103. Oja P and others: Feasibility of an 18-month physical training program for middle-aged men and its effects on physical fitness, *Am J Public Health* 64:459, 1975.

104. Oldridge NB: Compliance of post-myocardial infarction patients to exercise programs, *Med Sci Sports Exer* 11:373, 1979.

105. Oldridge NB: Compliance and exercise in primary and secondary prevention of coronary heart disease: a review, *Prev Med* 11:56, 1982.

106. Oldridge NB: Compliance and dropout in cardiac rehabilitation, *J Cardiac Rehabil* 4:166, 1984.

107. Oldridge NB and Spencer J: Exercise habits and perceptions before and after graduation or dropout from supervised cardiac exercise rehabilitation, *J Cardiopulm Rehab* 5:313, 1985.

108. Oldridge NB and others: Noncompliance in an exercise rehabilitation program for men who have suffered a myocardial infarction, *Can Med Assoc J* 118:361, 1978.

109. Oldridge NB and others: Compliance in exercise rehabilitation, *Phys Sports Med* 7:94, 1979.

110. Oldridge NB and others: Predictors of dropout from cardiac exercise rehabilitation: Ontario exercise-heart collaboration study, *Am J Cardiol* 51:70, 1983.

111. Oldridge NB and others: Cardiac rehabilitation after myocardial infarction, *JAMA* 260:945, 1988.

112. Oscai LB and others: Normalization of serum triglycerides and lipoprotein electrophoretic patterns by exercise, *Am J Cardiol* 30:775, 1972.

113. Oscai LB: The role of exercise and weight control, *Exer Sport Sci Rec* 1:103, 1973.

114. Ott CR and others: A controlled randomized study of early cardiac rehabilitation: the sickness impact profile as an assessment tool, *Heart Lung* 12:162, 1983.

115. Palac RT and others: Risk factors related to progressive narrowing in aortocoronary vein grafts studied 1 and 5 years after surgery, *Circulation* 66(suppl 1):1, 1982.

116. Palatsi I: Feasibility of physical training after myocardial infarction and its effect on return to work, morbidity and mortality, *Acta Med Scand* 599:1, 1976.

117. Paterson DH and others: Effects of physical training on cardiovascular function following myocardial infarction, *J Appl Physiol* 47:482, 1979.

118. Pozen MW and others: A nurse rehabilitator's impact on patients with myocardial infarction, *Med Care* 15:830, 1977.

119. Rahe RH and others: Brief group therapy in myocardial infarction rehabilitation: three- to four-year follow-up of a controlled trial, *Psychosom Med* 41:229, 1979.

120. Rahimtoola SH: A consensus on coronary bypass surgery, *Arch Intern Med* 94:272, 1981.

121. Rajagopalan B and others: Alterations of skeletal muscle metabolism in humans studied by phosphorus 31 magnetic resonance spectroscopy in congestive heart failure, *Am J Cardiol* 62:53E, 1988.

122. Rechnitzer PA: The effects of training: reinfarction and death—an interim report, *Med Sci Sports Exer* 11:382, 1979.

123. Rechnitzer PA and others: The effect of exercise prescription in the recurrence rate of myocardial infarction in men (abstract), *Am J Cardiol* 47:419, 1981.

124. Rechnitzer PA and others: Relation of exercise to the recurrence rate of myocardial infarction in men: Ontario Exercise Heart Collaborative Study, *Am J Cardiol* 51:65, 1983.

125. Redwood DR and others: Circulatory and symptomatic effects of physical training in patients with coronary artery disease and angina pectoris, *N Engl J Med* 286:959, 1972.

126. Rentrop KP and others: Effects of intracoronary nitroglycerin infusion on coronary angiographic patterns and mortality in patients with acute myocardial infarction, *N Engl J Med* 311:1457, 1984.

127. Rigo P and others: Hemodynamic and prognostic findings in patients with transmural and nontransmural infarction, *Circulation* 51:1064, 1975.

128. Rod JL and others: Symptom-limited graded exercise testing soon after myocardial revascularization surgery, *J Cardiac Rehabil* 2:199, 1982.

129. Roman O and others: Cardiac rehabilitation after acute myocardial infarction: 9-year controlled follow-up study, *Cardiology* 70:223, 1983.

130. Russell RO and others: Unstable angina pectoris study group: unstable angina pectoris: national cooperative study group to compare surgical and medical therapy. II. In-hospital experience and initial follow-up results in patients with one, two, or three-vessel disease, *Am J Cardiol* 42:839, 1978.

131. Sable DL and others: Attenuation of exercise conditioning by beta-adrenergic blockade, *Circulation* 65:679, 1982.

132. Sanmarco ME and others: Atherosclerosis: its progression and regression, *Primary Cardiology* July/August:51, 1978.

133. Sanmarco ME and others: Abnormal blood pressure response and marked ischemic ST-segment depression as predictors of severe coronary artery disease, *Circulation* 61:572, 1980.

134. Selvester R and others: Exercise training and coronary artery disease progression, *Ann NY Acad Sci* 301:495, 1978.

135. Shapiro S and others: Return to work after first myocardial infarction, *Arch Environ Health* 24:17, 1972.

136. Shaw LW: Effects of a prescribed supervised exercise program on mortality and cardiovascular morbidity in patients after a myocardial infarction: The National Exercise and Heart Disease Project, *Am J Cardiol* 48:39, 1981.

137. Shephard RJ and others: The influence of an employee fitness and lifestyle modification program upon medical care costs, *Can J Public Health* 73:259, 1982.

138. Sidney KH and Shephard RJ: Attitudes toward health and physical activity in the elderly. Effects of a physical training program, *Med Sci Sports* 8:246, 1976.

139. Sim DN and others: Investigation of the physiologic basis for increased exercise threshold for angina pectoris after physical conditioning, *J Clin Invest* 54:763, 1974.

140. Sinoway LI: Effect of conditioning and deconditioning stimuli on metabolically determined blood flow in humans and implications for congestive heart failure, *Am J Cardiol* 62:45E, 1988.

141. Sinoway and others: An intensive cardiovascular rehabilitation program for patients with disabling angina and diffuse coronary artery disease, *J Cardiopulm Rehab* 7:425, 1987.

142. Stamford BA and others: Task specific changes in maximal oxygen uptake resulting from arm versus leg training, *Ergonomics* 21:1, 1978.

143. Stein RA and others: Clinical values of early exercise testing after myocardial infarction, *Arch Intern Med* 140:1179, 1980.

144. Stern MJ: Psychosocial adaptation following an acute myocardial infarction, *J Chronic Dis* 29:513, 1976.

145. Stern MJ and Cleary P: The National Exercise and Heart Disease Project: long-term psychological outcome, *Arch Intern Med* 142:1093, 1982.

146. Stern S and others: Clinical outcome of silent myocardial ischemia, *Am J Cardiol* 61:16F, 1988.

147. Streja D and others: Moderate exercise and high density lipoprotein-cholesterol, *JAMA* 242:2190, 1979.

148. Sullivan MJ and others: Exercise training in patients with severe left ventricular dysfunction: hemodynamic and metabolic effects, *Circulation* 78:506, 1988.

149. Szklo M and others: Survival of patients with nontransmural myocardial infarction: a population-based study, *Am J Cardiol* 42:648, 1978.

150. Tatman D and others: Exercise conditioning and early return to work after coronary bypass surgery (abstract), *Med Sci Sports Exer* 113:133, 1981.

151. Theroux P and others: Prognostic value of exercise testing soon after myocardial infarction, *N Engl J Med* 301:341, 1979.

152. Thompson PD and Keleman MH: Hypotension accompanying the onset of exertional angina, *Circulation* 52:28, 1975.

153. Vermeulen A and others: Effects of cardiac rehabilitation after myocardial infarction: changes in coronary risk factors and long-term prognosis, *Am Heart J* 105:798, 1983.

154. Wallace C: Evaluation of a cardiac exercise programme: a pilot study, *N Zealand J Physiother* 15:8, 1987.

155. Weiner DA and others: ST-segment changes post-infarction: predictive value for multi-vessel coronary disease and left ventricular aneurysm, *Circulation* 58:887, 1978.

156. Weiner DA and others: Identification of patients with left main and three-vessel coronary disease with clinical and exercise test variables, *Am J Cardiol* 46:21, 1980.

157. Wenger NK: Rehabilitation of the patient with acute myocardial infarction: early ambulation and patient education. In Pollack ML and Schmidt DH, editors: *Heart disease and rehabilitation,* Boston, 1979 Houghton Mifflin Co.

158. Wenger NK: Research related to rehabilitation, *Circulation* 60:1636, 1979.

159. Wenger NK and others: Cardiac conditioning after myocardial infarction: an early intervention program, *Cardiovascular Rehabil Q* 2:17, 1971.

160. Wilhelmsen L and others: A controlled trial of physical training after myocardial infarction: effects of risk factors, nonfatal reinfarction, and death, *Prev Med* 4:491, 1975.

161. Williams DO and others: Intravenous recombinant tissue-type plasminogen activator in patients with acute myocardial infarction: a report from the NHLBI thrombolysis in myocardial infarction trial, *Circulation* 73:338, 1986.

162. Williams RS and others: Physical conditioning augments the fibrinolytic response to venous occlusion in healthy adults, *N Engl J Med* 302:987, 1980.

163. Wilmore J and others: Validity of skinfold and girth measurements for predicting alterations in body composition, *J Appl Physiol* 29:313, 1970.

164. Wohl AJ and others: Cardiovascular function during early recovery from acute myocardial infarction, *Circulation* 56:931, 1977.

165. Young DT and others: A prospective controlled study of in-hospital myocardial infarction rehabilitation, *J Cardiac Rehabil* 2:32, 1982.

# CHAPTER 10

# The Beneficial Effects of Aerobic Exercise for Patients with Coronary Artery Disease

*Raymond L. Blessey*

It has been emphasized in several of the preceding chapters that many factors contribute to coronary disease. It follows therefore that the treatment of coronary artery disease should be multifaceted, including life-style modifications that include changes in diet, prescriptions for medication, and a program of exercise therapy to reduce risk factors. It is inappropriate to think that any of the previously mentioned treatment approaches by itself could be the panacea for coronary artery disease.

The value of exercise for coronary patients is often questioned, and skeptics continue to state that there is no "definitive proof" that exercise is beneficial to the coronary patient in terms of prolonging life or "preventing" a repeat myocardial infarction. This negative view of the value of exercise stems from a limited perspective and, in fact, is poorly founded. The "definitive" lack of proof is not available for a number of reasons, including the following:

(1) it is virtually impossible to design and implement a study that "proves" that exercise therapy significantly reduces the coronary death rate and the repeat infarction rate because of the large number of subjects needed, and (2) previous attempts at proving or disproving the protective effect of exercise have often used less than adequate exercise intensity and duration and have not properly handled the problem with "crossover" in the treatment and control groups. Furthermore, the skeptic's view of exercise for coronary patients is shortsighted because the benefits of properly designed exercise programs are not limited to reducing mortality and morbidity and, as mentioned earlier, treatment of the coronary patient should be multifaceted.

Our view regarding the benefits of aerobic exercise for the coronary patient is that there is more than adequate clinical evidence and literature to support it as one of several essential treatment modalities. The keys to achieving beneficial results are the design and implementation of an aerobic exercise program that is appropriate in terms of intensity, duration, and frequency (see Chapter 9). The box on p. 186 lists the ranges of exercise intensity, duration, and frequency and the various modes of exercise we have used with our patients in the past 20 years.

This chapter is designed to discuss the various well-documented, beneficial effects of aerobic exercise for coronary patients. In addition, there will be some discussion regarding the need to study further the effects of long-term regular exercise in certain specific areas.

## AEROBIC EXERCISE AND RISK FACTOR REDUCTION

Several major factors associated with an increased risk for the development and progression (worsening) of coronary disease can be modified by consistent aerobic exercise programs.

---

### Summary of aerobic exercise programs used for coronary patients

**Exercise mode**

Walking, jogging, cycling, aerobic dancing, cross-country skiing, roller skating, rope jumping, trampoline, swimming, arm cranking, rowing, circuit weight training

**Exercise intensity**

65% to 95% of patient's maximum heart rate

**Exercise duration**

30 to 60 minutes

**Frequency**

3 to 6 days per week

---

### Serum lipid levels and exercise

The beneficial effect of aerobic exercise on serum lipids in normal subjects has been well documented.[47,116] Studies indicate that when the training intensity is sufficient to result in a significant increase in the $\dot{V}_{O_{2max}}$, there is an associated increase in the HDL-cholesterol (HDL-C) of at least 10% to 15% and a decrease in triglyceride values of 16% to 20%.[51,105] A systematic analysis of 95 studies of exercise effects on lipid values (from 1955 to 1983) by Tran and others[106] indicated that there is a significant relationship between the degree of body-weight change that occurred with training and the changes in lipid values, including total cholesterol (TC), triglycerides, and total cholesterol/HDL ratios (TC/HDL). Wood and others[117] found similar decreases in triglycerides and increases in HDL-C, $HDL_2$-C, and $HDL_3$C in dieters versus exercisers during a 1-year follow-up period. Both analyses found a correlation between the amount of exercise (total distance run or total hours of exercise) and the degree of change in HDL-C, $HDL_2$-C, TC, LDL-C and TC/HDL ratio.

There have also been similar studies involving patients with known coronary disease. Both Hartung[48] and Streja[102] found significant increases in HDL-C values after training. Hartung also observed a significant correlation ($r = 0.79$, $p < 0.05$) between the change in HDL-C value and $\dot{V}_{O_{2max}}$.[48] Heath[49] found a significant correlation between change in $\dot{V}_{O_{2max}}$ and both HDL-C and LDL-C values and that the patients with the lowest HDL-C values and highest LDL-C values showed the greatest degree of change with training.

Both Oschrin[80] and Erkelens[33] documented increased HDL-C values of 11% to 14% above pretraining values after 6 months of training. The major difference in the results of these two studies is that Oschrin also reported triglyceride values that were 34% lower after training ($p < 0.05$). The higher training intensity (mean of 83% of maximum heart rate) and greater frequency of training (mean of 5.1 days per week) in our patients and thus greater total caloric expen-

diture probably are responsible for the different findings in the posttraining triglyceride values. Ballantyne's findings[2] were very similar to those of Oschrin, with the additional observation that LDL values were significantly lower after training. A summary of these six studies is given in Table 10-1.

We have also investigated the relationship between various levels of aerobic exercise and HDL values in patients with documented coronary artery disease. Our study involved 98 men, divided into three groups: (1) inactive patients, (2) patients performing up to 96 minutes of aerobic exercise per week, and (3) patients performing more than 120 minutes of exercise per week.[41] Both exercising groups demonstrated significant decreases in serum triglyceride values and increases in high-density lipoptrotein values. However, although there was a trend for a greater magnitude of change in the patients performing a longer duration of exercise, the difference between the two subgroups' pretraining and posttraining values ($n = 10$ in each group) was not statistically significant.

There is also evidence that when the exercise training stimulus in coronary patients fails to alter $\dot{V}_{O_{2max}}$, it fails to alter lipid values as well.[105] Furthermore, ongoing cigarette smoking, beta blockers, and thiazides either block or diminish the beneficial effects of training on serum lipid levels in coronary patients.[23,56] An extensive review of this topic and an in-depth history of the literature are available in an article by Durstine and Haskell.[28]

In summary, the literature indicates that adequate training intensity and duration will beneficially alter HDL-C values in coronary patients[106] and, in certain subsets of patients, will decrease LDL-C and triglyceride levels. There are epidemiological and angiographic studies indicating that higher HDL values and lower triglyceride values are associated with a decreased likelihood of progression of coronary artery disease.[75,95] Additional studies are needed to investigate whether the magnitude of the changes that occur in serum lipids in exercising coronary patients is likely to affect the probability of disease progression. However, there is some preliminary evidence from Schuler and others[97] suggesting that the combination of intense physical exercise and low-fat diet alters the likelihood of progression and, in some cases, actually results in regression of the disease process.

### Aerobic exercise and hypertension

Consistent long-term aerobic exercise can result in at least a 10 to 20 mm Hg decrease in both resting and exercise (at a given submaximal workload) blood pressure of hypertensive subjects.[13,14,17,89] Boyer and Kasch's study[14] is especially impressive, because it involved 23 hypertensive men whose resting blood pressure did not respond to medical therapy alone. After 6 months of aerobic exercise combined with medical therapy, these investigators reported a mean decrease in resting systolic and diastolic blood pressures of

**Table 10-1.** Summary of training effects on serum lipids in coronary patients

| Author/year | n | Training average duration (months) | Percent change in total cholesterol | Percent change in HDL cholesterol | Percent change in LDL cholesterol | Percent change in triglycerides |
|---|---|---|---|---|---|---|
| Streja, 1979[102] | 32 | 3 | +4.7* | +9.7* | +6.6 | −8.0 |
| Hartung, 1981[48] | 18 | 3 | −2.0 | +15* | −5.7 | −8.1 |
| Erkelens, 1979[33] | 18 | 6 | −5.0 | +14.0* | — | −6.0 |
| Oschrin, 1982[80] | 17 | 6 | −3.0 | +11.0* | −3.0 | −34* |
| Heath, 1983[49] | 10 | 7 | −8.0† | +11.0* | −9.0† | −13* |
| Ballantyne, 1982[2] | 19 | 6 | −3.0 | +14.0‡ | −7.0* | −22† |

*$p < 0.05$
†$p < 0.01$
‡$p < 0.001$

14 and 12 mm Hg respectively. It is important to note that the improved blood pressures in these men were not associated with a significant decrease in body weight or sodium intake. Krotkiewski[65] also reported significant decreases in the blood pressures of obese hypertensive subjects after physical training that was not associated with decreases in body weight or body fat. In fact, the greatest reduction in both the systolic and diastolic blood pressures in those obese subjects occurred in the group patients with the least change in body weight and body fat. On the other hand, Gilders's group[40] found that mild hypertensives and normotensives do not exhibit a reduction in ambulatory pressures after aerobic training.

What are the mechanisms through which aerobic exercise modifies systolic and diastolic blood pressure? This is an area that definitely requires further study. Björntorp[5] has concluded from his work that a decrease in the sympathetic nervous system activity via a decrease in plasma norepinephrine levels is the major mechanism through which physical training mediates its antihypertensive effect. A number of other investigators have drawn a similar conclusion.[27,46,108] Other mechanisms postulated to play a role in blood pressure reduction after training include decreased sodium reabsorption associated with lowered serum insulin levels[8,66] and decreased blood volume.[108]

We have noted a sharp reduction in the blood pressures of our hypertensive coronary patients involved in long-term regular physical training. The changes in these patients are not unlike those reported in the hypertensive subjects discussed above. A recent study of 125 cardiac rehabilitation participants with hypertension at Duke University Medical Center supports our clinical impression.[74] After training, the mean diastolic blood pressure decreased from 98 to 80 mm Hg, and 73% of these patients achieved a diastolic pressure below 90. In this study, unlike those cited earlier, the decreased blood pressures were associated with decreased weight loss and sodium intake.

How important is the control of hypertension in the prevention of cardiovascular mortality and morbidity? This

was the focus of the Hypertension Detection and Follow-up Program Study involving 10,940 participants.[34] The conclusion of this 5-year randomized prospective trial was that effective management of hypertension has great potential for reducing mortality for the large numbers of individuals with elevated blood pressure, and even for those with mild hypertension. In addition, there are data from the Mayo Clinic indicating that effective treatment of hypertension improves the survival of patients with known coronary artery disease.[21] The survival rates at 1, 5, and 10 years for 300 patients (with angina pectoris or who had an MI) treated for hypertension was 91%, 82%, and 74% and in the untreated patients 76%, 65%, and 41% respectively. Based on this data and that of the Hypertensive Detection and Follow-up Study, hypertension is a major prognostic variable, and thus therapy aimed at modifying the degree of hypertension is definitely in the patient's best interest.

### Aerobic exercise and glucose intolerance

The data from the Framingham, Massachusetts study suggest that diabetic men and women have two to three times the risk of developing coronary artery disease as their nondiabetic counterparts.[57] Furthermore, the diabetic patient has a higher risk of more rapid progression of coronary disease,[91] multiple myocardial infarctions,[24] and a higher mortality rate from coronary disease[64] than the nondiabetic patient. Thus the goal of modifying the risk factor of glucose intolerance by exercise and other therapies appears to be indicated for the patient with known coronary artery disease, as well as for the patient with multiple risk factors for the disease.

Glucose intolerance has been shown to be associated with obesity and a sedentary life-style.[22,72] Thus, physical training would appear to have a positive effect on the tendency toward glucose intolerance, and, in fact, studies have shown that serum insulin levels are reduced during oral glucose tolerance tests in obese men after training.[7] More importantly, studies of subjects with documented chemical diabetes by Saltin and others[93] demonstrated that after 3 to

6 months of aerobic exercise, the glucose tolerance levels of these subjects were normalized (Fig. 10-1). Ruderman and others[91] suggested that the improvement in glucose disappearance rate found in the intravenous glucose tolerance tests of adult-onset diabetics after training was attributable to either an enhanced sensitivity to endogenous insulin or a decreased or diminished "anti-insulin" factor.

In those coronary patients who perform regular aerobic exercise we have frequently noticed a decreased need for insulin or oral medication. A study by Björntorp and others[6] of post-MI patients on a regular training program supports our clinical findings in that there are noted lower serum insulin levels after a glucose challenge in the trained patients presumably because of an increased insulin sensitivity at the cellular level. These improved results were associated with significantly decreased serum triglycerides and body fat levels.

In summary, aerobic exercise has been shown to be effective in altering several of the major risk factors for coronary disease[69] including low serum HDL-C levels, high LDL-C levels, hypertriglyceridemia, hyperglycemia, and arterial hypertension. More significantly, several of these risk factors have also been shown to be related to risk of coronary disease progression[84] and coronary artery bypass graft occlusion.[81]

## AEROBIC EXERCISE AND IMPROVEMENT IN PHYSICAL WORK CAPACITY OF CLIENTS WITH KNOWN CORONARY ARTERY DISEASE

In the 1950s, exercise therapy was used primarily to help the coronary patient overcome the detrimental effects of prolonged bed rest. In the early and middle 1960s, several of the more "aggressive" centers began to use exercise therapy for the purpose of conditioning the coronary patient, with the overall aim of returning the individual to a more active life-style. Formal studies documenting the beneficial effects of physical training for coronary patients began appearing in the literature in the early mid-1960s.[4,50,77,110] Frick and Katila,[36] reporting on seven coronary patients exercised for 1 to 2 months three times per week, concluded that after training (1) the stroke volume was improved during exercise, (2) the heart volume was unchanged, (3) the arterial blood lactate levels during exercise were reduced, (4) the exercise tolerance was improved, and (5) there was some evidence suggestive of increased coronary flow. These same authors cautioned, however, that there was a "need for proper selection of patients and close medical supervision during training."

Since the early 1960s, when it became clear that coronary patients are capable of responding appropriately to exercise training, clinicians and researchers have continued to ask

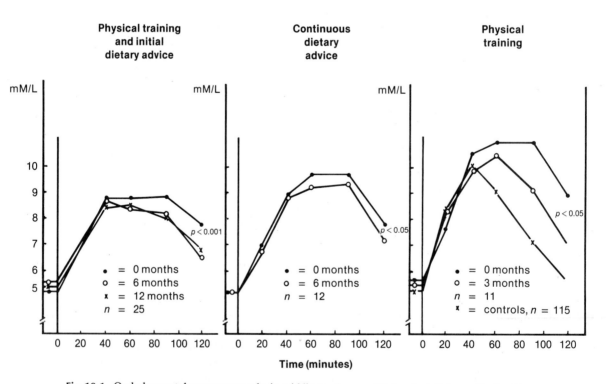

Fig. 10-1. Oral glucose tolerance test results in middle-aged men with chemical diabetes. Notice that physical training by itself and in combination with dietary advice had significantly improved glucose tolerance test results. (From Saltin B and others: Physical training and glucose tolerance in middle-aged men with chemical diabetes, *Diabetes* 28 [suppl 1]:30, 1979.)

two major questions. What degree of improvement in maximum aerobic capacity is it reasonable to expect in the coronary patient? What are the mechanisms through which coronary patients improve their aerobic capacity? Not surprisingly, these two questions are closely related. Based on a review of the literature and 21 years of clinical experience, it is my opinion that the major variable that determines the coronary patient's adaptations to training is the training stimulus—that is, training intensity, duration, frequency, and period of time the program is carried out (see Chapter 9). To a lesser extent, the degree of coronary disease and left ventricular dysfunction and the use of beta-adrenergic blocking agents such as sectral, atenolol, and timelol may influence the coronary patient's responses to long-term regular training.

The results of Detry and others[25] are representative of most of the earlier studies on the hemodynamic consequences of physical training in coronary patients. After 12 patients (six with angina, six after myocardial infarction without symptoms) underwent exercise training for 45 minutes three times per week for 3 months, Detry and others reported a 22.5% improvement in $\dot{V}o_{2max}$. The exercise intensity used in this study was not specified. The results of this study indicated that the classic posttraining bradycardia at rest and at a given submaximal workload was attributable to peripheral changes (i.e., increased ateriovenous differences), and not related to changes in left ventricular function (i.e., increased stroke volume or ejection fraction). Many clinicians continue to believe that the only mechanism through which coronary patients improve their aerobic capacity is the increased extraction of oxygen by the trained skeletal muscle. However, in the late 1970s there were several studies published that challenged the conclusions of Detry and others.

Patterson and others[82] studied two groups of coronary patients randomly assigned to either a low-intensity or a high-intensity exercise program. The high-intensity group exercised for 30 to 45 minutes at workloads equivalent to 65% to 80% of their $\dot{V}o_{2max}$. As expected, the high-intensity group showed the classic changes in aerobic capacity over the course of the 1-year study. More importantly, however, the high-intensity group demonstrated improvements (10% increase in stroke volume) in ventricular function that did not appear until the last 6 months of training. Patterson's results suggest that to stimulate central cardiac adaptations to exercise training in coronary patients, it is important to evaluate the patients over a period longer than 2 to 3 months as most of the previous studies had done. Shortly after Patterson published his results, Jensen and others,[53] using radionuclide ventriculography, reported improvements in exercise left ventricular ejection fractions in a subset of coronary patients trained for 3 to 9 months (mean of 6 months) at an intensity equivalent to 65% to 85% of maximal oxygen uptake.

Hagberg and others[43] documented impressive changes in left ventricular function after training in a group of coronary patients as well. Once again, the training program was carried out over a period of 12 months, with the last 6 months of training consisting of exercise sessions 50 to 60 minutes in duration at 70% to 90% of $\dot{V}o_{2max}$, four to six times per week. These patients had a mean increase in their aerobic capacity of 39% and demonstrated significant increases in stroke volume at both a given submaximal workload and the same relative workload (i.e., same percent of $\dot{V}o_{2max}$). The authors concluded that these results demonstrated that "if training is continued and progressively increased in intensity, duration and frequency, some patients with coronary artery disease can, over 12 months, have improved cardiac function as reflected in an increase in stroke volume and stroke work." Posttraining improvement in left ventricular function, as evidenced by improvement in exercise ejection fraction and the systolic blood pressure and end-systolic volume relationship, was reported by Ehsani and others[30] after 12 months of intense exercise. The beneficial changes were not seen in a group of patients with comparable maximal base-line exercise capacities who did not exercise. These studies support the earlier statement that training stimulus is in fact the key variable in determining the cardiac patient's adaptations to long-term regular aerobic exercise.

What about the influence of the degree of coronary disease and left ventricular dysfunction on the patient's ability to respond to training? In patients with normal or near normal ventricular function, both Patterson[82] and Jensen[53] found no correlation between the degree of improvement in aerobic capacity and the baseline ejection fraction. We have also reported on a subset of patients with good ventricular function but with severe coronary disease (three with severe double-vessel, five with triple-vessel disease) who have trained for and completed numerous marathon (26.2 mile) runs.[11] Several of these patients had limiting exertional angina before initiating their training program. Thus it has been our observation that severe coronary artery disease and angina do not necessarily prevent patients from training to high levels of fitness.

Our experience with a group of patients with poor ventricular function who underwent a training program for 12 to 42 months, demonstrating the classic training responses and no evidence of deterioration in their clinical status or ventricular function, has also been reported.[68] Both Letac[70] and Conn[20] have confirmed our finding that exercise training is safe in this population of patients and that they respond appropriately to regular exercise. Arvan's results[1] suggest that patients with the combination of poor left ventricular function and exercise ischemia do not respond to 12 weeks of exercise training to the same degree that patients with only poor ventricular function do. However, there is evidence that patients with poor ventricular function, angina, and history of congestive heart failure do show favorable responses to exercise training secondary to both increases in maximum cardiac output and increased arterial-venous oxygen differences, but that these changes require a minimum of 75 days of training before they are measurable.[103] In these patients, once again, it appears that the variables of the training stimulus and the duration of the exercise program (weeks or months) are critical.

The effect of beta blockers on coronary patients' ability to improve their aerobic capacity has been studied.[71,78,83] It is difficult, however, to draw any general conclusions because of the variety of training programs used, the individual patient's sensitivity to the drug, and the variety of dosages used. The results of both Obina[78] and Pratt[83] suggest that certain coronary patients on beta blockers can significantly increase their aerobic capacity. In fact, Pratt reported that a group of patients receiving 120 to 240 mg of propranolol per day were able to increase their $\dot{V}o_{2max}$ by 46% 3 months after training, compared with a group of clinically matched patients not receiving propranolol who demonstrated a 27% improvement in their aerobic capacity. Pratt's data may be somewhat misleading because of the self-selected nature of the patient population.

In summary, it is clear from the literature that coronary patients can significantly improve their aerobic capacity. The degree of improvement that occurs appears to be primarily related to the training stimulus and perhaps secondarily related to the clinical status and medical therapy of the client. In addition, it is evident from the literature that coronary patients continue to improve their aerobic capacity over extended periods of time (years) provided that an adequate training stimulus is used. The specific type of cardiovascular adaptations that occur in coronary patients may vary, again, depending on the training stimulus and the duration of the exercise program. The key point, however, is that no matter what specific physiological adaptations take place in the trained coronary patient, an increased aerobic capacity means a greater reserve for both recreational and occupational activities and therefore the potential for a greater quality of life.

## EXERCISE TRAINING AND IMPROVEMENT OF ISCHEMIC SIGNS AND SYMPTOMS

A relatively high percentage of patients referred to our centers for rehabilitation have stable exertional angina pectoris despite medical or surgical intervention. In fact, we are seeing increasing numbers of postbypass patients who have had a return of their exertional angina. In addition, we see a significant number of patients with a combination of coronary artery and peripheral artery disease who are primarily limited by their claudication symptoms.

### Exercise training and angina patients

In the early 1970s we had a patient enter our outpatient cardiac rehabilitation program with the primary diagnosis of angina pectoris. At the time, this gentleman was 64 years of age and had sought medical attention because of exertional chest pressure that was progressive in nature. The patient was limited to walking slowly with his dog two or three blocks at a time because of his symptoms. He underwent exercise testing and angiography at another facility. On his exercise test he demonstrated both symptoms and electrocardiographic changes consistent with myocardial ischemia at a relatively low workload and myocardial oxygen demand. Fortunately, on his ventriculogram he had evidence of normal left ventricular function at rest with an ejection fraction of 75%. His left ventricular end-diastolic volume and pressures were both elevated, however, being 149 m/m$^2$ and 18 mm Hg, respectively. The results of his angiography were not quite so encouraging. His angiogram findings were as follows:

*Left main artery:* no significant lesions

*Left anterior descending artery (LAD):* 90% occlusion proximally; 95% occlusion distal to the first septal perforator and diagonal; diffuse distal disease extending throughout the course of the LAD; 95% occlusion in the proximal portion of the diagonal artery

*Circumflex artery:* 90% occlusion of the midportion, distal to the take-off of the main marginal artery

*Right coronary artery (RCA):* 50% to 60% lesions proximally; complete (100%) obstruction of the distal RCA

In summary, this patient had triple-vessel coronary artery disease, and he was told by the surgeons that he was not a candidate for bypass surgery because both the LAD and RCA had distal lesions and were therefore not suitable for grafting. Furthermore, he was not a candidate for beta-receptor blocking agents because of an inherent resting and exercise bradycardia. In essence, he was told to go home, take it easy, use nitroglycerin as needed, and not to make any long-range plans. Despite this advice from an outside facility, he entered our rehabilitation program shortly after his angiogram. Using an individualized exercise program that initially involved walking up to his angina threshold, this patient began to make improvements in his exercise capacity. In fact, within 4 months after initiating exercise therapy, he began a walk-jog program and was eventually able to progress to a continuous jog. Provided that the patient warmed up sufficiently and jogged at a reasonable pace, he was eventually asymptomatic with exercise. He went on to participate in numerous 10-km runs and half-marathon runs. In addition, he completed over 20 marathon runs during his 9-year involvement with our program. The dramatic changes in the exertional symptoms of this patient and many others like him raise several questions in the minds of clinicians. What are the mechanisms that allow patients with exertional angina to significantly improve their exercise capacity? Furthermore, what allows certain subsets of these initially symptomatic patients to eventually exercise to considerably higher levels of exertion and not perceive angina? (See Chapter 7).

We examined the exercise test data on the previously referred-to patient and 17 others with documented coronary disease who were either on no medication or the same medication throughout the course of a 20-month training program.[10] This particular group of patients was exercised at their angina threshold for 60 to 300 minutes per week. After training, nearly half (44%) of the patients demonstrated higher rate-pressure products (RPP) at the onset of angina and 56% had higher maximum RPP on their maximal exercise tests. Several of them demonstrated higher maximum RPP after training because they were asymptomatic. Unfortunately, there were more questions than answers raised by this study. We were unable to predict which patients were likely to improve their angina threshold or become asymptomatic based on their angiography, training program, or initial exercise test results. In addition, the specific mechanisms leading to improvement of symptoms were not studied.

There is considerable controversy in the literature regarding the adaptations that occur in the symptomatic coronary patient after training. The earlier studies explained the beneficial effects of physical training on exertional angina in terms of the relationship between the RPP (indicator of myocardial oxygen demand) and a given external workload;[18,36,110] that is, after training, angina patients were able to exercise at a higher workload before reporting angina because of the lower RPP at comparable pretraining workloads. Therefore it was concluded that the patients' symptoms improved at a given workload because of a lower level of myocardial oxygen demand and not because of any change in myocardial oxygen delivery. However, the more recent work of Clausen and others[19] made it evident that not all patient's symptomatic improvement could be explained by the RPP changes at a given workload. They noted that, after training, a subset of patients exercised to significantly higher RPPs before reporting angina. They speculated that an improvement in myocardial oxygen supply caused by increased vascularization or increased content of oxidative enzymes in myocardial muscle cells might have explained these changes. These authors also cautioned that using the RPP alone as an indicator of myocardial oxygen demand ($M\dot{V}o_2$) may be misleading. RPP does not take into account the left ventricular end-diastolic volume, which is another determinant of $M\dot{V}o_2$.

After studying symptomatic coronary patients, both Sim and Neill[100] and Redwood and others[87] have theorized that after training, the improved symptoms could be explained by increased myocardial oxygen supply. Other mechanisms that have been considered in explaining the adaptation to exercise training in angina patients include (1) a higher threshold for perception of exertional angina, (2) improved left ventricular function with decreased exercise end-diastolic volumes, and (3) enhanced mechanical efficiency.[26] In addition, Ehsani and others[29] have shown prolonged high-level exercise training results in a reduction in myocardial ischemia (as indicated by ECG changes) at the same or higher RPPs. Froelicher[38,39] has published results of preexercise and 1-year postexercise Thallium studies of patients with exercise-induced angina and/or ischemic ST changes. His data indicate that in these patients (with or without bypass surgery), exercise training can lead to improved myocardial perfusion based on computerized Thallium ischemia scores. Ehsani and Froelicher's findings raise the point again that perhaps some of the variation in the mechanisms through which the patient improves angina is related to the training stimulus and the length of the training program. Finally, Rizi and others[88] have speculated that transient coronary spasm superimposed on a high-grade arterial obstruction was responsible for "walk-through" angina in a patient they studied. This raises questions about the influence of changes in the coronary vasomotor tone on posttraining symptoms. Up to now there have been no studies dealing with this phenomenon.

Does exercise training angina patients with the lower extremities (trained limbs) influence their angina threshold during performance of upper-extremity exercise (untrained limbs)? This was the basis for study by Thompson and others[104] involving a total of 15 patients—four trained with the arms, seven trained with the legs, and four served as controls. The exercise training program was 8 weeks in duration. In summary, they reported that the posttraining angina threshold (absolute workload) was enhanced primarily because of a lower rate-pressure product at a given workload. These authors concluded that it is therefore not necessary to use upper-extremity exercise as part of the total exercise rehabilitation program to improve the upper-extremity angina threshold. Our clinical impression goes along with their findings regarding the carry-over effect between trained and untrained limbs or extremities; however, using more aggressive exercise programs of longer duration, we have noticed a greater degree of symptomatic improvement specific to the trained muscle group, not explained entirely by a decreased rate-pressure product, and therefore have used upper-extremity exercise training in addition to lower-extremity training when indicated. Additional studies involving larger patient populations and longer training programs are needed for further investigation.

## Exercise therapy in the treatment of peripheral vascular disease

Claudication pain manifested as burning or numbness in the feet, pain in the "calf" (gastrocnemius and soleus muscles), or (in some cases) hip discomfort can be more limiting to the coronary patient than angina pectoris. Claudication symptoms are ischemic in nature, that is, attributable to an imbalance between oxygen supply and demand and, as a result, precipitated by exertion and relieved promptly by rest. Patients with these symptoms tend to want to avoid exertion and therefore are somewhat difficult to motivate to exercise regularly. However, these patients often respond favorably to exercise therapy in a relatively short period of time. According to the Framingham statistics,[58] approximately one fourth of coronary artery disease patients suffer from claudication. Approximately 5% to 10% of all the coronary patients referred to our centers report claudication symptoms.

Foley[35] was probably the first to document a beneficial effect of exercise training for patients with advanced peripheral vascular disease in the lower extremities. Since that time, there have been other reports on the favorable responses to exercise training in patients with claudication symptoms; however, the explanations for the symptomatic improvement in these patients remain controversial. Zetterqvist,[119] after studying nine patients with claudication who were treated with a combination of a daily walking program and isotonic exercise for 3 to 4 months, reported a 73% increase in the walking tolerance of his study population. He used venous occlusion plethysmography to evaluate arterial inflow capacity and, basing his views on the posttraining results, did not see any evidence of improved regional arterial circulation despite considerable clinical improvement. He concluded that the major mechanism for improvement was more efficient distribution of blood flow to the exercising muscle. Finally, he speculated that increased concentration of the oxidative enzymes and increased mechanical efficiency may have accounted for some of the increased functional capacity. Larsen and Larsen[67] reported that a subset of patients with claudication did demonstrate significant improvement in calf-muscle blood flow during exercise. Their findings have been supported by Skinner and Strandness.[101] Saltin,[92] after reviewing the literature, concluded that the reasons for improved walking tolerance in these patients include any and possibly all of the following: (1) improved mechanical efficiency, which lowers the oxygen demand during walking, (2) enhanced anaerobic energy yield, and (3) increased oxygen supply to the working muscle. Finally, the literature does not support the hypothesis that severe proximal stenosis or resting claudication symptoms prohibit patients from responding favorably to exercise therapy.[32,54]

Hall's findings[44,45] suggest that exercise training by itself may not be the ideal therapy for claudication patients. He has documented improved muscle blood flow using Doppler studies (arm/ankle index) in patients treated with the combination of high complex carbohydrates, high-fiber, low-fat diet, and exercise training. The improvement in walking time and maximum metabolic equivalent level was associated with a decrease in the serum cholesterol and triglyceride levels of 28% and 32%. Earlier investigators have reported increased blood flow both at rest and during reactive hyperemia in patients treated with the combination of exercise training and vitamin E.[32]

In summary, aerobic exercise is effective in improving the exercise capacity of patients with exertional angina and ischemic ST changes. This improvement in ischemic threshold appears to be attributable to a number of factors. First, after training, the myocardial oxygen demand as a given exercise level (as measured by the heart rate and systolic blood pressure) is lower, and therefore the likelihood of an imbalance between $M\dot{V}O_2$ demand and supply is reduced. Furthermore, there seems to be a subset of patients who, after training, are able to achieve higher rate-pressure products with few or no symptoms, apparently as a result of better oxygen supply to the myocardium.

The coronary patient who is limited by symptoms of peripheral vascular disease also often dramatically improves his or her exercise tolerance after training. The mechanisms that allow these patients to improve after training include more efficient distribution of cardiac output to the working muscle, improved oxygen extraction of the trained muscle, and improved blood supply to the previously ischemic muscle as a result of improved collateral circulation.

## EXERCISE AND CORONARY MORTALITY AND MORBIDITY: DOES EXERCISE PROVIDE A PROTECTIVE EFFECT?

The preceding sections in this chapter discussed the documented benefits of long-term regular aerobic exercise in risk factor reduction, improvement in maximum aerobic capacity, and relief or improvement in exertional angina, ischemic ST changes, and claudication. As was mentioned earlier, there has not as yet been definitive proof through a randomized prospective trial that exercise significantly influences the mortality and morbidity of coronary patients. Below are several of the major reasons why the previous studies have not reported a significant protective effect of exercise:

1. The need for large randomized sample groups because of the relatively low mortality and morbidity and because of the various subsets of coronary patients
2. High drop-out rates in exercising groups
3. Improper handling of crossover in the control and treatment groups
4. Use of low-intensity and short-duration exercise programs
5. Treatment of a multifaceted disease with a single intervention (i.e., exercise)

After one reviews the above list, it becomes apparent that there are both inherent problems with the disease (i.e., multifaceted, relatively low mortality and morbidity, and various subsets of patients) and problems with study design that have clouded the results of previous trials. Table 10-2 summarizes the results of the major studies that have previously examined the value of exercise in reducing coronary morbidity (reinfarction) and mortality (attributable to all causes and cardiac death specifically). A careful review of this table reveals that there has been a consistent trend toward a lower recurrence rate (reinfarction or death) in the

**Table 10-2.** Summary of major studies on exercise and coronary mortality and morbidity (1968-1978)

| Authors/year | Follow-up period (years) | Number of patients in exercise group | Exercise group | | | Control group | | |
|---|---|---|---|---|---|---|---|---|
| | | | Recurrence and mortality (%/year) | Mortality (%/year) | Cardiac mortality (%/year) | Recurrence and mortality (%/year) | Mortality (%/year) | Cardiac mortality (%/year) |
| Bruce (1974)[15] | up to 4.0 | 195 | 10.3 | 3.1 | — | — | 11.2 | — |
| Gottheiner (1968)[42] | 5.0 | 1103 | — | 0.88 | 0.72 | — | 4.8 | — |
| Kavanagh and others (1975)[62] | 2.0 | 31 | 2.3 | 2.3 | 5.0 | — | — | — |
| Kentala (1972)[63] | 2.0 | 77 | 7.1 | 5.8 | 8.6 | 6.8 | 6.2 | — |
| Rechnitzer and others (1972)[85] | 7.0 | 68 | 5.0 | 3.6 | — | 14.3 | 9.0 | — |
| Sanne (1972)[96] | 1.9 | 158 | 6.6 | 3.8 | 2.9 | 12.5 | 8.8 | 8.3 |
| Wilhelmsen and others (1975)[113] | 4.0 | 158 | 8.4 | 4.4 | 3.6 | 10.0 | 5.6 | 5.3 |

exercise groups with the exception of Kentala's data.[63] However, the differences in the recurrence rates between the treatment and control groups, more often than not, have not been found to be statistically significant. Once again, the lack of statistically significant differences can be explained, at least in part, by the factors listed earlier.

The National Exercise and Heart Disease Project was the most recent randomized controlled trial attempted in this country.[76] Further discussion of this project is warranted because it is the largest randomized trial of its kind completed in the United States. This trial was originally designed to randomize some 4000 participants to provide a large enough number of treatment and nontreatment subjects to produce statistically significant results. However, because of a lack of funding, only 651 men between 30 and 64 years of age and with a previous documented MI were randomized into either the exercise or the nonexercise group.[99] The number of actual randomized subjects is equivalent to 16% of the desired number, and thus the study had limited probability of demonstrating statistically significant differences between the two randomized groups.

Moreover, the exercise program for the treatment group appeared to barely meet the "minimum" intensity recommendations of most authorities in the field. During the first 8 weeks of the study, the subjects exercised three times per week for 24 minutes—4 minutes at four different exercise stations (treadmill, bicycle, arm ergometer, and shoulder wheel). Thereafter the participants completed 15 minutes of continuous aerobic exercise followed by 25 minutes of "games" three times per week. It is assumed that the relatively mild exercise program was implemented by the investigators to minimize the problem of subject dropout.

The study also had problems with crossover between the two groups. By the end of 2 years, 23% of the exercising group reported that they had discontinued regular exercise and 31% of the nonexercising group stated that they were exercising regularly. However, because this crossover was ignored in analysis of the data an obvious bias existed against the positive effects of exercise.

Despite the problem of a less than aggressive exercise program and crossover, there were some encouraging findings from the study. The mortality in the exercise group (4.3%) was 37% lower than that in the nonexercise group (6.1%). This difference was not statistically significant because of the relatively small group size; however, if this difference had been seen in a study population of 1400, the lower death rate would have been significant. In addition, the exercise group had a death rate from cardiovascular causes of 1.9% versus 4.3% in the nonexercise group. Furthermore, of the nine deaths related directly to recurrent MI, eight occurred in the control group and one in the treatment group (p <0.05). Also of note was that men in the exercise group with a peak systolic blood pressure of 140 mm Hg or greater in the final stage of their entry exercise test had a statistically significant (p <0.05) lower death rate than their counterparts in the control group. There were no statistically significant differences between the two groups in morbidity though the exercise group had 31% fewer events.

In 1988 Oldridge and others[79] published their results of a meta-analysis of the combined results of the randomized clinical trials that involved 4347 patients. This analysis was done in an attempt to overcome the problem of the relatively small sample size that existed in all previous clinical trials. Their findings included a statistically lower cardiovascular death rate in the rehabilitation group but no difference in nonfatal MIs. Table 10-3 summarizes the cardiovascular death rate and nonfatal recurrent infarction rate in all 10 studies analyzed.

**Summary**

In summary, despite a number of design problems and relatively small sample size, the data from The National Exercise and Heart Disease Project are somewhat encouraging in regard to the protective effects of exercise on mortality and morbidity. At the very least, the data from this study suggest that the protective effect may be more significant in certain subsets of post-MI patients. It is unfortunate that this project was unable to randomize an

**Table 10-3.** Summary: cardiovascular death rate and nonfatal recurrent infarction rate in 10 randomized clinical trials*

| | Number of events/number of patients | | | |
| | Cardiovascular death | | Nonfatal recurrence | |
| Author/year | Treatment | Control | Treatment | Control |
|---|---|---|---|---|
| Kentala, 1972[63] | 8/77 | 10/81 | 6/77 | 4/81 |
| Wilhelmsen, 1975[113] | 28/158 | 33/157 | 25/158 | 28/157 |
| Kallio, 1979[56] | 35/188 | 55/187 | 34/188 | 21/187 |
| Shaw, 1981[99] | 14/323 | 20/328 | 15/323 | 11/328 |
| Carson, 1982[16] | — | — | 11/141 | 10/152 |
| Rechnitzer, 1983[85] | 15/379 | 13/354 | 39/379 | 33/354 |
| Roman, 1983[90] | 13/93 | 24/100 | 9/93 | 8/100 |
| Vermeulen, 1983[111] | 2/47 | 5/51 | 4/47 | 9/51 |
| World Health Organization, 1984[118] | 84/705 | 88/655 | 88/705 | 58/655 |
| Marra, 1985[73] | 5/81 | 4/80 | 5/81 | 9/80 |

*Adapted from Oldridge NB and others: Cardiac rehabilitation after myocardial infarction: combined experience of randomized clinical trials, *JAMA* 260:945, 1988.

adequate number of subjects, since it is unlikely that the funding agencies will support similar projects in the future.

Dr. Terence Kavanagh,[62] director of the largest cardiac rehabilitation program in the world, published data on the influence of exercise compliance on the prognosis in men with a previous myocardial infarction. Although this was not a randomized trial, the data are very impressive and warrant further discussion at this point. Kavanagh's study involved a consecutive series of 620 men referred to the Toronto Rehabilitation Center after a documented MI. These men were followed for a mean of 36 months to assess which were the most important prognostic indicators of cardiac events (death, reinfarction). The goal of the exercise program was to complete 3 miles in 30 to 36 minutes, five times per week. Of the study subjects 505 were exercising three times per week and 78 of the remaining 105 men were following through twice per week.

During the follow-up period, there were 23 cardiac deaths and 21 recurrent MIs. Risk ratios were calculated for the various factors believed to influence prognosis. Patients with an elevated cholesterol value (≥270 mg/dl) had a risk ratio of 1.98. In other words, patients with elevated cholesterol levels had nearly twice the risk of a future coronary event as those with a lower value. Cigarette smokers had a risk ratio of 1.93. Exercise noncompliance, on the other hand, had a risk ratio of 22.6, meaning that those who did not continue to comply with the exercise program had nearly 23 times the chance of suffering a second coronary event.

In fact, exercise noncompliance was the major prognostic factor, even more important than the presence of more than 2 mm of ST-segment depression on the initial exercise test, age, hypertension (≥150/110 mm Hg), persistent angina, evidence of ventricular aneurysm, or enlarged heart on the radiograph. Once again, these data very definitely indicate that exercise compliance dramatically lowers the probability of repeat coronary events.

If one interprets the data from The National Exercise and Heart Disease Project and The Toronto Rehabilitation Center as evidence that exercise training decreases the probability of future coronary events in post-MI patients, then the question becomes: Through which mechanism or mechanisms does exercise provide its protective effect? Following are several mechanisms through which exercise may theoretically influence the prognosis of the coronary patient:

1. Alteration of the normal rate of progression of coronary atherosclerosis through risk factor reduction and other mechanisms
2. Improvement in the myocardial oxygen supply and demand balance partly as a result of increased collateral circulation or increased size of the lumen of the coronary vessels
3. Decreased tendency to form coronary thrombi because of increased fibrolytic activity
4. Decreased coronary vasomotor tone resulting in decreased tendency toward coronary spasm

Does risk factor reduction influence the progression of atherosclerosis as suggested above? Barndt and others[3] have demonstrated that reduction of serum cholesterol and triglycerides and blood pressure in hyperlipidemic patients can result in regression of early femoral atherosclerosis over a 13-month period of follow-up. Blankenhorn,[9] after further analyzing the data on these patients with early femoral lesions, reported that the percent change in atherosclerosis was highly correlated with the serum triglyceride level in type-IV hyperlipidemic patients; that is the lower the serum triglyceride level, the greater the degree of regression. The earlier studies on atherosclerotic changes in the coronary arteries conflict somewhat partly because of the failure either to control some of the major risk factors or to attempt aggressive risk factor reduction. Furthermore, these studies have involved subjects with clinical manifestations of the disease and therefore a more advanced degree of atherosclerosis. It is possible that factors such as ulceration, hemorrhage, calcification, and thrombosis may influence the course of the disease as much as, if not more than, the major risk factors such as smoking and hypertension. However, Sanmarco and others[95] have reported on 38 men with advanced coronary atherosclerosis studied with serial angiography. They found that changes in coronary lesions are directly related to the risk factors of cigarette smoking and serum HDL cholesterol levels, as well as the age of the patient at the onset of his clinical manifestation of coronary disease. After reviewing his data, Sanmarco[94] stated that "a program consisting of diet modification, regular exercise, cessation of cigarette smoking, and control of blood pressure and hyperlipidemia will at least stabilize the disease process in some patients and offers the greatest chance of reducing cardiovascular morbidity and mortality." The data of Selvester and others[98] suggest that both cigarette smoking and exercise training are related to progression in coronary lesions. In those patients who were nonsmokers and complied with high levels of exercise training, 20% of their vessels demonstrated progression (worsening) of disease over a course of 18 months, whereas nonsmokers who were inactive demonstrated progression in 30% of their vessels. The more recent work by Raichlen[84] cited earlier supports the concept that progression of coronary disease is related to blood pressure, cigarette smoking, control of diabetes, and exercise habits. Thus it appears that risk factor reduction through exercise and other intervention is worthwhile and may help to stabilize coronary disease.

Thus far, the other "mechanisms" listed previously have not been studied. Specifically, no studies are available on the influence of exercise training on the size of the coronary vessels or on vasomotor tone. In addition, the studies on exercise training and collateralization have been inconclusive. Williams and others[115] have reported that regular aerobic exercise over a 10-week period in healthy adults 25 to 69 years of age can enhance fibrinolysis in response to thrombotic stimuli. They concluded that the augmented fibrinolytic response to venous occlusion "could be an important mechanism in the beneficial effect of habitual physical activity on the risk of cardiovascular disease." Further study is needed to see if the coronary patient demonstrates a similar tendency toward enhanced fibrinolysis and what influence it has on future coronary events.

## PSYCHOLOGICAL EFFECTS OF EXERCISE TRAINING

Kavanagh and others[60] have studied the effects of exercise training on depression in coronary patients after myocardial infarction and have noted reduced depression scores after training. The control group in this study did not demonstrate a similar trend. In a group of coronary long-distance runners, posttraining depression scores and psychological profiles were dramatically improved.[47] Based on our and others' observations, much of the postevent (MI,

surgery, or onset of angina) depression seen in coronary patients is a result of fear over loss of life and, just as important, loss of ability to "safely" participate in various recreational and everyday activities. Once the coronary patient realizes that through a program of exercise rehabilitation he or she can become (in most cases) more active than he or she was before the event, much of the depression and fear is overcome.

Finally, Blumenthal and others[12] have published a preliminary report on the effects of regular exercise (jogging) on type A behavior as assessed by the Jenkins Activity Survey in 10 healthy adults. These authors reported a significant reduction in the survey scores after training. Coronary patients at our centers in Los Angeles are currently participating in a study, under the direction of Dr. Alan Abbott, designed to investigate whether exercise and rehabilitation efforts in general influence type A behavior as assessed by both the Jenkins Activity Survey and a structured interview.

As was mentioned earlier, no single intervention by itself should be considered the panacea for coronary disease, since its clinical course appears to be influenced by multiple factors. Exercise therapy is, however, an essential component of rehabilitation and therapy for the coronary patient. Its potential benefits include improvement in aerobic and physical work capacity, risk factor reduction, improvement or relief of effort, angina and claudication discomfort, and reduction in postevent depression. In addition, there is evidence indicating that exercise training can slow the progression of coronary disease and reduce the likelihood of future coronary events. To be truly effective, a therapeutic exercise training program must be designed to include adequate intensity, duration, and frequency and the program must be ongoing. Finally, therapists must expend a great deal of effort and creativity to ensure the highest possible exercise compliance rate of his or her patient population.

## REFERENCES

1. Arvan S: Exercise performance of the high risk acute myocardial infarction patient after cardiac rehabilitation, *Am J Cardiol* 62:197, 1988.
2. Ballantyne BS and others: The effects of moderate physical exercise on the plasma lipoprotein level subfractions of male survivors of myocardial infarction, *Circulation* 65:932, 1982.
3. Barndt R Jr and others: Regression and progression of early femoral atherosclerosis in treated hyperlipoproteinemic patients, *Ann Intern Med* 86:139, 1977.
4. Barry AJ and others: Effects of physical training in patients who have had myocardial infarctions, *Am J Cardiol* 17:1, 1966.
5. Björntorp P: Hypertension and exercise, *Circulation* 4(suppl 3):56, 1982.
6. Björntorp P and others: Effects of physical training on the glucose tolerance, plasma insulin and lipids, and on body composition in men after myocardial infarction, *Acta Med Scand* 192:439, 1972.
7. Björntorp P and others: Physical training in human hyperplastic obesity. IV. Effects on the hormonal state, *Metabolism* 26:319, 1977.
8. Björntorp P: Effects of physical training on blood pressure in hypertension, *Eur Heart J* 8(suppl B):71, 1987.
9. Blankenhorn DH: The rate of atherosclerosis change during treatment of hyperlipoproteinemia, *Circulation* 57:355, 1977.

10. Blessey R and others: Therapeutic effects and safety of exercising coronary patients at their angina threshold, *Med Sci Sports Exer* 11:110, 1979 (abstract).

11. Blessey R and others: Angiographic, clinical, and exercise test data in marathoning coronary patients (abstract), *Med Sci Sports Exer* 13:131, 1981.

12. Blumenthal JA and others: Effects of exercise on the type A (coronary prone) behavior pattern, *Psychosom Med* 42:289, 1980.

13. Bonanno J and others: Effects of physical training on coronary risk factors, *Am J Cardiol* 33:760, 1974.

14. Boyer JL and Kasch FW: Exercise therapy in hypertensive men, *JAMA* 211:1668, 1970.

15. Bruce RA: The benefits of physical training for patients with coronary heart disease. In Ingelfinger FJ and others, editors: *Controversy in internal medicine, II,* Philadelphia, 1974, WB Saunders Co.

16. Carson P and others: Exercise after a myocardial infarction: a controlled trial, *JR Coll Physicians Lond* 16:141, 1982.

17. Choquette G and Ferguson RJ: Blood pressure reduction in borderline hypertension following physical training, *Can Med Assoc J* 108:699, 1973.

18. Clausen JP and others: Physical training in the management of coronary artery disease, *Circulation* 40:143, 1969.

19. Clausen JP and others: Heart rate and arterial blood pressure during exercise in patients with angina pectoris, *Circulation* 53:436, 1976.

20. Conn EH and others: Exercise responses before and after physical conditioning in patients with severely depressed left ventricular function, *Amer J Card* 49:296, 1982.

21. Conolly DC: Treatment of hypertension improves survival in patients with coronary heart disease (abstract), *Circulation* 64(suppl 4):300, 1982.

22. Cooper KH and others: Physical fitness levels versus selected coronary risk factors, *JAMA* 236:166, 1978.

23. Cowan GO: Influence of exercise on high density lipoproteins, *Am J Cardiol* 52:13B, 1983.

24. Dash E and others: Cardiomyopathic syndrome due to coronary disease. II. Increased prevalence in patients with diabetes mellitus: a matched pair analysis, *Br Heart J* 39:740, 1977.

25. Detry JM and others: Increased arteriovenous oxygen difference after physical training in heart disease, *Circulation* 44:109, 1971.

26. Dressendorfer RH and others: Therapeutic effects of exercise training in angina patients. In Cohen LS and others, editors: *Physical conditioning and cardiovascular rehabilitation,* New York, 1981, John Wiley & Sons.

27. Duncan JJ and others: The effects of aerobic exercise on plasma catecholamines and blood pressure in patients with mild essential hypertension, *JAMA* 254:2609, 1985.

28. Durstine LJ and Haskell WL: Effects of exercise training on plasma lipids and lipoproteins, *Exer and Sport Sci Rev* 22:477, 1994.

29. Ehsani AA and others: Effect of 12 months of intense exercise training on ischemic ST-segment depression in patients with coronary artery disease, *Circulation* 46:1116, 1981.

30. Ehsani AA and others: Improvement of left ventricular contractile function by exercise training in patients with coronary artery disease, *Circulation* 74:351, 1986.

31. Ekroth R and others: Physical training of patients with intermittent claudication: indications, methods, and results, *Surgery* 84:640, 1978.

32. Erickson B and others: Maximal flow capacity before and after training. In Larsen MA and Malmborg RO, editors: *Coronary heart disease and physical fitness,* Baltimore, 1971, University Park Press.

33. Erkelens DW and others: High density lipoprotein cholesterol in survivors of myocardial infarction, *JAMA* 242:2185, 1979.

34. Five-year findings of the hypertension detection and follow-up program. I. Reduction in mortality of persons with high blood pressure, including mild hypertension, *JAMA* 242:2562, 1979.

35. Foley WT: Treatment of gangrene of the foot and legs by walking, *Circulation* 15:689, 1957.

36. Frick WH and Katila M: Hemodynamic consequences of physical training after myocardial infarction, *Circulation* 37:192, 1968.

37. Frick MH and others: The mechanism of bradycardia evoked by physical training, *Cardiologia* 51:46, 1967.

38. Froelicher V and others: A randomized trial of exercise training in patients with coronary heart disease, *JAMA* 252:1291, 1984.

39. Froelicher V and others: A randomized trial of exercise training after coronary bypass surgery, *Arch Intern Med* 145:689, 1985.

40. Gilders RM, Voner C and Dudley, GA: Endurance training and blood pressure in normotensive and hypertensive adults, *Med Sci Sports Exer* 21:629, 1989.

41. Goeransson C and Peppy M: *Effects of exercise on lipids and lipoproteins of men with coronary artery disease,* master's thesis, Los Angeles, 1979, University of Southern California, School of Physical Therapy.

42. Gottheiner V: Long-range strenuous sports training for cardiac reconditioning and rehabilitation, *Am J Cardiol* 22:426, 1968.

43. Hagberg JM and others: Effects of 12 months of intense exercise training on stroke volume in patients with coronary artery disease, *Circulation* 67:1194, 1983.

44. Hall JA and others: Effects of diet and exercise on peripheral vascular diseases, *Phys Sports Med* 10:90, 1982.

45. Hall JA and others: Effects of an intensive short-term diet and exercise program on patients with peripheral vascular disease (abstract), *Med Sci Sports Exer* 14:179, 1982.

46. Hartley LH and others: Multiple hormonal responses to graded exercise in relation to physical training, *J Appl Physiol* 33:602, 1972.

47. Hartung H and others: Relation of diet to high density lipoprotein cholesterol in middle-age marathon runners, joggers and inactive men, *N Engl J Med* 302:357, 1980.

48. Hartung GH and others: Effect of exercise training on plasma high density lipoprotein cholesterol in coronary disease patients, *Am Heart J* 101:181, 1981.

49. Heath GW and others: Exercise training improves lipoprotein lipid profiles in patients with coronary artery disease, *Am Heart J* 105:889, 1983.

50. Hellerstein HK and others: Reconditioning of the coronary patient: preliminary report. In Likoff W and Moyer JH, editors: *Coronary heart disease,* New York, 1963, Grune & Stratton, Inc.

51. Huttunen JK and others: Effect of moderate physical exercise on serum lipoprotein levels. A controlled clinical trial with special reference to serum high-density lipoproteins, *Circulation* 60:1220, 1979.

52. Jennings G and others: The effects of changes in physical activity on major cardiovascular risk factors, hemodynamics, sympathetic function, and glucose utilization in man: a controlled study of four levels of activity, *Circulation* 73:30, 1986.

53. Jensen D and others: Improvement in ventricular function during exercise studied with radionuclide ventriculography after cardiac rehabilitation, *Am J Cardiol* 46:770, 1980.

54. Jonason T and others: Effect of physical training on different categories of patients with intermittent claudication, *Acta Med Scand* 206:253, 1979.

55. Kahrs SJ and others: Effects of exercise training and diet modification on serum lipids and lipoproteins in coronary artery disease patients treated with thiazides, *Clin Card* 8:636, 1985.

56. Kallio V and others: Reduction in sudden deaths by multifactorial intervention program after acute myocardial infarction, *Lancet* 2:1081, 1979.

57. Kannel WB and McGee DL: Diabetes and cardiovascular risk factors: the Framingham Study, *Circulation* 59:8, 1979.

58. Kannel WB and others: Intermittent claudication: incidence in the Framingham Study, *Circulation* 41:875, 1970.

59. Kavanagh T: Intervention studies in Canada: primary and secondary intervention. In Pollack ML and Schmidt DH, editors: *Heart disease and rehabilitation,* Boston 1979, Houghton Mifflin Co.

60. Kavanagh T and others: Depression after myocardial infarction, *Can Med Assoc J* 113:23, 1975.

61. Kavanagh T and others: Depression following myocardial infarction: the effects of distance running, *Ann NY Acad Sci* 301:1029, 1978.

62. Kavanagh T and others: Prognostic indexes for patients with ischemic heart disease enrolled with an exercise-centered rehabilitation program, *Am J Cardiol* 44:1230, 1979.

63. Kentala E: Physical fitness and probability of physical rehabilitation after myocardial infarction in men of working age, *Ann Clin Res 9* (suppl 1), 1972.

64. Kessler II: Mortality experience of diabetic patients: a 26-year follow-up study, *Am J Med* 51:715, 1971.

65. Krotkiewski M and others: Effects of long-term physical training on body fat, metabolism, and blood pressure in obesity, *Metabolism* 21:650, 1979.

66. Krotkiewski M and others: Effects of physical training on andrenergic sensitivity in obesity, *J Appl Physiol* 55:1811, 1983.

67. Larsen MA and Larsen OA: Effect of training on the circulation in ischemic muscle tissue: observations of calf muscle blood flow in patients with intermittent claudication. In Larsen MA and Malmborg RO, editors: *Coronary heart disease and physical fitness,* Baltimore, 1971, University Park Press.

68. Lee AP and others: Long-term effects of physical training on coronary patients with impaired ventricular function, *Circulation* 60:1519, 1979.

69. Leon AS: Effects of exercise conditioning on physiologic precursors of coronary heart disease, *J Cardiopul Rehab* 11:46, 1991.

70. Letac B and others: A study of left ventricular function in coronary patients before and after physical training, *Circulation* 56:375, 1977.

71. Malmborg R and others: The effect of beta blockage and/or physical training in patients with angina pectoris, *Curr Ther Res* 16:171, 1974.

72. Mann GU and others: Exercise to prevent coronary heart disease: an experimental study of the effects of training on risk factors for coronary disease in man, *Am J Med* 46:12, 1969.

73. Marra S and others: Long term follow-up after a controlled randomized post myocardial rehabilitation program: effects on morbidity and mortality, *Eur Heart J* 6:656, 1985.

74. Mau HS and Wagner ED: Cardiac rehabilitation effects on exercise and diet on blood pressure (abstract), *Circulation* 64 (suppl 4):275, 1981.

75. Miller H and others: Troms heart study: HDL and coronary artery disease: a prospective case control study, *Lancet* 2:965, 1977.

76. Naughton J: The National Exercise and Heart Disease Project: the pre-randomized exercise program, *Cardiology* 63:352, 1978.

77. Naughton J and Balke B: Effect of physical training on work capacity in post-myocardial infarction patients, *J Sports Med* 4:185, 1964.

78. Obina R and others: Effect of a conditioning program on patients taking propranolol for angina pectoris, *Cardiology* 64:365, 1979.

79. Oldridge NB and others: Cardiac rehabilitation after myocardial infarction: combined experience of randomized clinical trials, *JAMA* 260:945, 1988.

80. Oschrin A and others: Effects of aerobic exercise training on lipids and lipoproteins in coronary artery diease patients. *Proceedings of the Ninth International Congress of the World Confederation of Physical Therapy,* Stockholm, May 1982, Legitimerade Sjukgymnastears Ikssorbune.

81. Palac RT and others: Risk factors related to progressive narrowing of aortocoronaryvein grafts studies 9 and 5 years after surgery, *Circulation* 66 (suppl 1):40, 1982.

82. Patterson DH and others: Effects of physical training on cardiovascular function following myocardial infarction, *J Appl Physiol* 47:482, 1979.

83. Pratt CM and others: Demonstration of training effect during chronic beta-adrenergic blockage in patients with coronary artery disease, *Circulation* 64:1125, 1981.

84. Raichlen JS and others: Risk factors and angiographic progression

of coronary artery disease (abstract), *Circulation* 66 (suppl 2):283, 1982.

85. Rechnitzer PA and others: Long-term follow-up study of survival and recurrence rate following myocardial infarction in exercising and control subjects, *Circulation* 43:853, 1972.

86. Rechnitzer PA and others: Relation of exercise to recurrence rate of myocardial infarction in men: Ontario Exercise-Heart Collaborative Study, *Am J Cardiol* 51:65, 1983.

87. Redwood RR and others: Circulatory and symptomatic effects of physical training in patients with coronary artery disease and angina pectoris, *N Engl J Med* 286:959, 1972.

88. Rizi HR and others: Walk-through angina phenomenon demonstrated by graded exercise radionuclide ventriculography: possible coronary spasm mechanisms, *Am Heart J* 102:292, 1982.

89. Roman O and others: Physical training program in arterial hypertension: a long-term prospective follow-up, *Cardiology* 67:230, 1981.

90. Roman O and others: Cardiac rehabilitation after myocardial infarction: nine-year controlled follow-up study, *Cardiology* 70:223, 1983.

91. Ruderman NB and others: The effect of physical training on glucose tolerance and plasma lipids in maturity-onset diabetes, *Diabetes* 28:89, 1979.

92. Saltin B: Physical training in patients with intermittent claudication. In Cohen LS and others, editors: *Physical conditioning and cardiovascular rehabilitation,* New York, 1981, John Wiley & Sons.

93. Saltin B and others: Physical training and glucose tolerance in middle-aged men with chemical diabetes, *Diabetes* 28:30, 1979.

94. Sanmarco ME and Blankenhorn DH: Atherosclerosis: its progression and regression, *Primary Cardiol* p 51, July-Aug 1978.

95. Sanmarco ME and others: Smoking and high density lipoproteins and coronary change in two and three-vessel disease (abstract), *Am J Cardiol* 41:423, 1978.

96. Sanne H: Preventive effect of physical training after a myocardial infarction. In Tibblin G and others, editors: *Preventive cardiology,* New York, 1972, John Wiley & Sons.

97. Schuler G and others: Progression of coronary artery disease in patients on low-fat diet and intensive physical exercise (abstract), *Amer J Card* 63:48, 1989.

98. Selvester R and others: Effects of exercise training on progression of documented atherosclerosis in men, *Ann NY Acad Sci* 302:495, 1977.

99. Shaw LW: Effects of a prescribed supervised exercise program on mortality and cardiovascular morbidity in patients after a myocardial infarction, *Am J Cardiol* 48:39, 1981.

100. Sim DN and Neill WA: Investigation of the physiological basis for increased exercise threshold for angina pectoris after physical conditioning, *J Clin Invest* 54:763, 1974.

101. Skinner JS and Strandness DE Jr: Exercise and intermittent claudication. II. Effect of physical training, *Circulation* 36:23, 1967.

102. Streja D and Mymin O: Moderate exercise and high density lipoprotein cholesterol, *JAMA* 242:2190, 1979.

103. Sullivan MJ and others: Exercise training in patients with severe left ventricular dysfunction: hemodynamic and metabolic effects, *Circulation* 78:500, 1988.

104. Thompson PD and others: Effect of exercise training on the untrained limb: exercise performance of men with angina pectoris, *Am J Cardiol* 48:844, 1981.

105. Thompson PD and others: Modest changes in high-density lipoprotein concentration and metabolism with prolonged exercise training, *Circulation* 78:25, 1988.

106. Tran ZV and Brammell HL: Effects of exercise training on serum lipid and lipoprotein levels in post-MI patients: a meta-analysis, *J Cardiopulm Rehab* 9:250, 1989.

107. Tran ZV and Weltman A: Differential effects of exercise on serum lipid and lipoprotein levels seen with changes in body weight: a meta-analysis, *JAMA* 254:919, 1986.

108. Urata H and others: Antihypertensive and volume-depleting effects of mild exercise on essential hypertension, *Hypertension* 9:245, 1987.

109. Urata H and others: Effect of mild aerobic exercise on serum lipids and apolipoproteins in patients with coronary artery disease, *Jpn Heart J* 28:27, 1987.

110. Varnauskas E and others: Haemodynamic effects of physical training in coronary patients, *Lancet* 2:8, 1966.

111. Vermeulen A and others: Effects of cardiac rehabilitation after myocardial infarction: changes in coronary risk factors and long-term prognosis, *Am Heart J* 105:798, 1983.

112. Waller BF and Roberts WC: Acceleration of coronary atherosclerosis in diabetes mellitus only with onset of diabetes less than 30 years of age: necropsy analysis of 275 diabetic patients (1100 arteries) aged 1 to 87 years and 242 age-matched control subjects, *Circulation* 64(suppl 4):80, 1981.

113. Wilhelmsen L and others: A controlled trial of physical training after myocardial infarction: effects on risk factors, nonfatal reinfarction, and death, *Prev Med* 4:491, 1975.

114. Williams RS: Exercise training of patients with ventricular dysfunction and heart failure. In Wenger N, editor. *Exercise and the heart,* Philadelphia, 1982, WB Saunders Co.

115. Williams RS and others: Physical conditioning augments the fibrinolytic response to venous occlusion in healthy agents, *N Engl J Med* 302:987, 1980.

116. Wood P and others: Plasma lipoprotein distribution in male and female runners, *Ann NY Acad Sci* 302: 748, 1978.

117. Wood P and others: Changes in plasma lipids and lipoproteins in overweight men during weight loss through diet as compared to exercise, *N Engl J Med* 310:1173, 1988.

118. World Health Organization: Rehabilitation and comprehensive secondary prevention after acute myocardial infarction, *EURO Rep Stud* 84:1, 1983.

119. Zetterqvist S: Effects of training in intermittent claudication: redistribution of blood flow due to training. In Larson OA and Malmborg RO, editors: *Coronary heart disease and physical fitness,* Copenhagen, 1971, Munkesgaard.

# Administrative Considerations

*Scot Irwin*

To initiate and maintain a cardiac rehabilitation program (phases I to III), specific administrative responsibilities must be complete. These responsibilities cover six broad areas: physician support, clinical knowledge and skills of the rehabilitation team members, communication procedures, space, equipment, and reimbursement. Clinical knowledge and skills for physical therapists have been discussed in the previous chapters. Each of these administrative responsibilities is subject to variations according to the clinical environment and thus require innovation and adaptability.

## PHYSICIAN SUPPORT

Each program needs a medical director or directors—preferably, one or more board-certified cardiologists. The medical director should have a well-established rapport with the facility administrator and potential referring physicians. The medical director has three major roles: referral, reinforcement of the rehabilitation philosophy, and supervision.

As a source of referral, the medical director should consider each of his patients as appropriate candidates for the program. The director should encourage other physicians to refer to the program by developing and distributing criteria and methods for admission. A director may quickly increase the referrals to the program through discussions with potential referring physicians. These discussions should provide a careful orientation to the program, explaining methods of referral, appropriate candidates, communication mechanisms, referring physician role, and program structure and goals. A sample written orientation guide is included as Appendix A of this chapter. Following a review of the material in Appendix A, a physician's referral for cardiac rehabilitation effectively clears a patient for participation in all aspects of the program. In other words, the referring physician does not and should not have to order each step of the program. However, he or she should be consulted before any exercise tests, and an additional referral for testing may be required.

Referral to the program can be facilitated by simplifying procedures. Phase I referral can be enhanced by using a check-off sheet in the coronary care unit (see Fig. 11-1). Phases II and III referrals are accomplished by using a form that can be completed and returned easily. An example is shown in Fig. 11-2.

A medical director should constantly reinforce the program's philosophy; a director who has few or no risk factors and who actively participates in the exercise program will make the program go and grow. The opposite is also true. If the medical director even suggests to patients that smoking, overeating, or not exercising is all right, the team's efforts at risk factor modification will not succeed. Reinforcement of the program philosophy is therefore a major responsibility of the medical director. In addition, director involvement in patient and team educational activities is essential. In my clinical experience, the cardiac rehabilitation programs that are most effective and have the greatest longevity are those with active, on-site, physician participation.

The third task of the medical director is to assist with supervision of the program. This task includes approving protocols, advising team members on patient medical problems, and making medication changes as necessary.

The following protocols need to be developed and approved by the medical director: resuscitation procedures (Appendix B, Fig. 11-3), consent forms for exercise tests and outpatient exercise programming (Appendixes C and D),

| CCU to Step-down transfer orders | | | |
|---|---|---|---|
| 1. Transfer to Step-down Unit | | | |
| 2. Diagnosis | | Condition | |
| 3. Telemetry | yes | no | |
| 4. Diet    a. Regular | No added salt | | Sanka |
| b. Sodium restricted to | | | grams |
| c. "Prudent" | | | |
| d. Other | | | |
| 5. TED hose | yes | no | |
| 6. IV | | | |
| 7. Initiate cardiac rehabilitation | | yes | no |
| 8. Medications | | | |
| a. NTG 1/150 g PRN angina | | | |
| b. Sedation | | | |
| c. Sleep | | | |
| d. Noncardiac analgesic | | | |
| e. Anticoagulant | | | |
| f. Antidysrhythmic | | | |
| g. Laxative | | | |
| h. Digoxin | | | |
| i. Propranolol (Inderal) | | | |
| j. Diuretic | | | |
| k. Other | | | |
| 9. Lab    a. PPT | q | | |
| b. PT | q | | |
| c. Other | | | |

**Fig. 11-1.** Sample transfer order sheet used to facilitate referral to cardiac rehabilitation (phase I).

exercise testing guidelines and protocols (Appendix E, Table 11-1), and all cardiac rehabilitation policies and procedures. All of these protocols are commonly a part of most programs except for the resuscitation procedures. The resuscitation procedures are critical to patient safety. In my opinion, a program that does not allow defibrillation by the team members involved in the exercise program is assuming an inordinate risk and liability. At some time, despite assessments, monitoring, and careful program design, a patient will go into ventricular tachycardia or ventricular fibrillation and require immediate resuscitation.

A second supervisory task of the medical director is to be familiar with all of the program participants' medical histories and problems. This knowledge allows the medical director to answer team members' questions about medical disorders (e.g., gout, pericarditis, arthritis, and diabetes) and their effects on disease progression, exercise tolerance, and exercise prescription.

Perhaps the medical director's most important task is to respond to the team members' objective findings by making medication adjustments as needed. For example, a patient 3 weeks into phase II develops serious ventricular dysrhythmias, and this information is communicated to the medical director. If there is no response to this new development,

```
                    CARDIAC REHABILITATION REFERRAL FORM

            Department of Physical Therapy and Rehabilitation


The following person has applied for entry into the

Cardiac Rehabilitation Program:

Mr.
Mrs.
Miss _____     Address: _____

Telephone
number:   H _____  B _____ Age: _____ Sex: __ M or __ F

Participation in this program requires referral by the attending physician.

If you wish the above person to enter the program, please complete the fol-

lowing information.  Thank you.


I am referring the above-named person for participation in the Cardiac

Rehabilitation Program.

Diagnosis: _____

           _____

Major symptoms: _____

                _____

Medication: _____

            _____

            _____

            _____

                         Signed _____ M.D.

Periodic progress reports will be sent to the referring physician.
```

**Fig. 11-2.** Outpatient referral form.

team member morale will fall and the program's effectiveness will be impaired. A strong medical director will make the appropriate medication changes or explain to the team members why medical intervention is not necessary.

Physician support and supervision is essential, and the key to that support comes from the program's medical director. The director's duties include being a referral source, medical advisor, and a program supervisor.

## CLINICAL KNOWLEDGE AND SKILLS OF THE TEAM

Several texts could be written describing the knowledge and skill required of each potential member of a cardiac rehabilitation team. That is not the intent of this section. If the philosophy of a cardiac program is the same as the one described in the first chapter of this text, the following knowledge and skills will be needed.

Team members with knowledge in the following areas are preferred: dietary content and food preparation, metabolism of cholesterol, medication interaction (effects and side effects), psychological manifestations of heart disease, community resources (financial, vocational) available to patients and their families, exercise training (methods and effects), and medical care.

Each team member should also be knowledgeable in educational methods and be trained and certified in cardiopulmonary resuscitation.

## COMMUNICATION PROCEDURES

There are three simple, but essential, communication procedures that will enhance the program's effectiveness and

CARDIOPULMONARY RESUSCITATION FLOW SHEET

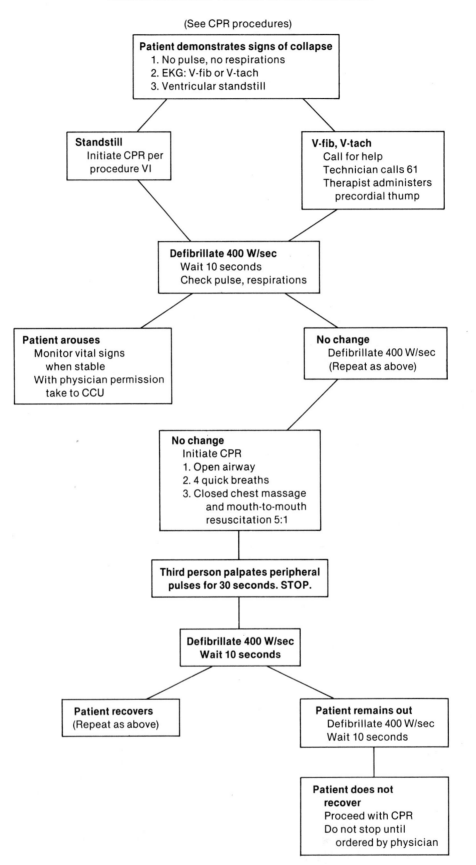

**Fig. 11-3.** Flow chart of resuscitation procedures.

**Table 11-1.** Treadmill protocols

| | Speed (mph) | Grade (%) |
|---|---|---|
| **Maximal Bruce Multistage protocol** | | |
| Stage I | 1.7 | 10 |
| Stage II | 2.5 | 12 |
| Stage III | 3.4 | 14 |
| Stage IV | 4.2 | 16 |
| Stage V | 5.0 | 18 |
| Stage VI | 5.5 | 20 |
| Stage VII | 6.0 | 22 |
| **Low-level protocol—submaximal** | | |
| Stage I | 1.7 | 0 |
| Stage II | 1.7 | 5 |
| Stage III | 1.7 | 10 |
| Stage IV | 2.0 | 12 |
| Stage V | 2.5 | 12 |

ensure safety. These procedures include physician contact, progress notes, and patient diaries.

A system for immediate physician contact is essential. As the previous chapters have demonstrated, complications can occur at any point in the patient's program (see Chapters 7 to 9). These complications are rarely life threatening or serious enough to require emergency procedures, but they may require medical intervention. Often, a simple change in frequency or dosage of a patient's medication will remedy a potentially serious complication. The therapist thus needs to have a direct line to the patient's physician or the program's medical director. Several physicians may be required, and priority order of contact should be established in a written policy and procedure.

Written progress reports about the patient's program progression and current exercise assessment should be sent to the patient's physician at least monthly (phases II and III). A sample progress report is presented in Fig. 11-4. Daily reports are required in phase I as part of the patient's inpatient medical record. We have found that it is effective and convenient to generate progress reports before a patient's appointment with the referring physician. We then have the patient carry the report to the physician's office. In addition, we encourage patients to take their exercise diaries (Fig. 11-5) with them when they visit their physician. A combination of monthly progress reports and exercise diaries ensures frequent written documentation of the patient's progress. This data sheet is also used for documentation to third-party reimbursement agencies.

The patient exercise diary is a crucial written communication for the physician, physical therapist, and patient (Fig 11-5). These diaries help to constantly update the therapist about the patient's home exercise sessions. Careful review of the diaries can help identify degree of compliance, current exercise intensity, and new signs or symptoms. Our thera-

pists are encouraged to check the diaries before each supervised session and to use the data from them to assess patient progression.

A combination of physician contact, progress notes, and patient diaries is key to good communication within the program. Without these communication procedures, patient compliance, physician referral, and therapist assessments will be less than optimal.

## SPACE

Cardiac rehabilitation programs have two major space requirements: an area for the exercise program (phases II and III) and an area for the educational sessions (phases I to III).

The educational area is situated best near the coronary care unit. An area large enough to accommodate the patients, their families, and audiovisual aids will suffice.

The space requirements for a cardiac rehabilitation program are often dependent on climate. Dry, temperate climates require less space because much of the exercise training can be conducted outdoors. Most regions are not fortunate enough to have that kind of climate, and space requirements can be a major block to development and implementation of a program.

The exercise program space is best situated within a gymnasium, but this is rarely available at a hospital. Space requirements for the exercise program should allow for enough equipment to have group exercise training sessions. Our facility has seven treadmills, two bicycle ergometers, and a seven-station Universal gym. This allows for seven patients to be treated simultaneously. The space is 30 by 30 feet.

## EQUIPMENT

Table 11-2 lists the approximate cost for the majority of equipment needed to conduct a cardiac rehabilitation program. Each piece of equipment has specific requirements that will make it useful to the program. These requirements and some helpful hints about purchases are found below.

### Radiotelemetry monitoring units

Radiotelemetry monitoring units should have an oscilloscope, strip chart recorder, and transmitters. The strip chart recorder should have memory capabilities so that dysrhythmias observed on the oscilloscope can be recorded on the strip chart. Group exercise sessions require at least enough telemetry channels to allow each patient to be monitored. These units will be the program's greatest equipment expense. Before including these units in your budget, check your hospital or clinic for outdated telemetry systems. Over the last few years, technological improvements have caused coronary care units to replace their telemetry systems. The old systems are usually quite adequate and will allay the expense of purchasing additional telemetry units.

```
CARDIAC REHABILITATION OUT-PATIENT PROGRESS REPORT

Name _____    Plan established  _____

Diagnosis  _____

Report period from   _____  to  _____

Current medications   _____

General information   _____

EXERCISE

a. Dates attended   _____
b. Frequency    Home _____/week       Hospital _____ /week _____/month
c. Maximum HR   _____
d. Average resting HR _____    Average exer. HR _____
e. Mode    Walk _____              Intensity  _____ mph _____ grade
           Walk-jog _____                     _____ miles
           Jog _____                          _____ minutes
           Stationary bicycle _____  Intensity _____ miles
           Arm bicycle _____                  _____ minutes
                                               _____ resistance
f. Dysrhythmias  none _____    other _____
g. Average resting BP _____    Average peak BP with exercise _____
h. BP response  adaptive _____    hypertensive _____  hypotensive _____
i. Symptoms  angina level _____    leg pain _____  dyspnea _____

    other _____


EDUCATION

Complete _____  Ongoing _____    Needs all sessions _____

ADHERENCE TO PROGRAM

Poor _____    Fair _____  Good _____    Next report _____

COMMENTS (indicate major changes)




Signed _____ PT    Date _____
```

Fig. 11-4. Sample progress report form.

### Treadmills

Treadmills should be able to be calibrated. They are more useful if they have the capability for fine speed and grade adjustments.

There are some details about treadmill purchases that it pays to watch out for. These include, but are not limited to, ensuring that the treadmills have (1) acceptable leakage currents, (2) adequate power sources, and (3) acceptable ceiling height.

### Bicycle ergometers and exercise bicycles

Bicycle ergometers should have workload indicators that are easily observed and calibrated. They should be durable, and their seats should be as comfortable as possible.

Exercise bicycles are simply stationary bicycles with resistance capabilities. Measurable workloads cannot be obtained, and they are generally less durable. These bicycles are adequate for patient use at home but rarely withstand the stresses of a busy outpatient cardiac program.

Name:_____ Month:_____ Hospital:_____ Medications:_____

_____

S.C.O.R.
(Specialized Coronary Outpatient Rehabilitation) _____
Exercise Diary

Prescription: Distance_____ mile(s)

Time:_____ minutes    Physical fitness stage:_____

Target heart rate:_____ bpm    Weight (end of month):_____

| Day | Rest. HR | Exercise mode | Distance (peak) | Time (peak) | Work load | W-U HR | Peak HR | C-D HR | Symptoms or remarks |
|-----|----------|---------------|-----------------|-------------|-----------|--------|---------|--------|---------------------|
| 1   |          |               |                 |             |           |        |         |        |                     |
| 2   |          |               |                 |             |           |        |         |        |                     |
| 3   |          |               |                 |             |           |        |         |        |                     |
| 4   |          |               |                 |             |           |        |         |        |                     |
| 5   |          |               |                 |             |           |        |         |        |                     |
| 6   |          |               |                 |             |           |        |         |        |                     |
| 7   |          |               |                 |             |           |        |         |        |                     |
| 8   |          |               |                 |             |           |        |         |        |                     |
| 9   |          |               |                 |             |           |        |         |        |                     |
| 10  |          |               |                 |             |           |        |         |        |                     |
| 11  |          |               |                 |             |           |        |         |        |                     |
| 12  |          |               |                 |             |           |        |         |        |                     |
| 13  |          |               |                 |             |           |        |         |        |                     |
| 14  |          |               |                 |             |           |        |         |        |                     |
| 15  |          |               |                 |             |           |        |         |        |                     |
| 16  |          |               |                 |             |           |        |         |        |                     |
| 17  |          |               |                 |             |           |        |         |        |                     |
| 18  |          |               |                 |             |           |        |         |        |                     |
| 19  |          |               |                 |             |           |        |         |        |                     |
| 20  |          |               |                 |             |           |        |         |        |                     |

*Continued.*

**Fig. 11-5.** Patient exercise diary and data recording sheet.

| Day | Rest. HR | Exercise mode | Distance (peak) | Time (peak) | Work load | W–U HR | Peak HR | C–D HR | Symptoms or remarks |
|-----|----------|---------------|-----------------|-------------|-----------|--------|---------|--------|---------------------|
| 21 | | | | | | | | | |
| 22 | | | | | | | | | |
| 23 | | | | | | | | | |
| 24 | | | | | | | | | |
| 25 | | | | | | | | | |
| 26 | | | | | | | | | |
| 27 | | | | | | | | | |
| 28 | | | | | | | | | |
| 29 | | | | | | | | | |
| 30 | | | | | | | | | |
| 31 | | | | | | | | | |

MONTHLY SUMMARY

Average resting heart rate =
Average peak heart rate =
Total days exercise =
Average peak interval = _____ miles
Average peak duration =
Total monthly mileage =

DEFINITIONS

Level of angina
$L_1$ mild discomfort
$L_2$ moderately painful
$L_3$ severe pain
$L_4$ intolerable

SOB—Shortness of breath
PVC—Premature ventricular contraction

Recommendations: _____

_____

_____

_____

**Fig. 11-5, cont'd.** Patient exercise diary and data recording sheet.

### Emergency equipment (crash cart—defibrillator)

The key requirement for emergency equipment is that it be mobile. The defibrillator should have enough extension cord to be able to reach any part of the exercise area. Battery-powered defibrillator units are available, but in my experience they are not reliable enough and tend to produce inadequate power outputs.

### REIMBURSEMENT

Before developing a program, it is helpful to discuss reimbursement with the major third-party agencies. Each state has its own guidelines for reimbursement of cardiac rehabilitation programs. If guidelines or procedures for reimbursement are not established in your state, then help develop them.

In my experience, all major third-party reimbursement agencies will pay for cardiac rehabilitation except Federal Employees Blue Cross-Blue Shield and Champus. Medicare reimbursement is limited to 12 weeks of outpatient care, and billing should be labeled as cardiac rehabilitation. Medicare will not pay for physical therapy for cardiac patients if the clinic or hospital has a separate cardiac rehabilitation unit.

| Table 11-2. Equipment list | |
|---|---|
| **Equipment** | **Approximate cost** |
| Radiotelemetry monitoring unit | $6000 per channel |
| Treadmill | $5000-8000 each |
| Bicycle ergometer | $750-1000 |
| Exercise bicycles | $300-500 |
| Arm ergometer/rowing ergometer | $600-800 |
| Defibrillator (400 W/sec) | $2000[+] |
| Crash cart and medications | $500[+] |
| Mobile standing-mercury sphyg-momanometers | $200 each |
| Stethoscopes | $40[+] each |
| Miscellaneous | Widely variable |
| Data board | |
| File cabinets | |

## SUMMARY

To facilitate cardiac rehabilitation program development several administrative procedures need to be established and controlled. This chapter is an endeavor to delineate some key administrative considerations and to highlight some potential problems. It may be helpful to identify one team member to coordinate these administrative procedures. Such a member should be responsible for ensuring physician support, clinical knowledge and skills of the team members, and communication mechanisms.

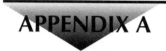

# APPENDIX A   *CARDIAC REHABILITATION PROGRAM (DEPARTMENT OF PHYSICAL THERAPY AND REHABILITATION)*

The Cardiac Rehabilitation Program consists of two phases: inpatient (after infarction, for example) and outpatient. The following is a general description of the program, along with other information of importance to physicians interested in entering their patients into the program.

**Inpatient phase.** A patient may enter the rehabilitation program only on his or her physician's referral. Optimally, this should coincide with the patient's transfer from the coronary care unit (CCU) to the step-down unit. Patients not having suffered an acute MI, but who are otherwise candidates (e.g., coronary prone, postbypass) for the program, may be referred at an appropriate time in their hospital course or as outpatients. The new transfer orders (CCU to step-down) have a check-off space for cardiac rehabilitation. Other inpatients may enter the program by ordering "cardiac rehabilitation" on the hospital chart order sheet.

Upon transfer to the step-down unit and initiation of rehabilitation, the patient is visited by the nurse coordinator, who introduces the patient to the inpatient educational program, discusses rehabilitation objectives, and explains the patient notebook used in the program. The inpatient educational program is 4 days long and repeats every 4 days Tuesday through Friday. Patients may enter this phase on any weekday.

While the patient is in the inpatient program, the following evaluation procedures constitute important "baseline" data on which each program is individualized.

1. Self-care monitor. This monitor provides a comprehensive evaluation of the patient's cardiac responses to normal activities. It monitors heart rate, blood pressure, ECG, symptoms, and heart sound changes while the patient is supine, sitting, standing, dressing, grooming, ambulating, and performing a Valsalva maneuver. A full interpretation of this evaluation, along with appropriate recommendations, is placed in the medical chart. The physician and therapist use the data and evaluation before allowing the patient to begin ambulating activities.

2. Based on the self-care monitoring results, the patient begins supervised ambulation in the hall. Supervision may consist of observing the heart rate and blood pressure and ECG monitoring as is indicated by the self-care evaluation. Patients are progressed according to their ability.

3. If the patient is to progress to the cardiac rehabilitation program as an outpatient, a low-level treadmill test is required. This is an important data base for devel-

oping low-level exercise training and as a final screening evaluation before discharge from the hospital. The protocol for this test is as follows:

| Stage | Speed (mph) | Grade (%) | Time (min) | Metabolic equivalents |
|-------|-------------|-----------|------------|-----------------------|
| 1 | 1.7 | 0 | 3 | 1-2 |
| 2 | 1.7 | 5 | 3 | 2-3 |
| 3 | 1.7 | 10 | 3 | 4 |

There are several predetermined termination points:

1. Attaining a heart rate of 130 bpm
2. Onset of angina
3. Inappropriate hypotensive or hypertensive blood pressure response
4. Coupled or tripled premature ventricular contractions
5. Multifocal premature ventricular contractions
6. ST-segment depression/elevation of 2 mm or more (net)
7. Completion of all three stages of the protocol

**Outpatient phase.** After discharge, the patient is scheduled for an outpatient supervised low-level exercise program. The goals of this aspect of the program are to gradually and safely progress the patient's activity tolerance and to give the physician objective feedback about the effects of the medical regimen. For example, routine monitoring will allow the physical therapist to give the physician input regarding dysrhythmia control or ventricular function. A referral from the physician and consent from the patient are required to enter this phase of the program.

Upon approval of the referring physician, approximately 6 to 8 weeks after the infarction the patient will be scheduled for a maximal exercise test. The report of this test is sent to the referring physician as are monthly progress notes regarding the patient's progression in the program.

After the maximal treadmill test, the patient's exercise program is revised according to the results of the test. A progress note indicating this revision is sent to the referring physician. Continuation with the program is subject to the referring physician's approval. The patient's educational program continues on an outpatient basis with expansion of the inpatient sessions.

---

# APPENDIX B    *CARDIOPULMONARY RESUSCITATION PROCEDURES CARDIAC REHABILITATION PROGRAM (DEPARTMENT OF PHYSICAL THERAPY AND REHABILITATION)*

All personnel involved in the exercise training portion of the cardiac rehabilitation program shall be trained and certified in basic life support by the American Heart Association.

Patient demonstrates abnormal cardiopulmonary distress requiring emergency procedures (Fig. 11-3).

## Assumptions

1. Witnessed arrest not on monitor
2. Defibrillator immediately available, turned on and functional
3. Physician not immediately available but on call

---

I. Definition of cardiac emergency
   a. Sustained ventricular tachycardia with hypotension
   b. Ventricular fibrillation
   c. Asystole
   d. Severe bradycardia

   e. Other (e.g., pulmonary emergency)

II. Standard precautions
   a. Defibrillator available and operational
   b. Full crash-cart equipment available
   c. All patients referred to the program by a qualified physician
   d. All patients have had a recent thorough cardiac examination, as well as treadmill testing

## Procedures

*Patient collapses*

III. Call for help; call and call code 7C, dial #61, and report "cardiac arrest"

IV. a. Shake and shout
   b. Check pulse and respirations: if no pulse, proceed to a precordial thump

c. Check pulse; if no pulse, defibrillate at 400 W/sec.

V. Wait 10 seconds; check pulse and respirations carefully; if still no response, defibrillate again

VI. Initiate cardiopulmonary resuscitation per American Heart Association Guidelines
 a. Open airway
 b. Four quick breaths
 c. Begin closed-chest massage and mouth-to-mouth resuscitation; team 5:1 when a third rescuer enters, one should feel for peripheral pulses, preferably femoral artery; or if the peripheral pulse is palpable,

maintain CPR for 30 seconds; discontinue CPR unless instructed otherwise

VII. Defibrillate at 400 W/sec and recharge
 a. Wait 10 seconds and review vital signs as in (V)

*Patient remains in state of emergency*

VIII. Defibrillate at 400 W/sec
 a. Wait 10 seconds and review vital signs as in (V)
 b. If no recovery, resume CPR as in (VI) until directed to discontinue by a physician

*Remember: Do not stop until requested to do so by a physician*

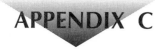

# APPENDIX C   *SPECIALIZED CORONARY OUTPATIENT REHABILITATION TREADMILL CONSENT FORM*

Name of
patient _____
Date and time of
patient's signature _____

I hereby authorize the Center to carry out the prescribed exercise stress testing and graded, monitored exercise indicated for me as the preliminary steps in a comprehensive cardiac rehabilitation program.

It is understood that I voluntarily enter into this program at the recommendation of my own physician and that the Center accepts me for the program only on my physician's recommendation and prescription.

In becoming a participant in this program, I agree to cooperate with the personnel at the Center and accept their recommendations pertaining to the amount of exercise prescribed. I further agree not to exceed these recommendations, and if I do so, it will be at my own risk.

I hereby consent to engage voluntarily in exercise stress testing to determine the state of my heart and circulation. The information thus obtained will help the physicians in prescribing an exercise program of activities in which I may engage.

The nature and purpose of the proposed testing and the procedures involved have been explained to me. There exists the rare possibility of a serious complication occurring during the tests and procedure. The risks, hazards, and

possible complications have been explained to me. These may include occasional induction of chest discomfort or pain, decrease in blood pressure, fainting, disorders of heart rhythm, and very rarely a heart attack or even death. Every effort will be made to minimize these by the preliminary examination and by continuous observation during stress testing and monitored exercise by the physician or therapist. Emergency equipment and trained personnel are available to deal with unusual situations that may arise. However, I understand more detailed information is available if I wish to discuss it.

Should any complications arise, I consent to whatever is necessary to correct the complication, including cessation of the program as it pertains to me.

The information that is obtained will be sent to my personal physician and will not be released to any other person without my expressed written consent. The information, however, may be used for a statistical or scientific purpose.

I certify that I have read all the foregoing consent form and that I fully understand its contents.

Signed: _____   Date: _____
      Patient

      _____   Date: _____
      Witness

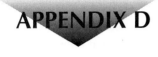 **APPENDIX D**   *INFORMED CONSENT OF OUTPATIENT CARDIAC REHABILITATION PROGRAM (DEPARTMENT OF PHYSICAL THERAPY AND REHABILITATION)*

**Purpose of the outpatient cardiac rehabilitation program.** The present cardiac rehabilitation program is designed to improve your physical exercise capacity and to reduce your level of physical impairment because of your heart condition. This program uses a form of physical exercise known as "aerobic" or "endurance" training, which has beneficial effects on cardiovascular performance. The program is expanding and will ultimately include additional areas such as nutritional and weight control education, vocational rehabilitation, psychological counseling, and other appropriate rehabilitative modalities.

Based on an "initial intake graded exercise test" you will begin at an appropriate level of physical exercise and then progress to more intense levels under skilled professional supervision. During the earlier stages of the program, especially if you are convalescing from a heart attack, you should attend three exercise sessions a week to closely supervise and evaluate your progress. In the later stages, as you become more familiar with the concept of aerobic training, heart rate response, and other important aspects of rehabilitative sessions, you will continue your exercise program at home on your own according to carefully planned exercise prescriptions. The graded exercise test at the end of convalescence and periodically throughout the year is the cornerstone of appraisal of "cardiovascular fitness."

Your doctor will receive periodic updates on your progress so that he may objectively prescribe medications and advise you regarding work, general daily activities, etc.

**Possible risks.** All possible precautions will be taken to avoid any complications of exercise. Strict adherence to your "exercise prescription" is essential to minimize any risks. We want you to understand however, that a small possibility still exists of your developing an abnormal blood pressure, dizziness or even fainting, or an irritable heart beat during exercise. Close monitoring (telemetry) and supervision generally precludes these complications leading to a serious event; however, a rare heart attack or heart arrest can occur

in such a program. Emergency equipment and trained personnel are available to deal with any situation that might arise.

**Advantages.** This program can benefit you in many ways, among which the most important are as follows:

1. To give you a carefully supervised progression of activity during your convalescence with important objective data feedback to your physician
2. To maximize your cardiovascular exercise capacity, as well as your overall physical conditioning
3. To provide you with a sound basis to maintain your level of cardiovascular conditioning over the years
4. To provide educational sessions and material regarding cardiovascular risk factors (diet, smoking, weight, etc.)
5. In some instances, to possibly reduce the quantity or types of medications

**Inquiries.** All questions about the rehabilitation program are welcome. If you have doubts or questions, please discuss them with us.

**Consent to participate.** Entry into this program requires your physician's referral. Participation in the rehabilitation program is voluntary. You are free to withdraw, if you so desire, at any point in the program.

I have read this form and understand the rehabilitation program in which I will participate. I realize that there is a remote possibility of a complication occurring during the exercise session, including heart attack and cardiac arrest, but I believe the benefits far exceed any risks. I consent to participate in this rehabilitation program.

_____   Date: _____
Signature
_____   Date: _____
Witness

# APPENDIX E    MAXIMAL SYMPTOM-LIMITED EXERCISE TEST PROTOCOL

**Definition.** A maximal symptom-limited exercise test is an electrocardiographically monitored evaluation of a person's maximum oxygen consumption during dynamic work (exercise) utilizing large muscle groups. It begins with submaximal exertion, allows time for physiological adaptations, and has progressive increments in workloads until individually determined end points of fatigue are reached or limiting symptoms or signs occur.

## Purpose

1. To establish the diagnosis or severity of coronary artery disease by observation of exercise-induced ECG changes. This may occur as confirmation of clinically suspected coronary artery disease or detection of latent coronary artery disease in asymptomatic persons.
2. To evaluate the functional cardiovascular capacity and reserve in response to exercise in patients with coronary artery disease for assessment of return to work or leisure activities and candidacy for exercise training programs.
3. To evaluate prescribed therapy as an objective measure of efficacy of medical or surgical intervention. This is particularly important in the assessment of the effect of a person's participation in an ongoing aerobic exercise program.
4. To serve as motivation and a stimulus to make needed changes in behavior or life-style (e.g., to stop smoking, alter diet, or adhere to an exercise program).

## Indications for procedure

1. Surgery after an MI or after coronary artery bypass graft; 4 or more weeks after either event in uncomplicated patients; greater than 4 weeks in patients with complications
2. Outpatient referral for admission to a cardiac rehabilitation program in a patient suspected of having coronary artery disease
3. Distinguishing angina from noncardiac chest pain
4. Development of a change in the patient's medical status that requires reevaluation of cardiovascular status (onset of hypertension, inability to maintain habitual exercise program because of onset of dyspnea, excessive fatigue, or angina), or evaluation of a change in medication
5. Ongoing periodic reevaluation of the patient's cardiac status and physical work capacity as part of a treatment program (e.g., exercise conditioning, surgery)
6. Assistance in determining whether a coronary patient can return to a particular type of vocational or recreational activity

## Personnel required for the procedure

1. Cardiac technician trained in the recognition of ECG dysrhythmias
2. Exercise tester, either physician or designated physical therapist or nurse, who is responsible for the actual conduction and preliminary interpretation of the test; this person is also responsible for supervision of the technician assisting in the test
3. Physician who will assume overall responsibility for the conduction, supervision, and interpretation of the evaluation; the physician will be in the immediate vicinity of the test area during the test, though he may designate responsibility for the conduction of the test to a specific staff member

## PROCEDURES FOR CONDUCTING A MAXIMAL SYMPTOM-LIMITED EXERCISE TEST
*Equipment and supplies required*

1. Disposable ECG electrodes
2. Conduction gel
3. Treadmill and treadmill speed- and grade-control unit
4. Alcohol swabs, razor, extrafine sandpaper for skin preparation
5. Stethoscope
6. Standing blood pressure apparatus
7. ECG recorder with oscilloscope
8. Defibrillator and crash cart
9. Stretcher
10. Linens: sheets, towels, pillow cases
11. Patient's medical chart
12. Treadmill data collection worksheet for maximal test
13. Treadmill consent form
14. ECG paper

*Preparation of patient*

1. The purpose and potential hazards of the test are explained to the patient and a consent form is signed (if necessary).
2. Before the test, a 12-lead ECG is performed on all patients and read before testing.
3. Preliminary information (name and dose of medications, patient's age, height, and weight) is obtained and recorded.
4. The patient is instructed to report any chest discomfort, dizziness, leg cramps, or any other unusual or discomforting sensations.

5. The patient is instructed to describe any angina in terms of levels:

   *Level 1:* Very mild sensation or initial perception of discomfort
   *Level 2:* Moderately uncomfortable sensation of greater intensity
   *Level 3:* Severe, chest discomfort
   *Level 4:* Intolerable chest pain

6. The exercise tester or technician demonstrates how to walk on the treadmill including getting on the treadmill and instructions not to grip the handrails during the test. (If balance support is necessary, the patient may rest two fully extended fingers on the handrail.)

7. Electrode placement. The patient is monitored simultaneously by a lead system using Y, X, $CM_4$, $MS_4$, $V_1$, and $V_5$ leads.

8. Women being tested should be wearing a bra to minimize interference on the ECG.

9. Emergency equipment. A defibrillator is in the room at all times and remains turned on throughout the test. A completely equipped crash cart is also present.

*STANDARD EVALUATIVE PROCEDURES FOR PRE-TESTING, TESTING, AND POSTTESTING (COMMON TO ALL PROTOCOLS INCLUDING LOW-LEVEL TESTING)*

1. Preliminary information (name and dosage of medications, patient's age, height and weight, etc.) is obtained and recorded on the raw data sheet.

2. Exercise procedures
   a. Heart rate, heart sounds, blood pressure, and symptoms are evaluated and recorded in the supine position for 2 consecutive minutes.
   b. *Special considerations:* Nonambulatory patients will not undergo supine positioning before or after exercise. Heart rate and blood pressure are measured and recorded after 1 minute of sitting. When expired, air measurements are to be performed with either the arm or leg ergometry tests; the patient will remain seated at rest for 3 minutes while gas collection and analysis are performed.
   c. 10-second breath-holding and 30 seconds of hyperventilation are performed by the patient in the sitting position with continuous ECG recording during both maneuvers.
   d. Heart rate and blood pressure are measured and recorded immediately after 1 minute of standing.
      *Special considerations:*
      (1) The attending measurements are not included in the arm and leg ergometry protocols.
      (2) When expired air measurements are to be performed, the patient will remain standing for 3 minutes while base-line measurements are performed.

3. Exercise procedures
   a. Heart rate and blood pressure measurements are taken during each minute of exercise and recorded.
   b. The time of onset of angina is recorded, as are changes in the severity of discomfort on a minute-by-minute basis. Recording of the angina levels is to continue after exercise until pain subsides completely.
   c. Continuous recording of ECG is with a paper speed of 10 mm/sec, except for last 10 seconds of each minute at 25 mm/sec, carried out for documentation of the type and frequency of dysrhythmias and the frequency of ectopic beats.

4. After exercise
   a. Immediately after exercise the treadmill speed and grade or the ergometer workload is reduced over a 30 to 60-second period.
   b. Heart rate and blood pressure are recorded every minute after exercise.
   c. Postexercise monitoring continues until the heart rate is within 15 to 25 bpm of the resting rate, the systolic blood pressure is within 20 mm Hg, dysrhythmias have stabilized, the patient is asymptomatic, and the net ST-segment depression or elevation is less than 1 mm above or below baseline measurements.
   d. When expired air collection is performed, gas sampling will continue for 5 minutes after exercise.
   e. In the intermittent ergometry tests, postexercise heart rate, blood pressure, and angina levels are recorded for the duration of the recovery intervals on a minute-by-minute basis.
   f. When expired air collection is performed as part of the intermittent tests, sampling will be discontinued at the end of each workload and resumed 1 minute before the beginning of the following workload.

*TEST CONDUCTION*

1. *Test protocol:* Bruce Multistage Continuous Protocol.

| Stage | Speed (mph) | Grade (%) | Time (min) | Metabolic equivalents |
|-------|-------------|-----------|------------|------------------------|
| 1 | 1.7 | 10 | 3 | 4-5 |
| 2 | 2.5 | 12 | 3 | 6-7 |
| 3 | 3.4 | 14 | 3 | 8-9 |
| 4 | 4.2 | 16 | 3 | 10-12 |
| 5 | 5.0 | 18 | 3 | greater than 14 |

2. Continuous ECG monitoring is done and heart rate, blood pressure, and a 10-second ECG strip recording are taken each minute of the test.

3. Upon reaching the designated end point of the test, one conducts a cool-down stage during which the treadmill speed and grade is reduced. (This may last up to 30

seconds.) At this point, the treadmill is turned off, and the patient is instructed to march in place on the treadmill while the heart rate, blood pressure, and continuous ECG are recorded for an additional 30 seconds. Thus the total time standing after exercise is 1 minute.

4. The patient then lies down, and the exercise tester again auscultates the chest for cardiac gallop rhythms, murmurs, etc.

5. Minute-by-minute heart rate, blood pressure, and ECG recordings are taken until values approximate resting pretest values. (Heart rate is within 15 bpm of resting value.) At this point, the patient is questioned regarding symptoms and is disconnected from the equipment and released if asymptomatic.

6. Continued monitoring is required if the patient demonstrates evidence of continuing ischemia or angina (persistent ST-segment depression or elevation), unstable dysrhythmia, or unusual signs or symptoms.

## ERGOMETRY TESTS
### Arm ergometry tests

1. Continuous protocol
   a. Initial workload not less than 150 kg
   b. A total of four or five workloads, each with a duration of 2 minutes
   c. Workload increments not less than 50 kg
   d. Crank speed 50 to 60 rpm
2. Intermittent protocol
   a. Initial workload not less than 150 kg
   b. A total of four or five workloads each 3 minutes in duration followed by 3-minute recovery periods
   c. Workload increments not less than 50 kg
   d. Crank speed of 50 to 60 rpm

### Bicycle ergometry tests

1. Intermittent protocol
   a. Initial workload not less than 150 kg.
   b. A total of four or five workloads, each 4 minutes long, followed by 4-minute recovery periods.
   c. Seat height adjusted so that there is no more than 5 to 10 degrees of flexion in the knee at the lowest point in the pedal resolutions.
   d. Workload increments should be 20% to 25% of the difference between the initial workload and the estimated maximal workload.
   e. Crank speed should be maintained at 50 to 60 rpm.
2. Care of equipment
   a. Dispose of all used electrodes, alcohol swabs, and packages.
   b. Change sheets and pillowcases on gurney.
   c. Turn off defibrillator.
   d. Return ECG leads, blood pressure cuffs, and stethoscopes to proper place.
   e. Turn off all equipment.

f. Check to ensure that there are adequate supplies of electrodes, swabs, and ECG paper; replace as necessary.

3. Charting
   a. Immediately upon completion of the test, the exercise tester should enter into the chart a preliminary interpretation of the test, which includes the following:
      (1) Date of test
      (2) Type of test
      (3) Minutes completed and limiting factor(s)
      (4) Resting heart rate and maximum heart rate achieved
      (5) Resting and maximum blood pressure values; comment whether hypoadaptive, normoadaptive, or hypertensive
      (6) Angina: level I to IV during or after exercise
      (7) Additional symptoms (e.g., nausea, ataxia, dizziness)
      (8) Dysrhythmias: comment on any dysrhythmias (e.g., supraventricular versus ventricular, number, type [multifocal, parasystolic, etc.], frequency, and when they occurred)
      (9) Auscultation findings: presence or absence of $S_4$, $S_3$, murmurs
      (10) Positive (+), negative (−), or indeterminate for ischemia and degree of ST-segment change (or R-wave amplitude change)
      (11) Maximal or submaximal test and assessment of physical working capacity and functional aerobic impairment (FAI)
      (12) Recommendations for additional monitoring or follow-up tests
   b. A formal interpretation of the test is made after complete data is reviewed and signed by the physician. This interpretation should be entered into the chart, along with sample ECG strips taken from the test.

## SPECIAL OBSERVATIONS, ASSESSMENTS, PRECAUTIONS
### Criteria for termination of test

1. Patient's report of fatigue that would make continued exertion uncomfortable:
   a. Patient's report of dizziness
   b. Increasing premature ventricular contractions (PVC) becoming multifocal
   c. Coupled PVCs or ventricular tachycardia (three PVCs in a row)
   d. Development of rapid atrial dysrhythmias
   e. Level III angina (scale of I to IV)
   f. A progressive fall in systolic blood pressure of 20 mm Hg or more in the presence of increased heart rate and workload
   g. Extreme hypertensive response (systolic 240/diastolic 130 mm Hg)

h. Severe musculoskeletal pain as in leg claudication
i. Uninterpretable ECG tracing
j. Patient signs such as cold and clammy skin, ataxic gait, or other signs of vascular insufficiency

2. If patient becomes moderately uncomfortable, from any cause

*Contraindications and precautions to exercise testing*

1. Contraindications
   a. Overt congestive heart failure
   b. Rapidly intensifying or unstable angina
   c. Recent acute myocardial infarction (less than 3 weeks)
   d. Dissecting aneurysm
   e. Second- or third-degree heart block
   f. Recurrent ventricular tachycardia
   g. Rapid atrial dysrhythmias
   h. Acute myocarditis or pericarditis
   i. Severe aortic stenosis
   j. Recent pulmonary embolus
   k. Acute infections or other active disease process

2. Precautions (attending physician to be consulted before beginning of test)
   a. Repetitive or frequent ventricular ectopic activity at rest (more than 10 PVCs/min)
   b. Resting hypertension (systolic 180/diastolic 110 mm Hg)
   c. Severe cardiomegaly
   d. Resting tachycardia of greater than 110 bpm or a recent change in cardiac symptoms

# Evaluation and Physical Treatment of the Patient with Peripheral Vascular Disorders

*Joanne R. Eisenhardt*

Peripheral vascular disease can be considered the "step-child" of cardiopulmonary care. Despite the significance of systemic vascular resistance and venous return to the function of the cardiopulmonary system, little emphasis has been placed on preventing or treating vascular problems until recently. Peripheral vascular disease was a neglected area in medicine until the work of Buergher[29] in the 1920s. Although "peripheral" in its purest sense refers to any vessel distal to the coronary arteries, unless otherwise specified, it is used in this chapter to refer to the vasculature below the aortoiliac bifurcation, since it is this portion of the circulatory system that is most vulnerable to disease and of most significance to physical therapists.

## RISK FACTORS

It is unknown what percentage of people actually has peripheral vascular disease (PVD). That the problem is widespread across sexual and cultural lines in American society, that it is exacerbated by other factors, and that it is functionally devastating if left untreated are well-established facts. Highly reliable, noninvasive tests for PVD have been compared with the more subjective symptom assessment and pulse palpations to show that symptoms alone underestimate PVD occurrence and pulses alone overestimate its incidence. It is suspected that over 10% of the elderly have large vessel arterial disease, 16% have small vessel disease, and at least 5% have a mixture of both problems.[49] Of the approximately 10% of PVD patients who undergo amputation, less than half ever become functional prosthetic wearers.[11,17,83,125,146]

Controlled studies have shown that diabetics, even those who are asymptomatic of peripheral neuropathies, have measurable arterial calcification.[44] At least 50% are diagnosed as having diabetic peripheral neuropathy, and some researchers believe that vascular disease is responsible for these neuropathological symptoms. Uncontrolled diabetes is believed to be a significant precursor to small vessel disease.[34,75,77] Researchers have also shown a high incidence of below-knee amputation as a result of small vessel disease in diabetics.[154] Furthermore, large vessel disease is seen in conjunction with small vessel obliteration in many diabetics; this combination significantly increases morbidity and mortality for these PVD patients.

Systolic hypertension and smoking are other significant risk factors for PVD. In a recent study of otherwise healthy elderly adults, 42% of those with essential hypertension were found to have lower extremity arterial disease. Hypertension is considered one of the strongest predisposers to large vessel arterial disease, especially in conjunction with one or more additional risk factors.[11,75,125,157] In particular, smoking aggravates hypertension by attenuating the therapeutic effects of beta blockers used to lower blood pressure.[165] Smoking also accelerates atherosclerosis by reducing high-density lipoproteins and elevating plasma fibrinogen concentration.[100] In diabetics, smoking increases the risk of above-knee amputation through the combination of large vessel occlusive disease and the destruction of distal runoff vessels.[154]

Other risk factors for PVD include elevated serum cholesterol (especially low density lipoproteins), elevated white blood cell count, fibrinogen greater than 4g/L and, in women, elevated triglycerides.[4,19] Low cardiac output may also be a predictor of severity in peripheral arterial occlusive disease.[84]

For all peripheral vascular diseases, age seems to be a predisposing factor. The impact of age alone is difficult to identify because of its overlap with other risk factors. One study found gradual increases in peripheral vascular resistance in healthy individuals up to the sixth decade of life.[86] Others document age dependence of arterial disease without any upper limit.[68,125,157] It is clear that advanced age in the presence of other risk factors such as diabetes or hypertension increases the incidence of PVD, but this may simply reflect the duration of a predisposing disease or behavior.

A person's activity level can influence several aspects of PVD. The sedentary individual aggravates his or her other risks of arterial disease by promoting obesity, low-density lipoprotein concentrations, and inefficient oxygen extraction by peripheral muscles. The person who stands for long hours encourages venous stasis and lymphedema through decreased muscle pumping, just as a patient on bed rest has an increased risk of venous disease as a result of stasis. At the other extreme, someone who denies the presence of PVD and continues to work past the point of pain invites tissue necrosis.[11]

The majority of risk factors for PVD are modifiable, with some changes in behavior actually reversing vascular damage. As therapists, we should strive to prevent PVD just as we work toward prevention of heart disease. Additionally, we should be alert for early evidence of vascular disease in all of our patients. Early identification and intervention in the form of treatment plus risk factor reduction can significantly reduce vascular morbidity.

## PHYSIOLOGY

To clarify some of the important concepts of function within the peripheral circulation, a brief presentation of some basic physiological principles follows.

### Flow controls

Possible bases of peripheral vascular problems can be identified through an analysis of Poiseuille's Law:

$$Q = \frac{K\Delta Pr^4}{Lh}$$

The $Q$ in the above equation represents blood flow, the critical concern of the circulatory system. The $K$ represents $\pi/8$, a constant that assumes laminar flow within a rigid pipe.

This, however, is not the case in vivo. Therefore, we must substitute for $K$ a Reynold's number specific to the blood vessel in question in order to get a more appropriate clinical analysis of blood flow. A Reynold's number is an index for indicating whether flow will be laminar or turbulent.[179] At high Reynold's numbers flows are turbulent, whereas at low Reynold's numbers flows are laminar. Turbulence increases at bifurcations and around plaques on vessel walls, facilitating the progression from small occlusions to larger ones by repeatedly traumatizing the vessel wall.

The pressure gradient along a vessel is represented by $\Delta P$. Normally, large vessels exhibit a Windkessel effect that provides accessory pumping of blood during systole and storage of blood (capacitance) during diastole (Fig. 12-1). Because of their wall properties, arteries are especially good accessory pumps, and veins are especially good reservoirs. When decreases in the elasticity of vessel walls, decreases in vascular tone, or buildup of hydrostatic pressure in surrounding tissues disrupt this Windkessel effect, the result is a decrease in the pressure gradient along the vessel, which in turn reduces flow within the vessel.

The radius, $r$, of the vessel has the greatest effect on flow. Temporary decreases in radius caused by increased vascular tone can be offset by the enhanced pressure gradient effect. However, when the vessel radius is reduced significantly (greater than 70%) by prolonged vasospasm, stenosis, or embolus, the resulting effects on the downstream flow can be severe enough to cause ischemic pain or even tissue necrosis.

The vessel length, $L$, changes slightly with each pulsation, but the average length remains constant. Loss of linear elasticity because of atherosclerosis will have a minimal impact on flow. Of greater concern is the length of a stenosis within a vessel. The longer the stenotic vessel segment, the greater the resistance to blood flow through that segment.[59]

The last element of flow control is the blood viscosity, $h$. In conditions such as polycythemia and sickle cell anemia, blood viscosity increases, thereby making it harder to perfuse peripheral vessels.

The tension in the vessel, discussed earlier in Chapter 4, is directly proportional to pressure and radius and inversely proportional to wall thickness. In peripheral vessels wall thickness is a minor consideration in comparison with either the pressure within the vessel or the vessel radius.[180] When arterial wall tension is reduced because of low pressure or

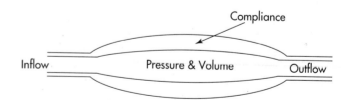

**Fig. 12-1.** Windkessel model of a blood vessel as a compliant compartment. (From Coleman TG: Mathematical analysis of cardiovascular function, *IEEE Trans Biomed Engr* 6(4), 1985. Used by permission.)

narrowing, the vessel can collapse. This is not a major problem for the veins because they derive most of their support from surrounding tissues, including adjacent arteries. This external support allows the venous system to function under low pressure; hence, a pressure gradient can be maintained between the arterial and the venous sides of the circulatory system.

### Local flow adjustments

Local flow adjustments can be made by changing the tone of the arterioles. Areas in need of increased flow (e.g., working muscle) can be supplied by relaxing those arterioles and constricting the arterioles of another area such as the gut. Variations in vascular tone are discussed in Chapter 4.

The size and quality of the distal runoff beds are also important to flow. If the cross-sectional area of the distal vasculature is large and has normal elasticity, blood flow through the proximal artery will be enhanced—even in the event of large vessel disease. However, the development of collateral circulation around a large vessel occlusion will be of limited value if the downstream circulation is unable to receive adequate flow from these collateral vessels. Stokes and others[155] report a very poor prognosis for angioplasties when distal runoff is impaired, and Brothers and Greenfield[32] have found progressive disease of outflow vessels to be the single most important cause of endarterectomy or prosthetic bypass graft failure.

Another local control of arterial flow is the buildup of metabolites such as lactic acid in the tissues. When exercising muscle produces metabolites faster than they can be removed by the blood stream, these substances act chemically on arterial smooth muscle to induce vasodilation. This is one of the mechanisms thought to be responsible for postocclusive and postexercise reactive hyperemia.

Local adjustments to venous flow are somewhat different from arterial flow adjustments since the major deterrent to flow is not vascular resistance but the force of gravity. For this reason the competence of the valves within the veins is critical. Without competent valves backflow can occur, resulting in increased distal venous pressure. Valves are positioned to facilitate proximal flow and to direct flow from the superficial veins, which lack soft tissue support and periarterial pulses, to the deep veins, which have significant soft tissue support, and associated arteries to facilitate venous return.[91,180] Precapillary vasoconstriction normally occurs upon standing and helps reduce the blood volume in the capillary beds and the venous system; hence, venous pressure increases due to gravity are somewhat relieved by this decrease in venous volume.[15] Muscular contractions and higher distal turgor (extravascular tissue pressure) can assist with venous return by reducing distal venous capacitance and maintaining a pressure gradient between distal and proximal venous structures. Gravity can also be used to enhance venous return simply by elevating the limb.

Movement of fluid through the lymphatic system depends totally on local flow regulation. This extremely low-pressure, low-velocity system is heavily influenced by muscle pumping action.[11] Additionally, changes in colloid osmotic pressure affect lymphatic drainage, with fluid moving toward areas of higher osmotic pressures. Lymphatic vessels are quick to collateralize after insult and can fully restore lymphatic drainage in as little as 8 days.[91] Failure of the lymphatic system in combination with inadequate scavenging of stagnating plasma protein by macrophages leads to lymphedema.[63] Mobility of lymphatic fluid in pitting (soft) edema is greater than in normal tissues and appears to be due to increased preload within the lymphatic system.[16,107] Brawny (hard) edema involves fibrosis and very limited mobility of lymphatic fluid.

## ARTERIAL DISORDERS

Although an exhaustive description of vascular pathological conditions is beyond the scope of this text, certain problems should be familiar to all therapists. Included here are those vascular conditions seen in patients who might logically be referred to physical therapists and those conditions that are common secondary diagnoses in patients referred to us for other problems.

### Arterial pathological conditions

Acute arterial problems are commonly related to trauma. Isolated arterial severance is surgically repaired and seen only in physical therapy if there are complications or associated injuries. More common are arterial compressions and soft tissue crush injuries involving multiple tissues. For example, Volkmann's ischemia or radial artery compression resulting from a distal humeral fracture creates a significant deformity of the hand if undetected, but it can be readily identified by coldness and pallor of the hand, coupled with sensory losses in the web space of the thumb. Information on this and other traumatic arterial problems can be found in orthopedics textbooks.

Arterial emboli most often occur at the femoropopliteal bifurcation, although they also occur at other bifurcations throughout the body. Most nontraumatic upper-extremity vascular deficits are related to arterial emboli. The heart is a common source of thromboemboli. Fat emboli may be seen a few days following fracture of the long bones of the body. Other sources of emboli include chronic ulcerative colitis, foreign bodies resulting from intravenous drug abuse, and aortic thrombi that break free and embolize.[13,17,91,159] The first symptom may be decreased sensation in the ischemic tissue that is followed by edema and ischemic muscle pain similar to that of a compartment syndrome. If left untreated, the embolic occlusion will progress to skin demarcation and tissue necrosis. Local systolic blood pressure of less than 40 mm Hg is considered significant for development of gangrene.[91]

Therapists working in areas where poisonous snakes are indigenous should be aware of the arterial compromise caused by snakebite. Progressive edema and discoloration of the limb from the wound site proximally may result in arterial occlusion if medication and cryotherapy do not effectively control the edema. In these cases, decreased skin temperature and abnormal blood flow evaluations would indicate the need for more aggressive action, i.e., fasciotomy.[50]

Some medications can have acute arterial side effects. Vascular spasms severe enough to cause gangrene can result from the use of ergotamines, drugs used to treat migraines. Affected persons are most often women in their mid-thirties.[178] On rare occasions, heparin can cause the formation of multifocal arterial thrombi with progressive pain, pallor, and pulselessness.[130] This is ironic since heparin is an anticoagulant drug used to treat conditions that give rise to these very symptoms.

Thromboangitis obliterans, or "Buergher's disease," is a disease of younger persons, predominantly male and almost exclusively smokers. This disorder usually begins in small, distal arteries and moves proximally. Complaints of coldness, numbness, and tingling may precede objective symptoms of decreased local systolic blood pressure, pulselessness, paralysis, and decreased skin temperature if there is no collateralization or, if collaterals are present, symptoms of intermittent claudication. This disease is treated symptomatically but all too often results in amputation.[17,55,91] Convincing the patient to stop smoking is paramount in the treatment of this disorder.

Progressive arterial occlusive disease (PAOD) is a chronic, progressive stenosis of the arterial walls. It is prevalent in the middle third of the femoral artery and the aortoiliac areas and is commonly associated with carotid artery stenosis and diabetes mellitus.[58,83,91,157] The relationship between diabetes and PAOD is so strong that, until recently, 50% to 70% of all amputations were performed on diabetics.[125,154] Aggressive intervention with percutaneous transluminal angioplasty and/or arterial bypass grafts at both above- and below-knee levels have decreased the amputation rates in diabetic and nondiabetic PAOD patients.[56,171] Although diabetic patients are more likely to develop PAOD, their disease progression compared to nondiabetics is debatable. Osmundson and others[116] report no greater risk of progression in diabetic patients postangioplasty, whereas Davies and others[54] found significantly greater risk of subsequent surgery and risk of death in diabetics postangioplasty. This may be because of the greater tendency toward distal, small vessel stenosis in diabetics that compromises the distal runoff of larger arteries and renders collateral circulation ineffective.[17,146,151] Diabetic neuropathy may be an early sign of arterial insufficiency since nerve tissue is very intolerant of ischemia.[34,44,77]

Commonly, the first symptom of PAOD is intermittent, exercise-induced pain in the area of ischemia (intermittent claudication). Whereas calf pain due to femoral artery occlusion is the most frequently recognized symptom, intermittent claudication may also be present in the low back with aortic occlusion, in the hip or buttock with iliac occlusion, or in the foot with tibial occlusion.[12,55,87] Motor nerve damage may compound the decrease in exercise tolerance through muscle denervation.[58,94] Symptoms may progress to pain at rest if ischemia is severe and can lead to tissue necrosis.

Primary Raynaud's disease is an idiopathic, intermittent, bilateral vasospasm usually seen in women and aggravated by cold or stress. The digits experience cycles of cyanosis followed by redness and reflex vasodilation. Those affected complain of pain and paresthesias in their hands, and occasionally one can see trophic changes such as hair loss or shiny, fragile skin on inspection of the hands and/or feet bilaterally. Superficial tissue necrosis may occur around nail beds. Deep tissue damage and amputation are rare.[17,55] Habitual smoking appears to sensitize Raynaud's sufferers to the vasoconstricting effects of nicotine.[72] Hyperreactivity of the central nervous system at rest has been documented in both primary Raynaud's disease and Raynaud's phenomenon associated with other diseases.[57,114,118]

A vasospastic arterial dysfunction similar to primary Raynaud's disease and seen in industrial workers is hand-arm vibration syndrome (HAVS), formerly known as vibration white finger disease. Workers with prolonged exposure to vibrating tools, especially if this occurs in conjunction with exposure to cold, frequently develop vasospasm with or without tingling, sensory losses along both median and ulnar distributions, and weakness of hand musculature. This problem is often confused with carpal tunnel syndrome because of its neurological symptoms, and the two problems occur simultaneously in some cases. Avascular necrosis of the carpal bones or degenerative joint disease of the wrist are less common components of this syndrome.[29,113,160] Vasospasm begins distally in one or more fingers and progresses proximally. Symptoms are usually more pronounced during the colder months of the year but may be seen year round in advanced cases. One or both hands may be affected, depending on the ergonomics of the tool in use. Sakakibara and others[136] have identified circulatory disturbances in the feet as well as the hands of workers with HAVS. The pathophysiology of HAVS is still under debate with some researchers proposing a central sympathetic etiology and others a local mechanical disorder.

### Arterial evaluation

Knowledge of the risk factors and symptoms of arterial disease makes the patient history a valuable assessment tool. Perhaps the two most important questions here, as in an orthopedic history, are "Where is the pain?" and "What makes it worse?" Ischemic pain will always present itself in the soft tissue served by the impaired artery. Treadmill testing, bicycle ergometry and six- or twelve-minute walk

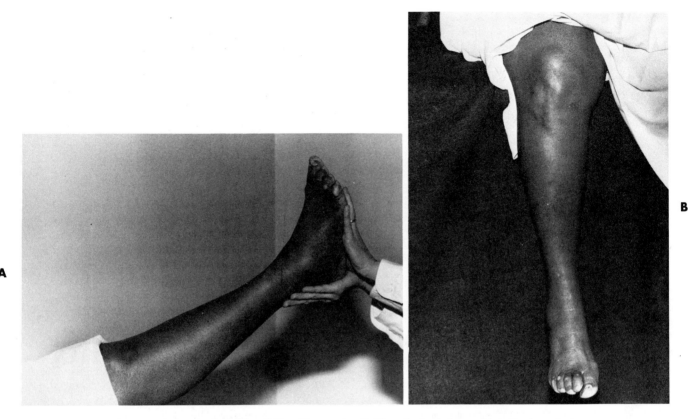

**Fig. 12-2. A,** Leg is elevated until blanching occurs. **B,** Then the leg is lowered into the dependent position, and rubor is observed and timed for its duration.

tests can be used to quantify intermittent claudication with an ambulatory distance of greater than 150 m being mild impairment, 50-150 m being moderate, and less than 50 m being severe.[8,175] There are four types of arterial pain that must be distinguished. The first and most common is intermittent claudication, a pain that is brought on by exercise and relieved by cessation of activity without a change in posture. The second, ischemic neuropathy, may be present when good collateralization around the blockage exists or when small vessel disease predominates. This produces paresthesias coupled with sudden, shocking pain. The third type, resting pain, is due to severe, uncollateralized occlusions that can cause constant pain at rest. This is intensified distally and is more pronounced at night when the legs are not dependent. The fourth, vasospastic pain, is a distal intermittent pain most often felt in one or both hands and aggravated by exposure to cold.[53,55,87,91,118,146,156] The rate of onset can be used to differentiate the cause of arterial pain. Acute arterial embolus is characterized by rapid onset of pain. More commonly, the occlusive process is gradual and chronic; pain increases as the disease progresses.

Both acute occlusion and vasospasm will produce noticeable pallor in the flow-deprived area, although vasospasm does produce an early episode of mottling or cyanosis first. Dependent cyanosis and blanching on elevation are signs of chronic occlusion. A reactive hyperemia test can be performed to subjectively assess flow through an extremity. One method of inducing reactive hyperemia is a postural challenge (Fig. 12-2). Sharp elevation of the limbs should produce complete blanching after at least one minute of elevation; blanching within 60 seconds is indicative of arterial disease. Once blanching has occurred, rubor (hyperemic flush) should appear and then fade within 2 to 3 minutes after lowering the limbs into a dependent position. With mild occlusion blanching requires nearly a full minute, and rubor persists less than 30 seconds; with moderate occlusion blanching is more rapid and rubor lasts up to 60 seconds; finally, with severe occlusion rubor is present at the onset of the test and further reactive hyperemia should not be attempted.[118,180] Prolonged rubor may be caused by diminished vasoconstriction of the microvasculature which is normally seen when a person moves from supine to sitting.[143,166,167] Reactive hyperemia can also be induced by occluding arterial flow with a cuff placed proximally and inflated to approximately 200 mm Hg for four minutes. This method, however, is quite painful even to normal individuals and is poorly tolerated by ischemic patients.

Visual inspection for trophic changes is a valuable evaluation tool, especially with moderate to severe arterial occlusions lacking collateralization. Chronic flow deprivation will cause muscle atrophy, hair loss, thick and down-curving nails, and dry skin. In extreme cases, dry

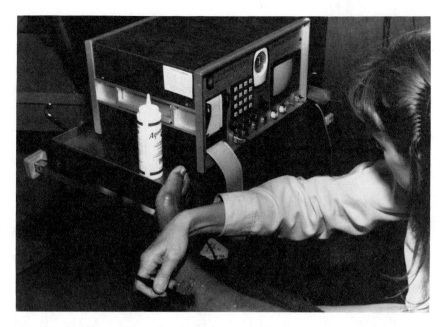

**Fig. 12-3.** Doppler ultrasound is used to obtain an accurate blood pressure in the posterior tibial artery.

gangrene will be present.[55,87] Ulcers caused by pressure on poorly vascularized areas (e.g., metatarsal heads, malleoli, lateral leg) are frequently seen by physical therapists. These ulcers can be either recent or long-standing problems, have an irregular border, have a high incidence of infection, and respond poorly to antimicrobial therapy.[6,41] Ulcers around the nail beds are generally due to severe vasospasm.[55]

Palpation of inadequately perfused tissues will reveal cold, dry skin and diminished or absent pulses in corresponding arteries. However, pulse palpation can be hard to quantify, lacks reliability from one clinician to the next, and has poor sensitivity. For these reasons, pulse palpation is now supplemented by methods of evaluation using noninvasive techniques such as ankle/arm blood pressure ratio (ankle/brachial index), Doppler velocimetry, and/or segmental blood pressure gradient. These are particularly preferred for early identification of asymptomatic arterial disease or for evaluation of patients whose pulses are severely obliterated.[30,48,97,137] By incorporating preexercise and postexercise ankle/brachial indexes, segmental blood pressures, or other special tests into the evaluation, therapists can obtain accurate and objective documentation on treatment effectiveness or disease progression in patients with vascular disease.[80,156]

Ankle/brachial indexes and segmental blood pressures are easy to obtain without special equipment. Segmental blood pressure measurement can identify sharp pressure drops along a limb and significant flow asymmetries from one limb to the contralateral limb. A drop of more than 20 mm Hg systolic pressure from one segment to the next is considered clinically significant. An ankle systolic pressure of less than 50 mm Hg[81] or a great toe pressure of less than 30 mm Hg[7] have been used to define chronic critical limb ischemia. An ankle/brachial index, which compares posterior tibial to brachial systolic pressure, is considered quite reliable with reported relative precision as high as 0.3%.[85,127] The accuracy of both ankle/brachial index and segmental blood pressure can be improved by using Doppler ultrasonography rather than the standard sphygmomanometer and stethoscope to obtain systolic pressures[156] (Fig. 12-3). Normally, ankle systolic pressure equals or exceeds brachial pressure. An ankle/brachial index of less than 0.97 is considered abnormal.[36] Severe ischemia is assumed with ankle/brachial indexes of 0.5 at rest and 0.15 after exercise.[11] Indices of 0.4 or less are generally considered indications for amputation. Doppler velocimetry can be used to assess blood flow both qualitatively and quantitatively by obtaining flow velocity curves along the arterial tree.[18,64,66,67,106,134,172,181] Normal flow velocities produce characteristic curves that change shape in the presence of either arterial occlusion or spasm. Additionally, the acceleration slope, half-width, and peak amplitude of the curve can provide semiquantifiable information on vessel perfusion (Fig. 12-4). The advent of laser Doppler flowmetry techniques has enhanced the quality of information obtained noninvasively. Photoplethysmography can be used to assess total blood volume in the digits and the change in volume with each pulse. This gives a comparative measurement of arterial flow, assuming one digit can be identified as "normal." However, there is no way to individually assess what constitutes normal digital flow. Photoplethysmographs (discussed later) are easy to perform, but they require special equipment and are hard to quantify.[68,91] Transcutaneous oxygen tension attempts to measure oxygen delivery to specific tissues. It, too, requires special equipment, and its reliability is questionable.[10,92,95,105,112,119]

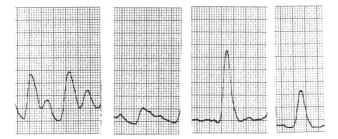

**Fig. 12-4.** *Left to right,* Normal arterial Doppler curve with a sharp acceleration slope, moderate half-width and dicrotic notch at approximately one third of peak height; vasospastic curve with less steep acceleration slope, saw-toothing downslope and wide half-width; inelastic curve showing steep upslope and downslope, high peak and no dicrotic notch; upstream occlusion showing slightly diminished upslope with low peak height and no dicrotic notch.

Raynaud's phenomenon is best measured by use of a cold provocation test. The hand or foot to be tested is placed in cold water (10° C to 15° C) for 1 to 10 minutes. Visible cyanosis or blanching indicates vasospasm.[128,162] Skin temperature can be measured over time to note the rate of digital rewarming after this procedure. Rewarming after cold provocation is significantly slowed in patients with either primary or secondary Raynaud's disease.[117] Savin and others[142] suggest that Doppler blood flow measurements through the brachial artery reflect changes in digital blood flow during cold provocation testing.

No single test for arterial insufficiency has been universally accepted nor has one grading system for arterial disease been espoused. A functional grading system is presented by Winsor and Hyman:[180]

Grade I    No functional limitations
Grade II   Ambulatory at least four blocks before onset of claudication
Grade III  Ambulatory less than four blocks before onset of claudication
Grade IV   Nonambulatory due to ischemic pain at rest

I strongly prefer the scoring system for arterial dysfunction developed by Walden and others[175] because it incorporates a variety of vascular tests into a single scoring system which indicates not only assessment of the arterial system but also completeness of the examination upon which that assessment is made. Only clinical judgments based on history, physical examination, and vascular laboratory tests provide the practitioner and the patient with the necessary information upon which to base treatment decisions.

### Arterial treatment

In planning treatments for patients with vascular disease, therapists must proceed in a pragmatic fashion. These patients generally have multiple diagnoses and may have socioeconomic constraints that preclude "ideal" therapeutic approaches. Young[151] has outlined an approach to vascular care that we, as therapists, can use as a model. First, the therapist should identify the system(s) involved. Is it a purely arterial problem or a mixed arterial-venous insufficiency? Second, the severity of the problem should be established. Do the symptoms warrant extensive therapy or even surgery? Given the time, money, and quality of life this patient may have to give up, is the "cost" of correcting the problem worth the benefit to this individual? Third, the therapist should estimate the patient's tolerance for treatment at the present time. Will the patient's cardiopulmonary status allow an extensive exercise program? Is there someone at home to assist with the recommended therapy? Fourth, priorities should be set based on the above concerns. Where can the therapist effect the greatest improvement with the least inconvenience to the patient and family?

The best "therapy" for all types of PVD is prevention. Appropriate exercise, healthy diet, and avoidance of smoking are preventive measures that cannot be overstressed. Once PVD has become established, these preventive measures can help reverse or retard many vascular disease processes. Everyone, but especially diabetics, should know the value of good foot care. Well-fitted shoes that provide pressure distribution across the soles and allow feet to breathe are an important consideration. Patients with arterial disease should be advised against wearing support hose since they further increase peripheral resistance to blood flow. Accommodative orthotics can be of value in redistributing pressure. Careful washing and drying of feet, especially drying between the toes, is imperative. Prevention of minor trauma includes not only careful pedicuring and avoidance of home remedies for corns, calluses, and athlete's foot, but also home and work safety. Small objects left on the floor can lead to serious problems if stepped on by bare feet. Low drawers left open, cluttered furniture with sharp corners, and objects dropped on unprotected toes cause many amputations each year.

For patients with mild arterial disease, exercise is considered an excellent therapy. The program of choice is walking at a steady pace up to, but not beyond, the point of pain. This program may take months to reach maximum effectiveness and must be continued to maintain those effects. It is known that regular exercise promotes collateralization of blood flow in animals. Conclusive evidence that this occurs in humans is lacking. It has been demonstrated that muscular efficiency improves with exercise, providing a higher functional level before claudication appears.[11,80,147,150,156,163]

Use of a small heel lift on the affected side can reduce oxygen demand in the gastrocnemius during exercise by creating a passive insufficiency of the muscle. However, this limits the effectiveness of push-off by that limb during gait.

It is questionable whether patients with more advanced arterial disease can be treated with exercise alone. However, many of these patients receive bypass grafts, and in those cases, exercise may maintain or improve distal runoff and retard occlusion of the graft. Since these are significant complications in bypass graft recipients, any improvements in these areas is welcomed.[46,47,101,115]

Exercise within pain-free limits has also been supported for patients with vasospastic arterial disease. Exercise, in conjunction with abstinence from smoking, is considered a very effective treatment for Raynaud's disease.[42] The addition of sympathetic antagonist activities such as biofeedback or relaxation techniques could prove useful to some patients.

There has been much discussion in years past about the use of Burgher or Burgher-Allen exercises for vascular patients. To date there is no evidence that these exercises improve either blood flow or muscle efficiency in poorly perfused lower extremities. Nonetheless, Kim and Ebel believe that they are beneficial to recover muscle tone and prepare for functional activities."

Patients who experience night pain or who are on bed rest for severe occlusive disease may obtain some relief by elevating the head of the bed several inches, thus maintaining the feet in a dependent position for gravity-assisted perfusion.[118] Bedridden patients must be watched carefully for pressure sores on the lower extremities and may require special protection of heels, malleoli, and fibular heads. If they are ischemic at rest, under no circumstances should patients be put on an exercise program, nor should they receive whirlpool treatments since whirlpool is very effective in turning dry gangrene into wet gangrene.

High voltage pulsed direct current stimulation (HVPC) has been given much attention recently in the treatment of arterial flow disorders, ischemic ulcers and acute trauma. Mohr and others[104] found increased flow velocities in rat hindlimbs immediately following HVPC application. Walker and others[176] compared flow effects of isometric contraction elicited by HVPC to voluntary isometric contraction and found isometric exercise to have a greater effect on flow velocity. Bettany and others[22] administered 120 Hz HVPC at voltages 10% below motor threshold levels to bluntly traumatized frog legs with significant reduction in edema formation. This study was followed up to assess the effect of different polarities of the active electrode. With cathodal HVPC, edema formation posttrauma was reduced.[161] With anodal HVPC, no treatment effect was noted.[61] Cathodal HVPC was also found effective in healing ischemic ulcers in patients with spinal cord injuries.[74]

Other forms of electrical stimulation have been used to treat problems related to arterial insufficiency. Both alternating and direct currents at low voltages have been used for treating ischemic ulcers. Carley and Wainapel[35] used low voltage direct current to facilitate wound healing, but it is unclear whether the beneficial effects were antimicrobial or circulatory. Others have documented both direct local tissue effects and circulatory improvements through the use of low-voltage electrical stimulation.[23] Transcutaneous electrical nerve stimulation (TENS) has been used to increase microcirculation in skin ulcers of various types[27] and to

improve local blood flow in ischemic skin flaps of reconstructive surgery patients.[90] Research has extended to spinal cord stimulation (SCS) to improve both flow velocity and pulse waveform in PAOD patients.[131] An overall limb salvage rate of 42% was obtained by Mingoli and others[103] in limb-threatening chronic ischemia. Of the limbs saved, 80% showed control of ischemic pain with SCS at one-year follow-up. Other researchers have demonstrated improved arterial flow in severe PAOD including patients with ischemic ulcers and gangrene.[138,153] A combination of electrical stimulation to the sympathetic trunk and ultrasound in liquid tomicide is reported to be effective in the treatment of suppurative wounds.[69]

Oxygen therapy shows potential benefit in the treatment of ischemia. Upson[168] reports that the use of hyperbaric oxygen on diabetic ulcers enhanced tissue repair and antimicrobial activity. Hyperbaric oxygen is also reported to have resolved ischemia in accidental arterial injection of oral methadone[2] and to have assisted in managing a nonhealing saphenectomy wound.[78] In a controlled study of the effects of 40% oxygen inhalation on skin microcirculation of toes in PAOD patients, both normal subjects and patients with moderate PAOD showed vasoconstriction, but microcirculation increased in patients having severe PAOD.[27]

In two studies diabetic plantar ulcers responded well to pressure redistribution by total contact casting, provided the patient's ankle/brachial index was at least 0.5.[28,149] Cardiosynchronous (R-wave triggered) circumferential limb compression is another form of pressure utilization that has shown increased arterial flow with lasting improvement in ischemic symptoms in clinical trials.[152] Negative pressure is also being investigated with two reports of improved arterial perfusion using vacuum compression therapy on lower limbs.[3,99] Various forms of pressure therapy continue to be studied with regard to treatment of chronic ischemic conditions.

Both hot and cold lasers have been used in the management of arterial problems. Gogia and others[70] demonstrated healing of a recalcitrant diabetic ulcer with iodine whirlpool followed by infrared (cold) laser. Various laser wavelengths have been used by vascular surgeons to perform atheroablations successfully, but one associated problem has been damage, including perforation, of the arterial wall.[139] Argon and yttrium-aluminum-garnet (YAG) lasers have been used independently and in conjunction with percutaneous transluminal angioplasty (PTA) for recanalization of segmental femoral and popliteal occlusions.[98]

Surgical approaches to relief of PAOD include sympathectomy, PTA, bypass grafting, thrombolysis and ultrasound angioplasty. Lumbar sympathectomy clinical trials have received mixed reviews due to limited long-term success rates.[79,173] Thrombolysis with urokinase appears to be a reasonable alternative to surgical thrombectomy according to a study by Janosik and others,[82] but this study is limited by its short (60 days) follow-up time. Ultrasound angioplasty appears promising as either an independent procedure or an adjunct to PTA.[9,139] However, more clinical trials are needed to support this treatment regimen. PTA is receiving wide support clinically, especially when used in the absence of diabetes or gangrene[51,52,135] Bypass procedures using either saphenous vein or prosthetic grafts remain the most common surgical interventions for PAOD, having broader applicability and generally lower restenosis rates than PTA or other angioplasty procedures.[122]

The physical therapist's role in postoperative care of bypass graft patients or vascular amputees is primarily to remobilize the patient and maximize function. Following grafting, patients should work on maintaining venous return with active muscle pumping and progress as quickly as feasible to weight-bearing ambulation to tolerance. These patients should avoid hip and knee flexion for some time postoperatively to reduce the risk of graft occlusion, especially if they receive femoral-popliteal bypass grafts. With vascular amputees, therapists must remember that the goals of surgery are pain relief and prevention of life-threatening sepsis. In many cases the remaining limb and the stump are arterially compromised to some extent. Aggressive stump wrapping may cause sloughing of the skin flap or conversion to a higher level of amputation; hence, stump wrapping before the flap is well healed should be avoided. Attempts at prosthetic wear must be made with serious concern for skin condition in the socket and energy demands on the opposite limb. In general, above-knee vascular amputees make poor prosthetic candidates and have low 5-year survival rates.[14,91]

Treatment of primary and secondary Raynaud's disease is a combination of preventive and symptomatic care. Patients presenting with vasospasm should avoid all precipitating factors such as exposure to cold, vasoconstrictive drugs and emotional stress. HAVS patients should avoid vibration exposure completely and permanently. Stress management, relaxation training, and thermal biofeedback have proved helpful in controlling vasospasm. Medications to reduce sympathetic activity or vascular smooth muscle contractility should be employed only when the severity of the symptoms outweigh the systemic side effects of these drugs.[1] TENS has been tried experimentally in Raynaud's patients with no clinically significant results.[108]

## VENOUS DISORDERS
### Venous pathological conditions

Treatment of acute venous disease is not generally within the scope of physical therapy. However, many of our patients are at risk for venous thromboses, making it necessary for us to be able to identify these problems. Differentiating superficial from deep thrombophlebitis is especially important. Superficial thrombophlebitis, caused by embolic occlusion of a surface vein, will cause inflammation with redness, warmth, and tenderness to palpation of the affected vein without demonstrable edema. It is rarely overlooked and

causes no serious circulatory deficit provided deep veins are patent. Deep vein thrombophlebitis, on the other hand, causes significant edema in addition to inflammatory signs. It is often "silent" until the thrombus embolizes and may be associated with reflex arterial spasm. Thrombophlebitis can be caused by trauma, muscle strain, blood dyscrasias, or prolonged bed rest.[17,55,151] A significant risk in patients with peripheral neurological diseases, thrombophlebitis must be differentiated from the peripheral neuropathy itself or from complications such as undetected fracture or osteoarthritis in the affected limb.[126]

Thrombophlebitis can result in chronic venous insufficiency (CVI) as can any other process that increases venous pressure, interferes with valve closure or disrupts normal muscle pump function in the lower extremity. Particularly important is the body's ability to shift venous flow from superficial to deep veins since the deep vessels carry approximately 85% of the total venous volume returning from the lower limbs. Deep vein insufficiency has been noted particularly in patients with posterior tibial vein reflux, emphasizing the importance of muscle pumping in the foot, lower leg, and the calf.[132] While superficial vein incompetence is the most common source of CVI, incompetent calf perforating veins can elevate distal venous pressures similarly to deep vein insufficiency.[5,183] This is probably due to the limited ability to move venous blood from superficial to deep veins and can complicate postthrombotic deep venous insufficiency.

Varicose veins (VV) may be either primary or secondary. They are thickened, tortuous veins caused by chronic valvular insufficiency. Although there is no demonstrated genetic defect responsible for VV, the problem does seem to be familial and is aggravated by obesity. Primary varicosity is usually bilateral, whereas unilateral occurrence tends to be caused by thrombophlebitis. If the deep veins are patent, superficial VV may be ligated without circulatory compromise.[17,55]

Even short periods of venous hypertension can cause decreases in microcirculation. When this is prolonged, as in CVI or VV, fluid filtration equilibrium can be disrupted with resultant edema formation. If not treated early and aggressively, this can progress to brawny edema, hyperpigmentation and, eventually, stasis ulcer development.[40,45,62,102]

Stasis ulcers may arise from occlusion of superficial veins or from prolonged standing in persons with venous valvular insufficiency. During exercise the deep veins are compressed by working muscle, shunting venous return to the superficial vessels. If these vessels cannot handle the increased flow demands, blood will pool in the veins around the ankle, and skin breakdown will occur. The same ulcers result when weak venous valves are deprived of assistive muscle pumping to keep blood flowing upward against gravity. This is commonly seen in persons whose occupations demand prolonged standing on hard surfaces. The progression of symptoms, if untreated, is dependent edema followed by skin discoloration just proximal to the medial malleolus, ulceration of this area, and finally, development of cellulitis in the foot and leg.[91]

### Venous evaluation

The history given by a patient with venous disease will be strikingly different from that of the patient with arterial disease. Pain may be similar to intermittent claudication and may be worse at night. However, this pain after exercise will not be relieved simply by cessation of activity. It will require, in addition, that the patient elevate his or her legs substantially, the source of venous claudication being an inability to handle the increased venous return occasioned by the exercise. More often, the venous patient will complain of aching or fatigue when standing, a discomfort that is relieved by light exercise or elevation of the legs. Night pain is of a cramping nature. The patient will likely report pedal edema that worsens as the day progresses and is gone by morning. There may be a history of acute thrombophlebitis or a family history of varicose veins.[17,55,180]

On inspection, acute thrombophlebitis may present a hot or swollen leg with local tenderness. However, deep vein thrombophlebitis may be asymptomatic except for sharp pain beneath the gastrocnemius muscle when the foot is dorsiflexed. This finding, a positive Homen sign, must not be confused with the discomfort of a tight heel cord. Visual inspection provides more reliable information on chronic venous disease, especially if the inspection is done with the patient standing (Fig. 12-5.) This position will intensify venous pressures and make abnormalities more clearly visible. Any cyanosis seen in standing can be readily reduced by elevating the legs. Skin discoloration is common just proximal to the medial malleolus; in more recent venous problems the skin will be purple, and for chronic problems the skin will be brown. Skin necrosis is possible with venous disease due to associated disruption of microcirculation. Stasis ulcers are usually located proximal to the medial malleolus and have smooth, well-defined borders. Wet gangrene with purulent, edematous lesions may be present in severe venous stasis or in milder disease with superimposed minor trauma.[55,118,151,180]

An exercise test similar to that used for testing arterial perfusion can be performed to differentiate deep and superficial venous insufficiency. The suspect limb is tightly wrapped with elastic bandages from ankle to groin to occlude the superficial veins. The patient then walks on a treadmill (or on level surfaces) at a brisk pace until discomfort, edema, or significant purple discoloration of the feet is noted (Fig. 12-6). If this fails to occur after an extended period of time, deep veins are considered patent. The shorter the exercise tolerance, the more deep vein involvement is suspected.[11]

Impedance plethysmography has been used for some time to study both arterial and venous flow volume, but it has only

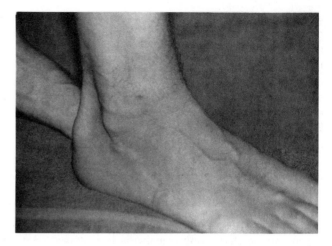

Fig. 12-5. Venous distention exhibited in standing.

recently entered the physical therapy clinic. Using one or two pairs of electrodes, one can measure changes in electrical impedance between the electrodes as volume within a limb changes (e.g., as entering arterial blood engorges an insufficient venous system). This technique has been combined with exercise to test the venous system under stress. However, van den Broek and others[169] found that passive external compression to the calf followed by strain gauge plethysmography performed in standing was a more reliable test for venous insufficiency. Photoplethysmography can also be used to measure venous emptying and venous reflux (Fig. 12-7).[88] Despite its semiquantitative nature, plethysmography in its various forms remains a popular tool for clinical evaluation of venous insufficiency because of its noninvasiveness and ease of application. Plethysmography has been criticized, however, for its inability to discriminate among varying degrees of venous disease.[109] Determining the venous refilling time by photoplethysmography significantly enhances the sensitivity and specificity of plethysmographic evaluation when using a 95% refilling time of less than 15 seconds as the definition of abnormal.[141] This decreased refilling time is caused by backflow from the proximal veins.

Venous Doppler velocimetry is used both qualitatively and semiquantitatively with the emphasis on deceleration slope (Fig. 12-8). Doppler velocimetry is particularly helpful in the identification of long-term deep vein insufficiency caused by acute thrombophlebitis.[89,110]

A grading system for venous disease has been established by the Ad Hoc Committee for Reporting Standards of the Society for Vascular Surgery and the International Society for Cardiovascular Surgery:[177]

Class 0 No clinical signs of CVI
Class 1 Mild swelling of the limb or dilated superficial veins
Class 2 Significant edema and/or hyperpigmentation
Class 3 Active or healed venous ulcers

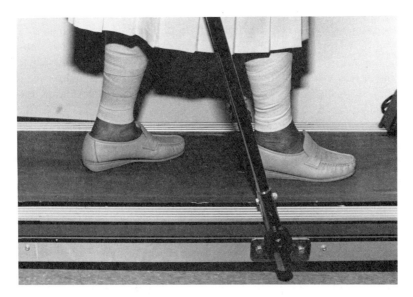

**Fig. 12-6.** Patient's legs are tightly wrapped to occlude the superficial veins. She then walks on the treadmill until pain, fatigue, or discoloration occurs.

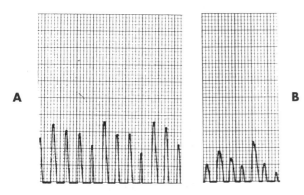

**Fig. 12-7. A,** Normal venous photoplethysmograph. **B,** photoplethysmograph showing venous occlusion.

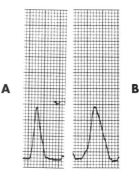

**Fig. 12-8. A,** Normal venous Doppler curve showing moderately steep downslope and moderate half width. **B,** Venous Doppler curve showing less steep downslope and wider half width of venous occlusion.

## Venous treatment

Acute thrombophlebitis in a superficial vein requires only rest, elevation, and warm soaks until symptoms are relieved. On the other hand, deep vein thrombophlebitis, carries the risk of long-term venous insufficiency if poorly managed. As soon as the patient is out of danger of embolization (usually 48 hrs after the onset of anticoagulant therapy), passive range of motion can begin to the affected limb. Ambulation with support hosiery begins as soon as the inflammation has cleared. Early exercise is thought to enhance fibrinolysis and to maintain patency of the deep veins. Patients should avoid sitting or standing for the duration of the subacute period to decrease venous stasis. High heels should be avoided, and patients should be encouraged to stretch heel cords regularly to lessen compression of the deep veins by the gastroc-soleus muscle group.[11,91]

It is generally accepted that patients with CVI should wear well-fitted support hosiery and perform frequent muscle pumping throughout the day. Hose should be donned before arising from bed in the morning, removed and reapplied once during the day, and worn until retiring in the evening.[11,91,118] Brown and Brown[33] found similar improvement in venous circulation in patients wearing heavy support stockings and those wearing sheer support stockings.

Intermittent pneumatic compression (IPC) is beneficial for patients whose edema cannot be controlled with support hose alone. IPC acts to correct venous reflux and lower venous pressures, which some researchers feel reduce reflex microvascular constriction in standing.[123,140] This resultant improvement in microcirculation may prevent stasis ulcers. Kristensen and others[93] did not see this increase in microcirculation when treating patients with compression bandaging.

Stasis ulcers, like ischemic ulcers, are approached in a variety of ways. Whirlpool has long been used for cleansing these open areas. It is now considered beneficial by some therapists to rinse the wound after whirlpool or to use rinsing alone to remove bacteria. Bohannon[26] reported a fourfold increase in bacteria removed by whirlpool-plus-rinse over whirlpool alone. Bactericidal and tissue healing effects of hyperbaric oxygen, cold laser, and electrical stimulation appear equally as effective on stasis ulcers as on ischemic ulcers. Direct current stimulation can be used for antimicrobial therapy. Electrical stimulation at suprathreshold levels has the added benefits of edema reduction and enhanced venous return resulting from muscle pumping.[35,70,129,168] Pulsed electromagnetic waves have been used experimentally on stasis ulcers with good results.[144] Weight reduction to relieve stress on the venous system is indicated if the patient is obese. Patients must remember to change the size of their support hose during weight loss programs to ensure continued proper compression.

An exercise program of ambulation or cycling is indicated to enhance muscle pumping of the lower limb and to increase subcutaneous blood flow.[124] Resisted plantarflexion exercises may be used even with patients who are nonambulatory to assist venous circulation. For patients who complain of night cramps or "restless legs," elevating the foot of the bed several inches can reduce discomfort by improving venous return while muscle pumping is inactive. This should be done cautiously, however, in patients at risk for right ventricular failure since it increases ventricular preload.

Any of the treatments discussed above for CVI can be applied to varicose veins. In advanced cases, VV may be ligated. Some vascular surgeons now support a less invasive surgical approach comprised of stab evulsion phlebotomy plus ligation of the most proximal source of venous reflux.[73] This more conservative approach can be performed as an outpatient surgery using regional anesthesia, allowing the patient to resume normal activities almost immediately.

## LYMPHATIC DISORDERS
### Lymphatic pathologic conditions

The most common disruption of lymphatic circulation is trauma as evidenced by the swelling associated with even minor injuries. In such circumstances, however, the lymphatic capillaries are quick to regenerate and require little therapeutic intervention. More germane to this text are the acute and chronic lymphedemas that do not resolve themselves.

Lymphangitis is an acute local inflammation that spreads from an area of cellulitis proximally along the lymph vessels toward the lymph nodes. It is often precipitated by trauma that results in infection of extravascular tissues around the site of injury. Red streaks develop as the infection moves proximally along channels of lymphatic drainage. These are accompanied by symptoms of sepsis (fever, aching, headache). The original area of cellulitis may progress to necrosis, or the entire process may become subacute with persistent swelling and inflammation of the cellulitic area and the involved lymph vessels.[11,55]

Chronic lymphedema can be either primary or secondary. In either case, an imbalance of filtration versus drainage exists. Capillaries become more permeable to fluid and proteins, causing an increase in tissue osmotic pressure. This further accelerates fluid movement into the tissue. The end result is painless edema of the dependent extremity.[55,180] Primary lymphedema is a hereditary predisposition to swelling that is treated symptomatically. Lymphedema caused by disease may be reversed by treating both the symptoms and the underlying problem. However, lymphedema caused by surgical excision of lymph nodes is not reversible and must be treated symptomatically.

It is lymphedema resulting from surgery, muscle paralysis, or severe CVI that therapists see most often. Edema of an extremity can cause paresthesias, fatigue, and either dependent, pitting edema or persistent, brawny edema. Lymphedema reduces range of motion and leads to soft tissue fibrosis if unresolved. It also predisposes the individual to trauma and infection.[11,55,118]

### Lymphatic evaluation

The patient with lymphedema will have either a history of cause (surgery, trauma, paralysis) or a familial predisposition for painless swelling of the dependent limb. Patients commonly seen in physical therapy tend to have either resection of lymph nodes necessitated by cancer or paralysis of a limb with loss of normal muscle pumping. Progression of symptoms will be pitting edema leading to fatigue or paresthesias followed by development of brawny edema and associated fibrosis. Often the patient is referred to physical therapy only after minor trauma to a chronically edematous limb has resulted in cellulitis and acute infection.

On visual inspection, the most significant finding is usually dependent edema. Differentiation of pitting from brawny edema can help establish the duration of the problem and rule out CVI as a cause. Pitting edema indicates venous swelling of short duration while hard, brawny edema

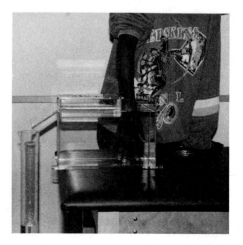

**Fig. 12-9.** Fluid displacement into a graduated cylinder is used to measure volume of an edematous hand.

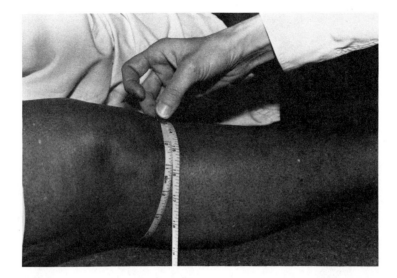

**Fig. 12-10.** Circumferential measurements of a limb are taken at 5 cm intervals.

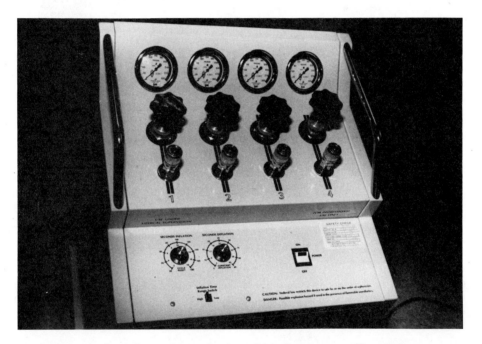

**Fig. 12-11.** Intermittent compression is useful in the treatment of lymphedema.

indicates chronic lymphatic insufficiency.[55,91] Red streaking proximally indicates lymphangiitis and requires immediate medical intervention.

Volumetric measurement is useful in the evaluation and quantification of lymphedema (Fig. 12-9). The water displaced into a graduated cylinder by the swollen hand or foot will be equal to the volume of the submerged segment. Although collection and measurement of displaced water are straightforward for the distal extremities, the therapist may have to be creative when doing volumetric testing of the entire limb. This is especially true for patients with limited mobility. One suggestion is to completely fill a whirlpool, allowing it to overflow into the floor drain when the patient's

extremity is placed in the tank. The volume of water needed to refill the tank after the limb is removed can then be measured to approximate the volume displaced. For those therapists who hesitate to create floods in their facilities, circumferential measurement offers an alternative. Although this provides only an indirect volumetric measurement, it is more feasible under a variety of situations. At 5 cm intervals along the affected extremity, measurements of circumference are taken (Fig. 12-10). This process can be made more time efficient by using string rather than a tape measure. At each measurement point, string is passed around the extremity and cut at the point where it meets itself. Each string is tagged and can be measured and recorded while the

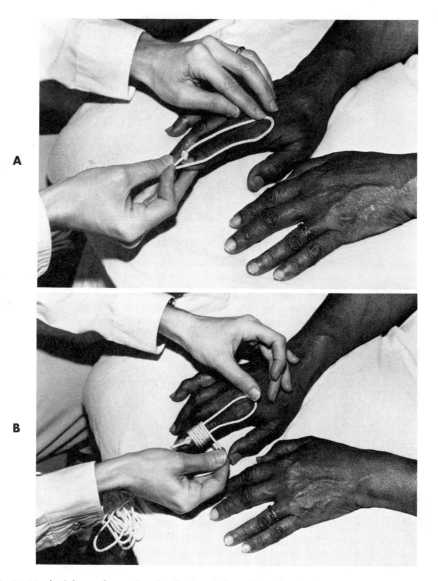

**Fig. 12-12. A,** A loop of smooth string is placed along the patient's finger with the open end of the loop toward the therapist. **B,** String is wrapped firmly around the finger from distal to proximal; the short end of the loop is then pulled to unwrap the finger from distal to proximal.

patient is being treated. This method also prevents cross-contamination from the tape measure in patients with open skin lesions.

### Lymphatic treatment

Skin care and avoidance of trauma are important for prevention of lymphangitis, cellulitis, and ulceration. Skin should be kept well lubricated and should not be exposed to strong soaps or detergents. Injections and blood pressure measurements should always be done on the unaffected side. If the limb is insensitive, special protection should be worn to prevent minor abrasions.[118]

Acute lymphangiitis may either precede or follow chronic lymphedema. In either case, the treatment is rest, elevation, moist heat, and antibiotics. If the patient is on a therapy program for lymphedema at the time of the infection, it should be discontinued until all symptoms of acute infection subside.

Lymphedema caused by trauma or radiation therapy can be controlled if the patient is willing to carry out the program over an extended period of time. Use of external intermittent compression in conjunction with a conscientious program of limb elevation and active muscle pumping produces good results if treatment is initiated early after the onset of edema (Fig. 12-11). Most commonly used are pneumatic boots or sleeves, but mercury pressure gradient equipment is also available.[120] Massage also can be used effectively if the skin of the affected extremity can tolerate it. Some patients may require compression bandaging or customized pressure garments to control edema between treatments.[11,91] When a pressure garment is used, it must be applied immediately after intermittent compression. Edema in the fingers is

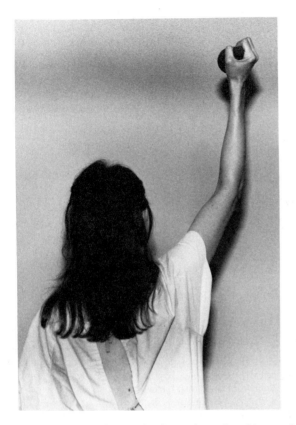

**Fig. 12-13.** Active muscle pumping in an elevated position can be used to treat lymphedema.

difficult to manage with standard compression sleeves. String wrapping (Fig. 12-12) can be used to provide external compression specifically to the fingers.

Patients who sustain significant damage to proximal lymphatic structures or who undergo surgical resection of lymph nodes are harder to treat and may need therapy indefinitely. Symptomatic control and prevention of injury are the primary goals in such situations. Avoidance of the dependent position is mandatory. Intermittent compression may be necessary on a daily basis. Maximum inflation pressures average 60 to 100 mm Hg, varying directly with the patient's diastolic blood pressure. Inflation time should be 3 times the deflation time with treatment durations up to 120 minutes, depending on the severity of the problem.[91] Exercise may not be of great value for chronic edema because it is the receiving end of the lymphatic system that is faulty. However, exercise is of therapeutic value immediately after surgery when recanalization and redistribution of lymphatic circulation are easiest to implement (Fig. 12-13).

A combination of skin care, massage, compression bandaging and exercise was used by Casley-Smith[38] with significant improvement over the first four weeks of therapy (limb volume decreases of 1.1 L in mild cases of edema, 1.3 L in moderate, and 3.7 L in severe) and continued gradual improvement over the next year of therapy. Bertelli and others[20] used compression garments alone to achieve 14.7%

edema reduction in postmastectomy patients over a six-month treatment period. They also noted patients who did not gain weight overall after surgery had nearly 25% edema reduction. Brennan[31] reported a 50% decrease in edema in postmastectomy patients using compression garments and pneumatic compression pumps. Pappas and O'Donnell[121] followed lymphedema patients on a program of high pressure (90 to 100 mm Hg) pneumatic compression, compression garments and skin care for 25 months on average. They found a full response in 53% of patients and a partial response in an additional 20%. The duration of lymphedema and subsequent subcutaneous fibrosis negatively affected response to treatment in this study, suggesting a benefit from early intervention in lymphedema progression. Surgical excision of subcutaneous fibrosis is indicated in patients with long-standing edema and fibrosis who do not respond to conservative measures.[158]

Current research efforts in the area of lymphedema treatment include the use of microwave diathermy and electrical stimulation. Chang and others[39] treated ninety-eight lymphedema patients with 75% of those patients achieving better than 50% edema reduction. The incidence and severity of secondary inflammation also decreased significantly. In another study by Ohkuma[111] thirty patients received both microwave diathermy and compression bandaging with twenty-four responding to treatment. Ten patients received only compression bandaging, six of whom showed slight decreases in edema. One patient received only diathermy and did not respond. A combination of electrically stimulated muscle pumping and compression garments was used by Bertelli and others[21] against a control of compression garments alone. Both groups achieved a 17% reduction in edema. Clearly, no final statement can be made at this time about the ideal approach to treatment of chronic lymphedema.

**ACKNOWLEDGMENT**

I would like to thank Henry C. Foehl for his editorial assistance in the preparation of this manuscript.

**REFERENCES**

1. Adee AC: Managing Raynaud's phenomenon: a practical approach, *Am Fam Physician* 47(4):823, 1993.
2. Adir Y and others: Hyperbaric oxygen therapy for ischaemia of the hand due to intra-arterial injection of methadone and flunitrazepam, *Eur J Vasc Surg* 5(6):677, 1991.
3. Agerskov K and others: External negative thigh pressure. Effect upon blood flow and pressure in the foot in patients with occlusive arterial disease, *Dan Med Bull* 37(5):451, 1990.
4. Agishi T and others: Improvement of peripheral circulation by low density lipoprotein adsorption, *Asaio Trans* 35(3):349, 1989.
5. Alam S and others: Hemodynamic assessment of chronic venous insufficiency, *Jap J Surg* 21(2):154, 1991.
6. Amin MM: Infected diabetic foot ulcers, *Am Fam Physician* 37(2):283, 1988.
7. Andersen HJ and others: The ischaemic leg: a long-term follow-up with special reference to the predictive value of the systolic digital blood pressure. Part I: No arterial reconstruction, *Thoracic Cardiovasc Surg* 37(6):348, 1989.
8. Arfvidsson B and others: Co-variation between walking ability and

circulatory alterations in patients with intermittent claudication, *Eur J Vasc Surg* 6(6):642, 1992.

9. Ariani M and others: Dissolution of peripheral arterial thrombi by ultrasound, *Circulation* 84(4):1680, 1991.

10. Bacharach JM and others: Predictive value of transcutaneous oxygen pressure and amputation success by use of supine and elevation measurements, *J Vasc Surg* 15(3):558, 1992.

11. Kim DDJ and Ebel A: Therapeutic exercise in peripheral vascular disease. In Basmajian JV, Wolf SL, editors: *Therapeutic exercise,* ed 5, Baltimore, 1990, Williams & Wilkins, p. 374.

12. Barker WF, editor: *Peripheral arterial disease,* ed 2, Philadelphia, 1975, WB Saunders Co.

13. Becquemin JP and others: Acute ischemia of the extremities and drug addiction, *J Mal Vasc* 11(1):35, 1986.

14. Beekman CE and Axtell LA: Prosthetic use in elderly patients with dysvascular above-knee and through-knee amputations, *Phys Ther* 67(10):1510, 1987.

15. Belcaro G and others: Skin flow and swelling in postphlebitic limbs, *Vasa* 18(2):136, 1989.

16. Benoit JN and others: Characterization of intact mesenteric lymphatic pump and its responsiveness to acute edemagenic stress, *Am J Phys* 257(6 Pt 2):H2059, 1989.

17. Berkow R, editor: *Merck manual of diagnosis and therapy,* ed 15, West Point, Pa, 1987, Merck Sharp & Dohme.

18. Bernstein EF, editor: *Noninvasive diagnostic techniques in vascular disease,* ed 3, St Louis, 1985, Mosby.

19. Berridge DC and others: Risk factors in patients with ischaemic rest pain of the lower limbs, *J Royal Coll Surg Edinburgh* 35(4):221, 1990.

20. Bertelli G and others: Conservative treatment of postmastectomy lymphedema: a controlled randomized trial, *Ann Oncology* 2(8):575, 1991.

21. Bertelli G and others: An analysis of prognostic factors in response to conservative treatment of postmastectomy lymphedema, *Surg Gynecol Obstet* 175(5):455, 1992.

22. Bettany JA and others: Influence of high voltage pulsed direct current on edema formation following impact injury, *Phys Ther* 70(4):219, 1990.

23. Biedebach MC: Accelerated healing of skin ulcers by electrical stimulation and the intracellular physiological mechanisms involved, *Acupunct Electrother Res* 14(1):43, 1989.

24. Bielski J: Balneoclimatic prevention and treatment of vascular disorders due to vibration at the forestry workers, *Int Arch Occup Environ Health* 60(2):125, 1988.

25. Bjrna H and Kaada B: Successful treatment of itching and atopic eczema by transcutaneous nerve stimulation, *Acupunct Electrother Res* 12(2):101, 1987.

26. Bohannon RW: Whirlpool versus whirlpool and rinse for removal of bacteria from a venous stasis ulcer, *Phys Ther* 62(3):304, 1982.

27. Bongard O and others: Effects of oxygen inhalation on skin microcirculation in patients with peripheral arterial occlusive disease, *Circulation* 86(3):878, 1992.

28. Borssen B and Lithner F: Plaster casts in the management of advanced ischaemic and neuropathic diabetic foot lesions, *Diab Med* 6(8):720, 1989.

29. Brammer AJ, Taylor W, and Lundborg G: Sensorineural stages of the hand-arm vibration syndrome, *Scand J Work Environ Health* 13(4):279, 1987.

30. Brearley S and others: Peripheral pulse palpation: an unreliable physical sign, *Ann Royal Coll Surg England* 74(3):169, 1992.

31. Brennan MJ: Lymphedema following the surgical treatment of breast cancer: a review of pathophysiology and treatment, *J Pain Symptom Mgt* 7(2):110, 1992.

32. Brothers TE and Greenfield LJ: Long-term results of aortoiliac reconstruction, *J Vasc Intervent Radiol* 1(1):49, 1990.

33. Brown JR and Brown AM: Office diagnosis of lower extremity venous insufficiency and treatment with the use of nonprescription support hose, *J Am Osteopath Assn* 92(4):459, 1992.

34. Cahill BE and Kerstein MD: Ischemic neuropathy, *Surg Gynecol Obstet* 165(5):469, 1987.

35. Carley PJ and Wainapel SF: Electrotherapy for acceleration of wound healing: low intensity direct current, *Arch Phys Med Rehab* 66(7):443, 1985.

36. Carter SA: Clinical management of systolic pressures in limbs with arterial occlusive disease, *JAMA* 207(10):1869, 1969.

37. Cartier, CJ: Pressure therapy using a mercury bath, *Phlebologie* 39(1):113, 1986.

38. Casley-Smith JR: Modern treatment of lymphedema. I. complex physical therapy: the first 200 Australian limbs, *Austral J Dermatol* 33(2):61, 1992.

39. Chang TS and others: Microwave: an alternative to electric heating in the treatment of peripheral lymphedema, *Lymphology* 22(1):20, 1989.

40. Cheatle TR and others: Skin microcirculatory responses in chronic venous insufficiency: the effect of short-term venous hypertension, *Vasa* 20(1):63, 1991.

41. Chesham JS and Platt DJ: Patterns of wound colonization in patients with peripheral vascular disease, *J Infect* 15(1):21, 1987.

42. Coffman JD: New drug therapy in peripheral vascular disease, *Med Clin North Am* 72(1):259, 1988.

43. Coffman JD: Pathogenesis and treatment of Raynaud's phenomenon, *Cardiovasc Drugs Therapy* 4(Suppl 1):45, 1990.

44. Corbin DO and others: Blood flow in the foot, polyneuropathy and foot ulceration in diabetes mellitus, *Diabetologia* 30(7):468, 1987.

45. Cordts PR and others: Physiologic similarities between extremities with varicose veins and with chronic venous insufficiency utilizing air plethysmography, *Am J Surg* 164(3):260, 1992.

46. Cormier JM and others: Limitations and results of revascularization of the lower extremities of diabetics, *J Mal Vasc* 10(4):287, 1985.

47. Courchia G and others: Preoperative measurement of peripheral vascular resistance, *J Mal Vasc* 13(1):27, 1988.

48. Criqui MH, Fronek A, and Klauber MR: The sensitivity, specificity, and predictive value of traditional clinical evidence of peripheral arterial disease: results from noninvasive testing in a defined population, *Circulation* 71(3):516, 1985.

49. Criqui MH and others: The prevalence of peripheral arterial disease in a defined population, *Circulation* 71(3):510, 1985.

50. Curry SC and others: Noninvasive vascular studies in management of rattlesnake envenomations to extremities, *Ann Emerg Med* 14(11):1081, 1985.

51. Dacie JE and Daniell SJ: The value of percutaneous transluminal angioplasty of the profunda femoris artery in threatened limb loss and intermittent claudication, *Clin Radiol* 44(5):311, 1991.

52. Dalsing MC and others: Limb salvage in high-risk patients with multisegmental disease, *Indiana Med* 82(9):700, 1989.

53. D'Amour ML and others: Peripheral neurological complications of aortoiliac vascular disease, *Can J Neurol Sci* 14(2):127, 1987.

54. Davies AH and others: The effect of diabetes mellitus on the outcome of angioplasty for lower limb ischaemia, *Diab Med* 9(5):480, 1992.

55. Delp MH and Manning RT, editors: *Major's physical diagnosis,* ed 9, Philadelphia, 1981, WB Saunders Co.

56. Dorros G and others: Below-the-knee angioplasty: tibioperoneal vessels, the acute outcome, *Cath Cardiovasc Diag* 19(3):170, 1990.

57. Engelhart M and Kristensen JK: Local and central orthostatic sympathetic reflexes in Raynaud's phenomenon, *Scand J Clin Lab Invest* (51(2):191, 1991.

58. England JD and others: Muscle denervation in peripheral arterial disease, *Neurol* 42(5):994, 1992.

59. Epstein SE, Cannon RO III, and Talbot TL: Hemodynamic principles in the control of coronary blood flow, *Am J Cardiol* 56:4E, 1985.

60. Ernest E: Physical exercise for peripheral vascular disease—a review, *Vasa* 16(3):227, 1987.

61. Fish DR and others: Effect of anodal high voltage pulsed current on edema formation in frog hind limbs, *Phys Ther* 71(10):724, 1991.

62. Fitzpatrick JE: Stasis ulcers: update on a common geriatric problem, *Geriatrics* 44(10):19, 1989.

63. Foldi E and others: The lymphedema chaos: a lancet, *Ann Plast Surg* 22(6):505, 1989.

64. Forsberg L, Norgren L, and Sjoberg T: Acceleration ratio measurements with ultrasound doppler in patients with occlusive arterial disease, *Acta Radiol [Diagn]* 26(2):121, 1985.

65. Freedman RR: Quantitative measurements of finger blood flow during behavioral treatments for Raynaud's disease, *Psychophys* 26(4):437, 1989.

66. Fremont RE: The clinical use and value of non-invasive diagnostic techniques in peripheral arterial occlusive disease, *Angiology* 26(9):650, 1975.

67. Fronek A, Coel M, and Bernstein EF: Quantitative ultrasonographic studies of lower extremity flow velocities in health and disease, *Circulation* 53(6):957, 1976.

68. Gavish B: Plethysmographic characterization of vascular wall by a new parameter—a minimum rise-time: age dependence in health, *Microcirc Endothelium Lymphatics* 3(3-4):281, 1986-87.

69. Gerasimov and others: Effectiveness of regional electric stimulation of the sympathetic ganglia in the treatment of suppurative wounds, *Klin Khirugiia* (1):4, 1992.

70. Gogia PP, Hunt BS, and Zinn TT: Wound management with whirlpool and infrared cold laser therapy, *Phys Ther* 68(8):1239, 1988.

71. Golden JC and Miles DS: Assessment of peripheral hemodynamics using impedance plethysmography, *Phys Ther* 66(10):1544, 1986.

72. Goodfield MJ and others: The acute effects of cigarette smoking on cutaneous blood flow in smoking and non-smoking subjects with and without Raynaud's phenomenon, *Brit J Rheum* 29(2):89, 1990.

73. Goren G: Primary varicose veins: hemodynamic principles of surgical care. The case for the ambulatory stab evulsion technique, *Vasa* 20(4):365, 1991.

74. Griffin JW and others: Efficacy of high voltage pulsed current for healing of pressure ulcers in patients with spinal cord injury, *Phys Ther* 71(6):433, 1991.

75. Gutherie RA, Gutherie D, and Hinnen D: Self-monitoring of blood glucose: an important adjunct to diabetes therapy, *Compr Ther* 12(1):62, 1986.

76. Hamalainen O and Kemppainen P: Experimentally induced ischemic pain and so-called diaphase fix current, *Scand J Rehab Med* 22(1):25, 1990.

77. Harati Y: Diabetic peripheral neuropathies, *Ann Intern Med* 107(4):546, 1987.

78. Horowitz MD and others: Hyperbaric oxygen: value in management of nonhealing saphenectomy wounds, *Ann Thoracic Surg* 54(4):782, 1992.

79. Huber KH and others: Sympathetic neuronal activity in diabetic and non-diabetic subjects with peripheral arterial occlusive disease, *Klinische Wochenschrift* 69(6):233, 1991.

80. Hummel BW and others: Reactive hyperemia vs. treadmill exercise testing in arterial disease, *Arch Surg* 113(1):95, 1978.

81. Jacobs MJ and others: Assessment of the microcirculation provides additional information in critical limb ischaemia, *Eur J Vasc Surg* 6(2):135, 1992.

82. Janosik JE and others: Therapeutic alternatives for subacute peripheral arterial occlusion. Comparison by outcome, length of stay, and hospital charges, *Invest Radiol* 26(11):921, 1991.

83. Jerntorp P, Ohlin H, and Almer LO: Aldehyde dehydrogenase activity and large vessel disease in diabetes mellitus, *Diabetes* 35(3):291, 1986.

84. Jivegard L and others: Cardiac output in patients with acute lower limb ischaemia of presumed embolic origin—a predictor of severity and outcome? *Eur J Vasc Surg* 4(4):401, 1990.

85. Johnston KW, Hosann MY, and Andrews DF: Reproducibility of noninvasive vascular laboratory measurements of the peripheral circulation, *J Vasc Surg* 6(2):147, 1987.

86. Kato M and others: Clinical studies on peripheral hemodynamics in arterial hypertension, *Angiology* 27(7):422, 1976.

87. Kelsey JR and Beard EF, editors: *Vascular insufficiency,* Springfield, Ill, 1969, Charles C Thomas Co.

88. Kempczinski RF, Berlatzsky Y, and Pearce WH: Semiquantitative photoplethysmography in the diagnosis of lower extremity venous insufficiency, *J Cardiovasc Surg* 27(1):17, 1986.

89. Kistner RL: Diagnosis of chronic venous insufficiency, *J Vasc Surg* 3(1):18S, 1986.

90. Kjartansson J and Lundeberg T: Effects of electrical nerve stimulation (ENS) in ischemic tissue, *Scand J Plastic Reconst Surg Hand Surg* 24(2):129, 1990.

91. Kottke FJ, Stillwell GK, and Lehmann JF, editors: *Krusen's handbook of physical medicine and rehabilitation,* ed 3, Philadelphia, 1982, WB Saunders Co.

92. Kram HB and others: Transcutaneous oxygen recovery and toe pulse reappearance time in the assessment of peripheral vascular disease, *Circulation* 72(5):1022, 1985.

93. Kristensen JK and others: A conventional compression bandage lacks effect on subcutaneous blood flow when walking and during passive dependence in chronic venous insufficiency, *Acta Dermato-Venereologica* 71(5):450, 1991.

94. Lachance DH and Daube JR: Acute peripheral arterial occlusion: electrophysiologic study of 32 cases, *Muscle Nerve* 14(7):633, 1991.

95. Linge K, Roberts DH, and Dowd GS: Indirect measurement of skin blood flow and transcutaneous oxygen tension in patients with peripheral vascular disease, *Clin Phys Physiol Meas* 8(4):293, 1987.

96. Marcus S and others: Raynaud's syndrome. Using a range of therapies to help patients, *Postgrad Med* 89(4):171, 1991.

97. Marinelli MR and others: Noninvasive testing vs. clinical evaluation of arterial disease, *JAMA* 241(19):2031, 1979.

98. Matsumoto T and others: Laser arterial disobstructive procedures in 148 lower extremities, *J Vasc Surg* 10(2):169, 1989.

99. McCulloch JM Jr and Kemper CC: Vacuum-compression therapy for the treatment of an ischemic ulcer, *Phys Ther* 73(3):165, 1993.

100. McGill HC Jr.: The cardiovascular pathology of smoking, *Am Heart J* 115(1):250, 1988.

101. Memsic L and others: Interval gangrene occurring after successful lower extremity revascularization, *Arch Surg* 122(9):1060, 1987.

102. Michel CC: Microvascular permeability, venous stasis and oedema, *Internat Angiol* 8(4 Suppl):9, 1989.

103. Mingoli A and others: Clinical results of epidural spinal cord electrical stimulation in patients affected with limb-threatening chronic arterial obstructive disease, *Angiol* 44(1):21, 1993.

104. Mohr T, Akers TK, and Wessman HC: Effect of high voltage stimulation on blood flow in the rat hind limb, *Phys Ther* 67(4):526, 1987.

105. Moosa HH and others: Transcutaneous oxygen measurements in lower extremity ischemia: effects of position, oxygen inhalation, and arterial reconstruction, *Surgery* 103(2):193, 1988.

106. Montani T and others: Arterial pulse wave velocity, fourier pulsatility index, and blood lipid profiles, *Med Sci Sports Exer* 19(4):404, 1987.

107. Mridha M and Odman S: Fluid translocation measurement. A method to study pneumatic compression treatment of postmastectomy lymphedema, *Scand J Rehab Med* 21(2):63, 1989.

108. Mulder P and others: Transcutaneous electrical nerve stimulation (TENS) in Raynaud's phenomenon, *Angiology* 42(5):414, 1991.

109. Neglen P and Raju S: Detection of outflow obstruction in chronic venous insufficiency, *J Vasc Surg* 17(3):583, 1993.

110. Norris CS and Darrow JM: Hemodynamic indicators of post-thrombotic sequelae, *Arch Surg* 121(7):765, 1986.

111. Ohkuma M: Lymphedema treated by microwave and elastic dressing, *Internat J Dermat* 31(9):660, 1992.

112. Olerud JE and others: Reliability of transcutaneous oxygen tension (TcPo$_2$) measurements in elderly normal subjects, *Scand J Clin Lab Invest* 47(6):535, 1987.

113. Olsen N: Vibration-induced white finger, *Dan Med Bull* 36(1):47, 1989.

114. Olsen N and Hansen SW: Vasomotor functions of skin microcirculation in vasospastic Raynaud's phenomena, *Acta Physiol Scand* 603(Suppl):101, 1991.

115. Ortenwall P, Lundstam S, and Risbery B: Prognostic value of consecutive peripheral pressure registration after reconstructive periphaal arterial surgery, *Acta Chir Scand* 153(10):587, 1987.

116. Osmundson PJ and others: Course of peripheral occlusive arterial disease in diabetes. Vascular laboratory assessment, *Diab Care* 13(2):143, 1990.

117. O'Reilly D and others: Measurement of cold challenge responses in primary Raynaud's phenomenon and Raynaud's phenomenon associated with systemic sclerosis, *Ann Rheum Dis* 51(11):1193, 1992.

118. O'Sullivan SB, Cullen KE, and Schmitz TJ: *Physical rehabilitation: evaluation and treatment procedures,* Philadelphia, 1981, FA Davis Co.

119. Padberg FT Jr and others: Comparison of heated-probe laser Doppler and transcutaneous oxygen measurements for predicting outcome of ischemic wounds, *J Cardiovasc Surg* 33(6):715, 1992.

120. Palmer A and others: Compression therapy of limb edema using hydrostatic pressure of mercury, *Angiology* 42(7):533, 1991.

121. Pappas CJ and O'Donnell TF Jr: Long-term results of compression treatment for lymphedema, *J Vasc Surg* 16(4):555, 1992.

122. Payne JS: Alternatives for revascularization: peripheral atherectomy devices, *J Vasc Nurs* 10(1):2, 1992.

123. Pekanmaki K, Kolari PJ and Kiistala U: Laser Doppler vasomotion among patients with post-thrombotic venous insufficiency: effect of intermittent pneumatic compression, *Vasa* 20(4):394, 1991.

124. Peters K and others: Lower leg subcutaneous blood flow during walking and passive dependency in chronic venous insufficiency, *Brit J Dermatol* 124(2):177, 1991.

125. Peterson CM, editor: *Diabetes management in the '80s,* New York, 1982, Praeger Publishers.

126. Pieri JB: The phlebologist confronted with the neurologic foot, *Phlebologie* 40(2):365, 1987.

127. Podhaisky H and Hansgen K: Effectiveness of angiology study methods in stage 1 arterial occlusive disease, *Z Gesamte Inn Med* 40(21):629, 1985.

128. Pyykko I and others: Cold provocation tests in the evaluation of vibration-induced white finger, *Scand J Work Environ Health* 12:254, 1986.

129. Read BV: Effect of high voltage pulsed stimulation on microvascular permeability to plasma proteins, *Phys Ther* 68(4):491, 1988.

130. Ribal JP, Glanddier G, and Gilbert M: White thrombus syndrome, *J Chir (Paris)* 122(6-7):375, 1985.

131. Roldan P and others: Hemodynamic changes from spinal cord stimulation for vascular pain, *Acta Neurochir [suppl] (Wein)* 39:166, 1987.

132. Rosfors S: Plethysmographic evaluation of volume changes of the foot and the distal calf in healthy subjects and in patients with distal venous pump dysfunction, *Vasa* 20(1):30, 1991.

133. Rosfors S and others: Severity and location of venous valvular insufficiency: the importance of distal valve function, *Acta Chir Scand* 156(10):689, 1990.

134. Rushmer RF, Baker DW, and Stegall HF: Transcutaneous doppler flow detection as a nondestructive technique, *J Appl Physiol* 21(2):554, 1966.

135. Saab MH and others: Percutaneous transluminal angioplasty of tibial arteries for limb salvage, *Cardiovasc Intervent Radiol* 15(4):211, 1992.

136. Sakakibara H and others: Circulatory disturbances of the foot in vibration syndrome, *Internat Arch Occup Environ Health* 63(2):145, 1991.

137. Sako Y: Clinical use of flow meters, *Angiology* 35(4):206, 1984.

138. Sampere CT and others: Spinal cord stimulation for severely ischemic limbs, PACE *Pacing Clin Electrophysiol* 12(2):273, 1989.

139. Sanfelippo PM: The role of lasers in the management of peripheral vascular disease, *Angiology* 40(11):982, 1989.

140. Sarin S, Scurr JH and Coleridge Smith PD: Mechanism of action of external compression on venous function, *Brit J Surg* 79(6):499, 1992.

141. Sarin S and others: Photoplethysmography: a valuable noninvasive tool in the assessment of venous dysfunction, *J Vasc Surg* 16(2):154, 1992.

142. Savin E and others: Blood flow through the brachial artery at different temperatures in patients with Raynaud's phenomenon, *Cor Et Vasa* 31(4):299, 1989.

143. Scheffler A, Jendryssek J and Rieger H: Redistribution of skin blood flow during leg dependency in peripheral arterial occlusive disease, *Clin Physiol* 12(4):425, 1992.

144. Seiller MJ and others: A portable pulsed electromagnetic field (PEMF) device to enhance healing of recalcitrant venous ulcers: a double-blind, placebo-controlled clinical trial, *Brit J Dermat* 127(2):147, 1992.

145. Shafer R, Shafer N, and Positano RG: The early diagnosis of peripheral vascular disease, *Clin Podiatr Med Surg* 4(3):729, 1987.

146. Shepard RJ: *Physical activity and aging,* London, 1978, Croom Helm, Ltd.

147. Sidoti SP: Exercise and peripheral vascular disease, *Clinics Pod Med Surg* 9(1):173, 1992.

148. Siegel RJ, Cumberland DC and Crew JR: Ultrasound recanalization of diseased arteries. From experimental studies to clinical application, *Surg Clinics N Am* 72(4):879, 1992.

149. Sinacore DR and others: Diabetic plantar ulcers treated by total contact casting, *Phys Ther* 67(10):1543, 1987.

150. Spitzner S, Bach R and Schieffer H: Walk training and drug treatment in patients with peripheral arterial occlusive disease stage II. A review, *Internat Angiol* 11(3):204, 1992.

151. Steinberg FU, editor: *Care of the geriatric patient,* ed 6, St Louis, 1983, Mosby.

152. Steinberg J: Cardiosynchronous limb compression: effects on noninvasive vascular tests and clinical course of the ischemic limb, *Angiology* 43(6):453, 1992.

153. Steude U, Abendroth D and Sunder-Plassmann L: Epidural spinal electrical stimulation in the treatment of severe arterial occlusive disease, *Acta Neurochir* 52(Suppl):118, 1991.

154. Stewart CP: The influence of smoking on the level of lower limb amputation, *Prosthet Orthot Int* 11(3):113, 1987.

155. Stokes KR and others: Five-year results of iliac and femoropopliteal angioplasty in diabetic patients, *Radiol* 174(3 Pt 2):977, 1990.

156. Strandness DE Jr.: Intermittent claudication, *Cardiovascular Clin* 3(1):54, 1971.

157. Sutton KC, Wolfson SK Jr, and Kuller LH: Carotid and lower-extremity arterial disease in elderly adults with isolated systolic hypertension, *Stroke* 18(5):817, 1987.

158. Talarico F and others: Fibrosclerotic lymphedema: pathophysiology and therapy, *Lymphol* 24(1):11, 1991.

159. Talbot RW and others: Vascular complications of inflammatory bowel disease, *Mayo Clin Proc* 61(2):140, 1986.

160. Taylor JS: Vibration syndrome: a missed diagnosis, *Occup Med: State of the Art Rev* 1(2):259, 1986.

161. Taylor K and others: Effect of a single 30-minute treatment of high voltage pulsed current on edema formation in frog hind limbs, *Phys Ther* 72(1):63, 1992.

162. Taylor W, Ogston SA, and Brammer AJ: A clinical assessment of seventy-eight cases of hand-arm vibration syndrome, *Scand J Work Environ Health* 12:265, 1986.

163. Todd GJ and others: Muscle high energy phosphates in chronic peripheral vascular disease, *J Surg Res* 44(3):277, 1988.

164. Trainor FS and Cole D: Noninvasive vascular testing in occupational medicine, *Clin Podiatr Med Surg* 4(3):753, 1987.

165. Trap-Jenson J: Effects of smoking on the heart and peripheral circulation, *Am Heart J* 115(1):263, 1988.

166. Ubbink DT and others: Posturally induced microvascular constriction

in patients with different stages of leg ischemia: effect of local skin heating, *Clin Sci* 81(1):43, 1991.

167. Ubbink DT and others: Microvascular reactivity differences between the two legs of patients with unilateral lower limb ischaemia, *Eur J Vasc Surg* 6(3):269, 1992.

168. Upson AV: Topical hyperbaric oxygenation in the treatment of recalcitrant open wounds, *Phys Ther* 66(9):1408, 1986.

169. van den Broek TA and others: Use of passive function testing in venous insufficiency: a prospective study, *Surg* 110(5):860, 1991.

170. Varon J and Gasman JD: Raynaud's disease: an update, *Hosp Pract (office ed)* 26(1):157, 1991.

171. Veith FJ and others: Changing arteriosclerotic disease patterns and management strategies in lower-limb-threatening ischemia, *Ann Surg* 212(4):402, 1990.

172. Vogelberg KH, Muhl M, and Kohler M: Doppler ultrasound determination of maximal blood flow velocity in the diagnosis of peripheral arterial occlusive diseases in diabetes mellitus, *Klin Wachenschr* 65(15):713, 1987.

173. Vulpio C and others: Lumbar chemical sympathectomy in end stage of arterial disease: early and late results, *Angiology* 40(11):948, 1989.

174. Wahlberg E and others: The influence of reactive hyperemia and leg dependency on skin microcirculation in patients with peripheral arterial occlusive disease (PAOD), with and without diabetes, *Vasa* 19(4):301, 1990.

175. Walden R and others: Scoring of vascular disease in the lower extremities, *J Cardiovasc Surg* 30:210, 1989.

176. Walker DC, Currier DP, and Threlkeld AJ: Effects of high voltage pulsed electrical stimulation on blood flow, *Phys Ther* 68(4):481, 1988.

177. Welkie JF and others: Hemodynamic deterioration in chronic venous disease, *J Vasc Surg* 16(5):733, 1992.

178. Wells KE and others: Recognition and treatment of arterial insufficiency from cafergot, *J Vasc Surg* 4(1):8, 1986.

179. West JB, editor: *Best and Taylor's physiological basis of medical practice,* ed 11, Baltimore, 1985, Williams & Wilkins Co.

180. Winsor T and Hyman C: *A primer of peripheral vascular diseases,* Philadelphia, 1965, Lea & Febiger.

181. Winsor T and others: Clinical application of laser doppler flowmetry for measurement of cutaneous circulation in health and disease, *Angiology* 38(10):727, 1987.

182. Wollersheim H and others: Laser Doppler evaluation of skin vasomotor reflexes during sympathetic stimulation in normals and in patients with primary Raynaud's phenomenon, *Internat J Microcirc: Clin Exper* 10(1):33, 1991.

183. Zukowski AJ and others: Haemodynamic significance of incompetent calf perforating veins, *Brit J Surg* 78(5):625, 1991.

# PART TWO

# *Pulmonary Physical Therapy and Rehabilitation*

# CHAPTER 13

# Respiratory Physiology

*Thomas H. Shaffer, Marla R. Wolfson, and Joan H. Gault*

The main function of the respiratory system is the exchange of gases such that arterial blood oxygen, carbon dioxide, and pH levels remain within specific limits throughout many different physiological conditions. The following five fundamental processes are involved in the maintenance of homeostasis:

1. Ventilation and distribution of gas volumes
2. Gas exchange and transport
3. Circulation of blood through the lungs
4. Mechanical interaction of respiratory forces that initiate breathing (respiratory muscles) and those that resist the flow of air (lung compliance and airway resistance)
5. Control and organization of respiratory movements

To appreciate the coordinated and integrated function of the entire respiratory system, it is essential to understand the functions of each of the five fundamental processes. In what follows we have attempted both to analyze and present each fundamental process individually and to discuss the integration and function of each of these processes with respect to the entire system.

Knowledge of respiratory physiology is paramount for proper diagnosis and effective treatment of pulmonary disease. With this in mind, we have presented basic scientific principles as viewed from the perspective of the physical therapist. The processes involved during normal respiration are described in detail in the following sections to establish a scientific basis for therapeutic interventions required for the patient with pulmonary disease.

## VENTILATION AND DISTRIBUTION
### Functional anatomy of the respiratory system

On gross inspection, each lung is cone shaped and covered by visceral pleura. The right lung is slightly larger than the left and is divided by the oblique and horizontal fissures into the upper, middle, and lower lobes. The left lung has two lobes, upper and lower, separated by an oblique fissure. The lobes are further subdivided into bronchopulmonary segments, each receiving a segmental bronchus and artery, and giving rise to a vein (Fig. 13-1).

The airways, pleura, and connective tissue of the lung are vascularized by the systemic circulation through the bronchial arteries. The bronchial veins bypass the pulmonary circulation and join the pulmonary veins to return blood to the heart. Alveoli are perfused by the pulmonary circulation.

The lungs and airways are innervated through the pulmonary plexus. Located at the root of each lung, this plexus is formed from branches of the sympathetic trunk and vagus nerve. Recently, a nonadrenergic, noncholinergic inhibitory nerve fiber has been identified in the airway

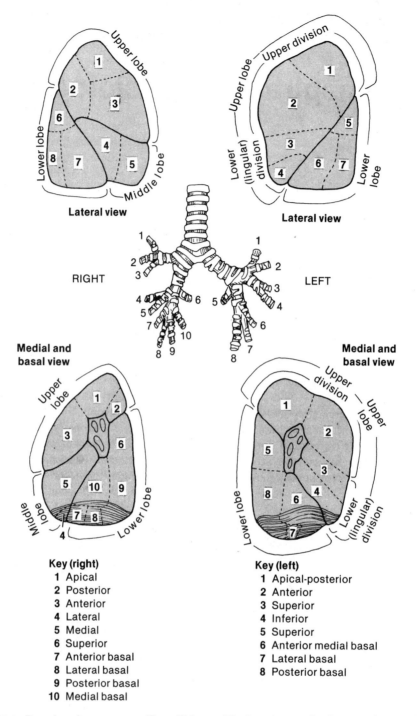

**Key (right)**
1 Apical
2 Posterior
3 Anterior
4 Lateral
5 Medial
6 Superior
7 Anterior basal
8 Lateral basal
9 Posterior basal
10 Medial basal

**Key (left)**
1 Apical-posterior
2 Anterior
3 Superior
4 Inferior
5 Superior
6 Anterior medial basal
7 Lateral basal
8 Posterior basal

**Fig. 13-1.** Bronchopulmonary tree. (From Fishman AP: *Assessment of pulmonary function,* New York, 1980, McGraw-Hill Book Co.)

smooth muscle. Sympathetic stimulation causes bronchodilatation and marginal vasoconstriction, whereas parasympathetic stimulation produces bronchoconstriction and indirect vasodilation.

The respiratory system is conceptually divided into two major divisions: (1) a *conducting portion,* which includes the nose, pharynx, larynx, trachea, bronchi, and bronchioles, and (2) a *respiratory portion,* consisting of the terminal portion of the bronchial tree and alveoli, the site of gas exchange (Fig. 13-2). The transitional zone, separating the conducting and respiratory portions, consists of the respiratory bronchioles.

In the conducting zone, air moves by bulk flow under the pressure gradients created by the respiratory muscles and the

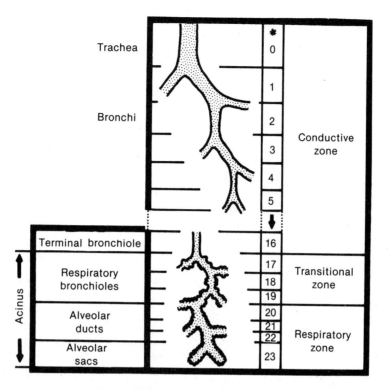

**Fig. 13-2.** Airway branching (Z-generation). (From Fishman AP: *Assessment of pulmonary function,* New York, 1980, McGraw-Hill Book Co.)

elastic recoil of the lung. The total cross-sectional area of the airways increases rapidly at the respiratory zone. Forward velocity of air flow therefore decreases, and the gases readily move by diffusion through the alveoli into the pulmonary capillaries. This is one example of the numerous histological (Fig. 13-3) and morphological alterations occurring throughout the respiratory system that provide for optimal ventilation and gas exchange.

Inspired air enters the body through the nose or mouth. Because of its architecture, large mucosal surface area, and fibrillae, the nose serves to filter, humidify, and warm or cool the air to body temperature. This process protects the remainder of the respiratory system from damage caused by dry gases or harmful debris. The gas then passes through the pharynx, where skeletal muscles contract during swallowing to prevent aspiration of food or liquid into the nose. The pharynx is essential for articulated speech and allows interaction between the sense of smell and taste; however, aside from serving as a conduit, it does not participate in respiration. Next, air travels through the larynx, in which the epiglottis acts as a valve to prevent particles of food from entering the trachea. The larynx, lined by a mucous membrane, is formed by cartilages that are connected by ligaments and moved by skeletal muscles. The most caudal cartilage, the cricoid, is of particular importance in ventilation. It is located at the upper end of the trachea and is the only complete cartilaginous ring around the trachea; as such,

it protects the trachea from dynamic compression during forced inspiration or expiration.

The trachea is generally considered to be the differentiating structure between the upper and lower airways. It is continuous with the larynx and is lined by a pseudostratified ciliated, columnar epithelium containing goblet cells and seromucinous glands. The latter structures produce a sol-gel mucous blanket in which the cilia are embedded. As the cilia beat, this mucous blanket is set into motion and carries unfiltered debris toward the pharynx. This process of mucociliary transport is one of the major defense mechanisms in the lung.

The trachea is formed by 16 to 20 horseshoe-shaped cartilaginous rings connected by smooth muscle that is interlaced with elastic fibers. The cartilage rings support the anterior and lateral walls of the trachea. The posterior wall consists of the tracheal muscle, a thin sheath of smooth muscle whose horizontal fibers bridge the opened ends of the cartilaginous rings. The trachea divides at the carina into the right and left main bronchi, which in turn branch in an irregular dichotomous pattern forming the lobar and segmental bronchi.

The left main bronchus branches at a more acute angle and is longer than the right main bronchus, which is more directly in line with the trachea. This relationship predisposes to aspiration of material into the right rather than the left lung. Bronchial walls consist of irregular plates of

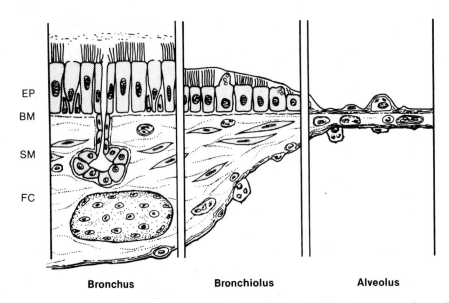

**Fig. 13-3.** Histological modification accompanying airway branching. *BM,* Basement membrane: *EP,* epithelial layer; *FC,* fibrous coating containing cartilage; *SM,* smooth muscle.

cartilage joined by circular bands of smooth muscle. The walls are lined with a continuation of the tracheal epithelium. With further bronchial divisions the cartilaginous plates become scant, and smooth muscle and elastic fibers become prominent with respect to lumen diameter. Cartilage and glands disappear and goblet cells decrease in number at the level of the bronchiole. In addition, the pseudostratified epithelium is replaced by a simpler ciliated cuboid cell epithelium. The bronchioles proximal to the emergence of alveoli are the terminal bronchioles. The transitional zone is demarcated by the appearance of alveoli in the walls of the respiratory bronchioles. The smooth muscle begins to spiral to the terminal bronchiole thereby fulfilling the supportive function provided by cartilage in the more proximal airways. Smooth muscle thins and cilia gradually disappear so that, by the final division, the respiratory bronchiole wall consists of a few strands of muscle and elastic fiber and is lined by a simple cuboid epithelium. Alveolar macrophages are found at this level and provide another defense mechanism by ingesting small unfiltered particles.

Alveolar ducts, completely lined with alveoli, are formed by the branching of the respiratory bronchioles (Fig. 13-2). This diversion demarcates the respiratory zone of the lung, where gas exchange occurs. The discontinuous wall of the alveolar duct is composed of elastic and sparse smooth muscle fibers. The lining is further reduced to a low cuboid epithelium. The alveolar duct gives rise to the alveolar sphincter, the final sections of smooth muscle, and terminates as simple alveoli and alveolar sacs that contain two or more alveoli.

Alveoli (Fig. 13-4) are small evaginations of the respiratory bronchioles, alveolar ducts, and alveolar sacs. Because adjacent alveoli share a common wall, their shape and dimensions vary depending on the arrangement of adjoining alveoli and on lung volume. This phenomenon, wherein an increase in volume in one alveolus will tend to increase the volume in the adjacent alveoli, is called "interdependence." A similar mechanism increases the lumen diameter of distal airways that are surrounded by and tethered to the alveoli. In addition, adjacent alveoli communicate through channels called "pores of Kohn" and with bronchioles through channels called "Lambert's canals." All these alveolar and airway architectural features contribute to the stability and uniformity of lung expansion.

The thin alveolar lining is particularly suited for gas exchange (Fig. 13-5). It consists of two types of cells: (1) type I alveolar cells, which are large flat cells composing most of the internal alveolar surface and (2) type II alveolar cells, which are less numerous, are ovoid, and are involved in the synthesis of surfactant, a substance that facilitates alveolar stability.

## Definition of ventilation and volumes

Ventilation is the cyclic process of inspiration and expiration whereby optimal levels of oxygen and carbon dioxide are maintained in the alveoli and arterial blood. Total ventilation ($\dot{V}_E$) is the volume of air expired each minute. It is the product of the volume of gas moved in and out of the alveoli ($V_A$) and airways with each breath ($V_D$), the tidal volume ($V_T$), and the number of breaths taken each minute, the respiratory rate ($f$). Therefore:

$$\dot{V}_E = V_T \times f$$

where $V_T = V_A + V_D$

The volume of alveolar gas ($V_A$) in the tidal volume represents the volume of fresh gas entering the respiratory zone with each breath. Alveolar ventilation, $\dot{V}_A = V_A \times f$, is extremely important because it represents the amount of

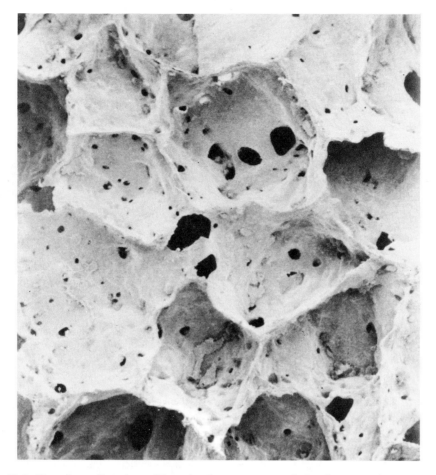

**Fig. 13-4.** Horse lung. Cut edges of interalveolar septa surround alveoli seen *en face*. Pores and alveolar epithelial cells are visible on the surfaces of the interalveolar septa, and pulmonary alveolar macrophages are seen in the alveoli. (Field width, 250 μm.) (From American Lung Association: *In defense of the lung*, New York, 1974, The Association.)

fresh air available for gas exchange per minute. Hyperventilation is defined as an increase in alveolar ventilation that decreases carbon dioxide levels below the normal limits ($Pco_2 = 40$ mm Hg)—that is, hypocapnia. Hypoventilation, in contrast, is defined as an increase in carbon dioxide (hypercapnia) levels caused by a decrease in alveolar ventilation. The oxygen tension of alveolar air is increased by hyperventilation and decreased by hypoventilation.

Total ventilation is the combined volume of gases moving through the conducting and respiratory zones of the lung each minute. It is described as:

$$\dot{V}_E = \dot{V}_D + \dot{V}_A$$

where $E$ is exhaled air, $D$ is dead space, and $A$ is alveolar air.

The terms used in the discussion of the dynamic process of ventilation are best understood with respect to static lung volumes and lung capacities (Fig. 13-6). Although these values are essentially anatomic measurements, alterations in lung volumes or capacities may reflect the effects of cardiopulmonary disease. In general, lung volumes are

subdivisions that do not overlap. Capacities include two or more primary volumes.

There are four primary lung volumes: (1) tidal volume, (2) inspiratory reserve volume, (3) expiratory reserve volume, and (4) residual volume. Tidal volume ($V_T$) is the volume of gas inspired or expired during each respiratory cycle. It reflects the depth of breathing and is comprised of the volume entering the alveoli ($V_A$) and the volume remaining in the airways ($V_D$). These values, when coupled with the respiratory frequency, are used to describe ventilation.

Reserve volumes represent the maximum volumes of gas that can be moved above or below a normal tidal volume. These values reflect the balance between lung and chest wall elasticity, respiratory muscle strength, and thoracic mobility. *Inspiratory reserve volume* (IRV) is the maximum volume of gas that can be inspired from the peak of a tidal volume. *Expiratory reserve volume* (ERV) is the maximum volume of gas that can be expired after a normal tidal expiration. Therefore reserve volumes are associated with the ability to

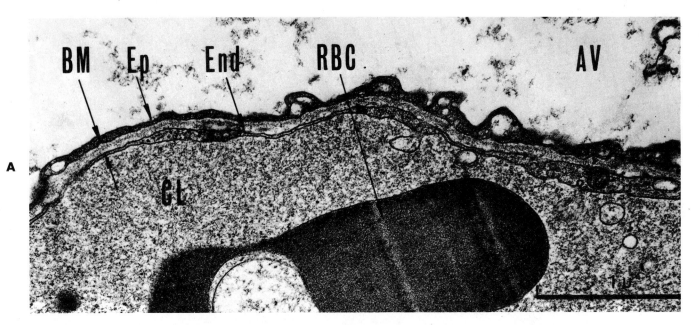

**Fig. 13-5. A,** Electron micrograph of the lung, showing the alveolocapillary region of the left lower lobe of a healthy 35-year-old man. (Courtesy AE Vatter, Department of Pathology, Webb-Waring Institute, University of Colorado Medical Center, Colo.)

increase or decrease the tidal volume. Normal lungs do not collapse at the end of the greatest expiration. The volume of gas remaining is called the *residual volume* (RV).

These four volumes can be combined to form four capacities: (1) total lung capacity, (2) vital capacity, (3) inspiratory capacity, and (4) functional residual capacity. *Total lung capacity* (TLC) is the amount of gas in the respiratory system after a maximal inspiration. It is the sum of all four lung volumes. *Vital capacity* (VC) is the maximum volume of gas that can be expelled from the lungs after a maximal inspiration. As such, the vital capacity is the sum of IRV + TV + ERV. *Inspiratory capacity* (IC) is the maximum volume of gas that can be inspired from the resting end-expiration level; therefore it is the sum of TV + IRV. *Functional residual capacity* is the volume of gas in the lungs when the respiratory system is at rest, that is, the volume in the lung at the end of a normal expiration. The size of the FRC is determined by the balance of two opposing forces: (1) inward elastic recoil of the lung tending to collapse the lung and (2) outward elastic recoil of the chest wall tending to expand the lung. Functional residual capacity is the volume of gas above which a normal tidal volume oscillates. A normal FRC avails optimal lung mechanics and alveolar surface area for efficient ventilation and gas exchange.

### Definition of dead space

Dead space ($V_D$) refers to the volume within the respiratory system that does not participate in gas exchange. It is composed of several components. *Anatomic dead space*

is the volume of gas contained in the conducting airways. *Alveolar dead space* refers to the volume of gas in areas of "wasted ventilation," that is, in alveoli that are *ventilated* but poorly or underperfused. The total volume of gas that is not involved in gas exchange is called the *physiologic dead space.* It is the sum of the anatomic and alveolar dead space. In a normal person, the physiologic dead space should be equal to the anatomic dead space. For this reason, some investigators refer to physiologic dead space as *pathologic dead space.*

Several factors can modify the dead-space volume. Anatomic dead space increases as a function of airway size. Because of the interdependence of the alveoli and airways, anatomic dead space increases as a function of lung volume. Similarly, dead space increases as a function of body height, bronchodilator drugs, diseases such as emphysema, and oversized artificial airways. In contrast, anatomic dead space is decreased by reduction of the size of the airways, as occurs with bronchoconstriction or a tracheostomy.

### Distribution of gas

Inspired air is not distributed uniformly throughout the lungs. One obvious explanation for this nonuniform distribution is the difference in size between the right and left lungs. Topographical differences in ventilation also occur within each lung. Because of intrapleural pressure gradients caused by gravitational, chest wall, and lung forces, the alveoli in dependent portions of the lung are smaller and more compliant than alveoli within less dependent segments. Therefore when breathing is around a normal functional

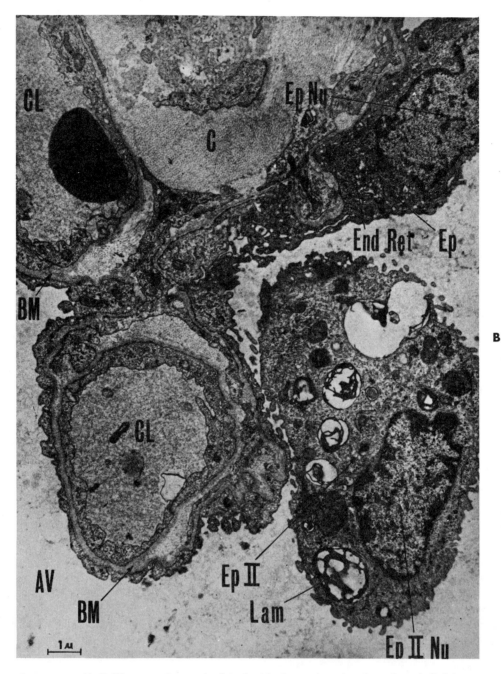

**Fig. 13-5, cont'd. B,** Electron micrograph of the healthy human lung (specimen from the left lower lobe of a 74-year-old man), showing alveolocapillary structures with large epithelial (type B, type II) cell containing cytoplasmic lamellar bodies. *AV,* Alveolar space; *BM,* basement membrane; *CL,* capillary lumen; *C,* collagen; *End,* endothelial cytoplasm; *End Ret,* endoplasmic reticulum; *Ep* (in **A**), epithelial cytoplasm, type II; *Ep* (in **B**), epithelial cytoplasm, *Ep Nu,* epithelial nucleus; *Ep II,* cytoplasm of alveolar epithelial cell, type II; *Ep II Nu,* nucleus of the alveolar epithelial cell, type II; *Lam,* lamellar body; *RBC* red blood cell. (Courtesy Robert L. Hawley, Mercy Institute of Biomedical Research, Denver, Colo.)

residual capacity, the dependent alveoli receive three times more inspired air than the independent alveoli do. For example, basilar ventilation exceeds apical ventilation with the subject sitting or standing. In the supine position, the posterior portion of the lung is better ventilated than the anterior portion. Similar ventilation inequalities exist in the lateral and Trendelenburg positions.

This relationship changes if breathing occurs at very high or low lung volumes. At high volumes, all alveoli become less compliant; therefore the volume changes tend to be

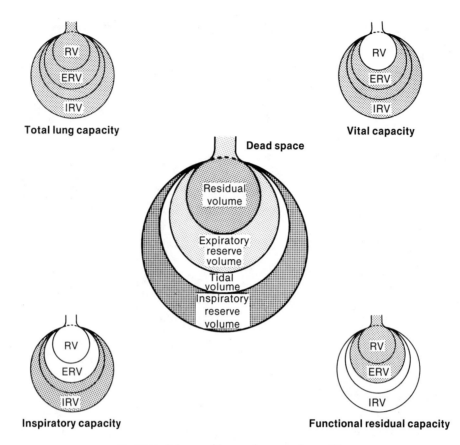

**Fig. 13-6.** Scheme of lung volumes and capacities.

similar. However, at low lung volumes, airways in the dependent portion close, and distribution of air to the dependent areas is prevented.

The distribution of gas is further altered by local factors in disease. Regional airway obstruction, abnormal lung or chest wall compliance, or respiratory muscle weakness may significantly increase the nonuniformity of air distribution in the lung. However, collateral ventilation between adjacent alveoli through the pores of Kohn, or between alveoli and respiratory bronchioles through Lambert's canals, may help ventilate lung regions behind occluded airways.

### Testing and evaluation

**Lung volumes and ventilation.** Lung volumes are measured by spirometry, inert gas dilution, nitrogen washout, and body plethysmography techniques. Because lung volumes are essentially anatomical measurements, they do not directly evaluate pulmonary function. However, changes in lung volumes are associated with respiratory pathologic conditions. For this reason these tests offer valuable information to assist in the diagnosis and management of patients with cardiopulmonary disease.

Spirometry is a traditional technique used to measure lung volumes and specific ventilatory capacities. As originally described in the mid-1800s by Hutchinson, the spirometer records changes in lung volumes from movement of a lightweight bell that is inverted over a water bath. The patient's breathing through a mouthpiece causes the bell to rise or fall. The change in volume is recorded on a variable-speed rotating drum of graph paper by corresponding movements of a pen (Figs. 13-7 and 13-8). Recent modifications of this system enable rapid collection of data by a computer. Tidal volume and expiratory and inspiratory reserve volumes are measured when one performs particular respiratory maneuvers from which inspiratory and vital capacity can be determined. Because the lung cannot be emptied by maximal expiration, other techniques must be employed to measure residual volume, functional residual capacity, and total lung capacity. Typically, the functional residual capacity is determined and residual volume is calculated. Once residual volume is calculated, one deduces the total lung capacity by adding the vital capacity and residual volume.

Closed-circuit helium dilution is commonly used to determine residual volume and functional residual capacity. This technique is based on the facts that (1) helium is an inert gas that is insoluble in blood and not found in the lungs and (2) consumed oxygen is replaced and carbon dioxide is removed from the spirometer and therefore the total volume of the system is constant. The patient breathes through a

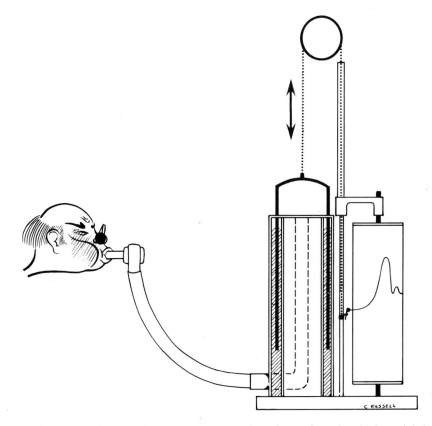

**Fig. 13-7.** A type of spirometer. Spirometers measure the volume of gas that the lungs inhale and exhale, usually as a function of time. They are used to measure the volume changes and flow rates of spontaneous breathing and various breathing maneuvers.

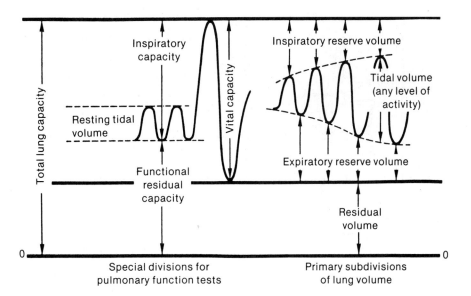

**Fig. 13-8.** Subdivisions of the lung volume. (Modified from Pappenheimer JR and others: *Fed Proc* 9:602, 1950.)

spirometer containing a known concentration of helium ($C_1$). After several minutes the concentration of helium in the lung and in the spirometer equilibrates ($C_2$). The final helium concentration ($C_2$) reflects dilution of the initial helium volume ($V_1$) by the volume of gas in the lungs ($V_2$). Therefore the unknown value ($V_2$) can be calculated:

$$C_1 \times V_1 = C_2 (V_1 + V_2)$$

or

$$V_2 = V_1 \left( \frac{C_1}{C_2} - 1 \right)$$

Body plethysmography utilizes Boyle's law ($PV = K$) in the determination of lung volume (Fig. 13-9). Basically, a subject sits in an airtight booth and breathes against a mouthpiece that is occluded at the lung volume to be measured. According to Boyle's law, pressure and volume change inversely in the lung as a result of respiratory efforts. Because the "body box" is sealed, opposite pressure and volume changes occur in the box. By measuring the pressure inside the box and the volume change in the box, one can calculate the lung volume as follows:

$$P_1 V = P_2 (V - \Delta V)$$

or

$$V = \Delta V \frac{P_2}{P_2 - 1}$$

where $P_1$ is end-inspiratory pressure: $P_2$ is end-expiratory pressure: $\Delta V$ is change in volume of box; and $V$ is unknown lung volume.

Ventilatory capacity is most commonly evaluated by the force vital capacity (FVC). The maximal voluntary ventilation (MVV) test requires that the patient breathe as deeply and rapidly as possible for 15 seconds. This test is often too fatiguing for patients, and comparable diagnostic information is readily gained from the forced vital capacity. However, assessment of respiratory muscle endurance is best made on the basis of tests such as the MVV.

The forced expiratory volume at 1 second ($FEV_1$) is the volume of gas forcibly expired in 1 second after maximal inspiration. It is recorded by a spirometer when the patient exhales as hard, as much, and as fast as possible from maximum lung volume. The change in volume occurring in the first second and the total volume exhaled (FVC) can be directly measured (Fig. 13-10) from the curve on the spirometer graph. The FVC is a measurement of the maximum volume output of the respiratory system. As such, the FVC reflects the integrity of all the components involved with pulmonary mechanics. The $FEV_1$ provides information about airway resistance and the elastic recoil of the lungs. In

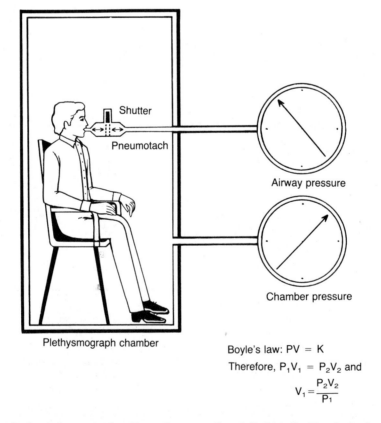

Boyle's law: $PV = K$

Therefore, $P_1V_1 = P_2V_2$ and

$$V_1 = \frac{P_2V_2}{P_1}$$

**Fig. 13-9.** Body plethysmography. (From Spearman C and Sheldon R: *Egan's fundamentals of respiratory therapy,* ed 4, St Louis, 1982, Mosby.)

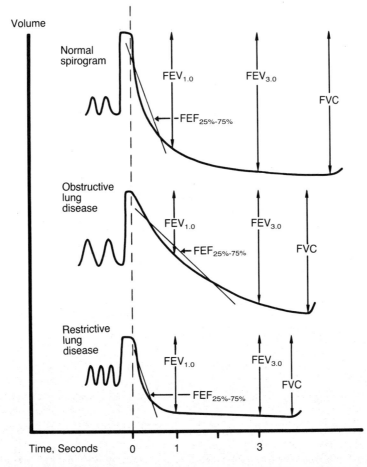

**Fig. 13-10.** Spirometric recording of forced expiratory volume (*FEV*) and forced vital capacity (*FEC*): normal, obstructive, and restrictive lung disease. (From Slonim NB and Hamilton LH: *Respiratory physiology,* ed 4, St Louis, 1981, Mosby.)

addition, the ratio of $FEV_1/FVC$ varies in the presence of a pathological condition. Therefore this test can help distinguish between obstructive and restrictive lung disease. In restrictive disease, the total lung capacity and the forced vital capacity are decreased. However, because the elastic recoil of the lungs may be increased in restrictive disease, the $FEV_1/FVC$ ratio may also increase. In contrast, increased airway resistance associated with obstructive lung disease decreases the $FEV_1$. The total lung capacity and functional residual capacity are typically increased as a function of airtrapping distal to the occluded airways. Therefore in obstructive lung disease the $FEV_1/FVC$ ratio is decreased.

Ventilation is commonly determined by measurement of the total volume of expired gas over a given duration. Typically the patient breathes through a mouthpiece for about 3 minutes, and the expired gas is shunted into a collecting bag. The total ventilation ($\dot{V}_C$) is determined when the total volume of gas is divided by the duration of the collecting period. Alternatively, minute ventilation can be determined by calculation of the tidal volume, wherein the total volume ($V$) is divided by the total number of breaths ($n$) and multiplied by the number of breaths per minute ($f$).

Therefore:

$$\dot{V}_E = V_T \times f$$

or

$$\frac{V}{n} \times f = V_E$$

Alveolar ventilation is calculated in two ways: (1) by subtracting dead-space volume from the tidal volume and (2) on the basis of $CO_2$ elimination by the lungs. Determination of dead space is discussed later. The second method measures alveolar ventilation from the concentration of $CO_2$ in expired gas. $CO_2$ is derived solely from alveolar air, since gas exchange does not occur in the conducting airways.

Inadequate alveolar ventilation is associated with faulty pulmonary mechanics and neural control and results in abnormal blood gas tensions.

**Distribution of gases.** Several techniques are employed to assess the distribution of inspired air. The three most commonly discussed tests are (1) single-breath nitrogen test, (2) multibreath nitrogen test, and (3) use of radioactive gases.

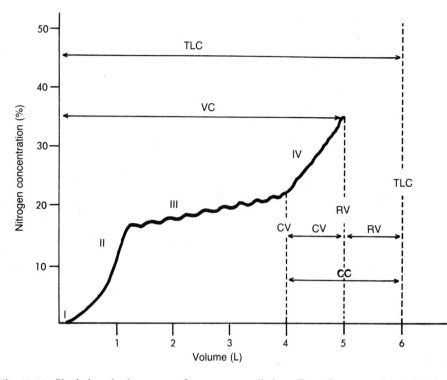

**Fig. 13-11.** Single-breath nitrogen test for uneven ventilation. (From Spearman C and Sheldon R: *Egan's fundamentals of respiratory therapy,* ed 4, St Louis, 1982, Mosby.)

The single-breath nitrogen test involves plotting the changing concentrations of nitrogen ($N_2$) in the expired gas after a maximal inspiration of 100% oxygen. As seen in Fig. 13-11, four phases are described. Phases 1 and 2 reflect gas expired from the dead space. Phase 3, the plateau phase, represents alveolar gas. In patients, the slope of phase 3 is steep, reflecting varying concentrations of nitrogen in the expired gas. This steep slope usually indicates that either the inspired oxygen was unevenly distributed or there are regional variations in the emptying rate of the alveoli. The abrupt rise in nitrogen concentration, phase 4, marks the onset of the "closing volume," the volume at which dependent airways close.

The multibreath nitrogen test records the nitrogen concentration at the end of each breath while the patient breathes 100% oxygen. A normal lung empties uniformly so that the nitrogen concentration decreases by the same proportion of each breath. In patients with lung disease, gross inequalities in ventilation dilute some alveoli before others; therefore a variable pattern of nitrogen concentration decrease occurs (Fig. 13-12).

Radionuclide tracers are used to demonstrate regional differences in ventilation. A volume of radioactive xenon is inspired from a spirometer and is carried to alveoli. A radioactive counter detects the gas and records the distribution through the lung.

Gross inequalities in ventilation are associated with many pulmonary diseases. Abnormalities in lung compliance, resistance, and collateral ventilation of alveoli obstructed by airway disease are associated with emptying and filling defects.

**Dead space.** Each component of respiratory dead space can be evaluated. Specific tests include (1) Fowler's single-breath nitrogen technique, which measures anatomical dead space, and (2) use of the Bohr equation to calculate physiological dead space. Total dead-space volume is estimated to be 1 ml for each pound of body weight.

The Fowler technique measures anatomical dead space through nitrogen concentration analysis of expired air after a single inspiration of 100% oxygen. The inspired gas enters the alveoli, and the last part of this tidal volume stays in the conducting airways (anatomic dead space). Nitrogen concentration begins to rise as the airways are cleared and alveolar gas is expired. The recorded volume to this point represents anatomical dead space.

The Bohr equation is used to calculate physiological dead space. This method requires analysis of the carbon dioxide ($CO_2$) in a collected volume of expired gas and of the $CO_2$ in the very end of the expired tidal volume. It is assumed that all the expired $CO_2$ is from the alveolar gas. Therefore:

$$V_D = \left( \frac{F_{A_{CO_2}} - F_{F_{CO_2}}}{F_{A_{CO_2}}} \right) \cdot V_T$$

In the normal lung, measurements derived from the Fowler technique and the Bohr equation should be equal. A difference reflects alveolar dead space.

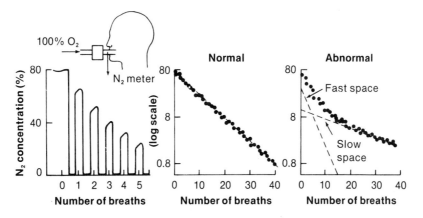

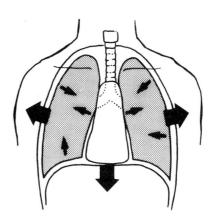

Fig. 13-12. Multibreath nitrogen washout test for determination of uneven ventilation. (From West JB: *Respiratory physiology,* ed 2, Baltimore, 1979, The Williams & Wilkins Co.)

In the normal population, variations in lung volumes and ventilatory capacity are associated with age, position, body proportions, obesity, and cooperation. Once these factors are considered, values that deviate from normal standards are usually indicative of a pulmonary disease. The aforementioned tests aid in the differential diagnosis and therapeutic recommendations in the presence of abnormal findings. For example, body plethysmography measures thoracic gas volume, whereas spirometry and gas dilution measure only ventilated lung volume. Disparity between thoracic gas volume and ventilated lung volume indicate gas that is trapped by airway obstruction. Furthermore, reversible airway obstruction, associated with asthma, is demonstrated by improved $FEV_1$ and FVC values after administration of a bronchodilator.

## MECHANICS OF BREATHING

The mechanics of breathing involve the respiratory muscle forces required to overcome the elastic recoil of the lungs and thorax, as well as frictional resistance to air flow through hundreds of thousands of conducting airways. The energy for ventilating the lungs is supplied by active contraction of the respiratory muscles, which are discussed in a subsequent chapter. This section discusses the elastic and nonelastic forces that resist movement of the lung and chest wall. We begin our discussion of pulmonary mechanics by considering the elastic nature of the lung.

### Elastic behavior of the respiratory system

Elasticity is the property of matter such that if we disturb a system by stretching or expanding it the system will return to its original position when all external forces are removed. Like a spring, the tissues of the lungs and thorax stretch during inspiration; when the force of contraction (respiratory muscular effort) is removed, the tissues return to their resting position. The resting position or lung volume is established when there is a balance of elastic forces. Under this condition, the elastic force of the lung tissues (Fig. 13-13) exactly equals those of the chest wall and diaphragm. This

Fig. 13-13. Balance of elastic forces in the lung at rest.

occurs at the end of every normal expiration, when the respiratory muscles are relaxed and the volume remaining in the lungs is the functional residual capacity (FRC).

The visceral pleura of the lung is separated from the parietal pleura of the chest wall by a thin film of fluid. In a normal person at the end of expiration, the mean pleural pressure is 3 to 5 cm $H_2O$ below atmospheric pressure. This pressure results from the equal and opposite retractive forces of the lungs and chest wall. Since there is no air movement at the end of expiration, gas throughout the lungs is in equilibrium with atmospheric air.

During inspiration, the inspiratory muscles contract, expanding the chest wall and lowering the diaphragm. Since the lungs tend to pull inward, this expansion results in a further reduction of pleural pressure. Therefore the more the chest wall is expanded during inspiration, the more subatmospheric is the resultant pleural pressure.

**Lung compliance.** If pressure is sequentially decreased (made more subatmospheric) around the outside of an excised lung, as shown in Fig. 13-14, the lung volume increases. When the pressure is removed from the lung, it deflates along a pressure-volume curve that is different from that during inflation. The difference between the inflation and deflation levels of the pressure-volume curve is called "hysteresis." The elastic behavior of the lungs is characterized by the pressure-volume curve. More specifically, the ratio of change in lung volume to change in distending pressure defines the compliance of the lungs. Although the pressure-volume relationship of the lung is not linear over the entire range, the compliance or slope ($\Delta V/\Delta P$) is linear over the normal range of tidal volumes beginning at functional residual capacity. Thus, for a given change in intrathoracic pressure, tidal volume will increase in propor-

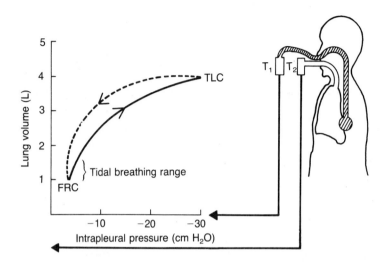

**Fig. 13-14.** Measurement of the pressure-volume curve of excised lung. (From Ruppel G: *Manual of pulmonary function testing,* ed 3, St Louis, 1982, Mosby).

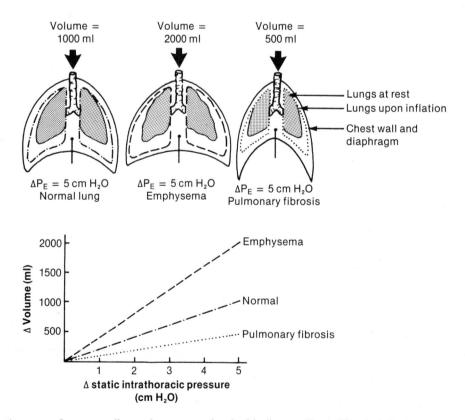

**Fig. 13-15.** Lung compliance changes associated with disease. (From Cherniack RM and others: *Respiration in health and disease,* ed 2, Philadelphia, 1972, WB Saunders Co.)

tion to lung compliance. As lung compliance is decreased, the lungs become stiffer and more difficult to expand. When lung compliance is increased, the lung becomes easier to distend, that is, more compliant.

Lung compliance and pressure-volume relationships are attributable to the interdependence of elastic tissue elements and alveolar surface tension. Tissue elasticity is dependent on the elastin and collagen content of the lung. A typical value for lung compliance in a young healthy adult would be 0.2 L/cm $H_2O$. This value is dependent on the size of the lung (mass of elastic tissue). As may be expected, compliance of the lung increases with development as the tissue mass of the lung increases.

In pulmonary fibrosis, collagen content is increased and lung compliance is reduced; in emphysema, elastin content is decreased (destruction of alveolar walls) and lung

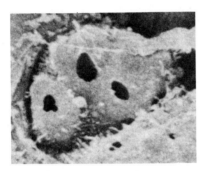

**Fig. 13-16.** Electron micrograph ($\times$ 10,000) of type II alveolar epithelial cell demonstrating presence of osmophilic lamellated bodies (LB). (From West JB: *Respiratory physiology,* ed 2. Baltimore, 1979. The Williams & Wilkins Co.)

compliance is increased as compared to normal (Fig. 13-15).

The surface-active material (surfactant) lining the alveoli of the lung has significant physiological function. Surfactant lowers surface tension inside the alveoli, thereby contributing to lung stability by reducing the pressure necessary to expand the alveoli. Alveolar type II cells (Fig. 13-16) contain osmophilic lamellated bodies that are associated with the transformation of surfactant. Impaired surface activity, as occurs in some premature infants, typically results in lungs that are stiff (low compliance) and prone to collapse (atelectasis).

**Chest wall compliance.** Like the lung, the chest wall is elastic. If air is introduced into the pleural cavity, the lungs will collapse inward and the chest wall will expand outward (Fig. 13-17). As previously discussed, there is a balance of elastic forces at rest (end of expiration) such that the lungs maintain a stable functional residual capacity (FRC) volume. In certain pathological conditions this balance of forces becomes disturbed. For example, as a result of destroyed elastic tissue in emphysema, the inward pull of the lungs is less than normal (increased compliance); therefore the chest wall is pulled out and the FRC is increased. In contrast, pulmonary fibrosis results in a greater elastic recoil than normal (decreased compliance), thereby pulling the chest wall inward and decreasing the FRC (Fig. 13-15).

Chest wall compliance and pressure-volume relationships are attributable to the elastic-tissue properties of the rib cage and diaphragm. A normal value for chest wall compliance in a healthy young adult would be 0.2 L/cm $H_2O$, approximately the same as lung compliance. Chest wall compliance may be decreased in kyphoscoliosis, skeletal muscle disorders, and abdominal disorders.

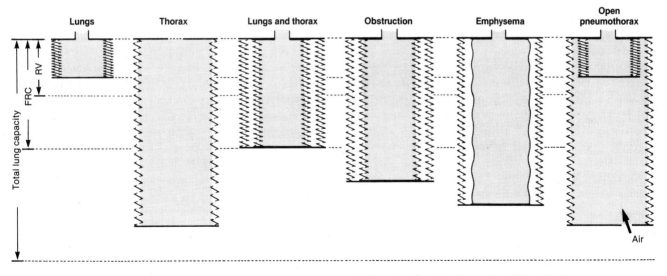

**Fig. 13-17.** Interaction of lungs and chest walls. *FRC,* Functional residual capacity; *RV,* residual volume. (Modified from Comroe JH Jr: *The lung,* ed 2, Chicago, 1962, Year Book Medical Publishers.)

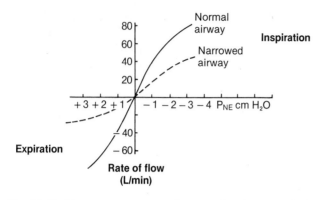

**Fig. 13-18.** Flow pressure curves for normal and narrowed airways. From Cherniack RM and others: *Respiration in health and disease,* ed 2, Philadelphia, 1972, WB Saunders Co.)

### Nonelastic behavior of the respiratory system

Nonelastic properties of the respiratory system characterize its resistance to motion. Because motion involves friction or loss of energy, whenever two surfaces are in contact, resistance to breathing occurs in any moving part of the respiratory system. These resistances would include frictional resistance to air flow, tissue resistance, and inertial forces. Lung resistance results predominantly (80%) from frictional resistance to air flow. Tissue resistance (19%) and inertia (1%) also influence lung resistance, but under normal conditions have a relatively small effect. Airflow through the airways requires a driving pressure generated by changes in alveolar pressure. When alveolar pressure is less than atmospheric pressure (during spontaneous inspiration), air flows into the lungs; when alveolar pressure is greater than atmospheric pressure, air flows out of the lungs. By definition, resistance to air flow ($R_A$) is equal to the pressure difference between alveolar and atmospheric pressure ($\Delta P$) divided by air flow $V$; therefore:

$$R_A = \frac{\Delta P}{\dot{V}}$$

Under normal tidal-volume breathing conditions, there is a linear relationship between airflow and driving pressure. As shown in Fig. 13-18, the slope of the flow-pressure curve changes as the airways narrow, indicating that the patient with airway obstruction has a greater resistance to air flow. Normal airway resistance in a young adult is approximately 1.0 cm $H_2O$/L/sec.

About 80% of the total resistance to air flow occurs in large airways to about the fourth to fifth generation of bronchial branching. Thus the finding that resistance to airflow is elevated in a patient usually indicates large-airway disease. Because the smaller airways contribute a small proportion of total airway resistance, they have been designated as the "short zone" of the lung, where airway obstruction can occur without easy detection.

**Mechanical factors influencing airway resistance.** The dimensions (length and cross-sectional area) of airways

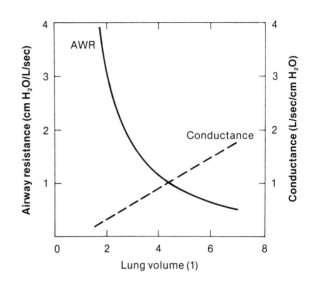

**Fig. 13-19.** Airway resistance and conductance as a function of lung volume. (From West JB: *Respiratory physiology,* ed 2, Baltimore, 1979, The Williams & Wilkins Co.)

are greatly influenced by lung volume. Small bronchi, bronchioles, and respiratory bronchioles have attachments to lung parenchyma so that with increases in volume, these airways are stretched. Like lung tissue, the airways are elastic. At high lung volumes, the pressure on the outer surface of the airway becomes more subatmospheric and transmural pressure (difference between inside and outside pressure of the airway) becomes greater. These pressure differences cause the airways to increase in cross-sectional area and decrease the resistance of airflow (Fig. 13-19).

During a forced expiration, dynamic compression of the airway can occur with a resulting increased resistance to airflow. Since smaller airways are more compressible than larger airways (no supporting cartilage in bronchiolar walls and beyond), smaller airways are more likely to collapse when the pressure outside the airway is greater than that inside (forced expiration) (Fig. 13-20). Further effort by the respiratory muscles produces no further increase in airflow. The increase in driving force is offset by dynamic compression of the airways. Patients with lung disease who have abnormal elastic and nonelastic properties of the lungs exhibit expiratory flow limitations at much lower levels of transmural pressure and lower lung volumes than that seen in normal subjects.

**Neural control of airway resistance.** The cross-sectional area of airways is also under control of airway smooth muscle tone, which results from constant parasympathetic impulses. Stimulation of parasympathetic cholinergic nerves causes contraction of airway smooth muscle with an increase in airway resistance, whereas sympathetic adrenergic stimulation causes relaxation with a decrease in airway resistance. Smooth muscle in large

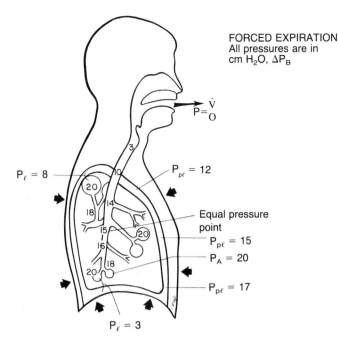

**Fig. 13-20.** Dynamic compression of the airways during forced expiration. (From Slonim NB and Hamilton LH: *Respiratory physiology,* ed 4, St Louis, 1981, Mosby.)

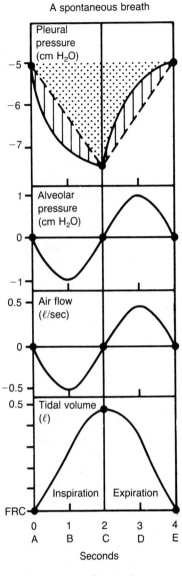

**Fig. 13-21.** Dynamic pressure: flow, volume recordings during quiet breathing. (From Moser K and Spragg RG: *Respiratory emergencies,* ed 2, St Louis, 1982, Mosby.)

airways has a more dense innervation than in small airways. Stimulation of vagal bronchioconstrictor fibers narrows the bronchioles, increases airway resistance, and decreases anatomical dead space, but enlarges the alveoli because of gas trapping.

**Airway obstruction.** Airway obstruction refers to a reduction in relative cross-sectional area of an airway resulting in an increase in airway resistance. The degree of severity of obstruction is also dependent on how diffusely the airways are involved. Finally, airway obstruction can be either partial or complete. Partial obstruction acts as a check valve by increasing resistance to air flow, impairing drainage of secretions, and reducing alveolar emptying to a greater degree during expiration. In complete airway obstruction there is no airflow or drainage of secretions.

### Testing and evaluation

The mechanical properties of the lung play an important role in established lung volume and the respiratory muscle force requirements for sustaining adequate alveolar ventilation. Like other pulmonary tests, the determination of lung mechanical properties is an important practical application of respiratory physiology for diagnosis and management of patients with lung disease.

**Lung compliance.** Lung compliance is a measure of the elastic properties of the lung and is defined as the change in lung volume per change in pressure across the lung.

To determine lung compliance, one first needs to measure intrapleural pressure. Clinically as well as experimentally, intrapleural pressure has been estimated by intraesophageal

measurements. This determination is accomplished when one has a subject swallow a small latex balloon attached to a catheter and pressure transducers. In addition, lung volume changes are determined by either spirometry or pneumotachography.

When lung compliance is measured during breathholding procedures (a subject breaths into or out of a spirometer in steps of 500 ml), the result is termed "quasi-static." Thus the ratio of the change in spirometer volume to the change in esophageal pressure provides an estimate of static lung compliance. It is also possible to measure lung compliance during quiet breathing. As shown in Fig. 13-21, there are two points in the respiratory cycle when airflow is zero: the end of inspiration and the end of expiration. Under these conditions all intrapleural pressure effort is associated with lung elastic forces. The change in tidal volume between these points per change in intrapleural (esophageal) pressure is a measure of dynamic lung compliance.

**Lung resistance.** Lung resistance is a measure of the nonelastic properties of the lungs and, accordingly, requires a dynamic measurement. Like compliance evaluations, intrapleural pressure measurements are required. In addition, simultaneous measurements of tidal volume and air flow are necessary (Fig. 13-21). As shown, intrapleural pressure reflects the forces required to overcome both elastic and nonelastic forces. The pressure required to overcome the elastic forces is represented by the dashed lines, whereas the additional pressure (that between 1 and 1′, 2 and 2′, etc., on the intrapleural pressure trace) is necessary to overcome tissue and airway resistance. Lung resistance (tissue and airway resistance) can therefore be determined at a specific point in the respiratory cycle (e.g., at point 1) as the change in pressure $(P_1 - P_{1'})$ divided by the airflow at that instant in time.

To measure airway resistance directly, we need to know alveolar pressure, since by definition this is the pressure difference between the alveoli and the mouth per unit of airflow. Alveolar pressure measurements (Fig. 13-21) require the use of a body plethysmograph (previously discussed in the measurement of functional residual capacity).

## GAS EXCHANGE AND TRANSPORT

Respiratory gas exchange takes place in the alveoli. Oxygen enters the blood from the alveolar air; carbon dioxide enters the alveolar air from the blood. There are several hundred million alveoli, which provide an enormous surface area (about the size of a tennis court) for such gas exchange. Blood flows through the walls of these alveoli in wide, short capillaries. It is as if a bubble of air were encased in a film of blood. The air and blood are separated by the thinnest of tissue barriers (less than 0.5 μm in width). These features make for rapid gas transfer between the air and blood.

### Respiratory exchange ratio

The volumes of oxygen and carbon dioxide that are exchanged depend on the metabolic activity of the tissues. During strenuous exercise the oxygen uptake by the blood may be 10 times the resting uptake. The volume of carbon dioxide that must be expired is correspondingly increased. Indeed there is a relationship between the oxygen uptake and the carbon dioxide output that depends on the type of fuel (glucose, amino acids, or fatty acids) being utilized in energy production. This relationship is known as the respiratory exchange ratio (R):

$$R = \frac{CO_2 \text{ output}}{O_2 \text{ uptake}}$$

The body normally uses a mixture of fuels; the exchange ratio is normally 0.8. When measured under basal conditions the ratio is termed the respiratory quotient (RQ).

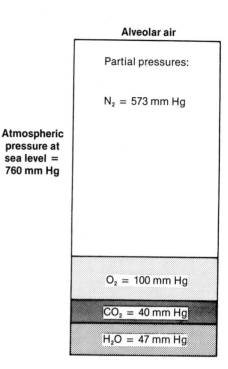

**Fig. 13-22.** Composition of alveolar air.

### Determinants of gas exchange

Gas exchange takes place in the alveolus by a process of diffusion. Diffusion is the random movement of molecules down their concentration gradient. The term "partial pressure" can be substituted for "concentration" when speaking of gas mixtures because the contribution of each gas to the total pressure of a gas mixture is directly proportional to the concentration of that gas in the mixture (Dalton's law). If the fractional concentration (F) of oxygen in a dry gas mixture is 21%, the partial pressure exerted by the oxygen is 21% of the total pressure. The total pressure of ambient (atmospheric) air is the barometric pressure. At sea level this is one atmosphere, or 760 mm Hg. The barometric pressure determines the total pressure of the air in the respiratory passages and the alveoli when the respiratory system is at rest.

Alveolar air is a mixture of nitrogen, oxygen, carbon dioxide, and water vapor (Fig. 13-22). The concentrations and consequently the partial pressures of these gases in the alveolar air differ considerably from their concentrations in the ambient air. In ambient air the water-vapor content (humidity) is variable. As the inspired air moves through the respiratory passages into the alveoli, it becomes fully saturated with water, and it is warmed to body temperature (37° C). Such air has a water vapor pressure of 47 mm Hg. The concentration of oxygen in the alveoli (about 14%) is much less than in ambient air (21%). Although the oxygen supply to the alveolus is periodically renewed during inspiration, oxygen is constantly removed from the alveolar air by the blood. The average partial pressure of oxygen in

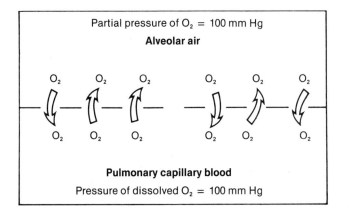

**Fig. 13-23.** Partial pressure of oxygen at an air-blood interface when the system is in equilibrium.

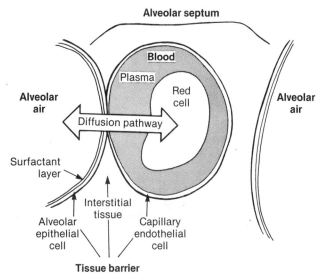

**Fig. 13-24.** Diffusion pathway for respiratory gases between alveolar air and pulmonary capillary blood.

alveolar air (PAo₂) at sea level is about 100 mm Hg. There is a negligible amount of carbon dioxide in ambient air and significant amounts (about 5.6%) in alveolar air because carbon dioxide is constantly being added to the alveolar air by the blood. During normal breathing the average partial pressure of alveolar carbon dioxide (PAco₂) is 40 mm Hg. If the carbon dioxide production by the tissues remains constant, a decrease in alveolar ventilation will result in an accumulation of carbon dioxide in the alveolus with an increase in its partial pressure. This is termed "hypoventilation." Conversely, an increase in alveolar ventilation will produce a decreased alveolar partial pressure of carbon dioxide.

When a liquid is exposed to a gas mixture, as pulmonary capillary blood is to alveolar air, the molecules of each gas diffuse between air and liquid until the pressure of the dissolved molecules equals the partial pressure of that gas in the gas mixture (Fig. 13-23). When equilibrium is achieved in the alveolus, the gas tensions in the end-pulmonary capillary blood are the same as the partial pressures of the gases in the alveolar air.

### Diffusion of respiratory gases

The diffusion pathway between air and red cells consists of both tissue and blood (Fig. 13-24). The tissue barrier, which is extremely thin, is made up of the surfactant lining the alveolus, the alveolar epithelium, the interstitial tissue, and the capillary endothelium. The blood barrier is made up of the plasma and the red cell membrane. Oxygen diffuses from alveolar air through the tissue and plasma into the red blood cell, where it combines with hemoglobin. The red blood cell also plays an important part in the handling of carbon dioxide. In the pulmonary capillary, carbon dioxide diffuses out of the red blood cell, through the plasma and the tissue barrier, into the alveolar air.

The rate of diffusion of a gas through a tissue barrier is dependent on several physical factors: the surface area (A) available for gas exchange; the thickness (T) of the tissue;

the partial pressure gradient across the tissue $(P_1 - P_2)$; and the diffusing constant (D) for the gas. The relationship of these factors is described in Fick's law:

$$\dot{V}_{gas} \propto \frac{A}{T} D \, (P_1 - P_2)$$

The alveolar surface area ranges from 50 to 100 square meters. However, for this surface to be available for gas exchange, blood must be flowing through the capillaries. At rest not all the pulmonary capillaries are open. During exercise additional capillaries are opened. In disease states alveolar walls may be destroyed (as in emphysema) or blood flow may be blocked by emboli.

Normally, the tissue barrier is extremely thin, but in disease states, such as pulmonary fibrosis, the interstitial tissues may be thickened. This widens the tissue barrier.

Not only is the direction of the partial pressure gradient the opposite for oxygen and carbon dioxide (from air to blood for oxygen, from blood to air for carbon dioxide), the gradient for oxygen (100 to 40 mm Hg) is also about 15 times that for carbon dioxide (44 to 40 mm Hg) (Fig. 13-25). Because carbon dioxide is more soluble than oxygen, the diffusing constant (D) for carbon dioxide is about 20 times that for oxygen. The net result of these two factors (partial pressure gradient and D) is that carbon dioxide diffuses across the tissue barrier more easily and faster than oxygen.

At the end of the diffusion pathway, oxygen enters the red blood cell and combines with hemoglobin. This chemical reaction influences the rate of transfer of oxygen from air to blood. A reduction in the volume of blood flowing through the capillary, a reduction in the red cell mass (anemia), or the presence of abnormal hemoglobin molecules, which do not readily combine with oxygen, will reduce the volume of oxygen taken up by the blood.

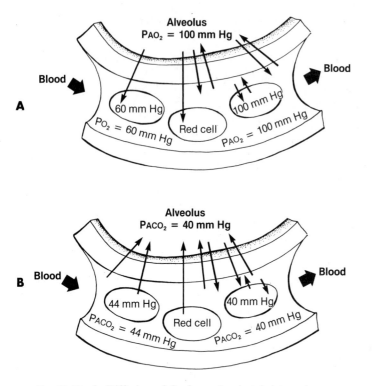

**Fig. 13-25. A,** Diffusion of $O_2$ from alveolar air into pulmonary capillary blood. **B,** Diffusion of $CO_2$ out of pulmonary capillary blood into alveolar air.

The normal transit time for blood through a pulmonary capillary is less than 1 second. The rate of diffusion for both oxygen and carbon dioxide is so rapid that equilibrium occurs in less than a fourth of that time. Even when the velocity of blood flow is increased, as occurs during exercise, there is ample time for equilibrium to be achieved. Only in disease states where the tissues are greatly thickened or the partial-pressure gradients are drastically reduced is equilibration incomplete between air and blood.

### Transport of gases

After the diffusion of oxygen from the alveolar air into the blood, oxygen is transported by the blood to the tissue capillaries. Here it diffuses out of the capillaries to the cells, which use it in the production of energy (ATP). The metabolic activity of the cells results in the production of carbon dioxide, which diffuses out of the cells into the tissue capillaries and is carried by the blood to the lungs, where it diffuses into the alveolar air and is expired.

As oxygen diffuses into the pulmonary blood, it is present as the dissolved gas. It quickly diffuses into the red blood cell, where it combines with hemoglobin to form oxyhemoglobin. It is in this form that all but about 1% to 2% of the oxygen is transported by the blood.

The red blood cell is an ideal transport mechanism for oxygen. Its biconcave shape gives it a large surface area; it is flexible and slips easily through narrow capillaries. Within the cell the hemoglobin molecules are densely packed. Also contained within the red blood cell are enzymes and agents, such as DPG (diphosphoglyceride), which aid in the rapid underloading of oxygen in the tissues.

Oxygen forms a reversible chemical combination with hemoglobin (oxyhemoglobin). When the hemoglobin is 100% saturated with oxygen, each molecule is capable of combining with four molecules of oxygen, or 1 gram of hemoglobin can combine with 1.34 ml of oxygen. This is the oxygen capacity of the blood:

$$O_2 \text{ capacity} = 1.34 \text{ ml } O_2 \text{ (gm Hb)}$$

It is the partial pressure of the dissolved oxygen molecules in the blood that primarily determines the volume of oxygen that combines with hemoglobin (percent hemoglobin saturation). The relationship is shown in the oxyhemoglobin dissociation curve (Fig. 13-26). As the partial pressure of dissolved oxygen ($Po_2$) increases, the percent saturation of hemoglobin increases. At the usual $Pao_2$ of arterial blood (100 mm Hg), the hemoglobin is about 97% saturated. Full saturation is achieved when the $Pao_2$ is in the range of 250 to 300 mm Hg. Such pressures are only produced when the individual breathes air enriched with oxygen. The actual volume of oxygen carried by the blood is termed the oxygen content. It depends upon the percentage saturation of the hemoglobin and the grams of hemoglobin available for oxygen transport:

$$O_2 \text{ content} = \% \text{ saturation of Hb } (O_2 \text{ cap}) + \text{ml dissolved } O_2$$

The volume of dissolved oxygen is not significant in the blood of an individual breathing room air.

The relationship of $Po_2$ to percent hemoglobin saturation produces an S-shaped curve. In the pulmonary capillaries the "loading" of oxygen onto the hemoglobin occurs in the flat portion of the curve. Dissolved oxygen tensions ranging from 90 to 110 mm Hg produce a hemoglobin saturation of about 97%. Increases of tension up to 135 mm Hg, such as might occur with hyperventilation, do not significantly increase this. Therefore the oxygen content of the blood does not increase with hyperventilation. In the tissue capillaries, where the "unloading" of oxygen from the hemoglobin takes place, the oxygen tensions are much lower (20 to 50 mm Hg). At these tensions the dissociation curve is steep. Relatively large volumes of oxygen are released with small decreases in tension. Hemoglobin unloads about 25% of its oxygen in the tissue capillaries. When a tissue is metabolically active, more oxygen is released or "extracted" from the hemoglobin.

An active tissue also produces more $CO_2$ and becomes acidotic, and the temperature of the tissue is raised. All these conditions increase the amount of $O_2$ released at any given $Po_2$. The oxyhemoglobin dissociation curve is said to be "shifted to the right."

The volume of oxygen delivered to the tissues depends not only on the oxygen content of the blood, but also on the

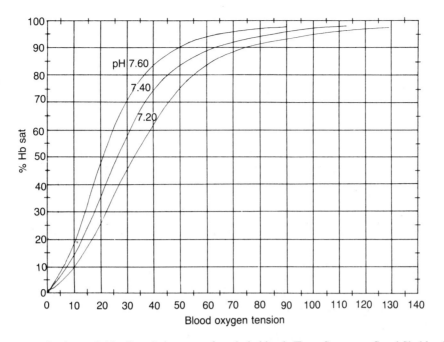

**Fig. 13-26.** Oxyhemoglobin dissociation curve for whole blood. (From Spearman C and Sheldon R: *Egan's fundamentals of respiratory therapy,* ed 4, St Louis, 1982, Mosby.)

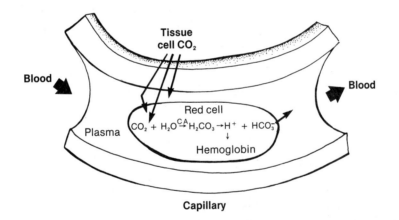

**Fig. 13-27.** Diffusion of $CO_2$ from tissue cell into tissue capillary blood. The major pathway for handling $CO_2$; the processing of $CO_2$ in the red cell in the presence of carbonic anhydrase (CA).

cardiac output. When the oxygen content of the arterial blood is reduced as a result of reduced oxygen tensions, a peripheral chemoreceptor reflex, triggered by the low oxygen tension, increases the cardiac output. Thus the oxygen supply to the tissues is increased.

Carbon dioxide is transported from the tissues to the lungs by way of the blood. Transport also involves the red blood cell. Carbon dioxide diffuses out of the tissue into the plasma and then into the red blood cell. Here it is processed (Fig. 13-27). $CO_2$, in the presence of the enzyme carbonic anhydrase, is rapidly hydrated into $H_2CO_3$. This latter compound quickly dissociates into $H^+$ and $HCO_3^-$. The bicarbonate ion then diffuses out of the red blood cell into the plasma. The hydrogen ion that remains within the red

blood cell is buffered by the hemoglobin. (Hemoglobin that has lost its oxygen is a better buffer than oxyhemoglobin.) About 65% of the carbon dioxide produced by the tissues is handled in this fashion, thus transported back to the lungs as bicarbonate.

Another 25% of the carbon dioxide entering the capillary combines with hemoglobin to form a carbamino compound. About 10% of the carbon dioxide remains as dissolved gas. It is the dissolved gas that produces the carbon dioxide tension of the blood.

Within the pulmonary capillaries the processes are reversed. $CO_2$ diffuses from the capillary blood into the alveolar air, and the chemical process within the red cell is reversed (Fig. 13-28). $H^+$ is released from the hemoglobin

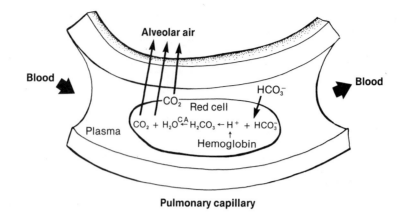

**Fig. 13-28.** Diffusion of $CO_2$ out of pulmonary capillary blood into alveolar air. Reversal of reactions seen in Fig. 12-31.

and $HCO_3^-$ diffuses into the red cell from the plasma. These combine to form $H_2CO_3$, which is rapidly dehydrated to $CO_2 + H_2O$, and the $CO_2$ diffuses out. The $CO_2$ dissociates from the hemoglobin. It is the average partial pressure of $CO_2$ within the alveolar air (determined by the alveolar ventilation) that determines the tension of $CO_2$ in the arterial blood.

### Testing and evaluation

The diffusing capability of the lung is known as the diffusing capacity ($D_{L\ gas}$). It is the measurement of the volume of a gas that diffuses into the blood per minute per millimeter of mercury partial pressure gradient. It differs for each gas, depending on the diffusing constant for the gas.

$$D_{L\ gas} = \text{ml of gas/min/mm Hg}$$

Clinically, carbon monoxide (CO) is used as the standard test gas. It measures the diffusing characteristics of the tissue component of the diffusion pathway. Because carbon monoxide combines 250 times more readily with hemoglobin than oxygen does, the diffusion of carbon monoxide into the pulmonary capillary is not limited by the blood flow. The patient breathes a very dilute mixture of known carbon monoxide concentration from a spirometer, holds his or her breath for 10 seconds, and then expels the mixture, and the carbon monoxide concentration in the expired air is measured.

$$D_{L_{CO}} = \frac{\text{vol of CO taken up by the blood/min}}{P_{ACO} - P_{aCO}}$$

where $A$ is the alveolus and $a$ is the artery. Again, because of the tremendous affinity of carbon monoxide for hemoglobin, all of the carbon monoxide entering the blood combines with the hemoglobin and no significant CO tension builds up. Thus the $P_{aCO}$ in the equation is zero.

The normal value for $D_{L_{CO}}$ is 25 ml/min/mm Hg. In exercise the $D_{L_{CO}}$ may be doubled as blood flow increases and capillaries are opened; in disease states, loss of surface area or thickening of the tissues may reduce the capacity to 4 to 5 ml.

## PULMONARY CIRCULATION

Blood flow through the alveolar capillaries is an integral part of gas exchange. The pulmonary circulation carries the entire output of the right heart through the lungs to the left heart (Fig. 13-29). The pulmonary blood vessels are short and wide compared to their systemic counterparts. Their walls, which contain far less smooth muscle than systemic vessels, are thin and compliant. Mixed venous blood flows from the right ventricle through the pulmonary artery and its branches into the pulmonary capillaries, which lie in the alveolar septa. The short, wide, intersecting capillaries maximize the exposure of the blood to the alveolar air. Finally, oxygenated blood is collected by the pulmonary veins and emptied into the left atrium. The veins are distensible and have the capacity to store an extra 300 to 500 ml of blood. Such storage occurs with a change in body position: with a change from standing to supine position, for example, blood is shifted out of veins in the lower extremities into the pulmonary veins.

At rest, some of the pulmonary capillaries are closed. When the cardiac output increases, as in exercise, closed capillaries are opened (recruitment) and those that were already open are distended. This increases the volume of blood exposed to alveolar air and increases the surface area available for gas exchange.

### Vascular mechanics

Resistance to blood flow through the short wide vessels is only about one tenth of that found in the systemic vessels. The differential pressure (between pulmonary artery pressure and left atrial pressure) needed to drive blood across the circuit is proportionately decreased (average, 15 mm Hg). When cardiac output increases, the compliant pulmonary vessels distend and resistance to blood flow actually drops.

Indeed, there are very few situations in which pulmonary vascular resistance increases. The lowest resistance is found at the FRC. Changes in the dimensions of the vessels during both deep inspiration and deep expiration cause increases in

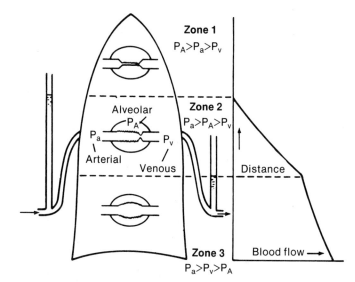

**Fig. 13-30.** Zones of West. (From West JB: *Respiratory physiology,* ed 2, Baltimore, 1979, The Williams & Wilkins Co.)

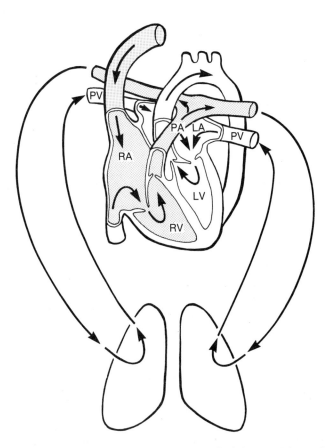

**Fig. 13-29.** The pulmonary circulation. *Shaded area,* Flow of unoxygenated blood. *RA,* Right atrium; *RV,* right ventricle; *PA,* pulmonary artery; *PV,* pulmonary vein; *LA,* left atrium; *LV,* left ventricle.

resistance. At high lung volumes the alveolar vessels are stretched and narrowed; at very low lung volumes the extra-alveolar vessels (small pulmonary arteries) narrow because of the elastic recoil of their walls, which are no longer pulled open by the lung parenchyma.

Active vasoconstriction will increase pulmonary resistance. Such vasoconstriction is produced chiefly by low alveolar oxygen tensions but also by high carbon dioxide tensions and acidosis. The response of the pulmonary vessels to the altered respiratory gases is in direct contrast to the response of systemic arterioles, which dilate when exposed to low interstitial oxygen tensions and high carbon dioxide tensions. When the alveolar gas changes are localized, blood is shunted away from these areas to alveoli that are better ventilated. However, when hypoventilation is generalized, the total pulmonary vascular resistance is increased. Pulmonary artery pressure rises (pulmonary hypertension), and so the work of the right ventricle is increased. In some cases right heart failure (cor pulmonale) develops.

Under normal circumstances sympathetic stimulation to the pulmonary vessels does not cause significant vasoconstriction. However, humoral substances such as histamine can cause vasoconstriction.

Blood flow is not evenly distributed to all alveoli. Flow through the pulmonary capillaries depends on the relation-

ship of alveolar air pressures to capillary hydrostatic pressures. Although the alveolar air pressures are essentially the same in all alveoli, the capillary pressures are varied. In an upright person the effect of gravity lowers the hydrostatic pressure of the blood as it rises above the level of the pulmonary artery and augments the pressures in vessels below the level of the pulmonary artery. The zones of West (Fig. 13-30) describe the pressure-flow relationships. In zone I, at the apex of the lung, there is no blood flow through the alveolar capillaries. Alveolar air pressures are greater than capillary hydrostatic pressures; the capillaries are compressed. By far the largest portion of the lung is zone II. Pulmonary arteriole pressures are greater here than alveolar air pressures, but pressure at the venous end of the capillaries is less than air pressure. Blood flow is determined by the pressure difference between the pulmonary arterioles and alveolar air. With advancement toward the more dependent portions of the lung, the intracapillary pressures increase and flow increases. In zone III, or the dependent portion of the lung, venous hydrostatic pressures exceed alveolar air pressures. Capillaries are wide open, and flow is unrestricted. In the normal lung, blood flow increases tenfold from apex to base in the upright person. In zone IV, which is only present in cases of interstitial edema or fibrosis, the tissue compresses the alveolar capillaries and reduces blood flow.

The pulmonary capillaries are more permeable to plasma proteins than systemic capillaries are. The protein content of the pulmonary interstitial tissue is 10 to 20 times that of systemic tissues. This increases the interstitial osmotic pressure and significantly alters the Starling forces (Table 13-1). Filtration occurs along the entire length of the alveolar capillary. In normal persons the alveolar epithelium is quite impermeable to small solutes. The filtered fluid does not enter the alveoli, but is carried away by the lymphatics. The

**Table 13-1.** Starling forces

| Pressure (mm Hg) | Promoting | |
|---|---|---|
| | Filtration | Reabsorption |
| Capillary hydrostatic | 10 | |
| Capillary osmotic | | 25 |
| Interstitial tissue | −4 | |
| Interstitial osmotic | 15 | |
| TOTAL | 29 | 25 |

lymphatics can handle up to 10 times the normal volume of lymph. When the rate of filtration increases above this, fluid accumulates in the interstitial tissue (pulmonary edema) and ultimately enters the alveoli.

### Matching of blood and gas

For ideal gas exchange, equal volumes of fresh air entering the alveoli should come into contact with equal volumes of blood flowing through the alveolar capillaries. In other words, alveolar ventilation ($\dot{V}_A$) should match the pulmonary blood flow ($Q$). The relationship of the two flows is the ventilation/perfusion ratio, or the $\dot{V}/\dot{Q}$ ratio. In the ideal matching of equal volumes of gas and blood, the ratio would be 1. However, when one is considering the lungs as a whole, the ratio is less than one. A normal alveolar ventilation of 4 L/min is usually matched with a 5 L/min cardiac output, which would give a $\dot{V}/\dot{Q}$ ratio of 4/5, or 0.8.

Usually $\dot{V}/\dot{Q}$ ratio is considered for various areas of the lungs and not for the lungs as a whole. Alveolar ventilation and blood flow vary independently throughout the lung. Ventilation of lung units depends on their compliance and the patency of the airways; blood flow is unequally distributed and is dependent on the principles described by the zones of West or the patency of blood vessels. In an upright person blood flow is less than ventilation at the lung apex because some of the capillaries are compressed (zone I of West). The $\dot{V}/\dot{Q}$ ratio is high. At the base of the lung, ventilation is three times greater but blood flow is 10 times greater than that at the apex. The $\dot{V}/\dot{Q}$ at the bases is low. In chronic obstructive pulmonary disease, large areas of the lung may have reduced ventilation because of the blockage of the bronchioles by secretions. Large areas of low $\dot{V}/\dot{Q}$ ratios results.

In areas of the lung with low $\dot{V}/\dot{Q}$ ratios, the renewal of the alveolar oxygen supply is sufficient to oxygenate adequately the blood flowing through the pulmonary capillaries. The end-capillary blood is not fully oxygenated. This is termed a "physiological intrapulmonary shunt" (Fig. 13-31). The poorly oxygenated blood from these areas mixes with blood from other better ventilated areas. The total oxygen content of the mixed blood is reduced. In lung disease the presence of large areas of the lung with low $\dot{V}/\dot{Q}$

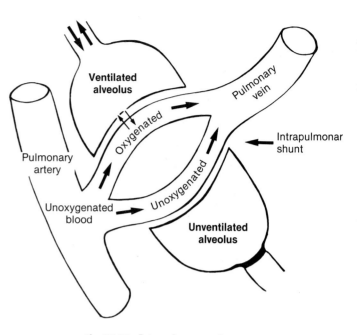

**Fig. 13-31.** Intrapulmonary shunt.

ratios is the most common cause of low arterial oxygen (hypoxemia). Although the carbon dioxide concentrations in the poorly ventilated alveoli are increased when mixing occurs with blood from other areas, the carbon dioxide tension of the final mixture in the aorta is usually within normal limits. This normal carbon dioxide tension occurs for two reasons: the venous-arterial gradient for carbon dioxide is small, and so there is only a small increase in $Pa_{CO_2}$ from the areas with low $\dot{V}/\dot{Q}$ ratios and a small decrease in $Pa_{CO_2}$ from the better ventilated areas. In addition, the neural respiratory controls adjust the alveolar ventilation to maintain a normal $Pa_{CO_2}$.

When ventilation exceeds blood flow, the $\dot{V}/\dot{Q}$ ratio is high. There is excess alveolar ventilation, and not all of the ventilated air takes part in gas exchange. This produces an "alveolar dead space" and is often termed "wasted" ventilation.

The end-pulmonary capillary blood from all areas of the lung mixes as it flows into the left side of the heart. Blood from areas with low $\dot{V}/\dot{Q}$ ratios has a lower oxygen tension than normal. It constitutes an "intrapulmonary" shunt. Such blood from low $\dot{V}/\dot{Q}$ areas lowers the oxygen tension in the final mixture, the aortic blood. A small amount of blood from bronchial and thebesian veins also flows directly into the pulmonary veins and the left side of the heart. This venous admixture also lowers the oxygen tension of the blood (Fig. 13-32). Because of these mixtures, the oxygen tension of the blood ejected into the aorta never equals the average alveolar oxygen tension. This difference is known as the "alveolar-arterial difference," or the "A-a gradient."

In normal persons the A-a gradient is small, amounting to about 6 to 10 mm Hg when room air is breathed. In persons with pulmonary disease, large areas with low $\dot{V}/\dot{Q}$ ratios may

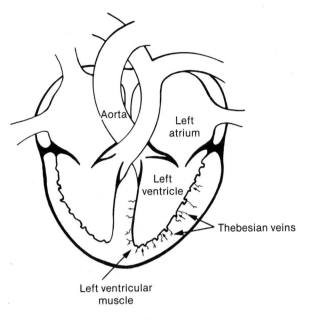

**Fig. 13-32.** Thebesian veins.

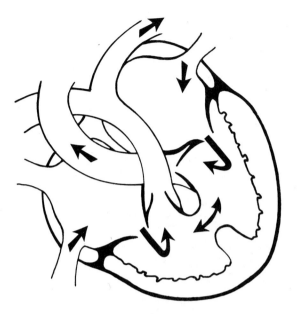

**Fig. 13-33.** Septal defect between the right ventricle and left ventricle.

be present, and the A-a gradient may be as much as 30 to 40 mm Hg in room air. In persons with congenital heart disease, abnormal openings in the atrial or ventricular septum may occur (Fig. 13-33). Large volumes of blood may be shunted directly from the right side of the heart into the left side, creating a large venous admixture, a large A-a gradient, and very low arterial oxygen tensions.

### Testing and evaluation

Examination of the arterial blood gases is a means of determining the overall adequacy of the gas-exchange mechanisms. Blood is obtained by arterial (radial, brachial, femoral) puncture. The oxygen tension ($Pa_{O_2}$) and the carbon dioxide tension ($Pa_{CO_2}$) are measured. The normal $Pa_{O_2}$ ranges from 90 to 110 mm Hg. A reduction in $Pa_{O_2}$ could be caused by reduced oxygen tension in the inspired air ($PI_{O_2}$), hypoventilation, inadequate diffusion across a thickened tissue barrier, low $\dot{V}/\dot{Q}$ ratios, or increased anatomical shunts (Fig. 13-34). If at the same time the arterial sample is taken, the alveolar oxygen tension ($PA_{O_2}$) is calculated by using the modified alveolar air equation, the A-a gradient can be determined. The modified alveolar air equation is as follows:

$$PA_{O_2} = PI_{O_2} - Pa_{CO_2} \, (1.25)$$

The arterial $P_{CO_2}$ is also very helpful. Since there is virtually no gradient for $P_{CO_2}$ between the alveolar air and the arterial blood, the arterial $P_{CO_2}$ represents the average alveolar $P_{CO_2}$. Normal $P_{CO_2}$ ranges from 38 to 42 mm Hg. A high arterial $P_{CO_2}$ (over 44 mm Hg) reflects a high alveolar $P_{CO_2}$ and is caused by hypoventilation; a low arterial $P_{CO_2}$ represents a low alveolar $P_{CO_2}$ and indicates hyperventilation.

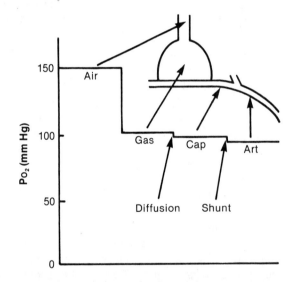

**Fig. 13-34.** Changes in the partial pressure of $O_2$ as oxygen moves from inspired air to the arterial blood. (From West JB: *Ventilation/blood flow and gas exchange,* ed 3, 1977, Blackwell Scientific Publications.)

## CONTROL OF BREATHING
### Automatic and voluntary mechanisms

Control of respiratory muscle activity arises from within the central nervous system. The rate and depth of respiration are regulated by two control systems—the automatic and the voluntary mechanisms—that usually interact with each other (Fig. 13-35). Both systems terminate in a final common pathway, comprised of the spinal motor neurons, that innervates the respiratory muscles. Any disease process that involves either the motor nerves or the respiratory muscles will interfere with both sets of controls.

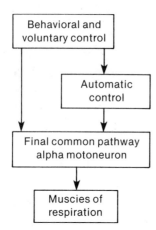

Fig. 13-35. Relationship between voluntary and automatic respiratory control pathways.

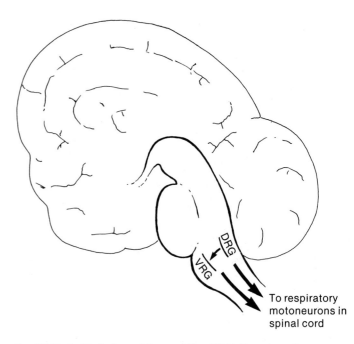

Fig. 13-36. Lateral view of the medulla. *DRG,* Dorsal respiratory group of neurons; *VRG,* ventral respiratory group of neurons.

The most important control system is the automatic mechanism that originates in the brainstem. It produces spontaneous, cyclical respiration. Voluntary or behavioral control, important during verbal communication, arises from the cerebral cortex. This control typically exerts a modifying influence on the automatic activity. However, there is a direct pathway from the cortex to the spinal motor neurons that can, on occasion, function independently of the automatic control system.

The spontaneous neuronal activity that produces cyclic breathing originates in the respiratory centers in the dorsal region of the medulla (Fig. 13-36). These neurons drive the ventral medullary centers. Together the centers drive contralateral respiratory muscles. Destruction of these medullary centers, associated with bulbar poliomyelitis, eliminates all automatic breathing, though voluntary respiratory activity is still possible. Breathing produced by the medullary centers is weak and irregular. When the activity of the two pontine centers (the apneustic and the pneumotaxic) is superimposed on that of the medullary centers, breathing becomes strong, regular, and effective. This activity is further modified by the central and peripheral chemoreceptors, peripheral reflexes from the lungs and other parts of the body, and by the cortical centers.

### Central and peripheral chemoreceptor mechanisms

The dominant normal regulation of the respiratory centers usually arises from the chemoreceptors. These mechanisms modify alveolar ventilation to ensure that the blood gases remain within normal limits. Of the two respiratory gases, carbon dioxide is most tightly controlled. The central chemoreceptors, which lie just below the surface of the ventrolateral aspects of the medulla, monitor the carbon dioxide levels of both the arterial blood and the cerebrospinal fluid. Carbon dioxide rapidly diffuses out of the cerebral capillaries into the interstitial tissue of the brain. It reacts with water to produce free hydrogen ions:

$$CO_2 + H_2O \rightarrow H_2CO_3 \rightarrow H^+ + HCO_3^-$$

It is the hydrogen ions that stimulate the central chemoreceptor cells, which in turn stimulate the medullary centers.

Thus a rise in $Pa_{CO_2}$ produces an increase in alveolar ventilation, which restores the $Pa_{CO_2}$ levels to the normal (40 mm Hg) range.

A second group of chemoreceptors, the peripheral chemoreceptors, are found in the carotid and aortic bodies that lie outside the walls of the carotid sinus and the aortic arch (Fig. 13-37). The carotid chemoreceptors are stimulated by low arterial oxygen tensions, high arterial carbon dioxide tensions, and acidosis. The stimulation is carried through the afferent sensory nerve (cranial nerve IX) to the brainstem. The medullary centers are stimulated, and ventilation is increased. The aortic chemoreceptors are not involved in ventilation, but produce reflex cardiovascular responses (i.e., stimulation increases the heart rate and raises the BP). In addition to responding to the same stimuli as the carotid chemoreceptors, they are also stimulated by a low oxygen content of the arterial blood.

The peripheral chemoreceptors demonstrate low-grade tonic activity, which contributes to normal ventilation. However, stimulation by arterial oxygen tensions below 60 mm Hg produces a strong respiratory drive. High arterial carbon dioxide tensions and acidosis act synergistically with low oxygen tensions. The reflex drive, from the carotid body in particular, can stimulate brainstem centers, which are depressed by narcotics or anoxia, into activity and thus maintain breathing. At high altitudes, when inspired oxygen tensions are reduced, peripheral chemoreceptor stimulation overrides the central chemoreceptor regulation. In such a situation a person may hyperventilate in an attempt to maintain normal arterial oxygen levels at

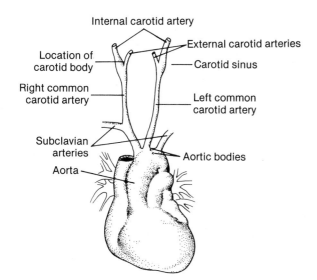

Fig. 13-37. The aortic and carotid bodies.

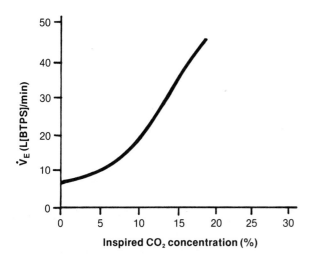

**Fig. 13-38.** Diagram of the ventilatory response to increase $CO_2$ concentrations in the alveolar air and in the arterial blood. *BTPS,* Body temperature, ambient pressure, saturated with water vapor. (Modified from Slonim NB and Hamilton LH: *Respiratory physiology,* ed 5, St Louis, 1987, Mosby.)

the expense of arterial carbon dioxide levels, which are reduced.

## Lung and peripheral reflex mechanisms

The lungs contain sensory receptors that stimulate reflex respiratory activity. Although these reflexes are not usually active, they can override the normal chemical control of breathing.

The longest known lung reflex is the Hering-Breuer reflex (inflation reflex), which is stimulated by inflation of the lung during inspiration. The reflex response is to inhibit inspiration. This reflex is too weak to control the depth of the tidal volume during normal breathing. It is only during very deep inspiration, under anesthesia, in newborns, or in some

patients with lung disease that the signals become strong enough to inhibit inspiration and thus regulate the depth of breathing.

A more important reflex is that produced by stimulation of the irritant receptors. This is one of the lung's defense mechanisms against noxious materials. The receptors lie in the epithelial lining of the airways. They are stimulated by inhaled particles, by irritant gases, or by excessive amounts of sticky mucus produced by the respiratory tract itself. The reflex response is a sneeze if the stimulus occurs in the upper airways or a cough if the stimulus is in the lower airways.

A less well-understood lung reflex is that produced by the "J receptors," which lie within the lung parenchyma. These are stimulated by interstitial edema and by some inhaled gases. The response is rapid, shallow breathing (tachypnea).

In asthma, pulmonary embolism, and heart failure, a frequent finding is a low $Pa_{CO_2}$. This is probably produced by the reflex hyperventilation caused by stimulation of either the irritant or the J receptors.

Stimulation of peripheral pain receptors will also produce reflex hyperventilation, accompanied by tachycardia and a rise in blood pressure. Visceral pain may produce the opposite effect: inhibition of breathing, a slow pulse, and a fall in blood pressure.

## Control mechanisms during exercise and sleep

The control of breathing during both sleep and exercise is worthy of further examination. During slow-wave sleep sensory stimuli are reduced, behavioral modifications are minimal, the central control mechanisms are depressed, and alveolar ventilation is reduced. The arterial $CO_2$ runs 2 to 3 mm Hg higher than in the waking state. The situation is very different during REM (rapid eye movement) sleep. Breathing becomes irregular. Muscular activity is greatly reduced; indeed, the skeletal muscles, including those of the larynx and pharynx, relax. This may produce upper airway obstruction and apnea. This type of apnea is termed "obstructive." Arousal occurs when the increasingly low $Pa_{O_2}$ and high $Pa_{CO_2}$ stimulate the carotid chemoreceptors. This type of "sleep apnea" is seen in all persons; however, it is especially frequent in older men. In patients with chronic obstructive pulmonary disease whose normal ventilation is severely reduced, further reduction attributable to apneic episodes may be extremely detrimental. If the depression of the central mechanisms is severe enough, a "central" type of sleep apnea may occur. Respiratory activity ceases until arousal occurs. This may be a cause of the sudden infant death syndrome.

During exercise the use of oxygen and the production of carbon dioxide increase. Yet the control of respiration is such that alveolar ventilation is correspondingly increased and the blood gas levels remain within normal limits, except during the most severe exercise. The central chemoreceptors are certainly involved in this control, as are peripheral reflexes from muscles and joints, but the whole picture is not clear;

perhaps other chemoreceptors, as yet undefined, in the lungs or the pulmonary vasculature are involved.

## Testing and evaluation

Evaluation of the central chemoreceptors involves breathing increasing concentrations of $CO_2$ in 100% $O_2$. As the concentration of inspired $CO_2$ is increased, ventilation should increase (Fig. 13-38). One can test the function of the peripheral chemoreceptor by having the person breathe gas mixtures with reduced oxygen concentrations. The difficulty with these tests is that so many other stimuli, such as auditory and visual, can alter respiration, and the pure effect of the altered respiratory gases may be obscured.

## SUGGESTED READINGS

Bouhuys A: *The physiology of breathing,* New York, 1977, Grune & Stratton, Inc.

Cherniack RM, Cherniack L, and Ziment J: *Respiration in health and disease,* ed 3, Philadelphia, 1983, WB Saunders Co.

Clausen JL, editor: *Pulmonary function testing: guidelines and controversies,* New York, 1982, Academic Press, Inc.

Comroe JH: *Physiology of respiration,* ed 2, Chicago, 1974, Year Book Medical Publishers.

Comroe JH and others: *The lung, clinical physiology and pulmonary function tests,* Chicago, 1962, Year Book Medical Publishers.

Fishman AP: *Assessment of pulmonary function,* New York, 1980, McGraw-Hill Book Co.

Green JF: *Fundamental cardiovascular and pulmonary physiology: an integrated approach for medicine.* Philadelphia, 1982, Lea & Febiger.

Kryger MH, editor: *Pathophysiology of respiration,* New York, 1981, John Wiley & Sons, Inc.

Scanlan C and others: *Egan's fundamentals of respiratory care,* St. Louis, 1994, Mosby.

Slonim NB and Hamilton R: *Respiratory physiology,* ed 5, St. Louis, 1987, Mosby.

Tisi GM: *Pulmonary physiology in clinical medicine.* Baltimore, 1980, The Williams & Wilkins Co.

Vander A, Sherman JH, and Luciana D: *Human physiology,* ed 3, New York, 1980, McGraw-Hill Book Co.

West JB: *Respiratory physiology: the essentials,* ed 4, Baltimore, 1990, The Williams & Wilkins Co.

West JB: *Pulmonary pathophysiology: the essentials,* ed 4, Baltimore, 1992, The Williams & Wilkins Co.

# CHAPTER 14

# Common Pulmonary Diseases

*Jan Stephen Tecklin*

To provide a rationale for therapeutic intervention and to understand the possible outcomes of that intervention, the physical therapist must know the basic features of the numerous lung diseases that afflict patients. This chapter presents both an overview of the major groups of pulmonary disorders and specific details about individual diseases and disorders.

## CHRONIC OBSTRUCTIVE DISEASES

The terms "chronic obstructive lung disease," "chronic obstructive pulmonary disease," "chronic airways obstruction," "chronic airflow obstruction," and other similar phrases describe a spectrum of diseases from pulmonary emphysema to chronic bronchitis but usually include some characteristics of each disorder. Reduction in expiratory flow rates is the consistent feature of disorders within this spectrum. Expiratory airflow reduction is caused by several pathophysiological factors and results in numerous signs and symptoms that are closely associated with the various diseases. Two other diseases are often included under the classification of chronic obstructive diseases—asthma and cystic fibrosis. Because it is episodic, asthma is not a classic chronic lung disease, but cystic fibrosis fits the group because of its chronic obstructive and progressive pattern.

### Pulmonary emphysema

Pulmonary emphysema actually includes several diseases that ultimately result in destruction of pulmonary structures, most notably alveolar walls distal to the terminal bronchiole. The disease is common: some studies have reported that as many as two thirds of all autopsies in men and one seventh of autopsies in women show clear signs of emphysema. Cigarette smoking is the clearest etiological agent for pulmonary emphysema. The most severe forms of emphysema are found in cigarette smokers; virtually any time more than mild effects of emphysema are found, the person was a smoker.

The pathogenesis of emphysema stems from either the lack of proteolytic enzyme inhibitors or an overabundance of proteolytic enzymes. In either case, enzymatic destruction of pulmonary architecture will occur. Alpha$_1$ antitrypsin deficiency is an inherited disorder that serves as a prototype for lung destruction caused by a deficiency in proteolytic enzyme inhibitors. As a result of the protease inhibitor absence, naturally occurring proteases (enzymes) destroy elastic tissue in alveolar walls, thereby causing larger than normal air spaces. The excessively large and ineffective air spaces are a hallmark of pulmonary emphysema. The second mechanism for emphysema is an overabundance of proteolytic enzymes. Cigarette smoke is thought to be the most common cause of this mechanism. As cigarette smoke is

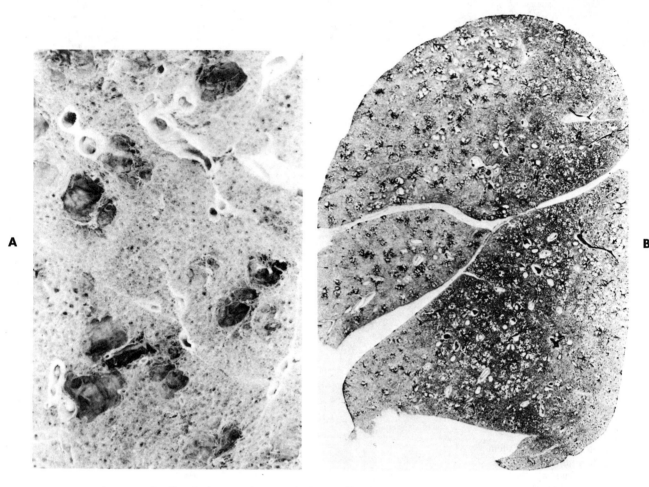

**Fig. 14-1. A,** Centriacinar emphysema: barium sulfate-impregnated lung. Enlarged, abnormal airspaces in center of lobules are surrounded by normal tissue. **B,** Centriacinar emphysema: paper-mounted lung section. (**B,** Courtesy of Dr. AA Liebow; **A** and **B** reproduced from Kissane JM: *Anderson's pathology,* ed 9, St Louis, 1990, Mosby.)

inhaled, an inflammatory response occurs within the airways. Neutrophils and macrophages, cells commonly active during the inflammatory process, are found in abundance in the airways of smokers. After participating in the inflammatory activity, these cells necrose, at which time they liberate proteolytic enzymes that digest and destroy lung parenchyma. Either or both of these mechanisms can exist in an individual, and when they exist together, a more severe form of the disorder is often found. This describes two common types of emphysema; identifications of other less common types follow.

The name of any particular type of emphysema is based primarily on the portion of the acinus or primary lobule that has been most affected by the disease. The acinus is the section of lung parenchyma supplied by an individual respiratory bronchiole. Centrilobular (centriacinar) emphysema is characterized by destruction of the more central portion of the acinus nearer to the respiratory bronchiole. Centrilobular emphysema is the dominant form associated with smoking. In this pattern of destruction, distal alveolar

septa are usually spared, and there is a classic pattern seen on histological specimens (Fig. 14-1). In panlobular (panacinar) emphysema, a more generalized, evenly distributed destruction of acinar elements is found (Fig. 14-2). This type of emphysema is more commonly associated with alpha₁ antitrypsin deficiency, although it coexists with centrilobular emphysema in some smokers. Panlobular emphysema also tends to be more evenly distributed throughout the lungs as opposed to centrilobular emphysema, which predominates in the upper lobes. Localized emphysema, also referred to as paraseptal or distal acinar emphysema, describes the disease in which a few local areas of the distal portions of the acinus, the alveolar ducts and sacs, are involved. The fourth major type of emphysema is paracicatricial, or irregular, emphysema which is also referred to as airspace enlargement with fibrosis. This disorder is usually adjacent to a previous pulmonary lesion that has healed by scarring, as might occur with pneumoconiosis or tuberculosis. Unless large areas of paracicatricial emphysema exist, there are usually no symptoms or major problems associated with the disorder.

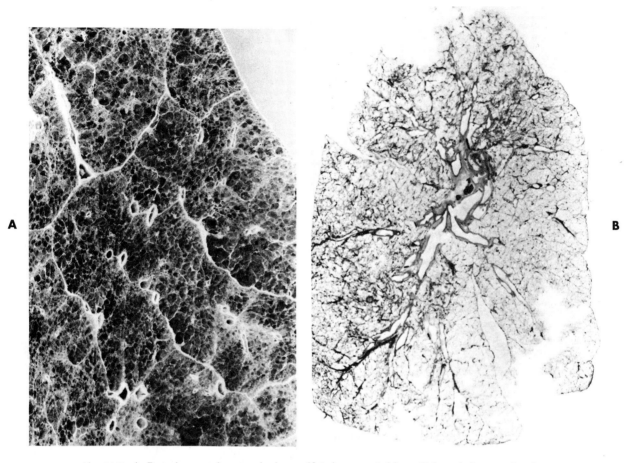

**Fig. 14-2. A,** Panacinar emphysema: barium sulfate-impregnated lung. Enlarged airspaces involve lobule uniformly. **B,** Panacinar emphysema: paper-mounted lung section. (**B** courtesy Dr. AA Liebow; **A** and **B** reproduced from Kissane JM: *Anderson's pathology,* ed 9, St Louis, 1990, Mosby.)

Most pathophysiological problems in emphysema are caused by the protease destruction of acinar support structures. With the loss of alveolar walls, large air spaces form from what had previously been small, effective alveoli. These air spaces have a reduced surface area for gas exchange, and their distention may have a negative effect on pulmonary perfusion. As elastic tissue within the alveolar walls and between respiratory bronchioles is destroyed, elastic recoil of the lung is lost along with radial traction. The former results in air-trapping; the latter causes early airway collapse during expiration, which contributes to air-trapping. These are the basic physiological changes caused by pulmonary emphysema.

Signs and symptoms of emphysema include dyspnea on exertion early in the disease, dyspnea at rest as the disease progresses, coughing, prolonged expiration, physical inactivity and resultant deconditioning, use of accessory inspiratory muscles, increased anteroposterior diameter of the thorax resulting from hyperinflation (barrel chest) with hyperresonance to mediate percussion, and a flattened diaphragm caused by the mechanical force of the hyperinflated lungs. Breath sounds are distant because of the hyperinflated thorax, but adventitious sounds such as wheezes and crackles are not extremely obvious. The patient often assumes a position of sitting and leaning forward on the arms to afford better mechanical advantage to the accessory inspiratory muscles despite the fact that the hyperinflated thorax offers little inspiratory reserve. This limited reserve is caused by a rib cage and inspiratory musculature that is in a position of virtual maximum inspiration at all times.

### Chronic bronchitis

Chronic bronchitis has been defined as a disorder in which a patient's cough is productive of sputum on most days for at least 3 consecutive months out of a year for at least 2 consecutive years. As with pulmonary emphysema, chronic bronchitis is more common in men and in individuals older than 40 years. The disease has a strong association with cigarette smoking, although a significant percentage of people with chronic bronchitis do not have a smoking history. Approximately 10% to 25% of adults are afflicted by chronic bronchitis.

The pathogenesis of chronic bronchitis is not fully elucidated, although a strong relationship to cigarette smoking is presumed. The notion is that smoking results in airway inflammation that, as a result of an unknown series of events, causes the specific pathological changes seen in mucous glands and epithelial goblet cells. Certain environmental factors, including heavy air pollution and industrial exposure to inhaled matter or fumes, will exacerbate the pathological response of mucous-producing cells.

The pathological changes associated with chronic bronchitis are found in the two sources of bronchial mucus—epithelial goblet cells and mucous-secreting bronchial glands. The glands produce almost all of the bronchial mucus, whereas, goblet cells are responsible for relatively little volume of mucus. The bronchial glands also produce serous fluid.

In people with chronic bronchitis there is an enlargement of the glands themselves (hypertrophy) and an increase in the number of mucous-secreting cells (hyperplasia). Several scientists have attempted to quantify the relationship of the gland size to the size of the bronchial wall. The Reid index is the most widely employed method of quantification. This index is determined by dividing the thickness of the bronchial mucous gland by the thickness of the entire bronchial wall. The Reid index for men with no sign of chronic bronchitis was in the vicinity of 25%, whereas those with the disorder had bronchial glands that were closer to 60% of the thickness of the bronchial wall (Fig. 14-3). As the mucous gland enlarges, the number and ratio of goblet cells in the respiratory epithelium increase. Although the normal ratio of goblet cells to ciliated cells in the larger airways is approximately 1:20, airways in some patients with chronic bronchitis have more goblet cells than ciliated cells. These pathological changes—along with the possible presence of chronic inflammatory cells, an increase in bronchial smooth muscle, possible atrophy in bronchial cartilage, and other less well-established changes—result in the pathophysiological changes associated with this disorder.

Airway obstruction and associated decreased expiratory flow rates are the major pathophysiological events that stem from chronic bronchitis. Obstruction of the airways is thought to occur from two major sources. The production of increased amounts of mucus will mechanically obstruct bronchi despite intact mechanisms of mucociliary clearance and coughing, which normally protect against airway obstruction. The second major cause of obstruction may be the increased size of the glands, which may increase the size of the bronchial wall causing reduction in the caliber of the bronchial lumen. In addition, possible inflammatory changes, bronchial smooth muscle hypertrophy, and loss of bronchial cartilage stability may add to the airway obstruction seen with chronic bronchitis. The airway obstruction is most clearly demonstrated by a decreased forced expiratory volume in 1 second ($FEV_1$) and by increased airway resistance. Unlike emphysema, chronic bronchitis results in little or no loss of radial traction on the distal airways or in decreased alveolar

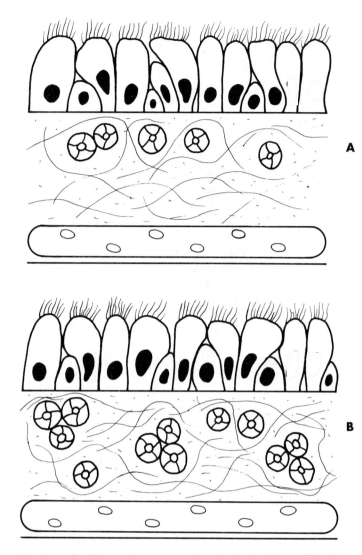

**Fig. 14-3. A,** Schematic representation of the Reid index (the normal relationship between the thickness of the submucosal gland layer and the thickness of the bronchial wall). **B,** Schematic representation of the changes in the bronchial submucosal gland layer that occur in chronic bronchitis. (From Whitcomb ME: *The lung: normal and diseased,* St Louis, 1982, Mosby.)

surface area. Chronic bronchitis is almost entirely a disease of mechanical obstruction of the airway.

Coughing is the hallmark symptom of chronic bronchitis. The cough begins slowly and worsens insidiously but steadily until there is mucous production. Coughing is often more pronounced during the winter months, but gradually it becomes almost constant. Exercise tolerance decreases slowly but steadily until the individual has virtually no physical reserve for times of stress. The course of chronic bronchitis is characterized by respiratory infections during which severe coughing, dyspnea, production of purulent secretions, and aberration in pulmonary gas exchange may require hospitalization. Prolonged expiration, wheezes and crackles during expiration, cyanosis, and peripheral edema

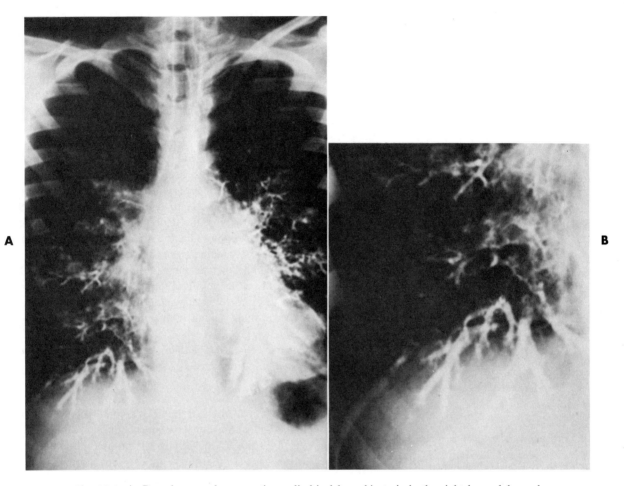

**Fig. 14-4. A,** Bronchogram demonstrating cylindrical bronchiectasis in the right lower lobe and varicose bronchiectasis in the left lower lobe. **B,** Close-up of the cylindrical bronchiectasis in the right lower lobe. (From Whitcomb ME: *The lung: normal and diseased,* St Louis, 1982, Mosby.)

are the classical physical features of the patient with chronic bronchitis.

Chronic bronchitis and emphysema often coexist in the same patient. This dual affliction is most commonly found in cigarette smokers. Since the larger airways and the distal air spaces and alveoli are affected by cigarette smoke, both processes of pathogenesis—mucous gland and goblet cell hypertrophy and hyperplasia and increased elastic tissue destruction caused by increased proteolytic enzyme—may coincide. When this dual destruction occurs, the patient is likely to develop the signs and symptoms of both disorders, although one often predominates.

### Bronchiectasis

Bronchiectasis is an abnormal dilation of a bronchus that is largely irreversible. It can occur following infection, aspiration, tumors or foreign bodies in the bronchi, or with abnormalities of the immune system. In addition, several genetic disorders are almost always associated with bronchiectasis. These disorders include cystic fibrosis, Kartagener syndrome, and the immotile cilia syndrome. Abnormali-

ties in ciliary removal of secretions are common to each of these disorders and probably cause the localized inflammation that results in bronchiectasis. Because of the many varied causes of bronchiectasis, it is difficult to offer specific figures on the prevalence of the disease. Some refer to bronchiectasis as acute versus chronic, others as obstructive versus nonobstructive, yet others describe bronchiectasis on the basis of its radiographic appearance—for example, saccular, cylindrical, or tubular (Fig. 14-4).

The pathogenesis of bronchiectasis is commonly related to the effects of either severe inflammation or bronchial infection. The infective episode results in a severe inflammatory reaction within the bronchi, thereby causing an exudative response by the mucous-secreting glands. As a result of the exudative response, viscous secretions accumulate that can completely obstruct airways distal to the point of exudation. As the obstruction becomes complete, atelectasis is likely to occur. In addition, the bronchus just proximal to the point of obstruction begins to dilate. This dilation is not dangerous, and obstruction is the major problem because it prevents distal air flow. The combination

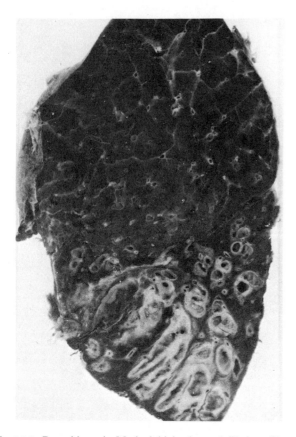

**Fig. 14-5.** Bronchiectasis. Marked thickening and dilation of lower lobe bronchi. (From pathological museum of University of Manchester, U.K. Reproduced from Kissane JM: *Anderson's pathology*, ed 9, St. Louis, 1990, Mosby.)

of obstruction and mucous secretion associated with the inflammatory response results in the accumulation of large amounts of secretion. The infection probably interferes with normal mucociliary function, and obstruction prevents adequate expiratory airflow to enable the patient to cough effectively and thereby remove the secretions. With secretions in place, there is a heightened chance for secondary infection, which is followed by greater exudation, additional secretion accumulation, and further weakening of the bronchial architecture. This cyclical process causes the copious secretions commonly found in people with bronchiectasis.

A classical pathological condition is associated with bronchiectasis. The dilated bronchi have obvious transverse ridges when examined grossly. In addition, there may be openings (bronchial pits) out of which several mucous glands empty. Inflammatory changes are often seen, since bronchiectasis is so often associated with infection. The inflammation may be acute, but chronic inflammation is more often the case. Most of the normally occurring bronchial wall elements—epithelium, cartilage, smooth muscle, and glands—have been replaced by fibrous tissue (Fig. 14-5). Physiological changes are most specifically related to the obstructive lesion. During early stages of the disease there is little or no pulmonary function abnormality. As obstruction becomes greater and as secretions develop, forced expiratory flow rates decrease. Pulmonary perfusion and ventilation are often severely reduced or absent in the area of bronchiectasis. These changes often cause ventilation/perfusion mismatching that produces hypoxemia. Bronchial artery hypertrophy is a feature of note. These small arteries enlarge as a result of an increased demand for localized bronchial blood flow. The high level of metabolic activity associated with chronic inflammation and infection and the replacement of normal tissue with fibrous tissue result in a need for increased bronchial circulation.

Regardless of the underlying cause of bronchiectasis, a chronic cough productive of copious amounts of sputum is the most common symptom. Radiographic changes most commonly include increased bronchial markings. Hemoptysis may be present in the form of blood-tinged sputum or in the form of frank hemorrhage. Foul-smelling breath is occasionally found. Other physical findings include low-pitched crackles, wheezes, and breath sounds with a loud, harsh character. Digital clubbing is common in long-standing bronchiectasis.

### Asthma

Asthma is one of the most common chronic disorders in the United States with estimates that 10 million individuals are afflicted, including 3.2 million children. Mortality associated with asthma, not considered a major issue in the past, appears to have increased during the 1980s. Adding to this increase is clear evidence of asthma mortality becoming a greater problem in the inner cities than elsewhere. Asthma is characterized by bronchial smooth muscle hyperreactivity in response to many external and internal stimuli. The hyperreactivity may be reversed, either with medication or spontaneously. The common "asthmagenic" stimuli include pollens, inhalants, foods, medications, dyes, air pollution, infection, cigarette smoke, exercise, and cold, dry inhaled air. Once the stimulus is encountered by the patient, a series of pathophysiological events results in classic signs and symptoms of asthma.

Unlike pulmonary emphysema, in which various types of the disease are based on pathological changes in tissue, a common categorization of asthma is by the origin of the offending stimuli. Extrinsic asthma is probably the most common form and is thought to be present in as many as 5% to 10% of children. As the name implies, the offensive agent that causes the acute episode of asthma is from a source external to the body. Common agents include inhaled allergens such as ragweed, grasses, and animal dander; other factors include foods, cigarette smoke, and medications. These agents are thought to bind with the immunoglobulin IgE on the surfaces of mast cells within the airways. This interaction results in a release of several mediators that cause certain predictable changes in airway physiology.

Intrinsic asthma is caused by factors from within the body including viral and bacterial respiratory tract infections, air pollution, and exposure to occupational fumes and dusts. Exercise-induced asthma is another category of the disorder. This type of asthma must receive particularly close attention by physical therapists who provide conditioning programs and other forms of continuous vigorous exercise for patients. The patient with exercise-induced asthma, usually a child, will have a sudden onset of symptoms following exercise for approximately 6 to 7 minutes at a heart rate of around 170 bpm. Upon cessation of exercise, the classical symptoms of asthma begin. Further study of the phenomenon has led to the finding that in addition to exercise, the loss of both heat and humidity across the bronchial epithelium causes symptoms that are virtually identical to exercise-induced asthma.

The precise pathogenesis of asthma has not been fully elucidated, but a few theories receive strong support. It is generally accepted that two related substances called cyclic AMP and cyclic GMP are largely responsible for tone in bronchial smooth muscles. When the levels of cyclic AMP are low, or when levels of cyclic GMP are high, there is a greater likelihood of smooth muscle spasm. One of two theories in current favor involves autonomic nervous system control of bronchial smooth muscle. Several mechanisms may function within this theory. Decreased beta-adrenergic airway receptor activity, increased cholinergic airway receptor activity, and liberation of specific neurotransmitters following sensory stimulation can all result in reduced levels of cyclic AMP, increased levels of cyclic GMP, contraction of bronchial smooth muscle, and the signs and symptoms of asthma.

In recent years great interest has developed in the role of inflammation as a major factor causing bronchial hyperreactivity. This theory of inflammation suggests that, in response to some stimulus, chemical mediators of inflammation are liberated from cells, probably mast cells, within the airway. These mediators—histamine, prostaglandin $D_2$, leukotriene $C_4c$, and others—cause inflammatory cells to migrate into the airways. These migrating cells include neutrophils, platelets, and macrophages, which respond to local inflammation by releasing additional substances that exert an injurious effect upon the airways. This inflammatory chain of events leads to abnormal smooth muscle tone and secretion of excess mucus, which are common causes of the pathophysiological events in asthma. Inhalation of allergens, smoke, dust, cold and dry air, infection, and exercise are all thought to contribute to this process.

The pathology in asthma includes bronchial smooth muscle contraction and hypertrophy, mucous secretion, and inflammation of the airways with edema. Several theories of bronchial smooth muscle spasm have been identified. In addition to muscle spasm, bronchial smooth muscle hypertrophy will occur over time. Large numbers of inflammatory cells are found in the airways of individuals with asthma. The inflammatory response of the airways in asthmatics includes heightened bronchial smooth muscle reactivity. In addition, both a direct and a reflex stimulation of bronchial smooth muscle contraction may be elicited. The excessive amount of bronchial mucus seen in patients with asthma is probably related to increased mucous gland size and production as a result of the periodic inflammatory changes within the airways. Also, the severe airway narrowing that accompanies asthma often reduces normal mucociliary clearance, thereby leading to excessive secretions.

Signs and symptoms of asthma include wheezing, dyspnea, and coughing that, in the early stages of the acute episode, is nonproductive. These symptoms are all related specifically to the severe airway obstruction caused by a combination of smooth muscle spasm, mucous secretions, and bronchial wall edema. The wheezing is often high-pitched and may occur during both the expiratory and inspiratory phase of breathing. Wheezing may be audible without a stethoscope. Breath sounds are usually distant and, in cases of severe airway obstruction, may be virtually absent as the patient moves too little air for sound to be effectively generated. Dyspnea, or labored breathing, is associated with tachypnea, rapid breathing, as the patient attempts to maintain minute ventilation in the face of severe expiratory obstruction. The airways widen normally during inspiration to allow the inflow of air. Normal airway narrowing during expiration is accentuated by obstruction, which prevents normal expiration. Gas that cannot be expired begins to accumulate in the lungs, and hyperinflation is the result. Hyperinflation is characterized physically by increased anteroposterior diameter of the chest, by a tympanic percussion note, and by limited movement of the ribs at the costovertebral joints during inspiration. Hyperinflation leads to mechanical flattening of the diaphragm, which makes inspiration more difficult (Fig. 14-6).

## Cystic fibrosis

Cystic fibrosis (CF) is the most common lethal genetic disorder affecting whites. It is characterized by widespread abnormalities in the exocrine glands with particular emphasis on bronchial mucous glands, the exocrine cells of the pancreas, and sweat glands. It is responsible for the majority of cases of severe chronic lung disease and bronchiectasis in children. Although commonly considered a pediatric disorder, because of advances in treatment and early diagnosis, CF has become a problem of young adults too. CF was recognized as a specific disease only in 1936 by Fanconi and until the 1950s most afflicted children died before 5 years of age.

CF is clearly a genetic disorder inherited in an autosomal recessive pattern. The gene for CF, inherited in a Mendelian recessive pattern, was recently identified on the long arm of chromosome 7. The major mutation associated with the gene responsible for CF has been defined and, in approximately 70% of cases, is the ΔF508. A protein, the cystic fibrosis transmembrane conductance regulator, is the product of this

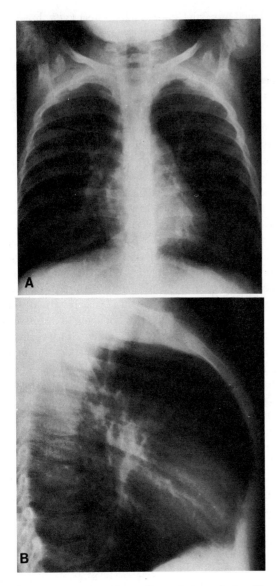

**Fig. 14-6. A,** Anteroposterior radiograph in patient with acute asthma. Note flattened hemi-diaphragms indicative of severe hyperaeration. **B,** Lateral view of same patient with acute asthma shows severe increase in anteroposterior diameter of thorax and flattened hemi-diaphragms. (From Burton GG and Hodgkin JE, editors: *Respiratory care: a guide to clinical practice,* ed 2, Philadelphia, 1984, JB Lippincott Co.)

gene and is thought to be a chloride channel. The abnormal function of the channel causes abnormal salt transport, which may be responsible for some of the basic defects in the organs involved in the disease. Identification of the gene will likely lead to improved and more accurate testing, counseling, and ultimately, treatment. When two individuals who are heterozygotes for CF (carriers) have a child, there is a 25% chance that the child will have CF, a 50% chance that the child will be heterozygous for the gene, and a 25% chance that the child will be completely free from the CF gene. Testing for the carrier or heterozygous state is now possible,

as is prenatal testing. However, due to numerous factors neither of these approaches has become standard, universal procedure. Approximately 1 in 1600 to 2000 live births among whites will result in a child with CF. Cystic fibrosis is much less common in blacks, with estimates of its prevalence in the 1 in 17,000 to 20,000 range, and it is rare in Asians. Other than the racial predilection, no clear geographic, environmental, socioeconomic, or cultural factor helps account for the distribution of CF.

Changes in CF include abnormal secretions from salivary, sweat, mucous, and pancreatic glands that may result in obstruction at the opening of the gland. Ciliary function in those with CF has been shown to be abnormal as has the physical and chemical nature of bronchial mucous secretions. Consistently high levels of sodium and chloride are found in sweat electrolytes of CF patients, and obstruction of the pancreatic ducts results in a loss of pancreatic digestive enzymes reaching the gastrointestinal tract. The increased viscous character of bronchial secretions along with the abnormal ciliary function in the airway cause secretion retention. This retention facilitates secondary infection, which may be in the form of pneumonia, bronchiolitis, or bronchitis. This infection, usually *Staphylococcus aureus* or *Pseudomonas aeruginosa,* becomes chronic and leads to bronchiectasis, pneumothorax, hemoptysis, and, ultimately, cor pulmonale and respiratory insufficiency.

The pathological condition associated with CF is almost always related to the effects of obstruction of the specific portion of the organ from which the exocrine secretions are liberated. In the pancreas, dilated pancreatic ducts become obstructed with concretions, as well as fibrous and inflammatory tissue. As the disease progresses, the exocrine portions of the pancreas are replaced with fat and fibrosis. Pulmonary lesions often begin with pneumonia in the neonate or acute bronchiolitis in the infant. Many pediatricians believe that an infant who has more than one episode of bacterial pneumonia should be considered at risk for CF. These acute infections are associated with complete plugging of small airways by inflammatory exudate and abnormal bronchial secretions (Fig. 14-7). As the child ages, the episodes of acute infection often become more frequent and the infection and inflammatory response caused by the infection becomes chronic. Pathological features of the chronic pulmonary lesions in CF begin to look much like chronic bronchitis as seen in adults. Mucous gland hypertrophy and hyperplasia are apparent. Increased mucous production along with the abnormal nature of mucus in CF result in massive amounts of mucus and extraordinary airway obstruction by those secretions. A concomitant increase in chronic infection within the airways and the development of bronchiectasis are common findings in teenagers and adults with CF. Bronchiectasis predisposes to further secretions, airway obstruction, and hemoptysis, which can be massive and often has a poor prognosis.

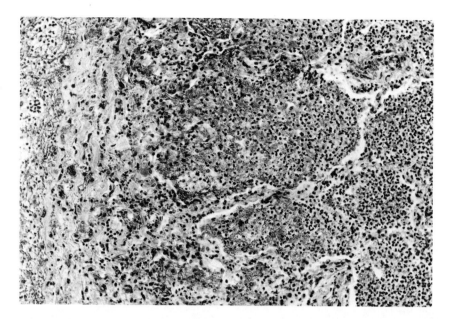

**Fig. 14-7.** Acute pneumonia in infant with cystic fibrosis. Note alveolar sac filled with purulent exudate and inflammatory cells. (From Kissane JM: *Anderson's pathology,* ed 9, St Louis, 1990, Mosby.)

The pathophysiology of CF is almost entirely related to the mucous obstruction of distal airways followed by the more proximal airways. It should be noted that the early pulmonary lesions associated with pneumonia, bronchiolitis, and acute bronchitis are usually reversible with treatment. As the chronic infection associated with CF becomes established, the obstruction becomes more generalized, less reversible, and causes more obvious physiological changes. This obstruction commonly leads to atelectasis, or loss of lung inflation, when the obstruction is complete. When obstruction is only partial, the excessive secretion acts as a "check valve" mechanism to allow air to enter but not exit the lung, thereby causing hyperinflation. The lack of proper ventilation accompanying both atelectasis and hyperinflation commonly results in lung areas that are poorly ventilated but normally perfused. The resulting mismatch in ventilation/perfusion ratio causes hypoxemia because of areas in which pulmonary blood flow is unable to perform gas exchange. Hypoxemia, which becomes more marked over years, is a strong stimulus for pulmonary artery vasoconstriction. This constriction causes pulmonary hypertension and, when severe enough over time, leads to cor pulmonale (also known as right ventricular failure). Like hemoptysis, cor pulmonale has a poor prognosis.

Because of the extreme variability in presentation of CF, the various pulmonary symptoms may occur in any of a myriad of combinations or may be absent. Early pulmonary signs and symptoms of CF are tachypnea, dyspnea, cough, wheezing, and fever in the infant who develops early pneumonia as the presenting aspect of CF. As the disease becomes more established, chronic coughing and production of copious amounts of thick, purulent mucus are the hallmark signs and symptoms. The patient with CF will wheeze, have crackles in many areas of the thorax, exhibit tachypnea, dyspnea, and throat-clearing. The physical habitus of the patient is typically one of cachexia resulting from the pancreatic insufficiency and the extreme caloric expenditure for coughing and breathing. The CF patient will have a barrel-chest appearance because of hyperinflation and will be lethargic, often anorexic, and cyanotic when hypoxemia is severe. Radiographic changes may include air-trapping and increased bronchial markings in a "honeycomb" pattern. Definable areas of atelectasis are not unusual and represent a major complication of CF. Areas of pneumonia are present on an intermittent basis, and cardiac enlargement is seen when right-sided heart failure becomes well established. Finally, occasional episodes of pneumothorax are seen.

In the early years of CF care, a majority of children died well before their teenage years. As comprehensive and aggressive care became routine in accredited CF treatment centers, the life span of these children increased. Today, adults with CF are common, and the various life decisions regarding career, family, and other personal goals must be made by this group of young adults with a disease that offers, at best, an uncertain future.

## INFECTIOUS DISORDERS

Infectious disorders of the pulmonary system represent an enormous group of diseases to which many patients are particularly susceptible. Respiratory tract infection can be caused by bacteria, viruses, fungi, and protozoa, each of

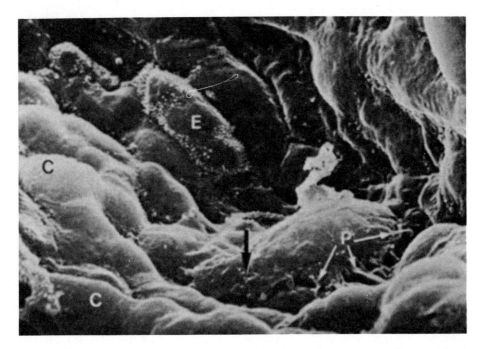

**Fig. 14-8.** Scanning electron micrograph of the alveolar surface demonstrating an alveolar macrophage. Numerous cytoplasmic extensions *(arrows)* and pseudopods *(P)* attach the cell to the alveolar surface. The bulging capillaries *(C)* and type II cells *(E)* are in the background. (From West JB: *Bioengineering aspects of the lung,* New York, 1977, Marcel Dekker, Inc.)

which has a multitude of subgroups. This portion of the chapter first reviews normal defense mechanisms against infection, then presents general characteristics of infections within the four specific categories noted above. It is beyond the scope of this text to offer a specific description of the great multitude of respiratory infections.

Defense mechanisms of the lungs can generally be grouped into those that provide protection against organisms and injurious material entering the respiratory tract, those that help clear organisms and injurious material from the respiratory tract, and cellular defenses. Protection of the upper airway against inhaled organisms or aspirated material is accomplished in two primary ways. First, the coordinated act of swallowing affords momentary closure of the upper airway by virtue of adduction of the vocal cords and movement of the epiglottis in a posterior and caudal direction. This closure protects against aspiration of food into the trachea. Nasal filtration is the second means by which the upper airway is protected. Vibrissae (nasal hairs) protect against the entrance of large particulate matter. The nasal turbinate bones provide an intricate network of surfaces onto whose epithelial surface organisms and other particulate matter impact during inspiration. In addition to filtering it, the nasal airway also warms and humidifies the inspired air.

Clearance of material from the respiratory tract is accomplished by two gross methods, coughing and sneezing, and by the mucociliary escalator that removes smaller particulate matter. Coughing is described in several other chapters, and sneezing is more reflexive than active.

Mucociliary clearance is accomplished by the coordinated action of the cilia found on the pseudostratified columnar epithelial cells of the airways. Cilia beat to propel a layer of mucus from distal to proximal in the respiratory tract. Once the mucus reaches a point above the vocal cords, it is usually swallowed or expectorated. As microorganisms and particulate matter impact upon the mucous layer, the material is swept along with the layer and is thereby removed from the respiratory tract.

The alveolar macrophage is the most notable cellular element of the pulmonary defense mechanisms (Fig. 14-8). It is an active cell that responds to the inhalation of organisms and particulate matter by isolating and then phagocytizing the material. Macrophages also appear to be involved in the inflammatory process and in the process of repair that follows acute injury or inflammation in the lungs. T and B lymphocytes play either a direct or indirect role in pulmonary defenses. T lymphocytes are responsible for cell-mediated immunity, which is the type of reaction associated with the immune system's attempt to protect against the tubercle bacillus, the microorganism responsible for tuberculosis. B lymphocytes produce immunoglobulins that are protective against certain bacterial infections. Immunoglobulins IgA, IgG, and IgM are active in respiratory tract infections and can be found in either the serum, the mucus, or both. Of these immunoglobulins, IgG probably plays the greatest role in preventing infection. Despite these defense mechanisms, the population is commonly vulnerable to infection of the respiratory tract. Although respiratory tract infections do not pose the major public health threat

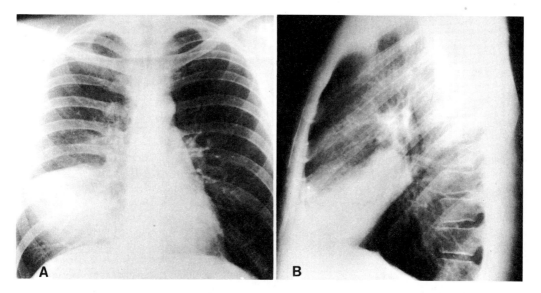

**Fig. 14-9.** Right middle lobe pneumonia. **A,** Posteroanterior projection showing the consolidation with its characteristic triangular configuration. The upper border is limited by the horizontal fissure and the lateral border by the oblique fissure. Note that the costophrenic angle is clear and the right heart border is obliterated (the so-called silhouette sign). **B,** Lateral view showing the roughly triangular opacity overlying the cardiac opacity. The upper margin of the consolidation is often more sharply outlined than in this case. (From Burton GG and Hodgkin JE, editors: *Respiratory care: a guide to clinical practice,* ed 2, Philadelphia, 1984, JB Lippincott Co.)

seen before the development of antimicrobials, they continue to be a major source of morbidity and mortality.

### Bacterial infections

Bacteria are microorganisms commonly found in one of three basic morphological shapes. The bacillus is a rod-shaped bacterium, the coccus is a round organism, and the spirochete is spiral. Bacterial infections of the respiratory tract have been categorized in different fashions. Categories include the type of disease (e.g., community-acquired versus chronic), the staining characteristics of the bacteria (e.g., gram negative versus gram positive), the morphology (e.g., baccilli versus cocci versus spirochete), and the area affected (e.g., airway versus alveoli). Once the basic type of bacterium is known, other tests of metabolic or biochemical function are employed to determine the specific type of infecting bacterium, such as *Staphylococcus aureus.*

Regardless of the type of bacteria or area of infection, acute inflammation and localized suppuration are consistent findings. Bacterial infections of the conducting airways are characterized by organisms that attach to epithelial cells and cause a localized inflammation (bronchitis or bronchiolitis) by liberating destructive toxins (e.g., *Bordetella pertussis*). As a result of the local inflammation, inflammatory exudate, which includes mucous secretions, cellular debris, and serous fluid, accumulates in the airways. The volume or viscosity of the exudate prevents removal by mucociliary mechanisms, and coughing becomes the effective means for removing the debris.

As infectious organisms reach the alveolar region, the infection is referred to as either lobar pneumonia or bronchopneumonia depending on the pattern of disease. Lobar pneumonia is generally agreed to involve all of one or more lobes of a lung. Its radiographic picture is usually one of uniformity of disease process (Fig. 14-9). Lobar pneumonia has four stages:

1. Edematous: vascular enlargement and alveolar exudate
2. Red hepatization: movement of erythrocytes, fibrin, and inflammatory cells into alveoli
3. Gray hepatization: movement of large numbers of alveolar macrophages into alveoli
4. Resolution: destruction and removal of exudate and rebuilding of normal architecture begins

Bronchopneumonia, also referred to as lobular pneumonia, is characterized by a patchy, inconsistent pattern of inflammation and exudation from the terminal bronchioles out into the alveolar tissue. Historically, bronchopneumonia has been referred to as atypical pneumonia. Bronchopneumonia occurs most commonly in individuals with underlying chronic diseases, in the elderly, and in infants and young children. The left box on p. 276 presents salient features about the most common bacterial infections of the lower respiratory tract.

### Viral infections

Viral infections of the respiratory tract are extremely common among all age groups. Despite their prevalence and great morbidity, in the healthy population there is relatively low mortality from these infectious agents. Viral respiratory illnesses have been categorized according to the portion of

## Characteristics of selected bacterial infections of the lungs

*Streptococcus pneumoniae*
- Common in very young, very old, and chronically ill patients
- A majority of cases are nonhospital acquired
- Complications include pleuritis, bacteremia, and empyema

*Staphylococcus aureus*
- Common bacterial complication of influenza
- Very prevalent, almost universal, pathogen in cystic fibrosis
- Purulent, hemorrhagic exudate
- Thrombosis in capillaries adjacent to alveoli
- Pneumothorax can occur

*Klebsiella pneumoniae*
- Most common in men over age 50
- Commonly associated with chronic illness, malignancy, alcoholism
- Highly cellular alveolar exudate with necrosis of alveolar wall
- Complications include bacteremia and bronchiectasis

*Escherichia coli*
- Seeds lung from initial site of gastrointestinal or urinary systems
- Bronchopneumonia characterized by edematous and hemorrhagic exudate
- Mortality is unusually high (greater than 50%)

*Haemophilus influenzae*
- Most commonly found in young children or older adults
- Also common as superimposed infection in patients with established chronic bronchitis
- Can exist as either a diffuse lung infection or in a discrete lobar or segmental pattern
- Mortality is usually well under 10%

*Legionella pneumophila*
- Organism isolated in 1976 following epidemic of lung infections following American Legion conference in Philadelphia
- Infection stems from contaminated water in cooling systems, evaporation units, and construction areas
- Alveoli are invaded by fibrin and purulent material including inflammatory cells
- Symptoms may be protracted over weeks

## Characteristics of selected viral infections of the lungs

Influenza
- Found worldwide, most common in winter months
- Ranges from asymptomatic to fatal
- Most common in very young and very old, as well as in those with chronic diseases
- Bronchiolitis, necrotic respiratory epithelium, congested interstitial space, and alveolar space filled with edema, inflammatory cells, and fibrin
- Secondary bacterial superinfection is common

Respiratory syncytial virus
- Common pathogen in infants and children
- Classic bronchiolitis picture in infants and classic picture of croup in older children
- Pneumonia is less common but occurs in infants and adults
- Bronchiolitis associated with predisposition to adult pulmonary disease

Adenovirus
- Several dozen species of this virus
- Causes pharyngitis and influenza symptoms in children
- Also affects immunocompromised and military base personnel
- Causes necrosis of bronchiolar and bronchial mucosa
- Alveolitis with fibrin, edema, and inflammatory cells along with interstitial edema
- Complications include bronchiectasis and bronchiolitis obliterans

Cytomegalovirus
- Common infection in neonates, although very few develop pneumonia
- Pneumonia common in immunosuppressed, including renal and bone marrow transplant patients and those with AIDS
- Varied pulmonary response: some show diffuse damage to epithelial cells in alveoli and bronchioles; others have hemorrhage, necrosis, and small nodular lesions
- Often associated with *Pneumocystis carinii* infection

the respiratory system affected by the infection. Upper respiratory infections usually refer to the area above the vocal cords, and lower respiratory infections include the area below the cords. The common cold is one very prevalent type of viral respiratory infection and may include sneezing, nasal discharge, sore throat, sinusitis, and obstruction of the nasal passages caused by edema. "Flu" is a second general type of respiratory tract viral infection and includes the well-known symptoms of general weakness and malaise, headache, fever, myalgia, and prostration. Bronchitis and viral pneumonia are the common lower respiratory tract infections caused by viruses. These syndromes are characterized respectively by productive coughing and by dyspnea and coughing.

Just as there are several groups of symptoms caused by viral infections, there are patterns of pathological changes that are not necessarily specific to any particular virus but may be common among several viruses. Acute inflammation of the bronchi and the bronchioles, seen in viral infections, results in focal areas of necrosis within the airway epithelium. Diffuse alveolar damage is another response to viral infection and is most commonly associated with viral pneumonias. Alveolar damage is associated with accumulation of inflammatory cells and exudate in the alveoli followed by the development of hyaline membranes and increased number and size of alveolar type II cells. Focal inflammatory and hemorrhagic lesions are a third pathologi-

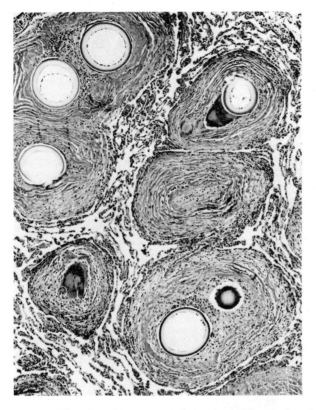

**Fig. 14-10.** Fibrotic pulmonary granulomas in reaction to fungal infection with chrysoporium parvum fungus. (From Kissane JM: *Anderson's pathology,* ed 9, St Louis, 1990, Mosby.)

cal response to viruses. This type of response is most commonly seen in immunocompromised patients.

The right box on p. 276 presents both the more common viral agents that infect the respiratory tract and the major features of the associated illnesses.

### Fungal infections

Fungi are organisms that exist in either a mold or a yeast form, each having pathogenic possibilities. Almost all human fungal infections are likely to result from exposure to naturally occurring fungi in either mold or yeast form. In addition to primary fungal infections, certain fungi are most commonly found in immunocompromised hosts. Candida albicans is such an opportunistic fungal infection and is likely to be found in patients receiving immunotherapy, those with immune disorders such as acquired immunodeficiency syndrome (AIDS), and patients with chronic diseases, including chronic lung disease, diabetes mellitus, renal failure, alcoholism, and drug abuse.

A granulomatous reaction is common to several of the major types of fungal infections, including histoplasmosis, coccidiomycosis, and blastomycosis. A granuloma is the body's reaction to the inhaled fungi and consists of an inflammatory response heralded by an accumulation of lymphocytes and macrophages at the site of the fungi. These

cells attempt to phagocytize and "process" the fungi, and in doing so a granuloma is formed. The granuloma is a collection of cells within the tissue that, in the case of fungi, often includes significant necrotic material. Within the granuloma, the various immune cells and their secretions, such as lysosomes and lymphokines, all combine in an effort to destroy the invading organism (Fig. 14-10).

In addition to granulomatous reactions, several types of fungal infections of the respiratory tract are said to be invasive. These infections are almost always found in immunocompromised hosts or in patients who have otherwise lost the mechanical and biological defense mechanisms against such infections. Some invasive fungi will enter the lung via aspiration from an oral lesion, whereas other fungi will seed the lung from a hematogenous spread. Pathologically, the fungi will invade the lung parenchyma by entering through the bronchial tree. Depending on the specific organism, there can be a necrotic inflammatory response within the alveoli, small bronchioles, and arterioles, or there may be nodules that develop around the fungal cells. The cells themselves may respond by developing either pseudohyphae or true hyphae, which are tube-like extensions of the fungal cells commonly found in the invaded tissue (Fig. 14-11).

The box on p. 279 lists the more common fungal diseases and several characteristics of each.

### Protozoan infections

Protozoa are parasitic organisms found more commonly outside of the United States with a few exceptions. The most notable of the exceptions is *Pneumocystis carinii,* a protozoan infection that is a primary disease of the lungs. Other parasitic diseases, including malaria, toxoplasmosis, trichomoniasis, and dirofilariasis (heartworm disease of dogs), are rarely seen in this country, although at least malarial lung is common in the tropics.

*Pneumocystis carinii* pneumonia is a disease seen almost exclusively in the immunocompromised patient. Individuals with leukemias or other types of malignancies, those taking immunosuppressive medications, those with collagen vascular disorders, and patients with AIDS are all at risk for *Pneumocystis carinii* pneumonia. Pathologically, *Pneumocystis carinii* pneumonia is characterized by a frothy exudate within the alveolar spaces along with alveolar macrophages and other cellular material and debris. The signs and symptoms are those of an acute pneumonia with high fever, dyspnea, coughing, and an alveolar pattern to the infiltrates as seen on radiograph. As the incidence of AIDS continues to increase, the likelihood of infections caused by *Pneumocystis carinii* also increases (Fig. 14-12).

### HIV AND THE RESPIRATORY SYSTEM

Human immunodeficiency virus (HIV) infection commonly results in pulmonary complications of both an infectious and noninfectious type. As a portal of entry for

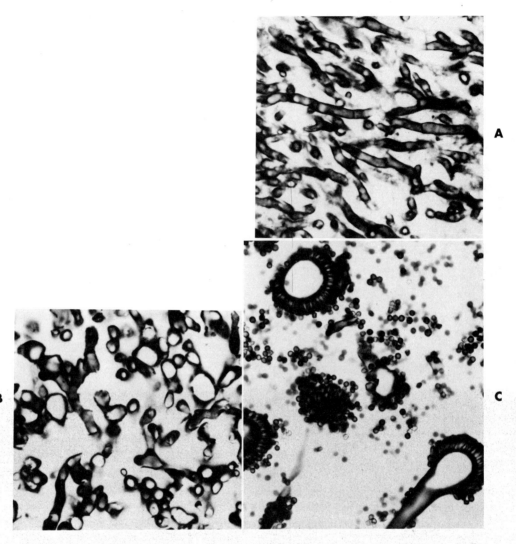

**Fig. 14-11.** Aspergillosis. **A,** Typical hyphae are uniform and septate and branch dichotomously. **B,** Bizarre, varicose hyphae in a pulmonary fungus ball. **C,** Fruiting heads and conidia in a pulmonary cavity. (Gomori methenamine-silver; ×760) (From Kissane JM: *Anderson's pathology,* ed 9, St Louis, 1990, Mosby.)

many infectious agents, the lungs are a common target for infection associated with HIV disease. In addition, numerous pulmonary disorders associated with HIV infection and AIDS are thought to be related to localized immunodeficiency and reduction of pulmonary defense mechanisms caused by HIV. HIV-1, the primary organism responsible for AIDS, has an affinity for cells with $CD_4$ molecules, particularly T lymphocytes and cells in the monocyte-macrophage group. $CD_4$ helper or inducer T-cells are responsible for many immune responses including immunoglobulin production, cytotoxic and suppressor cell activity, production of lymphokines, and others. Interference with or damage to these T-cells, as occurs with HIV-1 infection, can severely impair the immune response of the infected individual. In addition, HIV infection is thought to interfere with monocyte/macrophage function which results in re-

duced immune protection and increased infectivity by certain microorganisms.

HIV-1 is thought to enter the lungs as an extracellular body through the alveolar capillary membrane, or it is brought to the lung by infected circulating cells through the pulmonary circulation. Once the virus is in the lung tissue it will likely infect pulmonary lymphocytes, alveolar macrophages, and polymorphonuclear leukocytes within the lung. The specific responses of each group of cells to the infection is beyond the scope of this chapter but the reader is referred to Agostini and others for a review. The general response of pulmonary infection by HIV-1 is to render the infected individual very susceptible to opportunistic pulmonary pathogens including *pneumocystis carinii (P. carinii), mycobacterium tuberculosis (M. tuberculosis), cryptococcus neoformans (C. neoformans), histoplasma capsulatum (H.*

## Characteristics of selected fungal infections of the lungs

*Histoplasma capsulatum*
    Found in soil, spores are inhaled
    Acute lung infection most common in infants and children
    Chronic pulmonary disease found in adults
    Granulomatous inflammatory response with necrosis
    Fever, cough, lymphadenopathy, infiltrates on radiograph
    Usually self-limiting disease
Coccidiomycosis
    Distributed in soil in Southwest United States, Central and
        South America
    Majority of infections are asymptomatic
    Lung involvement includes cough, chest pain, dyspnea,
        and flu-like symptoms of malaise, fever, and headache
    More severe cases include pneumonia with infiltrates
        evident on radiograph
    Necrotizing granuloma that may include central suppura-
        tion
Aspergillosis
    Exists in three forms: saprophytic, invasive, allergic
    Saprophytic form results in mycetoma (fungus ball) growth
        in lung tissue
    Allergic form causes inflammation with eosinophils
    Invasive form almost always in individuals with immune
        dysfunction: fever, dyspnea, dry cough, infiltrates
    Invades through bronchial wall into alveoli and vascula-
        ture
    Can result in bronchopneumonia and arterial occlusion
    Invasive form has poor prognosis
*Candida albicans*
    Almost always found in immunocompromised hosts
    Very common infections in the mouth
    Lung involvement uncommon but severe, usually associ-
        ated with disseminated, hematogenous spread of or-
        ganism
    Necrotic nodules with pseudohyphae common to he-
        matogenous spread to the lungs
    Inflammatory response is limited because of poor immune
        response of patient

*capsulatum), candida, aspergillosis, and various bacterial pneumonias.*

### Common infections in HIV

*P. Carinii.* This organism is classified as a fungus and as a parasite. It is the most common serious complication of AIDS with a prevalence of up to 75%. Although thought to be an airborne organism, infection with *P. carinii* is believed to be due to a preexisting, latent infection reactivated by the immunosuppression associated with AIDS. Alveolar filling with *P. carinii* and its debris results in abnormal gas exchange leading to hypoxemia and hypercapnia. Interstitial inflammation often results in reduced lung compliance.

Infection with *P. carinii* always occurs in immunosup-pressed hosts and is a late feature in AIDS. Patients who develop *P. carinii* often have a $CD_4$ lymphocyte level at about 10% of the normal level. Respiratory failure is a common finding and those patients with advanced AIDS often have a steady, progressive course to a respiratory death.

Treatment of *P. carinii* includes cotrimoxazole, a relatively new combination drug, and pentamidine, a medication known for years to be effective against the organism. Prevention of *P. carinii* through chemoprophylaxis is recommended and aerosolized pentamidine or cotrimoxazole are suggested for all patients with HIV whose level of peripheral $CD_4$ lymphocytes reaches $200/mm^3$ as compared to a normal level of 800-1200 cells/$mm^3$.

*M. tuberculosis.* Tuberculosis, for centuries a disease of the poor, has seen a recent rise in prevalence because of its association with AIDS. Tuberculosis is an infection that becomes an active clinical disease primarily in the presence of impaired cellular immunity, as occurs in HIV infection. *M. tuberculosis* is almost always acquired through inhalation of the organism into the lung. About half of those who inhale *M. tuberculosis* will develop infection, but of those infected individuals, only about 10% develop active disease throughout their lifetime. Protection against active disease is normally provided via cellular immunity. When cellular immunity is deficient or has been suppressed, as in HIV infection, active *M. tuberculosis* may occur via newly acquired organisms or through reactivation of previously acquired organisms. The latter mode of occurrence is more probable in the United States, and *M. tuberculosis,* with greater virulence than most other common opportunistic infections, is often the first major latent pathogen to be reactivated during the immunosuppression associated with AIDS.

There are two general clinical patterns of infection with *M. tuberculosis* in individuals with HIV, depending upon the level of immunosuppression. When infection develops late in the course of AIDS, the advanced immunosuppression results in negative tuberculin skin response, disease external to the lungs, and atypical radiographic patterns. Among these radiographic patterns are diffuse lower-lobe disease as compared to the more common cavitary upper-lobe disease in non-HIV associated *M. tuberculosis.* Infection early in the course of AIDS is more like typical tuberculosis with positive skin-test reaction, increased frequency of upper-lobe disease, and reduced likelihood of extrapulmonary manifestations.

Diagnosis of *M. tuberculosis* is made by culture, isolation, and identification of the organism from sputum, biopsy, lavage, or needle aspirate from suspicious areas including bronchi, lymph nodes, and bone marrow.

Treatment is commonly begun when any strain of mycobacterium is found, without waiting for specific identification as *M. tuberculosis.* The three or four recommended medications include isoniazid, rifampin, pyrazinamide, and, when drug resistance is suspected, ethambutol may be added. Using this four-medication regimen for at

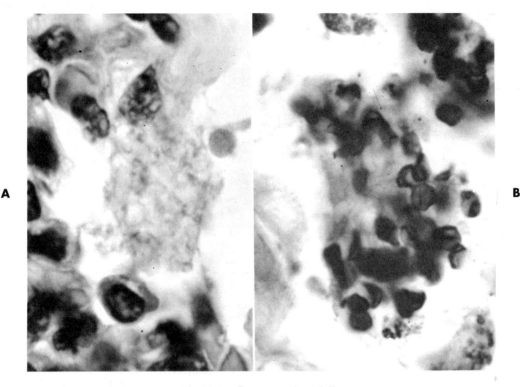

**Fig. 14-12.** *Pneumocystis carinii.*

least six months has been effective for HIV-related pulmonary tuberculosis.

***C. neoformans.*** Cryptococcosis is a fungal infection most commonly caused by *C. neoformans* and although it usually manifests as meningitis, pulmonary involvement is very common and often coexists with neurological disease. The fungus is common in the environment and has been found in fruit skins, milk, soil, and excreta of chickens and pigeons. Infection in humans is thought to occur when small organisms, liberated from environmental sources, are inhaled into the respiratory tract. The fungus can infect healthy individuals but is more common as an opportunistic infection.

Clinical findings include fever and cough. Pathologic findings have been described as interstitial pneumonias and granulomatous disease. Diagnosis depends upon isolating *C. neoformans* from sputum, bronchial lavage or pleural fluid, and biopsy of the site suspected to be involved.

Treatment includes administration of amphotericin-B, triazole, fluconazole, and itraconazole each alone or in varying combinations. Lifelong maintenance therapy is required for individuals with AIDS because relapses of cryptococcosis are frequent. Prognosis for cryptococcosis for persons with AIDS is almost uniformly poor with survival often less than one year.

***H. capsulatum.*** Histoplasmosis is a disease caused by the fungus *H. capsulatum* that exists in the soil and in the body in yeast form, with infection common in the lungs. The fungus is found in temperate climatic zones where it flourishes in soil associated with bird feces. When soil is disturbed, many spores become airborne to be inhaled into the respiratory tract where they transform to the yeast form and a parasitic invasion is complete. Hematogenous spread occurs to many other organs.

Fever and weight loss are the most common symptoms, with dyspnea and cough typical in those with pulmonary infection. Diagnosis is by isolation of *H. capsulatum* from culture or by radioimmunoassay of *H. capsulatum* antigen in urine or serum of patients with AIDS. As with cryptococcosis, amphotericin-B is the drug of choice.

***C. albicans* and *A. fumigatus.*** Candidiasis, commonly caused by *C. albicans,* and aspergillosis, commonly caused by *A. fumigatus,* are common fungal diseases found in patients with HIV infection. However, the incidence of pulmonary disease caused by these fungi is very low, with the possible exception of terminal infection.

***Hospital-acquired bacterial infection.*** Staphylococcal and gram-negative bacteria are the most frequently identified hospital-based infections of the lungs and are customarily developed late in the course of disease. The morbidity and mortality of these infections in individuals with AIDS are often great.

***Community-acquired bacterial infection.*** *H. influenzae* and pneumococcus are the most common bacterial pathogens encountered in individuals infected with HIV prior to the definitive diagnosis of AIDS. The features of infection with these bacteria are similar for the normal and immunocompromised populations.

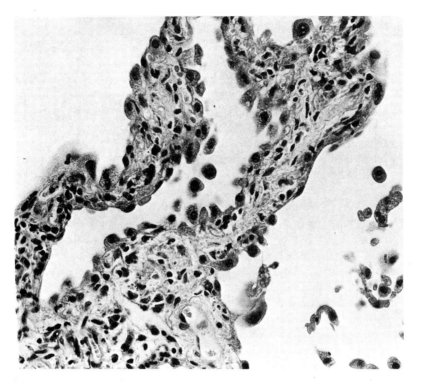

**Fig. 14-13.** Chronic interstitial pneumonia. Alveolar walls are fibrotic and contain predominantly mononuclear inflammatory cells. Alveolar epithelium is hyperplastic. Loss of capillaries in fibrotic septa is one factor contributing to abnormal gas exchange in this process. (From Kissane JM: *Anderson's pathology,* ed 9, St Louis, 1990, Mosby.)

## INTERSTITIAL PULMONARY FIBROSIS

Several dozen lung diseases have fibrosis as a major feature of their pathology. Some of these are discussed under the section on environmental disorders, but a large percentage of pulmonary fibrosis is considered to be idiopathic. This section discusses the major characteristics of the idiopathic forms of pulmonary interstitial fibrosis in which the major pathology exists with the walls of the alveoli.

Unknown interstitial lung diseases account for as many as 10,000 hospital admissions each year according to some sources. The prevalence of the disorder is between 5 and 10 cases per 100,000 people. Many different names have been used to describe the disease including Hamman-Rich syndrome, idiopathic fibrosing alveolitis, idiopathic pulmonary fibrosis, and diffuse interstitial pulmonary fibrosis.

Among the postulated reasons for the development of idiopathic interstitial pulmonary fibrosis are cigarette smoking, genetic predisposition, an association with other chronic diseases such as the collagen vascular diseases, and viral infection. In addition to the above possibilities, the immune system may play an important role in this disease process.

One proposed mechanism for fibrosis suggests lodging of antigen-antibody compounds in the pulmonary capillaries. On an acute basis, the response to these compounds will be an activation of the complement system and an attraction to the site of numerous alveolar macrophages. These responses are consistent with a generalized pulmonary inflammatory response to the antigen-antibody compounds. The complement system functions to enhance the inflammatory response, and the macrophages release their various factors that stimulate fibroblast activity at the site of the many antigen-antibody reactions. As fibrotic material is deposited within the capillaries and alveolar septa, the classic pathological changes associated with pulmonary fibrosis begin. This fibrotic response can become chronic as plasma cells that participate in the inflammatory process differentiate into B-lymphocytes that produce antibodies. These newly produced antibodies will bind with the initial antigen to form more antigen-antibody compounds, which continues the process that ultimately leads to pulmonary fibrosis.

The most striking pathological change in idiopathic interstitial pulmonary fibrosis is replacement of finely structured alveolar walls with dense fibrous tissue (Fig. 14-13). Presumably, the replacement of air-filled lung by fibrous tissue causes the increased lung weight found with massive fibrosis. The lung surface and the adjacent areas of pleural tissue appear to have nodular lesions, which are probably manifestations of large areas of fibrosis and scarring. Histological specimens may show accumulation of inflammatory cells in the remaining alveoli. These cells and accompanying edema are particularly striking in acute interstitial fibrosis and inflammation. Also, as the amount of fibrous deposition within the alveolar septa increases, the septa, or walls between the alveoli, become thick and cause predictable physiological changes.

Pathophysiological changes are those of classic pulmonary restrictive diseases. Loss of lung volume, found by spirometry or plethysmography, is related to the loss of alveolar architecture caused by the inflammation and subsequent fibrosis. Diffusion capacity is reduced because of (1) the increase in alveolar septal size, (2) the greater distance across which gas exchange must occur, and (3) the interference with gas exchange caused by the massive amount of fibrotic tissue. In addition to the diffusion block, the actual loss of capillaries because of their ablation by the process of fibrosis will reduce pulmonary perfusion, thereby reducing gas exchange. As with many disorders of gas exchange, the abnormality will be exacerbated when the patient exercises. Patients with interstitial fibrosis are hypoxemic, which may be the result of ventilation/perfusion abnormalities that occur once alveolar patency and ventilation are lost. If fibrosis is severe, it may affect not only pulmonary capillaries but larger pulmonary arterioles as well. Should this situation arise, it is another probable cause of hypoxemia in patients with idiopathic interstitial fibrosis.

Progressive dyspnea is the cardinal sign of idiopathic interstitial pulmonary fibrosis. Dyspnea progresses insidiously and may be associated with mild weight loss and exhaustion with little exertion. As the fibrosis progresses, dyspnea and exhaustion increase and the patient becomes incapacitated, finding it extremely difficult to perform even the most routine tasks of daily living. If the disease has an acute onset, the patient will be extremely ill and may require hospitalization. The majority of patients with interstitial fibrosis exhibit progressive deterioration of their pulmonary status, and death within 5 to 6 years is common.

## PULMONARY EMBOLISM

When large or small particles of any kind enter the venous circulation, the matter will likely lodge in the pulmonary circulation. The size of the matter determines whether it will be trapped in the smaller pulmonary capillaries, the pulmonary arterioles, or in the larger pulmonary arteries. Insofar as pulmonary perfusion is generally greatest to the lower lobes, there is a statistically greater likelihood of the embolic material lodging within the lower lobe pulmonary circulation.

The most common form of pulmonary embolism occurs following the development of deep vein thrombosis in the lower extremity. Veins in the calf are most often the site of thrombosis, with the iliac and femoral veins next in incidence. Thrombosis occurs as a result of a number of circumstances. Changes in local venous hemodynamics resulting in venous stasis are one of the most common causes of thrombosis. Reduced cardiac output, increased platelet count, clotting disorders, and certain medications, including oral contraceptives, are also known predisposing factors for deep vein thrombosis. Many patients seen in physical therapy, particularly those who are postoperative and those who are immobile, are at great risk for thrombosis and subsequent pulmonary embolism. Deep vein thrombosis is known to be a major complication of spinal cord injury, and physical therapists must be aware of its signs and symptoms.

A massive pulmonary embolism may cause sudden, acute chest pain and marked dyspnea. This clinical syndrome, which can be fatal, is usually associated with an embolism that lodges either at the bifurcation of the pulmonary trunk or in one of the more proximal branches of the large pulmonary arteries. A smaller pulmonary embolism can result in a localized pulmonary infarction when the blood supply to the alveoli is interrupted and leads to a collapse of the alveolar walls. This situation is not as common as one would expect because of the rapid and effective collateralization of the pulmonary circulation. When infarction occurs, the alveoli walls undergo necrosis, but the intact bronchial artery circulation causes a hemorrhagic appearance to the infarcted area. In some instances, emboli attach to the arterial wall and undergo fibrosis and canalization in which blood flow is restored by a channel that forms through the embolus. Finally, smaller emboli are often destroyed by protective enzymes released within the pulmonary vasculature.

Numerous other sources of pulmonary emboli exist. Among these are air embolism occurring when a large amount of air is introduced into the vasculature, usually through trauma or iatrogenic means. Bone marrow embolism and fat embolism are relatively common forms of pulmonary embolism and are most commonly seen following massive trauma. Amniotic fluid may be introduced into the circulation around the time of delivery, and this material can become a pulmonary embolus. Also, various material such as needles, cotton, tubing, and pieces of catheters have been documented as entering the pulmonary circulation.

## PULMONARY EDEMA

Pulmonary edema involves a significant increase in extravascular water entering either the interstitial spaces of the lung or the alveoli. Two general causes of this condition have been identified, with numerous disorders capable of contributing to these two causes. The first cause occurs when the pressure within the pulmonary capillary system increases to the point where water is forced to leave the circulation. The second cause is the loss of integrity of the pulmonary capillary endothelial cells, which permits fluid to escape from the vasculature. Of course, a combination of the two causes can also occur.

Four Starling forces are responsible for pressure changes resulting in movement of fluid out of the vasculature into the interstitium and alveoli. Specifically, an increase in the intravascular hydrostatic pressure forces fluid from the capillaries into the lung tissue. Also, increasing the extravascular colloid osmotic pressure or decreasing the intravascular colloid osmotic pressure will each cause fluid to leave the pulmonary capillary and enter the interstitial space or the alveoli. Left heart failure, myocardial infarction, and mitral valve disease such as stenosis are among the common causes of pulmonary edema resulting from increased capillary hydrostatic pressure. They also represent the causes of pulmonary edema that a physical therapist is likely to encounter.

Loss of integrity of the capillary endothelial cells occurs with microvascular injury that results in increased permeability of the capillary cells. Many agents are responsible for this type of endothelial cell change including:

Gases—toxic levels of oxygen, sulfur dioxide, noxious fumes
Liquids—aspirated salt or fresh water (drowning)
Microorganisms—viruses
Medications—bleomycin, cytoxan, methotrexate, phenylbutazone, colchicine
Shock and trauma

Pathological changes in the lung include obvious edema fluid in the alveolar spaces. Other changes in lung tissue will depend on the specific pathogenesis of the edema.

Signs and symptoms include dyspnea on exertion that can progress to dyspnea at rest, orthopnea or inability to assume a supine position as a result of dyspnea, nonproductive cough, and crackles, wheezes, and various heart murmurs when the edema is caused by heart failure.

## OCCUPATIONAL LUNG DISEASES

Occupational lung diseases have been known to exist for thousands of years and were recognized as a hazard of the mining industry as early as the first century AD. Today we can discuss three primary groups of occupational hazards that can lead to various types of pulmonary pathological conditions. The three groups include mineral dust inhalation, organic dust inhalation, and inhalation of toxic fumes. An overview of each group follows.

### Mineral dusts

**Silica dust.** Inhalation of silica dust is one of the most common forms of occupational exposure to minerals. The crystalline form of silica is often a byproduct of industries that include such activities as quarry work, sandblasting, making pottery, and stone masonry. Silica is also a constituent of other types of inhalants, such as coal, copper, and tin that are part of the mining industry. In the United States and in other industrialized nations, the incidence of silicosis, the primary disease caused by silica inhalation, has been declining. Mining is the major industry with workers at risk.

Silicosis is characterized by an onset as long as 15 to 25 years following initial exposure to the dust. Hard nodules are deposited throughout the pulmonary parenchyma and may also be found in the peribronchiolar and perivascular

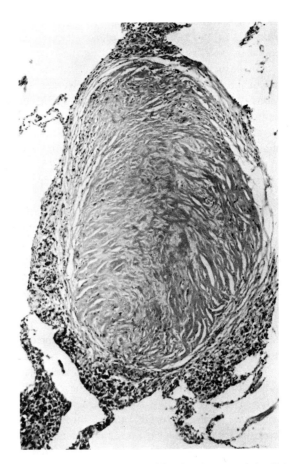

**Fig. 14-14.** Hyaline nodule in silicosis. Center of hyalinized collagen is enclosed by mantle of dust. (From Kissane JM: *Anderson's pathology,* ed 9, St Louis, 1990, Mosby.)

regions. The solitary nodules range from 5 to 10 mm and are usually found in "simple silicosis." When small nodules combine to form larger nodules of several centimeters, "complicated" or "conglomerate" silicosis is said to exist. The nodules appear histologically as layers of collagen fibers arranged in whorl-like patterns and are found in lymph nodes, as well as the lungs (Fig. 14-14). The pathogenesis of the nodules is not completely understood, although there is general agreement that a reaction of the pulmonary alveolar macrophage that leads to increased fibroblast activity may be responsible for the development of the nodule.

Symptoms depend largely on the type of lesion. Simple silicosis is often asymptomatic or may involve minor symptoms such as a dry cough and mild dyspnea. Complicated silicosis usually involves serious symptoms including severe pulmonary restriction and reduced lung volumes, hypoxia, severe dyspnea, and a predisposition to tuberculosis. This tendency for infection with the tubercle bacillus may relate to an injury to alveolar macrophages brought about by the inhaled silica dust.

**Coal worker's pneumoconiosis.** Coal worker's pneumoconiosis (CWP), commonly referred to as black lung disease, is endemic to the coal-mining regions of the world, including the United States, the United Kingdom, and Germany. Many factors have a major impact on the likelihood of developing CWP, including the type of coal being mined, the particular job of the worker, the concentration of coal dust, and whether the worker smokes cigarettes. When coal has a greater degree of silica crystal within its composition, as occurs with anthracite coal, there is a greater probability of CWP.

Small black macules or areas of discoloration comprise the basic lesion of simple CWP (Fig. 14-15). These discolorations are found most commonly in the upper lobe regions and in their simple form are not palpable upon manual examination by pathologists. When CWP is accompanied by silicosis, the lesions are then black macules and palpable because of the silicosis that accompanies the CWP. As with silicosis, CWP is also found in a more involved or complicated form. When this form is encountered, there are large black lesions that often reach several centimeters in diameter and may accumulate. Collagen is found in these lesions, which are often referred to as progressive massive fibrosis and, like complicated silicosis, create a predisposition to infection with tuberculosis.

The pathogenesis of simple CWP is related most specifically to the quantity of coal dust and the level of quartz (silica) in the dust. The dust is deposited within the lung parenchyma and phagocytized. Unlike silicosis, however, there is little tendency for fibrosis. Complicated CWP with its progressive massive fibrosis has been studied in an attempt to ascertain the etiology of this form of the disease. It appears that infection with the tubercle bacillus is one of the major features leading to the progression of simple CWP to the severe, complicated form.

As with silicosis, patients with simple CWP are often either asymptomatic or exhibit only mild symptoms. Conversely, the patient with complicated CWP and progressive massive fibrosis is likely to have a severe restrictive and obstructive defect. A form of pulmonary emphysema resembling centrilobular emphysema occurs in complicated CWP, and a form of chronic bronchitis is also common, with the secretions produced being obviously black.

**Asbestosis.** Asbestos and its fibrous and heat-resistant properties have been known for many thousands of years. Asbestos is a naturally occurring mineral found in several different chemical forms. Chief deposits of asbestos mined for industrial use are in the Ural Mountains in the former USSR, in Quebec province in Canada, in Zimbabwe, and in the People's Republic of China. Asbestos is used in building materials because of the strength afforded by its fibrous physical characteristics when added to a mixture of concrete. Concrete is then formed into sheets or molded into tiles, shingles, and pipes. Asbestos is commonly used in automotive applications when a high degree of friction resistance is required. Additionally, asbestos is used in industrial building and shipbuilding applications for thermal insulation, fire-

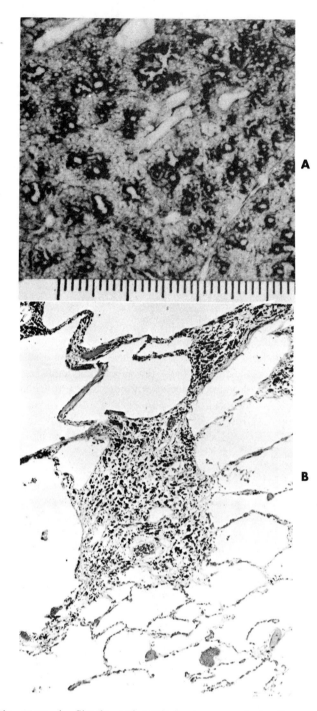

**Fig. 14-15. A,** Simple coal worker's pneumoconiosis. Paper-mounted lung section shows black dust deposits outlining respiratory bronchioles. **B,** Microscopic appearance of dust macule in coal worker. (**A,** Preparation by Prof J Gough.) (From Kissane JM: *Anderson's pathology,* ed 9, St Louis, 1990, Mosby.)

proofing, and soundproofing. The recent increase in the number of cases of asbestos-related lung disease is thought to result from shipbuilding applications during World War II and building applications during the 1950s. There is a long latency period before the development of symptoms caused

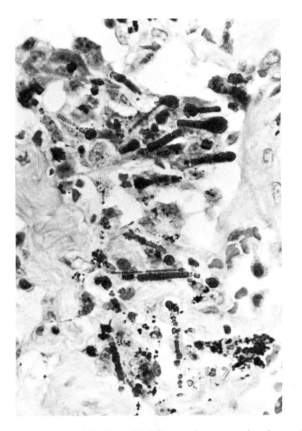

**Fig. 14-16.** Asbestosis. Interstitial fibrous tissue contains dust and asbestos bodies. (From Kissane JM: *Anderson's pathology,* ed 9, St Louis, 1990, Mosby.)

by inhalation of asbestos. Lung diseases caused by asbestos include pleural effusions and plaque development, asbestosis, and asbestos-related malignancies.

The pathogenesis of asbestosis is similar to that for silicosis—macrophage engulfing of the fiber with resultant fibrous tissue deposition. As the asbestos fibers enter the bronchioles and alveolar ducts, an inflammatory response ensues, and the pulmonary and alveolar macrophage responds by attempting to engulf the invading fiber. The macrophage secretes a substance that both attracts and stimulates activity of fibroblasts. As the collagen tissue is deposited within the respiratory bronchioles and alveolar ducts, a nonspecific lesion develops in a nonuniform and patchy distribution. Asbestosis lacks the specificity of the black macule seen in CWP and the nodular lesions that occur in silicosis. As exposure becomes more long term, the asbestos fibers invade the pulmonary interstitium, and interstitial fibrosis is stimulated. True asbestosis is diagnosed when a histological specimen shows interstitial fibrosis, and fibers of asbestos are identified (Fig. 14-16). As the disease process progresses, small cysts result in a "honey-comb" appearance of lung parenchyma. Massive areas of fibrosis (larger than 1 cm) have also been noted. Pleural involvement is relatively common in asbestosis. Thickening and fibrosis

of the visceral pleura is a common finding, and pleural effusions and calcification of pleural plaques are seen.

Physiological changes are those of restrictive lung disease. Lung volumes are reduced, and diffusion capacity for carbon monoxide is abnormally low, indicative of a diffusion block caused by fibrosis. Emphysema, chronic bronchitis, and other aspects of chronic obstructive diseases are missing.

Two types of malignancies are commonly associated with exposure to asbestos. Pulmonary carcinoma is encountered in asbestos-exposed individuals with up to 15 times the prevalence as in the general population. Cigarette smoking heightens this risk substantially. Malignant mesothelioma, usually a very rare tumor in the general population, is the second type of malignancy associated with asbestos exposure. This pleural tumor is thought to be derived from the serosal lining of the pleura, and asbestos is its most important cause.

### Organic dusts

Inhalation of organic material associated with various occupations often results in a hypersensitivity pneumonitis. This pneumonitis, also referred to as extrinsic allergic alveolitis, is caused by either a microorganism or an animal or insect protein in almost all cases. Some specific organic material and the associated causative agent include:

Moldy hay (farmer lung)—*Micromonospora faeni*
Mushroom compost (mushroom-worker lung)—*Thermopolyspora polyspora*
Bird droppings (pigeon-breeder lung)—pigeon serum
Moldy cork (suberosis)—*Penicillium frequentous*
Moldy barley (malt-worker lung)—*Cryptostroma corticale, Aspergillus clavatus*
Insect dust (miller lung)—*Sitophilus granarius* (wheat weevil)

When exposed to material to which they are allergic, individuals with hypersensitivity pneumonitis will show an immediate type I hypersensitivity reaction; many have a delayed reaction whose immune response type is controversial. Some authors suggest a type III reaction in which immunoglobulins (antibodies) attach to receptor sites on the antigens causing this large antigen/antibody molecule to become lodged in small vessels. The lodged particle causes a local inflammatory response that activates the complement system to enhance the inflammatory reaction. Others suggest a type IV cell-mediated immune reaction in which a granulomatous response occurs as T lymphocytes attempt to engulf and destroy the antigenic material.

Regardless of the controversy regarding immune pathogenesis, the pathological condition is agreed on. Upon exposure of the lungs to the offending antigen, an acute inflammatory lesion is the predominant feature. Inflammatory infiltrate with lymphocytes, plasma cells, and eosinophils is found within the alveolar septa and around the bronchioles. In a large percentage of cases, findings consistent with bronchiolitis obliterans and mild interstitial fibrosis are evident. Small granulomas are also found at the site of the offending antigen in most cases. As the disorder becomes chronic and as exposure continues for longer periods of time, the pathological features assume a character similar to idiopathic interstitial pulmonary fibrosis (Fig. 14-17).

Pathophysiological changes will vary with the phase of exposure. In the acute phase changes are of the obstructive pattern, including decreased flow rates and dynamic volumes along with a tendency toward hypoxemia. As chronic exposure occurs, a more restrictive pattern emerges, including reduced lung volumes and a diffusion block.

In the acute phase, signs and symptoms commonly include flu-like symptoms of malaise, fever, dyspnea, coughing, and possible wheezing if there is a component of reversible airway disease. The more chronic characteristics include anorexia and weight loss, chronic cough, dyspnea, and deteriorating pulmonary status by pulmonary function testing including spirometry, lung volumes, and arterial blood gas values.

## Toxic fumes and gases

Numerous fumes and gases have been found to be pathogenic. Some examples of such occupational materials and their potential side effects follow:

Cadmium—alveolitis and pulmonary emphysema
Mercury—pulmonary edema and hyaline membranes
Zinc—alveolar and interstitial damage
Oxygen—thickened alveolar septa and hyaline membranes
Ozone—inflammation of the airways
Sulfur dioxide—bronchitis and increased mucus secretion
Chlorine—irritation in upper airway, pulmonary edema
Ammonia—effects vary with severity of exposure

## PLEURAL DISEASES
### Pleural effusion and pleurisy

There are relatively few diseases that specifically affect the pleural tissue and pleural space. Normally there is a small volume (approximately 5 ml) of pleural fluid with relatively few cells found in that fluid. The pleural fluid serves the

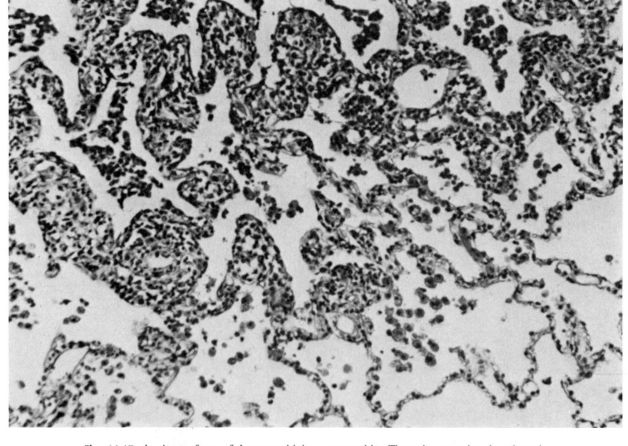

**Fig. 14-17. A,** Acute form of hypersensitivity pneumonitis. There is extensive lymphocytic infiltration of alveolar walls, which appear considerably thickened. Alveolar spaces contain lymphocytes, plasma cells, and macrophages. (×120.)       *Continued.*

purpose of lubricating the sliding of visceral against parietal pleural, thereby assisting in the mechanics of breathing. The most common disorder of the pleura, pleural effusion, occurs when an increased volume of fluid occurs, as is often the case when the vascular pressures associated with congestive heart failure result in transudation of fluid into the pleural space. The normally serous fluid may become hemorrhagic or suppurative. The majority of cases in the hemorrhagic category result from surgery, thoracic trauma, and neoplasms. In the suppurative group the pleural effusion is more properly termed "empyema" and is most commonly associated with tuberculosis and bacterial infection.

Numerous conditions and diseases will predispose to and cause pleural effusions. In addition to cardiac failure, renal failure and cirrhosis of the liver are common causes of transude fluid accumulation in the pleural space. Exudative effusions, which include suppurative effusions, are classically seen in infectious diseases of many types, in neoplastic disease, and (of special importance to physical therapists) in patients with collagen vascular disorders. Hemorrhagic effusions, in addition to the causes stated above, can also result from pulmonary infarction and tuberculosis. The pathogenesis of each type of effusion is related to the ongoing pathological process and its tendency to cause transudate, exudative, or hemorrhagic pleural fluid accumulation.

Once the pleural effusion is established, a local inflammatory response of the pleural surfaces will occur—pleuritis or pleurisy. The inflammatory response leads to cellular infiltration of the fluid within the pleural space and the development of fibrinous exudate among the surfaces of the involved pleura. The fibrinous response may cause significant local fibrosis that leads to scarring and pleural adhesions. Only rarely do the adhesions progress to calcifications.

Signs and symptoms usually suggest a rapid or sudden onset of the disease. Pain is the cardinal symptom, ranging from dull and nonspecific to knifelike and extremely localizable. Pain may be associated with deep breathing and coughing at first and may ultimately be present with quiet breathing. Doorstop breathing is seen with pleurisy because as the patient inspires, the sudden pain causes immediate cessation of inspiratory effort much as a door suddenly stops upon hitting a doorstop. Auscultation will often show

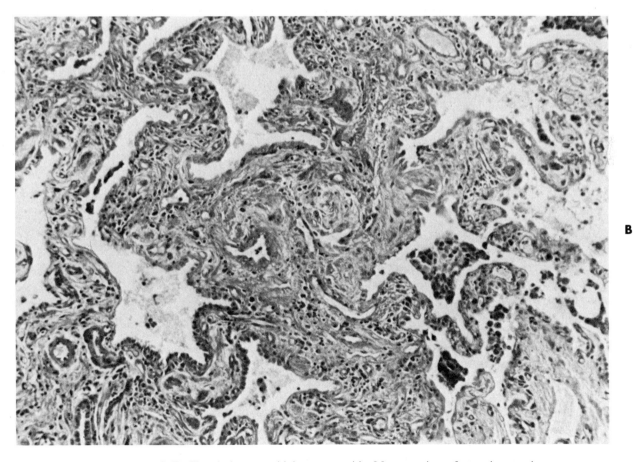

B

**Fig. 14-17, cont'd. B,** Chronic hypersensitivity pneumonitis. Most prominent feature is extensive fibrosis involving alveolar walls and peribronchial tissue. Many alveolar spaces are completely obliterated. Some dilated alveolar spaces contain clusters of macrophages. (×90). (From Middleton E and others, editors: *Allergy: principles and practice,* ed 3, St Louis, 1988, Mosby.)

reduced breath sounds and a characteristic pleural friction rub that has been described as a creaking sound as though two pieces of rough leather were rubbed over one another.

### Pneumothorax

A pneumothorax is said to exist when free air leaks into the pleural space between the visceral and parietal pleura. Pneumothoraces are often categorized on the basis of the general mechanism responsible for the disorder. Traumatic pneumothorax can occur following a multitude of injuries including automobile accidents, gunshot wounds, knife wounds, and other modes of thoracic trauma. Iatrogenic pneumothorax occurs with various types of cardiac and pulmonary surgeries and biopsies. Mechanical ventilation and associated high positive inspiratory pressures are well-known causes of pneumothorax. Induced or artificial pneumothorax is of historic interest since it was commonly applied for treatment of pulmonary tuberculosis. Spontaneous pneumothorax, also referred to as secondary pneumothorax, is seen in many pulmonary diseases that are not associated with trauma. Some of these diseases include asthma, cystic fibrosis, pulmonary emphysema, pneumoconiosis of many types, infections, malignancies, and empyema. Tension pneumothorax is worthy of special note. This situation occurs when the air leak responsible for the pneumothorax is such that a check-valve mechanism permits air to enter but not exit the pleural space. As air accumulates in the pleural space, it may compress the ipsilateral lung, the mediastinum, and ultimately the contralateral lung. Tension pneumothorax is life threatening. When pneumothorax is accompanied by hemorrhage into the pleura, usually caused by trauma, a hemothorax or hemopneumothorax is said to exist. Similarly, when traumatic rupture of the thoracic duct allows lymphatic drainage material to enter the pleural space, again usually with trauma, a chylothorax exists.

The pathogeneses of both traumatic and iatrogenic pneumothoraces are usually obvious. Secondary pneumothorax usually occurs when one or more of several conditions exist. Diseases that weaken the structural integrity of the pleural tissue surely place the patient at risk for pneumothorax. When those diseases are associated with increased intrapulmonary pressures, such as occurs in severe asthma, the risk for pneumothorax is greatly increased. In addition, diseases that destroy lung parenchyma and diseases that cause cysts or bullae are common causes of pneumothorax. Patients with pulmonary emphysema and cystic fibrosis have the type of parenchymal destruction that predisposes them to pneumothorax.

Signs and symptoms of pneumothorax are varied depending on such factors as the mechanism, severity of disease, and size of accumulation. Small pneumothoraces may be asymptomatic, particularly if they develop insidiously, which enables the patient to accommodate to the physiological changes. With a large, rapidly developing pneumothorax,

the patient might experience a sudden sharp pain and severe dyspnea. Coughing may occur but is not a classical symptom. A large pneumothorax will often cause a mediastinal shift to the contralateral hemithorax (Fig 14-18). This shift can be palpated by finding the trachea. In addition, auscultation of the large pneumothorax will result in diminished or distant breath sounds. Mediate percussion will usually show a tympanic note resulting from the air accumulation in the pleural space. The individual with concomitant severe lung disease, such as emphysema or cystic fibrosis, will often be severely ill, and signs and symptoms will be severe and pronounced. In situations involving a hemopneumothorax, shock is another possible complication, particularly with massive blood loss into the thoracic cavity. A well-known example of this last scenario occurred in 1981 when President Reagan suffered a gunshot wound in which a small artery in the thorax was involved and resulted in massive hemorrhage into his chest cavity.

## ATELECTASIS

Although not a disease itself, atelectasis is such a common finding in many diseases and is so commonly treated by various techniques of physical therapy that it merits description. Atelectasis is a state of lung tissue characterized by loss of volume resulting from a lack of expansion of gas exchange areas of lung tissue. Numerous pathological conditions and mechanical circumstances can lead to atelectasis.

Primary atelectasis is a term used to describe a condition in which lack of expansion occurs because of incomplete

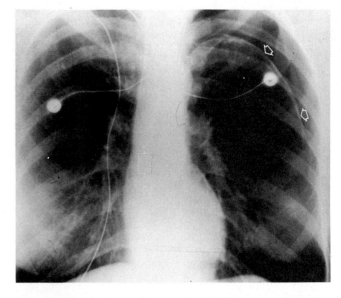

**Fig. 14-18.** Simple pneumothorax on the left. The characteristic thin white line representing the visceral pleura is readily identified *(open white arrows)*. (From Civetta JM, Taylor RW, and Kirby RR: *Critical care,* Philadelphia, 1988, JB Lippincott Co.)

inspiration. When an insufficient volume of air is inspired, alveoli will not become fully expanded. Patients who develop primary atelectasis are those with neurological, muscular, and skeletal disorders that either restrict thoracic expansion or prevent the development of adequate negative inspiratory pressure. In each of these states, the patient will fail to expand the lungs, and primary atelectasis is likely to follow. Of course, this group represents a large population commonly treated by physical therapists.

In addition to the inability to generate adequate inspiratory volume or pressure, reduced alveolar surface tension can result in a form of primary atelectasis. Low alveolar surface tension is maintained by the phospholipid material called "surfactant." Several major disorders are characterized by ineffective or absent surfactant. Adult respiratory distress syndrome, which follows severe trauma, surgery, and certain diseases, is thought to be caused by a loss of pulmonary surfactant resulting in massive areas of microatelectasis. Similarly, respiratory distress syndrome of prematurity is caused by surfactant that has not yet reached the correct chemical composition because of the prematurity of the infant. The baby is unable to maintain alveolar expansion because of the ineffective surfactant.

Secondary, or obstructive, atelectasis is a common finding in patients with other pulmonary disorders. Airway obstruction caused by copious or inspissated secretions, severe bronchial smooth muscle spasm, or significant edema of the bronchial wall and epithelium in patients with either acute or chronic obstructive lung disease are each capable of producing obstructive atelectasis. Foreign body aspiration is another common cause of atelectasis in children.

Patients who have undergone thoracic surgery present a special problem regarding atelectasis. These individuals usually have aspects of both primary and obstructive atelectasis. The primary atelectasis accrues from the pain encountered as they attempt to inspire spontaneously following discontinuation of mechanical ventilation. The obstructive aspect relates to the irritating effects on the respiratory epithelium of the commonly employed anesthetic gases and irritation by the cuff of the endotracheal tube. As a result of these predisposing factors, as many as 50% to 60% of thoracic surgery patients will develop postoperative atelectasis.

The pathophysiological mechanism of obstructive atelectasis is rather straightforward. When complete obstruction is encountered in a bronchus that supplies air to a normally perfused area of lung parenchyma, the gas within the alveoli distal to the obstruction is absorbed into the pulmonary circulation. This process of absorption is usually not immediate, but takes several hours or more. Once all alveolar gas has been absorbed into the circulation, the alveoli, now devoid of gas, will collapse in a fashion similar to a balloon that has lost its air.

Compression of the lung or of a bronchus is another common pathogenesis for obstructive atelectasis. These situations are often called extraluminal obstruction since the obstructing material is not found within the bronchial lumen. Children born with abnormalities of the great vessels will often have atelectasis because the pulmonary artery is in an abnormal position or the aorta can mechanically compress and obstruct a major airway. In adults tumors are a common cause of both extraluminal and intraluminal obstruction that leads to recurrent atelectasis. Bronchogenic carcinoma and other types of tumor can cause recurrent atelectasis, which should be carefully evaluated by the physician.

When atelectasis occurs normal lung function ceases. Gas exchange is obviously lost because of the inability to ventilate past the point of obstruction. Lung mechanics are ineffective because of an extraordinary decrease in lung compliance in the area to be expanded. Pulmonary perfusion is altered because the localized hypoxia causes a reflex vasoconstriction in the pulmonary vasculature to move blood from the ineffective lung tissue. In addition, it has been suggested that alveolar macrophage activity, mucous clearance, and other types of defense mechanisms may be ineffective in atelectasis.

Signs and symptoms of atelectasis may include cough, fever, sputum production, and crackles or wheezes. Physical signs include shift of the mediastinum to the ipsilateral side, a dull percussion note of the region of collapse, diminished or absent breath sounds, and reduced thoracic movement in the involved hemithorax. Radiographic views usually demonstrate a definable area of radiopacity in the portion of lung that lacks expansion (Fig. 14-19).

## ACUTE RESPIRATORY FAILURE

Acute respiratory failure can be defined in functional terms as a pathophysiological process interfering with gas exchange in a manner that threatens life. It may similarly be defined as a process that results in the inability to extract oxygen from inspired gas or to eliminate carbon dioxide from the lungs, or both. Finally, acute respiratory failure has been described in terms of arterial blood gas values. A partial pressure of arterial oxygen ($Pa_{O_2}$) of 50 mmHg or less or a partial pressure of arterial carbon dioxide ($Pa_{CO_2}$) of greater than 50 mmHg are values commonly associated with acute respiratory failure. When considering arterial blood gas values, one must recall that various factors, particularly age, will reduce arterial oxygen in the elderly. Clearly, acute respiratory failure can be subdivided into those instances caused by carbon dioxide abnormalities and those caused by deficits in oxygen.

### Hypercapnic respiratory failure

Hypercapnic respiratory failure is determined primarily by reduced tidal volume or respiratory rate, each of which will reduce minute ventilation, or by increased physiologic

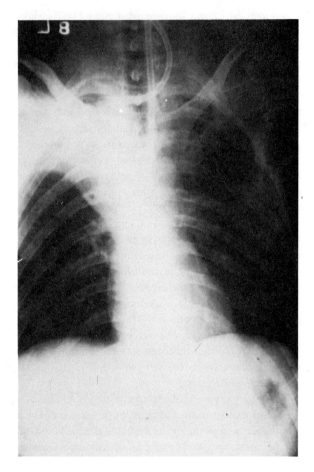

**Fig. 14-19.** Radiograph illustrating right upper lobe atelectasis.

dead space, areas of the lung that are well ventilated but poorly perfused with blood.

**Reduced minute ventilation.** Central nervous system disorders can reduce minute ventilation via depression of the respiratory center of the medulla. Accidental overdoses of sedatives, suicide attempts, and excess use of "street" drugs are all causes of respiratory depression. Diseases of the central nervous system, including tumors, vascular insufficiency, and infections can also have similar depressant effects on the respiratory center.

Neuromuscular diseases, which are seen commonly in physical therapy, can produce a rapid or slow reduction in minute ventilation. Most of these diseases, myopathy, spinal cord injury, amyotrophic lateral sclerosis, poliomyelitis, and Guillan-Barre syndrome, interfere with some link in the chain of events that ultimately produce contraction of the inspiratory muscles, primarily the diaphragm. Paresis and paralysis lead to reduced chest wall and lung compliance, thereby increasing the physical work of breathing and further reducing minute ventilation.

Thoracic cage disorders, like neuromuscular diseases, are very common in physical therapy and can lead to reduced minute ventilation and respiratory failure. Primary disorders of the thoracic cage include scoliosis and kyphoscoliosis,

ankylosing spondylitis, and rheumatoid arthritis to name a few. Secondary thoracic cage disorders may result from many of the central nervous system and neuromuscular diseases noted above. Thoracic compliance and lung compliance are both reduced, often to a severe degree, in each of the categories. With reduced compliance, work of breathing increases and $CO_2$ retention often follows.

**Increased physiologic dead space.** Physiologic dead space can be thought of as areas of the lung that are well ventilated but poorly perfused; hence, much of the ventilation to those areas is "wasted." That is, the well-ventilated areas add little to gas exchange for lack of adequate perfusion. Nonetheless, energy is required to ventilate the physiologic dead space even though neither oxygen gain nor carbon dioxide removal occurs. A point exists when the energy expended to maintain the ventilation is greater than can be sustained. Beyond that point, inadequate ventilation caused by extensive physiologic dead space can lead to acute respiratory failure of the hypercapnic variety. Hypercapnic respiratory failure secondary to increased physiologic dead space is common in chronic obstructive pulmonary diseases including chronic bronchitis, late in pulmonary emphysema, cystic fibrosis, and others.

### Hypoxemic respiratory failure

Although hypoxemia is a common feature in hypercapnic respiratory failure, it may exist in relatively pure form as hypoxemic respiratory failure. Two patterns of hypoxemic respiratory failure are common. One pattern involves patients whose hypoxemia responds well to administration of supplemental oxygen. In this group of patients, there is a significant rise of from 2 to 5 mm Hg in arterial oxygen tension per percent increase in $Fio_2$. The pathophysiology for this response is thought to be areas of the lung that are poorly ventilated but well perfused, thereby producing shunts in which the perfusion has no access to oxygen from the alveolar gas. Pneumothorax, severe and acute asthma, and obstructive pneumonia may precipitate this type of hypoxemic respiratory failure.

Hypoxemic respiratory failure may alternatively take a course in which supplemental oxygen has virtually no effect on the arterial oxygen tension. This pattern occurs in patients with adult respiratory distress syndrome. This is a very serious disorder caused by an unusual group of events including chest trauma, septicemia, fat embolism, oxygen toxicity, drug overdose and others. The severe hypoxemia is thought to be due to pulmonary edema and widespread atelectasis, which may be secondary to damage to the Type II pneumocytes which produce surfactant. Other theories of causation include a severe inflammatory reaction, microvascular thrombosis, and extensive activation of the complement system within the lung.

These are common patterns of hypoxemic respiratory failure. The several physiologic mechanisms that result in hypoxemia are shown in Table 14-1.

**Table 14-1.** The five causes of hypoxemia and example, method of determination, and results of oxygen therapy for each cause

| Cause | Example | Determination | Results of oxygen therapy |
|---|---|---|---|
| Decreased oxygen intake | High altitude, rebreathing expired air | Low ambient inspired oxygen, no oxygen gradient | Rapid increase in $Pao_2$ |
| $\dot{V}/\dot{Q}$ ratio imbalance | Chronic obstructive pulmonary disease | Oxygen gradient, correction of $Pao_2$ with 100% oxygen | Moderately rapid increase in $Pao_2$ |
| Shunt | Adult respiratory distress syndrome, ventricular septal defect, pulmonary arteriovenous fistula | Oxygen gradient, incomplete correction of $Pao_2$ with 100% oxygen | Moderately rapid, variable increase in $Pao_2$ depending on size of shunt |
| Diffusion impairment | Interstitial pneumonia, scleroderma | Normal oxygen gradient at rest; increased gradient with exercise | Moderately rapid increase in $Pao_2$ |
| Hypoventilation | Chronic obstructive pulmonary disease, drug overdose, cerebrovascular accident | Hypercapnia | Early increase in $Pao_2$; variable later response |

## BIBLIOGRAPHY

Agostini C and others: HIV-1 and the lung, state of the art, *Am Rev Respir Dis* 147:11038, 1993.

Bass J and others: Control of tuberculosis in the United States, 146:1623, 1992.

Burton GG, Hodgkin JE, and Ward JJ, editors: *Respiratory care: a guide to clinical practice,* ed 3, Philadelphia, 1991, JB Lippincott Co.

Dail DH and Hammar SP, editors: *Pulmonary pathology,* New York, 1988, Springer-Verlag.

Fishman AF, editor: *Pulmonary diseases and disorders,* ed 2, New York, 1988, McGraw.

Harvey AM and others, editors: *The principles and practice of medicine,* ed 22, Norwalk, Conn, 1988, Appleton & Lange.

Kissane JM, editor: *Anderson's pathology,* ed 9, St Louis, 1990, Mosby.

Murray JF and Mills J: Pulmonary infectious complications of human immunodeficiency virus infection, part 1, *Am Rev Respir Dis* 141:1356, 1990.

Murray JF and Mills J: Pulmonary infectious complictions of human immunodeficiency virus infection, part 2, *Am Rev Respir Dis* 141:1582, 1990.

Purtilo DT and Purtilo R: *A survey of human diseases,* ed 2, Boston, 1989, Little, Brown & Co.

Robins SL and Kumar V, editors: *Basic pathology,* ed 4, Philadelphia, 1987, WB Saunders Co.

Snider GL: Emphysema: The first two centuries—and beyond, part 1, *Am Rev Respir Dis* 146:1334, 1992.

Snider GL: Emphysema: The first two centuries—and beyond, part 2, *Am Rev Respir Dis* 146:1615, 1992.

Spencer H, editor: *Pathology of the lung,* ed 4, Elmsford, NY, 1984, Pergamon.

Thurlbeck WM, editor: *Pathology of the lung,* New York, 1988, Thieme Medical Publishers.

# CHAPTER 15

# Age-Related Changes in the Cardiopulmonary System

*Claire Peel*

## ADAPTATIONS IN THE CARDIOPULMONARY SYSTEM WITH AGING

As individuals age, normal physiological adaptations occur in the cardiovascular and pulmonary systems. Knowledge of these changes is important because of the growing number of older persons in the population who are served by physical therapy. Physical therapists are not only involved in the management of older persons with primarily musculo-

skeletal or neurological dysfunction, they also organize and direct general exercise programs designed to prevent deterioration of function. The purpose of this chapter is to discuss the changes that occur with aging in cardiovascular and pulmonary structure and function. Implications for the physical therapy management of older persons also are presented.

Identifying adaptations that result solely from the aging process is difficult, because both asymptomatic disease and physical deconditioning are common in older persons. The incidence of cardiac disease, including those persons without overt signs or symptoms, has been estimated to be as high as 60%.[42] Physical deconditioning occurs in part because older persons are often encouraged not to perform vigorous physical activities. To study age-related changes only, subjects need to be carefully screened for the presence of cardiopulmonary disease, and physical activity levels need to be documented. When changes associated with disease and deconditioning are not present, the remaining age-related changes do not appear to limit significantly most normal activities.

In designing physical therapy care plans for older persons, cardiovascular and pulmonary function need to be considered. Understanding the normal, expected changes in clinical measurements is necessary in order to identify abnormal values and to be able to establish realistic treatment goals. Another factor to consider is the increased variability in both resting measurements and in responses to stress that occurs with aging. Because of the wider range of physical characteristics, individualized programs are essential to challenge adequately and safely each patient.

This chapter begins with a discussion of structural and functional changes that occur in the cardiovascular system, followed by a discussion of changes that occur in the pulmonary system. Special considerations for exercise testing and for prescribing exercise for older patients are then presented, followed by a discussion of adaptations that result from performing regular physical exercise. The chapter

**Table 15-1.** Age-related changes in submaximal and maximal exercise responses

|  | Submaximal exercise | Maximal exercise |
|---|---|---|
| Oxygen consumption | — | ↓ |
| Heart rate | — | ↓ |
| Cardiac output | ↓ | ↓ |
| Stroke volume | ↓ | ↓ |
| a-$\tilde{V}O_{2diff}$ | ↑ | ↓ |
| Lactate | ↑ | ↓ |
| Blood pressure | ↑ | ↑ |

— = no change; ↑ = increases with aging; ↓ = decreased with aging.

## Age-related structural changes in the cardiovascular system

**Heart**
*Myocardium*
Increased wall thickness
Accumulation of lipofuscin
Increase in elastin, fat, and collagen
*Endocardium*
Thickened areas composed of elastic, collagen and muscle fibers
Fragmentation and disorganization of elastic, collagen and muscle fibers
*Conduction system*
Atrophy and fibrosis of left bundle branches
Decrease in number of SA-node pacemaker cells
*Valves*
Thickening and calcification

**Vasculature**

Increased size (primarily of proximal vessels)
Increased wall thickness (primarily of distal vessels)
Increase in connective tissue and lipid in subendothelial layer
Atrophy of elastic fibers in media layer
Disorganization and degeneration of elastin and collagen

concludes with a discussion of the influence of age-related cardiopulmonary changes on the general physical therapy management of geriatric patients.

## CARDIOVASCULAR SYSTEM

Structural adaptations occur in the heart and peripheral vasculature that may or may not be related to observed, functional changes that reflect cardiovascular status. In most healthy older persons, the cardiovascular system functions adequately at rest and during low-intensity exercise, but a decrease in maximal exercise capacity occurs. Because of this age-related decrease in maximal capacity, a given level of submaximal work becomes relatively more stressful.

In this section structural changes in the heart and vasculature are discussed first, followed by functional changes at rest and with activity. The section concludes with a discussion of the regulation of the cardiovascular system in response to varied stresses.

### Structural changes

**Heart.** Morphological, or structural, changes occur with aging in cardiac muscle, the endocardium, the conduction system, and in cardiac valves (Table 15-1). Left ventricular wall thickness increases slightly; the increase has been estimated to be approximately 30%.[26,42] This mild hypertrophy is most likely related to changes in the arterial system that produce increased resistance to ventricular outflow.[54] Within the cardiac muscle cells, there is an accumulation of lipofuscin,[45,60] a brown pigment that reflects oxidized lipid derived from the digestion of cell membranes.[9] Its accumulation tends to occur in cells that are subjected to chronic, low-grade injury.[9] Functional implications of this change are unknown. Foci of fibrosis, elastic tissue, fat, and collagen also are increased in the myocardium.[83,84] These changes may relate to the development of a stiffer, less compliant ventricle.

In the endocardium, thickened gray-white areas develop, which occur focally in the right atrium and ventricles and diffusely in the left atrium.[49] Histologically these thickened areas consist of a proliferation or hypertrophy of elastic,

collagen, and muscle fibers.[49] Degenerative changes described as fragmentation and disorganization of fibers appear in the hypertrophied tissue. Fat infiltration and a loss of cohesion of collagen and elastic fibers have been reported in the subendocardium. Mechanical factors determined by blood flow patterns appear to contribute to these changes.

Collagen and fat deposition occurs in specific areas of the conduction system.[59] Atrophy and fibrosis tend to occur in the left bundle branches, with a partial loss of proximal connections between the left fascicles and the main bundle. The infiltration of tissue in this area may produce dysrhythmias or heart block. Age-related changes do not appear to occur in the AV node and bundle of His.[35] Around age 60 the number of pacemaker cells in the sinoatrial (SA) node begins to decrease. By age 75 less than 10% of the pacemaker cells present in young adults may remain.[83] These changes in the SA node and the conduction system may contribute to the high incidence of ECG abnormalities seen in older persons.

The cardiac valves become thickened and calcified with aging. Nodular thickenings appear along the closure lines of the AV valves and along the attachments of the aortic cusps.[60,83] Common clinical effects of valvular calcification include mitral valve incompetence, aortic stenosis, and systolic murmurs. The cause appears to be related to mechanical factors, because the earliest calcium deposits occur at sites of highest expected mechanical stresses.[61] In addition, both systolic and diastolic blood pressures tend to be higher in older persons with mitral valve calcification.[61]

**Vasculature.** Structural changes in blood vessels vary, depending on the region of the body and on the proximal or distal relationship of that vessel to the heart (Table 15-1). Changes are most prominent in the thoracic aorta compared with other parts of the body and in the left coronary arteries compared to the right coronary arteries.[89] Chronic mechanical stresses may be greater for these parts of the vasculature.

With aging, blood vessels tend to become dilated and to increase in wall thickness. Proximal arteries are more prone to dilation, and peripheral arteries are more prone to develop wall thickening.[46] The dilation is especially prominent in the thoracic aorta, whose volume has been estimated to increase fourfold from age 20 to age 80.[42]

Wall thickness increases because of an increase in connective tissue and lipid in the subendothelial layer.[84] The media layer shows atrophy of elastic fibers and increased calcification.[35] In addition, diffuse increases in collagen occur throughout vessel walls.

These changes make older vessels less compliant, or more stiff, compared with younger ones. With the decrease in compliance, the pressure required to change volume is increased. The increase in size of the thoracic aorta is thought to be a compensatory mechanism for the increased stiffness. A larger aorta can more readily accept the stroke volume ejected from the left ventricle, avoiding excessively high pressures. Even though the vessel walls become thicker, there appears to be disorganization and degeneration of the elastin and collagen, with a decrease in tensile strength.[46] Consequently, arterial wall tissue may become weaker with age.

### Resting cardiovascular function

In normal, healthy older persons, age-related changes in cardiovascular function usually are not apparent when at rest. The two most common changes detected by routine clinical measurements occur in blood pressure (BP) and electrocardiography (ECG). Resting BP increases with age, with the increase more prominent for systolic BP, compared with diastolic BP (Fig. 15-1).[38] The increase occurs at least partially because of changes in the vascular system, which include an increased stiffness of the ascending aorta and a decrease in size of the peripheral vascular bed.[38,54] Both changes increase the resistance to ventricular outflow. The increased vascular load can produce decreases in both stroke volume (SV) and cardiac output (CO) and contribute to the mild ventricular hypertrophy.[63] Blood pressure also appears to become more variable within an individual with age. Because of the age-related "normal" increase in BP and the increased variability in measured values, identifying persons with hypertension is often difficult. The increases in BP with age may not be a natural consequence of aging, as these changes are not seen in all populations. Studies of persons living in the Solomon Islands and on Indian reservations have reported either no or minimal increases in BP with age.[18,56] The life-styles of both of these populations differ

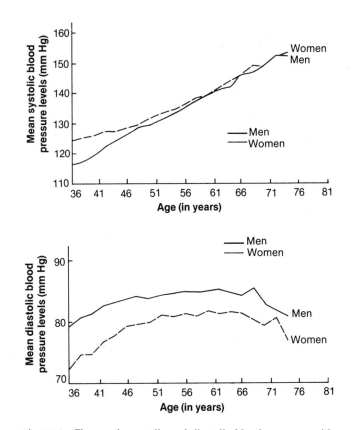

**Fig. 15-1.** Changes in systolic and diastolic blood pressures with age. (Adapted from Kannel WB and Gordon T: Evaluation of cardiovascular risk in the elderly: the Framingham study, *Bull NY Acad Med* 54:579, 1978.)

from populations of other studies in both diet and physical activity levels and in the lack of processed foods and modern conveniences.

A high incidence of resting ECG abnormalities has been reported. In a group of 2482 elderly patients, left axis deviation was recorded in 51%, ST-segment changes in 16%, atrial premature beats in 10%, first-degree heart block in 9%, atrial fibrillation in 8%, and ventricular premature contractions in 6%.[26] Resting heart rate (HR) does not usually change, but there appears to be a decrease in the normal HR variations related to the respiratory cycle and in spontaneous variations in HR during a 24-hour period.[17,40] In addition, intrinsic HR, or the HR after blocking the autonomic nervous system innervation to the heart, decreases.[45,68] These changes may relate to changes in SA-node tissue, decreased responsiveness of autonomic cardiovascular reflexes, or decreased sensitivity to catecholamines.[40] Functional consequences of these changes are unknown.

Age-related changes in cardiac muscle function include increases in the time to develop peak tension and in the time for relaxation.[43,44] These changes may be related to inhibition of calcium transport or alterations in calcium stores.[28] The slower relaxation time most likely contributes to the decreases that occur in diastolic filling rate. It has been estimated that, by age 70, the filling rate is approximately one half of that of a 35-year-old.[28,68] Consequently, relatively more ventricular filling occurs later during diastole.

The atrial contribution to diastolic filling appears to increase with age.[51] This change is most likely a compensatory mechanism to maintain adequate ventricular filling. In addition to the prolonged relaxation time, ventricular filling may be affected by changes in the mitral valve and in ventricular compliance. Both age-related thickening and calcification of the mitral valve and decreases in ventricular compliance increase resistance to flow of blood into the left ventricle. The changes in diastolic filling rate probably do not significantly affect resting function but may limit cardiac output during vigorous exercise.

### Cardiovascular responses during exercise

Age-related changes in the cardiovascular responses to exercise differ, depending on whether the exercise is performed at a submaximal or a maximal level of intensity (Table 15-1). For submaximal exercise the relationship between oxygen consumption ($\dot{V}o_2$) and HR is similar for old and young persons of comparable fitness levels.[86] In older persons SV (and consequently CO) tends to be lower for submaximal work. To maintain the same level of $\dot{V}o_2$ the arterial-venous oxygen difference (a-$\tilde{v}o_{2diff}$) increases.[73] Blood levels of lactate also tend to be higher during submaximal exercise in older persons, which may reflect a relatively higher generation of energy from anaerobic sources.

During maximal exercise, HR and $\dot{V}o_2$ are lower in older persons. The magnitude of the decrease in maximum HR is variable, and often is not as high as predicted by the commonly used formula, 220 – age.[5,25] One reason for the variability is that subjects may not be stressed to maximal levels in some of the reported studies. Reasons for the lower maximum HR are not known, but may include decreased compliance of the left ventricle (which prolongs diastolic filling time), decreased intrinsic HR, decreased input to the pacemaker cells, decreased sensitivity of the heart to catecholamines, or a combination of these factors.

The decreased maximum $\dot{V}o_2$ ($\dot{V}o_{2max}$) results from a decrease in maximum a-$\tilde{v}o_{2diff}$, and possibly a decrease in maximum CO. Maximum a-$\tilde{v}o_{2diff}$ tends to be lower in the elderly because of lower arterial oxygen saturation, lower hemoglobin levels, and a relatively greater increase in skin blood flow. Several studies have reported values for maximum CO for older persons that are 20% to 30% lower than values for younger persons.[14,37,77] These studies used invasive technology and possibly individuals with asymptomatic heart disease. The decrease in CO resulted primarily from a decrease in maximum HR, with less of a decrease in SV.[14,37] Ejection fraction during maximal exercise also has been reported to decrease with age, from approximately 84% at 35 years of age to 76% at 71 years of age.[86]

A recent study reported that CO during maximal exercise was maintained in older active individuals who had been carefully screened to rule out the presence of cardiovascular disease.[64] This study involved 61 volunteers without cardiovascular disease as determined by maximal treadmill ECG and thallium scans. The results of this study showed that maximum HR decreased, but that maximum CO was maintained by a compensatory increase in SV. It has been speculated that decreases in maximum $\dot{V}o_2$ and HR may be true age-related changes, but that decreases in maximum SV may be related to the presence of asymptomatic heart disease.

Blood pressure tends to be higher in older persons during both submaximal and maximal exercise.[20] Maximum systolic blood pressure levels of 217 and 206 mm Hg for older men and women respectively, compared with 180 mm Hg for young subjects, have been reported.[68] Higher BP responses are usually associated with higher levels of myocardial oxygen consumption, or cardiac work. The rate-pressure product (RPP), or product of HR and SBP, is used to estimate myocardial oxygen consumption. Because of the lower HR values for older persons performing maximal exercise, the RPP values may be similar for old and young persons. The causes of higher BP values during exercise are probably similar to those at rest and relate to the decreased compliance of the arterial system.

Because older persons tend to have increases in subcutaneous fat, skin blood flow during exercise may constitute a greater percentage of maximum CO. Visceral blood flow, in absolute units, is probably similar for old and young persons.[68] Because of the lower maximum CO in older persons, however, visceral flow represents a higher percentage of the total CO. Consequently, the proportion of blood flow to active skeletal and cardiac muscle may be decreased during maximal exercise.

An important implication of the age-related decrease in maximal exercise capacity is the effect on relative exercise intensity for submaximal work. A given level of submaximal exercise utilizes a greater percentage of maximal capacity, and consequently becomes more stressful. Because most activities of daily living are performed at submaximal work levels, these activities pose relatively greater stresses. Older persons may discontinue some of these activities, losing independence, or continue to perform activities that present excessive cardiovascular stresses and are unsafe.

### Regulation of cardiovascular function

With aging, the cardiovascular system loses some of its ability to rapidly adapt to varied stimuli. Baroreceptor sensitivity decreases, as demonstrated by changes in HR and BP responses to orthostasis, cough, and a Valsalva maneuver.[67,69,83,85] For example, in response to moving from supine to standing, the increase in HR is 10 to 15 beats per minute (bpm) less in older versus younger persons.[67] Blood pressure decreases with this maneuver, often producing symptoms of dizziness, weakness, and confusion.[68] The HR response to coughing is used as an index of the capacity for cardiac acceleration. The response to forceful coughing decreases in both magnitude and rate of response with increasing age.[85] This adaptation may also be related to the decrease in baroreceptor sensitivity.

With aging, the responsiveness of the heart and vasculature to beta-adrenergic stimulation also decreases.[89] This change involves decreases in the ability of the heart to increase rate and contractility and of the arterial system to vasodilate. The effects of this decreased responsiveness are most apparent during stressful physical activities. This adaptation partially explains the lower maximum HR and SV values during exercise in older persons. Many older persons compensate for this by an increase in end-diastolic volume during high-intensity exercise, which produces increases in SV.[64]

When beginning exercise, it takes older persons a longer time to reach steady state levels of HR, BP and ventilation.[72] It also takes older persons longer to recover form exercise. The longer recovery time may be related to a greater dependence on anaerobic energy sources or to a slower dissipation of heat. Consequently, the slowed rate of response for older persons needs to be considered in designing exercise programs.

### Summary

Structural changes, primarily in connective tissue, occur with aging in the myocardium, cardiac valves, and peripheral vasculature. The locations of these changes suggest that chronic mechanical stresses may be a causal factor. The result is a less compliant cardiovascular system. Functional consequences include an increase in BP, a mild left ventricular hypertrophy, and a decrease in the rate of diastolic filling. An increase in the size, primarily in the proximal part of the vasculature, compensates partially for the decreased compliance of blood vessels.

In most older persons, changes in resting cardiovascular function do not produce noticeable signs or symptoms. A decrease in maximal exercise capacity, or $Vo_{2max}$ occurs, which results from decreases in maximum HR, SV and a-$\tilde{v}o_{2diff}$. The lower values for maximal exercise are at least partially related to the decreased responsiveness to beta-adrenergic stimulation. With a lower maximal capacity, activities performed at submaximal exercise levels become relatively more stressful.

The decreases in cardiovascular reserve capacity seen in elderly persons may be at least partially attributed to undiagnosed coronary artery disease or to physical deconditioning. Healthy older persons who have remained active demonstrate smaller decreases in maximum CO and $Vo_2$ compared to older sedentary persons.[42] Consequently, persons should be encouraged to remain active and to maintain a low cardiovascular disease risk profile as they become older.

## PULMONARY SYSTEM

As individuals age, structural changes occur in the chest wall, lung tissue, and pulmonary blood vessels. Changes also occur in the regulation of respiration. These changes influence lung function, as indicated by altered lung volumes, flow rates, and other tests of pulmonary function. Limitations resulting from these changes may not be evident at rest but may become apparent with physical activity. In comparison to younger persons, the pulmonary system, rather than the cardiac system, is often the factor limiting vigorous exercise in older persons.

### Chest wall

With aging, changes occur in the thoracic spine and costovertebral joints that are similar to age-related changes throughout the musculoskeletal system. There is an increase in the cross-linking of collagen fibers, which increases tissue stiffness and resistance to movement.[34] Range of motion of the costovertebral joints decreases. Changes in the thoracic vertebrae include decreases in the elasticity of cartilage, in the collagen of the annulus fibrosis, and in water content of the nucleus pulposa.[48] The intervertebral disc becomes flattened and less easily moved. The compliance, or the change in volume for a given change in pressure, of the chest wall is decreased.[50]

These connective tissue changes produce alterations in posture and in the work of breathing. Postural changes include an increase in thoracic kyphosis and a shortening of the thoracic spine.[48] The anteroposterior diameter of the thoracic cavity increases. Because of the decreased compliance, there is an increase in the pressures that are necessary to move air in and out of the thoracic cavity. Consequently, the work of the respiratory muscles during breathing increases.

### Lung tissue

Structural changes in the conducting system are minimal and probably of little functional significance. The size of the large airways does not change,[68] but a decrease in the elasticity of the bronchial cartilage has been reported.[90] An increase in the number of bronchial mucous glands, with a thickening of the mucous layer, has also been reported.[90]

Important changes occur in the elastic fibers of the lung parenchyma, or supportive network. There is a decrease in the number and thickness of elastic fibers that are oriented radially to small airways.[88] Because these fibers function to maintain airway patency, there is increased resistance to airflow, especially when breathing at low lung volumes. The change is reflected by the age-related decreases in FVC, $FEV_{1.0}$, $FEF_{25\%-75\%}$, and $FEF_{200-1200ml}$ (Fig. 15-2).[52,75] The changes in $FEF_{25\%-75\%}$ are usually more pronounced compared with the other values, possibly because this test reflects flow rates at relatively low lung volumes.

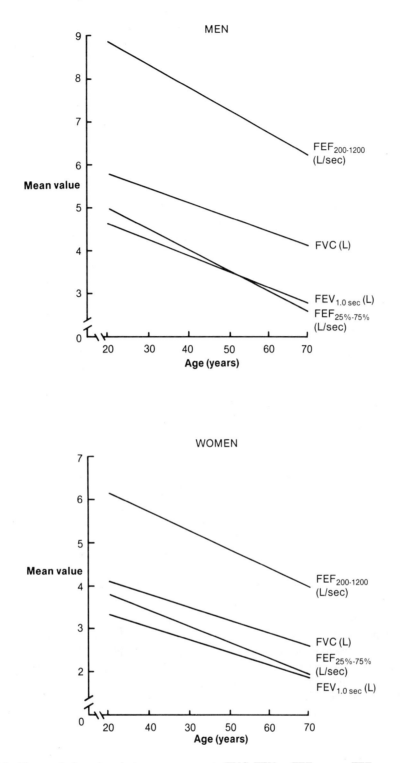

**Fig. 15-2.**  Changes in forced expiratory measurements (FVC, $FEV_{1.0}$, $FEF_{200-1200}$, $FEF_{25\%-75\%}$) with age for male and female subjects. (From Morris JF, Koski A, and Johnson LC: Spirometric standards for healthy nonsmoking adults, *Amer Rev Respir Dis* 103:63, 1971.)

A progressive loss of the elastic recoil of the lungs begins around age 25.[81] The lungs are stretched during inspiration, and the resulting recoil forces that occur during expiration are decreased. Consequently, more air is retained in the lungs at the end of expiration. The decrease in elastic recoil is reflected by an increase in residual volume (RV), or the air remaining in the lungs after a maximal expiration (Fig. 15-3).[12,36] Total lung capacity (TLC) does not change

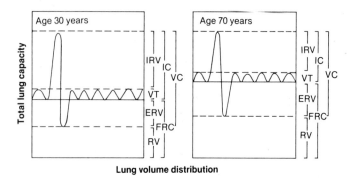

**Fig. 15-3.** Changes in lung volumes with age. (Reproduced with permission from Shapiro BA, Harrison RA, and Walton JR: *Clinical application of blood gases,* ed 3, Chicago, 1982, Year Book Medical Publishers.)

significantly with aging. Because TLC is the sum of RV and vital capacity (VC), VC decreases with age. Functional residual capacity (FRC), or the air left in the lungs after a normal expiration, may increase slightly or may not change. FRC is determined by a balance between the inward elastic recoil of the lungs and the outward elastic recoil of the chest wall. Similar decreases in both of these opposing forces explain the minimal changes in FRC.

The loss of elastic recoil also produces an increase in closing volume, or the volume of the lung at which dependent airways begin to close.[4,47] In young persons the closing volume is approximately 10% of VC. Closing volume increases to approximately 40% of VC as individuals approach 65 years of age.[87] As closing volume approaches or exceeds FRC, inspired air is preferentially distributed to the upper regions of the lungs. Because blood flow remains higher in the lower regions, an imbalance between ventilation and perfusion occurs. Ventilation/perfusion ($\dot{V}/\dot{Q}$) mismatch contributes to alterations in arterial oxygen values.

The functional units of the lung, alveoli, and alveolar ducts become larger with aging.[79] The changes occur uniformly throughout the lungs, in contrast to nonuniform, destructive changes that occur with emphysema.[88] Because of the increased size, additional time is needed for mixing between inspired air and alveolar air. Alterations in mixing time are demonstrated by having old and young persons breathe oxygen. When older persons breathe oxygen, there is a delay in the maximal level of oxygen saturation of arterial blood compared with younger persons.[12] A consequence of inadequate mixing is lower arterial oxygen values.

Even though the total amount of lung tissue does not appear to change with aging, there is a decrease in the surface area that is available for gas exchange. The surface area decreases from approximately 75 m$^2$ in a young adult to 65 m$^2$ for persons of 70 years of age.[79] The result is a decrease in the diffusing capacity, which also contributes to lower arterial oxygen values.

## Pulmonary vasculature

With aging, the intima layer of blood vessels becomes thicker with increased fibrosis, and vessel walls lose elasticity.[82] There is a decrease in the number of pulmonary capillaries, decreasing the amount of lung surface area that is covered with capillaries.[12] The decrease in capillary surface area correlates with a decrease in diffusing capacity.[15]

The decrease in the alveolar-capillary interface, in combination with the $\dot{V}/\dot{Q}$ mismatch, produces changes in blood gas values. There is a decrease in the arterial partial pressure of oxygen (Pao$_2$) of approximately 4 mm Hg per decade.[12] Arterial oxygen saturation decreases, and the alveolar-arterial oxygen difference increases.[78] The arterial partial pressure of CO$_2$ does not change significantly.[80]

## Respiratory muscles

Many changes occur with aging in skeletal muscle function, including a decrease in fiber size and number and a decreased capability of the neuromuscular junction to transmit nerve impulses.[80] These changes may be primarily related to inactivity rather than to aging. The diaphragm, which remains active throughout life, undergoes only minimal age-related changes.[80] As chest wall compliance increases with age, the respiratory muscles must exert higher forces to achieve similar changes in thoracic volume.

Because of the increase in RV, the resting position of the diaphragm is altered (Fig. 15-4). The normally domeshaped diaphragm becomes flattened by the additional air in the lungs. Consequently, the maximal excursion of the muscle decreases, making it less efficient in moving air into the lungs. To compensate, accessory breathing muscles are recruited, especially when older persons perform physical activities.

The strength of the diaphragm appears to decrease slightly with age, as indicated by measurements of mouth occlusion pressures. A 24% decrease in mean maximal static inspiratory pressure was reported in a comparison of an older (ages 55 to 75 years) versus a younger (ages 20 to 29 years) group of subjects.[58] The endurance of the respiratory muscles may also decrease with age, as indicated by decreases in maximal voluntary ventilation (MVV).[68] The decreased resting length of the diaphragm may contribute to the changes in strength and endurance. Other contributing factors may include changes in the neuromuscular junction and in phrenic nerve conduction velocity.

## Regulation of respiration

The respiratory system of control consists of peripheral and central chemoreceptors, a central nervous system integrator, and the respiratory neuromuscular system. The central chemoreceptors are primarily responsive to high levels of CO$_2$ (hypercapnia) and the peripheral chemoreceptors to low levels of O$_2$ (hypoxia). The ventilatory responses to hypercapnia and hypoxia decrease with ag-

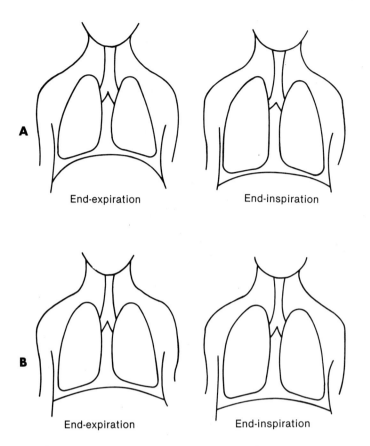

**Fig. 15-4.** Typical changes in the position of the diaphragm from end-expiration to end-inspiration in a 20-year-old person (**A**) versus a 70-year-old person (**B**).

ing.[10,41,58] The decrease may result from altered perception of $CO_2$ levels, poor central integration, decreased neural outflow to the respiratory muscles, or decreased muscular response. The expected increase in heart rate with hypoxia also appears to be decreased.[41] Because of these changes, older persons may have an impaired ability to adjust to hypoxic and hypercapnic disease states. In addition, the typical diagnostic signs of hypoxia, tachycardia, and increased ventilation may be absent.

Older individuals may be less able to protect large airways from obstruction and be more susceptible to aspiration pneumonia because of decreases in cough and laryngeal reflexes. Older persons demonstrate less of a response to inhaled ammonia, which is used as a cough stimulus.[62] In addition, older individuals tend to cough less than younger individuals.[62] Mean tracheal mucous velocity also has been reported to be slower in older persons.[30] The influence of these changes on the incidence of airway obstruction and on the recovery of older persons from pulmonary infections is unknown.

### Ventilatory responses during exercise

In moving from rest to exercise, gas exchange tends to improve because of an improvement in the matching of ventilation and perfusion. In persons of all ages, there is more uniform distribution of ventilation, as well as an increase in pulmonary artery pressure, which increases blood flow to the lungs.[68,87] Consequently, the abnormalities in ventilation and perfusion described in older persons at rest should not worsen during activity.

During progressive exercise, the pattern of increasing ventilation differs between young and old men (Fig. 15-4).[21] At low workloads older persons tend to increase ventilation by increasing tidal volume (TV) rather than breathing frequency (fb). As higher levels of ventilation are needed, fb increases. In contrast, younger men show higher breathing rates with lower tidal volumes. In older persons, the initial increase in TV may serve as a compensatory mechanism, allowing an improvement in airflow. Breathing at high lung volumes decreases the resistance to inspiratory flow and improves elastic recoil. The increased elastic recoil improves expiratory flow. Increasing TV at low workloads may be a disadvantage because of an associated onset of dyspnea. As TV approaches 50% to 60% of VC, dyspnea tends to occur. Considering that older persons have lower vital capacities, TV may reach this level at relatively low work levels.

With aging, the ventilatory requirements during activities increase. A greater ventilation is needed for a given workload and for a given level of oxygen consumption in older persons compared to younger persons (Fig. 15-5).[21,57] This change may result partially from age-related changes in structure that result in altered gas mixing and $\dot{V}/\dot{Q}$ mismatching. In addition, as maximal aerobic capacity decreases, older persons may rely more on anaerobic metabolism, with the additional $CO_2$ produced serving to increase ventilation. The rate of change of exercise ventilation has been estimated to be approximately 5% per decade.[21,55]

An additional consideration is the increase in the oxygen cost of breathing during exercise because of the age-related increases in chest wall stiffness. In young persons the oxygen cost of breathing during maximal exertion is approximately 10% of maximum oxygen consumption.[6] In older persons the energy cost of breathing increases, and maximum oxygen consumption decreases. Consequently, the amount of oxygen remaining for cardiac and skeletal muscle activity is lessened, decreasing maximal work capacity.

### Summary

Age-related structural and functional changes in the pulmonary system are summarized in Table 15-2. With aging, the chest wall becomes less compliant, requiring increased respiratory muscle force for a given change in lung volume. The lungs become more compliant, losing some of their ability to recoil passively during expiration. Consequently, there is an increase in the amount of air retained in the lungs after maximal expiration, and the diaphragm is flattened into a less advantageous position for function. Changes in elastic fibers also produce increases in small airway resistance.

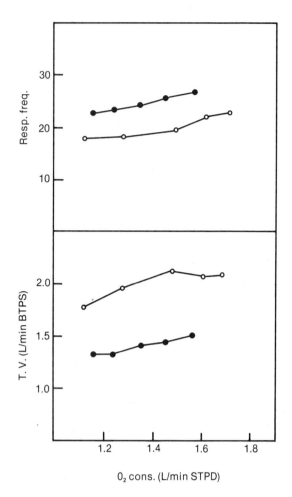

**Fig. 15-5.** Changes in tidal volume and respiratory frequency with progressive exercise in old and young subjects. (From deVries HA and Adams GM: Comparison of exercise responses in old and young men: II. Ventilatory mechanics, *J Gerontol* 27:350, 1972.)

**Table 15-2.** Age-related structural and functional changes in the pulmonary system

| Structural changes | Functional consequences |
|---|---|
| **Thorax** | |
| Increased stiffness of costovertebral joints | Increased kyphosis |
| Decreased compliance of chest wall | Increased work of breathing |
| **Respiratory muscles** | |
| Decreased resting length | Decreased mouth occlusion pressures |
| | Decreased MVV |
| **Lung tissue** | |
| Increased size of alveoli and alveolar ducts | Less efficient mixing of alveolar and inspired air |
| | Decreased surface area for diffusion |
| Decreased number and thickness of elastic fibers | Increased resistance to flow in small airways |
| | Decreased $FEV_{1.0}$, FVC, $FEF_{200-1200 ml}$, $FEF_{25\%-75\%}$ |
| | Decreased elastic recoil |
| | Decreased VC, increased RV |
| | Change in resting length of respiratory muscles |
| | Increased closing volume, and redistribution of inspired air |
| **Vasculature** | |
| Decreased number of pulmonary capillaries | Decreased diffusing capacity |
| | Increased A-a $O_2$ gradient |
| | Decreased $PaO_2$ $O_2$ sat |
| | $\dot{V}/\dot{Q}$ mismatch |

Structural changes in the alveoli and in capillaries decrease the alveolar-capillary interface, decreasing diffusing capacity and contributing to a $\dot{V}/\dot{Q}$ imbalance. Consequently, arterial oxygen partial pressure and saturation are decreased.

The changes described occur in normal, healthy persons and are similar to the changes that occur with some pulmonary diseases. For healthy older persons, the limitations primarily occur with vigorous activity, though the decreased responsiveness may be important during acute respiratory infections. For older persons with pulmonary disease, the combination of age-related and disease-related changes may severely impair lung function both at rest and with mild activity. When treating older persons with disease, the changes that naturally occur with aging need to be considered in formulating realistic treatment goals and in interpreting pulmonary function test results.

## CONSIDERATIONS FOR EXERCISE TESTING AND PRESCRIPTION FOR THE ELDERLY PATIENT

There appears to be an increased interest of older persons in participating in regular exercise programs. The specific goals of the individual need to be considered, as older persons vary in their purposes for starting an exercise program. Some are more interested in improving cardiorespiratory fitness, whereas others primarily seek health benefits. For healthy individuals who wish to begin a low-intensity exercise program, a thorough medical evaluation and stress test may not be needed. Persons who wish to begin a moderate- to high-intensity program, who have a history of cardiopulmonary disease, or who have signs or symptoms of disease, need a medical evaluation including an exercise stress test. Because of the variability in fitness levels and life-styles among older persons, it is important that the prescribed exercise program be appropriate to the individual. Group exercise programs are good for socialization, but often some participants are overstressed, whereas others are understressed. Ideally, exercise programs should be developed based on the individual's goals and objectives.

## Exercise testing

Purposes of exercise testing include determining the individual's capacity to perform exercise and determining safe levels of exercise. Interpretation of exercise test results in older patients is often difficult because of the inability to distinguish between age-related benign changes and pathological changes. The high incidence of ECG abnormalities both at rest and during exercise in older persons contributes to the difficulty in test interpretation. In a sample of approximately 2500 older persons, 57% demonstrated ECG abnormalities at rest.[26] Approximately 30% of 65-year-olds develop signs or symptoms of myocardial ischemia during vigorous exercise.[70] In determining the clinical significance of documented abnormalities, additional factors need to be considered, including the intensity and duration of the exercise test, the methods of collecting data, and the life-style and medical history of the patient. To ensure a safe and effective exercise prescription, abnormal findings should not be ignored. For questionable findings, additional evaluation or consultation may be indicated in lieu of preventing the patient from beginning an exercise program.

The method and protocol for exercise testing depend primarily on the purpose of the test. Because of the increased incidence of cardiovascular disease in older persons, the safety of performing graded exercise tests is often a concern. The risk of testing asymptomatic, healthy persons of age 65 has been speculated to be no greater than the risk of testing younger persons with symptoms of cardiovascular disease.[68] This risk is one episode of ventricular fibrillation per 30,000 tests, and one death per 150,000 tests.[68] Recent reports document both the safety and efficacy of exercise testing for older persons with signs or symptoms of cardiovascular disease.[29,53] In a study of 153 patients aged 65 years or greater, exercise stress testing to 85% of maximum HR was associated with a sensitivity of 85%, a specificity of 56% and a predictive value of 86%.[53] In these two reports, involving a total of 257 patients performing either symptom-limited maximal exercise tests or exercise to 85% of predicted maximum HR, there were no incidences of complications that required medical intervention.

Many older persons are not able to exercise to high enough levels to demonstrate a plateau in oxygen consumption with increasing workload. Maximal tests in older persons are more often symptom limited by shortness of breath, fear of overexertion, muscular weakness, or ECG abnormalities. If the primary purpose of performing a test is to identify abnormalities that may occur with increased activity, the patient should be stressed to his or her symptom-limited maximal level because many abnormalities are detected only during high-intensity effort.

Submaximal exercise tests are safer and more comfortable, but may not be of sufficient intensity to identify abnormalities. The error in predicting maximum $\dot{V}O_2$ from results of submaximal tests increases with age because the variability in maximum HR values increases and mechanical efficiency decreases.[71] Because of the high prediction error, documenting workload and/or $\dot{V}O_2$ at a specific submaximum HR, rather than extrapolating to a predicted maximum HR, provides more accurate information. This type of data is useful to compare changes within an individual as the result of exercise training.

The type of activity to be used during testing depends on the musculoskeletal and neurological status of the patient and on the anticipated exercise prescription. For persons with poor balance, the cycle ergometer offers a stable sitting position. An additional advantage is that BP can be easily monitored. Disadvantages of using a cycle ergometer include an unfamiliar movement pattern for many older adults and the possibility that exercise level may be limited by poor quadriceps muscle strength and endurance, rather than by the cardiovascular system. The treadmill provides an activity that is familiar and functional. Handrails should be available for support and balance, but should not be used if energy expenditure is predicted from the workload performed. Progressively increasing grade of walking, rather than speed, is easier for most older persons. Step ergometers can also be used with older subjects. These ergometers are inexpensive and portable, but may not be practical for patients with poor balance or with musculoskeletal limitations. For older persons with physical limitations, a stepping test performed sitting in a chair has been designed.[74] Ideally, the testing mode should be similar to the training mode to identify the optimal training prescription.

If possible, older persons should be able to practice on the equipment to be used for testing. A practice session is especially important for sedentary persons who are not accustomed to exercising. If the test is to involve collection of expired air, then practice using this equipment also is important. Many older persons, especially those with dentures, have difficulty maintaining an adequate seal when using a mouthpiece. Hearing and visual abnormalities should be identified, so that modifications can be made to assure a valid test result.

## Exercise prescription

Many of the principles for designing exercise programs for middle-aged, sedentary adults can be applied to designing programs for older adults.[2] Because of the age-related changes in exercise responses, there are areas that require modification. The exercise program should be comprehensive and should include activities based on the functional needs of the patient. Activities to increase or maintain muscle strength and endurance and flexibility need to be included. The program should be designed to stress the patient in a safe way and to provide enjoyment.

In designing the aerobic exercise component, additional time needs to be allowed for warm-up and cool-down activities. A longer time period is needed for older persons to adjust to exercise or to reach a physiological steady state, and a longer time period is needed to recover from exercise. Reasons for slower adjustment most likely relate to the decreased responsiveness of the cardiovascular system to catecholamines, and to decreased fitness levels. Five- to ten-minute periods of warm up and cool down are recommended, with a 20- to 30-minute period at the training HR or workload. Intensities of 60% to 75% of maximum HR, or 40% to 70% of maximum $Vo_2$ have been suggested to elicit aerobic training adaptations in older persons.[45,73] Though lower than the intensity recommended for young adults, this level may promote better compliance to the program, especially in sedentary older persons. Progression should be slow, with special attention to potential musculoskeletal problems, as older persons tend to be more prone to injuries. A minimum frequency of three sessions per week has been recommended.[45] Because older persons can often benefit from daily activities, a 6 day program, alternating aerobic, strengthening, and flexibility exercises, may be optimal.

Older persons tend to be less tolerant of the heat than younger persons. Causes include increased subcutaneous fat and possible atrophy of sweat glands.[45] Consequently, older persons need to be monitored closely for signs and symptoms of heat stress. In addition, education on prevention and management of heat stress is indicated.

For older persons who have been sedentary most of their lives, encouragement and supervision are essential. Many of these persons may be self-conscious about exercising and fearful of overexertion. Education on proper techniques, methods of monitoring intensity, and signs and symptoms of overwork will assist to minimize these concerns. Close supervision during the initial part of the program will facilitate compliance and ensure appropriate responses to the program. As patients gain skill in self-monitoring and progression, the amount of supervision can be decreased.

## BENEFITS OF PERFORMING REGULAR EXERCISE

During the past 5 to 10 years, many studies have been published documenting the effects of regular physical exercise in the older population. Most of these studies have involved healthy volunteers who are in the age range of 60 to 70 years. Recently, there have been a few reports of exercise studies involving the frail elderly or older persons with chronic diseases. The purpose of this section is to describe the results of some of these studies. Responses to both resistive, or strengthening exercise, and aerobic, or endurance exercise, are discussed.

### Studies involving independent older persons

Studies of healthy older persons can be divided into two categories based on the type of activities performed during training: 1) programs to increase aerobic capacity, or cardiorespiratory fitness, and 2) programs to increase muscle strength. In general, the results of programs are similar and indicate that older healthy persons can increase aerobic capacity and muscle strength by performing an appropriate program of regular exercise.

Table 15-3 provides a summary of selected studies that have been published during the past 10 years, and documents the results of aerobic exercise training. The subjects were healthy men and women, primarily 60 to 70 years of age. Most exercise programs were conducted 3 or 4 times each week, with sessions varying from 20 to 60 minutes in length. Several studies included a low-intensity training period for several months, followed by a higher-intensity training period.[22,32,66] (This strategy allows older sedentary persons time to accommodate gradually to the exercise stress, and most likely minimizes the risk of injury during the high-intensity training period.) One study compared low-intensity training at 40% of maximum heart rate reserve (HRR) to moderate-intensity training at 60% of maximum HRR, and found comparable results.[24] Most studies report that subjects participated with enthusiasm, and that compliance was excellent.

As noted in Table 15-3, all studies report an increase in maximum oxygen consumption, with average increases ranging from 11% to 30%. This result is similar to results of studies performed using young persons as subjects, and reflects differences in the intensity, duration, and frequency of exercise of the varied programs. A decrease in resting HR and BP is reported in one study, with no change reported in another study.[16,76] A decrease in blood cholesterol is reported in one study, with no change reported in another study.[8,24] Of particular interest is the study by Ehsani and others that reports increases in ejection fraction during exercise, and an increase in peak stroke volume.[22] The exercise prescription for this study was relatively intense, involving five, one-hour sessions per week, at an intensity up to 80% of maximum oxygen consumption. Subjects also performed brief periods of exercise at intensities up to 90% of maximum oxygen consumption during the final months of the program. The changes documented are most likely related to the program's high intensity, and to the 1-year duration of the program.

These studies indicate that older, healthy persons respond to aerobic training in a manner similar to younger persons. The exercise prescriptions used in the reported studies are similar to those recommended for healthy middle-aged adults. The major differences are longer periods for warm up and cool down. For older persons, a major benefit of exercise training is the lower physiological responses during submaximal exercise, which is the level that most activities of daily living are performed.

Results of studies of subjects performing strength training programs are summarized in Table 15-4. As noted in these studies, both older men and women are able to safely perform strength training with supervision. Studies report

**Table 15-3.** Studies of aerobic training in healthy older adults

| Source | Sex/age | Type of program | Duration | Results |
|---|---|---|---|---|
| Seals[66] | M,F/60-69 yrs | Low intensity for 6 months followed by high intensity for 6 months 3x/week 20-45-min. sessions walk/jog/cycle | 1 year | ↑ $\dot{V}_{O_{2max}}$—30% ↓ submaximal exercise HR, BP |
| Cunningham[16] | M/55-65 yrs | 70% of maximum HRR* 3x/week 30-min. sessions walk/jog | 1 year | ↑ $\dot{V}_{O_{2max}}$—11% No change in resting BP or HR |
| Blumenthal[8] | M,F/60-83 yrs | 70% of maximum HRR 3x/week 60-min. sessions walk/jog/cycling | 4 months | ↑ peak $\dot{V}_{O_2}$—12% ↓ cholesterol ↓ DBP |
| Foster[24] | F/67-89 yrs | 60% of maximum HRR, 40% of maximum HRR 3x/week 100 kcal expended per session walk | 10 weeks | ↑ $\dot{V}_{O_{2max}}$—15-21% No changes in blood cholesterol, maximal or lactate, maximum RPP |
| Hagberg[32] | M,F/70-79 yrs | 50-85% $\dot{V}_{O_{2max}}$ 3x/week 40-min. sessions walk/jog | 26 weeks | ↑ $\dot{V}_{O_{2max}}$—22% ↓ submaximal exercise HR, RPE |
| Steinhaus[76] | M,F/55-70 yrs | 65-80% of $HR_{max}$ 3x/week 60-min. sessions walk/jog | 4 months | ↑ $\dot{V}_{O_{2max}}$—27% ↓ resting HR, SBP |
| Ehsani[22] | M/60-70 yrs | 60-80% $\dot{V}_{O_{2max}}$ 5x/week 60-min. sessions walk/run/cycle | 11.8 months | ↑ $\dot{V}_{O_{2max}}$—23% ↑ ejection fraction during exercise ↑ peak SV |
| Kohrt[39] | M,F/60-71 yrs | 80% of $HR_{max}$ 4x/week 45-min. sessions walk/jog | 9-12 months | ↑ $\dot{V}_{O_{2max}}$—24% |
| †Coggan[13] | M,F/60-70 yrs | 80% $HR_{max}$ 4x/week 45-min. sessions walk/jog | 9-12 months | ↑ Type IIa fibers; ↑ area of Type I, IIa fibers; ↑ capillary density ↑ oxidative enzymes |

*HRR = $HR_{max} - HR_{rest}$; Training HR = .70 (HRR) + $HR_{rest}$
†Subjects in this study were a subset of a larger sample described by Kohrt.[39]

high subject compliance with few incidences of musculoskeletal discomfort. Although methods of evaluation of muscle strength differ in the reported studies, both increases in the maximum amount of weight lifted, and in peak torque measured with an isokinetic dynamometer are reported. Of particular interest are the increases in muscle size reported in two of the studies. These studies confirm that older persons retain the capacity for muscle hypertrophy. Although older persons typically begin strengthening programs at lower levels than younger persons, they appear to show similar increases when adaptations are expressed as percent changes.

**Studies involving older persons living in extended care facilities**

Older persons living in extended care facilities typically either are unable to walk or have difficulty walking. There are multiple causes, yet one contributing factor is physical deconditioning. Sauvage and others conducted a study to evaluate the effects of an aerobic and strengthening exercise program in older male nursing-home residents.[65] Subjects were selected who could ambulate independently, but who demonstrated both lower-extremity muscle weakness, and gait and balance difficulties. The exercise program was 12 weeks in duration, with 3 sessions per week. At each session,

**Table 15-4.** Studies of strength training in healthy older subjects

| Source | Sex/age | Type of program | Duration | Results |
|---|---|---|---|---|
| Aniansson[3] | M,F/63-86 yrs | 40-min. sessions<br>2x/week<br>Resistance provided by elastic bands | 10 months | ↑ isokinetic strength: 10-13%<br>↑ area of Type IIa fibers |
| Fontera[27] | M/60-72 yrs | 80% of 1RM<br>3x/week<br>Knee flexors and extensor | 12 weeks | ↑ 1RM: 10%<br>↑ isokinetic strength: 10%<br>↑ $\dot{V}o_{2max}$: 6% |
| Charette[11] | F/69 yrs | 65-75% of 1RM<br>3x/week<br>7 lower extremity muscle groups | 12 weeks | ↑ 1RM: 28-115%<br>↑ area of Type II fibers |
| Grimby[31] | M/78-84 yrs | Isometric, eccentric, concentric knee extension | 25 sessions | ↑ maximal torque<br>↑ EMG during eccentric activity |

subjects performed 20 minutes of stationary cycling at 70% of maximum HR and resistive exercises for major muscle groups of the lower extremities. Subjects improved in muscle strength, endurance, and gait velocity, but did not improve in aerobic capacity or balance. The authors considered the changes to be clinically meaningful, and speculated that a program of longer duration or greater intensity possibly could be more effective.

The effect of strength training in reversing muscle weakness in older men who lived in a nursing home was reported recently.[23] In this study, older men and women, with an average age of 90 years, participated in an eight-week program of high-intensity resistance exercise. The subjects performed knee extension exercises 3 times each week at an intensity of 80% of 1RM. Subjects demonstrated a threefold to fourfold increase in the amount of weight that could be lifted. In addition, mid-thigh muscle area increased 9% and gait speed increased 48%. The investigators concluded that supervised resistance exercise was not only safe, but also effective in increasing strength and function in older persons in their ninth and tenth decades of life.

Both of these studies demonstrate that supervised exercise programs are feasible in the population of older persons living in long-term care facilities. In both studies, improvements were demonstrated in walking, which is an important functional activity. For subjects to maintain improvements, exercise needs to be performed on a regular basis. An ideal situation would be for extended care facilities to provide exercise equipment and assistance, including creating an atmosphere to motivate clients.

### Studies involving older persons with cardiovascular disease

Cardiac rehabilitation programs can provide older persons with cardiovascular disease opportunities to improve functional capacity and to minimize dependence and dis-ability. In addition to their cardiovascular disease, these individuals often are deconditioned and have other chronic diseases. Therefore, it is a challenge to the health care professional to provide safe and effective exercise programs.

The question has been asked as to whether older persons receive similar benefits from exercise training as middle-aged individuals. A study by Ades and Grunvald compared a group of older persons, with an average age of 68 yrs, to a group of younger persons, with an average age of 52 years.[1] Subjects had experienced coronary events and entered a 12-week cardiac rehabilitation program. The program included three, one-hour sessions per week, with treadmill and cycle ergometry exercise performed at 75% to 85% of the maximum HR value from the initial treadmill test. Peak oxygen consumption was lower in the older group at the beginning of the program. At the end of the 12 weeks, the increases in peak $\dot{V}o_2$ were similar for the two groups, 27% for the older group and 23% for the younger group. The results of this study indicate that although older persons may be less fit than younger persons, the relative improvements with exercise training are similar.

The role of regular exercise for persons with hypertension also has been studied using older persons as subjects. Hagberg and others compared moderate-intensity training (73% of $\dot{V}o_{2max}$) to low-intensity training (53% $\dot{V}o_{2max}$) in older persons with hypertension.[33] Subjects trained for 9 months, 3 times per week. Subjects in the low-intensity group walked for one-hour sessions, and subjects in the moderate-intensity group trained for 45 to 60 minutes, using fast walking, jogging, cycle ergometry, and treadmill walking. The results indicated an increase in $\dot{V}o_{2max}$ in the moderate-intensity training group of 28%, with no significant change in the low-intensity group. Diastolic BP decreased 11 to 12 mm Hg in both groups. Systolic BP decreased 20 mm Hg in the low-intensity group, and only 8 mm Hg in the moderate-intensity training group. The investigators concluded that low-intensity exercise may be more beneficial than moderate-intensity exercise for older persons with hypertension.

Considering the high incidence of cardiovascular disease in the elderly, cardiac rehabilitation programs need to design ways to meet the unique needs of older clients. Focus should be on improving performance in functional activities, and on education so that clients can continue program activities in their home environments. The goals should include methods to maximize physical independence and minimize disability that results from deconditioning, cardiovascular disease, and other chronic diseases.

## CONSIDERATIONS FOR GENERAL PHYSICAL THERAPY MANAGEMENT OF THE ELDERLY PATIENT

The age-related adaptations described have implications for the therapist who is evaluating and treating older persons with primarily orthopedic and neurological problems. Many older patients referred for physical therapy are deconditioned because of sedentary life-styles or confinement to bed for medical problems. Many of these patients may also have asymptomatic cardiac or pulmonary disease that has not presented problems because of the lack of stress associated with an inactive life-style. Since most physical therapy care plans include an exercise component, it is important that these patients be monitored closely and progressed appropriately.

In the evaluation process information provided by the patient can supply important clues to cardiopulmonary status. Questions relating to previous episodes of cardiac or pulmonary dysfunction and to specific symptoms (such as shortness of breath, chest pain, dizziness, or palpitations) should be asked. The patient's past and current medications often reveal a history of cardiopulmonary abnormalities. The patient's past and present activity levels need to be considered to define a safe and reasonable initial level of exercise. Heart rate, BP, and respiratory rate should be documented at rest and in response to activity. If definite abnormal signs, such as hypertension, hypotension, or an irregular pulse, are noted or if symptoms of shortness of breath, dizziness, or chest pain with activity occur, the patient should be referred for further cardiopulmonary evaluation. If abnormal values are documented inconsistently, with no or minimal symptoms, then the patient can be observed carefully before referring for a more extensive medical evaluation.

Assessing an older person's risk for developing coronary artery disease can also be done as a part of the evaluation process. The importance of selected risk factors appears to change with age. Cigarette smoking, total cholesterol, and glucose tolerance tend to decrease in importance as risk factors in individuals over 60 years of age.[91] A risk-factor profile for geriatric patients has been constructed from data collected from individuals between the ages of 50 and 82

years.[38] This profile includes high-density and low-density lipoprotein values, systolic BP, ECG evidence of left ventricular hypertrophy, and diabetes. Risk-factor profiles can be used to identify patients at high risk for developing signs and symptoms of disease and to design educational programs to provide information on ways to modify risk factors.

In designing treatment programs, the lower maximal exercise capacity of this population needs to be considered. For example, the activity of walking using a three-point gait pattern involves minimal to moderate stresses for most young and middle-aged persons, but may stress older persons close to their maximal capacities. Consequently, the higher relative stress for submaximal activities needs to be considered. In addition, the magnitude and rate of regulatory responses are decreased in older persons. Dizziness and fainting may occur if patients are moved too quickly from supine to sitting or standing. Patients can wear lower-extremity support garments or perform isometric contractions of lower-extremity muscles to minimize the effects of orthostatic hypotension. Educating patients about signs and symptoms of activity intolerance is important because then patients can report relevant information to their therapists.

In designing long-term care plans, the older patient's regular physical activity pattern needs to be addressed. If activities can be performed safely, older persons should be encouraged to maintain or to increase activity levels. It is likely that older active persons are able to perform daily functional activities with less stress than older sedentary persons. A life-style that includes regular physical activity may allow independent living throughout life and minimize disability resulting from cardiovascular and pulmonary diseases.

## SUMMARY

The process of aging appears to cause some inevitable adaptations in the cardiopulmonary system. The most apparent changes involve connective tissue structures and produce increases in stiffness of the myocardium, lungs, and blood vessels. Lung volume and hemodynamic measurements reflect these changes. The regulatory functions of both the pulmonary and cardiovascular systems also experience changes, including decreases in both magnitude and rate of response to specific stimuli. Impaired regulatory function may be related to problems with aspiration and orthostatic hypotension that are common in the elderly. Activity-related changes are most apparent during vigorous activities, reflecting a decrease in cardiopulmonary reserve capacity.

The changes in the cardiopulmonary system that occur with aging are similar to those that occur with physical deconditioning and with some diseases. The age-related changes are opposite to those that result from aerobic exercise training. Therefore, by remaining active throughout life and by maintaining a low risk-factor profile for heart and lung diseases, individuals minimize some of the age-related changes. Healthy life-style patterns need to be developed early in life and maintained throughout life. By including education and appropriate activity prescription into care plans, therapists can hopefully effect the incidence of physical disability in the geriatric population.

## REFERENCES

1. Ades PA and Grunvald MH: Cardiopulmonary exercise testing before and after conditioning in older coronary patients, *Am Heart J* 120:585, 1990.
2. American College of Sports Medicine: *Guidelines for exercise testing and prescription,* ed 3, Philadelphia, 1986, Lea & Febiger.
3. Aniansson A and others: Effect of a training programme for pensioners on condition and muscular strength, *Arch Gerontol Geriatr* 3:229, 1984.
4. Anthonism NR and others: Airway closure as a function of age, *Respir Physiol* 8:58, 1969/70.
5. Astrand PO: Aerobic capacity in men and women with special reference to age, *Acta Physiol Scand* 49 (Suppl 169):1, 1960.
6. Astrand PO and Rodahl K: *Textbook of work physiology,* St Louis, 1977, McGraw-Hill Book Co.
7. Barry AM and others: The effects of physical conditioning on older individuals. I. Work capacity, circulatory-respiratory function and work electrocardiogram, *J Gerontol* 21:182, 1966.
8. Blumenthal JA and others: Cardiovascular and behavioral effects of aerobic exercise training in healthy older men and women, *J Gerontol* 44(5):M147, 1989.
9. Cawson RA and others: *Pathology: The mechanisms of disease,* ed 2, St Louis, 1989, Mosby.
10. Chapman KR and Cherniack NS: Aging effects on the interaction of hypercapnia and hypoxia as ventilatory stimuli, *J Gerontol* 42:202, 1987.
11. Charette SL and others: Muscle hypertrophy response to resistance training in older women, *J Appl Physiol* 70 (5):1912, 1991.
12. Chebotarev DF, Korkushko OV, and Ivanov LA: Mechanisms of hypoxemia in the elderly, *J Gerontol* 29:393, 1974.
13. Coggan AR and others: Skeletal muscle adaptations to endurance training in 60- to 70-yr-old men and women, *J Appl Physiol* 72(5):1780, 1992.
14. Conway J, Wheeler R, and Hammerstedt R: Sympathetic nervous system activity during exercise in relation to age, *Cardiovasc Res* 5:577, 1971.
15. Crapo RO and Morris AH: Standardized single breath normal values for carbon monoxide diffusing capacity, *Am Rev Respir Dis* 123:185, 1981.
16. Cunningham DA and others: Exercise training of men at retirement: A clinical trial, *J Gerontol* 42(1):17, 1987.
17. Davies HEF: Respiratory changes in heart rate, sinus arrhythmia in the elderly, *Gerontol Clin* 17:96, 1975.
18. DeStephano F, Coulehan J, and Kennethewiant M: Blood pressure survey on the Navajo Indian reservation, *Amer J Epidemiol* 109:335, 1979.
19. deVries HA: Physiological effects of an exercise training regimen upon men aged 52-88, *J Gerontol* 25:325, 1970.
20. deVries HA and Adams GM: Comparison of exercise responses in old and young men. I. The cardiac effort/total body effort relationship, *J Gerontol* 27:344, 1972.
21. deVries HA and Adams GM: Comparison of exercise responses in old and young men. II. Ventilatory mechanics, *J Gerontol* 27:349, 1972.
22. Ehsani AA and others: Exercise training improves left ventricular systolic function in older men, *Circulation* 83:96, 1991.
23. Fiatarone MA and others: High-intensity strength training in nonagenarians, *JAMA* 263:3029, 1990.
24. Foster VL and others: Endurance training for elderly women: Moderate vs low intensity, *J Gerontol* 44(6):M184, 1989.
25. Fox SM, Naughton JP, and Haskell WL: Physical activity and the prevention of coronary disease, *Ann Clin Res* 3:404, 1971.
26. Frisch C: Electrocardiogram in the aged: an independent marker of heart disease, *Am J Med* 70:4, 1981.
27. Frontera WR and others: Strength conditioning in older men: skeletal muscle hypertrophy and improved function, *J Appl Physiol* 64(3):1038, 1988.
28. Gerstenblith G and others: Echocardiographic assessment of a normal adult aging population, *Circulation* 56:273, 1977.
29. Glover DR, Robinson CS, and Murray RG: Diagnostic exercise testing in 104 patients over 65 years of age. *Eur Heart J* 5(Suppl E):59, 1984.
30. Goodman RM and others: Relationship of smoking history and pulmonary function tests to tracheal mucous velocity in nonsmokers, young smokers, ex-smokers, and patients with chronic bronchitis, *Am Rev Respir Dis* 117:205, 1978.
31. Grimby G and others: Training can improve muscle strength and endurance in 78- to 84-yr-old men, *J Appl Physiol* 73(6):2517, 1992.
32. Hagberg JM and others: Cardiovascular responses of 70- to 79-yr-old men and women to exercise training, *J Appl Physiol* 66(6):2589, 1989.
33. Hagberg JM and others: Effect of exercise training in 60- to 69-year old persons with essential hypertension, *Am J Cardiol* 64:348, 1989.
34. Hall DA: *The aging of connective tissue,* New York, 1976, Academic Press.
35. Hutchins GM: Structure of the aging heart. In Welsfeldt ML, editor: *The aging heart,* New York, 1980, Raven Press.
36. Jones RL and others: Effects of age on regional residual volume, *J Appl Physiol* 44:195, 1978.
37. Julius S and others: Influence of age on the hemodynamic response to exercise, *Circulation* 36:222, 1967.
38. Kannel WB and Gordon T: Evaluation of cardiovascular risk in the elderly: the Framingham study, *Bull NY Acad Med* 54:573, 1978.
39. Kohrt WM and others: Effects of gender, age, and fitness level on response of $\dot{V}o_{2max}$ to training in 60-71 yr olds, *J Appl Physiol* 71(5):2004, 1991.
40. Kostis JB and others: The effect of age on heart rate in subjects free of heart disease, *Circulation* 65:141, 1986.
41. Kronenberg RS and Drage CW: Attenuation of the ventilatory and heart rate responses to hypoxia and hypercapnia with aging in normal man, *J Clin Invest* 52:1812, 1973.
42. Lakatta EG: Hemodynamic adaptations to stress with advancing age, *Acta Med Scand* 711 (suppl):39, 1985.
43. Lakatta EG, Gerstenblith G, and Angell CS: Prolonged contraction duration in aged myocardium, *J Clin Invest* 55:61, 1975.
44. Lakatta EG and Yin FCP: Myocardial aging: functional alterations and related cellular mechanisms, *Am J Physiol* 242:H927, 1982.
45. Landin RJ and others: Exercise testing and training of the elderly patient. In Wenger NK, editor: *Exercise and the heart,* ed 2, Philadelphia, 1985, FA Davis Co.
46. Learoyd BM and Taylor MG: Alterations with age in the viscoelastic properties of human arterial walls, *Circ Res* 18:278, 1966.
47. LeBlanc P, Ruff F, and Milic-Emill J: Effects of age and body position on "airway closure" in man, *J Appl Physiol* 28:448, 1970.
48. Lewis CB: *Aging: the health care challenge,* Philadelphia, 1985, FA Davis Co.
49. McMillan JB and Lev M: The aging heart. I. Endocardium, *J Gerontol* 14:268, 1959.
50. Mittman C and others: Relationship between chest wall and pulmonary compliance and age, *J Appl Physiol* 20:1211, 1965.
51. Miyatake K and others: Augmentation of atrial contraction to left ventricular inflow with aging as assessed by intracardiac doppler flowmetry, *Am J Cardiol* 53:586, 1984.
52. Morris JF, Koski A, and Johnson LC: Spirometric standards for healthy nonsmoking adults, *Amer Rev Respir Dis* 103:57, 1971.
53. Newman KP and Phillips JH: Graded exercise testing for diagnosis of coronary artery disease in elderly patients. *Southern Med J* 81(4):430, 1988.
54. Nichols WW and others: Effects of age on ventricular-vascular coupling, *Am J Cardiol* 55:1179, 1985.
55. Norris AH, Shock NW, and Yiengst MJ: Age differences in ventilatory

and gas exchange responses to graded exercise in males, *J Gerontol* 10:145, 1955.

56. Page LB, Damon A, and Moellerlag RC: Antecedents of cardiovascular disease in six Solomon Island societies, *Circulation* 49:1132, 1974.

57. Patrick JM, Bassey EJ, and Fentem PH: The rising ventilatory cost of bicycle exercise in the seventh decade: a longitudinal study of nine healthy men, *Clin Sci* 65:521, 1983.

58. Peterson DD and others: Effects of aging on ventilatory and occlusion pressure responses to hypoxia and hypercapnia, *Amer Rev Respir Dis* 124:387, 1981.

59. Pomerance A: Cardiac pathology in the elderly. In Noble RJ and Rothbaum DA, editors: *Geriatric cardiology,* Philadelphia, 1981, FA Davis Co.

60. Pomerance A: Pathology of the myocardium and valves. In Caird Fl, Dalle JLC, and Kennedy RD, editors: *Cardiology in old age,* New York, 1976, Plenum Press.

61. Pomerance A, Darby AJ, and Hodkinson HM: Valvular calcification in the elderly: possible pathogenic factors, *J Gerontol* 33:672, 1978.

62. Pontoppidan H and Beecher HK: Progressive loss of protective reflexes in the airway with the advance of age, *JAMA* 174:2209, 1960.

63. Raven PB and Mitchell J: The effect of aging on the cardiovascular response to dynamic and static exercise. In Weisfeldt ML, editor: *The aging heart,* New York, 1980, Raven Press.

64. Rodeheffer RJ and others: Exercise cardiac output is maintained with advancing age in healthy human subjects: cardiac dilation and increased stroke volume compensate for diminished heart rate, *Circulation* 69:203, 1984.

65. Sauvage LR and others: A clinical trial of strengthening and aerobic exercise to improve gait and balance in elderly nursing home residents, *Am J Phys Med Rehabil* 71:333, 1992.

66. Seals DR and others: Endurance training in older men and women. I. Cardiovascular responses to exercise, *J Appl Physiol* 57(4):1024, 1984.

67. Shannon RP, Minaker KL, and Rowe JW: Aging and water balance in humans, *Semin Nephrol* 4:346, 1984.

68. Shephard RJ: *Physical activity and aging,* ed 2, Rockville, Md, 1987, Aspen Publishers.

69. Shimada K and others: Age-related changes of baroreflex function, plasma norepinephrine, and blood pressure, *Hypertension* 7:113, 1985.

70. Sidney KH and Shephard RJ: Attitudes towards health and physical activity in the elderly: effects of a physical training programme, *Med Sci Sports Exer* 8:246, 1977.

71. Sidney KH and Shephard RJ: Maximum and submaximum exercise tests in men and women in the seventh, eighth and ninth decades of life, *J Appl Physiol* 43:280, 1977.

72. Skinner JS: The cardiovascular system with aging and exercise. In Brunner D and Joki E, editors: *Medicine and sport, vol 4, Physical activity and aging,* Basel Switzerland, 1970, Karger.

73. Skinner JS: Importance of aging for exercise testing and exercise prescription. In Skinner JS, editor: *Exercise testing and exercise prescription for special cases,* Philadelphia, 1987, Lea & Febiger.

74. Smith EL and Gilligan C: Physical activity prescription for the older adult, *Phys Sports Med* 11:91, 1983.

75. Sparrow D and Weiss ST: Pulmonary system. In Rowe JW and Besdine RW, editors: *Geriatric medicine,* ed 2, Boston, 1988, Little, Brown & Company.

76. Steinhaus LA and others: Aerobic capacity of older adults: A training study, *J Sports Med Phys Fitness* 30:163, 1990.

77. Strandell T: Circulatory studies on healthy old men, *Acta Med Scand* 176:205, 1964.

78. Tenney SM and Miller RM: Dead space ventilation in old age, *J Appl Physiol* 9:322, 1956.

79. Thurlbeck WM and Anges GE: Growth and aging of the normal lung, *Chest* 67:35, 1975.

80. Timiras PS: *Physiological basis of geriatrics,* New York, 1988, Macmillan Publishing Co.

81. Turner JM, Mead J, and Wohl ME: Elasticity of human lung in relation to age, *J Appl Physiol* 25:664, 1968.

82. Wagenvoort CA and Wagenvoort N: Age changes in muscular pulmonary arteries, *Arch Path* 79:524, 1965.

83. Wei JY: Heart disease in the elderly, *Cardiovasc Med* 9:971, 1984.

84. Wei JY: Cardiovascular, anatomic, and physiologic changes with age, *Top Genatr Rehabil* 2(1):10, 1986.

85. Wei JY, Rowe JW, and Kestenbaum AD: Post-cough heart rate response: influence of age, sex, and basal blood pressure, *Am J Physiol* 245:R18, 1983.

86. Weisfeldt ML, Gerstenblith ML, and Lakatta EG: Alterations in circulatory function. In Andres R, Bierman EL, and Hazzard WR, editors: *Principles of geriatric medicine,* New York, 1985, McGraw-Hill, Inc.

87. West JB: *Respiratory physiology—the essentials,* ed 2, Baltimore, 1979, Williams & Wilkins.

88. Wright RR: Elastic tissue of normal and emphysematous lungs, *Amer J Pathol* 39(3):355, 1961.

89. Yin FCP: The aging vasculature and its effect on the heart. In Weisfeldt ML, editor: *The aging heart,* New York, 1980, Raven Press.

90. Zadai CC: Pulmonary physiology of aging: the role of rehabilitation, *Top Geriatr Rehabil* 1(1):49, 1985.

91. Zadai CC: Cardiopulmonary issues in the geriatric population: implications for rehabilitation, *Top Geriatr Rehabil* 2:1, 1986.

# CHAPTER 16

# Pulmonary Pharmacology

*David Arnall*

## RESPIRATORY DRUGS

There are several classes of medication commonly used in the treatment of patients with respiratory disease. These groups of medications consist of the following:

1. Sympathomimetics
2. Methylxanthines
3. Mucolytics and expectorants
4. Corticosteroids

Sympathomimetics are largely employed as bronchodilators using a beta-adrenergic receptor model to elicit this effect. Methylxanthines are used as bronchodilators improving ventilation by preventing the destruction of cyclic adenosine 3′, 5′-monophosphate (cAMP) thus prolonging its half life and in turn permitting it to carry out its role as a second messenger for a longer period of time. Methylxanthines also act as diaphragmatic muscle stimulants improving respiratory efforts and reducing the fatigue of respiratory muscles in patients with chronic obstructive pulmonary disease. Mucolytics and expectorants are prescribed by the physician to help clear the bronchopulmonary tree of tenacious mucous plugs, thus allowing better airflow mechanics and reducing airway obstruction. Corticosteroids are important members of the pharmacological armamentarium which the physician employs to give relief to those in respiratory distress. These medications are antiinflammatory agents with an impressive ability to reduce swelling, inflammation and pain. All of these medications have an important place in the treatment of patients with asthma, bronchitis, bronchiectasis, emphysema, cystic fibrosis and several other pulmonary diseases.

## SYMPATHOMIMETICS: HOW DO THESE DRUGS WORK?

The pharmacological management of pulmonary disease such as the chronic obstructive pulmonary diseases (emphysema, bronchitis, asthma, and bronchiectasis) is based in part on the knowledge that the lung has specific cell-surface receptors that mediate bronchoconstriction and bronchodilation. These receptors are referred to as alpha and beta adrenergic receptors. The beta adrenergic receptor populations are divided into two subpopulation types and are designated as beta-1 adrenergic receptors and beta-2 adrenergic receptors.

These adrenergic receptors are external cell-surface membrane bound structures, which when stimulated by a receptor-ligand interaction, initiate cellular events that are specific to that receptor subpopulation. The ligand that bonds to the external cell membrane receptor may be an endogenous hormone such as epinephrine or norepinephrine. Drugs may appear, structurally, to resemble the endogenous catecholamines and therefore have the ability to act as a ligand and bind to the adrenergic receptors.

The drugs that interact with the adrenergic receptor may either be stimulatory (i.e., act as an agonist) or inhibitory (i.e., act as an antagonist). Agonist drugs bind to the receptor and initiate the same intracellular events that the catecholamines stimulate. The antagonist medications will bind to the receptor and prevent the activation of the adrenergic receptor. Thus it is important to understand what biochemical events each receptor subpopulation orchestrates.

The beta-2 receptors are found in great numbers in the bronchopulmonary tree. They mediate bronchodilation and vasodilation with bronchodilation being of greater importance when speaking of lung function and health. For the purposes of this chapter, the main focus is on the beta-2 agonist in the sympathomimetic class of drugs.

## ACTIVATION OF THE BETA ADRENERGIC RECEPTOR

The transmembrane signaling carried out by adrenergic receptors is based on the premise that ligands (a first messenger) like the catecholamines, epinephrine and norepinephrine, bind to external cell membrane receptors and cause a second messenger inside the cell milieu to initiate intracellular events. This premise presumes a communicating link between the first messenger-receptor complex and the activation of the second messenger in the cell's cytoplasm. Research has born out the fact that there is indeed a first messenger, a receptor, a communicating protein called the $G_s$ protein, and a cytoplasmic second messenger called cAMP.

**The ligand.** The ligand might be any number of molecules such as: (1) the catecholamines, epinephrine and norepinephrine; (2) pharmacological agents that act as agonists meaning that they stimulate the adrenergic receptors like the catecholamines; (3) pharmacological agents that act as antagonists binding to the external cell membrane receptor and blocking the activation of the second messenger.

**The receptor.** The receptor has recently been shown to consist of hydrophobic and hydrophilic polypeptide sections. The hydrophobic polypeptide moieties are constructed such that the cylindrically shaped peptides fold back and forth across the entire width of the lipid bilayer seven times, forming a tubelike pore structure through the membrane. These hydrophobic segments are connected one to another by a hydrophilic strand on both the extracellular and intracellular sides of the receptor pore. It is the current thinking that the actual binding site for the ligand is located just inside the pore-shaped receptor on the extracellular side of the membrane.

**The $G_s$ protein.** The $G_s$ protein is located on the inner surface of the cell's lipid bilayer membrane. It is not certain at this time whether the $G_s$ protein is physically associated with the beta adrenergic receptor on the cytoplasmic side of the membrane or whether it is located at a distant site from the receptor. The model for $G_s$ that is currently in use is called the Collision Model. It suggests that when an agonist binds to the beta adrenergic receptor, the $G_s$ protein diffuses through the lipid bilayer and collides with the beta receptor activating the $G_s$ protein. The functional outcome of the activation of the $G_s$ protein is the creation of a second messenger (cAMP) and the activation of intracellular chemical pathways.

The $G_s$ protein consists of three subunits: the $alpha_s$, beta, and gamma subunits. The importance of each of these subunits will become apparent. Once the membrane bound beta receptor has actively bound an agonist and the $G_s$ protein collides with the receptor, the $alpha_s$ subunit of $G_s$ will break away from the beta-gamma dimer. Guanine triphosphate (GTP), a high energy nucleotide, then binds to the $alpha_s$ subunit to form an $alpha_s$ * GTP complex. This complex then associates with the catalytic C subunit of adenyl cyclase to form the $alpha_s$ * GTP * C complex. Adenyl cyclase is an enzyme that breaks high energy bonds, converting adenosine triphosphate (ATP) to the nucleotide called cyclic adenosine monophosphate (cAMP). Once the $alpha_s$ * GTP * C complex is formed, it activates the catalytic C subunit of adenyl cyclase. Cyclic adenosine monophosphate is created from an ATP molecule and it is this cyclic nucleotide that acts as a second messenger. Therefore, the presence of the $alpha_s$ * GTP * C complex describes the "on" or active phase of the $G_s$ protein. The "on" phase essentially is the period during which the intracellular biochemical pathways are being activated by the second messenger, cAMP.

The $alpha_s$ subunit possesses intrinsic GTP-ase enzymatic activity meaning that $alpha_s$ will be able to convert its GTP to guanine diphosphate (GDP). Once $alpha_s$ * GTP is converted to $alpha_s$ * GDP, the stimulatory capabilities of the alpha subunit to activate more catalytic C units of adenyl cyclase wane. The $alpha_s$ * GDP condition actually causes the dissociation from the catalytic C subunit. In other words, the change of state to $alpha_s$ * GDP signals the beginning of the transition from the "on" phase to the "off" or deactivated phase of the $G_s$ protein. Once the alpha subunit is in the $alpha_s$ * GDP state, it has a high bonding affinity for the beta-gamma dimer. As the three subunits reorganize into the trimeric $G_s$ protein, the stimulatory capability of the $G_s$ protein is in the "off" phase (i.e., it is quiescent and will not activate the catalytic C subunit of adenyl cyclase). During this "off" phase, no cAMP is being made and the biochemical pathways are not activated.

In summary, the physical state of the $G_s$ protein describes whether it is "on" or "off." If the trimer has separated into an $alpha_s$ unit and the beta-gamma unit, it is in the "on" state and cAMP is being made actively. If all three subunits are associated with each other, the $G_s$ protein is in the "off" state and no cAMP is being made. The "on" or "off" state of the $G_s$ protein is wholly dependent on beta receptor activation or deactivation. Additionally, the creation or destruction of cAMP is wholly dependent on the activity of the $G_s$ protein. Because of this close linkage of the receptor-ligand complex to the presence of the cAMP nucleotide, complex chemical events can and do lead to complex cellular outcomes, such as bronchodilation.

There is another mechanism by which the cellular levels of cAMP are regulated. An enzyme called phosphodiesterase destroys cAMP, and once the second messenger is no longer present in the cytosol, the biochemical pathways cease to be activated.

All of this information becomes important when you attempt to understand how chemical events such as beta adrenergic receptor stimulation, the eventual formation of cAMP, and the chemical activation of biochemical pathways can actually cause a physical/mechanical event such as bronchodilation. To date, research has been unsuccessful at determining the exact mechanism of action for bronchodilation. However, there are some plausible hypotheses.

One possible explanation is that bronchodilation occurs permissively or passively, secondary to the uncoupling of the interaction between myosin and actin. If no interaction between the contractile proteins were permitted, then passive smooth muscle dilation would be possible. Blocking the activation of an enzyme called myosin light chain kinase (MLCK) prevents the phosphorylation and activation of myosin light chain ($MLC_{20}$). Without the activation of $MLC_{20}$ through phosphorylation, interaction between the actin and myosin filaments will not occur. Additionally, interference with the rise in intracellular calcium just prior to contraction and the inhibition of the formation of the calcium-calmodulin complex that activates MLCK will inhibit contraction and permissively allow smooth muscle dilation to occur. These theoretical constructs need additional research to confirm which mechanism is at work.

## THE SYMPATHOMIMETIC FAMILY OF DRUGS

The sympathomimetic family of medications comprises a large class of natural and synthetic drugs. As a group these medications dominantly have beta adrenergic effects. However, a small number of these medications can also stimulate alpha adrenergic receptors—a receptor type that has not been discussed but that can be viewed as having opposite effects to the beta adrenergic receptors.

The sympathomimetics are widely prescribed because of their usefulness as beta-1 or beta-2 adrenergic agonists (i.e., they mimic some of the actions and the same side effects are observable when patients are given one of the catecholamines, epinephrine and norepinephrine). Some of the sympathomimetics are selective as to which beta receptor they will stimulate. These medications are called beta selective sympathomimetics and they represent a very important and useful subgroup of drugs in this class. Several sympathomimetics have the ability to stimulate both beta receptor types (i.e., they have mixed effects and are referred to as nonselective beta adrenergic drugs).

Those medications that have an affinity for binding to beta-1 receptors are medications that will affect cardiac function. These medications stimulate the heart such that stroke volume and heart rate are increased. Because these medications have a dramatic impact on the heart, the beta-1 drugs are considered to have inotropic and chronotropic effects. Medications with beta-1 effects must be cautiously given to patients because of their potentially harmful side effects such as tachyarrhythmias and hypertension.

For the purposes of this chapter, sympathomimetic medications are largely important for their beta-2 effects. Beta-2 adrenergic stimulation causes bronchodilation. The sympathomimetics with beta-2 actions or that are beta-2 selective in their effects become an extremely important class of drugs because they have very little effect on the heart and act primarily in the lungs. This is important if you want to bronchodilate a patient who has some accompanying heart condition that will be made worse if a nonselective beta adrenergic drug is administered.

## SPECIFIC SYMPATHOMIMETIC AGENTS
### Catecholamines

The two major catecholamines that are used in pulmonary medicine are epinephrine hydrochloride and isoproterenol hydrochloride. Epinephrine is a natural or endogenously produced catecholamine, but it is also synthetically produced, whereas isoproterenol is completely a synthetic analog.

*Epinephrine hydrochloride (also known as adrenalin)*
  Generic Name: epinephrine HCl, adrenalin
  Trade Name: Sus-Phrine

Epinephrine is a mixed adrenergic agonist with alpha, beta-1 and beta-2 effects. In the human body this catecholamine is produced by the adrenal medulla and circulates in the blood stream. It is the hormone that is secreted when a person is faced with a "fight or flight" situation. This hormone, whether naturally or synthetically produced, possesses a 50:50 alpha to beta effect (i.e., it stimulates alpha and beta receptors with equal potency). Therefore, it has very strong beta-1 effects that cause an increase in the strength of heart muscle contractions (increased inotropy) and an increase in heart rate (increased chronotropy). Its beta-2 effects stimulate significant bronchodilation. Its alpha-adrenergic effect is seen in the strong peripheral vasoconstriction that it exerts. Because of the wide number of organ systems that are affected by the administration of epinephrine and because it stimulates the adrenergic receptors nonselectively, physicians do not like using epinephrine unless other drugs of choice have proven ineffective at breaking a persistent or intractable bronchoconstriction. It is of interest to note that epinephrine is one of the active ingredients in Primatene Mist and Bronkaid Mist—two over-the-counter nonprescription medications that are used to break bronchoconstriction.

The biologic half life of epinephrine is short (a few minutes) because there are at least two major enzyme systems, the monoamine oxidase (MAO) system and the catechol-o-methyltransferase (COMT) system, that quickly break down this hormone.

***Side effects.*** Hypertension, headaches, increased nervousness and anxiety, tachycardia, angina, cardiac dysrhythmias, and palpitations.

In individuals with impaired cardiac perfusion, the patient may suffer angina. Epinephrine stimulates the heart to work harder, causing an increased myocardial oxygen demand, increases in the ventricular wall tensions, increases in the rate-pressure product, etc. Since the heart's work is increased when this medication is given, there is a dramatic rise in myocardial oxygen demand that may instigate an angina attack secondary to an under-perfused, hypoxemic myocardium in a person with impaired endocardial perfusion.

*Therapeutic uses.* Infrequently used. Pulmonary uses would be for the relief of bronchoconstriction.

### Isoproterenol hydrochloride
Generic Name: isoproterenol HCl
Trade Name: Isuprel, Medihaler-Iso

Isoproterenol potently stimulates both the beta-1 and beta-2 adrenergic receptors. It is therefore a nonselective beta agonist and has cardiac and pulmonary effects. The beta-1 stimulation causes the heart to beat faster (increased chronotropy) and to beat with greater force (increased inotropy). The beta-2 stimulation causes powerful bronchodilation. Even though isoproterenol has been used for a long time, there is the unattractive therapeutic side effect of driving the heart to work harder and faster. Because of the beta-1 component of this drug, many physicians are rightfully concerned about using this drug to treat bronchoconstrictive events in older patients. Certainly its use in patients with a known cardiac history would be contraindicated. The clinical use of isoproterenol has fallen off dramatically because of these untoward effects. Therefore, the pharmaceutical research chemists have developed over the years a number of very fine sympathomimetics that are beta-2 selective. Most of these newer generation drugs have either no effect or only a small effect on beta-1 receptors, and consequently beta-2 selective drugs have become the drugs of choice in treating the pulmonary patient.

*Side effects.* Palpitations, headaches, tachycardia, tremors, dizziness, and cardiac dysrhythmias.

*Therapeutic uses.* Infrequently used. Pulmonary uses would be for the relief of bronchoconstriction.

## Noncatecholamines

There are a number of noncatecholamines that are wholly beta adrenergic in their actions. Many of them are beta-2 selective, meaning they have small to no beta-1 actions. These agents are entirely synthetic drugs.

### Metaproterenol sulfate
Generic Name: metaproterenol sulfate
Trade Name: Alupent, Metaprel

This medication is considered to be a beta-2 selective agonist with some minor beta-1 activity. It has a chemical structure that makes it less easily broken down by the catechol-o-methyltransferase system, and therefore its biologic half life is approximately 3-4 hours—significantly longer than the catecholamines. This medication is taken orally in pill form, inhaled as a vaporized mist from a metered-dose inhaler, or taken as a syrup preparation for the treatment of small children.

*Side effects.* Tremors, nervousness, dizziness, anxiety, insomnia, hypertension, and tachycardia.

*Therapeutic uses.* Metaproterenol is used in the treatment of acute bronchoconstriction caused by acute asthma. It is also used by many athletes to prophylactically stall the onset of exercise-induced asthma. This medication is used in the treatment of all of the chronic obstructive pulmonary diseases for the purposes of dilating the bronchi and enhancing the clearance of mucous secretions. Whenever a patient is being posturally drained and percussed to help clear the mucous secretions from the bronchopulmonary tree, it is imperative to first give the bronchodilators via small volume nebulization (SVN). Optimal dilation assists the mucociliary elevator to clear mucous plugs from the bronchial passageways and logically should follow SVN treatment.

### Albuterol
Generic Name: albuterol or salbutamol
Trade Name: Proventil, Ventolin

This medication is a beta-2 selective drug with some beta-1 effects when the drug is taken in higher-than-normal doses. This medication is used extensively in an aerosolized form and is administered by the patient using a metered-dose inhaler. This self-administered type of delivery is desirable for the asthmatic patient because it can be delivered directly into the lungs onto the bronchial membranes to relieve bronchoconstriction. Using a metered-dose inhaler provides a fast-acting route of administration producing the desired bronchodilatory effects within a few seconds to a couple of minutes, and the medication can be delivered as soon as the bronchoconstrictive symptoms begin to occur. The medication is also made in pill form and as a syrup for use with pediatric patients.

*Side effects.* Anxiety, nervousness, headache, insomnia, dizziness, and irritability.

*Therapeutic uses.* This medication is commonly used for reversing bronchoconstriction in patients with acute asthma or in patients with the chronic obstructive pulmonary diseases. Albuterol is also a favorite drug used by aerobic athletes who are plagued with exercise-induced asthma (EIA) and typically must worry about EIA during exercise bouts in dry, cold air. Many will either carry it with them during their exercise routines or will preventively use it immediately before exercise to forestall the onset of EIA.

One very new beta-2 selective agonist, *pirbuterol* or *Maxair* by its trade name, is almost the same as albuterol. It is given by a metered-dose nebulizer and has the same side effects as the other beta-2 selective medications.

### Isoetharine hydrochloride
Generic Name: Isoetharine hydrochloride
Trade Name: Bronkosol, Bronchometer

Isoetharine is perhaps more commonly known by its trade name Bronkosol. Bronkosol is a beta-2 selective medication with relatively little beta-1 cardiac side effects. It is one of the earliest beta-2 selective drugs introduced on the market that continues to be used widely in the treatment of bronchoconstriction in patients with chronic obstructive pulmonary diseases. This medication is packaged for patient use in a hand-held, metered-dose nebulizer and is also used when small volume or SVN nebulization is given to patients in the acute care and home health settings.

*Side effects.* Nervousness, tremors, headaches, and nausea.

*Therapeutic uses.* It is used for its bronchodilatory effects in patients who have emphysema, chronic bronchitis, asthma, and bronchiectasis. This medication is rapidly oxidized when exposed to water or air. This oxidative chemical change will cause the patient's sputum to be tinged a pink to red color, making it falsely appear that the patient is bleeding in the lungs. At times the patient may need to be reassured that the color change in the sputum is only a chemical change in the drug.

### Terbutaline sulfate
Generic Name: terbutaline sulfate
Trade Name: Bricanyl, Brethaire, Brethine

This medication is a beta-2 selective bronchodilator that enjoys wide use among patients with any bronchoconstrictive or obstructive pulmonary disease. This medication is not easily broken down or metabolized by the catechol-o-methyltransferase system and thus has a relatively long half life of 4-6 hours. This medication is available as a pill, as an injectable medication for intramuscular administration, and as an aerosol form for inhalation.

*Side effects.* Nausea, vomiting, nervousness, headaches, tremors, dizziness, and anxiety.

*Therapeutic uses.* Terbutaline is used in the treatment of chronic obstructive pulmonary diseases to help bronchodilate the patient, enhance the removal of secretions, and to reverse airflow limitations associated with these pulmonary diseases. This drug is also useful in the treatment of status asthmaticus.

### Bitolterol mesylate
Generic Name: bitolterol mesylate
Trade Name: Tornalate

Bitolterol mesylate is a relatively new beta-2 selective sympathomimetic drug. It is a unique medication in that it is taken as a "prodrug." A drug that is complexed with another chemical group or moiety will often survive the body's degradation/detoxification processes for a longer period of time and is called a prodrug. The prodrug is not the actual active drug agent but rather a combination drug. The added chemical group—the "pro" portion of the drug—protects the basic drug molecule from being easily biotransformed to an intermediate molecule that may have a reduced biologic activity. Research chemists have frequently developed these prodrugs such that when the liver or other detoxification systems biotransform the prodrug, the drug portion of the prodrug is liberated by cutting off the protecting moiety, the "pro" portion of this macromolecule. In this fashion a drug will reach its intended target without being chemically altered and the "pro" molecule can then be disposed of as a useless chemical intermediate.

Bitolterol mesylate is available as an inhaled aerosol delivered by a metered-dose inhaler. It is biotransformed into the active drug by endogenous enzymes in the lung that cleave the "pro" portion of the drug, releasing the biologically active drug, a drug now called terbutylnorepinephrine. The biologic half life for this medication is approximately 4-6 hours.

*Side effects.* Tremors, anxiety, headaches, restlessness, and insomnia.

*Therapeutic uses.* This medication is used to bronchodilate the bronchopulmonary tree. However, it also has another unique action in that it stimulates the mucociliary elevator to clear secretions more quickly from the lung.

## METHYLXANTHINES

The methylxanthines consist of three, well-known compounds: caffeine, theophylline, and theobromine. The methylxanthines are natural alkaloids found in a wide variety of plants around the world. For centuries, these compounds have been distilled from plant sources for human consumption because of their stimulatory effects. In most cultures today, one of the methylxanthines, caffeine, is a socially accepted central nervous system stimulant.

The methylxanthines exert a wide variety of stimulatory effects on the central nervous system, on bronchial smooth muscle, on skeletal muscle, on the peripheral fat pads, and on the glomerular filtration rate of the kidney. Despite the wide array of biochemical effects in the body, the methylxanthines are largely used for their bronchodilatory effects.

The exact mechanism of action for methylxanthine-mediated bronchodilation is not completely understood. It is known that the methylxanthines do stimulate significant increases in the cellular levels of cyclic adenosine monophosphate (cAMP) and cyclic guanine monophosphate (cGMP). Both nucleotides are known to be involved with smooth muscle dilatation (i.e., cAMP is involved with bronchodilation and cGMP is known to be involved with vasodilation as in the case of the nitrate drugs [nitroglycerin]).

The rise in the cellular concentration of these nucleotides is thought to be due to the inhibitory effects of the methylxanthines on the actions of the phosphodiesterases. Phosphodiesterases are responsible for the destruction of the cyclic nucleotides, cAMP and cGMP. Hence, if these enzymes can be inhibited, then there will be an obligatory rise in the cellular levels of the cyclic nucleotides. Since these cyclic nucleotides act as second messengers turning on cell biochemical pathways, the increases of these nucleotides secondary to methylxanthine use could explain the significant bronchodilation these drugs produce. Also, it is suspected that the methylxanthines may increase the amount of circulating epinephrine which, as has been already pointed out, is a very strong sympathomimetic with substantial bronchodilatory effects. It is also known that the methylxanthines block the vascular receptors for adenosine, a chemical responsible for smooth muscle contraction. If these receptors are blocked, then smooth muscle dilation is permissively allowed.

Another well known pulmonary effect of theophylline is its apparent ability to increase the diaphragm's capacity to work. The exact mechanism is not understood, but the overall net effect of theophylline ingestion is the diaphragm's ability to resist fatigue and to elicit greater contractile force. This becomes important to the chronic obstructive pulmonary disease patient who, because of declining lung compliance and poor thoracic cage mechanics, already expends more energy to breathe than a healthy individual.

*Theophylline*
Generic Name: theophylline
Trade Name: Theo-Dur, Slo-Bid, Theo-24, Slo-Phyllin and others

Theophylline and the various salts of theophylline such as aminophylline have a narrow therapeutic range (i.e., the blood levels of theophylline must fall between a specific high and low blood concentration in order to elicit the desired result of bronchodilation without causing any toxic signs or symptoms). Serum concentrations of theophylline must be carefully monitored. The therapeutic range for theophylline is between 10-20 micrograms of theophylline per milliliter of blood (µg/ml). Because of this very narrow therapeutic range, the physician will take blood samples to determine if the dosing schedule for a particular patient is keeping the blood levels of theophylline within the prescribed high and low ranges. When the blood levels rise above the therapeutic range, the patient can experience seizures and a host of other symptoms. Consequently, pharmaceutical companies have made a number of theophylline preparations that are timed release and may only have to be given 1-2 times per day. Timed-release medications are ideal for patients with normal hepatic and renal function because a sustained level of blood theophylline can be maintained over time without the bother of keeping to a rigorous dosing schedule. However, in a patient with poor renal and hepatic function, the dose of theophylline will not be eliminated from the body as quickly, and therefore toxicity becomes particularly worrisome.

*Side effects.* Nervousness, insomnia, headaches, seizures, tachycardia, cardiac dysrhythmias, nausea, anorexia, and vomiting.

*Therapeutic uses.* It is used in the symptomatic relief of bronchospasm associated with the chronic obstructive pulmonary diseases. In addition, it is given to these patients to enhance the diaphragm's force of contraction and reduce the fatigue of breathing. It is given prophylactically to prevent the onset of dyspnea and shortness of breath associated with bronchoconstriction.

Most methylxanthine drugs that are being prescribed for treating bronchospastic episodes in the chronic obstructive pulmonary diseased patient and in the acute asthmatic patient are theophylline salt derivatives. They are structurally almost identical and have the same medical properties and nearly the same side effects. Some of these drugs are aminophylline, enprofylline, and dyphylline. The other two main members of the methylxanthine family, caffeine and theobromine and any of its derivatives, are not generally used for the treatment of bronchospasm. Caffeine has an alternate use in that it is prescribed for infants to stimulate a higher respiratory rate, produce a larger tidal volume, and enhance the survival rate of the infant. The serious use of theobromine as a pulmonary drug is unknown.

## MUCOLYTICS AND EXPECTORANTS

**Mucolytics.** Tenacious mucous secretions in the lung create airflow obstruction and serve as a reservoir for infection. Mucous plugs that obstruct bronchial airflow, as in the case of static asthmaticus, can be life threatening.

Increased mucus production results from physical irritation to the bronchopulmonary passages. As a defense mechanism against the irritating effects of inhaled smoke, fumes, and gases, or in response to bacterial or viral infections, the mucin secreting glands, the goblet cells, often become hyperactive. Chronic irritation may lead to the hypertrophy and hyperplastic expansion of the number of mucin secreting glands in the area of the irritation.

Several diseases are characterized by increased production of mucus, which complicates the patient's recovery. Asthma, bronchitis, bronchiectasis, emphysema, tuberculosis, pneumonia, and cystic fibrosis are notorious for excessive production of mucus. Excess mucus production is also part of the clinical picture of a number of occupational diseases such as asbestosis, silicosis, and coal workers pneumoconiosis to name but a few.

Clearance of secretions from the bronchial passages and keeping the bronchopulmonary tree patent is one of the main charges of the cardiopulmonary physical therapist. To help accomplish this important task, a drug called N-acetylcysteine was developed and is virtually one of only two mucolytic preparations being used today.

*N-acetylcysteine*
Generic Name: N-acetylcysteine
Trade Name: Mucomyst, Airbron, Parvolex, Mucosol

N-acetylcysteine helps to thin mucus secretions by breaking the disulfide bonds of mucus, a glycoprotein. These bonds give mucus its characteristic thick and viscous nature. When the disulfide bonds are broken, the mucus is thin and watery in its consistency.

N-acetylcysteine is usually given by inhalation. It is

mixed with a volume of sterile saline and administered to the patient via a small-volume nebulizer. As with any inhaled nebulized drug designed to dilate the bronchi and clear it of secretions, the cardiopulmonary physical therapist would follow up this treatment with deep breathing and coughing exercises, postural drainage and percussion, or some exercise routine designed to assist the mucociliary elevator in moving the secretions out of the lung toward the esophagus. Thinner secretions are cleared more efficiently by the mucociliary elevator.

***Side effects.*** This medication has the odor of rotten eggs. Its offensive smell may nauseate some patients and cause them to vomit. This medication has relatively few significant side effects.

***Therapeutic uses.*** N-acetylcysteine is used to thin mucous secretions that obstruct airflow and cause the patient to be short of breath and possibly hypoxemic.

Another rather unusual but medically important use of N-acetylcysteine is its use in the treatment of acetaminophen overdose. The various trade names for acetaminophen in the United States and Canada are Datril, Panadol, Tylenol, Atasol, Campain, and Robigesic. Children or adults who overdose on acetaminophen may experience severe liver damage. A 5% solution of N-acetylcysteine is given orally as an antidote to help prevent liver damage. N-acetylcysteine forms a conjugate with the oxidized metabolite of acetaminophen that makes it more easily disposed of by the liver and the kidneys.

*Recombinant human deoxyribonuclease I*
   Abbreviated Name: rhDNase

For many years, scientists have sought new forms of treatment for adults and children with cystic fibrosis. Physical therapy, antibiotic drugs, and nutritional support and supplementation have been the mainstays of medical treatment. The persistent killer of patients with cystic fibrosis has almost always been loss of pulmonary function (a declining $FEV_1$ and FVC) and respiratory failure secondary to mucous obstruction and superimposed bacterial superinfections. In large part this has been due to poor nutritional state and mucous secretions that became reservoirs for persistent and recurring bacterial infections. Although cystic fibrosis involves multiple organ systems, death is usually due to pulmonary complications.

One of the clinical features of this disease is the production of thick, tenacious pulmonary secretions that obstruct airflow in and out of the lung. A good deal of the palliative therapy for these patients has focused on the removal of these secretions. It appears that, in part, the reason the mucous secretions are so thick is the presence of deoxyribonucleic acid (DNA) mixed in with the mucal glycoproteins. The source of the DNA is believed to be the neutrophil, a phagocytic cell responsible for cleaning up damaged tissues, a condition that would be part and parcel of the inflamed and infected tissues of a chronically involved cystic fibrosis patient.

A logical way to break up these thick secretions would be the use of a deoxyribonuclease, the enzyme that cuts apart the DNA strands interspersed with the mucus. Experiments beginning in the 1950s and continuing today have used this lytic enzyme as a possible interventional form of treatment. New technology and the principles of genetic engineering have now created a drug called recombinant human deoxyribonuclease I or rhDNase. The drug cleaves the DNA strands and in effect thins the mucous secretions. This permits the mucociliary elevator to clear more effectively the mucous secretions from the lung, causes the airflow mechanics to greatly improve, and increases the pulmonary function of the cystic fibrosis patient. Since this medication has been genetically engineered to be a human deoxyribonuclease, the opportunity of the patient to mount a cell-mediated immune defense against this proteinacious enzyme is greatly reduced.

Although the experimental results are not complete at this time and experimentation continues, rhDNase holds great promise as a mucolytic drug that will greatly improve the quality of life for the cystic fibrosis patient. The prolongation of life is the hoped for outcome for this patient group.

**Expectorants.** Expectorants are designed to increase the removal of mucin from the respiratory tract. These drugs stimulate the goblet cells to hyperactively produce more mucin than normal. The extra mucin possibly has a higher water content and is therefore more easily moved along toward the esophagus by the mucociliary elevator. The mucociliary elevator begins at the trachea and can be found in the lungs down to the thirteenth or fourteenth generation of the bronchopulmonary tree. It acts as a removal system through the action of ciliated cells that sweep and cleanse the lungs of all pollutants that have been trapped in the mucous layer. The higher water content of the mucin probably helps move the tenacious mucin plugs out of the lungs as the mucus blanket is swept up and out of the lungs to the esophagus. These medications consist of a number of members listed below:

*Guaifenesin*
   Generic Name: guaifenesin
   Trade: Name: Robitussin, Breonesin
*Iodinated glycerol*
   Generic Name: iodinated glycerol
   Trade Name: Organidin, Isophen Elixir
*Terpin Hydrate*
   Generic Name: terpin hydrate

## CORTICOSTEROIDS

Adrenocorticosteroids are drugs that are made naturally by the adrenal cortex or that are produced synthetically for the purposes of treating a variety of inflammatory conditions. Three important, naturally occurring corticosteroids are cortisol, cortisone, and corticosterone. These steroids are classified as glucocorticoids because in addition to their antiinflammatory capabilities they also influence carbohydrate, lipid, and protein metabolism. Aldosterone, another natural corticosteroid, is called a mineralocorticoid because it exerts a significant influence on sodium, potassium and water homeostasis in humans.

Synthesis of the adrenocorticosteroids requires cholesterol as the basic intermediate. The adrenal cortex utilizes both exogenous (dietary) sources of cholesterol and endogenous cholesterol manufactured in the liver to synthesize the corticosteroids.

The corticosteroids, whether natural or synthetic, are used in pulmonary medicine because of their antiinflammatory effects. A general overview of glucocorticoid effects will be given to underscore the importance of this class of drug in the treatment of acute and chronic pulmonary diseases.

Glucocorticoids inhibit the release of arachidonic acid from membrane-bound phospholipids. Arachidonic acid is the substrate that the cyclooxygenase pathway uses to make prostaglandins and thromboxanes, and the lipoxygenase pathway uses it to produce leukotrienes. Since prostaglandins, leukotrienes, and thromboxanes are all mediators of inflammation, the inhibition of their formation reduces the chance for the development of inflammation.

Glucocorticoids also inhibit the release of migration-inhibition factor from macrophages. When the macrophage releases migration-inhibition factor, the macrophages in the area of the inflammation are prevented from leaving the injury site. Hence, if the glucocorticoids can block the release of this factor, the macrophages can move away from the injury site and there will be less inflammation.

Glucocorticoids reduce the permeability of capillaries by reducing the amount of histamine release and bradykinin formation. This happens in part because glucocorticoids stabilize the membranes of mast cells and prevent them from degranulating and releasing histamine. If the permeability of the vascular bed is reduced, then swelling is reduced and the migration of neutrophils into the area of injury is slowed.

Glucocorticoids stabilize the membranes of intracellular lysosomes such that they do not rupture as easily and spill their proteolytic enzyme contents. This preserves the integrity of the cell and prevents the release of chemotactic signals that would normally attract a vigorous neutrophil invasion. Neutrophils are notorious for aggressive phagocytosis. They often kill healthy cells in addition to phagocytically clearing dead and dying cells. This unfortunate lack of discrimination causes the level of chemotactic signals to be much higher than necessary.

Glucocorticoids inhibit the release of interleukin-1 (IL-1) by macrophages. The release of IL-1 promotes the activation of the $T4^+$ Helper cells ($CD4^+$) and acts as a chemotactic signal, stimulating fibroblast proliferation and the expansion of the neutrophil population (neutrophilia). Blocking the release of IL-1 blocks a number of factors influencing inflammation.

It should be apparent why corticosteroids are a mainstay in the pharmacological armamentarium of the physician. They effectively suppress inflammation at numerous chemi-

cal and tissue sites. Suppression of inflammation is very important in the treatment of chronic obstructive pulmonary diseases (COPD). In addition to smoking, recurrent bacterial and viral infections are some of the main root causes of chronic bronchitis. Infections set off intense inflammatory reactions as does cigarette smoke. In the case of the patient with emphysema, chronic cigarette smoke exposure elicits an intense inflammatory reaction causing a significant loss of alveolar-capillary surface area due to fibronecrotizing processes. As is evident, inflammation is an important variable to control with any pulmonary patient.

**Corticosteroid drugs.** There are only a small number of corticosteroids that are used in an inhaled or nebulized form. The ideal pulmonary steroid would be one that is easily used by the patient as a nebulized medication, does not elicit serious side effects in the upper or lower respiratory tracts, has good antiinflammatory capabilities, and that remains in the bronchopulmonary tree and does not measurably cross over into the systemic circulation. The great advantage of the inhaled corticosteroids is that they are delivered directly to the site of need in very small doses and, in the recommended dosing ranges, do not cross over into the systemic circulation. The nebulized corticosteroids are a vast improvement over the oral or injected medications because of little to no systemic effects.

*Triamcinolone acetonide*
   Generic Name: triamcinolone acetonide
   Trade Name: Azmacort

This synthetic medication is used primarily to reduce the inflammation and tissue swelling that are clinical features of asthma. It also reverses the increased permeability and leakiness of capillaries at or near the site of inflammation and stabilizes the lysosomes in cells. Since swelling and inflammation are reduced with the use of this medication, it helps to open the bronchial passageways. The inhaler is designed to deliver about 100 micrograms of triamcinolone per puff; as with all nebulized types of medications, the patient should be warned against abusive use of this medication. The patient is told to use the inhaler 3-4 times per day and to breathe in only 2 puffs per dosing time.

*Side effects.* There are relatively few side effects, though there may be some irritation to the mucosal lining, especially when the patient is sensitive to the medication, in which case it is advised that the patient discontinue use. Mucosal membrane irritation and hoarseness of the voice may occur but can be reduced or eliminated by rinsing the mouth and gargling with water after each administration. As with all corticosteroids there is the chance of bronchospasm especially if the patient is hypersensitive to corticosteroids.

*Therapeutic uses.* Suppression of inflammation secondary to the acute and chronic pulmonary diseases. This medication is used frequently to reduce the bronchial inflammation of asthma.

*Beclomethasone dipropionate*
Generic Name: beclomethasone dipropionate
Trade Name: Beclovent, Vanceril

Like all of the corticosteroids, this medication suppresses inflammation. It also inhibits the migration of neutrophils, decreases swelling by decreasing the permeability of capillary beds near the site of inflammation, and stabilizes the lysosomes of cells. Since it is delivered by a metered-dose inhaler, the overall daily dose is small and, consequently, will not have systemic effects. The inhaler delivers approximately 42 micrograms per puff with the recommended daily adult dose being 2-4 puffs, 3-4 times per day.

*Side effects.* Hoarseness, irritation to the mucosal lining and bronchospasm secondary to a hypersensitivity reaction to the medication. Many of the contact discomfort type of side effects can be eliminated by washing the mouth out and gargling with water after each administration.

*Therapeutic uses.* Suppression of inflammation especially associated with the chronic obstructive pulmonary diseases.

*Flunisolide*
Generic Name: flunisolide
Trade Name: Aerobid

This drug suppresses inflammation and inhibits the migration of neutrophils to the site of the injury. It also reverses capillary leakiness and therefore reduces swelling. This medication is taken at low doses with the patient taking 2 puffs twice daily. The inhaler meters out about 250 micrograms of flunisolide with each puff.

*Side effects.* Hoarseness, sore throat, irritation to the mucosal lining and bronchospasm secondary to a hypersensitivity reaction to the medication. Many of the contact discomfort type of side effects can be eliminated by washing the mouth out and gargling with water after each administration.

*Therapeutic uses.* Suppression of inflammation especially associated with the chronic obstructive pulmonary diseases and acute asthma.

There is a fourth corticosteroid by the name of dexamethasone sodium phosphate known as Decadron by its trade name. It is given by a metered-dose nebulizer at 100 micrograms per puff. However, this medication is not prescribed nearly as often as flunisolide, triamcinolone, or beclomethasone. It shares nearly the same side effects as the other inhaled forms of the corticosteroids.

*Cromolyn sodium*
Generic Name: cromolyn sodium, disodium cromoglycate
Trade Name: Intal, Intal Spincaps, Nalcrom

Cromolyn sodium is not a corticosteroid nor does it belong in any of the classes of drugs already discussed. Although it is an uncategorized drug, it is an important member of the pulmonary drug family. It was developed in the mid-1960s and marketed in the early 1970s as a drug for asthmatics. There were high expectations for this medication because initially it was hoped that it would be a replacement therapy for the corticosteroids. However, it did not have all of the actions of corticosteroids and hence did not replace these drugs in the treatment of COPD or acute asthma.

Cromolyn sodium appears to be able to stabilize the bronchial mast cell so that it does not degranulate and release histamine, one of the mediators of tissue inflammation and swelling. It appears to be highly specific for bronchial mast cells as it does not stabilize the membranes of mast cells from other organ systems.

Cromolyn sodium is used prophylactically *before* an asthma attack begins. It is designed to prevent the onset of inflammatory symptoms; once those symptoms have begun, it does not reverse them and is useless in the management of that particular bronchospastic episode. Cromolyn sodium is useful in preventing additional asthmatic attacks once the person has already become sensitized to some antigen (i.e., once there has been an antigen-IgE interaction).

The medication is dispensed in two forms for pulmonary inhalation. An early method of dispensing the medication to the patient used a Spin-Haler. A Spin-Haler is a device that crushes or punctures the capsule containing the medication. The powder is then blown out of the Spin-Haler directly into the patient's lungs and is topically deposited onto the bronchial membranes. A more recent and more convenient method involves the use of a metered-dose nebulizer that dispenses a liquid form of cromolyn sodium. If a patient is using the metered-dose nebulizer the normal dosing is prescribed at 2 puffs every four hours.

*Side effects.* Bronchospasm, coughing and choking after inhaling the powder form of the drug, sneezing and upper airway irritation.

*Therapeutic uses.* For the prophylactic prevention of bronchospasm, shortness of breath and wheezing associated with an asthmatic attack.

## SUGGESTED READING

Adelstein RS and others: Phosphorylation of smooth muscle myosin light chain kinase by the catalytic subunit of adenosine 3′:5′ monophosphate-dependent protein kinase, *J Biol Chem* 253(23):8347, 1978.

Aitken ML and others: Recombinant human DNase inhalation in normal subjects and patients with cystic fibrosis, *JAMA* 267(14):1947, 1992.

Baer CL and Williams BR: *Clinical Pharmacology and Nursing,* ed 2, Springhouse, PA, 1992, Springhouse Publishers.

Bukowskyj M and others: Theophylline reassessed, *Ann Intern Med* 101:63, 1984.

Ciccone CD: *Pharmacology in Rehabilitation,* Philadelphia, 1990, F. A. Davis Publishers.

Collins S: Recent perspectives on the molecular structure and regulation of the B$_2$-adrenoceptor, *Life Sci* 52:2083, 1993.

de Lanerolle P: Airway smooth muscle and asthma, *Am J Respir Cell Mol Biol* 7:565, 1992.

de Lanerolle P and Paul RJ: Myosin phosphorylation/dephosphorylation and regulation of airway smooth muscle contractility, *Am J Physiol* 261:L1, 1991.

Gerthoffer WT: Regulation of the contractile element of airway smooth muscle, *Am J Physiol* 261:L15, 1991.

Gilman AG, Rall TW, Nies AS, and Taylor P, editors: *Goodman and Gilman's the pharmacological basis of therapeutics,* ed 8, New York, 1990, McGraw-Hill Publishers.

Hassan E: The future role of theophylline, *J Cardiopulm Rehabil* 11(6):350, 1991.

Hubbard RC and others: A preliminary study of aerosolized recombinant human deoxyribonuclease I in the treatment of cystic fibrosis, *New Engl J Med* 236:812, 1992.

Levitzki A and others: The signal transduction between B-receptors and adenylyl cyclase, *Life Sci* 52:2093, 1993.

Losavio AS and Kotsias BA: Effect of aminophylline on the contraction threshold of rat diaphragm fibers, *J Appl Physiol* 71(4):1409, 1991.

Nijkamp FP: B-Adrenergic receptors in the lung: an introduction, *Life Sci* 52:2073, 1993.

Ramsey BW and others: Efficacy and safety of short-term administration of aerosolized recombinant human deoxyribonuclease in patients with cystic fibrosis, *Am Rev of Respir Dis* 148:145, 1993.

Rossing TH and others: Emergency therapy of asthma: comparison of the acute effects of parenteral and inhaled sympathomimetics and infused aminophylline, *Am Rev Respir Dis* 122:365, 1980.

Sigrist S and others: The effect of aminophylline on inspiratory muscle contractility, *Am Rev Respir Dis* 126(1):46, 1982.

Skorodin MS: Pharmacotherapy for asthma and chronic obstructive pulmonary disease—current thinking, practices and controversies, *Arch Intern Med* 153:814, 1993.

Tattersfield AE: Clinical pharmacology of long-acting B-receptor agonists, *Life Sci* 52:2161, 1993.

van Breeman C and Saida K: Cellular mechanisms regulating $[Ca^{2+}]_i$ smooth muscle, *Ann Rev Physiol* 51:315, 1989.

Vaz Fragoso CA and Miller MA: Review of the clinical efficacy of theophylline in the treatment of chronic obstructive pulmonary disease, *Am Rev Respir Dis* 147:S40, 1993.

Verberne AAPH and Kerrebijn KF: Effects of $B_2$-receptor agonists on airway responsiveness, *Life Sci* 52:2181, 1993.

# CHAPTER 17

# Respiratory Muscle

*Physiology, evaluation, and treatment*

*Marla R. Wolfson and Thomas H. Shaffer*

The respiratory muscles, like the heart, form an organ system that acts as a pump.[74] The movement of air in and out of the gas-exchange units of the lung is accomplished by the action of the respiratory pump. Because of the vital importance of the respiratory muscles, the aim of this chapter is to provide a synthesis of what is currently known of respiratory muscle function, which may be of direct help or interest to the student of pulmonary physical therapy. Of course, it includes a section on muscle mechanics, but this is placed in proper perspective for understanding how the respiratory muscles move and how airflow ensues. Furthermore, we have described the most recent techniques for assessing respiratory muscle function and training methods and for assessing the effect of lung and neuromuscular

disease and musculoskeletal dysfunction on respiratory muscles. Finally, we present a current review of training studies and their effects on cardiopulmonary function; respiratory muscle strength, endurance, and fatigue; and on exercise tolerance.

## RESPIRATORY MUSCLE MECHANICS
### Description of muscle function

The overall goal of the respiratory muscles is to pump gas into and out of the lungs in a coordinated and rhythmic manner. By convention, three groups of skeletal muscles have been related to respiratory function: (1) diaphragm, (2) rib cage muscles (including the intercostal and accessory muscles), and (3) abdominal muscles. More recently, airway smooth muscle has been added to this list based on its ability to alter the diameter and rigidity of the airway and thus affect airflow.[20,30,65] Although the significant differences between skeletal and smooth respiratory muscles are important to effective ventilation, a complete discussion is beyond the scope of this chapter. Therefore the discussion of respiratory muscles will be limited to those skeletal muscles that make up the respiratory pump. Most of the information on muscle function is summarized from the work of Campbell and co-workers.[25]

During quiet breathing, the primary muscle responsible for ventilation is the diaphragm. Although not essential for breathing, it is the principal muscle of inspiration. The diaphragm's contribution to tidal volume has been estimated to be two thirds in the sitting and standing positions and three fourths or greater in the supine position. Traditionally, the diaphragm has been described as a single large, thin sheet of skeletal muscle that separates the thoracic from the abdominal cavity (Fig. 17-1). The diaphragm is further defined by the origins of the muscle fibers. Fibers originating from the lumbar vertebral region constitute the crural part of the diaphragm; those originating from the lower six ribs give rise to the costal diaphragm. The costal and crural fibers

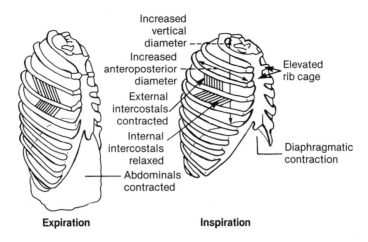

**Fig. 17-1.** Illustration of diaphragmatic contraction, elevation of the rib cage, and function of the intercostals. (From Guyton AC: *Textbook of medical physiology,* Philadelphia, 1971, WB Saunders Co.)

converge and form a central tendon: the insertion of the diaphragm. Its alpha motor neurons leave the spinal cord in the anterior roots of the third to fifth cervical segments and run downward in the phrenic nerve. According to the conventional viewpoint, the mechanical action of the diaphragm stems from a single functional entity that is attached all around the circumference of the lower thoracic cage. Contraction of the muscle pulls down the central part, compresses the viscera, displaces the abdomen outward, and lifts the rib cage. The inspiratory movement of the diaphragm decreases intrapleural pressure, which inflates the lungs, and increases intraabdominal pressure, which displaces both the abdomen and rib cage. Recent observations indicate that the diaphragm consists of two distinct muscles that correspond to the previously described costal and crural regions. Supportive evidence for this theory includes differing embryological origins, fiber types, and innervation of these muscles. According to this viewpoint, the mechanical action of the diaphragm is a result of two force generators. This theory proposes that, since the costal diaphragm inserts into the rib cage, and the crural diaphragm attaches only to the central tendon, net rib cage displacement during inspiration would be determined by the relative strength of contraction of each muscle. This theory is presented in detail by De Troyer and Loring.[36]

Also active during inspiration, the external intercostal muscles elevate the anterior portion of the rib cage and pull it upward and outward (Fig. 17-1). The intercostal nerves, which innervate these muscles, leave the spinal cord from between the first through the eleventh thoracic segments. In addition, other accessory muscles come into play during vigorous breathing including the sternocleidomastoid and scalene muscles in the neck, the muscles of the shoulder region, and the pectoral muscles.

Expiration is a passive process during quiet breathing and occurs because of the elasticity of the lung and chest wall. As breathing becomes more vigorous, as in exercise, or labored, as in respiratory disease, expiration is no longer a passive process. The internal intercostal muscles and abdominal muscles contract to increase intrapleural and intraabdominal pressure during expiration. The internal intercostal muscle group, like the external intercostal muscles, is innervated by the intercostal nerves. The abdominal muscles are innervated by nerve fibers that originate in the lower six thoracic and first lumbar segments of the spinal cord. Normally, the abdominal muscles are regarded as powerful expiratory muscles whose action increases the intraabdominal pressure to force the diaphragm cephalad. However, Grimby and associates[44] have demonstrated the role of the abdominal muscles in certain inspiratory maneuvers.

## Intrinsic properties of the respiratory pump

As previously discussed, the respiratory pump is composed of numerous skeletal muscle groups. Like other skeletal muscle, respiratory muscle force depends on muscle length and velocity of shortening. In the respiratory system, force-length relationships can be expressed indirectly as pressure-volume curves, whereas force-velocity relationships are described in terms of pressure-flow curves. Such curves describe the overall behavior of the respiratory pump yet do not provide direct information concerning the intrinsic properties of individual respiratory muscle groups.[34]

In confirmation of these principles, Rohrer[90] and Rahn and associates[88] have experimentally demonstrated that maximal inspiratory pressure diminishes as lung volume increases, whereas maximal expiratory pressure increases. Furthermore, studies involving maximal flow efforts have shown that the maximal pressure developed by the respiratory system decreases as flow increases.

**Table 17-1.** Properties of muscle fibers

| Naked eye | Microscopic | Histochemical | Contractile properties |
|---|---|---|---|
| Red | High myoglobin content<br>Rich in sarcoplasm<br>Many mitochondria | High oxidative activity<br>Low phosphorylase | Slow |
| White | Lower myoglobin content<br>Less sarcoplasm<br>Fewer mitochondria | Low oxidative activity<br>High phosphorylase | Fast |

Modified from Campbell EJM, Agostoni E, and Davis JN: *The respiratory muscles*, Philadelphia, 1970, WB Saunders Co.

## Cell biology of the respiratory muscles

The respiratory muscles are striated and microscopically classified into two muscle fiber groups, fast and slow. In general, fast muscle fibers are white, and slow muscle fibers are red. The description of skeletal muscle as slow-twitch or fast-twitch is a relative designation applicable only within a single species. For example, muscles of smaller animals are usually faster than similar muscles of larger animals.[25] Table 17-1 shows a simplified classification of muscle fiber properties. Precise correlation of microscopic, histochemical, and contractile characteristics has not been established. Early studies of the histochemical properties of muscle fibers reported that the oxidative capacity, and therefore the resistance to fatigue, of the ventilatory muscles increases greatly from midgestation to early childhood.[60] Based on studies of muscle fibers that were obtained at autopsy and frozen before analyses, Keens and others[60] demonstrated that premature infants have less than 10% high-oxidative, slow-twitch fibers in the diaphragm as compared with 55% found in the adult diaphragm. More recent studies have challenged these findings by demonstrating that most fibers of the premature baboon diaphragm have high oxidation capacity and many mitochondria.[76] Although the discrepancy between these studies may be species related, Maxwell and others[75] suggest that the differences are likely to be a result of the degradation of oxidative enzyme activity caused by frozen storage.

Age-related differences in the baboon diaphragm fibers have been reported.[76] In comparison with fibers in the full-term baby or adult, the diaphragm in the premature baboon has fewer contractile proteins per fiber area and poorly developed sarcoplasmic reticulum. Physiological findings of lower-developed force-per-area and longer contraction and relaxation times of the premature baboon diaphragm have been related to these histochemical differences. Fatigability studies have shown that the immature fibers recover rapidly from fatigue caused by isometric contractions.[76] However, although the premature diaphragm was found to be less fatigable than those of older animals during prolonged isometric contractions, it failed to fully relax following loaded isotonic contractions. Subsequently, the premature diaphragm contracted from progressively

shorter lengths and, according to the length-tension relationship, developed less tension.

Sieck[101] and Watchko[108] have demonstrated that while specific force (peak tetanic force output normalized for muscle cross-sectional area) of diaphragmatic fiber increases with postnatal age, fatigue resistance decreases with increasing age. They also found that in addition to oxidative capacity of the muscle (as reflected by increased succinic dehydrogenase activity), fatigue resistance could be related to myosin heavy chain [MHC] phenotype such that neonatal MHC appears to impart a greater degree of fatigue resistance than adult isoforms. As such, fatigue resistance of the respiratory muscle during development may relate to the balance between the energetic demands of the muscle contractile properties and the oxidative capacity of the muscle. Furthermore, major developmentally related structural changes of the chest wall have important functional implications for respiratory pump efficiency and function.

From infancy to maturity the orientation of the ribs changes from horizontal to a progressive downward sloping, wherein the adult pattern is reached by 10 years of age. Marked developmental changes in chest-wall ossification occur during the first 3-6 years with sternal and rib ossification continuing through the second decade of life. Intercostal and diaphragmatic muscle mass increase in direct proportion to body weight. These changes in ossification and muscularization are reflected in changes in the mechanical properties of the chest wall with growth. With aging, chest wall compliance progressively decreases with associated increases in ossification. A functional disadvantage of a highly compliant chest wall relative to the lung is a lowered resting end expiratory volume, thereby compromising the length-tension characteristics of the respiratory muscles. As opposed to the mechanical advantages afforded by the oblique orientation of the rib cage and dome-shaped diaphragm of the adult, the horizontal rib cage orientation and flattened diaphragm present mechanical disadvantages to the newborn. In this regard, only the pump handle effect assists rib cage motion in the newborn and the respiratory muscles must shorten to a greater extent to move the chest wall. In addition, because of the high cartilage to bone ratio and incomplete bone mineralization, chest wall compliance during early development is relatively higher than that of the adult and, more importantly, significantly greater than the compliance of the lungs. Therefore, a large portion of the pressure-effort generated by the diaphragm may be dissipated through pulling the rib cage, rather than fresh air, inward. On these bases it has been suggested that the ventilatory muscles of newborns experience relatively greater loads than those in the adult and are thus more susceptible to fatigue than those of older subjects, a factor that may contribute to the respiratory problems of preterm neonates.

## RESPIRATORY MUSCLE BLOOD FLOW

This section summarizes salient aspects of the control of respiratory muscle blood flow and the relationship between respiratory muscle blood flow and respiratory muscle fatigue. A comprehensive bibliography relating to this topic has been presented by Supinski.[105]

Blood flow has been found to directly affect the susceptibility of the respiratory muscles to fatigue. Although the exact cellular mechanisms involved in diaphragmatic fatigue are not fully understood, there is evidence that the lack of oxygen subsequent to blood flow inadequate to meet metabolic demands may cause a shift to anaerobic pathways of high-energy phosphate compound generation. This leads to increased lactic acid accumulation, reduction in the force-generating capability, and early fatigue of the diaphragm.

Diaphragmatic blood flow is affected by a variety of mechanical, neural, and humoral factors. Mechanical factors include those forces that distend or compress the microvasculature and thus affect vascular resistance. Reductions in arterial pressure, lengthening of muscle fibers, and high abdominal/pleural pressure ratios will decrease diaphragmatic blood flow.

Blood flow to the diaphragm is exceedingly well regulated. During cardiogenic shock, a progressively larger portion of the cardiac output is directed to the diaphragm at the expense of flow to other organs. During strenuous rhythmic contractions, neural (i.e., axonal reflexes, sympathetic efferents) and humoral (i.e., lactate, potassium, hydrogen ions, prostaglandins) vasoregulatory systems cause vasodilation, preserve blood flow, and thus support the increased metabolic demands of the diaphragm. In the presence of increased metabolic demands, the diaphragm increases oxygen extraction, thus widening the arteriovenous oxygen gradient. Bellemare and others[18] suggested that the observed positive correlation in the dog between diaphragmatic hyperemia following contraction and the intensity of contraction indicates repayment of an oxygen debt; moreover, this finding suggests an inadequate blood flow/metabolic need relationship during the preceding period of strenuous diaphragmatic activity. Therefore in the presence of high levels of demand, oxygen needs may be met by a combination of increased extraction and blood flow. Postcontraction hyperemia may provide a compensatory mechanism for muscle recovery if metabolic demands are not met; however, its overall effectiveness may be limited since postcontraction hyperemia may compromise blood flow to other organs and present systemic pathophysiological sequelae.

Vasoactive drugs have been shown to alter diaphragmatic blood flow through various mechanisms. For example, isoproteronol increases blood flow by reducing the critical closing pressure of the vascular bed, making it possible for perfusion driving pressure and blood flow to be increased at any arterial pressure. Similarly, amrinone increases blood flow; however, this drug has no effect on closing pressure but rather acts directly to decrease vascular resistance.

## EVALUATION AND CLINICAL DIAGNOSIS OF RESPIRATORY MUSCLE PERFORMANCE

Performance of any muscle can be assessed by its strength, endurance, and inherent ability to resist fatigue. Determination of these characteristics provides sensitive indexes to respiratory muscle function. In addition, assessment of chest wall motion may provide insight into respiratory muscle performance.

### Respiratory muscle strength

The strength of the respiratory muscle contraction is directly related to the intrinsic muscle properties. The pressures generated within the respiratory system depend on the forces generated during muscle contraction and on the elastic properties of the lung and chest wall. Thus respiratory muscle strength has been defined as the maximum or minimum pressure developed within the respiratory system at a specific lung volume.[24,31]

Inspiratory and expiratory muscle strength are determined by measurement of the maximum static inspiratory (MSIP) and expiratory (MSEP) pressures. Both MSIP and MSEP are measured as the static pressures developed at the mouth at a given lung volume. The subject's lung volumes are determined by a volume plethysmograph. The subject breathes through a mouthpiece attached to a pressure tap and a shutter. The maximum static pressures are generated against a closed shutter during inspiratory and expiratory maneuvers. These measurements are commonly made over the range of the vital capacity at intervals of 20% of total lung capacity. Each maneuver is sustained for 3 to 5 seconds, and both MSIP and MSEP are correlated to the particular lung volume.[69] A typical relationship is shown in Fig. 17-2. These pressures are reduced with muscular weakness and fatigue and are increased with strength training.

Diaphragmatic strength can be estimated by measurement of the transdiaphragmatic pressure ($P_{di}$). Maximal $P_{di}$ is measured during maximal diaphragmatic contraction.[92] The ratio of $P_{di}/P_{di\ max}$ at various lung volumes or maneuvers can be used to assess the strength of diaphragmatic contractions. Similarly, the ratio of inspiratory mouth pressure ($P_m$) to $P_{m\ max}$ (maximal inspiratory mouth pressure) can be utilized

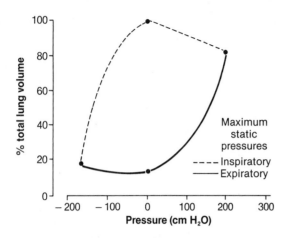

**Fig. 17-2.** Maximum inspiratory and expiratory pressures as a function of lung volumes. (Modified from Leith DE and Bradley M: *J Appl Physiol* 41:508, 1976).

to quantitate the combined strength of the inspiratory muscle groups.[94]

## Respiratory muscle endurance

The endurance capacity of the respiratory muscles depends on the mechanics of the respiratory system and the energy availability of the muscles. The endurance of these muscle groups is defined as the capacity to maintain maximal or submaximal levels of ventilation under isocapnic conditions.[39,69] The endurance capacity is standardized by (1) maximal ventilation for a specific duration of time, (2) ventilation against a known resistance, or (3) sustained ventilation at a given lung volume.[46,69]

The endurance of ventilatory muscles as a group is determined with respect to a specific ventilatory target (tidal volume × respiratory rate) and the time to exhaustion.[69] During this procedure of hyperpnea, a partial rebreathing system is used to maintain oxygen and carbon dioxide levels so they are relatively constant. Fig. 17-3, *A*, details one such system; simpler modifications of this system have been used for purposes of training (Fig. 17-3, *B*). A sequence of maximal ventilatory targets and the time to exhaustion are measured and correlated (Fig. 17-4). This relationship is geometric, and its asymptote has been defined as the sustainable ventilatory capacity (SVC). This value is one criterion of ventilatory muscle endurance but may be further standardized as a fraction of the 15-second maximal voluntary ventilation.

Inspiratory muscle endurance is measured when one breathes against inspiratory resistive loads, such as a narrow-bore tube, and gauged by the pressures generated at the mouth ($P_m/P_{m\ max}$) or across the diaphragm ($P_{di}/P_{di\ max}$).[92,94] The subject is instructed to breathe through a known, usually large, resistance and generate a constant, target $P_m$ but allowed to choose his or her own tidal volume or frequency. The endurance time is determined at the point

of exhaustion or inability to generate the target $P_m$. Likewise, the measurement of $P_{di}$ during these maneuvers allows assessment of diaphragmatic endurance. Roussos and Macklem[92] (Fig. 17-5) have shown that a $P_m/P_{m\ max}$ of 60% or less can support indefinite cyclical ventilation and that the diaphragm can generate 40% of its maximum pressure indefinitely. At these levels fatigue is prevented, and complete recovery from the inspiratory effort occurs during expiration.

## Respiratory muscle fatigue

The respiratory muscles, like any other skeletal muscle, fatigue when the rate of energy consumption exceeds the rate of energy supplied to the muscle. Depletion of the energy stores within the muscle subsequently leads to its failure as a force generator.[34] Diaphragmatic, and other inspiratory muscle fatigue, is an important potential clinical problem because it is the final common pathway toward respiratory failure. The psychological and physiological factors[97] contributing to respiratory muscle fatigue are depicted in Fig. 17-6. Muscle fatigue also accounts for exercise intolerance, which is increased in patients with lung disease, in those with neuromuscular and musculoskeletal disorders, and in those being weaned from mechanical ventilators. Decreased muscle strength or endurance in these patients may lead to premature onset of respiratory muscle fatigue. Abnormal chest wall and lung mechanics, as well as abnormal lung volumes, compromise the pressure-generating capabilities of the inspiratory muscles.[88]

The diagnosis of the onset of respiratory muscle fatigue assumes critical importance since it is this end point that measures strength, endurance, and response to training programs. Ventilatory muscle fatigue may be assessed clinically. Though histochemical and biochemical changes also provide indexes of fatigue, these are not used clinically because of the accompanying difficulties and potential complications when inspiratory muscle tissue samples are obtained.

## DETERMINANTS OF RESPIRATORY MUSCLE FATIGUE

Because respiratory muscle fatigue results in inadequate transpulmonary pressure development, it is thought to be the proximate cause of respiratory failure. Although the etiology of respiratory muscle fatigue is multivariant,[93] regulation of the respiratory muscle nutrient/demand ratio is the critical factor in preventing fatigue.

Respiratory patterns influence the potential for respiratory muscle fatigue. High inspiratory/expiratory timing ratios present insufficient time for blood flow to replenish metabolites and remove catabolites. As such, the muscle nutrient/demand ratio becomes imbalanced, and fatigue may result.

Asynchronous respiratory muscle activity potentiates fatigue. For example, in quadriplegia, where the rib cage

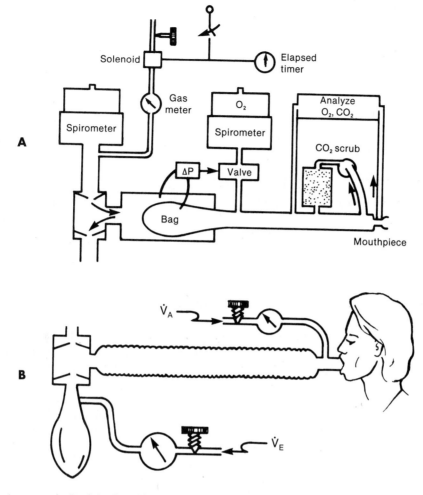

**Fig. 17-3. A,** Partial rebreathing system for endurance testing. **B,** Simplified partial rebreathing system for endurance training. (Modified from Leith DE and Bradley M: *J Appl Physiol* 41:508, 1976.)

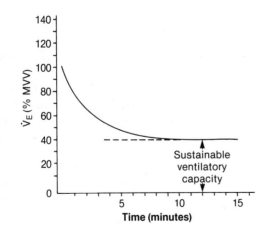

**Fig. 17-4.** Sustainable ventilatory capacity (SVC) defined as asymptote of the relationship between maximal ventilation performance ($\dot{V}_E$), expressed as a percentage of maximum voluntary ventilation (MVV), and the time to exhaustion. (Modified from Leith DE and Bradley M: *J Appl Physiol* 41:508, 1976.)

muscles are relatively inactive, the diaphragm is presented with greater force-generation demands and may be subject to early fatigue. In contrast, because the flattened diaphragm of the patient with emphysema is placed at a mechanical disadvantage, its force-generation capabilities may be compromised; therefore demands on the inspiratory rib cage muscles may be increased, thereby predisposing these muscles to fatigue.

The rate and extent of muscle shortening influence the threshold for fatigue. Because rapid diaphragmatic contractions consume more nutrients than slow contractions, patients with high breathing frequencies are susceptible to respiratory muscle fatigue. Similarly, energy expenditure is directly correlated to muscle shortening. This suggests that patients with large tidal volumes and greater muscle shortening may experience early respiratory muscle fatigue.

Nutrition and muscle use are important determinants of respiratory muscle fatigue. Malnutrition may cause mineral and electrolyte deficiencies and reduce the mass and force-generating capabilities of the respiratory muscles.

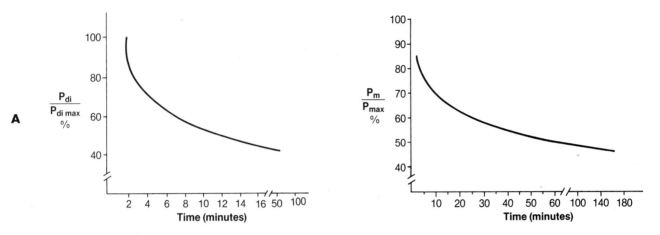

**Fig. 17-5.** Diagram of, **A,** transdiaphragmatic pressure ($P_{di}$) expressed as a fraction of maximum inspiratory pressure at functional residual capacity (FRC) ($P_{di}/P_{di\ max}$) as a function of time and, **B,** mouth pressure ($P_m$) as a percentage of maximum inspiratory pressure at FRC ($P_{max\ \%}$) plotted as a function of time. (Modified from Roussos C and others: *J Appl Physiol* 46(5):897, 1979.)

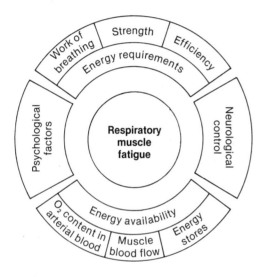

**Fig. 17-6.** Factors associated with respiratory muscle fatigue. (From Shaffer TH, Wolfson MR, and Bhutani VK: *Phys Ther* 61:12, 1711, 1981.)

Disuse atrophy as a result of prolonged mechanical ventilation presents similar structural and functional impairements. These factors compromise respiratory muscle force reserve and predispose the debilitated or recently ventilator-weaned patient to early respiratory muscle fatigue.

### Clinical evaluation of respiratory muscle fatigue

**Inspection and palpation.** Inspection of the thoracic cage may reveal out-of-phase and incoordinated chest wall movements, which produce combined or alternating diaphragmatic and intercostal breathing patterns. An inward movement of the costal margins (Hoover's sign) is observed in fatiguing patients with chronic obstructive pulmonary disease (COPD). Inward inspiratory motions of the abdomen may often predict severe respiratory failure. Palpation of the

chest wall and neck allows evaluation of increased activity of the accessory respiratory muscles. Although these are important clinical signs and are commonly associated with an increased respiratory load, these signs are difficult to measure and are neither specific nor sensitive indicators of fatigue.

**Lung volumes.** The values of total lung capacity (TLC) and residual volume (RV) are governed by elastic recoil of the lung chest wall and the respiratory muscle force. Thus, at total lung capacity the inspiratory muscle forces are most active, whereas at residual volume the expiratory muscle groups are predominant.

**Chest wall motion.** The dimensional changes of the rib cage and abdomen are measured with magnetometers or respiratory inductive plethysmography, which are useful for coordination of clinical observations.[64] These data may be used to infer lung volume displacements rather than respiratory muscle group activity. The subtle, mechanical signs of fatigue include (1) rapid, shallow respiratory cycles, (2) paradoxical movements, and (3) alternation between predominantly abdominal movement and rib cage movement during inspiration.

Studies of adults with COPD demonstrated asynchronous motion of the rib cage and abdomen in that outward motion of the abdomen preceded that of the rib cage during inspiration.[99] This can be analyzed by plotting rib cage against abdominal movement during a tidal breath and evaluating the phase angle of the resultant Lissajous loop.[2,64] Adults in respiratory failure demonstrate full-blown paradoxical motion, with the abdomen moving inward during inspiration.[99] A similar population demonstrated indrawing of the rib cage during inspiration, which has been explained to be the result of the impaired mechanical leverage of a flattened diaphragm and loss of apposition between the chest wall and diaphragm.[42]

The duration and the nature of paradoxical motion during

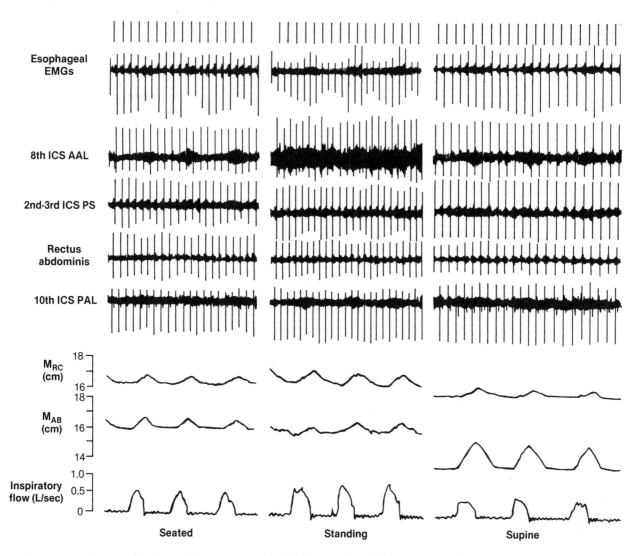

**Fig. 17-7.** Esophageal electromyographs of diaphragmatic activity. *AAL,* Anterior axillary line; *ICS,* intercostal space; *M_{AB},* abdominal displacement; *M_{RC},* rib cage displacement; *PAL,* posterior axillary line; *PS,* posterior scapular.

inspiration may have an impact on overall respiratory function. Age-related differences in chest wall compliance and configuration impose different working conditions for the respiratory muscles across development. Because the rib cage of the infant is much more compliant relative to that of the adult,[41] a large portion of the pressure effort generated by the diaphragm may be wasted in pulling the rib cage, rather than fresh air, inward. This pattern is exacerbated by elevated elastic and resistive pulmonary loads associated with bronchopulmonary dysplasia.[5,110] In addition, the horizontal orientation of the ribs and flattened diaphragm in the infant, as opposed to the mechanical advantages afforded by the oblique orientation of the rib cage and dome-shaped diaphragm of the adult,[49,66] require more shortening of the respiratory muscles to move the chest wall. Although it is erroneous to attribute abdominal motion exclusively to the diaphragm and rib cage motion to the intercostal muscles,

alterations in timing or pattern of chest wall motion may reflect the ability of the respiratory muscles to function efficiently as a pump.

**Pressures.** The pressures generated at the mouth ($P_m$), esophagus ($P_{es}$), stomach ($P_g$), and the difference between $P_{es}$ and $P_g$ (which is termed $P_{di}$) can be measured during ventilatory maneuvers. Although useful, these pressure measurements require that the patient swallow an esophageal balloon. This may be an uncomfortable, or even impossible, procedure for a person with severe dyspnea. These maneuvers have been described earlier and when repeated at intervals may be utilized to predict fatigue.

**Electromyography.** The electromyograph (EMG) presents an exceedingly complicated signal of motor-unit behavior during muscle contractions.[15] However, it has been recognized as a valuable predictor of muscle activity, timing, and fatigue.[45,83] As shown in Fig. 17-7, EMG activity of

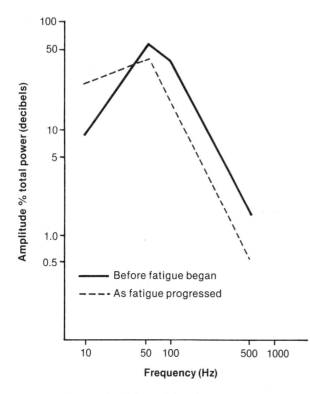

**Fig. 17-8.** Changes in high- and low-frequency components of EMG activity during diaphragmatic muscle fatigue. (Modified from Derenne J-PH, Macklem PT, and Roussos C: *Am Rev Respir Dis* 118(1-3):119, 373, 581, 1978.)

**Table 17-2.** Primary pulmonary disease affecting respiratory muscle function

| Adult | Pediatric |
|---|---|
| **Obstructive diseases** | |
| Asthma | Asthma |
| Bronchitis | Meconium aspiration |
| Emphysema | Amniotic fluid aspiration |
| Aspiration syndrome | Bronchiolitis |
| Bronchiolitis | Cystic fibrosis |
| Tumor | Congenital disorders of larynx and trachea |
| **Restrictive diseases** | |
| *Alveolar* | |
| Pneumonia | Hyaline membrane disease |
| Pulmonary edema | Atelectasis |
| Adult respiratory distress syndrome | Pneumonia |
| *Interstitial* | |
| Interstitial fibrosis | Bronchopulmonary dysplasias |
| Connective tissue disorders | Connective tissue disorders |
| | Cystic fibrosis |
| *Vascular* | |
| Thromboembolic disease | Persistent pulmonary hypertension of newborn |
| Pulmonary hypertension | |
| *Pleural* | |
| Pleural effusion | Pleural effusion |
| Mesothelioma | Chylothorax |

From Shaffer TH, Wolfson MR, and Bhutani VK: *Phys Ther* 61 (12):1711, 1981.

individual respiratory muscles can be associated with specific respiratory maneuvers and body positioning. Diaphragmatic EMG is obtained by electrode placement at sites with minimal or poor intercostal activity during inspiration. These sites are (1) the tenth intercostal space in the midaxillary line by needle electrodes, (2) the seventh, eighth, and ninth intercostal spaces in the midclavicular line by surface electrodes, and (3) the esophagus.[45] Diaphragmatic and intercostal muscle EMG activity are observable primarily during inspiration, as indicated by inspiratory flow and by chest wall and abdominal displacement. Inasmuch as quiet expiration is passive, there is no expiratory muscle EMG activity.

More recently, investigators have studied the frequency of respiratory muscle EMG activity.[96] Power-density spectral analysis of the frequency components has been used for assessment of the power of the myoelectric signal. Studies have shown that the diaphragmatic EMG spectrum is concentrated in the bandwidth of 25 to 250 Hz. Analysis of these EMGs has been used to make an early diagnosis of the onset of diaphragmatic fatigue. Characteristic patterns of electrical activity have been observed on the EMG of a fatiguing skeletal muscle. Similar shifts in the power spectrum of the EMG have been observed during diaphragmatic fatigue.[45] These observations (Fig. 17-8) document the onset of fatigue through (1) increased amplitude of low-

frequency (20 to 46.7 Hz) components, (2) decreased amplitude of high-frequency (150 to 350 Hz) components, and (3) decreased ratio of high to low (H:L ratio) frequency components. The H:L ratio is independent of respiratory muscle force and begins to decrease long before the muscle reaches its limit of endurance.[63]

The other aspects of EMG power spectrum also need to be considered for the evaluation of fatigue. These include (1) the maximum amplitude of the power spectrum, (2) the area under the amplitude-frequency curve, (3) the first movement of inertia, and (4) the centroid frequency. Which of these factors is the best predictor of respiratory muscle fatigue still needs to be evaluated.

## RESPIRATORY MUSCLE FUNCTION IN DISEASE

One of the major problems associated with respiratory management is the maintenance of adequate alveolar ventilation. Patients with primary pulmonary, neuromuscular, or musculoskeletal disease are at risk for respiratory failure. Respiratory muscle strength may be normal or increased in patients with primary pulmonary disease (Table 17-2) yet insufficient to overcome increased respiratory loads. In patients with neuromuscular or musculoskeletal disease (Table 17-3), inadequate respiration results from

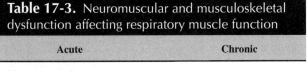

**Table 17-3.** Neuromuscular and musculoskeletal dysfunction affecting respiratory muscle function

| Acute | Chronic |
|---|---|
| **Neuromuscular** | |
| Spinal cord transection | Spastic quadriplegia |
| Guillain-Barré syndrome | Hemiplegia |
| Botulism | Cerebral palsy |
| Cholinergic poisoning | Parkinsonism |
| Poliomyelitis | Multiple sclerosis |
| Tetanus | Spina bifida |
| Diaphragmatic paralysis | Myasthenia gravis |
| Congenital diaphragmatic | Muscular dystrophy |
|   paralysis | Diaphragmatic fatigue |
| |   of prematurity |
| | |
| **Musculoskeletal** | |
| Crush injury of chest | Kyphoscoliosis |
| Postcardiothoracic surgery | Ankylosing spondylitis |
| | Pectus excavatum |

Modified from Shaffer TH, Wolfson MR, and Bhutani VK: *Phys Ther* 61 (12):1711, 1981.

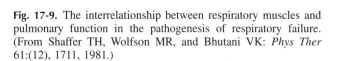

**Fig. 17-9.** The interrelationship between respiratory muscles and pulmonary function in the pathogenesis of respiratory failure. (From Shaffer TH, Wolfson MR, and Bhutani VK: *Phys Ther* 61:(12), 1711, 1981.)

primary muscle dysfunction, immobility, or respiratory center abnormalities. Regardless of the predisposing factors, respiratory muscle fatigue ensues, and although the clinical course may differ (Fig. 17-9), respiratory failure can result.

Although patients can usually be classified as having either primary pulmonary, neuromuscular, or musculoskeletal disease, mixed problems are commonly seen. For example, immobility and bulbar involvement associated with neuromuscular or musculoskeletal disease (typically leading to restrictive lung disease) may cause ineffective coughing, aspiration syndrome, or mucous plugging, airway obstruction results and so obstructive lung disease is diagnosed.[51] This further increases the demand on the respiratory muscles, which are already insufficient.

In critically ill patients in whom the work of breathing is high, the presence of diaphragm fatigue may have a considerable impact on treatment and specifically, the requirement for mechanical ventilation. Ideally, treatment of skeletal muscle fatigue involves rest of the muscles; total respiratory muscle fatigue, therefore, may be best treated by complete unloading or use of the mechanical ventilator. However, diagnosis of total respiratory muscle fatigue as compared to central respiratory fatigue is difficult to definitively diagnose.[17] Therefore, the conservative approach in treatment prior to complete ventilator support includes supplemental oxygen, which reduces central respiratory drive; use of bronchodilators, which diminishes airway resistance; and patient triggered ventilatory support so that the respiratory muscle workload is greatly diminished and the muscles can rest, while physiological gas exchange is maintained. Chronic night-assisted ventilation is a common form of respiratory muscle rest therapy[32,47] and has

reportedly led to improved inspiratory muscle strength and more stable resting lung volume and arterial blood chemistry.[26,28,38,40,54]

## TRAINING PROGRAMS AND PHYSIOLOGICAL RESPONSES
### General considerations and categories

Exercise programs have long been advocated as a therapeutic procedure for patients with respiratory dysfunction. Assessment of the efficacy of these programs has typically focused on changes in spirometric variables of lung function or on psychological advantages of rehabilitation training programs. However, unlike training programs for the physically healthy population, limited quantitative physiological data are available for assessing programs for the respiratory impaired. This dearth of information may be a function of several variables, including complicating health factors, ambiguous programming and assessment methods, and patient and personnel logistics within a predominantly outpatient population.

Nonetheless, exercise is a critical component in the care plan of the respiratory impaired. If the long-term goal of rehabilitation is to return to or to maintain maximal functional level, the student of pulmonary physical therapy should be capable of designing, administering, and reevaluating a rehabilitation program, and assessing the efficacy of this program for the population toward which it is intended.

To this end, the purposes of this section are as follows:

1. Compare and contrast effects of exercise in the normal and respiratory-impaired populations.
2. Highlight assessed rehabilitation programs with respect to pulmonary function, hemodynamics, cardiovascular function, respiratory muscle strength, fatigue, endurance, and exercise tolerance.

Exercise programs take on many forms, but for convenience they can be divided into two groups: general (systemic) and specific (localized training of respiratory muscles). General programs include activities using extremity muscles in addition to respiratory musculature with or without supplemental oxygen.[23,27,29,33,62,112] Almost all combinations of exercise have been studied: general conditioning, including treadmill and bicycling, breathing exercises, and psychological support; bicycling and treadmill or treadmill alone[6,16,50,86,88,113]; treadmill and breathing exercises, calisthenics, gymnastics, and swimming, and patient education for children;[52] jogging for adolescents;[109] and walking.[103,106] These programs have been designed to improve the physiological factors of pulmonary function, strength, endurance, cardiac function, and exercise tolerance, as well as nonphysiological factors, such as cooperation and psychological well-being.

Alternatively, specific training refers to exercises primarily involving and emphasizing ventilatory muscle groups. Diaphragmatic training alone or with incentive spirometry has been recommended in patients with chronic obstructive pulmonary disease.[9] In these patients, a flattened, depressed diaphragm was observed to have limited respiratory excursions and consequently made a minimal contribution to ventilation. Use of a Gordon-Barach belt and diaphragmatic breathing with active abdominal contraction during expiration is designed to cause a cephalic displacement of the diaphragm.[9] As the diaphragm lengthens, the abdominal and inspiratory rib cage musculature shortens. Length-tension relationships are optimized, providing increased contraction and pressure change for improved diaphragmatic respiration.[43] However, substantial data are scant and of questionable support for this modality as an independent means to enhance respiration.[27] Pursed-lips breathing, the pattern of exhaling through the mouth against the pressure of pursed lips, is used spontaneously by some patients and often is taught to other patients as one facet of breathing retraining.[56,82] Pursed-lips breathing is believed to prevent airway closure and provide relief to some patients from unpleasant sensations associated with breathing.

Ventilatory muscle strength training (VMST) has been shown to increase isometric pressures generated by inspiratory and expiratory muscles.[69] For example, maximum static inspiratory and expiratory pressures (MSIP and MSEP) are performed on the spirometer against a closed shutter at 20% intervals over the range of vital capacity. Each maneuver is sustained for 3 to 5 seconds, and the performance is repeated so that the exercise lasts ½ hour a day. Finally, positional change alone (from supine to prone) has been shown to improve thoracoabdominal synchrony in preterm infants by increasing the mechanical leverage of the diaphragm through the area of apposition.[111]

Ventilatory muscle endurance training (VMET) helps develop the capacity for sustaining higher levels of ventilation for relatively long periods of time, approximately 15 minutes. Leith and Bradley[69] described VMET as sustained ventilation achieved 3 to 5 times, until exhaustion, interspersed with recovery intervals of unspecified duration. Each episode lasted 12 to 15 minutes; the duration of the session was 45 to 60 minutes, 5 days a week. Normocapnic hyperpnea was achieved with a partial rebreathing system. Use of a breathing bag provided visual biofeedback to the patient, and the $CO_2$ scrubber was adjusted to maintain a normal end tidal $CO_2$. Both VMST and VMET are current approaches in exercise programs and areas of active research in pulmonary rehabilitation.

Other unique collaborative therapeutic approaches to training may be required when respiratory problems are caused or complicated by nonrespiratory disabilities. For example, children with cerebral palsy are extremely vulnerable to respiratory disease because of shallow, irregular respirations and ineffectual cough.[22,91] Although respiratory functions are impaired in these children, concomitant decreased efficiency and poor coordination of the breathing mechanisms further jeopardize ventilatory capacity.[21] In addition, impaired neuromotor control is often coupled with reduced physical activity, which by itself is another respiratory disease risk factor.

### Effect of training programs on pulmonary function

Respiratory muscles, like other skeletal muscles in the normal population, improve their efficiency after training. This improvement is reflected in improved breathing function. Training effects on pulmonary ventilation are associated with a decrease in rate and an increase in depth of breathing.[57] In the trained subject these changes are noticed at rest and during heavy exercise as well.

Pulmonary function response to general training programs for patients with COPD is reviewed by Shaffer and co-workers.[97] In general, no significant change was seen in most pulmonary function variables. A decreased respiratory rate with a deeper breathing pattern was noted.[81,106,112] One investigator suggested that a more efficient breathing pattern resulted, whereas others described a task-specific improvement in ventilation. A few studies found an increase in forced vital capacity (FVC), which may have reflected a reduction in air trapping;[103] additionally, improvements in maximal voluntary ventilation and inspiratory capacity are reported.[16] High pretraining values for specific and static lung compliance decreased (although not significantly) toward normal after training.[6] In addition, a trend toward improved dynamic compliance and reduced respiratory work has been reported as a result of training.[113]

Less information is available about the effects of specific training programs on pulmonary function.[61] Furthermore, conflicting results are reported, with some studies reporting improvement in lung volumes and maneuvers[19,69,91] and others reporting no significant change after training.[58,80] Lane[67] weight-trained the diaphragm of nonintubated patients with acute spinal injury and found a significant increase in vital capacity and a decrease in the average hospital stay.

Mechanisms for pulmonary function improvement after specific training programs have been suggested. Postural compensation (forward leaning upon respiratory stress) compresses the abdomen. Because of mechanical relationships, the diaphragm is stretched upward, and this stretching facilitates the length-tension relationship, thereby increasing the capacity of the diaphragm to generate tension. Alternatively, research on animals possibly indicates a neurophysiological mechanism by which costovertebral joint mobilization may stimulate joint mechanoreceptors. This information may be processed through the medullary-pontine "rhythm generator" to influence the respiratory pattern.[98]

### Effect of training programs on hemodynamics and cardiopulmonary function

Training programs improve certain hemodynamic and cardiopulmonary functions in the normal population. Maximum oxygen consumption ($\dot{V}_{O_2\,max}$), oxygen extraction (a-$\tilde{v}_{O_2}$), cardiac output, and stroke volume increase, whereas resting heart rate is found to decrease after training. In general, oxygen consumption ($\dot{V}_{O_2}$) and $\dot{V}_{O_2\,max}$ are used to evaluate the effectiveness and intensity of training, since they reflect a change in cardiac output and oxygen extraction by the tissues.

Oxygen consumption increases linearly as a function of escalating workloads and becomes stable with maximal work, the point of $\dot{V}_{O_2\,max}$. Thereafter, the oxygen needs of the muscle are not met by the cardiovascular-respiratory system, and the energy for increased work is derived from anaerobic metabolism. Lactic acid accumulation results. Therefore a higher $\dot{V}_{O_2\,max}$ implies increased oxygen use by the peripheral musculature at maximal loads with associated increments in a-$\tilde{v}_{O_2}$ and decrements in exercise blood lactate levels. As such, an objective indication of a training effect is an increase in $\dot{V}_{O_2\,max}$. Furthermore, in the normal population, the rate of change of $\dot{V}_{O_2}$ at each level of exercise is not physiologically altered by mild training once the exercise is learned, whereas $\dot{V}_{O_2\,max}$ increases. General training programs are known to produce slower heart rates regardless of the exercise employed. The reasons for this are unclear; however, it has been suggested that general muscle training

may alter autonomic control, levels of circulating catecholamines, stroke volume, or the integrating ability of the central nervous system. Increases in stroke volume are also associated with training. These increases are related to increased ventricular volume or bradycardia. Finally, cardiac output increases parallel the increase in $\dot{V}_{O_2\,max}$ in response to training.[95]

Research of general training programs in patients with COPD report changes in some of the aforementioned parameters. Several studies demonstrated a decrease in $\dot{V}_{O_2}$ at each level of exercise, relating this finding to improved coordination and exercise efficiency.[6,86] One group of investigators reported that the greater the initial exercise load (higher $\dot{V}_{O_2}$), the greater the decrease in $\dot{V}_{O_2}$ at a given exercise level after training.[106] They suggest that this relationship emphasizes the importance of beginning exercises at the highest safe level. Increases in $\dot{V}_{O_2\,max}$ and a-$\tilde{v}_{O_2}$ values are also reported.[33,86] These findings are most probably related to improved oxygen extraction capacity of the muscles or oxygen delivery to the muscle (i.e., elevated myoglobin concentration or increased number of capillaries per skeletal muscle fiber).

Conflicting data are reported as to changes in heart rate and cardiac output after general training. Some studies report decreases in heart rate, whereas others found no significant change in either parameter. It may be that severely disabled pulmonary patients are unable to reach the level of activity needed to induce a training effect.[29] This has been related to the low level of peripheral activity resulting from the high oxygen cost of breathing, at rest, for patients with COPD. This factor might also explain why no increase in stroke volume was found as a result of a general training program in the COPD population. These findings seem to support the possibility that increased work tolerance in these patients is most probably attributable to improved oxygen extraction by exercising muscles.

Finally, little is known about general training program effects on gas transport in the respiratory-impaired population. One study reports smaller alveolar/arterial oxygen gradients and improved venous admixtures, implying improved ventilation/perfusion relationships.[113] Oxygen-assisted exercise increased arterial oxygen ($P_{O_2}$) values while the pH remained stable because of the supplemental oxygen, which reduced exercise-induced lactic acidosis.[23] Furthermore, blood lactate levels have been reported to decrease in another study.[113] This decrease may demonstrate the training effects of producing a more efficient capillary blood supply, providing additional oxygen to the muscle, and thereby reducing anaerobic metabolism.

In contrast to the data for general training programs, relatively little is known about the effects of specific training programs on hemodynamic and cardiopulmonary parameters in the population with COPD. Reports include increases in $\dot{V}_{O_2\,max}$ and maximal exercise heart rate and are associated with the higher exercise levels that were attained.[19] Recruitment of low-oxidative, high-glycolytic, fast-twitch muscle fibers at higher levels of exercise may explain reported increases in postexercise blood lactate levels.[19] Other studies propose improvement in aerobic capacities yet report insignificant changes.[58] This dearth of information is not surprising because specific training techniques are relatively new. This is an area of active investigation, and one would expect more definitive forthcoming data.

### Effect of training programs on respiratory muscle strength, endurance, fatigue, and exercise tolerance

The training response of respiratory muscle is similar to that of skeletal muscle. Muscles respond differently to exercises oriented to improving strength as compared with improving endurance. One important difference is that strengthening exercises produce mostly muscle hypertrophy, whereas endurance exercises increase the vascularity of muscle fibers.[57] The reason for this difference is not as yet fully understood.

As mentioned previously, respiratory muscle strength is defined as the maximum and minimum static pressures measured at the mouth attributable to the muscular effort needed to produce the change, whereas ventilatory muscle endurance may be defined and measured as the capacity for sustaining high levels of ventilation under isocapnic conditions for relatively long periods. Diaphragmatic fatigue is defined as the point at which the diaphragm is unable to sustain a predetermined level of transdiaphragmatic pressure. Exercise tolerance is the ability to exercise without discomfort. Strength, endurance, fatigue, and dyspnea play a role in determining an exercise tolerance level.

Limited quantitative data are available on respiratory muscle strength and endurance response to a general exercise program in the population with COPD. Some studies attribute an increase in exercise tolerance to psychological components of improved motivation and a sense of well-being and confidence.[1,62,73,81,112] Several studies allude to improved neuromuscular coordination as the causative factor.[29,86,91] Reported stride-length increments and improvements in specific exercises used in general training programs may demonstrate improved neuromuscular coordination and efficiency of movement. Recent studies demonstrate that nonspecific upper body exercise, such as swimming and canoeing, is effective in improving respiratory muscle endurance in children with cystic fibrosis.[58]

Specific training programs are reported to affect respiratory muscle strength and endurance, as well as exercise tolerance. Leith and Bradley[69] trained normal volunteers according to the VMET and VMST methods previously described. They concluded that VMST improved strength whereas VMET improved endurance. A similar study of children with cystic fibrosis reported increased endurance and exercise tolerance after 4 weeks of training.[58] After training with inspiratory flow-resistive loads, quadriplegic, muscular dystrophy, cystic fibrosis and COPD patients are reported to demonstrate improvement in ventilatory muscle strength and endurance[3,4,8,37,46,68,70,89]; in addition, dyspnea in other patients disappeared during routine daily activities.[7,87] Specific weight training in healthy subjects, such as use of weights placed on the abdomen, does not increase maximal shortening, velocity of shortening, or strength of the diaphragm.[80] Postural compensation, such as forward leaning, provides relief of dyspnea in patients with COPD.[100] This modality may be an effective means to increase exercise tolerance by maximizing the diaphragmatic length-tension relationship and enhancing full synergistic cooperation of the inspiratory muscles.

Respiratory muscle fatigue has not been assessed after a general training program. Several studies suggest that dyspnea curtails activity levels of patients with COPD before respiratory muscle fatigue occurs. It is unclear whether the physiological or psychological components of dyspnea or general debilitation characterized by early extremity skeletal muscle fatigue limits exercise tolerance.

A few studies indicate that specific training programs increase respiratory resistance to fatigue. Reported improvements in endurance after VMET suggest that fatigue is delayed.[58] Animal studies demonstrate delayed onset of fatigue with strength and endurance training associated with increases in cellular oxidative capacity, mitochondrial enzymes, and capacity for fatty acid oxidation.[59,71] Recruitment of other inspiratory muscles is suggested to prevent fatigue when one is breathing against a resistive load. By monitoring the abdominal pressure, investigators noticed that the diaphragm and intercostal muscles contributed alternately in time.[94] Recovery may occur during the alternate rest periods, possibly postponing the onset of fatigue. Although reduced accessory inspiratory muscle EMG activity is noted during forward leaning, patients utilizing this form of postural compensation experience relief of dyspnea.[100] It seems that the force generated by these muscles may be more effectively applied to the rib cage in this position. It is suggested that by stabilization of the upper extremities and use of the reverse action of the muscle, synergy of the inspiratory muscle may be enhanced, and overall respiratory muscle fatigue may thereby be reduced. Hyperinflation through intermittent positive-pressure mechanical ventilation is often recommended as a therapeutic modality in primary pulmonary disease and respiratory dysfunction caused by neuromuscular and musculoskeletal disease.[35,104] This technique is reported to improve ventilation and gas exchange either by improving pulmonary compliance or by preventing atelectasis. When intermittent positive-pressure ventilation is used in patients with respiratory muscle weakness, the work of breathing required to overcome the elastic forces of the lung is reduced, and therefore oxygen consumption is decreased. Ultimately, respiratory muscle fatigue may be prevented.

## PHARMACOTHERAPEUTIC APPROACHES TO RESPIRATORY MUSCLE FATIGUE

Therapeutic intervention in respiratory muscle fatigue includes agents that may improve respiratory muscle contractility by two major mechanisms: (1) agents that improve excitation-contraction coupling and (2) agents that improve diaphragmatic blood flow.

Intropic agents have been introduced for the management of respiratory muscle fatigue. The most intensely used agents, methylxanthines (i.e., theophylline, caffeine, enprofylline), appear to augment diaphragmatic contractility by increasing cystosolic calcium either by facilitating calcium influx from the extracellular space and/or by augmenting release of calcium sequestered in the sarcoplasmic reticulum. Physiologic markers of the therapeutic effectiveness have been identified in both adult[55,102] and neonatal animal preparations and, to a more limited degree, in humans. In this regard, transdiaphragmatic pressure in both fresh and fatigued adult muscle was augmented by up to 25% by a therapeutic concentration of theophylline (10-15 mg/ml).[10,84,85,107] Studies in neonates are conflicting with several studies indicating no improvement in diaphragmatic contractility or fatigue resistance in newborn piglets[78,79] as compared to improvements in mouth occlusion pressure and increased diaphragmatic excursion in preterm infants.[45,46] Whether these effects are species related or represent differences between a central or peripheral effect of the agent remains unclear. With respect to calcium flux and excitation-contraction coupling, the diaphragm resembles cardiac more so than skeletal muscle. In this regard, digoxin has recently been shown to have strong inotropic effects on diaphragmatic contractility in adult animals[12] and humans[11] but no effect in normal neonatal swine.[77]

The second approach in pharmacotherapy in respiratory muscle fatigue involves agents which act on the circulatory system to increase respiratory blood flow. While limited information exists in humans, Aubier[13] demonstrated that increases in diaphragmatic blood flow due to infusion of dopamine (10 mcg/kg/min) are associated with an increase in diaphragmatic mechanical output as reflected by an increase in transdiaphragmatic pressure development following electrophrenic stimulation. This response was repeatable and reversible with the reinitiation/cessation of the circulatory stimulus.

Parenthetically, the role of respiratory muscle inotropes and circulatory agonists in the management of critically ill patients with respiratory failure presents a potential paradox. Although it can be argued that augmentation of diaphragmatic tension has potential benefit in the short term, this approach might increase respiratory muscle energy expenditure and inadvertently lead to more serious and long-term

problems. Fatigue is generally thought to act as a protective mechanism to prevent muscle injury. As such, pharmacotherapy, as well as dynamic neuromusculoskeletal intervention, must be balanced with consideration to the role of rest and the maintenance of an effective energetic supply to demand relationship so as to achieve and maintain physiologic gas exchange.

## REFERENCES

1. Agle DP and others: Multidiscipline treatment of chronic pulmonary insufficiency. I. Psychologic aspects of rehabilitation, *Psychosom Med* 35:41, 1973.
2. Agostoni E and Mogroni P: Deformation of the chest wall during breathing efforts, *J Appl Physiol* 21:1827, 1966.
3. Aldrich TK: Respiratory muscle fatigue. In Belman MJ, editor: Respiratory muscles: function in health and disease, *Clin Chest Med* 9(2):225, 1988.
4. Aldrich TK and Karpel JP: Inspiratory resistive training in respiratory failure, *Am Rev Respir Dis* 131:461, 1985.
5. Allen J and others: Thoracoabdominal synchrony in infants with air-flow obstruction, *Am Rev Resp Dis* 1374:379, 1988.
6. Alpert JS and others: Effects of physical training on hemodynamics and pulmonary function at rest and during exercise in patients with chronic obstructive pulmonary disease, *Chest* 66:647, 1974.
7. Anderson JB and others: Resistive breathing in severe chronic obstructive pulmonary disease: a pilot study, *Scand J Respir Dis* 60:151, 1974.
8. Asher MI and others: The effects of inspiratory muscle training in patients with cystic fibrosis, *Am Rev Respir Dis* 126:855, 1982.
9. Astrand PO and Rodahl K: *Textbook of work physiology,* New York, 1977, McGraw-Hill Book Co.
10. Aubier M and others: Aminophylline improves diaphragm contractility, *N Engl J Med* 305:249, 1981.
11. Aubier M and others: Effects of digoxin on diaphragmatic strength generation, *J Appl Physiol* 61:1767, 1986.
12. Aubier M and others: Effects of digoxin on diaphragmatic strength generation in patients with chronic obstructive pulmonary disease during acute respiratory failure, *Am Rev Resp Dis* 135:544, 1987.
13. Aubier M and others: Dopamine effects on diaphragmatic strength during acute respiratory failure in chronic obstructive pulmonary disease, *Ann Intern Med* 110:17, 1989.
14. Barach AL and Seaman W: Role of diagram in chronic pulmonary emphysema, *NY State J Med* 63:415, 1963.
15. Basmajian JV: *Muscles alive,* Baltimore, 1978, Williams & Wilkins.
16. Bass H, Whitcomb JF, and Folman R: Exercise training: therapy for patients with chronic obstructive pulmonary disease, *Chest* 57:116, 1970.
17. Bellemare FD and Bigland-Ritchie B: Central components of diaphragmatic fatigue assessed by phrenic nerve stimulation, *J Appl Physiol* 62:1307, 1987.
18. Bellemare FD and others: The effect of tension and pattern of contractions on the blood flow of the canine diaphragm, *J Appl Physiol* 54:1597, 1983.
19. Belman MJ and Mittman C: Ventilatory muscle training improves exercise capacity in chronic obstructive pulmonary disease patients, *Am Rev Respir Dis* 121:273, 1980.
20. Bhutani VK, Koslo RJ, and Shaffer TH: The effect of tracheal smooth muscle tone on neonatal airway collapsibility, *Pediatr Res* 20:492, 1986.
21. Bjure J and Berg K: Dynamic and static-lung volumes of school children with cerebral palsy, *Acta Pediatr Scand* 204(suppl):35, 1970.
22. Blumberg M: Respiration and speech in the cerebral palsied child, *Am J Dis Child* 89:48, 1955.

23. Bradley BL and others: Oxygen-assisted exercise in chronic obstructive lung disease, *Am Rev Respir Dis* 118:239, 1978.

24. Byrd RB and Hyatt RL: Maximal respiratory pressures in obstructive lung disease, *Am Rev Respir Dis* 98:848, 1968.

25. Campbell EJM, Agostoni E, and Davis JN: *The respiratory muscles,* Philadelphia, 1970, WB Saunders Co.

26. Carroll N and Branthwaite MA: Control of nocturnal hypoventilation by nasal intermittent positive pressure ventilation, *Thorax* 43:349, 1988.

27. Casciari RJ, Fairshter RD, and Morrison JT: Effects of breathing retraining in patients with chronic obstructive pulmonary disease, *Chest* 79:393, 1981.

28. Celli B and others: A controlled trial of external negative pressure ventilation in patients with severe chronic airflow obstruction, *Am Rev Respir Dis* 140:1251, 1989.

29. Chester EH and others: Multidisciplinary treatment of chronic insufficiency. III. The effect of physical training on cardiopulmonary performance in patients with chronic obstructive pulmonary disease, *Chest* 72:695, 1977.

30. Coburn RF, Thortin D, and Arts R: Effect of trachealis muscle contraction in tracheal resistance to airflow, *J Appl Physiol* 32:397, 1972.

31. Cook CD, Mead J, and Orzalesi MM: Static volume-pressure characteristics of the respiratory system during maximal efforts, *J Appl Physiol* 19:1016, 1964.

32. Cropp A and Dimarco AF: Effects of intermittent negative pressure ventilation on respiratory muscle function in patients with severe chronic obstructive pulmonary disease, *Am Rev Respir Dis* 135:1056, 1987.

33. Degre S and others: Hemodynamic responses to physical training in patients with chronic lung disease, *Am Rev Respir Dis* 110:395, 1974.

34. Derenne J-PH, Macklem PT, and Roussos C: The respiratory muscles: mechanics, control, and pathophysiology, *Am Rev Respir Dis* 118(1-3):119, 373, 581, 1978.

35. DeTroyer A and Drisser P: The effects of intermittent positive pressure breathing on patients with respiratory muscle weakness, *Am Rev Respir Dis* 124:132, 1982.

36. DeTroyer A and Loring SH: Action of the respiratory muscles. In Fishman AP, Macklem PT, and Mead J, editors: *Handbook of physiology: the respiratory system,* ed 3, Bethesda, Md, 1986, American Physiological Society.

37. DiMarco AF and others: Respiratory muscle training in muscular dystrophy, *Clin Res* 30:427A, 1982.

38. Ellis ER and others: Treatment of respiratory failure during sleep in patients with neuromuscular disease. Positive-pressure ventilation through a nose mask, *Am Rev Respir Dis.* 135:148, 1987.

39. Freedman S: Sustained maximum voluntary ventilation, *Respir Physiol* 8:230, 1970.

40. Garay SM, Turino GM, and Goldring RM: Sustained reversal of chronic hypercapnea in patients with alveolar hypoventilation syndromes. Long-term maintenance with long-term non-invasive mechanical ventilation, *Am J Med* 70:269, 1981.

41. Gerhardt T and Bancalari E: Chest wall compliance in full-term and premature infants, *Acta Pediatr Scand* 69:359, 1980.

42. Gilmartin JJ and Gibson GJ: Mechanisms of paradoxical rib cage motion in patients with chronic obstructive pulmonary disease, *Am Rev Respir Dis* 134:683, 1986.

43. Goldman M and Mead J: Mechanical interaction between diaphragm and rib cage, *J Appl Physiol* 35:197, 1973.

44. Grimby G, Goldman M, and Mead J: Respiratory muscle action inferred from rib cage and abdominal V-P partitioning, *J Appl Physiol* 41:739, 1976.

45. Gross D and others: Electromyogram pattern of diaphragmatic fatigue, *J Appl Physiol* 46(1):1, 1979.

46. Gross D and others: The effect of training on strength and endurance of the diaphragm in quadriplegia, *Am J Med* 68:27, 1980.

47. Guitierrez M and others: Weekly cuirass ventilation improves blood gases and inspiratory muscle strength in patients with chronic airflow limitation and hypercarbia, *Am Rev Resp Dis* 138:617, 1988.

48. Guslits BG and others: Diaphragmatic work of breathing in premature human infants, *J Appl Physiol* 62(4):1410, 1987.

49. Guyton AC: *Textbook of medical physiology,* Philadelphia, 1971, WB Saunders Co.

50. Hale T, Spriggs J, and Hamley EJ: The effects of an exercise regime on patients with lung malfunction, *Br J Sports Med* 11:181, 1977.

51. Harrison BDW and others: Respiratory failure in neuromuscular diseases, *Thorax* 26:579, 1971.

52. Heimlich D: Evaluation of a breathing program for children, *Respiratory Care* 20:64, 1975.

53. Heyman E and others: The effect of aminophylline on the excursions of the diaphragm in preterm neonates, *Acta Pediatr Scand* 80:308, 1991.

54. Hoeppner VH and others: Nighttime ventilation improves respiratory failure in secondary kyphoscoliosis, *Am Rev Respir Dis* 129:240, 1984.

55. Howell S and Roussos C: Isoproterenol and aminophylline improve contractility of fatigued canine diaphragm, *Am Rev Respir Dis* 129:118, 1984.

56. Ingram RH and Schilder DP: Effect of pursed lips expiration on the pulmonary pressure-flow relationship in obstructive lung disease, *Am Rev Respir Dis* 96:381, 1967.

57. Johnson WR and Buskirk ER: *Science and medicine of exercise and sport,* ed 2, New York, 1974, Harper & Row.

58. Keens TG and others: Ventilatory muscle endurance training in normal subjects and patients with cystic fibrosis, *Am Rev Respir Dis* 116:853, 1977.

59. Keens TG and others: Cellular adaptations of the ventilatory muscles to a chronic increased respiratory load, *J Appl Physiol* 44(6):905, 1978.

60. Keens TG and others: Developmental pattern of muscle fibers types in human ventilatory muscles, *J Appl Physiol* 44:909, 1978.

61. Kigin CM: Breathing exercises for the medical patient: the art and the science, *Phys Ther* 70:700, 1990.

62. Kimbel P and others: An in-hospital program for rehabilitation of patients with chronic obstructive pulmonary disease, *Bull Am Coll Chest Physicians* 60:6, 1971.

63. Kogi K and Hakamada T: Slowing of surface electromyogram and muscle strength in muscle fatigue, *Rep Instit Sci Labour* 60:27, 1962.

64. Konno K and Mead J: Measurement of the separate volume changes of rib cage and abdomen during breathing, *J Appl Physiol* 22:407, 1967.

65. Koslo RJ, Bhutani VK, and Shaffer TH: The role of tracheal smooth muscle contraction on neonatal tracheal mechanics, *Pediatr Res* 20:1216, 1986.

66. Krahl VE: Anatomy of the mammalian lung. In Fishman AP, Macklem PT, and Mead J, editors: *Handbook of physiology: respiration,* ed 1, Bethesda, Md, 1964, American Physiological Society.

67. Lane C: *Inspiratory muscle weight training and its effect on the vital capacity of patients with quadraplegia,* (thesis), Boston, Mass, 1982 Northeastern Univ.

68. Larson JL and others: Inspiratory muscle training with a pressure threshold breathing device in patients with chronic obstructive pulmonary disease, *Am Rev Resp Dis* 138:689, 1988.

69. Leith DE and Bradley M: Ventilatory muscle strength and endurance training, *J Appl Physiol* 41:508, 1976.

70. Levine S, Weisser P, and Gillen J: Evaluation of a ventilatory muscle endurance training program in the rehabilitation of patients with COPD. *Am Rev Respir Dis* 133:400, 1986.

71. Lieberman DA, Maxwell LC, and Faulkner JA: Adaptation of guinea pig diaphragm muscle to aging and endurance training, *Am J Physiol* 222(3):556, 1972.
72. Lopes JM and others: The effects of theophylline on diaphragmatic fatigue in the newborn (abstract), *Pediatr Res* 16:355A, 1982.
73. Lustig FM, Haas A, and Castillo R: Clinical and rehabilitation regime in patients with chronic obstructive pulmonary disease, *Arch Phys Med Rehabil* 53:315, 1972.
74. Macklem PT: Respiratory muscles: the vital pump, *Chest* 78:753, 1980.
75. Maxwell LC, Kuehl TJ, and McCarter RJM: Temporal changes after death in primate muscle oxidative enzyme activity, *Am Rev Resp Dis* 130:1147, 1984.
76. Maxwell LC and others: Development of histochemical and functional properties of baboon respiratory muscles, *J Appl Physiol* 54(2):551, 1983.
77. Mayock DE, Standaert TA, and Woodrum DE: Effects of digoxin on diaphragmatic contractility in the piglet, *Pediatr Res* 25(3):271, 1989.
78. Mayock DE, Standert TA, and Woodrum DE: Effect of methylxanthines on diaphragmatic fatigue in the piglet, *Pediatr Res* 32:580, 1992.
79. Mayock DE and others: Effect of aminophylline on diaphragmatic contractility in the piglet, *Pediatr Res* 28:196, 1990.
80. Merrick J and Axen K: Inspiratory muscles function following abdomen weight exercises in healthy subjects, *Phys Ther* 61:651, 1981.
81. Moser KM and others: Results of a comprehensive rehabilitation program, *Arch Intern Med* 140:1597, 1980.
82. Mueller RE, Petty TL, and Filley GF: Ventilation and arterial blood gas changes induced by pursed lips breathing, *J Appl Physiol* 28:784, 1970.
83. Muller N and others: Respiratory muscle fatigue in infants, *Clin Res* 25:714A, 1977.
84. Murciano D and others: Effects of long-term theophylline administration on dyspnea, arterial blood gases, and respiratory muscle performance in COPD patients, *Am Rev Respir Dis* 134:4A150, 1986.
85. Murciano D and others: A randomized controlled trial of theophylline in patients with severe chronic obstructive pulmonary disease, *N Engl J Med* 329:1521, 1989.
86. Paez PN and others: The physiologic basis of training patients with emphysema, *Am Rev Respir Dis* 95:944, 1967.
87. Pardy RL and others: The effects of inspiratory muscle training on exercise performance in chronic airflow obstruction, *Am Rev Respir Dis* 123:426, 1981.
88. Rahn H and others: The pressure volume diagram of the thorax and lung, *Am J Physiol* 146:161, 1946.
89. Reid WD and Warren CPW: Ventilatory muscle strength and endurance training in elderly subjects and patients with chronic airflow limitation: a pilot study, *Physio Canada* 36:305, 1984.
90. Rohrer F: Der Zusammenhang der Atemkrafte und ihre Abhangigkeit von Dehnungzustand der Atmungsorgane, *Pflugers Arch Ges Physiol* 165:419, 1916.
91. Rothman JG: Effects of respiratory exercises on the vital capacity and forced expiratory volume in children with cerebral palsy, *Phys Ther* 58:421, 1978.
92. Roussos CS and Macklem PT: Diaphragmatic fatigue in man, *J Appl Physiol Respir* 43:189, 1977.
93. Roussos C and Macklem PT: Inspiratory muscle fatigue. In Fishman AP, Macklem PT, and Mead J, editors: *Handbook of physiology: the respiratory system,* ed 3, Bethesda, Md, 1986, American Physiological Society.
94. Roussos C and others: Fatigue of inspiratory muscles and their synergistic behavior, *J Appl Physiol* 46(5):897, 1979.
95. Scheuer J and Tipton CM: Cardiovascular adaptations to physical training, *Ann Rev Physiol* 39:221, 1977.
96. Schweitzer TW and others: Spectral analysis of human inspiratory diaphragmatic electromyograms, *J Appl Physiol* 41:152, 1979.
97. Shaffer TH, Wolfson MR, and Bhutani VK: Respiratory muscle function, assessment, and training, *Phys Ther* 61:12, 1711, 1981.
98. Shannon R: Respiratory pattern changes during costovertebral joint movement, *J Appl Physiol* 48:862, 1980.
99. Sharp JT and others: Thoracoabdominal motion in chronic obstructive pulmonary disease, *Am Rev Respir Dis* 115:47, 1977.
100. Sharp JT and others: Postural relief of dyspnea in severe chronic obstructive pulmonary disease, *Am Rev Respir Dis* 122:201, 1980.
101. Sieck GC, Mazar A, and Belman JM: Changes in diaphragmatic EMG spectra during hypercapneic loads, *Respir Physiol* 61.
102. Sigrist S and others: The effect of aminophylline on inspiratory muscle contractility, *Am Rev Respir Dis* 126:46, 1982.
103. Sinclair DJM and Ingram CG: Controlled trial of supervised exercise training in chronic bronchitis, *Br Med J* 280(6213):519, 1980.
104. Sinha R and Bergofsky EH: Prolonged alteration of lung mechanics in kyphoscoliosis by positive pressure hyperinflation, *Am Rev Respir Dis* 106:47, 1972.
105. Supinski G: Control of respiratory muscle blood flow, *Am Rev Respir Dis* 134:1078, 1986.
106. Unger KM, Moser KM, and Glansen P: Selection of an exercise program for patients with chronic obstructive pulmonary disease, *Heart Lung* 9:68, 1980.
107. Vires N and others: Effects of isolated diaphragmatic fibers: A model for pharmacological studies on diaphragmatic contractility, *Am Rev Respir Dis* 133:1060, 1986.
108. Watchko JF and others: Diaphragmatic electromyogram power spectral analysis during ventilatory failure in infants. In Gennnser G and others, editors: *Fetal and neonatal physiological measurements. III. Proceedings of the third international conference on fetal and neonatal physiologic measurements,* Malmo, Sweden Flenhags, Tryckeri, 1989.
109. Wilbourn K: The long distance runners, *Runner's World,* Aug 1978.
110. Wolfson MR and others: The mechanics and energetics of breathing helium in infants with BPD, *J Pediatr* 104(5):752, 1984.
111. Wolfson MR and others: Effect of position on the mechanical interaction between the rib cage and abdomen in preterm infants, *J Appl Physiol* 72:1032, 1992.
112. Woolf CR: A rehabilitation program for improving exercise tolerance of patients with chronic lung disease, *Can Med Assoc J* 106:1289, 1972.
113. Woolf CR and Suero JT: Alterations in lung mechanics and gas exchange following training in chronic obstructive lung disease, *Dis Chest* 55:37, 1969.

# CHAPTER 18

# Respiratory Evaluation

*Nancy Humberstone and Jan Stephen Tecklin*

## RESPIRATORY EVALUATION

The physical therapy evaluation of patients with pulmonary disease has two parts. Part one includes clinical signs and symptoms gathered through the history and chest examination. Part two completes the evaluation through objective assessment of the arterial blood gases, pulmonary function tests, chest radiography, graded exercise tests, and bacteriological studies. With the information and data collected from the evaluation, the physical therapist can assess physical dysfunction and identify treatment goals and therapeutic approaches to meet those goals.

Although this chapter presents aspects of the chest evaluation, a complete physical therapy evaluation for the patient with respiratory problems must also include musculoskeletal, neuromuscular, developmental, and other aspects of a traditional evaluation.

## History

The history provides important background information that often has a direct impact on the current condition and physical problems of the patient. General questions should include information about the individual's past medical and surgical history, particularly items that relate to the pulmonary problem for which physical therapy has been recommended. These items might include details of past illness, surgeries, allergies, and other illnesses or traumas that might interfere with physical rehabilitation. The therapist should also ask questions specific to the pulmonary system including items about smoking, cough, dyspnea, orthopnea, sputum productivity, pain, and others.

The therapist should investigate the patient's physical capacity through questions regarding activities of daily living, ambulation and its endurance in both time and distance, ability to ascend/descend stairs, employment and its physical demands, and the presence of any regular program of exercise or leisure physical activity.

Finally, the social history should be identified. Particularly important are issues of family support, current and future living arrangements and possible assistance, the use of habitual drugs such as alcohol, and any other related information that may be deemed useful in the physical rehabilitation of the patient.

### Chest examination

The chest examination is administered by almost all health care professionals providing services to the patient with pulmonary disease. Although the examination may be conducted in a similar manner by all, the objectives for the examination may differ.

The physical therapist has four objectives for the chest examination. First, the therapist identifies the pulmonary problems acknowledged by the patient. Often the problems uppermost in the patient's mind are the cardinal symptoms of pulmonary disease: dyspnea, cough sputum, and chest pain.[9] Second, the therapist assesses the coexisting signs of pulmonary disease. For example, the therapist identifies the patient's symptom of chest pain. Through further evaluation the therapist determines that the pain is localized to a small area of chest wall, exquisitely tender to palpation, associated with both a grating sound during breathing and a shallow, door-step breathing pattern, and aggravated by coughing and respiratory movements. At this point the coexisting signs suggest the presence of a rib fracture. Third, the therapist determines the need for further evaluative procedures when the results of the chest examination are unclear. In the preceding example, further evaluation by chest radiography not only may confirm the assessment by the therapist but may also localize the problem anatomically. Fourth, the therapist identifies treatment goals and formulates a plan to track progress toward realizing the identified goals. Using the previous example, the therapist identifies pain reduction and improved ventilation as treatment goals. Pain reduction could be monitored by palpation, and improvement in ventilation could be monitored through auscultation.

Despite any difference in objectives, the chest examination administered by any health care professional should be reliable and valid. For the examination to be reliable and valid, the examiner must have intact sensory apparatus and well-developed observational skills; the patient must follow directions exactly; and the examination room must be warm, well lit, and quiet.

## COMPONENTS OF THE CHEST EXAMINATION

The chest examination has four components: inspection, auscultation, palpation, and percussion.

### Inspection

The inspection phase of the chest examination documents the clinical characteristics associated with the presenting symptoms. During inspection the therapist detects problems previously unidentified. The results of the inspection determine what other components of the examination are necessary.

Part 1 of the inspection consists of evaluation of the patient's general appearance. In part 2 the therapist closely inspects the head and neck. The therapist inspects the chest in parts 3 and 4 and evaluates the breath, speech, cough, and sputum in part 5.

**1. Evaluation of general appearance.** In evaluating the general appearance of the patient, the therapist assesses the state of consciousness in reference to seven somewhat ill-defined and often overlapping stages.[24] Following are the seven stages of consciousness from highest to lowest level:

1. Alert
2. Automatic
3. Confused
4. Delirious
5. Stuporous
6. Semicomatose
7. Comatose

The alert patient is oriented, attends to the therapist's instructions, and cooperates in carrying them out. The automatic patient is irritable, shows impaired judgment, and retains instructions poorly. The confused patient is disoriented, illogical, and able to respond to simple commands only. The delirious patient is totally irrational, often agitated,

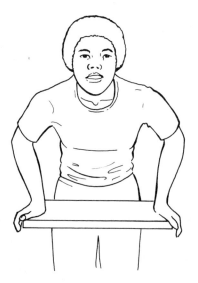

**Fig. 18-1.** The forward bent or professorial posture.

sometimes hostile, and generally uncooperative. The stuporous patient is unresponsive to the environment and often incontinent. The semicomatose patient is unconscious but rouses to painful stimuli. The comatose patient is both unconscious and unarousable.

The therapist evaluates body type as normal, obese or cachectic. In assessing posture, the therapist takes particular note of any spinal malalignment or unusual postures. In this part of the examination, the therapist documents kyphosis, scoliosis, and forward bent or professorial posture (Fig. 18-1).

During the extremity evaluation the therapist notes nicotine stains on the fingers, digital clubbing, painful swollen joints, tremor, and edema. Nicotine stains suggest a history of heavy smoking and are important in the evaluation of the unconscious patient. Clubbing of the fingers or toes is associated with cardiopulmonary and small bowel disease.[21] Painful swollen joints may indicate pseudohypertrophic pulmonary osteoarthropathy rather than the osteoarthritis or rheumatoid arthritis more familiar to physical therapists. The presence of asterixis (flapping tremor of the wrists when the arms are extended) may suggest hypercapnia.[5] Bilateral pedal edema suggests right-sided heart failure.

To complete the evaluation of the patient's appearance, the therapist notes all equipment used in managing the patient. For example, the use of a cardiac monitor, a Swan-Ganz catheter, or an intraaortic balloon pump suggests potential or actual cardiac rhythm disturbances, or hemodynamic or cardiac output problems respectively.

**2. Specific evaluation of head and neck.** In evaluating the head and neck, the therapist assesses the face to detect signs of distress, oxygen desaturation, carbon monoxide poisoning, or hypertension. The therapist completes this part of the evaluation by observing the neck veins to detect signs of elevated central venous pressure. Table 18-1 presents guidelines for the recognition and interpretation of clinical

**Table 18-1.** Guidelines for the recognition and interpretation of the clinical signs associated with evaluation of the head and neck

| Characteristic evaluated | Clinical sign | Interpretation |
|---|---|---|
| Facial expression | Alae nasi flaring | Severe distress |
| | Dilatation of pupils | |
| | Sweating | |
| | Pallor | |
| Color of mucous membranes | Blue | Severe arterial oxygen desaturation |
| Facial color | Plethoric | Possible hypertension |
| | Cherry red | Possible carbon monoxide poisoning |
| Size of neck veins | Distended above clavicle when sitting | Central venous pressure may exceed 15 cm $H_2O$ |

signs associated with the evaluation of the head and neck.

**3. Evaluation of the unmoving chest.** When examining the chest, the physical therapist evaluates the condition of the skin and the shape and symmetry of the chest. Inspecting the skin ensures documentation of incisions, scars, and trauma. Evaluating the shape of the chest permits documentation of congenital defects like pectus carinatum, pectus excavatum, or Harrison's sulcus.[8] Evaluating the chest in both the anteroposterior and transverse planes facilitates identification of the barrel-chest abnormality, a feature of obstructive lung disease. A barrel chest exists when the anteroposterior diameter is greater than or equal to twice the transverse diameter.[17]

Therapists next evaluate rib angles and intercostal spaces. Normally, rib angles measure less than 90° and attach to the vertebrae at an angle of about 45°. The spaces between them are broader posteriorly than anteriorly. Widening of the rib angles and broadening of the anterior intercostal spaces suggests hyperinflation of the lungs.

Evaluating the musculature around the chest may reveal bilateral trapezius muscle hypertrophy, which may be associated with chronic dyspnea. Finally comparing the symmetry of the hemithoraces permits detection of abnormalities like apical retraction.

**4. Evaluation of the moving chest.** Evaluation of the moving chest begins with assessment of the ventilatory rate, which normally ranges from 12 to 20 breaths per minute. This normal, or eupneic, pattern of breathing supplies one breath for every four heart beats. Tachypnea refers to a ventilatory rate faster than 20 breaths per minute. Bradypnea refers to a ventilatory rate slower than 10 breaths per minute. Fever affects ventilatory rate by adding four breaths per minute for every one Fahrenheit degree of fever.[23]

Next, the therapist evaluates the ratio of inspiratory and expiratory time, the I:E ratio. Normally, expiration is twice as long as inspiration, giving a ratio of 1:2. In obstructive lung disease reports of I:E ratios of 1:4 are common.

When evaluating the moving chest, one also evaluates the noise of breathing. Detection of *stridor*, a crowing sound during inspiration, suggests upper airway obstruction. Stridor may indicate laryngospasm. Another noise detected during inspiration is stertor. *Stertor* is a snoring noise created when the tongue falls back into the lower palate. Stertor may be heard in patients with depressed consciousness. During expiration one may also hear grunting sounds, particularly in children with pulmonary disease. Expiratory *grunting* may be a physiological attempt to prevent premature airway collapse. *Gurgling* sounds heard during both ventilatory phases are often called "death rattles."

The therapist then evaluates the pattern of breathing. This pattern reflects not only the rate but also the depth and regularity of the ventilatory cycle. Some commonly encountered ventilatory patterns appear in Table 18-2.

After evaluating the pattern and noise of breathing, the therapist evaluates the symmetry and synchrony of ventilation. The timing and relative motion of one hemithorax to the other and to the abdomen is compared during both tidal and deep breathing. One may find asymmetrical, asynchronous chest motion during deep breathing in hemiplegia. In patients with flail-chest deformity, expansion of one part of the chest may occur simultaneously with retraction of the other, a condition creating the basis for a paradoxical breathing pattern also known as *Pendelluft* ("pendulum air"). In chronic obstructive lung disease, the chest and abdomen may move as a unit, hence the term "en bloc" motion. At least one exploratory study suggests that asynchronous, or seesaw, motion between the rib cage and the abdomen has prognostic significance.[16]

Next to be evaluated are the muscles of breathing. Gross observation permits detection of deviations from the normal, diaphragmatic breathing pattern used by men and children and the costal breathing pattern used by women. Close inspection facilitates detection of accessory inspiratory or expiratory muscle activity. Moreover, careful observation of the intercostal spaces may reveal inspiratory retraction associated with decreased pulmonary compliance[7] or expiratory bulging associated with expiratory obstruction.[17]

**5. Evaluation of speech, breath, cough, and sputum.** Inspection of the chest continues with evaluation of speech, breath, cough, and sputum. Conversation with the patient facilitates recognition of various speech patterns or breath problems. Limited word patterns, frequently interrupted for breath, are known collectively as "dyspnea of phonation." Poor voice-volume control is associated with muscular incoordination and can be found in central nervous system disorders like cerebral palsy. Bad breath detected during the conversation may indicate anaerobic infection of the mouth or respiratory tract.[16]

After evaluating speech and breath, one identifies the characteristics of the cough. The therapist determines if

**Table 18-2.** Breathing patterns commonly encountered in the assessment of patients with respiratory problems

| Pattern of breathing | Description |
| --- | --- |
| Apnea | Absence of ventilation |
| Fish-mouth | Apnea with concomitant mouth opening and closing; associated with neck extension and bradypnea |
| Eupnea | Normal rate, normal depth, regular rhythm |
| Bradypnea | Slow rate, shallow or normal depth, regular rhythm; associated with drug overdose |
| Tachypnea | Fast rate, shallow depth, regular rhythm; associated with restrictive lung disease |
| Hyperpnea | Normal rate, increased depth, regular rhythm |
| Cheyne-Stokes (periodic) | Increasing then decreasing depth, period of apnea interspersed; somewhat regular rhythm; associated with critically ill patients |
| Biot's | Slow rate, shallow depth, apneic periods, irregular rhythm; associated with central nervous system disorders like meningitis |
| Apneustic | Slow rate, deep inspiration followed by apnea, irregular rhythm; associated with brainstem disorders |
| Prolonged expiration | Fast inspiration, slow and prolonged expiration yet normal rate, depth, and regular rhythm; associated with obstructive lung disease |
| Orthopnea | Difficulty breathing in postures other than erect |
| Hyperventilation | Fast rate, increased depth, regular rhythm; results in decreased arterial carbon dioxide, tension; called "Kussmaul breathing" in metabolic acidosis; also associated with central nervous system disorders like encephalitis |
| Psychogenic dyspnea | Normal rate, regular intervals of sighing; associated with anxiety |
| Dyspnea | Rapid rate, shallow depth, regular rhythm; associated with accessory muscle activity |
| Doorstop | Normal rate and rhythm; characterized by abrupt cessation of inspiration when restriction is encountered; associated with pleurisy |

cough is persistent, paroxysmal, or occasional; dry or productive; and finally notes the circumstances associated with the onset or cessation of the cough. Identifying the characteristics of the cough, as well as the conditions associated with it, enables the therapist to interpret its significance (Table 18-3). Assessing the voluntary cough permits evaluation of its constituent parts and its sequencing as well. For example, the cough of a surgical patient is often associated with a poor inspiratory effort followed by negligible abdominal muscle compression. These findings contribute to a "poor" nonproductive cough. They provide important clues for the treatment plan.

Sputum evaluation often follows cough assessment. The source of the sputum sample and the quantity of expectorate raised per day should be noted. Normally, persons are unaware of the 100 ml of mucus raised daily. Conscious awareness of any sputum production is significant. In addition to quantity, the color and consistency of any sputum raised should be evaluated. Table 18-4 presents some guidelines for evaluating sputum samples.

The inspection phase of the chest examination closes with a brief evaluation of the abdomen to detect any impedance to diaphragmatic descent such as ascites, pregnancy, or a paralytic ileus.

Further evaluation of the signs and symptoms discussed during inspection occurs during the second phase of the chest examination, auscultation.

## Auscultation

Generally, the findings of auscultation are used to identify various approaches needed for treatment. When areas of the lung are found to be poorly ventilated, the therapist might choose breathing exercises in an attempt to increase local ventilation. Similarly, specific activities for secretion removal should be considered when secretions are identified by adventitious sounds such as wheezes or crackles.

**The stethoscope.** Readiness for auscultation requires preparation of the equipment, the patient, and the therapist. The stethoscope, designed as a simple tube by Laennec, a French physician in the mid-nineteenth century, is the only equipment necessary for auscultation. The stethoscope should have binaural earpieces connected to a removal diaphragm by tubing of sufficient length to permit examination of the patient in either supine or seated position. Improper tubing—such as tubing used for Foley catheters—may not conduct sound adequately to permit valid and reliable evaluation of all sounds produced.

Two styles and several sizes of earpieces are available to ensure comfortable fit. Earpieces may be made of hard, molded plastic or soft, flexible plastic. Directing the earpieces forward into the external auditory canals ensures proper position. Occasional wiping with conventional alcohol maintains earpiece cleanliness.

Most agree that the diaphragm rather than the bell chestpiece most accurately transmits higher frequency tones such as bronchial breath sounds. The bell may be more accurate at transmitting low frequency sounds such as wheezes, also called rhonchi, heard in the more central, larger airways. Prolonged use or frequent cleaning may break the diaphragm. Although exposed x-ray film can temporarily substitute for a broken diaphragm, manufacturers suggest that sounds are less accurately assessed with this

**Table 18-3.** Guidelines for evaluating cough

| Cough characteristics | Associated features | Interpretation |
|---|---|---|
| Nonspecific | Sore throat, runny nose, runny eyes | Acute lung infection; tracheobronchitis |
| Productive | Preceded by an earlier, painful, nonproductive cough associated with an upper respiratory infection | Lobar pneumonia |
| Dry or productive | Acute bronchitis | Bronchopneumonia |
| Paroxysmal; mucoid or blood-stained sputum | Flulike syndrome | *Mycoplasma* or viral pneumonia |
| Purulent sputum | Sputum formerly mucoid | Acute exacerbation of chronic bronchitis |
| Productive for more than 3 months consecutively and for at least 2 years | | Chronic bronchitis |
| Foul-smelling, copious, layered purulent sputum | Long-standing problem | Bronchiectasis |
| Blood-tinged sputum | Month long | Tuberculosis or fungal infection |
| Persistent, nonproductive | | Pneumonitis, interstitial fibrosis, pulmonary infiltrates |
| Persistent, minimally productive | Smoking history, injected pharynx | "Smoker's cough" |
| Nonspecific, minimal hemoptysis | Long standing | Neoplastic disease |
| Nonproductive | Long standing; dyspnea | Mediastinal neoplasm |
| Brassy | | Aortic aneurysm |
| Violent cough | Sudden; onset at the same time as signs of asphyxia; localized wheezing | Aspiration of foreign body |
| Frothy sputum | Worsens in supine position; dyspnea | Heart failure, pulmonary edema |
| Hemoptysis | Sudden; simultaneous dyspnea; pleural effusion | Pulmonary infarct |

Adapted from Fishman AP: *Pulmonary diseases and disorders*, vol. 1, New York, 1980, McGraw-Hill Book Co.

substitute and strongly urge their customers to order appropriate replacements. Stethoscopes equipped with both diaphragm and bell have a valve that may be turned toward either the bell or diaphragm to listen.

Preparing the patient for auscultation involves teaching the importance of deep breathing through the mouth and of reporting dizziness or undue fatigue during the deep breathing.

**Nomenclature.**[1] *Breath sounds* are generated by the vibration and turbulence of airflow into and out of the airways and lung tissue during inspiration and expiration. *Normal breath sounds* can be divided into four specific sounds—tracheal, bronchial, bronchovesicular, and vesicular. Each of the four is considered normal when heard over a specific region of the thorax. However, if heard in a region not normally expected, each is considered abnormal. *Tracheal breath sounds* are high-pitched, loud, and sound like wind blowing through a pipe. There is a distinct absence of sound during the transition from inspiration to expiration. This sound is auscultated normally over the trachea alone, and is not particularly important to the physical therapist. *Bronchial breath sounds* are heard normally adjacent to the sternum around the areas of the major airways, and are similar to tracheal sounds with the exception that bronchial sounds are not as loud. When heard in another area of the lungs, bronchial sounds usually indicate consolidated lung

**Table 18-4.** Guidelines for evaluation of sputum samples

| | |
|---|---|
| Source | Upper airway |
| | Lower airway |
| Quantity | Milliliters or cupsful per day |
| Color | Red: Blood |
| | Rust: Pneumonia |
| | Purple: Neoplasm |
| | Yellow: Infected |
| | Green: Pus |
| | Pink: Pulmonary edema |
| | Flecked: Carbon particles |
| Consistency | Thin, watery |
| | Gritty |
| | Thick, mucous |
| | Layered |

tissue, tissue that is fluid-filled, compressed, or airless due to atelectasis. *Vesicular breath sounds* are low-pitched, muffled, and have been described as a rustling sound similar to a gentle breeze through the leaves of a tree. Inspiration with vesicular sounds is louder, longer, and higher in pitch than expiration which is heard for only a brief period. Vesicular breath sounds are considered normal over all areas of the lung except areas noted for tracheal and bronchial sounds. Vesicular breaths can be abnormal by their diminution or absence. These abnormal situations are likely to occur when underlying lung tissue is poorly ventilated, or when extensive hyperaeration reduces the transmission of vesicular sounds from the lung tissue. *Bronchovesicular sounds,* as one might expect, combine characteristics of bronchial and vesicular sounds. Inspiration and expiration are heard for similar times, at the same pitch, and with a slight break between the two phases. This sound is normal when heard adjacent to the sternum at the costosternal border, at the angle of Louis, and between the scapulae from about T3 through T6.

*Voice sounds* reflect the ability of lung tissue to transmit spoken or whispered sound to the thoracic wall to be heard through the stethoscope. All voice-generated sounds, whether whispered or spoken, should be evaluated as decreased, normal, or increased. Bronchophony, egophony, and pectoriloquy are voice sounds. *Bronchophony* characterizes a voice sound in which the intensity and clarity of a repeated sound, usually "ninety-nine," will be heard distinctly through the stethoscope. This finding indicates that underlying lung tissue is relatively airless and therefore transmits the sound more distinctly than through air-filled lung. *Egophony* is similar to bronchophony in that egophony is an increase in intensity and clarity of spoken sound. Egophony further includes a change in the character of the sound, typically from a spoken "EEEE" to an auscultated "AAAA." This "EE to AA change" is also related to sound transmission through airless lung. The final speech sound, *whispered pectoriloquy,* describes how a whispered sound, usually "one-two-three," responds with consolidated lung tissue. The whispered sound is not heard through normal air-filled lung tissue, but is heard distinctly through the stethoscope with airless or consolidated lung.

There are two categories of commonly heard adventitious sounds: crackles, previously called rales (French *râles*), and wheezes, previously called rhonchi. Crackles are defined as nonmusical sounds whose further subclassification serves no useful purpose. Inspiratory crackles or rales may be heard throughout inspiration or only at its termination. Inspiratory crackles are common at the bases of the lungs in an erect subject. Crackles may represent the sudden opening of airways previously closed by gravity and therefore may be a sign of abnormal lung deflation.[14,22] Expiratory crackles or rales are rhythmical and nonrhythmical. Rhythmical crackles may indicate the reopening of previously closed airways. Nonrhythmical sounds are generally low pitched and occur throughout the ventilatory cycle. They may represent fluid in the large airways.

Wheezes, or rhonchi, are both continuous and musical. Wheezes are probably produced by air flowing at high velocities through apposed airways. Their pitch varies directly with the velocity of airflow. Wheezes may be monophonic or polyphonic and may be heard in either inspiration or expiration. Inspiratory wheezes unaccompanied by expiratory wheezes are usually monophonic. These rarely occurring wheezes suggest that the airway is rigid. Inspiratory wheezes may be caused by stenosis produced, for example, by bronchospasm or foreign-body impaction. End-inspiratory wheezes occur when the inspiratory traction forces, initially insufficient to allow some airways to open, are suddenly overcome. This results in high-velocity airflow across the still apposed airway lumens producing a musical sound of short duration. Expiratory wheezes are encountered more frequently. They tend to be low pitched and polyphonic and may reflect unstable airways that have collapsed. Expiratory wheezes are associated with diffuse airway obstruction. Monophonic expiratory wheezes occur when only one airway reaches the point of collapse. The bagpipe sign describes a persistent monophonic wheeze occurring at end expiration.[7]

Other adventitious sounds detected during auscultation include rubs and crunches. Rubs are coarse, grating, leathery sounds occurring with either the ventilatory or the cardiac cycle. Pleural rubs are heard concurrently with the ventilatory cycle, whereas pericardial rubs are heard during the cardiac cycle. Rubs generally indicate inflammation. Crunches are crackling sounds heard over the pericardium during systole. Detection of such crunches suggests the presence of air in the mediastinum, called mediastinal emphysema.

**The examination.** With the above descriptions in mind, the therapist compares the quality, intensity, pitch, and distribution of the breath and voice sounds of homologous bronchopulmonary segments of the anterior, lateral, and posterior aspects of the chest. Fig. 18-2 presents one method of sequential auscultation of the chest. Following are the steps for this method of auscultation:

1. Instruct the patient to sit forward (where sitting is not possible, place patient in side-lying position).
2. Expose the anterior chest sufficiently to permit evaluation of the upper and middle lung zones.
3. Remind patient to breathe in and out through the mouth.
4. Evaluate at least one breath in each pulmonary segment, comparing the intensity, pitch, and quality of the breath sounds heard between the right and left lungs.
5. Proceed craniocaudally in a systematic manner.
6. At the completion of the examination of the anterior chest, readjust draping to cover the anterior chest and expose the back (Fig. 18-2, *B*).
7. Proceed as in step 1. Close gown. Indicate you are finished, and instruct the patient to relax.

**Interpretation of the examination.** On completing auscultation, the therapist must record and interpret the findings in a nomenclature acceptable to the institution.

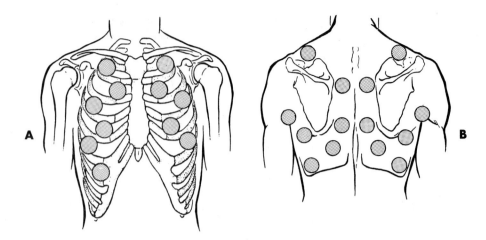

**Fig. 18-2.** One method of auscultating the chest. **A,** The chest. **B,** The back. (From Buckingham EB: *A primer of clinical diagnosis,* ed 2, New York, 1979, Harper & Row, Publishers, Inc.)

Table 18-5 presents some guidelines for the documentation and interpretation of breath sounds.

Normal breath and voice sounds in all bronchopulmonary segments suggest a normal examination. If inspection was also normal and the patient denied all pulmonary symptoms, one considers the chest examination normal and further evaluation is deferred. If breath sounds are abnormal or if adventitious sounds are present, the examination findings are abnormal but at this point inconclusive. Generally, decreased or absent breath sounds or inspiratory crackles suggest reduced ventilation. Crackles during both ventilatory cycles suggest impaired secretion clearance. Monophonic, biphasic wheezing suggests stenosis or bronchial smooth-muscle spasm. Polyphonic wheezing suggests diffuse airway obstruction. The absence of crackles and wheezes does not, however, ensure the absence of acute disease because patients with chronic obstructive lung disease may have hyperinflation so severe that adventitious sounds cannot be heard through the excessive air in the lungs.

In summary, auscultation either confirms the findings of inspection or identifies for the physical therapist areas of impaired ventilation or impaired secretion clearance. In addition, auscultation and changes in the findings provide important feedback about the effectiveness of a treatment program in resolving pulmonary problems.

### Palpation

In general, palpation refines the information gained previously. It further evaluates any thoracoabdominal asymmetry or asynchrony detected during inspection through evaluation of the mediastinum and evaluation of chest motion. It detects signs of increased work of breathing by palpation of the scalene muscles and evaluation of the diaphragm. It provides information concerning the amount of air in the chest through evaluation of fremitus, and finally it further describes chest pain through palpation of the painful area.

**Evaluation of the mediastinum.** Fig. 18-3 presents one method of evaluating the mediastinal position by tracheal location. Following are the steps for this method of evaluating the mediastinum:

1. Place the patient in the sitting or recumbent position.
2. Flex the neck slightly to relax the sternocleidomastoid muscles.
3. Position the chin in the midline.
4. Place the top of the index finger in the suprasternal notch medial to the left sternoclavicular joint.
5. Push inward toward the cervical spine.
6. Repeat from step 4 to evaluate along the right sternoclavicular joint.

Another equally acceptable method consists of either palpating or auscultating the point of maximal impulse of the heart. This point is normally located in the fifth intercostal space in the midclavicular line (5 ICS MCL).

Shifts in the mediastinum occur when intrathoracic pressure or lung volume is disproportionate between the hemithoraces. The mediastinum shifts toward the affected side when lung volume is unilaterally decreased. The mediastinum shifts toward the unaffected side or contralaterally when pressure or volume is unilaterally high. Mediastinal shifts to the right because of pressure exerted by the ascending aorta may be seen in the elderly. Table 18-6 provides some examples of problems that result in mediastinal shifts. This evaluation informs the examiner of the consequences of any disproportionate expansion detected during inspection.

**Evaluation of chest motion.** Palpation also permits comparative evaluation of upper, middle, and lower lobe expansion during quiet and deep breathing. In each case the

**Table 18-5.** Guidelines for the documentation and interpretation of auscultated sounds

| Type of sound | Nomenclature | Interpretation |
|---|---|---|
| Breath sound | Normal | Normal, air-filled lung |
| | Decreased | Hyperinflation in chronic obstructive pulmonary disease |
| | | Hypoinflation in acute lung disease, e.g., atelectasis, pneuomothorax, pleural effusion |
| | Absent | Pleural effusion |
| | | Pneumothorax |
| | | Severe hyperinflation |
| | | Obesity |
| | Bronchial | Consolidation |
| | | Atelectasis with adjacent patent airway |
| | Crackles | Secretions, if biphasic |
| | | Deflation, if monophasic |
| | Wheezes | Diffuse airway obstruction, if polyphonic |
| | | Localized stenosis, if monophobic |
| Voice sound | Normal | Normal, air-filled lung |
| | Decreased | Atelectasis |
| | | Pleural effusion |
| | | Pneumothorax |
| | Increased | Consolidation |
| | | Pulmonary fibrosis |
| Extrapulmonary adventitious sounds | Crunch | Mediastinal emphysema |
| | Pleural rub | Pleural inflammation or reaction |
| | Pericardial rub | Pericardial inflammation |

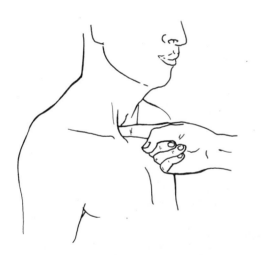

**Fig. 18-3.** Palpation of the mediastinum. (From Cherniack RM and others: *Respiration in health and disease,* ed 2, Philadelphia, 1972, WB Saunders Co.)

**Table 18-6.** Conditions associated with shifts of the mediastinum

| | Direction of shift | |
|---|---|---|
| Condition | Ipsilateral | Contralateral |
| Atelectasis | + | |
| Lobectomy | + | |
| Pneumonectomy | + | |
| Pleural effusion | | + |
| Pneumothorax | | + |
| Herniation of abdominal viscera | | + |

therapist compares the timing and extent of movement of each hand. Lobar motion is considered normal when each hand moves the same amount at the same time. One method of evaluating chest motion appears in Figs. 18-4 to 18-6.[9]

Following are the steps for palpating the lobes:

**Upper lobe motion**

1. Face the patient.
2. Instruct the patient to turn his or her face away from yours.
3. Drape to expose the upper lobes of both lungs.
4. Place the palms of the hand firmly over the anterior aspect of the chest from the fourth rib cranially.
5. Hook the fingers over the upper trapezii.
6. Stretch the skin downward until the palms are in the intraclavicular areas.
7. Draw skin medially until the tips of the extended thumbs meet in the midline.
8. Relax the elbows and shoulders.
9. Instruct the patient to inspire.
10. Allow your hands to reflect the movement of the lobe of the lung underneath.

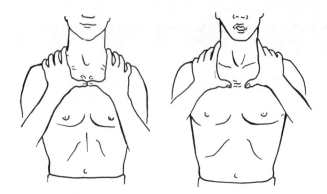

**Fig. 18-4.** Palpation of upper lobe motion. (From Cherniack RM and others: *Respiration in health and disease,* ed 2, Philadelphia, 1972, WB Saunders Co.)

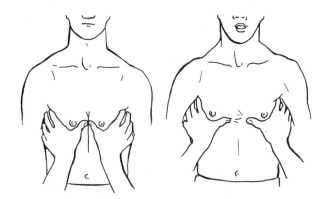

**Fig. 18-5.** Palpation of right middle and left lingula lobe motion. (From Cherniack RM and others: *Respiration in health and disease,* ed 2, Philadelphia, 1972, WB Saunders Co.)

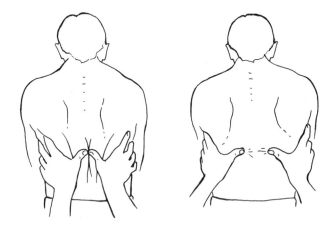

**Fig. 18-6.** Palpation of lower lobe motion. (From Cherniack RM and others: *Respiration in health and disease,* ed 2, Philadelphia, 1972, WB Saunders Co.)

**Right middle and left lingula lobe motion**

1. Face the patient.
2. Instruct the patient to turn his or her face away from yours.

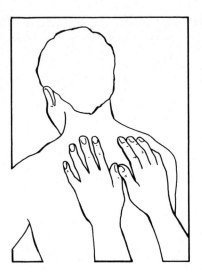

**Fig. 18-7.** Palpation of tactile fremitus.

3. Drape to expose the right middle lobe of left lingula with males (may permit light clothing on females).
4. Hook fingers over posterior axillary folds.
5. Place palms firmly against chest wall.
6. Draw skin medially until the tips of the extended thumbs meet in the midline.
7. Relax the elbows and shoulders.
8. Instruct the patient to inspire.
9. Allow your hands to reflect the movement of the lobe of the lung underneath.

**Lower lobe motion**

1. Position patient with his or her back toward you.
2. Drape to expose back.
3. Hook fingers around the anterior axillary fold.
4. Draw skin medially until extended thumbs meet at the midline.
5. Relax the elbows and shoulders.
6. Instruct the patient to inspire.
7. Allow your hands to reflect the movement of the lobe of the lung underneath.

This phase of palpation allows the therapist to localize any disproportionate expansion observed during inspection. For example, if inspection reveals asymmetrical chest expansion, palpation may not only localize the problem to the right upper lobe but also uncover a resultant ipsilateral shift of the mediastinum. Together these signs suggest that the problem is either a loss of right upper lobe lung volume or a volumetric gain in the left upper lobe.

**Evaluation of fremitus.** Fremitus is the vibration produced by either the voice or secretions and transmitted to the chest wall, where it is detected by the hand, that is, tactile fremitus. Fig. 18-7 presents one method of evaluating fremitus.

Following are the steps for performing this method of palpating the fremitus:

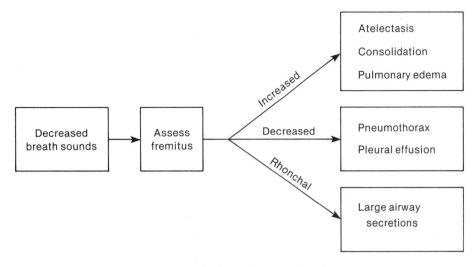

**Fig. 18-8.** Role of fremitus assessment in further defining the sign of decreased breath sounds. In the example, if breath sounds are decreased and fremitus is increased, alveolar airlessness is most likely caused by atelectasis, consolidation, or pulmonary edema. If both breath sounds and fremitus are decreased, pneumothorax or pleural effusion may be most likely. Rhonchal fremitus suggests large airway secretions.

1. Place palms lightly in symmetrical areas of the chest, or alternatively place the hypothenar eminence of each hand over symmetrical areas of the chest.
2. Instruct the patient to say "99."
3. Compare the intensity of the vibrations detected by each hand in the apical, anterior, lateral, and posterior areas of the chest.

Other methods for evaluation of fremitus are by substitution of the hypothenar eminences, or fingertips for the palms.[6]

The therapist evaluates fremitus by comparing the intensity of the vibrations detected by each hand during quiet breathing and speech. A normal evaluation occurs when equal and moderate vibrations are perceived during speech. Fremitus is abnormal when it is increased, decreased, or present during quiet breathing. Increased fremitus suggests a loss or decrease in ventilation. Decreased fremitus suggests a gain in the amount of air within the chest. "Rhonchal fremitus" is the term describing vibrations detected during quiet breathing.

Evaluation of fremitus permits the therapist to locate secretion problems or to define further the decreased breath sounds found during auscultation (Fig. 18-8).

**Evaluation of scalene muscles.** Palpation also permits specific evaluation of muscle activity identified grossly during inspection. One method of detecting activity of the scalene muscles is presented in Fig. 18-9.

Following are the steps for performing this method of palpating scalene muscle activity:

1. Position the patient with his or her back toward you.
2. Place thumbs over spinous process so that fingers reach around to the anterolateral aspects of the neck.

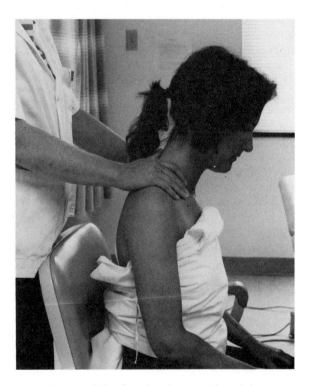

**Fig. 18-9.** Palpation of scalene muscle activity.

3. Evaluate the area during at least two resting respiratory cycles to detect activity of the scalenes.

Normally, the scalene muscles are inactive during quiet breathing. Palpation of scalene muscle activity indicates that the tertiary muscles of inspiration are functioning and therefore the work of breathing is increased.

**Evaluation of chest pain.** Palpation also permits assessment of chest pain. The results of this assessment determine

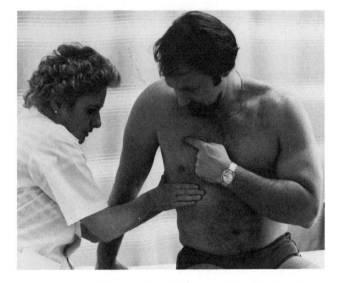

**Fig. 18-10.** Palpation of painful areas of the chest wall.

**Table 18-7.** Guidelines for identifying the probable source of chest pain

| Symptom characteristics | Effective stimulus | Anatomical source |
|---|---|---|
| Sharp<br>Superficial<br>Burning<br>Precisely localized | Fine touch<br>Pinprick<br>Heat<br>Cold | Skin |
| Dull or sharp<br>Intermediate depth<br>Aching<br>Generally localized | Movement<br>Deep pressure | Chest wall |
| Dull<br>Deep<br>Aching<br>Diffuse, vaguely<br>localized | Ischemia<br>Distention<br>Muscle spasm | Thoracic viscera |

Adapted from Edmeads J and Billings RF: Neurological and psychological aspects of chest pain. In Levene DL, editor: *Chest pain: an integrated diagnostic approach*, Philadelphia, 1977, Lea & Febiger.

**Table 18-8.** The segmental innervation of the chest and abdomen

| Cord segments | Structure |
|---|---|
| T1-T4 | Mediastinal contents; heart, aorta, pulmonary vessels |
| T3-T8 | Descending aorta |
| T4-T8 | Esophagus |
| T3-T5 | Trachea and bronchi |
| T7-T9 | Upper abdominal viscera |
| C5-T1 | Chest wall; apical parietal pleura |
| T2-T8 | Remainder parietal; upper pericardial pleura |
| T6-T8 | Peripheral diaphragm |
| C3-C5 | Central diaphragm; lower pericardial pleura |
| T2-T10 | Intercostal muscles; ribs |
| C5-T1 | Pectoral muscles |
| C3-C4 | Skin overlying shoulders |
| T1-T2 | Upper arms, inner surface |
| T3-T8 | Skin on chest wall |

Adapted from Edmeads J and Billings RF: Neurological and psychological aspects of chest pain. In Levene DL, editor: *Chest pain: an integrated diagnostic approach*, Philadelphia, 1977, Lea & Febiger.

the safety of continuing further evaluation or treatment. In addition, palpation facilitates identification of those characteristics associated with the pain for more complete and effective communication with the attending physician. One method of evaluating chest pain is illustrated in Fig. 18-10.

Following are the steps for performing this method of palpating the chest wall:

1. Request the patient to describe the type, extent, distribution, characteristics of onset, and characteristics of diminution of the pain.
2. Request the patient to point to the painful area. Expose the area and drape accordingly.
3. Starting distant from the painful area identified, palpate the ribs and intercostal spaces by pressing downward firmly.
4. Determine the effect of deep breathing and coughing on the pain.
5. Determine the effect of breath holding and ipsilateral arm motion on the pain.

Palpation provides information regarding the source of chest pain, which may be caused by musculoskeletal problems, coronary artery disease, malignancy, cervical disk or nerve root disease, thoracic outlet syndrome, shoulder-hand syndrome, herpes zoster, or pulmonary embolism.[20] Identifying the probable anatomical source of chest pain requires associating the type of pain and its stimulus (Table 18-7).

Matching the sensory distribution of the pain to the appropriate anatomical structure may also help the therapist identify the anatomical source of the pain. Table 18-8 presents the segmental innervation of the structures of the chest and abdomen. Fig. 18-11 illustrates the distribution of the cervical and thoracic dermatomes.

Exquisite localized tenderness accompanied by grating during the ventilatory cycle characterizes the pain associated with rib fracture. Subluxation of the costal cartilage generates local tenderness over the intercostal space and suggests intercostal fibrositis. Pleuritic pain is sharp, usually localized, and aggravated by breathing and coughing. Pleuritic pain is often associated with bacterial pneumonia, but when accompanied by hemoptysis and restricted activity, it may indicate pulmonary embolism.

Chest wall pain resulting from musculoskeletal problems is common. This pain is usually nonsegmental, localized to the anterior chest and aggravated by deep breathing. Chest wall pain is usually unrelated to exercise and differs from

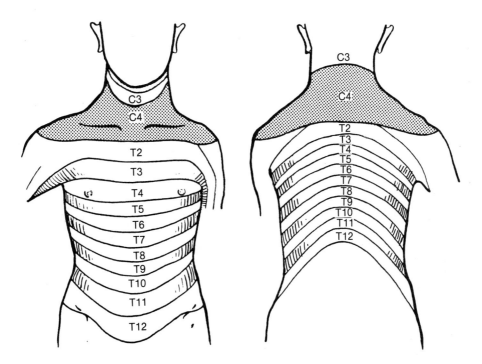

**Fig. 18-11.** Cervical and thoracic dermatomes. (From Cherniack RM and others: *Respiration in health and disease,* ed 2, Philadelphia, 1972, WB Saunders Co.)

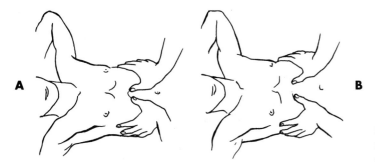

**Fig. 18-12.** Palpation of diaphragmatic motion. **A,** At rest. **B,** At the end of a normal inspiration. (From Cherniack RM and others: *Respiration in health and disease,* ed 2, Philadelphia, 1972, WB Saunders Co.)

angina pectoris. Angina is a viselike, crushing, midline pain that radiates to the jaw and arm and is aggravated by an exercise. Chest pain from an undiagnosed tumor is commonly associated with other pulmonary symptoms such as cough and hemoptysis. Disk and nerve root pain follow dermatome distribution.

**Evaluation of diaphragmatic movement.** During the last phase of palpation, movement of the diaphragm is evaluated as normal or abnormal. Fig. 18-12 presents one method of evaluating diaphragmatic motion.

Following are the steps for performing this method of palpating diaphragmatic motion:

1. Direct the patient to assume the supine, flat position.
2. Drape to expose the costal margins of the anterior chest.

3. Stand beside the patient.
4. Place both hands lightly over the anterior chest wall with thumbs over costal margins so that the tips almost meet at the xiphoid.
5. Instruct the patient to take a deep breath.
6. Allow thumbs to move with the breath.

Motion of the normal diaphragm results in equal, upward motion of each costal margin. Inward motion of the costal margins during inspiration has been associated with a poor prognosis for the survival of patients with chronic obstructive lung disease.[15]

### Percussion

Percussion is the fourth and final part of the chest examination. It enables the therapist to associate any symptoms and signs previously uncovered with changes in lung density. In addition, it enables the therapist to establish the borders of abnormally dense lung areas and normally occurring organs. Finally, percussion allows the therapist to evaluate the extent of diaphragmatic motion.

**Evaluation of lung density.** In assessment of lung density any of three sounds or notes may be produced.[1] A normal note is produced when resonant lung of normal density is percussed. A dull note is soft, brief, high pitched, and thudlike. It can be simulated by percussion of the liver or the thigh. A tympanic note, on the other hand, is loud, lengthy, low pitched, and hollow. It can be simulated by percussion of the empty stomach.

Normally dense, resonant lung can be found from the clavicle to the sixth rib anteriorly, the eighth rib laterally, and the tenth rib posteriorly (Fig. 18-13).

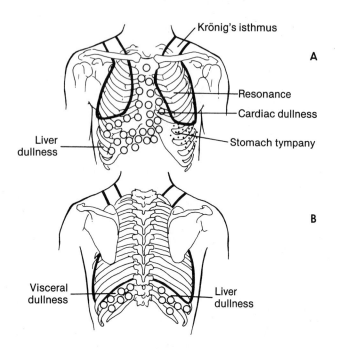

**Fig. 18-13.** Normal resonance pattern of the chest. **A,** Anteriorly. **B,** Posteriorly. *Circles,* Areas of dullness; *small dots,* tympanic areas.

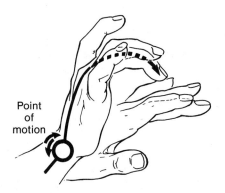

**Fig. 18-14.** The correct hand position for percussion. (From Buckingham EB: *A primer of clinical diagnosis,* ed 2, New York, 1979, Harper & Row, Publishers, Inc.)

Fig. 18-14 presents the correct hand position for percussion. One technique for examining lung density is presented in Fig. 18-15.

Following are the steps for performing this technique for evaluating lung density:

1. Position the patient supine for evaluation of the density of the upper and middle lobes and sitting for evaluation of the lower lobes.
2. Expose the suspicious area and drape accordingly.
3. Lightly place the terminal phalanx of the middle finger of the nondominant hand between the ribs of the area to be evaluated.
4. Lift the rest of the middle finger, as well as the others, from the surface of the chest.

5. Using the wrist as the fulcrum, strike the middle finger of the nondominant hand in rapid succession, recoiling instantly after each blow.
6. Percuss the unaffected lungs before percussing the affected lung wherever possible, proceeding from apex to base, and right to left in 2-inch intervals.
7. Compare the pitch of the sound produced during percussion, and its intensity and duration.
8. Notice the limits of the abnormality both vertically and horizontally.

In a normal evaluation the resonance is similar across homologous lung segments. Moreover, to be normal, the resonance must extend throughout the anatomical limits of the lungs.

Abscesses, tumors, cysts, and areas of atelectasis and pneumonia produce changes in lung resonance. To be detected in this manner, however, the lesion must be at least 2 or 3 cm in diameter and no more than 5 cm in depth.[23]

Lung borders are affected by volume changes in either the abdomen or lungs. Abnormally high lung bases are associated with increased abdominal volume as is seen in pregnancy and ascites. Abnormally low lung bases are associated with increased lung volumes as is typical in chronic obstructive lung disease.

**Evaluation of diaphragmatic excursion.** Percussion also quantifies diaphragmatic motion. Evaluating diaphragmatic excursion requires that the patient be seated. After exposing the posterior thorax, the therapist percusses the rib interspaces from apex to base. When dullness is encountered, the therapist stops percussing and asks the patient to exhale fully. The examiner uses percussion to track the motion of the diaphragms, marking the limit of their ascent. The patient then inspires fully. Once again, diaphragmatic motion is tracked by percussion and the limit of descent is identified. Diaphragmatic excursion is the distance traveled between maximal inspiration and maximal expiration.

Diaphragmatic excursion is normally from 3 to 5 cm and is commonly decreased bilaterally in chronic obstructive lung disease.

## LABORATORY EVALUATION

In addition to the chest examination, the complete clinical evaluation of a pulmonary patient requires interpretation of arterial blood gases, pulmonary function tests, chest radiographs, exercise tests, and bacteriological tests. Interpretation of arterial blood gases permits assessment of oxygenation, ventilation, and acid-base balance.

### Arterial blood gases

**Assessment of oxygenation.** Oxygenation is adequate when the partial pressure of oxygen in the arterial blood, $Pao_2$, is sufficiently intense to bind most of the hemoglobin with a net quantity of oxygen fast enough to meet tissue needs.[12] Aberrations in $Pao_2$ reflect abnormal oxygenation, also known as "hypoxemia." The therapist may suspect

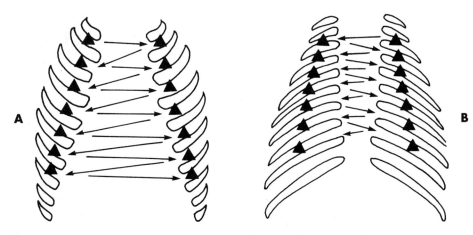

**Fig. 18-15.** Technique for evaluating lung density. **A,** Anteriorly. **B,** Posteriorly.

**Table 18-9.** Examples of estimated arterial oxygen tensions in persons over 60 years of age

| Age (years) | Pao$_2$ (mm Hg) |
|---|---|
| 60 | 80 |
| 65 | 75 |
| 70 | 70 |
| 75 | 65 |
| 80 | 60 |
| 85 | 55 |

Adapted from Shapiro BA and others: *Clinical interpretation of blood gases*, Chicago, 1977, Year Book Medical Publishers.

**Table 18-10.** Criteria for interpreting the severity of acute hypoxemia

| Pao$_2$ (mm Hg) | Interpretation |
|---|---|
| 60-80 | Mild hypoxemia |
| 40-60 | Moderate hypoxemia |
| <40 | Severe hypoxemia |

Adapted from Shapiro BA and others: *Clinical interpretation of blood gases*, Chicago, 1977, Year Book Medical Publishers.

hypoxemia when inspection reveals any of the following clinical signs: pallor, cyanosis, skin coolness, or unexplained behavioral changes. A blood gas report of a low Pao$_2$, that is less than 80 mm Hg (the lower limit of normal), may confirm clinical suspicions. In persons over 60 years of age, however, lower oxygen tensions are acceptable if they do not exceed an additional 1 mm decrement in oxygen tension for each year of age over 60.[25] Examples of some estimated arterial oxygen tensions in persons over 60 years of age are in Table 18-9. Criteria for interpreting the magnitude of acute hypoxemia are presented in Table 18-10.

Regardless of its severity, arterial hypoxemia suggests abnormal cardiopulmonary function. Hypoxemia is often the earliest sign of atelectasis, embolism, or infiltrate. In response to hypoxemia, the body increases total ventilation. However, this increase in total ventilation is minimally effective at improving oxygenation because it may cause a simultaneous increase in oxygen consumption because of increased energy cost of breathing at higher rates. Persistent arterial hypoxemia may also increase cardiac output, though this response may be more common in stagnant and anemic hypoxemia than in hypoxic hypoxemia.[12]

The most effective method of correcting arterial hypoxemia is oxygen therapy. Oxygen therapy is adequate when

normal arterial oxygen tensions are approximated. Arterial hypoxemia is overcorrected when the arterial oxygen tension exceeds the upper limit of the normal range, 100 mm Hg.

**Assessment of ventilation.** Assessment of ventilation requires evaluation of alveolar ventilation, which is reflected by the arterial carbon dioxide tension, Paco$_2$. Under normal or steady-state conditions, the relationship between carbon dioxide production and elimination results in Paco$_2$ of 35 to 45 mm Hg. When the lungs eliminate carbon dioxide faster than the body produces it, the arterial carbon dioxide tension decreases. Conversely, when carbon dioxide production exceeds elimination, Paco$_2$ increases.

Arterial pH is inversely related to the Paco$_2$, and acute changes in Paco$_2$ have a predictable impact on pH. Generally, in acute situations every 10 mm Hg decrease in Paco$_2$ increases pH by approximately 0.10 units. Conversely, a 20 mm Hg increase in Paco$_2$ decreases arterial pH by approximately 0.10 units.[25]

The relationship between minute ventilation and alveolar ventilation additionally allows the therapist to predict how changes in the rate and depth of breathing, that is, the minute ventilation, will affect the Paco$_2$ and therefore the pH. Table 18-11 illustrates these relationships.

Ventilation is abnormal when the Paco$_2$ falls out of the normal range. Hyperventilation exists when the Paco$_2$ is not only less than normal, but also less than the clinically

**Table 18-11.** Approximate relationship among minute ventilation ($Pa_{CO_2}$), and acid base status (pH)

| Minute ventilation | $Pa_{CO_2}$ (mm Hg) | pH |
|---|---|---|
| Normal | 40 | 7.40 |
| Twice normal | 30 | 7.50 |
| Four times normal | 20 | 7.60 |

Adapted from Shapiro BA and others: *Clinical interpretation of blood gases*, Chicago, 1977, Year Book Medical Publishers.

**Table 18-12.** Conditions associated with primary acid-base disturbances of metabolic origin

| Acid-base disturbances | Clinical problem |
|---|---|
| Metabolic acidosis | Renal failure |
| | Ketoacidosis |
| | Lactic acidosis |
| | Shock |
| | Severe diarrhea |
| | Dehydration |
| | Poisoning: alcohol, paraldehyde |
| | Acetazolamide therapy (Diamox) |
| | Ammonium chloride |
| | Pancreatic drainage |
| | Ureterosigmoidostomy |
| Metabolic alkalosis | Hypokalemia |
| | Hypochloremia |
| | Vomiting |
| | Nasogastric suction |
| | Steroid therapy with Cushing's disease |
| | Aldosteronism |

tolerable lower limit of 30 mm Hg.[25] This condition is commonly called "respiratory alkalosis." If accompanied by a simultaneous increase in pH, it is called "respiratory alkalemia." Pain and pulmonary emboli often induce respiratory alkalemia. Hypoventilation exists when the $Pa_{CO_2}$ exceeds not only the upper range of normal but also the clinically tolerable limit of 50 mm Hg.[25] This condition is called "respiratory acidosis" and implies acute ventilatory failure. When pH is simultaneously decreased, it is called "respiratory acidemia." Acute airway obstruction may induce acute alveolar hypoventilation.

When hypoventilation or hyperventilation is not associated with acute changes in pH, that nonassociation may indicate that the condition is chronic. In chronic alveolar hyperventilation, for example, the pH falls within the range of normal. The reason is that the kidneys have had time to compensate for the increased elimination of carbon dioxide by increasing their elimination of bicarbonate, $HCO_3$. Similarly, in chronic alveolar hypoventilation the normality of the pH is obtained by counteraction of the acid gain from ventilatory failure with reduced bicarbonate excretion by the kidneys. Chronic alveolar hypoventilation is most usually associated with chronic obstructive pulmonary disease.

**Assessment of acid-base balance.** A complete interpretation of arterial blood gases requires evaluation of the acid-base status in addition to evaluation of the respiratory status. The preceding section described the relationship between minute ventilation, $Pa_{CO_2}$, and pH. This section describes the additional impact of metabolic factors on pH.

Metabolic factors directly influence the pH because of the action of the kidneys on the serum bicarbonate. As the serum bicarbonate increases or decreases from its normal range of 22 to 28 milliequivalents per liter (mEq/L), the pH becomes more alkalotic or acidotic respectively. When the bicarbonate concentrate is less than 22 mEq/L, the pH is less than 7.30, and the alveolar ventilation ($Pa_{CO_2}$) is normal, the problem is uncompensated, or primary, metabolic acidemia.

When the serum bicarbonate concentration is more than 28 mEq/L, the pH is greater than 7.50, and the alveolar ventilation is normal, the acid-base problem is uncompensated or primary metabolic alkalemia. Table 18-12 presents some conditions known to be associated with primary acid-base disturbances.

Because the lungs compensate for metabolic disturbances, changes in alveolar ventilation often occur simultaneously with acid-base problems. For example, the lungs will hyperventilate to assist in correcting metabolic acidemia or hypoventilate to assist in correcting metabolic alkalemia.

Further analysis of blood gas aberrations is beyond the scope of this chapter. However, a description of the role of blood gases in cardiopulmonary physical therapy is essential. Clinicians use arterial blood gases to determine the need for physical therapy intervention, to generate appropriate therapeutic regimens, and to monitor treatment effectiveness. For example, postoperative atelectasis and mild hypoxemia, despite routine nursing care, warrant cardiopulmonary physical therapy. The effectiveness of this and any other therapy may be reflected by changes in arterial oxygen tension.

### Pulse oximetry

Pulse oximetry is a recently developed technology that permits noninvasive determination of oxyhemoglobin saturation of arterial blood (%$SpO_2$). It is a rapid, noninvasive, and inexpensive procedure. The technique has become prevalent in critical care for adult and pediatric use, in general hospital care, during exercise testing and training sessions, and for research. A physical therapist will have regular occasion to use the information provided by pulse oximetry during many different types of exercise testing and training sessions in addition to the above scenarios.

Pulse oximetry determines arterial oxygen saturation through a probe that passes two different wavelengths of light through a pulsating arterial bed. Probes are available to fit the finger, ear, foot, and nose. Each wavelength is subject to variable absorption due to differing levels of oxyhemoglobin and deoxyhemoglobin in the arterial pulsation. A

**Table 18-13.** The relationship between predicted ventilatory function and respiratory impairment

| Percent impairment | Percent predicted ventilatory function |
|---|---|
| 0 | >85 |
| 20-30 | 70-85 |
| 40-50 | 55-70 |
| 60-90 | 55 |

Adapted from American Medical Association, Committee on Rating of Mental and Physical Impairment: Guidelines to evaluation of permanent impairment: the respiratory system, *JAMA* 194:919, 1965.

**Table 18-14.** Conditions associated with abnormal ventilatory regulation

Chronic hypoxemia
Encephalitis
Bulbar palsy
Cerebrovascular disease
Parkinsons' disease
Anemia
Tabes dorsalis
Hypothyroidism
Carotid body endarterectomy
Familial dysautonomia
Idiopathic hypoventilation
Obesity
After adult respiratory distress syndrome
Athleticism
Narcotic addiction
Chronic obstructive pulmonary disease

Adapted from Wanner A: Interpretation of pulmonary function tests. In Sackner MA, editor: *Diagnostic techniques in pulmonary disease*, Part 1, New York, 1980, Marcel Dekker, Inc.

photodetector, which measures the wavelengths after they pass through the vascular bed, produces an electrical signal that estimates the oxyhemoglobin saturation of arterial blood ($\%SpO_2$). A recent review demonstrated variable accuracy of the devices. In general, the accuracy is greater at oxyhemoglobin saturations greater than 80%.[19]

Difficulty with pulse oximetry and loss of accuracy occurs with severe anemia, motion of the probe, darkly pigmented skin, poor perfusion with reduced vascular pulsation, and certain vascular dyes.[19]

### Pulmonary function tests

Pulmonary function tests (PFTs), in a general sense, can evaluate virtually every physiological aspect of breathing from respiratory muscle function, to the diffusion of gas across the alveolar wall, to the neurological control mechanisms that drive the process of breathing. PFTs serve as a diagnostic guide, assist in the formulation of specific treatment plans, and can prognosticate outcomes. This same information can help both the physician and the physical therapist identify realistic therapeutic goals and measure the effect of therapeutic intervention appropriate to the pulmonary problem identified and the level of respiratory impairment present.

**Guidelines for interpretation of pulmonary function tests.** Pulmonary function tests evaluate ventilatory mechanics, ventilatory regulation, and airway responsivity. Spirometry, performed today using electronic devices, as opposed to the previous use of water-sealed systems, is the most common approach to PFTs and should be among the laboratory evaluations available to patients. Forced vital capacity maneuvers are the most often used technique for examining various aspects of pulmonary function.

Ventilatory mechanics assessment includes measurement of lung volumes and flow rates. The measured values facilitate the categorization of the patient's response into one of two patterns—restrictive or obstructive. Examination of lung volume measurements will identify a restrictive pattern. Active lung volumes, those measured by direct patient effort, and static lung volumes, those measured by gas diffusion techniques, are typically measured. The specific volumes and capacities (a capacity is composed of more than one

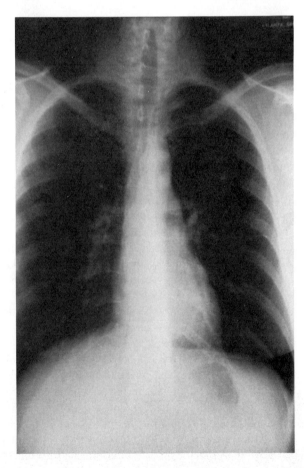

**Fig. 18-16.** A chest radiograph where the soft tissue, heart and hilar structures, diaphragms and lungs are all normal.

volume) and the basis for their measurement are presented in Chapter 13. In general terms, a reduction of all lung volumes and capacities is associated with restrictive disorders. Some of these disorders, such as interstitial pulmonary

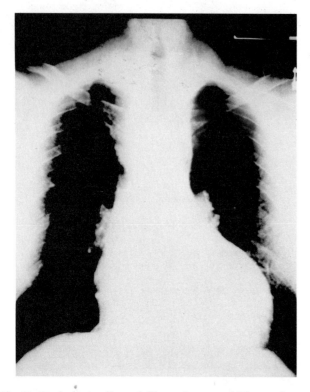

**Fig. 18-17.** A chest radiograph illustrating normal hilar configuration.

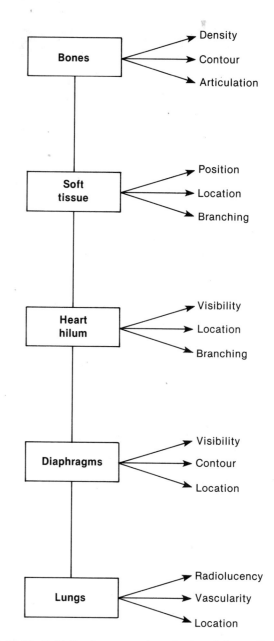

**Fig. 18-18.** Guideline for systematic evaluation of chest radiograph. Boxes identify structures, and arrows indicate criteria for each assessment.

fibrosis, commonly restrict the expansion of lung tissue. Other disorders, such as severe kyphoscoliosis or hypertrophic burn scars, restrict chest wall expansion. Their causes and treatment vary, but the underlying effect is a diminution in lung volume. Measurement of flow rates (see Chapter 13) indicates the general condition of the airways. Reduced flow rates are commonly associated with an obstructive pattern often accompanied by *increased* static volumes, such as residual volume, and increased capacities such as total lung capacity. The increased lung volumes and capacities are due to hyperaeration of the lungs, commonly found in conjunction with severe airways obstruction.

Assessment of ventilatory mechanics also permits evaluation of the effectiveness of therapy, the general progression of the disease process, and the determination of pulmonary impairment. By administering tests of ventilatory mechanics before and immediately after a physical therapy treatment, one can objectively assess the effect of that treatment. Serial tests, administered over several months and years, demonstrate the stability or instability of the disease process. Finally, by comparing a patient's actual performance to the predicted performance, the extent of permanent respiratory impairment can be estimated. Table 18-13 presents some guidelines recommended for this estimation.

When used to assess ventilatory regulation, PFTs enable the laboratory to examine the effect of hypoxic or hypercapnic stimuli on the rate and depth of breathing. Normally,

either type of stimulus will produce hyperventilation. Conditions associated with regulatory dysfunction are listed in Table 18-14.

Bronchial provocation tests, virtually never performed by a physical therapist but of great importance to those who work with patients with asthma, document the response of the airways to a suspected allergen. A normal, or nonresponsive test is one in which inhalation of the suspected allergen fails to induce a decrease in expiratory flow rates. The response associated with asthma is a diminution in expiratory flow rates of >15% of the initial value.

**Table 18-15.** The radiographic signs of collapse associated with specific lobes of the lung

| Lobe | Radiographic sign |
|---|---|
| Left upper lobe | Elevated left hilum<br>Ipsilateral tracheal shift<br>Bowing of major fissures |
| Left lingula | Slight left hilar displacement downward obliteration of left heart border |
| Left lower lobe | Left hilar displacement downward<br>Elevated left hemidiaphragm<br>Major fissure displacement caudally<br>Triangular opacity adjacent to spine |
| Right upper lobe | Elevated right hilum<br>Ipsilateral tracheal shift<br>Minor fissure displacement upward |
| Right middle lobe | Slight right hilar displacement downward<br>Obliteration of right heart border<br>Minor fissure displacement downward |
| Right lower lobe | Right hilar displacement downward<br>Elevated right hemidiaphragm<br>Major fissure displacement caudally<br>Triangular radiopacity adjacent to spine |

Adapted from Felson B and others: *Principles of chest roentgenology: a programmed text*, Philadelphia, 1965, WB Saunders Co.

## Chest radiography

Clinicians involved in pulmonary care frequently encounter chest radiographs taken to update the condition of their patients. The therapist uses this information to modify the physical therapy program to reflect any changes documented. Because resources for the interpretation of radiographs are not always readily available, physical therapists should develop a familiarity with the basic principles of radiology. An understanding of those principles can be acquired quickly through programmed learning.[11]

**Evaluation of the chest radiograph.** Interpretation of the chest radiograph involves evaluating the bones, soft tissue, heart and hilar structures, the diaphragm, and the lungs.

First, one evaluates the dense radiopaque bony structures. Normally, the ribs are uniformly dense, their margins are smooth and free of deformity, and they articulate with thoracic vertebrae only.

Next, the soft tissue of the neck and chest wall is evaluated. Here one examines the position of the trachea, carina, and mainstem bronchi. Normally, the tracheal shadow falls in the midline, the carina overlies the fourth thoracic vertebrae, and the right mainstem bronchus branches slightly higher and more vertically than the left mainstem bronchus. Fig. 18-16 presents a chest radiograph in which the bones and soft-tissue structures are all normal.

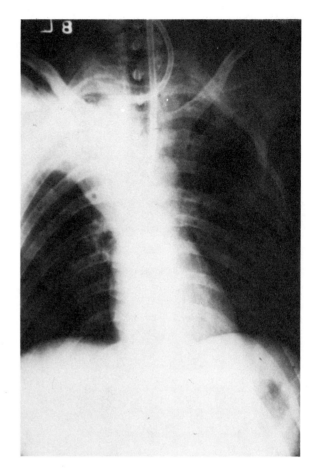

**Fig. 18-19.** A chest radiograph illustrating a right upper lobe collapse.

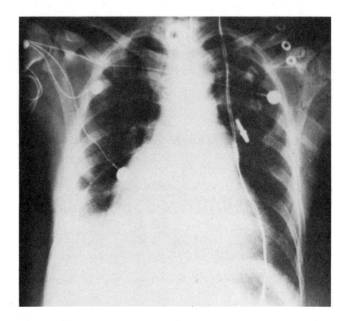

**Fig. 18-20.** A chest radiograph illustrating a right lower lobe collapse.

**Table 18-16.** The silhouette signs associated with various labor pneumonias

| Silhouette sign | Site of pneumonia |
| --- | --- |
| Loss of aortic knob or appendage | Left upper lobe |
| Loss of left ventricular border | Left lingula |
| Loss of left hemidiaphragm | Left lower lobe |
| Loss of right heart border; loss of ascending aorta | Right upper lobe |
| Loss of most of right heart border | Right middle lobe |
| Loss of right hemidiaphragm | Right lower lobe |

Adapted from Felson B and others: *Principles of chest roentgenology: a programmed text*, Philadelphia, 1965, WB Saunders Co.

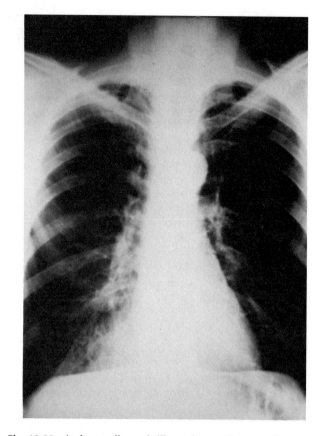

Fig. 18-22. A chest radiograph illustrating a silhouette sign at the right lower lobe.

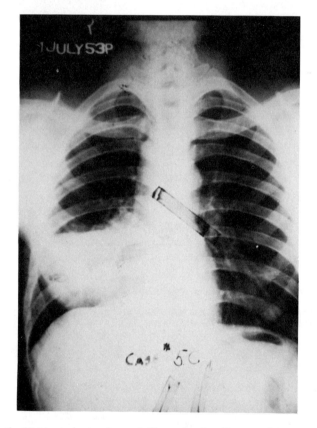

Fig. 18-21. A chest radiograph illustrating the silhouette sign at the right middle lobe.

Evaluation of the heart and hilar structures follows the soft-tissue evaluation. Normally, the borders of the right atrium, superior vena cava, aortic knob, aortic appendage, and left ventricle are visible, and the left hilum is higher than the right. Fig. 18-17 illustrates the normal relationship between the left and the right hilum.

Next, one evaluates the diaphragms. Normally, both diaphragms are visible and well rounded. They lie at the level of the tenth rib posteriorly, and the right diaphragm is about one interspace higher than the left. Both costophrenic angles (CPA) should be clear and sharp. In Fig. 18-16 the diaphragms are also normal.

To summarize, interpreting the chest radiograph requires a systematic evaluation of the structures contained within. Fig. 18-18 summarizes this evaluation by relating the structure evaluated to the criteria for its assessment. Abnormal chest radiographs require further examination to determine their impact on the physical therapy program.

**Guidelines for interpretation of abnormal chest radiographs.** Radiographic abnormalities commonly encountered in respiratory treatment include changes in the size, shape, or density of the lungs, heart, or diaphragms. Changes in the size of the lungs usually indicate a loss of lung volume and may indicate atelectasis. Additional signs of atelectasis include any of the following: displacement of the transverse or oblique fissures, nonuniform radiolucency, vascular crowding, displacement of the hilum toward the collapsed side, tracheal or hemidiaphragmatic shift toward the collapsed side, or inequality of intercostal spaces. The radiological characteristics associated with atelectasis of specific lobes are summarized in Table 18-15. Fig. 18-19 illustrates right upper lobe collapse, where the minor fissure is displaced upward and the right middle and lower lobes are more radiolucent than the left. Fig. 18-20 illustrates right

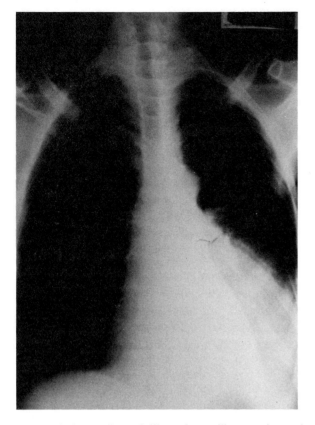

**Fig. 18-23.** A chest radiograph illustrating a silhouette sign at the left lower lobe.

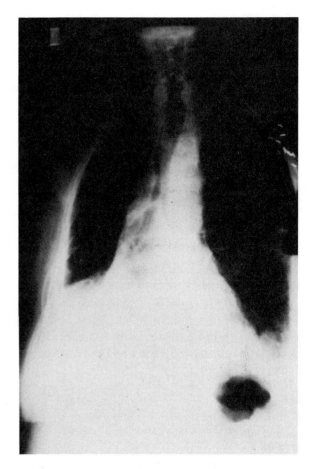

**Fig. 18-24.** A chest radiograph illustrating a left pneumothorax and a left pleural effusion.

lower lobe collapse, where the major fissure is displaced caudally and the right hilum is displaced downward.

Changes in the normal shape of the heart or diaphragms usually indicate that a border formed by the abutment of structures of unlike density has been obliterated. The change in shape induced by the loss of a border is called the "silhouette sign." In the absence of signs of atelectasis, the silhouette sign is closely associated with lobar pneumonia. Table 18-16 associates some silhouette signs with the probable site of the responsible lobar pneumonia. Figs. 18-21 to 18-23 present chest radiographs with silhouette signs suggesting pneumonia of the right middle lobe, right lower lobe, and left lower lobe respectively.

Changes in lung density occur in pneumothorax. Additional radiographic signs of pneumothorax include failure of the vascular markings to extend to the chest wall and the existence of an extreme radiolucency between the termination of the vascular markings and the chest wall. Fig. 18-24 presents a radiograph of a left pneumothorax.

The radiological characteristics associated with pleural effusion also include failure of vascular markings to extend fully to the chest wall. However, pleural effusion also blunts the costophrenic angles and may be associated with the presence of an air-fluid level. Fig. 18-24 is also an example of a left pleural effusion.

In summary, interpretation of a chest radiograph helps the therapist differentiate atelectasis and pneumonia. In addition, the skill assists in locating problems and directing treatment anatomically.

## Graded exercise tests

As in cardiac disease, exercise testing facilitates the diagnosis of respiratory disease, assists in quantifying disability, provides an appropriate basis for exercise prescription, and permits objective evaluation of general progress. In patients with lung disease, however, limited exercise tolerance may be the result of impaired oxygen transport, impaired pulmonary circulation, metabolic disturbances or disturbances of respiratory regulation, and/or the sensation and result of impaired cardiac function.[4]

The role of the physical therapist in exercise testing and prescription is described elsewhere in this book. Because the principles and practice of exercise testing and prescription do not differ greatly in pulmonary disease, the subject will not be discussed further here except to note that patients with known pulmonary hypertension or whose arterial oxygen tension is less than or equal to 50 mm Hg at rest, generally require oxygen supplementation for both initial testing and subsequent training.[27]

**Table 18-17.** Characteristics of the infective process associated with the staining properties of sputa

| | Characteristics of infective process | | | |
|---|---|---|---|---|
| Staining property | Type of infection | Probable infecting organism | Most probable type of pneumonia | Potential complications |
| Gram positive | Primary | *Pneumococcus* | Lobar | Empyema, bacteremia, meningitis |
| | Secondary | *Staphylococcus* | Lobar | Empyema, bronchopleural fistula, pyopneumothorax, bacteremia |
| Gram negative | Secondary | *Klebsiella* | Upper lobes | Suppuration, destruction of lung tissue, bacteremia |

Adapted from Cherniack RM and others: *Respiration in health and disease*, ed 2, Philadelphia, 1972, WB Saunders Co.

## Bacteriological and cytological tests

Therapists may be requested to obtain from their patients sputum samples for cytological or bacteriological evaluation. The validity and reliability of the results of these tests depend largely on the collection technique used when the specimen is obtained.

**Technique for specimen collection.** Appropriate collection technique requires no preparation beyond assurance that the patient's nasopharynx and oropharynx are free of contaminants. The therapist therefore directs the patient to clear the nose and throat and rinse the mouth thoroughly before expectorating the sputum sample. The therapist then directs the patient to inhale maximally and cough forcefully, expectorating secretions into a sterile receptacle. This process may be repeated as many as five times on five successive days for cytological evaluations. Bacteriological evaluations, however, require fewer samples.

**Clinical significance of test results.** Bacteriological evaluation of the sputum sample ensures the institution of appropriate antibiotic therapy by allowing identification of the infecting organism and the antimicrobial drug to which the organism is sensitive. This knowledge, along with the symptoms and signs of the disease, provides valuable clues concerning the pneumonic process and its potential complications. Table 18-17 demonstrates how, if the staining property and type of infection are known, one can predict the probable infecting organism, type of pneumonia, and its potential complications.

Cytological evaluation contributes to the differential diagnosis. For example, the discovery of lymphocytes in the sputum supports the differential diagnosis of tuberculosis. The discovery of erythrocytes supports the diagnosis of pneumonia. The discovery of malignant cells supports the diagnosis of carcinoma.

## REFERENCES

1. American College of Chest Physicians, American Thoracic Society, Joint Committee on Pulmonary Nomenclature: Pulmonary terms and symbols, *Chest* 67:583, 1975.
2. American Medical Association, Committee on rating of mental and physical impairment: Guidelines to evaluation of permanent impairment: the respiratory system, *JAMA* 194:919, 1965.
3. Banaszak EF and others: Phonopneumography, *Am Rev Resp Dis* 107:449, 1973.
4. Berglund E: Limiting factors during exercise in patients with lung disease, *Bull Europ Physiopath Resp* 15:15, 1979.
5. Bouchier IAD and Morris JS: *Clinical skills,* London, 1976, WB Saunders, Ltd.
6. Buckingham EB: *A primer of clinical diagnosis*, ed 2, New York, 1979, Harper & Row.
7. Burnside JW: *Adam's physical diagnosis,* ed 15, Baltimore, 1974, The Williams & Wilkins Co.
8. Chamberlain WN and Ogilvie C: *Symptoms in clinical medicine: an introduction to medical diagnosis,* ed 9, Chicago, 1974, Year Book Medical Publishers.
9. Cherniack RM and others: *Respiration in health and disease,* ed 3, Philadelphia, 1983, WB Saunders Co.
10. Edmeads J and Billings RF: Neurological and psychological aspects of chest pain. In Levine DL, editor: *Chest pain: an integrated diagnostic approach,* Philadelphia, 1977, Lea & Febiger.
11. Felson B and others: *Principles of chest roentgenology: a programmed text,* Philadelphia, 1965, WB Saunders Co.
12. Filley FG: *Acid base and blood gas regulation,* Philadelphia, 1971, Lea & Febiger.
13. Fishman AP: *Pulmonary diseases and disorders,* vol I, New York, 1980, McGraw-Hill Book Co.
14. Forgacs P: Lung sounds, *Br J Dis Chest* 63:1, 1969.
15. Gilbert R and others: Clinical value of observations of chest and abdominal motion in patients with pulmonary emphysema, *Am Rev Resp Dis* 119:155, 1979.
16. Lorber P: "Bad breath": presenting manifestation of anaerobic infection, *Am Rev Resp Dis* 112:875, 1975.
17. Malasanos L and others: Health assessment, ed 4, St Louis, 1989, Mosby.
18. McKusick VA and others: Acoustic basis of chest examination: studies made by means of sound spectography, *Am Rev Resp Dis* 72:12, 1955.
19. Mengelkoch LJ, Martin D, and Lawler J: A review of the principles of pulse oximetry and accuracy of pulse oximeter estimates during exercise, *Phys Ther* 74:40, 1994.
20. Miller RD: The medical history. In Sackner MA, editor: *Diagnostic techniques in pulmonary disease,* Part 1, New York, 1980, Marcel Dekker, Inc.
21. Mills P: *The significance of physical signs in medicine,* London, 1971, HK Lewis & Co, Ltd.

22. Nath AR and Capel LH: Inspiratory crackles and mechanical events of breathing, *Thorax* 29:695, 1974.

23. Prior JA and Silberstein JS: *Physical diagnosis: the history and examination of the patient,* ed 5, St Louis, 1977, Mosby.

24. Roddie IC and Wallace WFM: *Physiology of disease,* Chicago, 1975, Year Book Medical Publishers.

25. Shapiro BA ed: *Clinical application of blood gases,* Chicago, 1988, Mosby-Year Book Medical Publishers.

26. Wanner A: Interpretation of pulmonary function tests. In Sackner MA, editor: *Diagnostic techniques in pulmonary disease,* New York, 1980, Marcel Dekker, Inc.

27. Woolf CR: A rehabilitation program for improving exercise tolerance of patients with chronic lung disease, *Can Med Assoc J* 106:1289, 1972.

# CHAPTER 19

# Respiratory Treatment

*Nancy Humberstone and Jan Stephen Tecklin*

## RESPIRATORY TREATMENT

Proper management of the patient with a pulmonary problem requires an understanding of both the physiological derangement present and the effectiveness of a given treatment within the context of that problem. Historically, the effects of various therapeutic measures were not validated by rigorous scientific evaluation.[100] As a result, therapists must be prepared to amend their thinking in response to the continual influx of new information.

This section reviews those therapeutic measures commonly administered by physical therapists to patients with pulmonary problems. The review both describes the therapeutic measure and discusses its effectiveness; that is, the treatment is described in relation to the therapeutic goal, and

documentation is presented to support the desired therapeutic effects.

To facilitate the resolution of pulmonary problems, physical therapists administer treatments to improve ventilation and increase oxygenation, to decrease oxygen consumption, to improve secretion clearance, to maximize exercise tolerance, and to reduce pain.

Because changes in the amount of effective ventilation are best reflected in the arterial carbon dioxide tension ($Pa_{CO_2}$), the most accurate measure of the effectiveness of treatments given to improve ventilation is the $Pa_{CO_2}$. The most accurate measure of the effectiveness of treatments administered to improve oxygenation is the arterial oxygen tension ($Pa_{O_2}$). Oxygen consumption is difficult to measure directly at bedside. Consequently, the effectiveness of treatments administered to reduce oxygen consumption is also assessed indirectly as a reduction in the symptoms exhibited during the performance of a given activity.

In clinical medicine, changes in secretion clearance are assessed directly by changes in the volume or the chemical composition of sputum expectorated and indirectly by changes in the chest examination, the arterial blood gases, or the chest radiograph. The effectiveness of treatments administered to improve secretion clearance should therefore be assessed through these means.

Exercise tolerance is most accurately assessed by graded exercise tests. Therefore these tests should be utilized to assess the effectiveness of treatments administered to improve exercise tolerance.

Perceived pain depends not only on the quality, quantity, and duration of noxious stimulation, but also on one's emotional reaction. Therefore treatments administered to relieve pain, if effective, should modify at least one of these characteristics.

If the intent of physical therapy is to attain any of the therapeutic goals identified above, the effectiveness of the treatment must be measured by the suggested criteria. These criteria should serve as guidelines for interpreting the reviews of treatment effectiveness that follow.

# INCREASING VENTILATION AND OXYGENATION

Alveolar ventilation depends on the magnitude of tidal volume and dead space.[18] Decreases in alveolar ventilation are the result of decreased tidal ventilation or increased dead space ventilation. Therefore physical therapy strategies administered to increase alveolar ventilation should increase tidal ventilation, decrease dead space ventilation, or both. If successful, these strategies should decrease the arterial carbon dioxide tension ($Paco_2$).

Physical therapy strategies that increase alveolar ventilation may also increase alveolar oxygen tension ($Pao_2$). Therefore strategies that increase tidal ventilation or decrease dead space ventilation should also improve oxygenation. If successful, these strategies should increase $Pao_2$. Measures that increase ventilation and oxygenation include positioning techniques and breathing exercises.

## Positioning techniques

Research with small numbers of patients indicates that postural changes may improve ventilation and oxygenation. In one study of five patients with adult respiratory distress syndrome, the prone position improved arterial oxygen tension.[71] Another study of six patients with adult respiratory distress syndrome had similar results.[25] Improvement in $Paco_2$ occurred whenever patients were turned from supine to prone. Turning from prone to supine, however, decreased arterial oxygen tension in 12 of 14 trials.

Lateral decubitus positioning also affects ventilation and oxygenation. In 1974 Zack and colleagues[106] studied the effect of decubitus postures on oxygenation. Their results suggest that patients with unilateral lung disease lying with the affected lung dependent had significant decreases in oxygenation. When the disease process affected both lungs equally, turning onto the left side impaired oxygenation more than turning onto the right. Later research explored the effects of decubitus postures on oxygenation after thoracotomy.[82] The results of this later research suggest that lying on the unaffected side provides better oxygenation than supine-lying. A comparison of oxygenation when the surgical side was either dependent or uppermost was inconclusive. These results thus indicate that changes in patient position may significantly alter arterial oxygenation.

Dean and Ross present a careful analysis of studies regarding body positioning and mobilization of the patient as a means to enhance oxygen transport.[22] They support the work on oxygenation and body position cited above and recommend using various position changes to improve the ventilation/perfusion relationship and to reduce the deleterious effects of bronchial secretions. In addition, they cite work that indicates that cardiovascular effectiveness can be increased by optimizing plasma volume, preserving the fluid volume-regulating mechanisms, reducing the work of the heart, and maintaining stable hemodynamic status. Dean and Ross present additional studies that support the use of aggressive mobilization. This is an approach generally agreed upon and employed by therapists working in cardiopulmonary care on the basis of anecdotal reports and individual successes with patients. The authors state that mobilization should be considered a primary intervention that can improve or stimulate deep breathing, secretion removal, and efficient myocardial performance and oxygen transport.[22]

The objective and possible outcomes of changes in patient position are summarized in Table 19-1.

## Breathing exercises

To achieve the goal of increased alveolar ventilation, therapists teach breathing exercises that presumably influence the rate, depth, or distribution of ventilation or muscular activity associated with breathing. Although these exercises may affect the variables in the desired way, they may not necessarily result in improved alveolar ventilation or oxygenation.[100] Moreover, they may have unexpected negative effects. For example, maximal inspiratory efforts in asthmatics may result in bronchoconstriction.[30]

The breathing exercises commonly administered to improve ventilation and oxygenation are diaphragmatic breathing, pursed-lips breathing, segmental breathing, low-frequency breathing, and sustained maximal inspiration breathing exercises. The effectiveness of these breathing exercises in treating ventilatory problems of the acutely ill has been reviewed extensively elsewhere.[28,48,107]

**Diaphragmatic breathing exercises.** The diaphragm is the principal muscle of inspiration. Historically, when muscles other than the diaphragm assumed a role in

**Table 19-1.** Objectives and potential outcomes of position changes

| | |
| --- | --- |
| Therapeutic objective | Alleviate dyspnea |
| Physiological objectives | Increase oxygenation |
| | Improve ventilation |
| Potential outcomes | |
| Prone | Increased arterial oxygen tension in bilateral lung disease |
| Supine | Decreased arterial oxygen tension in bilateral lung disease |
| Lateral | Decreased arterial oxygen tension lying on the affected lung in unilateral lung disease |
| | Decreased arterial oxygen tension lying on the left side in bilateral lung disease |
| | Improved arterial oxygen tension lying on the unoperated side after thoracotomy (relative to supine) |

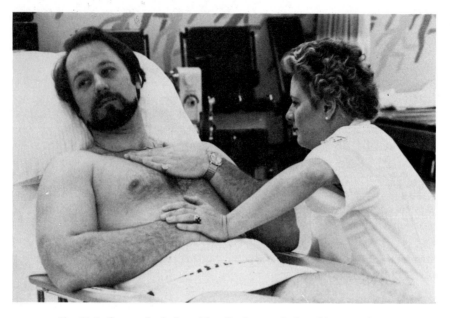

**Fig. 19-1.** One method of teaching diaphragmatic breathing exercises.

inspiration, therapeutic efforts were directed toward restoring a more normal, diaphragmatic pattern of breathing. The return to diaphragmatic breathing was thought to relieve dyspnea.

Diaphragmatic breathing exercises allegedly enhance diaphragmatic descent during inspiration and diaphragmatic ascent during expiration. Diaphragmatic descent is assisted by directing the patient to protract the abdomen gradually during inhalation. One assists diaphragmatic ascent by directing the patient to allow the abdomen to retract gradually during exhalation or by directing the patient to contract the abdominal muscles actively during exhalation. Although the exact techniques used to teach diaphragmatic breathing vary, in principle they are similar. That is, they all indicate that the patient should assume a comfortable position, usually one half to three quarters upright sitting, before beginning. In addition, they recommend that the patient's hips and knees be flexed to relax the abdominal and hamstring muscles respectively. Diaphragmatic breathing exercises are then taught. One method of teaching diaphragmatic breathing exercises is shown in Fig. 19-1.

Following are the steps for teaching diaphragmatic breathing exercises.

1. Place the patient's dominant hand over the mid-rectus abdominis area.
2. Place the patient's nondominant hand on the mid-sternal area.
3. Direct the patient to inhale slowly through the nose.
4. Instruct the patient to watch the dominant hand as inspiration continues.
5. Encourage the patient to direct the air so that the dominant hand gradually rises as inspiration continues.

6. Caution the patient to avoid excessive movement under the nondominant hand.
7. Apply firm counterpressure over the patient's dominant hand just before directing the patient to inhale.
8. Instruct the patient to inhale as you lessen your counterpressure as inspiration continues.
9. Practice the exercise until the patient no longer requires manual assistance of the therapist to perform the exercise correctly.
10. Progress the level of difficulty by sequentially removing auditory, visual, and tactile cues. Thereafter, progress the exercise by practicing seated, standing, and walking.

Diaphragmatic breathing exercises have also been administered to eliminate accessory muscle activity and to strengthen the diaphragm. In the past, increased diaphragmatic strength was assumed when increased resistance to abdominal protraction was tolerated. However, recent evidence may indicate that in normal subjects this assumption may be invalid.[62] Moreover, the inference that strong diaphragms increase ventilation has not been validated. Current efforts at respiratory muscle strengthening are not specific to the diaphragm, but address the inspiratory muscles as a functional group as discussed in Chapter 17.

The validation of diaphragmatic breathing exercises is the objective of much research. One study explored the effect of diaphragmatic breathing on the ventilation of erect normal subjects, two of whom were physical therapists and were presumably well trained in the technique.[84] The results suggested that diaphragmatic breathing increased lower lung zone ventilation when certain subjects inhaled diaphragmatically after a maximal exhalation. This effect, however, was limited to the physical therapists, an indication that proper execution of diaphragmatic breathing may require substantial training. Later research repeated the above study using different instrumentation and an experimental group of subjects with chronic obstructive pulmonary disease.[79] The results of this subsequent study supported the previous findings of improved lower lung zone ventilation only in well-trained, normal subjects inhaling after a maximal expiration.

This failure of diaphragmatic breathing to alter the distribution of ventilation in chronically obstructed patients has been corroborated in later studies.[11,33] However, its effect in normal subjects continues to be unclear.[11,78]

The effect of diaphragmatic breathing on oxygenation is also unclear. An early study reported significant improvement in arterial oxygen saturation during diaphragmatic breathing in selected subjects.[63] Sinclair[85] later failed to substantiate such improvement. Recent evidence, however, suggests that diaphragmatic breathing may affect oxygenation indirectly by altering regional pulmonary perfusion.[41]

The effect of diaphragmatic breathing on the mobility of the diaphragm is also controversial. Early research reported no increase in diaphragmatic motion whether normal subjects[98] or patients with chronic obstructive lung disease[85] breathed diaphragmatically. However, the recent report of improved diaphragmatic excursion in selected patients has fueled the controversy.[31]

Finally, and perhaps most notably, although the literature has frequently associated a reduced rate of postoperative pulmonary complications with breathing exercises,[92,95,102] the exact contribution of diaphragmatic breathing to this association has yet to be described.

Diaphragmatic breathing exercises will continue to be used as research progresses. The objectives and potential outcomes of diaphragmatic breathing are summarized in Table 19-2.

**Pursed-lips breathing exercises.** Pursed-lips breathing is another method suggested for improving ventilation and oxygenation. This breathing pattern, often used spontaneously by patients with chronic obstructive lung disease, was first recommended for therapeutic use in this country around 1935.[81] Since that time the technique has enjoyed wide popularity for the relief of dyspnea. Two methods of pursed-lips breathing have been reported. One method advocates passive expiration,[63] whereas the other recommends abdominal muscle contraction to prolong expiration.[101] Because abdominal muscle contraction and excessively prolonged expiration may promote airway collapse,[10,44] contemporary applications of this technique usually encourage passive expiration only.

Following are the steps for one method of teaching pursed-lips breathing:

1. Position the patient comfortably.
2. Review the objectives of the exercise: relief of dyspnea or improved ventilation.
3. Explain that the benefit of the technique varies among subjects.
4. Explain why abdominal muscle contraction is undesirable.
5. Place your hand over the mid-rectus abdominis area to detect activity during expiration.
6. Direct the patient to inhale slowly.
7. Instruct the patient to purse the lips before exhalation.
8. Instruct the patient to relax the air out through the pursed lips and refrain from abdominal muscle contraction.
9. Direct the patient to stop exhaling when abdominal muscle activity is detected.
10. Progress the intensity of the exercise by substituting the patient's hand for yours, removing tactile cues, and having the patient perform the exercise while standing and exercising.

How this pattern of breathing affects ventilation and oxygenation has been the object of research since the mid 1960s. Thoman and colleagues[91] studied the effect of pursed-lips breathing on ventilation in subjects with chronic obstructive lung disease. They found that this breathing pattern significantly decreased the respiratory rate and increased the tidal volume. In addition, pursed-lips breathing improved alveolar ventilation, as measured by $Paco_2$, and enhanced the ventilation of previously underventilated areas. The authors postulated that these beneficial effects might be attributed solely to slowing the respiratory rate.

Further research was prompted by the clinical observation that, with pursed-lips breathing, the symptomatic relief of dyspnea occurs before changes in ventilation.[43] Ingram[43] explored the short-term effects of pursed-lips breathing, which was found to reduce both the peak and mean expiratory flow rates. Moreover, those who claim to benefit from this technique obtained a greater reduction in "nonelastic" resistance across the lung than those who denied such benefit.

A later study reported significant decreases in respiratory rate during simulated pursed-lips breathing.[1] However, these

**Table 19-2.** Objectives and potential outcomes of diaphragmatic breathing exercises

| | |
|---|---|
| Therapeutic objectives | Alleviate dyspnea |
| | Reduce the work of breathing |
| | Reduce the incidence of postoperative pulmonary complication |
| Physiological objectives | Improve ventilation |
| | Improve oxygenation |
| Potential outcomes | Eliminate accessory muscle activity |
| | Decrease respiratory rate |
| | Increase tidal ventilation |
| | Improve distribution of ventilation |
| | Decreased need for postoperative therapy |

**Table 19-3.** The objectives and potential outcomes of pursed-lips breathing exercises

| | |
|---|---|
| Therapeutic objectives | Alleviate dyspnea |
| | Increase tolerance |
| Physiological objectives | Increase alveolar ventilation |
| | Increase oxygenation |
| | Reduce the work of breathing |
| Potential outcomes | Elimination of accessory muscle activity |
| | Reduced respiratory rate |
| | Increased arterial oxygen tension |
| | Decreased carbon dioxide tension |
| | Increased exercise tolerance |

reductions in respiratory rate were associated with reduction of tidal volume. Moreover, the study could not substantiate improvements in alveolar ventilation or oxygenation despite a decrease in physiological dead space.

Mueller and colleagues[65] reevaluated the effect of pursed-lips breathing on ventilation and oxygenation. Their results supported the previous findings of decreased respiratory rate and increased tidal volume. Moreover, they found that these effects persisted during exercise. At rest, pursed-lips breathing consistently improved alveolar ventilation and oxygenation, whereas during exercise the effect could not be sustained. Finally, like Ingram,[43] Mueller and others reported a positive association between symptomatic relief and magnitude of objective improvement.

Later research evaluated the effect of pursed-lips breathing on exercise tolerance in patients with severe chronic obstructive pulmonary disease.[15] The study reported that pursed-lips breathing improved exercise tolerance without incurring increased metabolic cost; that is, it improved performance without increasing the respiratory rate or decreasing the $Pao_2$.

This discussion indicates that research has failed to explain fully the symptomatic benefits some patients ascribe to pursed-lips breathing. At the very least, pursed-lips breathing appears to reduce the respiratory rate without compromising minute ventilation. It may also improve ventilation and oxygenation not only during rest, but also during exercise.

Physical therapists should continue to teach pursed-lips breathing exercises to patients complaining of dyspnea. The objectives and potential outcomes of this therapy are presented in Table 19-3.

**Segmental breathing exercises.** Segmental breathing is the third exercise used to improve ventilation and oxygenation. This exercise, also known as localized breathing, presumes that inspired air can be directed to a predetermined area.[75]

This treatment has been recommended to prevent the accumulation of pleural fluid, to reduce the probability of atelectasis, to prevent the accumulation of tracheobronchial secretions, to decrease paradoxical breathing, to prevent the panic associated with uncontrolled breathing, and to improve chest mobility.

Although contemporary methods of administering segmental breathing exercises differ from those described earlier,[36] their rationale is essentially the same. Each technique uses manual counterpressure against the thorax to encourage the expansion of a specific part of the lung.

Following are the steps for one method of administering segmental breathing exercises:

1. Identify the surface landmarks demarcating the affected area.
2. Place your hand or hands on the chest wall overlying the bronchopulmonary segment or segments requiring treatment.
3. Apply firm pressure to that area at the end of the patient's expiratory maneuver. (Pressure should be equal and bilateral across a median sternotomy incision.)
4. Instruct the patient to inspire deeply through his or her mouth attempting to direct the inspired air toward your hand, saying, "Breathe into my hand."
5. Reduce hand pressure as patient inspires. (At end inspiration, the instructor's hand should be applying no pressure on the chest.)
6. Instruct the patient to hold his or her breath for 2 to 3 seconds at the completion of inspiration.
7. Instruct the patient to exhale.
8. Repeat sequence until patient can execute breathing maneuver correctly.
9. Progress the exercises by instructing the patient to use his or her own hands or a belt to execute the program independently.

Evaluation of the effectiveness of segmental breathing begins with validation of its underlying premise that ventilation can be directed to a predetermined area.

In 1955, Campbell and Friend[14] studied the effect of lateral basal expansion exercises on ventilation. They concluded that this type of segmental breathing exercise failed to improve ventilation in patients with emphysema. A more recent study also failed to find any change in the distribution of ventilation when subjects with lung restriction breathed segmentally.[59]

Nonetheless, another study reported that, in a population of patients at high risk for the development of pulmonary complications, those treated with segmental breathing exercises suffered fewer postoperative pulmonary complications than those not similarly treated.[95] Because more than one type of breathing exercise was administered, the exact contribution of segmental breathing to this beneficial effect is uncertain. This meager evidence may indicate that the effect of segmental breathing exercises on ventilation is still unclear.

There is a lack of persuasive objective evidence linking

**Table 19-4.** Objectives and potential outcomes of segmental breathing exercises

| | |
|---|---|
| Therapeutic objective | Alleviate dyspnea |
| Physiological objectives | Increase alveolar ventilation<br>Increase oxygenation |
| Potential outcomes | Prevent accumulation of pleural fluid<br>Prevent accumulation of secretions<br>Decrease paradoxical breathing<br>Decrease "panic"<br>Improve chest mobility |

**Table 19-5.** Objectives and potential outcomes of both low-frequency and sustained maximal inspiration breathing

| | |
|---|---|
| Therapeutic objective | Alleviate dyspnea |
| Physiological objectives | Increase ventilation<br>Increase oxygenation |
| Potential outcome | Slow respiratory rate |

segmental breathing and other therapeutic effects identified in the introduction. The therapeutic benefits are still uncertain. The objectives and potential outcomes thought to be associated with segmental breathing are listed in Table 19-4.

**Low-frequency breathing exercises.** Several researchers report that slow, deep breathing improves alveolar ventilation and oxygenation. However, the improvement reported seems to be sustained only as long as the low-rate breathing pattern is maintained. The objectives and potential outcomes of low-frequency breathing are presented in Table 19-5.

**Sustained maximal breathing exercises.** Breathing exercises during which a maximal inspiration is sustained for about 3 seconds have also been associated with improved oxygenation.[99] The objectives and potential outcomes of sustained maximal inspiration breathing are also presented in Table 19-5.

## REDUCING OXYGEN CONSUMPTION

The amount of oxygen consumed in a given activity depends, in part, on the type of work performed. To sustain work, the oxygen supply must meet the oxygen demand. When the supply of oxygen cannot be expanded to meet work requirements, continued work depends solely on the reduction of oxygen demand. Theoretically the physical therapist can reduce oxygen demand by eliminating all work extraneous to the desired activity.

Following are several strategies for reducing oxygen consumption:[86]

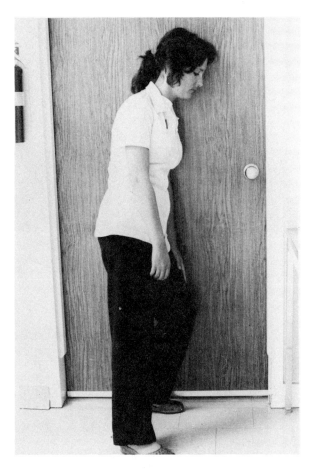

Fig. 19-2. The forward-leaning posture.

1. Reduce basal metabolic rate.
2. Minimize unsupported body position.
3. Minimize extrabasal body function.
4. Minimize antigravity work.
5. Minimize work to accelerate or decelerate body parts.

Physical therapy treatments administered for this purpose pursue these strategies by adjusting either the work of breathing or general body work.

## REDUCING THE WORK OF BREATHING
### Breathing exercises

The work of breathing may be reduced by either reducing the rate or depth of ventilation or by eliminating accessory muscle activity. Because the breathing exercises previously discussed have been associated with both the elimination of accessory muscle activity and the slowing of the respiratory rate, they are often incorporated in programs designed to reduce the work of breathing. Because they have been discussed previously, they are not discussed here.

### Forward-leaning postures

The forward-flexed posture shown with the individual leaning against a wall for support in Fig. 19-2 is also

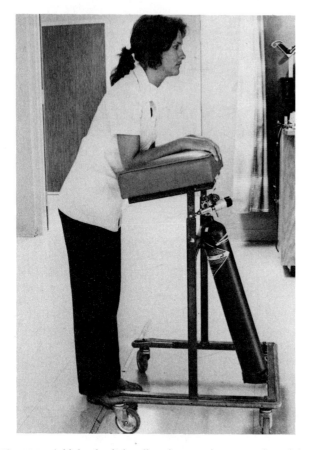

**Fig. 19-3.** A high-wheeled walker that permits assumption of the forward-leaning posture.

recommended to reduce the work of breathing.[5] In patients who are unable to tolerate functional walking in the forward-flexed posture, a high walker may be adapted to permit forward leaning, thereby eliminating sufficient work to permit the desired activity (Fig. 19-3).

The effectiveness of these treatments in reducing the work of breathing has not been substantiated objectively. It has been based largely on anecdotal observations that they eliminate accessory muscle activity. More objective evaluation is needed to substantiate this clinical observation.

## REDUCING GENERAL BODY WORK
### Relaxation exercises

Relaxation is the treatment most frequently administered to reduce general body work. The following steps present one method of facilitating total body relaxation:

1. Minimize auditory and visual distractions.
2. Position the patient in a posture that provides maximal support and minimal discomfort.
3. Direct the patient to refrain from generating mental images.
4. Instruct the patient to contract and then relax the major muscle groups of the lower extremities proceeding distally to proximally.

**Table 19-6.** Objectives and potential outcomes of treatment programs designed to reduce oxygen consumption

| | |
|---|---|
| Therapeutic objective | Improve the quality of life by increasing functional activity tolerance |
| Physiological objective | Reduce the oxygen consumption associated with a given activity |
| Potential outcomes | Elevate the dyspnea threshold for a given activity<br>Broaden the functional activity tolerance<br>Improve the quality of life<br>Elevate the functional activity tolerance |

5. Proceed as above, relaxing the major muscle groups of the upper extremities.
6. Monitor relaxation periodically by moving the limbs or palpating muscle tension.
7. Provide appropriate feedback or cues.
8. Contract then relax each accessory muscle of inspiration and expiration.
9. Direct the patient to inhale slowly and deeply and then "relax" the air out.
10. Monitor relaxation of specific respiratory muscles by palpation.
11. Progress the exercise by proceeding with self-monitoring.

Advance the exercise as tolerated by requiring relaxation while seated, while standing, and while ambulating.

This method incorporates the principles of relaxation as described by Benson[8] and Jacobsen.[45] Other authors have attempted to demonstrate therapeutic effects of relaxation techniques on children with asthma and of meditation on physiologic changes in normal subjects. Changes in various lung function tests have been absent or minimal, but reports of subjective well-being are common.[7,27]

### Work adjustment

Another method of reducing general body work uses the strategies presented previously to modify the conditions of work. For example, if a patient wants to perform all oral hygiene activities independently but becomes dyspneic standing at the sink, the therapist may eliminate the unnecessary work done by standing erect and direct the patient to assume the seated position.

Treatments administered to reduce oxygen consumption by a decrease in the work of breathing or general work, though apparently sound and widely practiced, require further objective evaluation. The objectives for and potential outcomes of treatments are summarized in Table 19-6.

## IMPROVING SECRETION CLEARANCE

Normal secretion clearance requires effective mucociliary transport and an effective cough. When either of these mechanisms functions improperly, secretions accumulate. Early clinical signs of accumulated secretions include changes in body temperature, respiratory rate, pulse, blood pressure, and breath sounds.[2]

The consequences of accumulated secretions include inflammation, infection, airway obstruction, atelectasis, and pneumonia. Identification and treatment of the underlying cause of the excessive secretions may help reduce the likelihood of these consequences.

Secretion accumulation may be caused either by impaired mucociliary transport or impaired cough. Impaired mucociliary transport results from altered ciliary function or altered mucous composition. Following are some causes of impaired mucociliary transport:

1. Hypoxia or hyperoxia
2. Cuffed endotracheal tube
3. Dehydration
4. Electrolyte imbalance
5. Infection
6. Loss of ciliated respiratory epithelium
7. Inhalation of dry gases
8. Cigarette smoke
9. Anesthetics and analgesics
10. Pollutants

Impaired cough may result from pain, weakness, incoordination, or structural abnormality.

Following are some conditions that may be associated with impaired cough:

1. Coma
2. Neuromuscular disease
3. Debilitation
4. Morphological abnormality
   a. Bronchiectasis
   b. Bronchomegaly
   c. Tracheomalacia
   d. Endotracheal tube
   e. Obstruction by tumor
5. Pain
   a. Associated with trauma
   b. Associated with incisions
6. Abnormal thoracic function
   a. Severe kyphoscoliosis
   b. Costovertebral arthritis
   c. Hypertrophic burn scars on thorax

Impaired secretion clearance is best treated by administration of the therapy most appropriate to the problem identified. Bronchial drainage enhances mucociliary transport. Hydration, humidity, aerosol, and drug therapy alter mucous composition, ciliary motility, or bronchial caliber. Where indicated, these treatments should precede bronchial drainage because thickened secretions moving slowly through constricted bronchi may not respond readily, if at all, to gravity. Physical therapy treatments that are administered

to improve an inadequate cough include positioning, forced expiration, pressure, manual ventilation, mechanical stimulation, and neuromuscular facilitation.

Improved secretion clearance may be inferred clinically from either increased volume or viscosity of secretions expectorated or from changes in the clinical signs associated with retained secretions.

### Classical bronchial drainage

The technique of bronchial drainage classically aligns the segmental bronchi with gravity.[64] In this way, theoretically, secretions accumulated in a bronchopulmonary segment move toward a central, segmental bronchus from which they can be removed by coughing and then easily expectorated. Figs. 19-4 to 19-6 illustrate the bronchial drainage positions for each bronchopulmonary segment of both lungs. Therapists commonly direct patients to maintain each posture for about 20 minutes and to cough before assuming a new position. If, however, the adjunctive techniques of percussion and vibration are administered simultaneously, the positions can be changed after approximately 2 minutes.

### Modified bronchial drainage

The following adverse physiological situations may be associated with various disease processes or may accompany bronchial drainage itself:

1. Increased intracranial pressure
2. Decreased arterial oxygen tension
3. Decreased cardiac output
4. Decreased forced expired volume in 1 second
5. Decreased specific airway conductance
6. Pulmonary hemorrhage

When these situations are present, the classical bronchial drainage positions should be modified. The following is an example of modified bronchial drainage. The positions described for the bronchial drainage of the lingula, right middle lobe, or lower lobes (except the superior segments) require elevation of the foot of the bed. This can increase venous return to the heart. In situations where this effect may be undesirable, the positions can be modified. One method of modifying these positions declines only the chest (Figs. 19-7 to 19-11). A different modification is required immediately after open heart surgery, when the chest itself must remain horizontal. Modified bronchial drainage, in this example, uses classical patient positioning in the horizontal position only.[39]

Finally, the modification of classical bronchial drainage positions to avoid adverse effects may require the avoidance of certain positions altogether. For example, in severe unilateral lung disease prolonged lying on the affected lung may be inadvisable.[106]

In the past 20 years bronchial drainage has been widely discussed. Researchers have studied the effects of bronchial drainage alone[4,26,46,55,57,104] and when augmented by per-

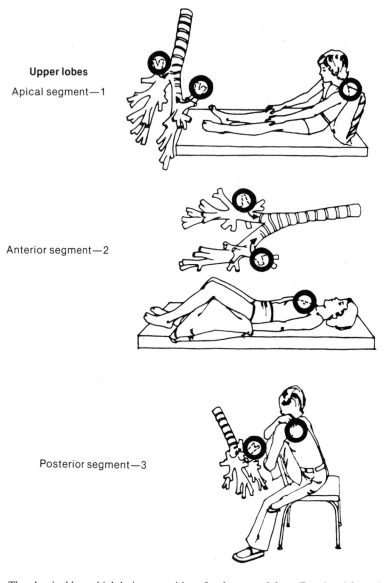

**Upper lobes**

Apical segment—1

Anterior segment—2

Posterior segment—3

**Fig. 19-4.** The classical bronchial drainage positions for the upper lobes. (Reprinted from *Segmental bronchial drainage slide chart,* New York, 1976, Breon Laboratories, Inc, with permission from the publisher.)

cussion,[29,46] vibration, or both.[13,40,70,89] Bronchial drainage has been evaluated by determining its effect on the transport of secretions in animals[63] and in humans.[6] Investigators have evaluated bronchial drainage in neonates,[29] children,[55] and adults. In addition, investigations have explored both the long-[26] and short-term[19] effects of drainage. The effects of drainage have been evaluated in a variety of conditions including chronic bronchitis,[13] cystic fibrosis,[57,77,89] respiratory failure,[58] and pneumonia.[32,55] Researchers have evaluated the effects of bronchial drainage in patients with acute exacerbations of chronic disease[4,13,67] and in patients with stable chronic disease.[6,26,90]

Bronchial drainage has also been evaluated according to its effects on sputum volume[4,57] and composition.[40] Its effects on the resolution of fever[4,26,32,55] have been exam-

ined. Its effect on forced expired volume in 1 second,[13,39,46,67] maximum midexpiratory flow rate,[89] and peak expiratory flow rates[89] has also been assessed. Other investigators have evaluated bronchial drainage according to its effect on lung compliance,[103] specific airway conductance,[67] vital capacity[67] functional residual capacity,[67] and oxygenation.[4,58,67,104] Finally, researchers have assessed bronchial drainage by evaluating its effect on the rate of postoperative pulmonary complications[56] and the length of hospital stay.[32]

Because these studies contain few similarities in experimental design, it is difficult to draw firm conclusions. At the very least, it appears that bronchial drainage augmented by percussion and vibration enhances mucociliary transport better than bronchial drainage alone. However, percussion

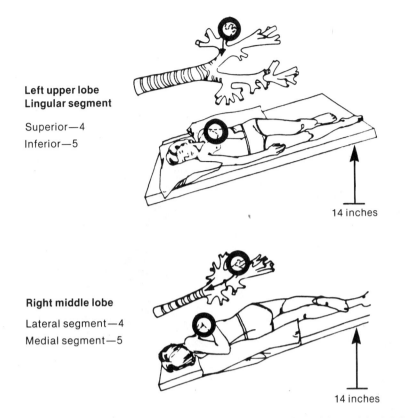

**Left upper lobe**
**Lingular segment**

Superior—4
Inferior—5

14 inches

**Right middle lobe**

Lateral segment—4
Medial segment—5

14 inches

**Fig. 19-5.** The classical bronchial drainage positions for the right middle lobe and the left lingula. (Reprinted from *Segmental bronchial drainage slide chart,* New York, 1976, Breon Laboratories, Inc, with permission from the publisher.)

may be associated with an immediate bronchospasm that lasts for 20 to 30 minutes. The onset of this transient bronchospasm may be avoided by administration of bronchodilators before treatment.[13] Bronchial drainage may be more effective with abundant secretions rather than scanty secretions.[66]

Although fatal hemoptysis has been associated with bronchial drainage administered to patients with end-stage disease,[35,87] the nature and frequency of this association is unclear. Physical therapists should exercise caution when administering bronchial drainage to any patient with end-stage disease until this association is clarified. Caution is also recommended when administering therapeutic percussion.

Following are some cardiovascular conditions in which caution in the application of therapeutic percussion has been recommended:

1. Chest wall pain
2. Unstable angina
3. Hemodynamic lability
4. Low platelet count
5. Anticoagulation therapy
6. Unstable or potentially lethal dysrhythmias

Following are some orthopedic conditions in which caution in the application of therapeutic percussion has been recommended:

1. Osteoporosis
2. Prolonged steroid therapy
3. Costal chondritis
4. Osteomyelitis
5. Osteogenesis imperfecta
6. Spinal fusion
7. Rib fracture or flail chest

Following are some pulmonary conditions in which caution in the application of therapeutic percussion has been recommended:

1. Bronchospasm
2. Hemoptysis
3. Severe dyspnea
4. Untreated lung abscess
5. Pneumothorax
6. Immediately after chest tube removal
7. Pneumonia or other infectious process
8. Pulmonary embolus

Following are some oncological conditions in which caution in the application of therapeutic percussion has been recommended:

1. Cancer metastatic to ribs or spine
2. Carcinoma in the bronchus
3. Resectable tumor

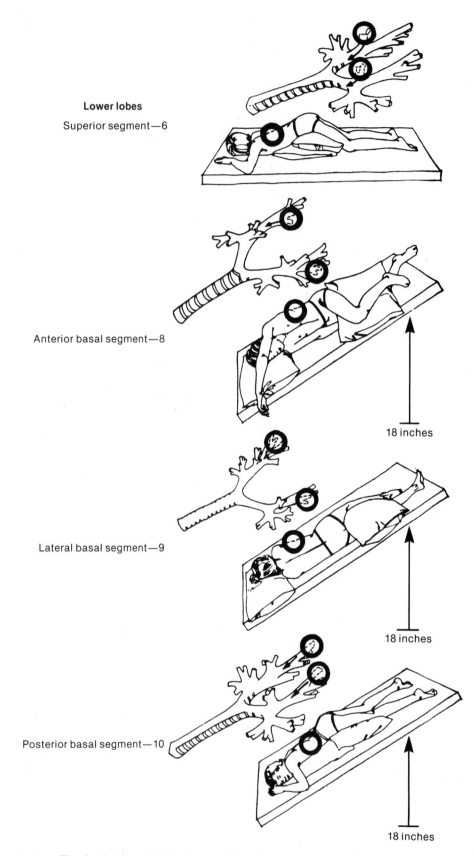

**Lower lobes**

Superior segment—6

Anterior basal segment—8

18 inches

Lateral basal segment—9

18 inches

Posterior basal segment—10

18 inches

**Fig. 19-6.** The classical bronchial drainage positions for the lower lobes. (Reprinted from *Segmental bronchial drainage slide chart,* New York, 1976, Breon Laboratories, Inc, with permission from the publisher.)

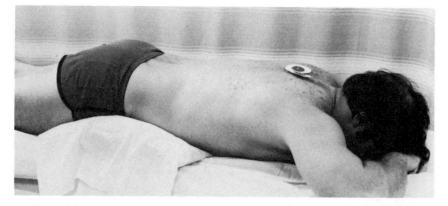

**Fig. 19-7.** Modification of the position classically recommended for bronchial drainage of the superior segments, both lower lobes.

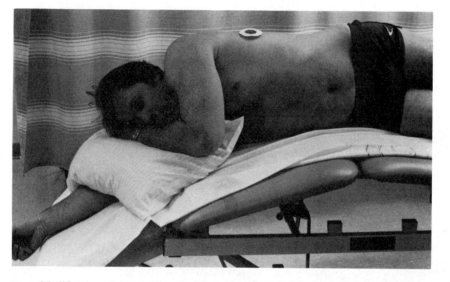

**Fig. 19-8.** Modification of the position classically recommended for bronchial drainage of the left lateral basal segment.

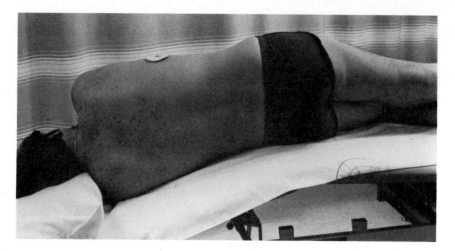

**Fig. 19-9.** Modification of the position classically recommended for bronchial drainage of the right lateral basal segment.

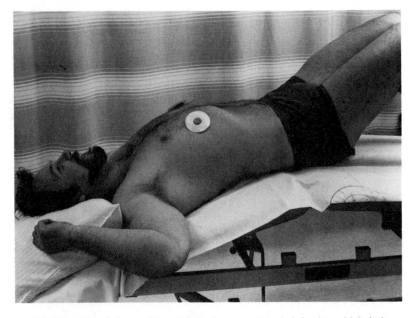

**Fig. 19-10.** Modification of the position classically recommended for bronchial drainage of the anterior basal segments, both lower lobes.

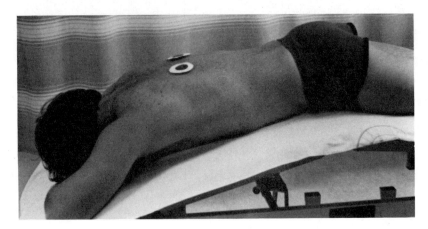

**Fig. 19-11.** Modification of the position classically recommended for drainage of both posterior basal segments.

Following are miscellaneous conditions in which caution in the application of therapeutic percussion has been recommended:

1. Recent skin grafts
2. Burns
3. Open thoracic wounds
4. Skin infection thorax
5. Subcutaneous emphysema head and back
6. Immediately after cataract surgery

The basis for the above recommendations is not always clear.

In summary, the conventional role of bronchial drainage and its adjunctive techniques of percussion and vibration is to facilitate clearance of excess secretions. This role is summarized in Table 19-7.

**Table 19-7.** Objectives and potential outcomes of postural drainage and adjunctive techniques like percussion and vibration

| | |
|---|---|
| Therapeutic objective | Eliminate retained secretions |
| Physiological objective | Improve mucociliary transport |
| Potential outcomes | Increase volume expectorated |
| | Improve clearance of thick secretions |
| | Reduce airway resistance |
| | Improve compliance |
| | Reduce the work of breathing |
| | Improve oxygenation and ventilation |
| | Reduce the rate of postoperative pulmonary complications |
| | Shorten hospitalization |

## ENHANCING MUCOCILIARY TRANSPORT

During the 1980s, several new approaches to classical bronchial drainage developed that employ various breathing maneuvers to mobilize and transport secretions. An important concept of these new approaches is that they can be performed by the patient alone, with no other individual required for the treatment. Significantly, the traditional manual techniques of percussion and vibration were deemed unnecessary in these techniques. The treatments were developed primarily for children and young adults with cystic fibrosis (CF), and the studies performed on the approaches have centered largely on the CF population. However, it seems reasonable that the approaches would be appropriate for all individuals with chronic lung disease productive of copious sputum.

### Autogenic drainage

Dab and Alexander introduced autogenic drainage and described the approach as follows:[20,21]

1. The patient is seated upright.
2. The patient breathes deeply at a "normal or relatively slow rhythm."
3. Secretions in the airway will move proximally as a result of the breathing pattern.
4. As secretions move into the trachea, they are expelled with a gentle cough or slightly forced expiration.

Dab and Alexander recommended a slightly forced expiration to expel secretions because the high transmural pressures that occur with coughing produce airway collapse, which reduces the effectiveness of coughing.[20,21]

### Forced expiratory technique

The forced expiratory technique (FET), was popularized by physiotherapists from the Brompton Hospital in London. Pryor and others began to employ the FET in the late 1970s and into the 1980s.[74] Independence or "self-treatment", as occurs with autogenic drainage, was the primary benefit experienced with the FET. Various investigators examined the clinical effects of the FET, with inconsistent results. Partridge and others believed that the lack of conclusive findings was because subsequent investigators misinterpreted the original description of the FET.[68] To prevent misinterpretation here, the following direct quote is from the original article about the FET.

The forced expiratory technique (FET) consists of one or two huffs (forced expirations), from mid-lung volume to low lung volume, followed by a period of relaxed, controlled diaphragmatic breathing. Bronchial secretions mobilized to the upper airways are then expectorated and the process is repeated until maximal bronchial clearance is obtained. The patient can reinforce the forced expiration by self-compression of the chest wall using a brisk adduction movement of the upper arm.[74]

The later paper by Partridge, attempting to clarify each segment of the FET, places significant emphasis upon huffing to low lung volumes in an effort to clear peripheral secretions. The term "from mid-lung volume" was clarified as a medium-sized inspiration that precedes the huffing. Recommendations were made that patients use the FET in gravity-assisted positions, and that pauses for breathing control and relaxation should be part of the overall approach.[68]

### Positive expiratory pressure (PEP) mask

An anesthesia face mask with a variable resistance one-way expiratory valve is the centerpiece of this technique. Resistance generated by the expiratory valve induces positive pressure within the airways. The pressure appears to stabilize smaller airways and prevents their collapse. By reducing or preventing small-airway collapse, the likelihood of peripheral air-trapping is decreased, which, most importantly, enhances the mobilization and removal of secretions. A period of PEP breathing through the mask is used, perhaps with the patient in classical gravity-assisted drainage positions,[38] followed by the FET and directed coughing to expel mobilized secretions.

## ENHANCING COUGH

A reflex cough has four phases: irritation, inspiration, compression, and expulsion. A voluntary cough does not require the first phase. To be effective either cough must generate enough force to clear secretions from the first through the seventh generation bronchi.[54] Decreased secretion clearance results when any phase of coughing fails to meet this objective.

The physical therapist improves an impaired cough by counseling the patient in proper cough technique and by administering treatments that either increase the volume inspired, augment the compression force generated, or elicit a cough reflex. Proper cough technique requires that the patient inspire maximally; close the glottis; "bear down" by tightening the abdominal, perineal, gluteal, and shoulder depressor muscles; and cough no more than two times during each expulsive, expiratory phase. Proper cough technique after surgery additionally requires the application of incisional splinting.

Following are techniques used to improve cough:

1. Positioning—sitting in the forward-leaning posture with the neck flexed, the arms supported, and the feet firmly planted on the floor promotes effective coughing[51] (Fig. 19-12).
2. Forced expiration or huffing—forceful rapid expiration, or huffing, may induce a reflex cough by stimulation of the pulmonary mechanoreceptors.
3. Pressure—pressure applied to the extrathoracic trachea may elicit a reflex cough. Pressure applied to the midrectus abdominis area after inspiration may improve cough effectiveness if the pressure is suddenly released. Pressure applied along the lower costal

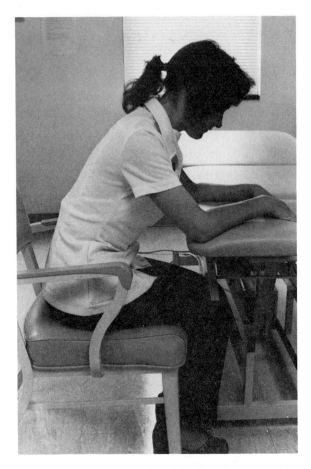

**Fig. 19-12.** The recommended position for effective coughing.

| **Table 19-8.** Objectives and potential outcomes of treatments administered to improve cough | |
| --- | --- |
| Therapeutic objective | Eliminate excessive retained secretions |
| Physiological objective | Increase the positive pressure developed during cough |
| Potential outcomes | Expectoration<br>Production of a reflex cough<br>Avoidance of cough complication<br>Elimination of the clinical signs of retained secretions<br>Appearance of a cough complication |

tary or reflex coughs are stronger than those voluntarily produced. Therefore patients who suffer from the following complications of cough should be taught controlled voluntary coughing or forced expiration to minimize the risk of complications:

1. Serum creatinine phosphokinase elevation
2. Rectus abdominis muscle rupture
3. Rib fracture
4. Pneumothorax
5. Fainting
6. Bradycardia
7. Vascular rupture
8. Heart block
9. Headache
10. Exhaustion
11. Vomiting
12. Urinary incontinence
13. Wound dehiscence
14. Sore throat

The physical therapy techniques administered to improve cough play a central role in the current practice of chest physical therapy. The objectives and potential outcomes of these techniques are summarized in Table 19-8.

## IMPROVING EXERCISE TOLERANCE

Patients with pulmonary disease often experience dyspnea on exertion. To avoid dyspnea, they may refrain from participating in any activity that precipitates this unpleasant sensation. The continued avoidance of activity may further decrease their exercise tolerance and, in turn, lower their dyspnea threshold. The physical therapy strategy most commonly used to break this vicious cycle is exercise. Because during exercise the work of breathing in patients with pulmonary disease may constitute a major portion of their oxygen consumption, the workload administered must be applied judiciously.[48]

### Exercise programs

Physical therapy programs administered to increase exercise tolerance vary widely. They may be formal, based

borders during exhalation may also improve the effectiveness of an impaired cough.

4. Manual ventilation—the high inspiratory flow rates produced by the forceful compression of a manual ventilator may stimulate the pulmonary mechanoreceptors and produce a reflex cough.[17]
5. Mechanical stimulation and suctioning—the direct application of mechanical stimulation to the airway may also induce a reflex cough.[93] However, if this direct stimulation fails to clear the airway, endotracheal suctioning is advisable.
6. Neuromuscular facilitation—the intermittent application of ice for 3 to 5 seconds along the paraspinal areas of the thoracic spine may also improve cough.[37] Because the application of ice has been associated with hypertension, candidates for this technique should be chosen carefully and monitored closely.

Although the literature describes several techniques to improve cough, few have scientifically evaluated cough effectiveness. Langlands[53] compared the effectiveness of voluntary and reflex coughs with forced expiration in a small population of normal subjects and patients with chronic bronchitis. The results of this study suggest that nonvolun-

on a strictly derived exercise prescription, or informal, started from an arbitrary point and progressed according to a patient's tolerance.[29] They may require special equipment like treadmills[72] or bicycle ergometers or merely require enough space to permit obstacle-free walking.[47] Participants may have either subacute pulmonary disease or chronic pulmonary disease of varying severity. Exercise may be administered while the patient breathes room air or supplemental oxygen.[9,12,97] Finally, completion of the programs may require several days, several months,[61] or as long as a year.[34]

Before administering any exercise program, the therapist must evaluate the medical history and the most recent clinical and laboratory data to identify any contraindications or precautions for exercise, as well as any indications for oxygen supplementation during exercise. The absolute and relative contraindications for any exercise testing are published elsewhere[3] and are not discussed here.

Following are some indications for oxygen-supplemented exercise[105]:

1. Right heart failure, cor pulmonale
2. Resting $PaO_2$ at 50 mm Hg
3. Inability to tolerate exercise while breathing room air
4. Oxygen desaturation during exercise while breathing room air

When patients tolerate 30 consecutive minutes of oxygen-supplemented exercise, one may progress the program by decreasing the level of supplemental oxygen.

Preparation for any exercise program also requires determining the degree of monitoring sophistication indicated to preserve the patient's safety. No formal guidelines that establish the monitoring requirements for informal exercise programs have been published; this determination must be made according to individual circumstances.

Final preparation for any exercise program requires that the therapist and patient identify a mutually acceptable goal for the program, develop a plan for periodically evaluating progress toward that goal, and, in asthmatics, discuss how the risk of exercise-induced bronchospasm[49] will be managed.

Bicycle ergometry to improve exercise tolerance is one technique that has been used successfully in formal programs. In addition to the preparation described above, a formal bicycle ergometry program requires a previously administered graded exercise test to determine the load at which the patient achieves his or her maximum oxygen consumption.

Following are steps for one method of implementing a conditioning program using bicycle ergometry:

1. Review the conditioning program with the patient. The review should include the purpose, expectations (risk to benefit), cost, and duration of the program (three 25-minute sessions per week for 4 weeks).

2. Differentiate between the roles and responsibilities of the patient and therapist.
3. Attach the ECG electrodes and obtain a base-line strip.
4. Measure the blood pressure with the patient lying supine and sitting.
5. Identify the symptoms that the patient should report immediately.
6. Direct the patient to mount the bicycle.
7. Cycle at 25 to 40 watts for 5 minutes to warm up.
8. Cycle at 75% of the previously determined maximum load.
9. Monitor the ECG every 5 minutes during the first exercise session and any time the patient reports chest pain, severe dyspnea, nausea, or palpitations.
10. Terminate the exercise in the presence of the following:
    a. Premature ventricular contractions in pairs, runs, or increasing frequency
    b. Atrial dysrhythmias: tachycardia, fibrillation, flutter
    c. Heart block, second or third degree
    d. Angina
    e. ST-segment changes of greater than or equal to 2 mm in either direction
    f. Persistent heart rate or blood pressure decline
    g. Elevation of diastolic pressure of more than 20 mm Hg greater than resting or more than 100 mm Hg
    h. Dyspnea, nausea, fatigue, dizziness, headache, blurred vision
    i. Intolerable musculoskeletal pain
    j. Heart rate greater than target
    k. Patent pallor, diaphoresis

Physical therapy can improve exercise tolerance. Six weeks of submaximal bicycle ergometry increased symptom-limited maximal oxygen uptake in 11 patients with moderate to severe chronic obstructive lung disease.[23] Vyas and colleagues[96] supported this finding, and Pierce's[72] research suggests that objective improvement is not specific to the bicycle but can also be associated with the treadmill.

The objectives and potential outcomes of physical therapy administered to improve exercise tolerance are summarized in Table 19-9.

## REDUCING PAIN

Pain is perceived when tissue is being damaged. The intensity of that perception depends on both the extent of tissue damage and the emotional reaction to the injury. To be effective, treatments administered to reduce pain must influence either the pathophysiological or the psychological aspects of pain, or both.

Physical therapists use many strategies in the management of pain. This section describes the use of one particular strategy, transcutaneous electrical nerve stimulation (TENS), in the management of the pain most frequently encountered in patients treated by chest physical therapists, postoperative pain.

**Table 19-9.** Objectives and potential outcomes of conditioning exercise administered to improve exercise tolerance

| | |
|---|---|
| Therapeutic objectives | Heighten dyspnea threshold<br>Increase exercise tolerance |
| Physiological objective | Improve maximum oxygen uptake |
| Potential outcomes | Increase walking, stepping, and cycling distance<br>Precipitation of dyspnea<br>Inability to progress breathing room air |

**Table 19-10.** Objectives for and potential outcomes of the postoperative application of transcutaneous electrical nerve stimulation (TENS)

| | |
|---|---|
| Therapeutic objective | Pain relief |
| Physiological objective | Physiological pain relief |
| Potential outcomes | Decreased narcotic requirement<br>No change of lower incidence of atelectasis<br>Increased forced vital capacity<br>Skin irritation<br>ECG or pacemaker interference |

### Transcutaneous electrical nerve stimulation (TENS)

TENS is a nonaddictive, noninvasive, non–habit-forming, relatively low-cost alternative to pharmaceutically induced analgesia for the management of acute postoperative pain. TENS may be most effective when a stimulator with dual-channel, variable voltage capability[80] applies a controlled, constant-current pulse[60] by way of crossed-channel electrodes.[80]

Ideally the electrodes would be placed close to the painful area[42,83] with the anode placed distally.[73] Because there may be some delay before the onset of the analgesia,[73] the stimulation would begin in the operating room and, ideally, be maintained constantly for at least 24[83] to 48[80] hours.

Because the only adverse effect associated with TENS is skin irritation,[52] any patient experiencing incisional pain may be a candidate for TENS. However, those who require electrocardiographic monitoring or artificial cardiac pacing should be offered other alternatives because TENS may affect monitoring feedback or pacemaker function.

Following is one method of administering TENS postoperatively:

1. Connect the leads to each channel according to the color code indicated on both the leads and the receptacles.
2. Abrade the electrode site with an alcohol scrub and then dry with gauze or clean toweling to lower skin resistance.
3. Coat electrodes with electrode gel.
4. Attach electrodes in crosswise fashion paraincisionally so that one electrode of channel 1 is, for example, on the upper right margin of the incision and the second electrode of channel 1 is on the lower left margin of the incision.
5. Secure electrodes in place with hypoallergenic tape.
6. Inform the patient and the nurse that you are initiating the treatment.
7. Instruct the patient to report any sensation perceived.
8. Ensure that the pulse rate is high.
9. Turn on the unit very slowly by increasing the intensity in both channels.

10. Continue to increase the intensity of both channels until a sensation is reported.
11. Increase the intensity slowly in both channels until the paraincisional area is numb: ideally this intensity should be below contractile threshold and be comfortable.
12. Maintain stimulation at this level until treatment ends.
13. Slowly decrease the intensity of stimulation in both channels until the unit is off.

Several investigators have evaluated the effectiveness of TENS in relieving postoperative pain. In their study of acute pain after thoracic and abdominal surgery, Hymes and others[42] reported a lower incidence of atelectasis in patients treated with TENS than in similar control groups. In addition, they discovered that TENS therapy was associated with reduced intensive care unit days and, for the most part, decreased length of hospital stay. In another study of acute pain, Vander Ark and McGrath[94] reported a high incidence of pain relief, 77% associated with TENS. They additionally noted that, in one third of the thoracic surgery patients studied, TENS lessened incisional pain by 50% and, as a result, obviated the need for analgesics. The finding that TENS decreased the narcotic requirement of postoperative patients was later supported by Rosenberg, Cutis, and Bourke,[76] whose research additionally uncovered a patient preference for TENS-induced analgesia over that which was pharmaceutically induced. This study could not, however, associate a lower incidence of atelectasis with TENS.

The impact of TENS on variables other than pain has also been explored. Noting that patients often associated a feeling of warmth with TENS, Dooley and Kasprak[24] examined the relationship between TENS and blood flow. Their results indicate that application of TENS along the peripheral nerve does not increase peripheral blood flow but TENS applied more centrally does. The effect of TENS on pulmonary function has also been explored. Stratton and Smith[88] reported higher forced vital capacities in patients treated with TENS after open thoracotomy than in a comparable control group.

This discussion suggests that TENS is an appropriate and effective therapeutic strategy for postoperative pain management. The objectives and potential outcomes of this treatment are summarized in Table 19-10.

## REFERENCES

1. Abboud RT and others: The effect of added expiratory obstruction on gas exchange in chronic airways obstruction, *Br J Dis Chest* 62:36, 1968.
2. Amborn SA: Clinical signs associated with the amount of tracheo-bronchial secretions, *Nurs Res* 25:121, 1976.
3. American College of Sports Medicine: *Guidelines for graded exercise testing and exercise prescription,* ed 2, Philadelphia, 1980, Lea & Febiger.
4. Anthonisen P and others: The value of lung physiotherapy in the treatment of acute exacerbations in chronic bronchitis, *Acta Med Scand* 175:715, 1964.
5. Barach AL: Chronic obstructive lung disease: postural relief of dyspnea, *Arch Phys Med Rehabil* 55:404, 1974.
6. Bateman JRM and others: Regional lung clearance of excessive secretions during chest physiotherapy in patients with stable chronic airways obstruction, *Lancet* 1(811):294, 1979.
7. Benson H: The physiology of meditation, *Sci Amer* 296:85, 1972.
8. Benson H: *The relaxation response,* New York, 1975, William Morrow & Co, Inc.
9. Block AJ and others: Chronic oxygen therapy treatment of chronic obstructive pulmonary disease at sea level, *Chest* 65:279, 1974.
10. Bolton JH and others: The rationale and results of breathing exercises in asthma, *Med J Aust* 2:675, 1956.
11. Brach BB and others: Xenon washout patterns during diaphragmatic breathing: studies in normal subjects and patients with chronic obstructive pulmonary disease, *Chest* 71:735, 1977.
12. Bradley BL and others: Oxygen assisted exercise in chronic obstructive lung disease, *Am Rev Respir Dis* 118:239, 1978.
13. Campbell AH and others: The effect of chest physiotherapy upon the FEV$_1$ in chronic bronchitis, *Med J Aust* 1:33, 1975.
14. Campbell EJM and Friend J: Action of breathing exercise in pulmonary emphysema, *Lancet* 19:325, 1955.
15. Casiari RJ and others: Effects of breathing retraining in patients with chronic obstructive pulmonary disease, *Chest* 79:393, 1981.
16. Chopra SK and others: Effects of hydration and physical therapy on tracheal transport velocity, *Am Rev Respir Dis* 115:1009, 1977.
17. Clemet AJ and Hubsch SC: Chest physiotherapy by the "bag squeezing" method: a guide to technique, *Physiotherapy* 54:355, 1968.
18. Comroe JH: *Physiology of respiration,* ed 2, Chicago, 1974, Year Book Medical Publishers.
19. Connors AF and others: Chest physical therapy: the immediate effect on oxygenation in acutely ill patients, *Chest* 78:L559, 1980.
20. Dab I and Alexander F: Evaluation of a particular bronchial drainage procedure called autogenic drainage. In Baran D, Van Bogaert E, editors: Chest physical therapy in cystic fibrosis and chronic obstructive pulmonary disease, Ghent, Belgium, 1977, European Press.
21. Dab I and Alexander F: The mechanism of autogenic drainage studied with flow-volume curves, *Monogr Paediat* 10:50, 1979.
22. Dean E and Ross J: Oxygen transport: The basis for contemporary cardiopulmonary physical therapy and its optimization with body positioning and mobilization, *Phys Ther Pract* 4:34, 1992.
23. Degre S and others: Hemodynamic responses to physical training in patients with chronic lung disease, *Am Rev Respir Dis* 110:395, 1974.
24. Dooley DM and Kasprak M: Modification of blood flow to the extremities by electrical stimulation of the nervous system, *South Med J* 69:1309, 1976.
25. Douglas WW: Improved oxygenation in patients with acute respir-atory failure: the prone position, *Am Rev Respir Dis* 115:559, 1977.
26. Emirgil C and others: A study of the long-term effect of therapy in chronic obstructive pulmonary disease, *Am J Med* 47:367, 1969.
27. Erskine J and Schonell M: Relaxation therapy in bronchial asthma, *J Psychosomatic Res* 23:131, 1979.
28. Faling LJ: Chest physical therapy. In Burton GG, Hodgkin JE, and Ward JJ, editors: *Respiratory care,* ed 3 Philadelphia, JB Lippincott, 1991.
29. Finer NN and Boyd J: Chest physiotherapy in the neonate: a controlled study, *Pediatrics* 61:141, 1977.
30. Gayrard P and others: Bronchoconstrictor effects of a deep inspiration in patients with asthma, *Am Rev Respir Dis* 111:433, 1975.
31. Gimenez M and others: Exercise training with oxygen supply and directed breathing in patients with chronic airway obstruction, *Respiration* 37:157, 1979.
32. Graham WCB and Bradley DA: Efficacy of chest physiotherapy and intermittent positive pressure breathing in the resolution of pneumonia, *N Engl J Med* 299:624, 1978.
33. Grimby G and others: Effects of abdominal breathing on the distribution of ventilation in lung disease, *Clin Sci Molec Med* 148:193, 1975.
34. Guthrie AG and Petty TL: Improved exercise tolerance in patients with chronic airway obstruction, *Phys Ther* 50:335, 1970.
35. Hammon WE and Martin RJ: Fatal pulmonary hemorrhage associated with chest physical therapy, *Phys Ther* 59:1247, 1979.
36. Harmony W: Segmental breathing, *Phys Ther Rev* 36:106, 1956.
37. Hedges J and Bridges CJ: Stimulation of the cough reflex, *Am J Nurs* 68:347, 1968.
38. Hofmyer JL, Webber BA, and Hodson ME: Evaluation of positive expiratory pressure as an adjunct to chest physiotherapy in the treatment of cystic fibrosis, *Thorax* 41:951, 1986.
39. Howell S and Hill JD: Chest physical therapy procedures in open heart surgery, *Phys Ther* 58:1205, 1978.
40. Huber AW and others: Effect of chest physiotherapy on asthmatic children, *J Allergy Clin Immunol* 53:109, 1974.
41. Hughes RC: Does abdominal breathing affect regional gas exchange? *Chest* 76:258, 1979.
42. Hymes AC and others: Acute pain control by electrostimulation: a preliminary report, *Adv Neurol* 4:761, 1974.
43. Ingram RH Jr and Schilder DP: Effect of pursed-lips expiration on the pulmonary pressure-flow relationship in obstructive lung disease, *Am Rev Respir Dis* 96:38, 1967.
44. Innocenti DM: Breathing exercises in the treatment of emphysema, *Physiotherapy* 52:437, 1966.
45. Jacobsen E: *Progressive relaxation,* Chicago, 1938, University of Chicago Press.
46. Kang B and others: Evaluation of postural drainage with percussion in chronic obstructive lung disease, *J Allergy Clin Immunol* 53:109, 1974.
47. Kass I and Rubin H: Chest physiotherapy for chronic obstructive pulmonary disease, *Postgrad Med* 48:145, 1970.
48. Keens TG: Exercise training programs for pediatric patients with chronic lung disease, *Pediatr Clin North Am* 26:517, 1979.
49. Khan AU and Olson DL: Physical therapy and exercise-induced bronchospasm, *Phys Ther* 55:878, 1975.
50. Kigin CM: Chest physical therapy for the postoperative or traumatic injury patient, *Phys Ther* 61:1724, 1981.
51. Lagerson J: The cough: its effectiveness depends on you, *Respir Care* 18:434, 1973.
52. Lampe GN: Introduction to the use of transcutaneous electrical nerve stimulation devices, *Phys Ther* 58:1450, 1978.
53. Langlands J: The dynamics of cough in health and in chronic bronchitis, *Thorax* 22:88, 1967.
54. Leith EE: Cough. In Hislop H and Sanger JO, editors: *Chest disorders in children,* New York, 1968, American Physical Therapy Association.

55. Levine A: Chest physical therapy for children with pneumonia, *J Am Osteopath Assoc* 78:101, 1978.

56. Lord GM and others: A clinical, radiologic, and physiologic evaluation of chest therapy *J Maine Med Assoc* 60:143, 1972.

57. Lorin MI and Denning CR: Evaluation of postural drainage by measurement of sputum volume and consistency, *Am J Phys Med* 50:215, 1971.

58. Mackenzie CF and others: Chest physiotherapy: the effect on arterial oxygenation, *Anesth Analg* 57:28, 1978.

59. Martin DJ and others: Chest physiotherapy and the distribution of ventilation, *Chest* 69:174, 1976.

60. Mason CP: Testing of electrical transcutaneous stimulators for suppressing pain, *Bull Prosthet Res* 25:38, 1976.

61. McGavin CR and others: Physical rehabilitation for the chronic bronchitic: results of a controlled trial of exercises in the home, *Thorax* 32:307, 1977.

62. Merrick J and Axen K: Inspiratory muscle function following abdominal weight exercises in healthy subjects, *Phys Ther* 61:651, 1981.

63. Miller WP: A physiological evaluation of the effects of diaphragmatic breathing training in patients with chronic pulmonary emphysema, *Am J Med* 17:471, 1954.

64. Motley JC: The effects of slow deep breathing on the blood gas exchange in emphysema, *Am Rev Respir Dis* 88:484, 1963.

65. Mueller RE and others: Ventilation and arterial blood gas changes induced by pursed-lips breathing, *J Appl Physiol* 28:784, 1970.

66. Murray JF: The ketchup-bottle method, *N Engl J Med* 300:1155, 1979.

67. Newton DA and Stephenson AL: Effect of physiotherapy on pulmonary function, *Lancet* 2(8083):228, 1978.

68. Partridge C, Pryor J, and Webber B: Characteristics of the forced expiratory technique, *Physiotherapy* 75:193, 1989.

69. Paul G and others: Some effects of slowing respiration rate in chronic emphysema and bronchitis, *J Appl Physiol* 21:877, 1966.

70. Pham QT and others: Respiratory function and the theological status of bronchial secretions collected by spontaneous expectoration and after physiotherapy, *Bull Pathophysiol Resp* 9:295, 1973.

71. Piehl MA and Brown RS: Use of extreme position changes in acute respiratory failure, *Crit Care Med* 4:13, 1976.

72. Pierce AK and others: Responses to exercise training in patients with emphysema, *Arch Intern Med* 173:28, 1964.

73. Pike PMG: Transcutaneous electrical stimulation: its use in the management of postoperative pain, *Anaesthesia* 33:165, 1978.

74. Pryor JA and others: Evaluation of the forced expiratory technique as an adjunct to postural drainage in treatment of cystic fibrosis, *Br Med J* 2:417, 1979.

75. Reed JMW: Localized breathing exercises in surgical chest condition, *Br J Phys Med* 16:111, 1953.

76. Rosenberg M and others: Transcutaneous electrical nerve stimulation for the relief of post operative pain, *Pain* 5:129, 1978.

77. Rossman CM and others: Effect of chest physiotherapy on the removal of mucus in patients with cystic fibrosis, *Am Rev Respir Dis* 126:131, 1982.

78. Roussos CS and others: Voluntary factors influencing the distribution of inspired gas, *Am Rev Respir Dis* 116:457, 1977.

79. Sackner MA and others: Distribution of ventilation during diaphragmatic breathing in obstructive lung disease, *Am Rev Respir Dis* 109:331, 1974.

80. Santiesteban AM and Sanders BR: Establishing a postsurgical TENS program, *Phys Ther* 60:789, 1980.

81. Schutz K: Muscular exercise in the treatment of bronchial asthma, *NY J Med* 55:635, 1935.

82. Seaton D and others: Effect of body position on gas exchange after thoracotomy, *Thorax* 34:518, 1979.

83. Shealy CM and Maurer D: Transcutaneous electrical stimulation for control of pain, *Surg Neurol* 2:45, 1974.

84. Shearer MC and others: Lung ventilation during diaphragmatic breathing, *Phys Ther* 52:139, 1972

85. Sinclair JD: The effect of breathing exercises in pulmonary emphysema, *Thorax* 10:246, 1955.

86. Slonim NB and Hamilton LH: Respiratory physiology ed 5, St Louis, 1987, Mosby.

87. Stern RC and others: Treatment and prognosis of massive hemoptysis in cystic fibrosis, *Am Rev Respir Dis* 117:825, 1978.

88. Stratton SA and Smith MM: Postoperative thoracotomy: effect of transcutaneous electrical nerve stimulation on forced vital capacity, *Phys Ther* 60:45, 1980.

89. Tecklin JS and Holsclaw DS: Evaluation of bronchial drainage in patients with cystic fibrosis, *Phys Ther* 55:1081, 1975.

90. Thacker WE: Postural drainage and respiratory control, London, 1947, Lloyd-Luke.

91. Thoman RL and others: The efficacy of pursed-lips breathing in patients with chronic obstructive pulmonary disease, *Am Rev Respir Dis* 93:100, 1966.

92. Thoren L: Post-operative pulmonary complication: observations on their prevention by means of physiotherapy, *Acta Chir Scand* 107:193, 1954.

93. Ungvarski P: Mechanical stimulation of coughing, *Am J Nurs* 71:2358, 1971.

94. Vander Ark GD and McGrath KA: Transcutaneous electrical stimulation in the treatment of postoperative pain, *Am J Surg* 130:338, 1975.

95. Vraciu JK and Vraciu RA: Effectiveness of breathing exercises in preventing pulmonary complications following open heart surgery, *Phys Ther* 57:1367, 1977.

96. Vyas MN and others: Response to exercise in patients with chronic airway obstruction: effects of exercise training, *Am Rev Respir Dis* 103:390, 1977.

97. Vyas MN and others: Response to exercise in patients with chronic airway obstruction. II. Effects of breathing 40 per cent oxygen, *Am Rev Respir Dis* 103:401, 1977.

98. Wade OL: Movements of the thoracic cage and diaphragm in respiration, *J Physiol* 124:193, 1954.

99. Ward RJ and others: An evaluation of postoperative respiratory maneuvers, *Surg Gynecol Obstet* 123:51, 1976.

100. Watts N: Improvement of breathing patterns. In Hislop HE and Sanger JO, editors: *Chest disorders in children,* New York, 1968, American Physical Therapy Association.

101. Westreich N and others: Breathing retraining, *Minn Med* 53:621, 1970.

102. Wiklander O and Norlin U: Effect of physiotherapy on postoperative pulmonary complications: a clinical and roentgenographic study of 200 cases, *Acta Chir Scand* 112:246, 1957.

103. Winning TJ and others: A simple clinical method of quantifying the effects of chest physiotherapy in mechanically-ventilated patients, *Anaesth Intensive Care* 3:237, 1975.

104. Winning TJ and others: Bronchodilators and physiotherapy during long-term mechanical ventilation of the lungs, *Anaesth Intensive Care* 5:48, 1977.

105. Woolf CR: A rehabilitation program for improving exercise tolerance of patients with chronic lung disease, *Can Med Assoc J* 106:119, 1972.

106. Zack MB and others: The effect of lateral positions on gas exchange in pulmonary disease, *Am Rev Respir Dis* 110:49, 1974.

107. Zadai CC: Physical therapy for the acutely ill medical patient, *Phys Ther* 61:1746, 1981.

# Physical Therapy for Patients with Cardiac, Thoracic, or Abdominal Conditions Following Surgery or Trauma

*P. Cristina Imle*

Pulmonary complications occur in up to 60% of patients who undergo cardiac, thoracic or upper abdominal surgery.[3,26,42] Trauma to the chest wall (or spine) also results in an increased incidence of lung pathology. Patients who smoke, are obese, elderly (over 70 years of age) or have preexisting lung disease are at greater risk of developing respiratory difficulties following surgery or trauma.[59,73,148,158] Chest physical therapy is advocated to prevent and treat pulmonary complications.[21,73,89,144] This chapter discusses the role of atelectasis and alveolar collapse related to surgery and trauma. It describes the components of chest physical therapy and the related literature on its efficacy in reversing these pulmonary complications. The use of common intensive care unit (ICU) equipment is presented along with its impact on physical therapy treatment. Traumatic injuries and cardiac, thoracic, or abdominal surgeries that are often associated with atelectasis and secretion retention are reviewed, as are methods of relieving postoperative pain. Although pediatric cardiac procedures are presented, physical therapy specific to this patient population is not addressed, but is covered in Chapters 25, 26 and 27. Some procedures and frequently used terms that are not defined in the chapter appear in the glossary (see pp. 605-608).

## POSTOPERATIVE PULMONARY COMPLICATIONS

Hypoxemia and impaired gas exchange can occur during general anesthesia and persist after surgery.[105] Atelectasis from progressive alveolar collapse was initially proposed as the mechanism behind these changes.[7] More recent studies suggest that atelectasis after surgery is due to a combination of many factors, including reduced arousal, decreased lung volumes and alveolar ventilation, altered pulmonary mechanics, impaired cough, and pain.[29] Decreases in surfactant and the effects of dry inhaled gases and tracheal tubes on ciliary action also have been implicated.[158] Pulmonary complications can occur from direct trauma to the lungs, increased pulmonary vascular pressures, or injury to the left phrenic nerve during thoracic or cardiac procedures.[36,73,77] Reports of decreased functional residual capacity (FRC), compression of dependent areas of the lung and diaphragmatic dysfunction are associated particularly with thoracic and upper abdominal surgery.[33,35,41,42,61,64,118,134]

### Chest physical therapy and bronchoscopy

Both chest physical therapy and bronchoscopy are advocated to treat atelectasis and secretion retention from lung injury and surgery. Two studies have evaluated physical therapy and bronchoscopy on the resolution of postoperative atelectasis.[72,99] Both authors conclude that in acute atelectasis, therapeutic bronchoscopy offers no demonstrable benefit over chest physical therapy. Three case studies have shown physical therapy superior to bronchoscopy in treating lobar collapse in ICU patients.[21,67] Physical therapy has advantages over therapeutic bronchoscopy, including fewer reported complications, decreased cost, and the need for less sedation. Also, chest physical therapy appears better able to clear peripheral secretions and is not limited by tracheal tube size. For these reasons, physical therapy is recommended as the treatment of choice for acute atelectasis; bronchoscopy should be reserved for patients who are unresponsive to or unable to tolerate chest physical therapy.[67] Precautions to physical therapy and modifications in treatment are addressed as they relate to specific diagnoses throughout this chapter.

### Pneumonia

Untreated atelectasis usually leads to clinical manifestations associated with bacterial pneumonia.[128] These symptoms include a positive sputum culture, fever, leukocytosis, and radiological evidence of infiltrates. The diagnosis of pneumonia is often difficult to make in postoperative patients in the ICU. Positive sputum cultures are common in patients requiring tracheal intubation but may not indicate lung pathology.[89,126] Oral or gastric secretions can contaminate expectorated sputum.[128] Both white blood cell and temperature elevation can occur from other causes after surgery or trauma, and infiltrates on chest radiograph may clear with chest physical therapy[89] as is shown in Case 1 on pp. 377-378.

It is generally maintained that the majority of postoperative pneumonias begin as atelectasis[128] and that retained lung secretions are a good culture medium for infection. If a pneumonia-like process is adequately treated by physical therapy early in its development, pneumonia may be prevented. However, well-established pneumonia does not usually benefit from chest physical therapy. Instead, appropriate antibiotic therapy along with systemic and local hydration are the recognized treatment for bacterial pneumonias.[92] Chest physical therapy may help some patients who have copious secretions while undergoing standard treatment for pneumonia.

## CHEST PHYSICAL THERAPY

Chest physical therapy is often advocated to prevent and treat atelectasis following trauma or surgery.[90,126,158] Although chest physical therapy has been used to improve respiratory function for more than a century,[111] its role in preventing postoperative pulmonary complications remains controversial. First, uniform agreement of what constitutes a significant respiratory complication after surgery is lacking.[73] Also, there is controversy over what component(s) of physical therapy best treat(s) atelectasis and secretion retention. Part of the confusion stems from a lack of standardization of what is meant by the term chest physical therapy, which is poorly defined in most studies. It is reasonable to expect that some measures directed at preventing atelectasis would differ from those aimed at treatment. Other discrepancies about the efficacy of physical therapy arise when study results pertaining to chronic lung disease are extrapolated to patients with acute pathology. Even when postoperative atelectasis is present, different physical therapy treatment may be indicated for the patient requiring mechanical ventilation or other medical support than the stable patient who is spontaneously breathing.

To avoid further confusion, the term chest physical therapy as used throughout this chapter, refers to the components shown in the box top left on page 379. To determine which treatment component(s) and modifications are indicated, careful assessment of the patient should precede each therapy session. Details on respiratory assessment are

---

**CASE 1    19-Year-Old Male Following Major Trauma**

A 19-year-old male was admitted by helicopter directly from the scene of an automobile accident. The patient was a passenger in a truck hit by a train. He arrived unconscious, with a right tension pneumothorax, absent bowel sounds and hematuria. Chest radiograph showed fracture of the first right and second left ribs. Minilaparotomy was positive, and the patient went to the operating room for placement of an intracranial pressure monitor (intracranial pressure = 9 mm Hg) and for laparotomy, which revealed a ruptured spleen and renal contusion.

The patient remained unconscious for 17 days because of cerebral contusion. Starting nine days after admission, *Pseudomonas aeruginosa* was grown for three successive days from tracheal cultures. Maximum daily temperature, white blood cell count and chest radiograph findings from the time of positive tracheal cultures are shown in Table 20-1.

Eleven days after admission, there was no obvious source for the leukocytosis and pyrexia, and the chest radiograph was not thought to be sufficient to account for these changes despite the positive tracheal cultures. On the twelfth day after admission, the morning chest radiograph showed development of fluffy infiltrates in the left lower lobe (LLL) and right middle and lower lobes (Fig. 20-1). These, and clinical examination, were thought to be compatible with a LLL pneumonia. Tobramycin and ticarcillin were suggested but not given, because, following 45 minutes of chest physical therapy (positioning, percussion, vibration, and airway suctioning), arterial oxygenation ($Pa_{O_2}$), total lung/thorax compliance, and temperature all improved significantly (Table 20-1). A repeat chest radiograph also showed improvement.

The leukocytosis and pyrexia decreased (Table 20-1) and the chest radiograph showed marked improvement by the following morning (Fig. 20-2). The patient had two further chest physical therapy treatments, on days 14 (Fig. 20-3) and 15 (Fig. 20-4). The chest radiograph confirmed complete resolution, and the patient was extubated on the seventeenth day after admission. The laboratory, chest radiograph, and clinical data strongly suggest that chest physical therapy had played a significant role in reversing this patient's pneumonia.

*Figures 20-1 to 20-4 for this case are on page 378.

**Table 20-1.** Maximum daily temperature ($T_{max}$), white blood cell count (WBC) and chest radiograph findings from a patient with signs and symptoms of pneumonia (see case study)

| Day from admission | $T_{max}$ (° F) | WBC | Chest radiograph |
|---|---|---|---|
| 9 | 101.6 | 24,600 | Clear |
| 10 | 101.8 | 33,800 | Clear |
| 11 | 102.6 | 37,400 | Slight infiltrate LLL* and RML* |
| 12 | 103 | 26,100 | Fig. 20-1 |
| **First chest physical therapy treatment given** | | | |
| 13 | 100.4 | 27,600 | Fig. 20-2 |
| 14 | 101.8 | 22,500 | Fig. 20-3 |
| 15 | 100.8 | 24,200 | Fig. 20-4 |

*LLL = left lower lobe; RML = right middle lobe.
Adapted from Mackenzie CF: Clinical indications and usage of chest physiotherapy. In Mackenzie CF, editor: *Chest physiotherapy in the intensive care unit*, Baltimore, 1989, Williams & Wilkins.

---

outlined in Chapter 18. Treatment goals for patients after surgery or injury to the heart, chest or upper abdomen are to assist in secretion removal, regain range of motion (ROM), restore mobility, prevent venous thrombosis, and to aid in pain management.[161] Along with the use of preoperative physical therapy, information on these treatment components is described.

### Preoperative physical therapy

The intent of preoperative education is to reassure the patient and allay anxiety, which may diminish pain and hasten recovery.[73] Information on chest physical therapy helps familiarize the patient with what will be expected and allows the therapist to establish realistic goals for treatment after surgery. Preferential preoperative education should be given to patients at increased risk for developing pulmonary complications after surgery. This includes patients with advanced age, poor nutrition or musculoskeletal disease, and those who smoke, are obese or produce excess secretions.[73] At times, treatment is needed before surgery to optimize lung function in patients with one or more of these conditions and atelectasis. Physical therapy in this situation differs very little from what is described below for patients with secretion retention following surgery or lung injury.

Structured preoperative training by nurses resulted in improved postoperative lung function when compared to a control group of patients undergoing abdominal surgery.[81] In earlier studies preoperative physical therapy was associated with a decreased incidence of postoperative pulmonary complications,[13,131,142,148,151] and hospital stay.[131] A recent report found no benefit from preoperative education and instruction in patients undergoing coronary artery

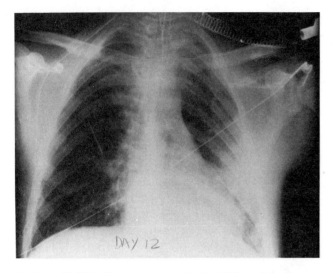

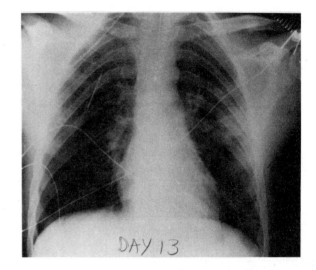

**Fig. 20-1.** Fluffy infiltrates are present in the left lower lobe, lingula, and right lower lobe developed on the twelfth day after admission. (From MacKenzie CF: Clinical indications and usage of chest physiotherapy. In MacKenzie CF, editor: *Chest physiotherapy in the intensive care unit,* Baltimore, 1989, Williams & Wilkins.)

**Fig. 20-2.** Marked clearing of the pneumonitis was evident on the day after chest physical therapy was given. (From MacKenzie CF: Clinical indications and usage of chest physiotherapy. In MacKenzie CF, editor: *Chest physiotherapy in the intensive care unit,* Baltimore, 1989, Williams & Wilkins.)

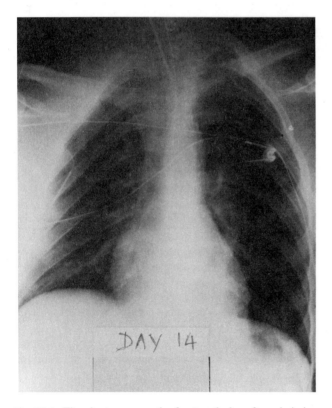

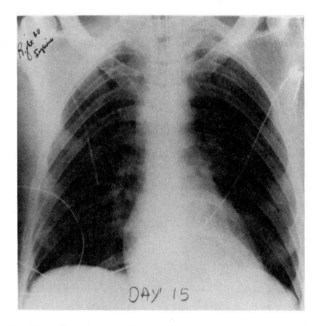

**Fig. 20-4.** Complete resolution of pneumonia occurred on the fifteenth day after admission. (From MacKenzie CF: Clinical indications and usage of chest physiotherapy. In MacKenzie CF, editor: *Chest physiotherapy in the intensive care unit,* Baltimore, 1989, Williams & Wilkins.)

**Fig. 20-3.** The chest x-ray on the fourteenth day after admission. (From MacKenzie CF: Clinical indications and usage of chest physiotherapy. In MacKenzie CF, editor: *Chest physiotherapy in the intensive care unit,* Baltimore, 1989, Williams & Wilkins.)

surgery.[144A] Reimbursement for preoperative physical therapy tends to make it the exception rather than the rule in the United States. When preoperative education and instruction are provided, it should include all components that are

pertinent to the individual patient (see the box top right on p. 379) and be coordinated with other clinicians involved in patient education.

## Positioning

This term refers to placing the body in one of 11 positions to achieve gravity assisted drainage of specific lung segments. These positions, shown in Chapter 19, are also

| Components of chest physical therapy |
| --- |
| Positioning<br>Manual techniques<br>   Percussion<br>   Vibration<br>Cough<br>Suctioning<br>Breathing exercises<br>Mobilization |

| Basic components of preoperative chest physical therapy |
| --- |
| Knowledge of:<br>   pertinent medical history<br>   laboratory values<br>   preoperative studies<br>Brief description of intended surgery<br>   including incision placement<br>Explanation of usual monitoring and support equipment*<br>   ECG leads<br>   endotracheal tubes<br>   chest tubes<br>   intravascular lines<br>   nasogastric tubes<br>Assessment<br>   chest exam with auscultation†<br>   musculoskeletal exam‡<br>Instruction in:*<br>   breathing exercises<br>   cough techniques<br>   range of motion and exercises§<br>   positioning<br>   manual techniques<br>   mobilization<br>Concerns of the patient |

\* See sections in this chapter for more details on these topics.

†If evidence of atelectasis or secretion retention is present during the preoperative assessment, the need for physical therapy treatment should be addressed.

‡A brief exam is performed, as needed, to assess preoperative ability.

§Range of motion is emphasized when appropriate; shoulder motion is stressed in patients undergoing thoracotomy or median sternotomy. Extremity exercises are appropriate for patients who are confined to bed or scheduled for saphenous vein graft.

referred to as bronchial or postural drainage. Alterations in cardiac[121] and respiratory function[119,164] normally occur with position changes and some persist beyond the period of adjustment. At resting tidal volumes, progressive airway collapse results from decreases in FRC and increases in closing volume when normal subjects are moved from sitting, to supine, to head-down.[27] Normally in sitting, both blood flow and ventilation are greater in the dependent lung zones and no significant changes in gas exchange occur between right and left decubitus positions.[100,164] In patients undergoing coronary artery bypass, FRC significantly improved in upright sitting and right side-lying compared to slouched sitting both before and after surgery.[74] No improvement in diaphragm function or respiratory pressures occurred with raising the head up 30° compared to flat in patients after thoracotomy for lung resection.[43]

When a unilateral lung condition[30,39,48,119,164] or pleural effusion[110,138] is present, most studies report improved arterial oxygenation and saturation when the patient is positioned with the "good lung down." This is the usual position for delivering chest physical therapy, with the involved lung zone uppermost. However, in some patients (with unilateral central airway lesions or effusions) improved gas exchange occurred when the lung with pathology was dependent.[15,16,96] It becomes more difficult to predict the best position for optimal lung function in patients with bilateral lung pathology. Ventilation and gas exchange also depend on the tidal volume and if there are spontaneous or ventilator delivered breaths.[18,43] Although placing the "good lung down" probably has advantages in most cases of unilateral lung disease, a patient's individual response to treatment cannot be presumed and should be continually assessed.

The effects of positioning may be responsible for the hypoxemia noted by some investigators during chest physical therapy,[23,51] particularly in patients with cardiovascular instability. Hypoxemia or decreased cardiac function are not routine findings during or after physical therapy treatment for acute lung pathology; nor were they reported in mechanically ventilated trauma patients who required positive and expiratory pressure (PEEP)[95] or who were spontaneously breathing,[90] but they may occur in individual situations. A regression analysis of the arterial oxygenation changes in a group of critically ill patients

during therapy showed that those with lower baseline values had a less dramatic fall in oxygenation during therapy.[154] These investigators suggest careful patient monitoring during treatment but that chest physical therapy need not be withheld in patients with $Pao_2 > 60$ mm Hg. A more conservative guide to prevent hypoxemia recommends that the fraction of inspired oxygen ($Fio_2$) be increased before and during postural drainage for patients in whom a drop in $Pao_2$ of 20 mm Hg is considered hazardous and that interruptions in PEEP should be avoided (see suctioning).[92] Monitoring of arterial saturation ($Sao_2$) provides the therapist with continuous feedback on a patient's response to treatment. The $Fio_2$ should be increased if the $Sao_2$ falls below 90% (corresponding to a $Pao_2$ of about 60 mm Hg) during chest physical therapy.[92]

There is some evidence supporting the use of prone positioning to improve oxygenation following acute lung injury.[84A] When indicated, many patients can be moved into the prone position. Before doing so, however, the physical therapist must have thorough knowledge of the patient's surgical procedures and associated injuries, and must ensure that all ICU lines, drains, and other equipment are functioning properly while the patient is prone.[18]

The majority of postural drainage positions involve turning the patient and tilting the bed head-down or into the Trendelenburg position. Repositioning patients after surgery or trauma is often painful and should be coordinated with adequate pain management, discussed later. The head-down position can be used without complication in many patients requiring intensive care. However, close monitoring of ECG, intravascular pressures and Sao$_2$ is recommended, particularly in cases of advanced age, brain injury or cardiac compromise.[47,53,90,92] In these patients there should be clear indications and expected benefits to physical therapy. When head-flat is substituted for head-down positioning, longer duration or multiple treatments may be needed to achieve the desired results. Many research clinicians use only bed-flat positioning (with or without turning) during chest physical therapy to minimize the need for equipment recalibration and the normal changes that occur when moving a patient head-down. In this chapter, the term positioning or postural drainage implies treatment to a specific area of the lung with pathology, including a head-down tilt when appropriate; positioning does not mean arbitrary side-to-side turning as part of a general postoperative routine to improve respiratory function. The latter falls under the description of mobilization and is discussed under that heading.

### Manual techniques

Percussion and vibration are two manual techniques used in conjunction with postural drainage. Both are thought to facilitate secretion clearance of both the large and small airways. Variation exists in applying manual techniques and research on the mechanism of action is lacking.[68] Percussion consists of rhythmic "clapping" with cupped hands, usually on bare skin, over the area of lung involvement and is performed during inspiration and expiration. It should not cause a slapping sound or exacerbate pain (see below). Manual percussion is applied at a rate of 100 to 400 times per minute and imparts between 2 to 4 foot-pounds or 58 to 65 Newtons of force.[40,53,108,156,162]

Complications attributed to percussion are rare. A single case of fatal pulmonary hemorrhage during positioning and "light" percussion is reported in a patient with squamous cell carcinoma and lung abscess[55] although the cause and effect are not clear since both lung abscess and malignancy increase the risk of spontaneous hemorrhage.[79] Increased bronchospasm is associated with percussion in some patients with chronic lung disease. When used to treat acute secretion retention, percussion has been used without complication in patients with lung contusion, subcutaneous emphysema, bronchopleural fistula, and multiple rib fractures. For patients with chest incisions, drainage tubes, or rib fractures, adequate analgesia is necessary to diminish pain, and manual techniques should be performed only by experienced personnel. Percussion (and most physical therapy techniques) should not be used in the case of an untreated pneumothorax or marked thrombocytopenia.[68]

Vibration differs from percussion in that it is performed during expiration. The force of vibration varies depending on the patient's condition and the therapist's bias. More vigorous forms are referred to as "rib springing" or "chest shaking." Some clinicians have used vibration together with hyperinflation, often termed "bag squeezing." This combination is not recommended as it causes fluctuations in thoracic pressure that adversely effect cardiac output[87] and intracranial pressure.[47] Frequencies of 12 to 20 Hertz are reported for manual vibration and about 2 Hertz for chest shaking.[4,51,147] Because of the shaking component of vibration, there is controversy as to whether this technique should be used on patients with rib, sternal, or thoracic spine fractures.[68,79]

Research of the efficacy of manual techniques in acute lung disease is lacking; however, in conjunction with positioning, they are successful in reversing or treating acute atelectasis.[20,56,95,99,144] Although not directly applicable to normal treatment of air-filled lungs, manual percussion was superior to either mechanical percussion or no manual technique in patients undergoing bronchopulmonary lavage for alveolar proteinosis.[57] Both percussion and vibration are thought to hasten the effects of postural drainage and may offer particular benefit in patients with acute atelectasis; when cooperation is decreased, mechanical ventilation is required or cough is impaired. In theory, a decreased chance for infection exists if secretions are removed expeditiously. There appears to be no benefit, and some disadvantages to using mechanical percussors or vibrators in patients after surgery or trauma.[68]

### Cough and suctioning

Both coughing and suctioning are used to clear upper airway secretions. It is generally agreed that removal of excess mucus is advantageous and some people suggest measuring sputum to assess chest physical therapy efficacy. Murray[109] proposed that at least 30 ml of sputum should be removed during physical therapy for treatment to be of benefit. However, there are many sources for error in measuring sputum volume and 30 ml has not been found to be an appropriate guideline when treating acute lung pathology. There are reports of atelectasis resolution and improved lung-thorax compliance when less than 30 ml of secretions are removed.[90,144] The area of the lung that is cleared of secretions (periphery versus central airways) is probably of greater significance than the volume removed.[89,90]

Coughing is very effective in removing secretions and foreign objects from the trachea and mainstem bronchi, but it produces little if any narrowing beyond four generations (trachea = 0).[135,136] A normal cough is composed of an inspiratory effort, glottic closure, contraction of the expiratory muscles and then opening of the glottis.[88] Forced expiration differs from a cough in that glottic closure does not occur. Other conditions that limit glottic closure (such as tracheal tubes) or limit inspiratory or expiratory function (such as neuromuscular disease or paralysis) diminish cough efficacy. Cough can also be suppressed volitionally because of pain or fear following surgery.[71] Effective pain management and discussion on the importance of clearing secretions may improve patient cooperation.

A variety of methods are described to facilitate cough in patients after surgery. (1) External tracheal compression and oropharyngeal suctioning can elicit a cough in patients with decreased levels of consciousness or cooperation. Because of associated complications, nasotracheal suctioning should be avoided in nonintubated patients. (2) "Huffing" consists of a single large inspiration, followed by short expiratory efforts that are interrupted with pauses. The glottis remains open during huffing, which reduces the potential for side effects that may occur from cough (bronchoconstriction, spasms of coughing, and marked swings in thoracic pressure or cerebral blood flow). (3) Vibration can mechanically stimulate a cough by oscillating secretions within the larger airways, and breathing exercises may be used to augment the inspiratory or expiratory component of cough.[71] (4) Forced expiratory technique FET is another method to clear bronchial secretions, particularly in persons with chronic lung disease.[115] This technique is described under breathing exercises.

When mechanical ventilation is required, suctioning is used to clear secretions from the upper airways. Guidelines for suctioning patients are shown in the box below, however, some procedures vary among institutions. Hypoxemia and cardiac dysrhythmia are two complications often associated with suctioning. These may be minimized by ensuring adequate oxygenation before suctioning. A variety of

---

### Guidelines for suctioning

Suctioning is a *sterile* procedure.

Gloves, mask and eye protection should be worn.

Catheter size should be ≤ one half the internal diameter of the artificial airway.

Negative pressure of 100-160 mm Hg is used to suction adults.

Using an occlusive port adaptor has advantages and minimizes disruption of mechanical ventilation.

Each pass of the suction catheter should last ≤ 15 seconds.

Supplemental oxygen should be given before and after each pass of the catheter.*

Patients who are breathing spontaneously should receive lung inflation with a resuscitator bag *before and after* each pass of the suction catheter.

Insert the sterile catheter into the airway *gently*.

Apply suction *only* while withdrawing the catheter.

Adapted from Imle PC and Klemic N: Methods of airway clearance: coughing and suctioning. In Mackenzie CF, editor: *Chest physiotherapy in the intensive care unit*, Baltimore, 1989, Williams & Wilkins.

*Patients receiving mechanical ventilation may not require changes in fraction of inspired oxygen.

---

methods have been investigated including insufflation, hyperventilation, hyperinflation and hyperoxygenation. Increasing the $F_{IO_2}$ prior to suctioning is indicated for patients with cardiac disease or signs of hypoxemia. Using an occlusive port adaptor is advantageous if ventilator flow rates are adequate; it helps to preserve PEEP, mean airway pressure and tidal volume, and increasing the $F_{IO_2}$ may not be necessary.[71] A suction catheter routinely enters the right mainstem bronchus. Cannulation of the left side is improved by using a curved tip catheter and may be beneficial when pathology is present in the left lung. Both mechanical trauma and bacterial contamination can occur from improper suctioning technique. Care is needed to prevent contamination when patients are suctioned in some of the postural drainage positions.[71]

### Breathing exercises

Encouraging patients to take deep breaths is a relatively easy and logical means to reverse the decrease in respiratory function that occurs after surgery. The main goals of breathing exercises for postoperative patients are to assist in lung reexpansion and removal of secretions, increase chest wall mobility, promote relaxation, and improve the pattern of breathing.[18,161] Localized or segmental breathing exercises are described in the literature (see Chapter 19), but research does not support their ability to alter regional lung ventilation.[54,101] However, the potential for benefit from breathing exercises should not be ignored; increases in inspired volume can improve alveolar ventilation and cough ability.

When compared to a control group, most studies demonstrate a decreased incidence of pulmonary complications when breathing exercises are included in physical therapy treatment after surgery.[14,28,106,123,149] Virtually all breathing exercises emphasize the inspiratory component of respiration; some also include expiration by instructing patients to exhale maximally before taking a deep breath.[32] However, many reports fail to describe adequately what is meant by the term, breathing exercises. Both inspiration and expiration are stressed in FET, which consists of periods of controlled breathing, thoracic expansion exercises (with or without manual techniques), followed by huffing at varying lung volumes. Appropriate postural drainage is used with FET and a minimum of 10 minutes is recommended in each position. Cough can be substituted for huffing at high lung volumes to clear the large airways and huffing at low lung volumes is thought to clear secretions from the smaller airways,[115] but effect beyond the fourth generation bronchi is lacking.[135,136] Studies are needed on the efficacy of FET for acute atelectasis, since most research has been done on patients with chronic lung disease. This technique incorporates all the components of chest physical therapy described so far, except suctioning, but cannot be used for uncooperative patients or those requiring mechanical ventilation.

## Mobilization

Patient mobilization is recommended to prevent postoperative pulmonary complications and to reverse the changes in respiratory function that accompany immobility.[29,70] Passive positioning is encouraged for patients restricted to bedrest; intravascular lines and life-sustaining equipment in the ICU rarely prevent careful turning.[70] When compared to supine, sitting upright (but not slouched) and standing are associated with improvement in virtually all respiratory parameters.[29,64,70,73] The upright position is advocated to counter the effects of reflex phrenic nerve inhibition,[29] surgical trauma,[26] and decreased diaphragm performance[42] that follows upper abdominal surgery. For these reasons, a timely progression to upright sitting, standing and ambulation is indicated as soon as is medically possible.

The beneficial effects of early patient mobilization are supported by most studies. Reduced postoperative fever and ICU stay are reported in patients who were turned every two hours after coronary artery bypass surgery.[17] Two studies have found early patient mobilization as effective as breathing exercises and incentive spirometry IS in similar patient populations.[32,75] An early mobilization program of sitting out of bed, progressing to walking, and then stair climbing, was as effective as pre- and postoperative physical therapy in preventing pulmonary complications after coronary artery surgery.[144A] Patients undergoing thoracotomy demonstrated no added benefit from positive expiratory pressure PEP to a physical therapy program that emphasized breathing exercises and mobilization.[44] Fewer pulmonary complications were reported after cholecystectomy in patients who received chest physical therapy that included bed mobility and ambulation[160] and no further benefit occurred when IS was used along with mobilization.[129]

Patients who are old (>65 years), obese, require prolonged mechanical ventilation (>24 hours) or lengthy ICU stay (>48 hours) are routinely excluded from studies assessing the efficacy of mobilization.[75,129] These are precisely the patients at greatest risk for developing postoperative pulmonary complications and who may most benefit from the other components of physical therapy treatment already described. From the literature, it is not always clear what is meant by the term "mobilization." In one study of patients undergoing coronary artery bypass grafting, mobilization included: active exercises of the upper and lower limbs, sitting in a chair (as soon as possible), ambulation on the second postoperative day, and stair climbing on the fourth.[75] Another article defines treatment only as "mobilization on the day of surgery."[129] In this chapter, mobilization refers to a progressively increased activity level, as allowed by the patient's condition, whether it be passive limb or position changes, supported sitting, transfers, independent sitting, standing, or ambulation.

## Other adjuncts used with physical therapy

None of the adjunct therapies described below are considered a part of chest physical therapy in this chapter.

Bronchodilators and mucolytic agents are sometimes administered along with physical therapy treatment in patients with chronic lung disease. There is little research to support their use in acute atelectasis. Inhaled medications tend to have little direct effect on collapsed airways since airflow, and therefore delivery to the atelectatic lung, is limited. Adequate humidification of inspired gases and systemic hydration are effective methods of liquefying secretions.[67] Modalities such as intermittent positive pressure breathing (IPPB), IS, continuous positive airway pressure (CPAP), and PEP have been proposed to assist deep breathing or prevent pulmonary complications. In nearly all studies, breathing exercises were found to be less costly and as effective or superior to IPPB.[5,14,67,130,149] Similarly, IS is reported as less expensive and at least as useful as IPPB in decreasing postoperative complications.[31,67,76,149,157] The results of these reports and other complications from IPPB have led to a marked decline in its use. There is one study on the successful use of lung inflation (to vital capacity or airway pressures of 40 cm $H_2O$) to reverse atelectasis during anesthesia (without PEEP) in adults with otherwise healthy lungs.[122] It is unclear if the intraoperative atelectasis recurred or if these results are applicable to the patients after surgery. Studies evaluating the use of CPAP and PEP after surgery are conflicting.[2,11,44,120,145] Optimal pressure, length and duration of treatment need to be established since improvement in FRC is lost within minutes of removing the facemask.[62,73,145]

## ICU MONITORS AND EQUIPMENT

It is common practice for patients who have had major surgery or trauma to spend some time in the ICU. Physical therapists who treat these patients should be familiar with the monitors, lines, pumps, drains and other support equipment that is regularly used in the ICU. Some devices that are routinely seen after abdominal, cardiac or thoracic surgery/injury are described along with modifications that may be needed during physical therapy treatment.

## Feeding tubes

Nasogastric tubes are commonly placed prior to surgery to prevent aspiration and because of decreased postoperative gastric motility. Oral gastric or nasogastric tubes are also used in emergency surgery to help evacuate stomach contents[52] and during recovery from posttraumatic paralytic ileus.[12] For trauma patients, the oral route may have the advantage of a decreased potential for sinus infections.[12] Feeding tubes are also used to provide supplemental enteral nutrition for patients unable to tolerate adequate oral intake. When the risk of aspiration is high or when long term tube feeding is expected, small bore tubes that terminate distal to the stomach are often used. Some tubes require endoscopic placement, whereas others are inserted percutaneously (such as gastrostomy tubes).

Physical therapists should note the type of feeding tube and where it terminates in the gastrointestinal tract prior to treatment. As a general rule to prevent aspiration, patients should not be positioned head-down for up to 30 minutes after a bolus gastric feeding. Continuous gastric feeding pumps should be stopped before chest physical therapy is begun. Some tubes require a flush with water to prevent clogging when they are stopped for a period of time. Feedings administered distal to the angle of Treitz in the jejunum can usually continue to run during physical therapy treatment, regardless of body position.[12,21]

## Chest tubes

Tube thoracostomy is often necessary after thoracic trauma since penetrating injuries, lung contusion, rib fractures, pulmonary lacerations, and vascular injuries lead to pneumothorax and hemothorax. Intrapleural and mediastinal drainage tubes are routinely placed after cardiothoracic surgery to aid in lung reexpansion. A subxiphoid incision, separate from the sternotomy incision, is used for mediastinal tubes. Hemothorax and pneumothorax are usually treated by inserting a drainage tube into the pleural cavity between the fourth or fifth intercostal space in the midaxillary line.[49,52,65,83] Alternately, pneumothorax may be ameliorated by placing a chest tube in the second intercostal space at the midclavicular line.[65] However, tubes placed anteriorly leave a visible scar and may imperil the heart on the left. Drains placed posteriorly are uncomfortable while lying supine or sitting, making midaxillary placement more desirable. Chest tube size is limited by the width of the intercostal space. Using the largest tube which can be easily accommodated is recommended since discomfort is not reduced with smaller gauged tubes; also drainage is enhanced and kinking is minimized.[49]

Thoracostomy tubes are sutured into place and connected to an underwater seal system, and suction drainage is often applied (15 to 40 cm $H_2O$).[49] Following insertion, a chest radiograph is used to confirm appropriate tube position and function. Chest tubes should not be kinked or clamped and the collection chambers should be kept upright, below the level of the chest. Thoracostomy tubes are usually left to water seal alone (without additional wall suction) once chest tube drainage is minimal, an air leak is not present, and the patient is breathing spontaneously. Chest tubes are also used in the treatment of bronchopleural fistulae and empyema.[49]

Patients with chest tubes can be mobilized. Transfers from bed to chair and short walks within the limits of the tubing are possible when wall suction is required. At the physician's discretion, chest tubes can be temporarily left to water seal to allow ambulation for greater distances.[70] Pain from the chest tube can lead to immobility and poor inspiratory effort. Physical therapy aimed at achieving normal shoulder and thoracic motion is often necessary following thoracostomy tube insertion and should be coordinated with adequate pain relief. Chest physical therapy to treat an underlying condition, such as atelectasis or lung abscess, is indicated to improve lung expansion and may assist pleural drainage. Manual techniques of percussion and vibration are used as needed in patients with chest tubes.

## Cardiac monitors, intravascular lines, and drains

Cardiac monitors rarely present a problem during physical therapy treatment. Electrode positioning may be altered to prevent artifact and allow optimal hand placement during manual techniques. Intravenous (IV) lines are not restrictions to physical therapy. To prevent dislodgement, the location of all IV lines should be noted and their patency checked before and after position changes. The presence of lines that monitor pulmonary artery (PA) and central venous pressure (CVP) are not contraindications to turning or mobilizing patients.[89] Waveforms should be checked after moving patients, but pressure readings displayed on the monitors normally vary with position changes, especially head-up and head-down. On occasion, PA lines may move within the heart, causing an abnormal waveform or dysrhythmia (usually premature ventricular contractions) when the patient is turned. If this occurs, physical therapy should be postponed until the line placement is checked. Transfers out of bed to a chair may be performed in patients with PA or CVP lines, unless the patients are hemodynamically unstable. Arterial lines are used to monitor blood pressure and to obtain blood gas samples. These catheters do not prevent physical therapy treatment, but flexion around the joint where an arterial line is inserted may interfere with accurate readings. Therapists should be aware that arterial pressure normally fluctuates with changes in body position and when the relationship between the transducer, catheter placement, and right atrium is altered.

Intraabdominal drains are used to remove fluid or air from the surgical site. The drains are usually connected to collection bags and may require suction. Care is required to prevent tension or dislodging of intraabdominal drains. Indwelling urinary catheters should not be pulled or kinked when patients are repositioned. Drainage collection bags always are kept below the bladder to prevent reflux and infection.

## Tracheal tubes

Tracheal tubes may be inserted into the trachea through the mouth (orotracheal), the nose (nasotracheal), or the anterior neck (tracheostomy). Patients with tracheal tubes should receive supplemental humidity. Naso- and orotracheal tubes pass through the vocal cords and are usually used after surgery when short-term ventilation is expected. Tracheostomy tubes are used in patients who require long-term ventilation or are unable to protect their airway. Tension or pressure on the tracheal tube must be avoided, but patients can be mobilized and turned prone, if necessary.[18]

## Intraaortic balloon counterpulsation (IABP)

The IABP is used to augment coronary artery perfusion and reduce afterload in some patients after cardiac surgery or myocardial infarction. It is inserted into the descending aorta through the femoral artery and is synchronized with the electrocardiogram (ECG) or arterial waveform. The balloon rapidly deflates just before ventricular systole and inflates immediately following aortic valve closure. Cardiac output and perfusion are improved while myocardial oxygen demand is decreased. In most cases, the IABP assists every heartbeat and then support is weaned as tolerated, down to every fourth beat, when the device is removed.[8] Physical therapy is performed on patients with IABP, when clear indications for treatment are present and vital signs are closely monitored. Increased heart rate or artifact during turning can effect IABP function that is regulated by the ECG. Patients with IABP can usually participate in range of motion and bed mobility, as long as hip flexion is kept to less than 70° near the site of insertion.[125]

Aside from the IABP, other means to assist cardiac or respiratory function have been developed. Extracorporeal membrane oxygenation (ECMO) can provide temporary respiratory support in adults for up to 48 hours. Longer periods of ECMO are associated with numerous complications. Methods to improve circulation and assist the heart are well described elsewhere[8] and newer types are evolving. Aside from supporting cardiac function in patients after bypass surgery, many of the ventricular assist devices are used as a bridge to cardiac transplantation (see Chapter 21).

## CARDIOTHORACIC SURGERY
### Incision placement

Although surgical practice may vary, a knowledge of the common types of incisions used in both cardiac and thoracic surgery are important to physical therapists. Two main incisions are used, the median sternotomy and the lateral thoracotomy, that may be performed through an anterolateral, midlateral (modified transaxillary), or posterolateral approach (see Fig. 20-5). Median sternotomy is used for most cardiac surgeries other than mitral valve replacement. The anterolateral thoracotomy is often used in trauma victims and in patients who are cardiovascularly unstable. The majority of pulmonary resections and esophageal operations traditionally are performed through a posterolateral thoracotomy.[82] A smaller midlateral incision has gained favor for pulmonary and hilar resections. Advantages to this incision are rapid access and closure, no cutting of major muscles and less postoperative discomfort.[82,104] Partial rib resection may accompany lateral thoracotomies.

More recently, technical improvements have allowed thoracoscopic surgery to be used for therapeutic and diagnostic procedures. Thoracoscopy results in markedly limited incision sites. Other advantages to thoracoscopic surgery include diminished intraoperative lung tissue injury and decreased postoperative pulmonary dysfunction, pain, and hospital stay.[84,141] Pain and analgesia associated with the different thoracic incision types are discussed on p. 398-399.

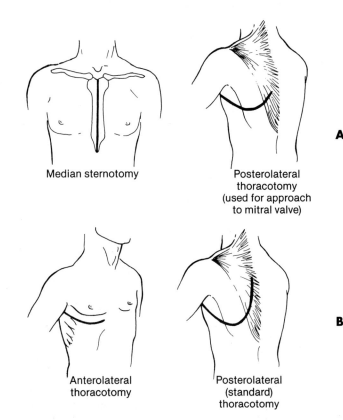

Median sternotomy

Posterolateral thoracotomy (used for approach to mitral valve)

**A**

Anterolateral thoracotomy

Posterolateral (standard) thoracotomy

**B**

**Fig. 20-5.** Cardiothoracic incisions. **A,** Common incisions used in cardiac surgery include the median sternotomy and the posterolateral thoracotomy (to replace some mitral valves). **B,** Common incisions performed to manage thoracic trauma and for pulmonary surgery include the anterolateral thoracotomy and the posterolateral thoracotomy. A median sternotomy (**A**) is used for most cardiac procedures and some pulmonary resections, particularly bilateral conditions.

## CARDIAC CONDITIONS

Not all operative procedures to the heart and great vessels require open-heart surgery. Some palliative and corrective techniques used on and around the heart are described. The use of hypothermia and cardiopulmonary bypass (CPB) are discussed along with preoperative studies commonly done before major heart surgery. Some operative techniques for treating congenital heart disease, coronary artery disease (CAD), ventricular aneurysms, and valvular disease are presented. Changes in respiratory function and chest physical therapy treatment that are specific to cardiac surgery are described.

### Preoperative investigations

Preoperative chest radiographs and ECG monitoring are standard for all patients. Other studies done prior to surgery vary depending on the underlying diagnosis. Stress testing is indicated for those with stable angina, asymptomatic patients following myocardial infarction (MI), or to determine the physiologic significance of coronary obstructions seen on angiography. Changes in symptoms, pulse, blood pressure,

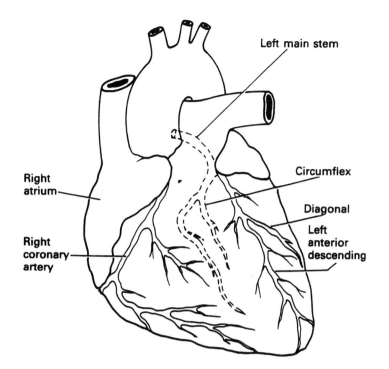

**Fig. 20-6.** Two coronary arteries arise from the aorta, the right and left main coronary artery. The latter is usually short and divides into the left anterior descending and circumflex arteries. In general, the right coronary, left anterior descending, and circumflex each supply perfusion to approximately one third of the heart, but variations often occur. The right main coronary artery bifurcates into the posterior descending artery and the atrioventricular branch (also called the posterior left ventricular branch). This anatomical situation is usually termed "right-dominant," depending on the amount of perfusion supplied by the right coronary artery. When the posterior descending artery arises from the circumflex artery, the system is referred to as "left-dominant." (From Burnand KG and Young AE: *The new Aird's companion in surgical studies,* New York, 1992, Churchill Livingstone.)

and ECG are documented during the stress test (also see Chapter 8).[153] The sensitivity and specificity of a stress test are improved with the use of thallium scanning or radionuclide ventriculography. For patients unable to exercise, thallium scintigraphy mimics the effect of blood redistribution seen with exercise by shunting blood away from myocardial regions perfused through ischemic vessels.[9] Echocardiography permits repeated noninvasive observation of cardiac anatomy and function. It is used to investigate most congenital and valvular defects and cardiac injury from trauma or infarct.[9,153]

In addition to the relatively noninvasive procedures just described, cardiac catheterization remains the mainstay of preoperative assessment for persons with CAD. Catheters inserted into arteries and veins can be introduced into all heart chambers where pressures and oxygen saturation are measured. Angiography is also performed by injecting radiopaque contrast material to evaluate coronary artery blood flow. Normal coronary artery anatomy is shown in Fig. 20-6. Angiography identifies the patient's coronary artery distribution and the exact site and degree of any lesions.

## CARDIAC PROCEDURES NOT REQUIRING CPB

Closed operations are used for some ventricular septal defects, patent ductus arteriosus (unresponsive to conservative therapy) and aortic coarctation. In the case of a common ventricle or with some ventricular septal defects, surgical correction in infancy is often too hazardous. Instead, palliative pulmonary artery narrowing or "banding" may be performed to decrease left-to-right shunting of blood. The ductus arteriosus allows the majority of blood that enters the pulmonary artery to bypass the lungs and flow into the aorta during fetal circulation (see Fig. 20-7). This duct normally closes within 12 hours of birth. However, persistent ductus arteriosus is a common congenital cardiac defect that requires a thoracotomy and surgical closure.[153]

Coarctation of the aorta can occur in isolation or along with other congenital abnormalities, such as a bicuspid aortic valve and beri aneurysms. The most common site of narrowing is just opposite the ductus arteriosus. Collateral circulation may develop to augment blood supply to the lower body and hypertension or some degree of heart failure may be present. Surgical repair involves a thoracotomy and

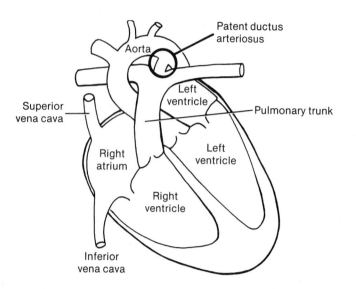

**Fig. 20-7.** Patent ductus arteriosus. Conduit between the pulmonary trunk and the aorta.

aortic cross clamping. The coarcted segment is resected, and an end-to-end anastomosis is usually performed. In adults, a prosthetic graft may be used when anastomosis is not possible, but this does not allow for natural growth and is not suitable for children.[46,153]

Acute cardiac tamponade restricts cardiac function and occurs from trauma (blunt or penetrating) after cardiac surgery or more rarely, from acute pericarditis. Cardiac function can also be limited by chronic constrictive pericarditis, which usually is of unknown etiology. Although pericardiocentesis may be used to drain fluid or blood from the pericardial space, an anterior thoracotomy or sternotomy is often needed for definitive treatment that consists of a pericardiectomy or pericardotomy.[9] Alternately, successful pericardotomy and almost complete pericardiectomy can be accomplished through thoracoscopy.[84]

Blunt cardiac trauma can result in relatively rare conditions such as cardiac rupture, septal tears, or traumatic rupture of a valve. The incidence of cardiac contusion varies between 20% to 70% in patients who sustain severe chest trauma. Diagnosis is difficult because cardiac enzymes may not be elevated[52] and, when elevated, may be due to other muscle injury.[153] Also ECG findings are nonspecific but include ST-T wave changes, axis shifts, bundle branch block, and hemiblock. Echocardiography is definitive when myocardial wall motion abnormalities occur with contusion.[52] Evidence suggests that patients with normal echocardiographic and ECG findings on admission after blunt chest trauma do not require ICU monitoring.[63] In other patients, hemodynamic and ECG monitoring is used to manage dysrhythmias that may arise. Chest physical therapy is indicated when retained secretions occur from chest injuries associated with myocardial contusion. In this situation, the therapist should closely monitor any changes in the ECG and other vital signs and modify treatment, if necessary.

## HYPOTHERMIA AND CPB FOR OPEN-HEART SURGERY

Many cardiac conditions that are now amenable to surgery, were not possible to correct in the past. The use of improved anesthesia techniques, hypothermia, and CPB have allowed increasingly complex surgical procedures to be performed on the heart. Systemic hypothermia reduces tissue metabolism and oxygen consumption, providing some degree of protection from ischemia to the myocardium, brain, and kidneys. During CPB, blood is drained either through a single cannula in the right atrium or separate cannulation of the superior and inferior vena cavae. Oxygenation and carbon dioxide removal are usually accomplished through membrane oxygenators (now preferred over bubble oxygenators). Then, for most types of cardiac surgery, blood is returned to the patient through cannulation of the distal ascending aorta (see Fig. 20-8).[9,153]

During CPB the myocardium is perfused through the coronary arteries, by blood flow into the aortic root, coronary ostia, and coronary sinus. However, coronary perfusion is interrupted for surgery to the left side of the heart, aortic valve replacement, and when a bloodless field is required (as in coronary artery or neonatal surgery). Ischemia is minimized by direct cannulation of the coronary ostia during aortic valve surgery or intermittent release of the aortic clamp during mitral valve or coronary surgery. In a moderately cooled, nonbeating heart, myocardial ischemia seems to be well tolerated for up to 15 minutes.[153]

Other techniques are used to allow longer periods of diminished perfusion while preserving myocardial function. Hypothermic intermittent ischemic arrest has been used for many years. It provides a quiet, bloodless field for up to 20 minutes, followed by an equivalent interval for reperfusion. Cold cardioplegic arrest induces rapid cardiac arrest that is usually supplemented by systemic and topical hypothermia. It allows improved myocardial protection and is used in the majority of cardiac operations performed today, including corrective congenital heart surgery in neonates and operations on the distal ascending aorta and aortic arch (where anastomoses must be performed without aortic crossclamping). Continuous warm cardioplegic arrest is a newer technique in which arrest is induced and maintained through a continuous infusion of a normothermic oxygenated substrate. The type of myocardial protection that is used for an individual patient depends on the type of intended surgery, the surgeon's choice, and the degree of preoperative ischemia.[9]

### Congenital heart defects

The techniques of CPB and hypothermia along with improved anesthesia and postoperative care have greatly improved the success of open-heart surgery to correct

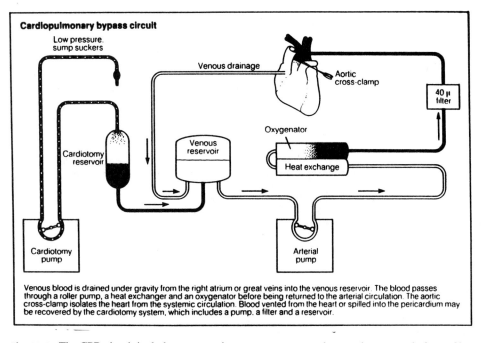

**Fig. 20-8.** The CPB circuit includes a reservoir, pump, oxygenator, heat exchanger, and often a filter to remove gaseous microemboli. (From Burnand KG and Young AE: *The new Aird's companion in surgical studies,* New York, 1992, Churchill Livingstone.)

congenital heart defects. Procedures for treating atrial and ventricular septal defects and tetralogy of Fallot are described. An atrial septal defect is an abnormal opening in the interatrial septum that allows a right-to-left shunting of blood. Surgery is usually advised if pulmonary blood flow is double systemic flow, as measured from oxygen saturation in the right atrium, pulmonary artery, and aorta. A median sternotomy is usually used and access is gained through a right atriotomy. The defect is then repaired by suturing or with a prosthetic patch graft.[46,153]

Ventricular septal defects may vary in size and location and may coexist with other lesions (see tetralogy of Fallot). The size of the intraventricular opening and the pulmonary vascular resistance determines the amount of left-to-right shunting of blood. Pulmonary vascular resistance normally falls within a few days after birth and the amount of systemic-to-pulmonary flow increases. A substantial number of ventricular septal defects close spontaneously so surgery is only performed during infancy if heart failure occurs. Otherwise, repair is deferred until after one year of age and is accomplished through a median sternotomy; a right ventriculotomy is performed and the placement of a prosthetic graft is often required. In some cases, palliative procedures (see pulmonary artery banding) may be used.[46,153]

Tetralogy of Fallot is a complex congenital heart condition that is composed of: a ventricular septal defect, anomalous position of the aorta, pulmonary stenosis, and right ventricular outflow obstruction, which leads to right ventricular hypertrophy (see Fig. 20-9). Cyanosis is usually present due to right-to-left shunting of blood that occurs

through the septal defect. A median sternotomy is used for total correction of this congenital defect. Access is gained through a right ventriculotomy; the infundibular defect is excised, a pulmonary valvotomy is performed and the ventricular septal defect is closed. An alternative approach that is used less often today, does not require CPB and open-heart surgery, but provides palliation until the child grows and surgical risk decreases. In such cases, a systemic-pulmonary shunt (usually between the subclavian artery to pulmonary artery) is created and total correction of the tetralogy of Fallot is delayed.[46,153]

### Coronary artery bypass surgery

Coronary artery bypass (CAB) surgery is performed on persons with CAD to relieve ischemia and intractable symptoms of angina (also see Chapter 2). Surgery may also be indicated to improve long-term survival by preserving left ventricular function and preventing MI (see the box on p. 388).[9] The success of percutaneous transluminal angioplasty (PTA) to dilate stenosed coronary arteries has markedly improved since its introduction in 1977. The more recent use of a stent during PTA to reduce vessel restenosis shows promise. When PTA fails and vessel occlusion occurs, MI and cardiac arrest may ensue, which require emergency CAB surgery.[9]

The operative technique of CAB surgery has become somewhat standardized, though individual variation exists because of patient needs and surgeon preference. There are three sources of grafts that are used to bypass stenosed coronary arteries. The greater saphenous vein graft (SVG)

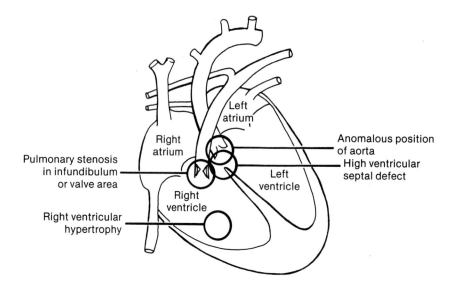

**Fig. 20-9.** Tetralogy of Fallot. *Left top,* Pulmonary stenosis in the infundibulum or valve area; *left bottom,* right ventricular hypertrophy; *right top,* anomalous position of the aorta; *right bottom,* high ventricular septal defect.

---

## Indications for coronary artery bypass surgery

### Clinical indications

Unstable or severe angina that is unresponsive to medical therapy

Postinfarction angina (<2-4 weeks post-MI)

Acute ischemia or hemodynamic instability following unsuccessful percutaneous coronary angiography

Acute evolving MI within 6 hours of onset of pain with/without failed PCA or thrombolytic therapy

Cardiogenic shock from acute MI

Ischemic pulmonary edema

Mechanical complications of MI

### Anatomic/physiologic indications

Stenosis >50% of left main CA

Three-vessel disease with impaired LV function

Three-vessel disease with normal LV function but inducible ischemia or physiologic testing

Two-vessel disease with significant proximal left anterior descending artery stenosis

Severely depressed LV function with evidence of reversible ischemia

Positive thallium imaging and angiographic abnormalities prior to major vascular surgery

CA anomalies with risk of sudden death

Significant CA stenosis during other cardiac operations

Adapted from Bojar RM: *Adult cardiac surgery,* Cambridge, 1992, Blackwell Scientific Publications.

---

was used almost exclusively for many years, but follow-up studies have demonstrated progressive occlusion of these grafts. The improved long-term survival, patency, and vessel autoregulation reported with internal mammary artery (IMA) grafts have made it the current procedure of choice. Because of the success of IMA grafts, using the right gastroepiploic artery has been investigated as an alternative. This artery is freed from the stomach and brought up through the diaphragm and pericardium. Although short-term patency is good, increased morbidity is a concern since a laparotomy is needed to access this artery.[9]

A median sternotomy is used for coronary artery bypass surgery. In most cases, one or both IMAs are then prepared, the pericardium is opened and hypothermia and CPB are initiated (as described above). Alternately, the greater saphenous vein is excised (usually before the sternotomy) or, if the right gastroepiploic artery is to be used, the chest incision is extended into the upper abdomen. Coronary arteriotomies are performed distal to the lesions and anastomoses are constructed using the IMA(s), often in a sequential manner. Proximal anastomoses to the ascending aorta are completed when SVGs or free IMA grafts are used. Cardiac function is resumed and CPB is weaned once systemic normothermia is achieved. Inotropic support is often required to obtain satisfactory cardiac output since left ventricular function is decreased. Some of the more common complications of coronary artery bypass surgery are listed in Table 20-2.[9]

### Ventricular aneurysms

Following an acute MI, about one quarter of patients will develop a thin-walled fibrous scar or localized area of paradoxical motion, termed a left ventricular aneurysm (LVA). This type of aneurysm is associated with a high mortality in patients who go on to develop congestive heart failure, ventricular dysrhythmia, or myocardial rupture. Resection of an LVA is often indicated in patients having angina or ventricular dysrhythmias, and more rarely, when

**Table 20-2.** Average incidence of common complications of coronary artery bypass surgery

| | |
|---|---|
| 30% | Atrial arrhythmias |
| 5% | Ventricular arrhythmias |
| 5% | Leg wound infections |
| 5% | Myocardial infarction |
| 5% | Respiratory failure |
| 3% | Sternal wound infections |
| 3% | Reoperation for mediastinal bleeding |
| 2% | Stroke |
| 2% | Gastrointestinal complications |
| 2% | Renal failure |

From Bojar RM: Coronary artery bypass surgery. In Bojar RM, editor: *Adult cardiac surgery*, Cambridge, 1992, Blackwell Scientific Publications. Reprinted by permission.

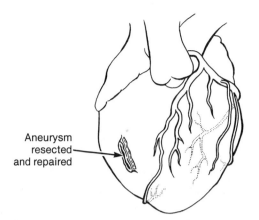

**Fig. 20-10.** Ventricular aneurysmectomy. Resected aneurysm with suture reinforcement.

mural thrombus is present.[9] Surgery is performed through a median sternotomy and CPB is instituted. The left ventricle is incised, any clots are removed, and the aneurysm is resected (see Fig. 20-10). After CPB is withdrawn, a temporary pacemaker electrode is usually inserted before the sternal incision is closed.[46] If the LVA is large, a pericardial or Dacron patch may be used to preserve the shape of the ventricle and improve function. Coronary bypass grafting to diseased vessels and mitral valve repair or replacement may be performed in addition to LVA resection.[9]

**Mitral valve disease**

Almost all cases of mitral stenosis are the result of rheumatic fever and occur more often in women. After the acute illness, years or decades may pass before the valve becomes progressively thickened and the commissures fuse. Symptoms include breathlessness (worse when recumbent), tiredness, atrial fibrillation, and systemic embolization.[153]

There are a variety of treatment options for mitral stenosis. CPB is avoided by use of either percutaneous balloon mitral valvotomy (PBMV) or closed mitral commissurotomy. For PBMV, a dilating balloon is passed from the femoral vein into the right atrium, through the atrial septum and across the mitral valve. The balloon is inflated and the adherent commissures opened. PBMV is also performed in a retrograde fashion, through the femoral artery, aortic valve, and mitral valve. Major complications from PBMV are rare although restenosis can occur. A left posterolateral thoracotomy is used for a closed mitral commissurotomy, which can produce excellent results in a select group of patients. Because concomitant subvalvular disease or induced mitral regurgitation cannot be treated by this procedure, it has been replaced with open commissurotomy in the United States. Open mitral commissurotomy requires CPB and is considered the procedure of choice for most patients with mitral stenosis. It provides direct visualization of the valve, allowing for a more precise commissurotomy.[9]

Acute causes of mitral regurgitation (MR) include papillary muscle rupture or endocarditis that may lead to acute pulmonary edema from the abrupt rise in left atrial and pulmonary venous pressures. Chronic MR is usually the result of degenerative, rheumatic, or ischemic etiologies. These patients may tolerate the progressive development of severe left ventricular overload for years. Decreased stroke volume leads to symptoms of marked fatigue and congestive heart failure that are exacerbated by exercise or the development of atrial fibrillation. Until the mid-1980s, mitral valve replacement was considered the usual procedure for treatment of MR. Growing evidence now supports using mitral valve reconstruction, when it is possible.[9]

Mitral valve replacement is indicated when the extent of the valve disease (stenosis or regurgitation) precludes commissurotomy or reconstruction. Mitral valve replacement requires CPB and is usually accomplished through a median sternotomy or, less often, using a posterolateral thoracotomy. A left atriotomy is performed, the mitral valve excised and a prosthetic valve sutured into place. The left atrium is then closed, CPB withdrawn, and a temporary pacemaker may be placed. Operative mortality of mitral valve replacement for MR is nearly twice that seen in patients undergoing valve replacement for mitral stenosis.[9,46] The surgical approach is similar for an open mitral commissurotomy or mitral reconstruction, which are well described elsewhere.[9]

**Tricuspid valve disease**

Tricuspid stenosis is usually a result of rheumatic disease, which also involves other heart valves. Tricuspid regurgitation most often occurs secondary to other cardiac disease that increases right ventricular pressure (systolic) and dilates the valve annulus. There is limited experience using percutaneous balloon valvotomy for tricuspid stenosis and commissurotomy is generally considered the procedure of choice. An annuloplasty is often indicated to avoid regurgitation (see Fig. 20-11). Most cases of tricuspid stenosis or regurgitation

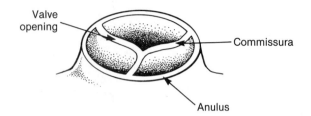

**Fig. 20-11.** Heart valve. Tricuspid valve showing commissura and surrounding fibrous anulus.

can be treated with commissurotomy and annuloplasty; tricuspid valves are replaced only in severe conditions. The procedure for tricuspid valve replacement is through a right atriotomy and may include permanent ventricular pacing, but is otherwise similar to that described for the mitral valve.[9,46]

### Aortic valve disease

Aortic stenosis occurs from congenital abnormality, rheumatic heart disease, or calcification. These conditions along with endocarditis and trauma also can cause aortic regurgitation. Surgery to treat aortic stenosis or regurgitation is principally indicated in patients with symptoms such as angina, heart failure, syncope or an episode of sudden death. Several reconstructive techniques can be used in some patients to restore aortic valve competence and avoid the need for valve replacement. Percutaneous balloon aortic valvuloplasty is a palliative procedure for stenosis that provides short-term improvement, but restenosis within one year is common. The techniques of aortic valve commissurotomy and valve debridement to treat stenosis have been supplanted by aortic valve replacement. Aortic valve replacement is performed through a median sternotomy, using CPB. An aortotomy is made and the damaged valve is excised. The replacement valve is inserted and sutured into place. Valve function is assessed before closing the aorta and CPB is withdrawn. A variety of sources have been used to replace the damaged aortic valve, including prosthetic, porcine, pulmonary autograft, and cryopreserved human homograft valves.[9,46]

### Chest physical therapy for adults after CPB

Whenever possible, patients should receive preoperative instruction in physical therapy as is outlined earlier in this chapter. Medication to minimize acute pain and reduce associated anxiety should be administered prior to physical therapy treatment. Because dysrhythmias routinely occur in patients after cardiac surgery (see Table 20-2), the physical therapist must be familiar with common ECG findings and pay close attention to any changes that may occur during treatment (see Chapter 5).

Technical advances of CPB and the use of membrane oxygenators have decreased the incidence of adult respiratory distress syndrome (ARDS) and some other pulmonary

**Table 20-3.** Changes in pulmonary function after CPB

| | |
|---|---|
| Alveolar-arterial oxygen difference | ↑* |
| Physiologic shunt | ↑ |
| Respiratory rate | ↑ |
| Tidal volume | ↓ |
| Minute ventilation | → |
| Alveolar ventilation | ↓ |
| Alveolar volume | ↓ |
| Static compliance | ↓ |
| Airways resistance | ↑ |
| Work of breathing | ↑ |
| Oxygen consumption | ↑ |
| Respiratory quotient | → |
| Physiological dead space | ↑ |
| Dead space/tidal volume ($V_D/V_T$) | → |
| Pulmonary vascular resistance | ↑ |

*↑ = increase; ↓ = decrease; → = no change.
From Edmonds LH: Effects of cardiopulmonary bypass on the lungs. In Fishman AP, editor: *Pulmonary diseases and disorders*, New York, 1980, McGraw-Hill. Reprinted by permission.

complications that occur after open-heart surgery. The effects of CPB on respiratory function are shown in Table 20-3. Most of these postoperative changes are small and begin to return to previous values after 48 hours.[77] Therefore, in many patients, breathing exercises, cough encouragement, range of motion, and maximal mobility (within limits that do not stress the heart) are adequate.[75] A recent study reports little added benefit from prophylactic use of the other components of chest physical therapy in patients who are adequately mobilized after routine CAB surgery.[144A] Different treatment may be indicated for patients with mobilization restrictions or those who require MV for more than 24 hours. For patients with preexisting lung dysfunction, even small changes in pulmonary function can lead to hypoventilation, atelectasis, pulmonary infection, hypoxia, and eventual respiratory failure.[77] To prevent secondary infection and its sequelae in these patients, postural drainage, percussion, vibration, and secretion clearance are often needed to clear retained secretions. Postural drainage positions can be modified and methods to minimize hypoxemia (described earlier) are used in patients who demonstrate significant dysrhythmia.[57,92]

Two other situations during cardiac surgery may complicate postoperative pulmonary dysfunction. Direct trauma to the lungs or airways, especially in patients who are anticoagulated, can lead to bleeding, atelectasis, ventilation-perfusion mismatch, and hypoxemia. Marked elevations in pulmonary venous pressures (during CPB or from left ventricular dysfunction) can cause hemorrhagic atelectasis and pulmonary edema.[77] Most patients with these conditions require mechanical ventilation for longer periods of time after surgery and the use of chest physical therapy is less well defined, particularly for patients who require postoperative use of an IABP or other ventricular assist device because of left ventricular dysfunction. Based on the author's experience, treatment with minimal modification (including postural drainage, manual techniques, and secretion clearance) can be performed with expected benefit to the patient who has evidence of bleeding from surgical trauma to the lungs but no significant cardiac compromise (see section on lung contusion). Patients with cardiogenic pulmonary edema and left ventricular dysfunction should have clear indications for chest physical therapy. Vital signs are monitored closely and changes in body position are accomplished slowly. Treatment in the head-down position can be counterproductive but problems are not reported with percussion and vibration. Because of potential complications, suctioning is performed only as needed and should occur through an occlusive port adaptor. The therapist should take measures to prevent hypoxemia (see Chapter 22) and allow adequate time for the patient to recover between each pass of the suction catheter.[71]

The use of SVGs or gastroepiploic grafts can impact on physical therapy treatment after CAB surgery. Although comparative studies are lacking, complications from retained secretions would likely increase after an upper abdominal procedure combined with open-heart surgery. The expected decrease in diaphragm function and additional postoperative pain would be significant (see related sections in this chapter). In addition to treatment for pulmonary secretions, lower-extremity pain occurs in patients after SVGs and may lead to decreased weight bearing and limit out-of-bed activities. Wrapping the lower limb with elastic bandages may help to minimize swelling and assist venous return. Range of motion exercises for the operative leg are often necessary to prevent joint limitations. Ankle exercises may be helpful in preventing phlebitis and improving venous return in patients who are confined to bed.

## THORACIC CONDITIONS

Thoracic injuries are the second leading cause of all trauma-related deaths.[65] Fifteen percent of patients admitted to the hospital with chest trauma required thoracotomy, while the remaining 85% needed resuscitation, chest tube insertion, and mechanical ventilation.[102] Persons sustaining penetrating chest injuries (such as gunshot wounds), tracheobronchial tears, or thoracic aorta rupture require thoracotomy, whereas rib fractures and lung contusion frequently require more conservative resuscitation. Unlike many other patients who require thoracic surgery, persons sustaining trauma are comparatively young (16 to 35 years old) and healthy.[89] However, injury to more than one body system is common, which can complicate both medical and surgical care and provide a challenge to physical therapists. Aside from thoracic injuries, surgery is often used to treat pulmonary tumors. Other less common indications for thoracotomy include lung or pleural space infection, acquired immune deficiency syndrome (AIDS), bullous emphysema, and thoracic aortic aneurysm. Physical therapy

treatment or precautions specific to these thoracic conditions are addressed.

### Tracheobronchial tears

Tracheobronchial tears occur with penetrating and blunt trauma. Lacerations due to penetrating injuries often occur with associated esophageal, carotid or jugular vessel disruption.[65] Tears from blunt trauma may be partial or complete and may occur at any level, though most occur in the mainstem bronchi. Hemothorax, pneumothorax, hemoptysis, and rib fractures accompany large lacerations, whereas mediastinal and subcutaneous emphysema occur with smaller tears. Bronchoscopy is done to confirm the diagnosis, but blood in the airway may preclude accurate bronchoscopic diagnosis.[52]

Surgical repair consists of an end-to-end anastomosis, or more rarely, a graft insertion. A thoracic incision is usually performed, but a cervical approach may be used, depending on the injury site. A double lumen endobronchial tube can be used perioperatively to facilitate ventilation and to prevent aspiration of blood into the uninjured lung.[52] Small tears are conservatively treated with airway management and thoracostomy tube drainage. Granulation tissue may narrow the bronchial lumen at the site of injury, facilitating atelectasis formation. Chest physical therapy is indicated to remove retained secretions and residual blood, thereby minimizing the risk of infection at the surgical site of repair. Patient mobilization is emphasized as are range of motion (ROM) exercises following thoracotomy. Also, methods to improve cough are used with patients who are spontaneously breathing since during healing, decreased cough reflex from diminished bronchial sensitivity is reported.[65]

### Chest wall fractures

Rib fractures are the most common blunt chest injury. Single rib fracture usually causes only minor discomfort and can be treated with analgesics and conservative therapy. More serious chest wall fractures, including scapular, clavicular, sternal or multiple rib fractures often lead to severe respiratory compromise. Vital capacity, FRC and cough ability are reduced, which leads to atelectasis, hypoxemia and pneumonia.[52,91] Flail chest, resulting in paradoxical motion of the chest, may also be present. Radiological evidence of flail chest is not always present and a 22% incidence of delayed diagnosis of this condition is reported.[85] Positive pressure ventilation is often needed to treat the inefficient breathing pattern of flail chest and to reverse the increased oxygen consumption and the work of breathing that occurs.[52] Mechanical ventilation also provides a form of internal pneumatic fixation to the unstable chest wall.[91] Surgical stabilization of fractured ribs is described but is rarely used, with the exception of some cases in which thoracotomy is necessary for other reasons, such as repair of bronchial or diaphragmatic tears.[49]

Aside from the application of transcutaneous nerve

stimulation (TENS) (see p. 398), physical therapy is not used to treat rib fractures. However, the decreased ventilation from pain and tracheobronchial injury or lung contusion that may accompany rib fractures, often results in secretion retention and atelectasis that are indications for chest physical therapy (see Case Study). The use of manual techniques for patients with rib fractures is controversial. Treatment including postural drainage and manual percussion is described on more than 300 patients with rib and chest wall fractures.[68,89] Also, no increase in the development of extrapleural hematomas is reported in patients with rib fractures who received manual percussion.[19] The use of gentle manual vibration rather than percussion over rib fractures has been recommended,[79] but studies comparing the two techniques are lacking.

### Lung contusion

Lung contusion is a bruising of the lung parenchyma by blunt trauma. The force of impact that occurs against the chest wall is transmitted to the lung, rupturing tissue, small airways, and alveoli. Lung contusion may be present as an isolated injury or occur along with bronchial tears, hemopneumothorax, multiple chest wall fractures, and flail chest. Lung contusion accompanied by flail chest is associated with a 42% mortality.[22] Acutely, lung contusion can be difficult to diagnose because signs of external injury may not be present. Crackles are heard during chest auscultation and bloody secretions are obtained when suctioning the tracheobronchial tree. The classic radiological pattern of nonsegmental infiltrates does not appear until 6 to 12 hours after injury and usually underestimates the extent of lung damage.[91,143] The resulting intravascular hemorrhage and parenchymal edema lead to decreased lung compliance, increased shunt, atelectasis, and hypoxemia. If left untreated, the bloody secretions also act as a good culture medium and will lead to infection, a common sequela of lung contusion. Traumatic lung cysts occur in the area of contusion and can become infected, causing lung abscesses if not adequately drained.[65,91]

Treatment of lung contusion depends on the extent of injury. Early tracheal intubation, positive pressure ventilation with PEEP, and chest physical therapy are associated with improved survival and reduced morbidity[65,132] from significant lung contusion. Chest physical therapy, including postural drainage, percussion, and suctioning to all involved lung segments is recommended.[65,90,91,132] Transbronchial spillage of bloody secretions from the area of contusion to the "good lung" is reported, particularly when coagulopathy occurs in conjunction with lung contusion. Careful suctioning during chest physical therapy can minimize such spillage and the need for further treatment to the "good lung" segments.[90] In severe cases where surgical resection of the damaged area is planned, physical therapy treatment is directed toward clearing secretions and preventing infection in the "good" or remaining lung.[68] A double lumen endobronchial tube can be used to prevent transbronchial spillage, and when independent lung ventilation is indicated, to reverse respiratory failure not responsive to conventional modes of therapy.[103] For patients with lung contusion who do not require ventilatory support, supplemental oxygen, pain relief, and early mobilization (including breathing exercises and encouragement to cough) may be sufficient to clear secretions and prevent infection.[91,143]

### Lung abscess, empyema, and bronchopleural fistula

Traumatic cysts may develop into lung abscesses in areas of contused lung. Lung abscesses can communicate with the tracheobronchial tree or rupture into the pleural space, causing an empyema. Empyema also occurs as a complication of pneumonia.[91] A bronchopleural fistula develops when an abscess drains into lung tissue and the pleural space, or when a traumatic tear allows for communication between a bronchus and the pleura. Bronchial tears are normally treated as previously outlined, however, a persistent leakage between the airway and the pleura often results in infection. Empyema is routinely treated with pathogen-specific antibiotics and drainage of the purulent fluid through an empyema tube inserted into the abscess cavity within the pleural space. Short rib resection may accompany tube placement. Unlike other thoracostomy drains, empyema tubes may be left in position for weeks or months and often are not connected to an underwater seal. Alternately, thoracotomy and decortication may be used to achieve more rapid resolution of empyema (see p. 395).[49,92]

Chest physical therapy is indicated to drain lung abscesses that communicate with the tracheobronchial airway.[91] Patients with empyema should be mobilized and breathing exercises may assist pleural drainage; other chest physical therapy is not necessary unless there is underlying lung pathology or loss of shoulder ROM. Chest physical therapy is used to treat lung secretions associated with bronchopleural fistula, but the therapist should minimize the time that a patient is positioned with the involved side uppermost since air leakage through the fistula may increase.[92] Hand position can be modified during manual techniques to prevent pain from cellulitis around the area of the drainage tube.[68] Newer forms of mechanical ventilation (pressure support, high frequency, or jet) may lessen fistula air loss and improve alveolar ventilation.[92]

### Adult respiratory distress syndrome

Adult respiratory distress syndrome (ARDS) is a severe form of acute respiratory failure that often accompanies trauma (particularly chest trauma), sepsis, and burns. Definition of this syndrome includes hypoxemia, diffuse infiltrates on chest radiograph, decreased lung compliance, and the absence of cardiac failure. Pulmonary edema is present due to a defect in endothelial permeability of the pulmonary microvessels. Management of ARDS is aimed at treating the noncardiogenic pulmonary edema. It consists of optimizing gas exchange with mechanical ventilation and PEEP. Also, administering fluids for resuscitation is warranted to maintain cardiac output. Clinical studies have not supported the use of corticosteroids and other antiinflammatory drugs in the treatment of ARDS.[112]

Chest physical therapy is not routinely used to treat ARDS but may be helpful in preventing secondary pulmonary complications and pneumonia.[49,89] However, an increase in lung compliance following chest physical therapy was reported in mechanically ventilated patients who had ARDS, lung contusion, atelectasis, or pneumonia from trauma.[94] A worsening of pulmonary edema can occur when PEEP is interrupted;[112] therefore, maintaining mechanical ventilation and suctioning through a port adaptor is recommended.[71]

## Ruptured thoracic aorta

Rupture of the thoracic aorta occurs from a rapid deceleration injury such as a plane crash or high-speed motor vehicle accident and is usually fatal. Although fractures of the first through third ribs are associated signs of severe blunt chest trauma and thoracic aorta rupture, external evidence of injury is not always present. For patients who survive the initial injury, diagnosis is confirmed by an erect chest radiograph, arteriography, chest computerized tomography, or transesophageal cardiography. The majority of tears occur in the descending thoracic aorta, most just distal to the left subclavian artery.[52] A double lumen endobronchial tube is used to facilitate lung deflation for improved surgical exposure and adequate lung reinflation afterwards. Repair is accomplished through a left thoracotomy where a graft is inserted after cross-clamping the aorta above and below the tear. When blood flow to the distal aorta is occluded during cross-clamping, complete motor paraplegia (near the T8 level) may occur due to poor spinal cord perfusion.[52] A shunt placed proximal and distal to the clamps provides improved caudal perfusion, but is time-consuming.[65] Bypassing the left side of the heart (left atrial to left femoral artery) is proposed as a means to preserve spinal cord perfusion and prevent paraplegia during aortic cross-clamping.[52] In all situations, thoracostomy drains are placed after surgery.

Physical therapy is indicated to clear retained secretions and improve shoulder and trunk motion following surgery. It is important to prevent pulmonary infection and subsequent seeding of the graft site, particularly in patients with concomitant lung contusion or multiple trauma.[65] Patients with weakness or paraplegia require complete spinal cord injury assessment and exercises appropriate to their level of function. Sensory sparing through the dorsal columns (vibration and position sense) may be present. Early patient mobilization after surgery is emphasized. However, it is imperative that the therapist pay close attention to decreases in blood pressure, respiratory function, and skin sensation that may occur with sitting in patients having spinal cord injury (SCI).[69]

## Thoracic spine injury

Trauma to the thoracic spine may occur independently or in conjunction with other chest injuries already discussed. Cardiovascular and respiratory changes accompany SCI, depending on the level of neurological deficit. Along with the obvious motor and sensory deficits in the lower limbs, a complete SCI above T6 disrupts sympathetic nervous system control, which can cause bradycardia, peripheral vasodilation, and hypotension. Left ventricular dysfunction and an altered vasovagal response may also be present.[69] The intercostal muscles (innervated by T1 to T11) and the diaphragm are the primary inspiratory muscles. The major expiratory muscles include the abdominals (innervated by T6 to L1) and the intercostals.[45] Therefore, reduced expiration and cough ability exist in most patients with thoracic neurological lesion; limited inspiratory function also occurs in those with upper thoracic SCI.

Physical therapy management is similar to that discussed under ruptured thoracic aorta. Cardiovascular compromise is more common following upper thoracic SCI, so close monitoring of vital signs is necessary during position changes and suctioning. Log rolling is used when turning patients with spinal injury.[69] Also, manual vibration or rib springing is not recommended when spinal instability is present.[68] Rigid body jackets are often used after surgery and to allow increased patient mobility. A hole cut in the orthosis over the epigastric area can improve diaphragmatic descent and respiration. Also most body jackets can be opened to allow skin access for manual techniques once the patient is positioned for postural drainage.[69]

## Ruptured diaphragm

Severe compression of the lower thorax or upper abdomen can rupture the diaphragm.[49] The vast majority of tears result from motor vehicle accidents, occur on the left side, and may involve the phrenic nerve.[25] Except in cases of penetrating trauma, a ruptured diaphragm is difficult to diagnose. Chest radiographs and peritoneal lavage are helpful, but herniation of viscera into the chest frequently is not present and positive lavage may not occur unless the patient is placed head-down. However, associated chest and abdominal injuries should lead to a high index of suspicion.[49,91] Surgical repair is usually through a thoracic approach, but an abdominal incision may be used, particularly for diaphragmatic tears from penetrating trauma.[12] Chest physical therapy may be indicated to treat associated lung injury or to clear retained secretions secondary to post surgical diaphragm weakness or phrenic nerve injury.

## Lung cancer

Smoking is the most common cause of lung cancer and there is growing evidence incriminating the effects of passive smoke exposure as well. Symptoms of primary lung cancer are cough, dyspnea, pleuritic pain, and hemoptysis; metastatic signs include weight loss, bone pain, and neurological symptoms. Diagnosis is made from chest radiographs and cytological examination using bronchoscopy or needle aspiration, depending on the lesion location. Lung cancers are generally categorized as small cell lung cancer (SCLC) (oat cell or intermediate cell type) or nonsmall cell cancer (NSCLC), which includes adenocarcinoma, squamous cell carcinoma, and undifferentiated large cell carcinoma. SCLC is associated with a very poor prognosis.[49,82] However, surgical resection is used along with multimodal therapy and in peripheral lesions without lymph node spread. NSCLC has a better potential for cure by resection, depending on size, location, and amount of lymph node involvement. Carcinoid tumors range from benign to highly malignant, with over 80% arising in the proximal bronchi. Metastatic tumors to the lung are common and surgical resection can result in significantly improved 5-year survival rates for several types of carcinomas or sarcomas.[49,82]

Overall, technological advances have improved patient selection and outcomes of surgery for lung cancer. These include less physiologically damaging incisions (median sternotomy and lateral thoracotomy), improved anesthesia with the use of double lumen endobronchial tubes, and the increasing use of parenchymal saving resections (sleeve, wedge and segmental).[82] Also, ventilation perfusion scans and computerized tomography provide better preoperative evidence of feasible tumor resection.[98] Historically, pneumonectomy was considered the optimal operation for lung cancer although it was associated with significant mortality and morbidity (see Fig. 20-12). Then lobectomy was found to result in similar outcomes and it became the operation of choice, whenever possible. Increased experience with sleeve and segmental resections generally has shown comparable long- and short-term tumor control and no advantage to resecting more than is required to remove the tumor and involved lymph nodes.[49,82] Recently, thoracoscopy has been used to remove small peripheral tumors and some deeper lesions,[141] but at the present time thoracoscopic resection of lung tumors demands a cautious approach and should only be considered as part of controlled clinical trials.[84] For the majority of patients with metastatic lesions, preserving as much lung tissue as possible is also the rule, making wedge or segmental resections the preferred surgical procedures.[49,82,98]

Following thoracotomy, physical therapy is needed to encourage active shoulder and arm ROM exercises, to prevent joint limitation, and to improve the function of accessory muscles of respiration. Shoulder exercises are particularly indicated when one or more shoulder girdle muscles has been divided.[82] Early ambulation is emphasized; most patients can be out of bed 12 hours after thoracotomy.[60] Postural drainage, manual techniques, and methods of secretion clearance are needed for most patients who require prolonged mechanical ventilation or when signs of atelectasis are present. Physical therapy should be

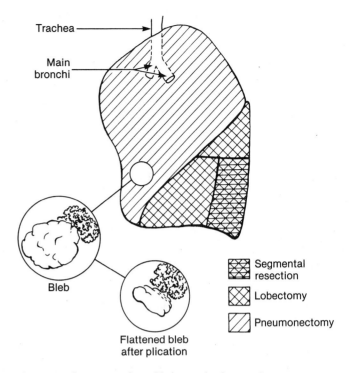

**Fig. 20-12.** Lung resections. Various selections and segments are plicated or removed for blebectomy, segmental resection, lobectomy, or pneumonectomy.

coordinated with optimal pain control.[49] Lying on the nonoperative side is contraindicated for the first ten days after pneumonectomy.[60,161]

### Acquired immunodeficiency syndrome (AIDS)

A dramatic increase in immunologically compromised patients has occurred mainly because of the expanding number of persons with AIDS. Kaposi's sarcoma and opportunistic infections including pneumonia (primarily *Pneumocystis carinii*), fungal infection (primarily *Aspergillus fumigatus*), and pulmonary tuberculosis are hallmarks of the disease and are associated with a high mortality. Along with medical treatment, palliative surgical procedures are often necessary. Chest tube insertion is used to treat air leaks, pneumothorax, and empyema that occur secondary to infection. Thoracoscopy or thoracotomy for pulmonary resection, thoracoplasty or, decortication may be necessary.[49,82,84] Chest physical therapy is indicated to abate secretion retention following thoracic surgery but is not specific to AIDS. Hemoptysis may occur, particularly in patients with opportunistic infections such as tuberculosis, lung abscess, and fungal infection. Scrupulous attention to infection control procedures is required when working with patients having AIDS.[49,82] See Chapter 22 for more information on treatment of patients with AIDS.

### Emphysematous blebs and bullae

Emphysema may occur from congenital or chromosomal abnormalities, but more commonly is due to the effects of cigarette smoking. Characteristic enlarged air spaces occur secondary to elastic tissue and alveolar wall destruction. The result is airway obstruction with impaired alveolar ventilation and gas exchange. Blebs are localized, subpleural areas of emphysema that attain significance with rupture, causing a pneumothorax. Bullae are larger areas of alveolar destruction, occurring deep within the lung parenchyma that may compress normal lung tissue.

Thoracic operations on patients with emphysema carry substantial risk. Therefore, surgery is aimed at removing blebs or bullae that impact on respiratory function. A posterolateral thoracotomy is usually used for patients with COPD although a median sternotomy may be favored for anterior or superior bullae. Chest physical therapy is important both before and after surgery for the patient with emphysema (see Chapter 22).[82] A minithoracotomy is the preferred approach for patients less than 40 years old, who do not have generalized bullous disease.[83] Thoracoscopy removal of blebs and bullae may offer major advantages over traditional surgery for patients with COPD as experience in this technique grows.[84]

### Pleural conditions

Most pathological conditions of the pleural space are treated with intercostal drainage. Needle aspiration may be successful in some cases, but chest tube insertion is preferred in most situations (see p. 383 on chest tubes). Pleurodesis, an obliteration of the pleural space, is used to prevent recurrence of pneumothorax, hemothorax, pleural effusion, or chylothorax. A chemical irritant is deposited into the pleural space through the chest tube by injection or thoracoscopy. Alternately, a thoracotomy is performed and a surgical pleurodesis is accomplished using a chemical irritant, by abrading the pleura with dry gauze or by stripping the parietal pleura from the lateral chest wall and superior mediastinum (pleurectomy).[49] Blebs and bullae may be excised along with an apical or complete pleurectomy.[83]

Decortication, which is used in the treatment of empyema, is often confused with pleurectomy. Infection causes pleural fluid to become more viscous, and fibrous tissue (cortex) progressively forms on the visceral and parietal pleura. The visceral cortex restricts lung movement, whereas the parietal cortex causes progressive contraction and immobility of the corresponding chest wall with an abscess cavity between the two. Decortication removes the abscess by stripping the cortex from the visceral pleura and excising the parietal pleura along with the cortex. This procedure is performed through a thoracotomy, or more recently, by thoracoscopy.[49,84] The success of pleurodesis and decortication depends upon the lungs' ability to expand and adhere to the chest wall. Reduced chest wall excursion also occurs with pleurodesis.[49] Therefore, chest physical therapy is directed towards breathing exercises, mobilizing the chest wall, and preventing secretion retention.[161]

### Thoracic aortic aneurysms

Thoracic aneurysms are rarer than abdominal aortic aneurysms (see p. 396). Aneurysms localized to the ascending aorta are due to degenerative connective tissue disease such as in Marfan's syndrome where concomitant aortic valve involvement causes cardiac failure from aortic insufficiency. Surgery is performed with CPB; the ascending aorta is replaced with a graft along with aortic valve replacement, as indicated. Aneurysms of the transverse aortic arch are invariably due to atherosclerosis and occur in people over 60 years old with associated coronary and cerebral vascular disease. Surgical treatment is complex and associated with high operative mortality. Most descending thoracic aneurysms also are due to atherosclerosis but are associated with significantly less operative risk. Surgery is performed through a left posterolateral thoracotomy and is similar to that for traumatic aortic rupture (see p. 393.)[140] Thoracoabdominal aneurysms are rare; surgical correction is complex and associated with a high mortality and incidence of paraplegia.[10,140]

Postoperative chest physical therapy treatment is not specific to aneurysm repair. However, there are precautions to preoperative coughing, postural drainage[161] (in the head-down position) and chest wall percussion or vibration. Because increased intraaortic pressure could lead to rupture, chest physical therapy techniques should be performed before surgery only with the express knowledge of the physician and clear indications for treatment.

## ABDOMINAL CONDITIONS

Pain and decreased diaphragmatic function are major contributors to the impaired respiratory function that occurs following abdominal surgery. In the past, upper abdominal operations have been associated with a postoperative pulmonary complication rate approaching 70%.[3,26,42] The type of incision is often thought to effect the pulmonary changes commonly seen after upper abdominal surgery, but studies are inconclusive.[10]

### Incision placement

Common placement of upper abdominal incisions is shown in Fig. 20-13.[10] Vertical (or longitudinal) incisions are often used in stomach, duodenal, and pancreas surgery. Exploratory laparotomy is performed through a vertical incision that can be extended to the xiphoid or pubis (and can encompass a median sternotomy). Gallbladder and some other biliary system surgery usually occur through a right subcostal incision though left subcostal placement allows splenic exposure (in nontrauma conditions). A combined right and left subcostal incision provides access for liver and spleen procedures, whereas a thoracoabdominal opening is used in liver and biliary surgery on the right and in esophageal and gastric surgery on the left.[10,46]

Over the past few years, laparoscopic surgery has replaced or supplemented many traditional abdominal

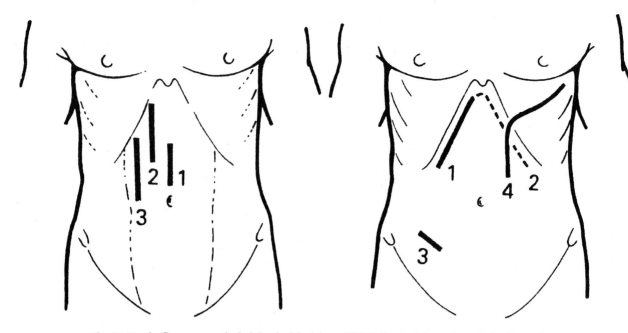

**Fig. 20-13. A,** Common vertical abdominal incisions. *(1)* Median incisions, through the linea alba, are relatively bloodless and provide rapid access to all four abdominal quadrants. *(2)* Paramedian incisions are made less than 1.5 cm lateral to midline. *(3)* Lateral paramedian incisions are performed about 3.5 cm from midline, over the rectus muscle and allow for improved postoperative wound stability. **B,** Oblique or subcostal abdominal incisions. The rectus muscles are cut with a right subcostal *(1)* or left subcostal *(2)* incision. These can be combined to form a bilateral costal (or rooftop) incision. The McBurney *(3)* incision is used for appendix surgery. A thoracoabdominal *(4)* incision can be made on either side and extends through the diaphragm muscle. (From Burnand KG and Young AE: *The new Aird's companion in surgical studies,* New York, 1992, Churchill Livingstone.)

procedures.[165] During laparoscopy, openings are made through the umbilicus and in the abdominal wall to insert various endoscopes and an insufflation device; the number of cannula used depends on the type of surgery and individual technique (see Fig. 20-14).

The use of laparoscopic techniques, same-day surgery, improved pain relief, and the routine use of early patient mobilization has changed the face of postoperative management for upper abdominal surgery.[10] Now, many patients are discharged home within a day of elective surgery and do not require physical therapy. However, internal surgical sites near the diaphragm markedly decrease respiratory function, even after laparoscopy.[35] Patients sustaining abdominal trauma or undergoing major vessel repair, hepatic, splenic, gastrointestinal, or renal surgery are at risk for developing postoperative pulmonary complications. Information on these procedures in adults is presented, while techniques specific to cardio-pulmonary transplants are discussed in Chapter 21.

### Abdominal aneurysms

Blunt abdominal aortic injury is uncommon[52] but the incidence of abdominal aortic aneurysms is increasing with most occurring in elderly (above 60 years old) male hypertensives who smoke. Dilation usually begins below the renal arteries and extends to the aortic bifurcation. Because

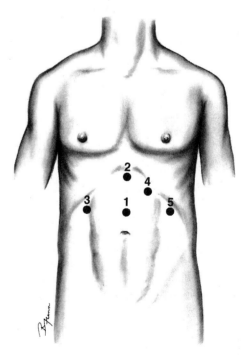

**Fig. 20-14.** The laparoscope is usually inserted near the umbilicus (point 1). Three small incisions for cannulas are often used but additional cannula sites may be necessary to obtain adequate exposure. (Frantzides C: *Laparoscopic and thorascopic surgery,* St. Louis, 1995, Mosby.)

the risk of rupture is considerable (as is the associated mortality), most abdominal aneurysms larger than 4 to 5 cm are electively repaired. The surgical approach varies with aneurysm location but often consists of a long vertical incision. The area of dilation is clamped above and below, the aneurysm sac opened, a graft inserted and the sac is closed over the graft.[10]

Postoperative atelectasis and pneumonia are relatively common and may be related to the age and smoking history of patients with abdominal aneurysm.[10,128] Chest physical therapy is not specific to aneurysm repair except as described earlier under thoracic aortic aneurysms (see p. 395).

## Splenic surgery

Most surgery to the spleen is due to trauma, spleno-megaly, malignancy, or hemolytic anemia. Rupture of the spleen is usually due to direct trauma to the left lower ribs, typically from a motor vehicle or bicycle accident. Peritoneal lavage is used to determine splenic injury. Although nonoperative management is considered in children, adults with splenic tears invariably require laparotomy.[10] As a result of overwhelming post-splenectomy infection, techniques of splenic conservation or splenorrhaphy are now favored over removal, whenever possible.[10,52] However, for treatment of hemolytic anemias, tumors, and some causes of splenomegaly, splenectomy is necessary. Surgical approach can be through a left subcostal, vertical or thoracoabdominal incision depending on the size of the spleen and reason for excision.[46] Laparoscopy has been used for diagnosis of splenic injury and, more recently, for splenectomy. Further experience is necessary to determine the role of laparoscopy in splenic surgery.[165]

Following splenectomy, patients have an increased risk of all forms of sepsis. The position of the left diaphragm next to the spleen and increased diaphragmatic pressure from splenomegaly may predispose patients to left basilar atelectasis and pulmonary infection that commonly occur after splenectomy.[10] A higher incidence of chest physical therapy directed towards left lower lobe pulmonary complications is reported in patients sustaining trauma.[89] Also, diaphragmatic dysfunction persists after upper abdominal surgery despite adequate pain management.[97] For these reasons, physical therapists should closely follow patients undergoing splenic surgery and pay particular attention to the left lower lobe. Early patient mobilization and breathing exercises may prevent postoperative pulmonary complications; postural drainage, manual techniques, and methods of secretion clearance are indicated to treat atelectasis and prevent infection.

## Hepatic surgery

Common causes of liver surgery are laceration from trauma and tumor resection. The normal liver has remarkable regenerative ability and can completely recover after major resection.[10] The recent development of vascular exclusion techniques, ultrasonic dissection, and biological glues have greatly reduced the blood loss and mortality associated with hepatic surgery. However, concomitant liver injury is responsible for a high percentage of deaths that occur from penetrating and blunt abdominal trauma. The operative goals are to control bleeding and to remove devitalized tissue.[152] Laparotomy may be extended to the chest through a median sternotomy for the life-saving placement of an atriocaval shunt to control hemorrhage.[6] Drains from the subhepatic and subphrenic spaces are often present after surgery.

Benign hepatic tumors may be resected because of risk of hemorrhage or when the possibility of malignancy cannot otherwise be excluded. Although the overall prognosis for primary malignant liver cancer remains poor, tumor resection is often associated with increased survival time. Liver transplant is currently considered in some cases. Limited surgical resection is also indicated for some secondary liver tumors, particularly metastases from colorectal cancer.[152]

Chest physical therapy can minimize the basilar atelectasis that is common after major liver surgery. Prolonged retraction on the lower ribs, manipulation of the diaphragm during surgery, and the anatomical position of the liver (under the diaphragm) may all contribute to postoperative secretion retention.[152] Chest physical therapy is similar to that described for splenic surgery, except that bilateral basilar atelectasis may occur due to the liver's location.

## Gastric, duodenal, and gallbladder surgery

In addition to operation for trauma or stomach cancer, treatment of ulcers makes up the majority of gastric and duodenal surgical procedures. Rupture of the stomach from blunt trauma is rare, but penetrating injury is not uncommon; many cases are managed by simple closure. Traumatic duodenal injuries occur more often and are associated with increased mortality when the pancreas is also involved. Surgery ranges from simple closure to complex reconstruction or, in rare instances, pancreatic-duodenectomy. Operative treatment for adenocarcinoma of the stomach depends on the location and lymph node involvement; a vertical or bilateral costal incision may be used. A total or partial gastrectomy is performed along with lymph node resection and appropriate reconstruction.[10]

Gastric and duodenal ulcers usually respond to medical treatment. When drug therapy fails, proximal gastric vagotomy or selective vagotomy is often performed since both are associated with fewer complications than truncal vagotomy with drainage and partial gastrectomy.[10] Experience in the successful use of laparoscopic and thoracoscopic vagotomy is growing. However, the increased operative time for highly selective vagotomy by laparoscopy limits its use over current traditional surgery.[165] Complications of gastrointestinal ulcers that require surgery include perforation and hemorrhage. Management of perforated duodenal ulcers ranges from simple closure using the omentum to truncal vagotomy and pyloroplasty.[10] There is a growing number of reports about successful laparoscopic treatment of some perforated duodenal ulcers, but the potential of this procedure needs further study.[165] Gastrointestinal hemorrhage from ulcers may be controlled by endoscopic treatment. However, surgery is often necessary and usually consists of oversewing the bleeding point combined with truncal vagotomy and pyloroplasty.[10]

Most gallbladder surgery is due to cholecystitis. Inflammation of the gallbladder is the result of stones, concentrated bile and secondary infection. Gall stones can be treated with dissolution therapy, lithotripsy, or cholecystectomy.[10] Although traditional laparotomy is still performed, laparoscopic cholecystectomy has become the procedure of choice for most patients with elective gallbladder disease. Also, the use of laparoscopic surgery to treat acute cholecystitis and other biliary tract pathology is growing and may reduce the need of open surgery for these conditions.[165]

Postoperative pain and the position of the diaphragm near the stomach and gallbladder contribute to the incidence of pulmonary complications after surgery. Compared to open surgery, laparoscopic surgery has reduced postoperative discomfort, but decreased diaphragm function still occurs.[35] In addition to pain relief, increased patient mobility along with breathing exercises and cough techniques are often needed to counter diminished respiratory function after surgery. Physical therapy treatment with postural drainage, percussion, and vibration should be reserved for patients with evidence of retained secretions.

### Renal surgery

Surgery is used to treat renal infections, tumors or stones, and upper urinary tract obstruction. In the past six years, extracorporeal shock-wave lithotripsy and endoscopic or percutaneous stone extraction has dramatically decreased the number of open operations for treatment of renal and ureteric stones.[10] However, surgery is necessary to prevent renal damage and ameliorate pelviureteric obstruction. Nephrectomy is indicated when infection or obstruction reduces overall renal function by less than 15%.[10] This surgery is usually performed through a subcostal or flank incision.[46] When renal tumors are present, a thoracoabdominal approach may be used and the kidney is removed along with perinephric fat, Gerota's fascia, and regional lymph nodes.[10] Blunt renal trauma is usually treated conservatively, with bedrest and transfusion,[10] except in the case of severe laceration or pedicle trauma (involving the kidney's blood supply) where nephrectomy is often required.[12]

Physical therapy treatment is not specific to renal surgery except in some transplant cases. However, diaphragm dysfunction is common due to the position of the kidneys; breathing exercises or out-of-bed mobilization, progressing to ambulation can be used to prevent secretion retention. Also, adequate pain control is important since the surgical incisions can be lengthy.

## PAIN MANAGEMENT

Pain reduction is a primary concern during the first few days after cardiac, thoracic, or upper abdominal surgery. In addition to its effects on other systems, postoperative pain is associated with a decrease in vital capacity and functional residual capacity (FRC), along with an increase in ventilation-perfusion mismatch, and alveolar-arterial oxygen tension difference.[139] If not ameliorated, these changes in respiratory function lead to hypoventilation, secretion retention, atelectasis, hypoxia, and pneumonia.[82] In the past, postoperative analgesia mainly consisted of oral or parenteral (intramuscular [IM] or IV) opiates. Although this regimen brought about some relief, respiratory depression often occurred with peak dosages and at other times, analgesia was inadequate. There have been many advances in the management of acute pain, such as occurs from surgery. Acute pain is comprised of both background and acute response pain. What the patient perceives at rest is termed background pain. Acute response pain is transient, occurring during activities such as deep breathing, coughing, dressing changes, and mobilization.[163] Adequate management of acute response and background pain allows for more normal movement to occur and may minimize the development of chronic symptoms such as myofascial pain.[116]

### Transcutaneous electrical nerve stimulation (TENS)

Since the 1970s, TENS has been used to manage both background and acute response pain. Two theories of action are that analgesia occurs from electrical interference with the spinal transmission of pain impulses and that electrical stimulation increases serotonin to centrally inhibit pain signal transmission.[163] Although some controversy surrounds its use, reported benefits of TENS include: a significant reduction in atelectasis and increased shoulder motion;[66] improved vital capacity;[1,146] improved FRC; and better maintenance of Pao$_2$.[1] Also, TENS is associated with reduced opiate use.[80,114,137] Clinical experience has shown that TENS has little beneficial effect on patients having multiple injuries and that better control of discomfort occurs in patients who can independently adjust the intensity. Thoracic placement of TENS electrodes may interfere with ECG monitoring. Also, the use of TENS is contraindicated in many patients with pacemakers.

### Patient-controlled analgesia (PCA)

Over the past few years, the use of PCA, epidural and subarachnoid opiates, interpleural local anesthetics, and peripheral nerve blocks has grown, becoming an area of subspecialty. A theoretical basis for PCA includes a more physiologic, rapid response and a patient-controlled system that provides more consistent therapeutic blood analgesic levels. Ideally, this method should decrease pain (or painful periods), anxiety, total analgesic use, complications of peak dosage, and nursing time while imparting a sense of control to the patient. However, successful use of PCA requires close physician-patient interaction and studies have not shown a consistent decrease in total narcotic use.[163] When compared to conventional IM analgesia, postoperative patients who used PCA have demonstrated earlier mobilization, improved cooperation with physical therapy, and a shortened hospital stay.[38] The use of PCA following thoracotomy is associated with a decrease in narcotic use, fever and respiratory complications,[86] and an increase in FRC when compared with IM therapy.[159] Although all reports on PCA are not favorable, it does have benefits over conventional parenteral regimens and has fewer side effects than epidural delivered narcotics.[163] Also, PCA is easily coordinated with chest physical therapy and efforts to increase patient mobilization.

## Epidural and subarachnoid analgesia

Since their introduction in 1979, epidural and subarachnoid delivered opiates have been widely used to manage postoperative pain. Epidural administration can be as a single dose, intermittent injection, or by continuous infusion. Segmental analgesia is achieved through binding the exogenously delivered opiates to receptors in the dorsal horn of the spinal cord.[37] Compared to IV delivery, smaller epidural doses can provide equal pain relief and fewer other associated responses (hormonal, metabolic and physiologic) in patients after thoracotomy.[127] Improved diaphragm function is reported using epidural analgesia following upper abdominal surgery.[97] Epidural catheters are generally placed at the interspace crossed by the middle dermatome of the surgical incision, allowing the drug to spread both cephalad and caudad. Because indwelling epidural catheters allow continuous or repeated opiate therapy, they are preferred over subarachnoid delivery when protracted analgesia is necessary. Yet, subarachnoid administration requires a smaller dosage, and the onset of analgesia is usually faster.[37]

Although good pain relief is achieved with their use, epidural analgesics may delay postoperative patient mobilization and early ambulation.[60] Other side effects from spinal narcotics include respiratory depression (from cephalad migration of the opiate to the brain stem), nausea, pruritus, urinary retention, and decreased gastrointestinal function.[37] To minimize some of these side effects, the epidural delivery of nonopiate analgesics is being investigated. Clonidine, an alpha-II agonist, has been studied with conflicting results in patients following thoracotomy and laparotomy.[50,113] Alpha-II agonists provide another option when narcotic use is contraindicated and may have an adjunct role to opiates. Complications of hypotension and sedation occur with epidural clonidine delivery.[117]

## Peripheral nerve blocks

Peripheral nerve blocks, including interpleural and intercostal nerve blocks, are well suited to patients having cardiothoracic surgery. In the classic approach, intercostal blocks (ICB) are performed posteriorly at the angle of the ribs, with the needle inserted just lateral to the sacrospinalis muscle. Alternately, local anesthetic drugs can be administered in the midaxillary, paravertebral, or parasternal region. ICB decreases pain and abnormal muscle activity (splinting), allowing for improved pulmonary function, gas exchange, and secretion clearance in postoperative patients without central respiratory depression (see Table 20-4).[34,107,124] The analgesia obtained from ICB enables patients to better tolerate early sitting and ambulation. However, the expertise required to perform ICB and the need to repeat the procedure are potential drawbacks.[150]

**Table 20-4.** Effects of ICB on pulmonary function in postoperative patients*

|  | Control | ICB |
|---|---|---|
| VC (1) | 36[a] | 75[a] |
|  | 55[b] | 60[b] |
|  | 25[c] | 56[c] |
| PEF (1/sec) | 39[a] | 82[a] |
|  | 50[b] | 60[b] |
|  | 32[c] | 57[c] |
| FEV$_1$ (1) | 32[a] | 76[a] |
|  | 55[b] | 63[b] |
|  | 30[c] | 60[c] |

Adapted from: Thompson GE, Hecker BR: Peripheral nerve blocks for management of thoracic surgical patients. In Gravlee GP and Rauck RL, editors: *Pain management in cardiothoracic surgery*, Philadelphia, 1993, J.B. Lippincott Co.

*Figures shown are the percent of presurgical baseline values for patients receiving intravenous or intramuscular opiates (control) compared with ICB. Measurements were taken within 24 hours after surgery and are significantly different. VC = vital capacity; PEF = peak expiratory flow rate; FEV$_1$ = forced expiratory volume in one second. (a) Mozell EJ and others: Continuous extrapleural intercostal nerve block after pleurectomy, *Thorax* 46:21, 1991. (b) Engberg G: Respiratory performance after upper abdominal surgery: a comparison of pain relief with intercostal blocks and centrally acting analgesia, *Acta Anesth Scand* 29:427, 1985. (c) Sabanathan S and others: Efficacy of continuous extrapleural intercostal nerve block on post-thoracotomy pain and pulmonary mechanics, *Br J Surg* 77:221, 1990.

## REFERENCES

1. Ali J, Yaffee C, and Serrette D: The effect of transcutaneous electric nerve stimulation on postoperative pain and pulmonary function, *Surgery* 89:507, 1981.
2. Andersen JB and others: Periodic continuous positive airway pressure, CPAP, by mask in the treatment of atelectasis, *Eur J Respir Dis* 61:20, 1980.
3. Anderson WA, Dorrett BE, and Hamilton GE: Prevention of postoperative pulmonary complications, *JAMA* 196:763, 1963.
4. Bateman JRM and others: Is cough as effective as chest physiotherapy in the removal of excessive tracheobronchial secretions? *Thorax* 36:683, 1981.
5. Baxter WD and Levine RS: An evaluation of intermittent positive pressure breathing in the prevention of postoperative pulmonary complications, *Arch Surg* 98:795, 1969.
6. Beal SL and Ward RE: Successful atrial caval shunting in the management of retrohepatic venous injuries, *Am J Surg* 158:409, 1989.
7. Bendixen HH, Headley-Whyte J, and Laver MB: Impaired oxygenation in surgical patients during general anesthesia with controlled ventilation, *N Engl J Med* 269:991, 1963.
8. Bojar RM: Circulatory assist devices. In Bojar RM, editor: *Adult cardiac surgery*, Cambridge, Mass, 1992, Blackwell Scientific Pulications.
9. Bojar RM, editor: *Adult cardiac surgery*, Cambridge, Mass, 1992, Blackwell Scientific Publications.

10. Burnand KG and Young AE, editors: *The new Aird's companion in surgical studies,* New York, 1992, Churchill Livingstone.

11. Campbell T, Ferguson N, and McKinlay RGC: The use of a simple self-administered method of positive expiratory pressure (PEP) in chest physiotherapy after abdominal surgery, *Physiother* 72:498, 1986.

12. Cardona VD and others, editors: *Trauma nursing from resuscitation through rehabilitation,* Philadelphia, 1988, W. B. Saunders Co.

13. Castello R and Haas A: Chest physical therapy: comparative efficacy of preoperative and postoperative in the elderly, *Archives Phys Med Rehab* 66:376, 1985.

14. Celli B, Rodriguez G, and Snider G: A controlled trial of intermittent positive pressure breathing, incentive spirometry, and deep breathing exercises in preventing pulmonary complications after abdominal surgery, *Am Rev Respir Dis* 130:12, 1984.

15. Chang SC, Shiao GM, and Perng RP: Postural effect on gas exchange in the patients with unilateral pleural effusions, *Chest* 96:60, 1989.

16. Chang SC, Shiao GM, and Perng RP: Effect of body position on gas exchange in patients with unilateral central airway lesions, *Chest* 103:787, 1993.

17. Chulay M, Brown J, and Summer W: Effect of postoperative immobilization after coronary artery bypass surgery, *Crit Care Med* 10:176, 1982.

18. Ciesla N: Postural drainage, positioning, and breathing exercises. In Mackenzie CF, editor: *Chest physiotherapy in the intensive care unit,* Baltimore, 1989, Williams & Wilkins.

19. Ciesla N and others: The incidence of extrapleural hematomas in patients with rib fractures receiving chest physical therapy (abstract), *Phys Ther* 76:766, 1987.

20. Ciesla ND, Klemic N, and Imle PC: Chest physical therapy to the patient with multiple trauma: two case studies, *Phys Ther* 61:202, 1981.

21. Ciesla ND: Chest physical therapy of the adult intensive care unit trauma patient, *Phys Ther Prac* 3:92, 1994.

22. Clark GC, Achecter WP, and Trunkey DD: Variables affecting outcome in blunt pulmonary chest trauma: flail chest v/s pulmonary contusion, *J Trauma* 28:298, 1988.

23. Connors AF and others: Chest physical therapy: The immediate effect on oxygenation in acutely ill patients, *Chest* 78:559, 1980.

24. Cooperman AM and others: Use of transcutaneous electrical stimulation in control of postoperative pain—results of a prospective, randomized, controlled study, *Am J Surg* 133:185, 1977.

25. Cox EF: Blunt abdominal trauma: a 5-year-analysis of 870 patients requiring celiotomy, *Ann Surg* 199:467, 1984.

26. Craig DB: Postoperative recovery of pulmonary function, *Anesth Analg* 60:46, 1981.

27. Craig DB, Wahba WM, and Don H: Airway closure and lung volumes in surgical positions, *Can Anaesth Soc J* 18:92, 1971.

28. Crawford BL, Blunnie WP, and Elliot AGP: The value of self-administered peri-operative physiotherapy, *Irish J Med Sci* 159:51, 1990.

29. Dean E: Invited commentary, *Phys Ther* 74:10, 1994.

30. Dhainaut JF and others: Improved oxygenation in patients with extensive unilateral pneumonia using the lateral decubitus position, *Thorax* 35:792, 1980.

31. Dohi S and Cold MI: Comparison of two methods of postoperative respiratory care, *Chest* 73:592, 1978.

32. Dull JL and Dull WL: Are maximal inspiratory breathing exercises or incentive spirometry better than early mobilization after cardiopulmonary bypass? *Phys Ther* 63:655, 1983.

33. Dureuil B and others: Diaphragmatic contractility after upper abdominal surgery, *J Appl Physiol* 61:1775, 1986.

34. Engberg G: Respiratory performance after upper abdominal surgery: A comparison of pain relief with intercostal blocks and centrally acting analgesica, *Acta Anesth Scand* 29:427, 1985.

35. Erice F and others: Diaphragmatic function before and after laparoscopic cholecystectomy, *Anesthesiology* 79:966, 1993.

36. Estenne M and others: Phrenic and diaphragm function after coronary artery bypass grafting, *Thorax* 40:293, 1985.

37. Ferrante FM and VadeBoncoure TR: Epidural and subarachnoid analgesia for thoracic surgery. In Gravlee GP and Rauck RL, editors: *Pain management in cardiothoracic surgery,* Philadelphia, 1993, J. B. Lippincott Co.

38. Finley RJ, Keeri-Szanto M, and Boyd D: New analgesic agents and techniques shorten postoperative hospital stay (abstract), *Pain* Suppl 2:S397, 1984.

39. Fishman AP: Down with the good lung, *N Engl J Med* 304:537, 1981.

40. Flower KA and others: New mechanical aid to physiotherapy in cystic fibrosis, *Br Med J* 2:630, 1979.

41. Ford GT and Guenter CA: Toward prevention of postoperative complications, *Am Rev Respir Dis* 130:4, 1984.

42. Ford GT and others: Diaphragm function after upper abdominal surgery in humans, *Am Rev Respir Dis* 127:431, 1983.

43. Fratacci MD and others: Diaphragmatic shortening after thoracic surgery in humans, *Anesthesiology* 79:654, 1993.

44. Frolund L and Madsen F: Self-administered prophylactic postoperative positive expiratory pressure in thoracic surgery, *Acta Anaesthesiol Scand* 30:381, 1986.

45. Fugl-Meyer AR: Effects of respiratory muscle paralysis in tetraplegic and paraplegic patients, *Scand J Rehabil Med* 3:141, 1971.

46. Fuller JR: *Surgical technology principles and practice,* ed 3, Philadelphia, 1994, W.B. Saunders Co.

47. Garradd J and Bullock M: The effect of respiratory therapy on intracranial pressure in ventilated neurosurgical patients, *Aust J Physiother* 32:107, 1986.

48. Gillespie DJ and Rehder K: Body position and ventilation-perfusion relationships in unilateral pulmonary disease, *Chest* 91:75, 1987.

49. Goldstraw P: The chest wall, lungs, pleura, and diaphragm. In Burnand KG and Young AE, editors: *The new Airs's companion in surgical studies,* New York, 1992, Churchill Livingstone.

50. Gordh T: Epidural clonidine for treatment of postoperative pain after thoracotomy: a double-blind, placebo-controlled study, *Acta Anaesthesiol Scand* 32:702, 1988.

51. Gormezano J and Brainthwaite MA: Pulmonary physiotherapy with assisted ventilation, *Anaesthesia* 27:249, 1972.

52. Grande CM, editor: *Textbook of trauma anesthesia and critical care,* St Louis, 1993, Mosby.

53. Gray L: Fatal pulmonary Hemmorrhage (letter), *Phys Ther* 60:343-344, 1980.

54. Grimby G: Aspects of lung expansion in relation to pulmonary physiotherapy, *Am Rev Respir Dis* 110:145, 1974.

55. Hammon WE and Martin RJ: Fatal pulmonary hemorrhage associated with chest physical therapy, *Phys Ther* 59:1247, 1979.

56. Hammon WE and Martin RJ: Chest physical therapy for acute atelectasis, *Phys Ther* 61:217, 1981.

57. Hammon WE, McCaffree R, and Cucchiara AJ: A comparison of manual to mechanical chest percussion for clearance of alveolar material in patients with pulmonary alveolar proteinosis (phospholipidosis), *Chest* 103:1409, 1993.

58. Hammon WE, Connors AF, and McCaffree: Cardiac arrhythmias during postural drainage and chest percussion of critically ill patients, *Chest* 102:1836, 1992.

59. Harman E and Lillington G: Pulmonary risk factors in surgery, *Med Clin North Am* 63:1289, 1979.

60. Hawthorne MH: Recognition of thoracic surgical complications: a nursing perspective. In Wolfe WG, editor: *Complications in thoracic surgery,* Baltimore, 1992, Mosby-Year Book.

61. Hedenstierna G: Gas exchange during anaesthesia, *Br J Anaesth* 64:507, 1990.

62. Heitz M, Holzach P, and Dittmann M: Comparison of the effect

of continuous positive airway pressure and blow bottles on functional residual capacity after abdominal surgery, *Respiration* 48:277, 1985.

63. Hiatt JR, Yeatman LA, and Childs JS: The value of echocardiography in blunt chest trauma, *J Trauma* 28:914, 1988.

64. Hsu HO and Hickey RF: Effect of posture on functional residual capacity postoperatively, *Anesthesiology* 44:520, 1976.

65. Hurn PD: Thoracic injuries. In Cardona VD and others, editors: *Trauma nursing from resuscitation through rehabilitation,* Philadelphia, 1988, W. B. Saunders Co.

66. Hymes AC, and others: Electrical surface stimulation for control of acute post-operative pain and prevention of ileus, *Surg Forum* 24:447, 1973.

67. Imle PC: Adjuncts to chest physiotherapy. In Mackenzie CF, editor: *Chest physiotherapy in the intensive care unit,* Baltimore, 1989, Williams & Wilkins.

68. Imle PC: Percussion and vibration. In Mackenzie CF, editor: *Chest physiotherapy in the intensive care unit,* Baltimore, 1989, Williams & Wilkins.

69. Imle PC: Physical therapy for acute spinal cord injury, *Phys Ther Prac* 3:1, 1994.

70. Imle PC and Klemic N: Changes with immobility and methods of mobilization. In Mackenzie CF, editor: *Chest physiotherapy in the intensive care unit,* Baltimore, 1989, Williams & Wilkins.

71. Imle PC and Klemic N: Methods of airway clearance. In Mackenzie CF, editor: *Chest physiotherapy in the intensive care unit,* Baltimore, 1989, Williams & Wilkins.

72. Jaworski A and others: Utility of immediate postlobectomy fiberoptic bronchoscopy in preventing atelectasis, *Chest* 94:38, 1988.

73. Jenkins SC: Pre-operative and post-operative physiotherapy—are they necessary? In Pryor JA, editor: *Respiratory care,* New York, 1991, Churchill Livingstone.

74. Jenkins SC, Soutar SA, and Moxham J: The effects of posture on lung volumes in normal subjects and in patients pre- and post-coronary artery surgery, *Physiotherapy* 74:492, 1988.

75. Jenkins SC and others: Physiotherapy after coronary artery surgery: are breathing exercises necessary? *Thorax* 44:634, 1989.

76. Jung R and others: Comparison of three methods of respiratory care following upper abdominal surgery, *Chest* 78:31, 1980.

77. Kaplan JA, editor: *Cardiac anesthesia,* Philadelphia, 1993, W.B. Saunders, Co.

78. Kigin CM: Chest physical therapy for the acutely ill medical patient. *Phys Ther* 61:1724, 1981.

79. Kigin CM: Advances in chest physical therapy. In O'Donohue WJ, editor: *Current advances in respiratory care,* Park Ridge, 1984, American College of Chest Physicians.

80. Kimball KL and others: Use of TENS for pain reduction in burn patients receiving travase, *J Burn Care Rehab* 8:28, 1987.

81. King I and Tarsitano B: The effect of structured and unstructured pre-operative training: a replication, *Nurs Res* 31:324, 1982.

82. King TC and Smith CR: Chest wall, pleura, lung, and mediastinum. In Schwartz SI and others, editors: *Principles of surgery,* ed 5, New York, 1989, McGraw-Hill Book Co.

83. Kirby TJ and Ginsberg RJ: Management of pneumothorax and barotrauma, *Clin Chest Med* 13:97, 1992.

84. Krasna MJ: Diagnostic and therapeutic thoracoscopy. In Zucker KA, editor: *Surgical laparoscopy update,* St. Louis, 1993, Quality Medical Publishing, Inc.

84A. Lamm WJ, Graham MM, and Albert RK: Mechanism by which the prone position improves oxygenation in acute lung injury, *Am J Respir Crit Care Med* 150:184, 1994.

85. Landercasper J, Cogbill TH, and Strutt PJ: Delayed diagnosis of flail chest. *Crit Care Med* 18:611, 1990.

86. Lange MP, Dahn MS, and Jacobs LA: Patient-controlled analgesia versus intermittent analgesia dosing, *Heart & Lung* 17:495, 1988.

87. Laws AK and McIntyre RW: Chest physiotherapy: a physiological assessment during intermittent positive pressure ventilation in respiratory failure, *Can Anaesth Soc J* 16:487, 1969.

88. Leith DE: Cough, *Phys Ther* 48:439, 1967.

89. Mackenzie CF, editor: *Chest physiotherapy in the intensive care unit,* Baltimore, 1989, Williams & Wilkins.

90. Mackenzie CF: Physiological changes following chest physiotherapy. In Mackenzie CF, editor: *Chest physiotherapy in the intensive care unit,* Baltimore, 1989, Williams & Wilkins.

91. Mackenzie CF: Respiratory management of trauma patients. In Grande CM, editor: *Textbook of trauma anesthesia and critical care,* St Louis, 1993, Mosby.

92. Mackenzie CF: Undesirable effects, precautions, and contraindications of chest physiotherapy. In Mackenzie CF, editor: *Chest physiotherapy in the intensive care unit,* Baltimore, 1989, Williams & Wilkins.

93. Mackenzie CF and Shin B: Cardiorespiratory function before and after chest physiotherapy in mechanically ventilated patients with post-traumatic respiratory failure, *Crit Care Med* 13:483, 1985.

94. Mackenzie CF and others: Changes in total lung/thorax compliance following chest physiotherapy, *Anesth Analg* 59:207, 1980.

95. Mackenzie CF, Shin B, and McAslan TC: Chest physiotherapy: the effect on arterial oxygenation, *Anesth Analg* 57:28, 1978.

96. Mahler DA and others: Positional dyspnea and oxygen desaturation related to carcinoma of the lung: up with the good lung, *Chest* 83:826, 1983.

97. Mankikian B and others: Improvement of diaphragmatic function by a thoracic epidural block after upper abdominal surgery, *Anesthesiology* 68:379, 1988.

98. Marincola FM and Mark JBD: Selection factors resulting in improved survival after surgical resection of tumors metastatic to the lungs, *Arch Surg* 125:1387, 1990.

99. Marini JJ, Pierson DJ, and Hudson LD: Acute lobar atelectasis: a prospective comparison of fiberoptic bronchoscopy and respiratory therapy, *Am Rev Respir Dis* 119:971, 1979.

100. Marti CH and Ulmer WT: Absence of effect of the body position on arterial blood gases, *Respiration* 43:41, 1982.

101. Martin CJ and others: Chest physiotherapy and the distribution of ventilation, *Chest* 69:174, 1976.

102. Mattox KL: Thoracic injury requiring surgery, *World J Surg* 7:49, 1983.

103. Miller RS and others: Synchronized independent lung ventilation in the management of a unilateral pulmonary contusion with massive hemoptysis. *J Tenn Med Assoc* 85:374, 1992.

104. Mitchell RL: The lateral limited thoracotomy incision: standard for pulmonary operations, *J Thorac Cardiovasc Surg* 99:590, 1990.

105. Moller JT and others: Hypoxaemia during anaesthesia—an observer study, *Br J Anaesth* 66:437, 1991.

106. Morran CG, and others: Randomized controlled trial of physiotherapy for postoperative pulmonary complications, *Br J Anaesth* 55:1113, 1983.

107. Mozell EJ and others: Continuous extrapleural intercostal nerve block after pleurectomy, *Thorax* 46:21, 1991.

108. Murphy M, Concannon D, and Fitzgerald MX: Chest percussion: help or hindrance to postural drainage? *Ir Med J* 76:189, 1983.

109. Murray JF: Ketchup-bottle method, *N Eng J Med* 300:1155, 1979 (editoral).

110. Neagley SR and Zwillich CW: The effect of positional changes on oxygenation in patients with pleural effusions, *Chest* 88:714, 1985.

111. Nicholson J: *A course of lessons on the art of deep breathing and giving physiological exercises to strengthen the chest, lungs, stomach, back, etc.,* London, 1890, Health Culture Co.

112. Perel A and Priel IE: Adult respiratory distress syndrome. In Grande CM, editor: *Textbook of trauma anesthesia and critical care,* St Louis, 1993, Mosby.

113. Petit J and others: Comparison of clonidine administered epidurally for postoperative analgesia, *Anesthesiology* 71:A647, 1989 (abstract).

114. Pike PM: Transcutaneous electrical stimulation: its use in management of postoperative pain, *Anaesthesia* 33:165, 1978.

115. Pryor JA: The forced expiration technique. In Pryor JA, editor: *Respiratory care,* New York, 1991, Churchill Livingstone.

116. Raj PP and Brannon JE: Analgesic considerations for the median sternotomy. In Gravlee GP and Rauck RL, editors: *Pain management in cardiothoracic surgery,* Philadelphia, 1993, J. B. Lippincott Co.

117. Rauck RL: Epidural clonidine. In Gravlee GP and Rauck RL, editors: *Pain management in cardiothoracic surgery,* Philadelphia, 1993, J. B. Lippincott Co.

118. Ray JF and others: Immobility, hypoxemia, and pulmonary arteriovenous shunting, *Arch Surg* 109:537, 1974.

119. Remolina C and others: Positional hypoxemia in unilateral lung disease, *N Engl J Med* 304:523, 1981.

120. Risksten SE and others: Effects of periodic positive airway pressure by mask on postoperative pulmonary function, *Chest* 89:774, 1986.

121. Rivara D and others: Positional hypoxemia during artificial ventilation, *Crit Care Med* 12:436, 1984.

122. Rothen HU and others: Re-expansion of atelectasis during general anaesthesia: a computed tomography study, *Br J Anaesth* 71:788, 1993.

123. Roukema J, Carol E, and Prins J: The prevention of pulmonary complications after upper abdominal surgery in patients with noncompromised pulmonary status, *Arch Surg* 123:30, 1988.

124. Sabanathan S and others: Efficacy of continuous extrapleural intercostal nerve block on post-thoracotomy pain and pulmonary mechanics, *Br J Surg* 77:221, 1990.

125. Sadowsky HS: Thoracic surgical procedures, monitoring, and support equipment. In Hillegass EA and Sadowsky HS, editors: *Essentials of cardiopulmonary physical therapy,* Philadelphia, 1994, W.B. Saunders Co.

126. Sales BO and others: Lower respiratory tract infections after abdominal operations: epidemiology and risk factors, *Eur J Surg* 158:105, 1992.

127. Salomaki TE and others: Epidural versus intravenous fentanyl for reducing hormonal, metabolic, and physiologic responses after thoracotomy, *Anesthesiology* 79:672, 1993.

128. Schwartz SI, Shires GT, and Spencer FC, editors: *Principles of surgery,* ed 5, New York, 1989, McGraw-Hill Book Co.

129. Schwieger I and others: Absence of benefit of incentive spirometry in low-risk patients undergoing elective cholecystomy, *Chest* 89:652, 1986.

130. Schypisser JP, Brandli O, and Meili U: Postoperative intermittent positive pressure breathing versus physiotherapy, *Am J Surg* 140:682, 1980.

131. Semanoff T, Kleinfeld M and Castle P: Chest physical therapy as a preventive modality in cardiac surgery patients, (abstract) *Arch Phys Med Rehabil* 62:506, 1981.

132. Shin B: Lung contusion. In Cowley RA and Dunham CM, editors: *Trauma care. Vol 1 Surgical management,* Philadelphia, 1987, Lippincott.

133. Shin B and others: Management of lung contusion, *Am Surg* 45:168, 1979.

134. Simmonneau G and others: Diaphragm dysfunction induced by upper abdominal surgery, *Am Rev Respir Dis* 128:899, 1983.

135. Smaldone GC and Messina MS: Enhancement of particle deposition by flow-limiting segments in humans, *J Appl Physiol* 59:509, 1985.

136. Smaldone GC and Messina MS: Flow limitation, cough, and patterns of aerosol deposition in humans, *J Appl Physiol* 59:515, 1985.

137. Solomon RA, Viernstein MC, and Lang DM: Reduction of postoperative pain and narcotic use by transcutaneous electrical nerve stimulation, *Surgery* 87:142, 1980.

138. Sonnenblick M, Melzer E, and Rosin AJ: Body positional effect on gas exchange in unilateral pleural effusions, *Chest* 83:784, 1983.

139. Spence AA and Smith G: Postoperative analgesia and lung function: a comparison of morphine with extradural block, *Br J Anaesth* 43:144, 1971.

140. Spencer FC: Diseases of great vessels. In Schwartz SI and others, editors: *Principles of surgery,* ed 5, New York, 1989, McGraw-Hill Book Co.

141. Stanley DG: Thoracoscopic lobectomy, *J Tenn Med Assoc* 85:463, 1992.

142. Stein M and Cassara FL: Pre-operative pulmonary evaluation and therapy for surgery patients, *JAMA* 211:787, 1962.

143. Stellin G: Survival in trauma victims with pulmonary contusion, *Am Surg* 57:780, 1991.

144. Stiller K and others: Acute lobar atelectasis, a comparison of two chest physiotherapy regimens, *Chest* 98:1336, 1990.

144A. Stiller K and others: Efficacy of breathing and coughing exercises in the prevention of pulmonary complications after coronary artery surgery, *Chest* 105:74, 1994.

145. Stock MC, Downs JB, and Corkran ML: Pulmonary function before and after prolonged continuous positive airway pressure by mask, *Crit Care Med* 12:973, 1984.

146. Stratton SA and Smith MM: Post-operative thoracotomy: effect of transcutaneous electric nerve stimulation on forced vital capacity, *Phys Ther* 60:45, 1980.

147. Sutton PP and others: Assessment of percussion, vibratory-shaking, and breathing exercises in chest physiotherapy, *Eur J Respir Dis* 66:147, 1985.

148. Tarhan S, Moffitt EA, and Sesson AD: Risks of anesthesia and surgery in patients with chronic bronchitis and chronic obstructive pulmonary disease, *Surgery* 74:720, 1973.

149. Thomas JA and McIntosh JM: Are incentive spirometry, intermittent positive pressure breathing, and deep breathing exercises effective in the prevention of postoperative pulmonary complications after upper abdominal surgery? A systematic overview and meta-analysis, *Phys Ther* 74:3, 1994.

150. Thompson GE and Hecker BR: Peripheral nerve blocks for management of thoracic surgical patients. In Gravlee GP and Rauck RL, editors: *Pain management in cardiothoracic surgery,* Philadelphia, 1993, J. B. Lippincott Co.

151. Thoren L: Post-operative pulmonary complications: observations on their prevention by means of physiotherapy, *Acta Chir Scand* 107:193, 1954.

152. Traynor O: Liver. In O'Higgins NJ, Chisholm GD, and Williamson RC, editors: *Surgical Management,* ed 2, Boston, 1991, Butterworth-Heinemann Ltd.

153. Treasure T: The heart and pericardium. In Burnand KG and Young AE editors: *The new Aird's companion in surgical studies,* New York, 1992, Churchill Livingstone.

154. Tyler E, Caldwell C, and Ghia JN: Transcutaneous electrical nerve stimulation: an alternative approach to the management of postoperative pain, *Anesth Analg* 61:449, 1982.

155. Tyler ML and others: Prediction of oxygenation during chest physiotherapy in critically ill patients, *Am Rev Respir Dis* Suppl 121: 218, 1980 (abstract).

156. Van der Schans CP, Piers DA, and Postma DS: Effect of manual percussion on tracheobronchial clearance in patients with chronic airflow obstruction and excessive tracheobronchial secretion, *Thorax* 16:448, 1986.

157. Van de Water JM and others: Prevention of postoperative pulmonary complications, *Surg Gynecol Obstet* 135:1, 1972.

158. Vickers MD: Postoperative pneumonias (editorial), *Br Med J* 284:292, 1982.

159. Wang CS and others: Efficiency of patient-controlled analgesia versus

conventional analgesia in patients after thoracotomy, *Ma Tsui Hsueh Tsa Chi* 29:604, 1991.

160. Warren CPW, Grimwood M: Pulmonary disorders and physiotherapy in patients who undergo cholecystectomy, *Can J Surg* 23:384, 1980.

161. Webber BA, editor: *The Brompton hospital guide to chest physiotherapy*, ed 4, Boston, 1980, Blackwell Scientific Publications.

162. White DJ, Mawdley RH: Effects of selective bronchial drainage positions and percussion on blood pressure and healthy human subjects, *Phys Ther* 63:300, 1983.

163. Wolman RL: Patient-controlled analgesia following thoracic surgery. In Gravlee GP and Rauck RL, editors: *Pain management in cardiothoracic surgery*, Philadelphia, 1993, J. B. Lippincott Co.

164. Zack MB, Pontoppidan H, and Kazemi H: The effect of lateral position on gas exchange in pulmonary disease: a prospective evaluation, *Am Rev Respir Dis* 110:49, 1974.

165. Zucker KA, editor: *Surgical laparoscopy update*, St Louis, 1993, Quality Medical Publishing, Inc.

# CHAPTER 21

# Physical Therapy in Heart and Lung Transplantation

*Barbara Bernard Butler*

By 1993 almost 26,000 cardiac and pulmonary transplantations had been reported throughout the world.[21A] With 5-year average survival rates ranging from 42% to 68% for patients with heart-lung, lung, and heart transplants,[26] many of these persons will return to a normal life-style including work, school, recreational, and avocational activities. They will need physical therapy to manage not only their cardiopulmonary status, but also the normal incidences of fractures, strains, musculoskeletal injuries, and neurological insults.

Therefore, the entry-level therapist needs practical knowledge of the impact and implications of the transplanted organ on the body, and theoretical and clinical understanding of the associated cardiopulmonary changes in order to educate and direct the patient, family, and other health care providers into the most effective treatment program.

This chapter is organized among the distinctive features of heart versus heart-lung versus lung transplant patients. The material is further organized under both pretransplant and posttransplant phases of care. Abbreviations used commonly in this chapter are presented in the box on p. 405.

## PHASE ONE: PRETRANSPLANT
### General information

The ultimate decision to transplant should be based on multiple clinical parameters including resting and active indices of cardiac, pulmonary, and hemodynamic function.

**Heart transplant.** In patients with chronic cardiac failure, the cardiac response to exercise limits exercise capacity because increasing cardiac output that occurs with exercise is inadequate to oxygenate the tissues.[58] In addition, respiratory muscle weakness,[36] diminished pulmonary perfusion causing ventilation/perfusion mismatch,[35] and reduced lung volumes[20] may be associated with congestive heart failure, further compromising oxygen supply to the tissues. Also, changes in autonomic nervous system responsiveness may alter the reflexive changes related to variations in posture during exercise.[28]

**Heart-lung transplant.** Most candidates for heart-lung transplants present symptoms including pulmonary edema,

## Indications for transplantation, and the organ(s) commonly used[29,26]

**Most common:**

| | |
|---|---|
| Cardiomyopathy | OHT |
| Coronary artery disease | OHT |
| Congenital heart disease children: | OHT, many |
| | HLT, some |
| | LT, rare |
| Congenital heart disease adult: | OHT |
| Cystic fibrosis | DLT > HLT |
| Eisenmenger's syndrome | HLT, more |
| | SLT or DLT, few |
| Chronic lung disease | DLT, SLT or HLT |
| Primary pulmonary hypertension | HLT, many |
| | DLT or SLT, few |
| Pulmonary fibrosis | SLT, most |
| | DLT, few |

**Less common:**

| | |
|---|---|
| Valvular heart disease, refractory dysrhythmias, Doxorubicin-induced cardiac toxicity, amyloidosis, Chagas' disease and cardiac tumors | OHT |
| Pulmonary thromboembolic disease, Wegener's Granulomatosis, sarcoidosis, histiocytosis X, bronchiectasis, lupus, scleroderma, hemosiderosis, lymphangiolyomyomatosis, acute respiratory failure, leiomyosarcoma of the pulmonary artery, inhalation and malignancy | SLT or DLT |
| Retransplantation | OHT, HLT, SLT or DLT |

**KEY:**
OHT: Orthotopic heart transplant.
HLT: Heart/lung transplant.
LT: Lung transplant.
DLT: Double lung transplant.
SLT: Single lung transplant.

elevated pulmonary arterial, capillary and venous pressures, and increased pulmonary vascular resistance.[55] The latter is associated with resting hyperventilation, excessive ventilation during exercise, and markedly inadequate cardiac output.[55,56]

**Lung transplant.** Transplant candidates with chronic lung disease, especially those with emphysema-related diseases, commonly have malnutrition and weight loss, probably because of increased energy demand.[17]

Preoperatively, pulmonary function tests show that SLT recipients tend to have severe restrictive changes, and DLT recipients commonly demonstrate a severe obstructive abnormality, with hyperinflation and a marked reduction in diffusion capacity.[38]

### Importance of exercise testing

Thorough cardiopulmonary exercise testing can determine exercise limitation. Algorithms, such as those developed by Eschenbacher,[12] interpret cardiopulmonary exercise tests by decision points that hinge on measurements of $\dot{V}O_2$ (oxygen consumption), $\dot{V}CO_2$ (carbon dioxide production), $\dot{V}E$ (minute ventilation), $Sao_2$ (oxygen saturation measured

by pulse oximetry), heart rate, and anaerobic threshold. The algorithms can identify and quantify the relative contribution of coexisting pulmonary and cardiac or circulatory problems to exercise limitation.[59]

Peak oxygen consumption ($\dot{V}O_2$ max) assesses cardiac reserve and peripheral adaptations to reduced cardiac output during exercise. It also provides objective assessment of functional capacity,[35] and may become a standard criterion for transplantation.[59]

Measurement of $\dot{V}O_2$ and $\dot{V}CO_2$ (carbon dioxide production) during exercise progression is used to estimate the anaerobic or ventilatory threshold, the point during exercise at which $\dot{V}CO_2$ rises disproportionately to the rise in $\dot{V}O_2$.[35,58]

The ventilatory response to submaximal exercise, the slope of line comparing minute ventilation to carbon dioxide production ($\dot{V}E/\dot{V}CO_2$), and arterial blood gas values are other useful values.[55,56]

As investigation continues, we expect more precise means of differentiating subgroups within the population of patients recommended for transplantation who would derive the greatest overall benefit from transplantation, and thus deserve higher priority.

## Assessing quality of life and the need for exercise

Fifty-two percent of heart transplant candidates are hospitalized at the time the donor organ becomes available, and 42% of these are on life support.[26] This hospitalization usually follows a prolonged period of severe illness and associated immobility that leads to deconditioning of various body systems, including the cardiovascular and muscular systems.[61]

Cardiovascular deconditioning is indicated by decreased exercise capacity, increased resting pulse rate, and orthostatic intolerance. The reduced cardiac reserve during rest and exercise probably results from a combination of impaired autonomic function and reductions in stroke volume, myocardial function, end-diastolic volume, and total heart volume.[40]

Muscular deconditioning becomes an issue and can exceed the severity of cardiovascular deconditioning, primarily when the lower extremity muscle mass is markedly diminished.[61] According to Appell, loss of the muscle's mitochondrial function and strength occurs most dramatically during the first week of immobilization. Muscles with slow, predominantly oxidative fibers are most susceptible to this atrophy, and the recovery time from atrophy is much longer than the total immobilization period.[1]

All lung transplant candidates are impaired in their conditioning for activities of daily living, and because of chronically debilitating illnesses, most have had steadily decreasing levels of activity for 1 to 4 years.[61]

Preoperative rehabilitation is controversial for patients with severe chronic obstructive pulmonary disease and possibly for other end-stage lung diseases. Williams states that ventilatory limitations prevent the imposition of sufficient exercise stress to stimulate muscular redevelopment.[61]

Exercise capacity is only one determinant of quality of life. "Adjustment to illness" questionnaires have demonstrated slightly greater feelings of social dysfunction in patients with heart failure compared with patients after transplantation.[52] The former group saw themselves as able to perform less activity, and their estimated metabolic equivalent levels were 5.3 versus 7.9, respectively. However, both groups had a similar intensity of general anxiety and depression. Notably, unexpected hospital days occurred more frequently after cardiac transplantation.

## Progression, expectations, and limitations

**Heart transplant.** According to Sullivan,[53] ambulatory patients with chronic heart failure who are stabilized by medical therapy can achieve a significant training effect from long-term exercise. Patients may start by walking half a block and progress to 1 or 2 miles; others may progress from 6 minutes of steady state, 20 watt submaximal bicycle exercise to a point of no evidence of anaerobic metabolism. Peripheral adaptations such as increases in muscle mass and vascularity, and in peak blood flow to the exercising lower extremity play important roles. Therefore exercise tolerance may be altered through training, independent of central hemodynamic limitations.

Patients with severe but medically stabilized congestive heart failure have achieved more than 50% of predicted maximal capacity and threefold to fourfold increases in left ventricular volumes, provided that mitral regurgitation can be minimized. Peripheral vasodilation and tachycardia normally associated with exercise can improve ejection fraction and cardiac output.[52] Factors, such as the effect of position on venous return and myocardial oxygen demand, suggest that upright would be the preferred position for exercise.[28,45]

However, there are limitations during exercise imposed by abnormal autonomic function that causes an inability to modulate heart rate, or by excessive ventilatory responses, such as exercise hyperpnea and exertional dyspnea, which may be the limiting symptoms.[2,36,54]

According to Mancini, a decline in exercise capacity does not signal a precipitous deterioration; however, a peak $\dot{V}o_2$ of 14 ml/kg/min or less (approximately 4 multiples of resting oxygen consumption [METS]) is a common criterion for acceptance for cardiac transplant.[35]

**Heart-lung and lung transplant.** According to Otulana,[40] the effects of deconditioning on the body's adaptive and homeostatic mechanisms vary depending on the nature and severity of the primary disease. Chronic lung diseases often produce an exaggerated tachycardia, excessive increase in pulmonary vascular pressures, poor oxygen delivery with exercise, diminished ventilatory capacity, and reduced inspiratory muscle strength. For example, advanced cystic fibrosis causes reduced work capacity, respiratory limitation, poor nutritional status, resting hypoxemia, and a reduced cardiac response due to secondary pulmonary hypertension.

**Lung transplant.** All lung transplant candidates are oxygen-dependent, desaturate with exercise, and have muscle weakness and posture deviations.[3]

The mean distance achieved on a 6-minute walk test averaged $353 \pm 39$ meters for lung transplant candidates; however, the level of disability in most patients precludes graded exercise studies.[61]

Candidates for single lung transplantation (SLT) are not comparable to double lung transplant (DLT) candidates with respect to anthropomorphic data; therefore, direct comparisons between these two groups should be used cautiously.[61]

## PHYSICAL THERAPY PROGRAM GUIDELINES FOR PRETRANSPLANT CARE

Initial physical therapy evaluation should include, as appropriate, cardiac, pulmonary, musculoskeletal, posture and flexibility screening. In addition, a 6-minute walk test at a self-determined pace is commonly employed to determine overall cardiopulmonary ability for ambulatory patients. Six minutes of steady-state cycle ergometry at 20 watts, if possible, and symptom-limited bicycle exercise with work rates continuously increasing at a rate of 15 watts per minute are used as well.

Physical therapy goals for heart or lung transplant candidates may include:

1. Increased cardiovascular endurance
2. Increased pulmonary hygiene
3. Improved breath control
4. Increased musculoskeletal strength
5. Improved posture and flexibility
6. Increased understanding of how to aid recovery after surgery
7. Increased knowledge of the changes secondary to transplantation

Some facilities require that heart or lung transplant candidates relocate to within a one-hour's distance of the transplant center, and participate in up to 90-minute exercise sessions at a frequency of 3 to 5 times per week.[3,61]

The preoperative exercise prescription may include warm-up stretches, treadmill, bicycle ergometry, light aerobic exercises, light weights, and cool-down stretches and relaxation, depending on the patient's exercise tolerance, physical capacity, and access to exercise equipment. Supplemental oxygen may be used during monitored exercise to maintain $Sao_2$ greater than 90%.[61]

Helpful education in preparation for thoracic surgery includes awareness of the postoperative pain-muscle tension cycle, which can increase discomfort and decrease pulmonary function. Patients can aid recovery beginning early after surgery through activities learned before surgery that include slow, rhythmic reaching, turning, bending and stretching of the trunk and all extremities frequently throughout the day. Exercise is often performed most easily shortly after receiving a dose of pain medication. The patient should be taught to move neither quickly nor jerkily, nor to remain rigidly stiff "to protect the incision." The patient should be taught to expect full shoulder and trunk range of motion immediately after surgery.

### Signs and symptoms of physiological compromise or fatigue

The physical therapist must be aware of the patient's current clinical physiological data and trends, including vital signs, arterial blood gases, blood analyses, invasive and noninvasive hemodynamics, blood glucose, radiographic findings, electrocardiographic findings, fluid and electrolyte balance, oxygen saturation, and other data.[46]

According to Sobush,[50] routine physiological responses to fatigue include changes in:

1. Blood pressure response pattern—hyper, hypo, or flat pulse pressure

2. Percentage heart rate capacity (compare resting, peak, and average values):

$$\frac{(\text{work HR} - \text{resting HR})}{(\text{max HR} - \text{resting HR})}$$

3. Cardiac output—evidence for decreases in central or peripheral parameters
4. Total peripheral resistance—can affect afterload or preload, and can influence blood pressure and $\dot{V}o_{2max}$
5. Respiratory rate
6. Tidal volume—changes in the relation of physiologic dead space volume to tidal volume with changes in respiratory rate
7. Ventilatory equivalent for oxygen or carbon dioxide—evidence for changes in central (respiratory drive) or peripheral (acidosis with anaerobic metabolism) parameters

A normal variation in heart rate occurs throughout an exercise session. However, in heart failure, only minimal and slowed changes in rate occur.[2]

Approximately 16% of patients with moderate to severe heart failure have an unusual periodic ventilatory response to exercise similar to the Cheyne-Stokes pattern. This abnormal pattern of breathing resolves following heart transplantation.[43]

A significant deterioration in maximal peak oxygen consumption is frequently a prelude to clinical decompensation in cardiopulmonary transplant candidates.[35]

Dyspnea and fatigue indicate the need for exercise termination.[52] One classification of symptom severity, graded on scales of 0 to 4, for three situations follows:[52]

Activity limitation:
    4 = bedridden
    3 = walking at home but less than one block
    2 = unlimited flat walking
    1 = unlimited routine activity
Orthopnea:
    4 = sitting to breathe
    3 = sleeping with three pillows or frequent paroxysmal nocturnal dyspnea
    2 = sleeping with two pillows or occasional paroxysmal dyspnea
    1 = sleeping with rare difficulty
Right-sided cardiac symptoms:
    4 = constant discomfort from splanchnic congestion or peripheral edema
    3 = frequent daily discomfort
    2 = discomfort several times weekly
    1 = rare discomfort

### SUMMARY OF ESSENTIAL POINTS FOR THE SUPERVISING CLINICIAN

- Decreased exercise capacity, increased resting heart rate, and orthostatic intolerance indicate cardiovascular deconditioning in either chronic heart failure or pulmonary disease.[40]

- In chronic heart failure, resting heart rate is higher than normal, modulation of heart rate during exercise occurs slowly, and peak heart rate is diminished.
- Overstress of perfusion will limit cardiac output.
- In chronic heart failure and pulmonary disease, attenuated or dampened pulmonary perfusion should be expected.
- Exertional dyspnea can be a limiting symptom during exercise for either chronic heart failure or lung disease.
- Overstress of ventilation will limit muscular development.
- During the stress of exercise, the upright position causes slightly less hemodynamic compromise than the supine position.
- Ensure that problems with malnutrition are being addressed to diminish the risk of further muscle catabolism during an exercise program.
- In chronic lung disease, diets high in fat and protein and low in glucose will result in lower $CO_2$ production, less risk of respiratory failure, and improved exercise tolerance.[17]
- Severe illness and immobility over an extended period will lead to muscle deconditioning, atrophy, and loss of vascularity; recovery time will be much longer than the total immobilization period.
- Markedly diminished muscle mass will cause exercise to be limited by peripheral rather than central factors, such as cardiac output.
- Exercise tolerance may be improved with training, independent of central hemodynamic limitations, and increased collateral blood flow by exercising leg muscles.
- Periodic steady power output, provided by an adequate mass of muscle fibers, can develop the utilization of oxygen by the periphery.

When developing an exercise prescription therapists should:

- Monitor changes in blood pressures, perceived exertion, arterial oxygen saturation, heart and respiratory rates, respiratory sounds and patterns
- Rely on measurements of oxygen uptake, not on target heart rates
- Use weight-bearing exercise for bone health when steroids are being used, and emphasize use of large muscle masses of the lower extremities for aerobic conditioning
- Note that sudden increase in minute ventilation without a corresponding increase in workload may indicate crossing of the anaerobic threshold

## PHASE TWO: POSTTRANSPLANT
### General information and descriptions

**Heart transplants.** According to the Eleventh Official Report of the International Society for Heart and Lung Transplantation (1994), almost 27,000 heart transplantations have been reported throughout the world.[21A] Recipients' ages range from newborn to 75 years old, with an average age of 45.[26] The donors' ages range from newborn to 70, but average 26 years. There is a marked male predominance in both cardiac recipients (81%) and donors (70%).

One-year survival rates vary depending on the age of the recipient, with patient groups aged 18 to 65 being 83%, aged 1 to 18 and over 65 being 79%, and under 1 year of age being 70%. The average 5-year survival rate for all age groups is 68%, and the 10-year survival rate is 56%.[26]

Heterotopic cardiac transplantation, in which the recipient retains the original heart and gains a donor heart, has remained very limited; orthotopic transplantation, in which the native heart is removed, is the norm.[29] Retransplantations numbering 577 have been reported with survival of 54% at 1 year, 49% at 2 years, and 48% at 3 years.[26]

**Heart-lung transplant.** Over 1550 heart-lung transplantations have been reported into persons aged newborn to 59 years, averaging 30 years. In contrast to the heart transplant group, 54% of recipients are female, and 20% are under age 18. Of the pediatric group, almost half have had a diagnosis of congenital heart disease. Average survival rates are 61% at 1 year, 46% at 5 years, and 42% at 10 years. Those with retransplantations have 37% and 34% survival rates at 6 months and 1 year respectively.[21A,26]

**Lung transplant.** Almost 1950 single lung transplants have been reported into an even ratio of males and females. Average recipient age is 47, with a range of a few days old to 70 years. Average survival rates are 73%, 67%, and 63% for 1, 2 and 3 years respectively; however, a large variation in survival is evident if patients are grouped by etiology. For example, one-year survival is 76% in persons with Alpha-1 Antitrypsin deficiency or Idiopathic Pulmonary Fibrosis, but only 63% with Primary Pulmonary Hypertension. Also, persons with emphysema have one year survivals of 87% with SLT, but only 58% with DLT! Those with SLT retransplantations have 48% and 39% survival rates at 6 months and 1 year respectively.[21A,26]

Double Lung Transplants (DLT) have been reported in almost 950 persons, of which almost 60% have been by the bilateral single technique, as opposed to an "en bloc" technique, because of significantly greater survival rates. Over 60% of pediatric cases have an etiology of Cystic Fibrosis. One-year survival is 78% in adults and 62% in children; 2-year survival is 55% for both groups.[21A,26]

Figures 21-1 through 21-4 indicate the sites of anastomoses in heart, heart-lung, and lung transplantation.

### General outcomes for transplant patients

The overall aim of organ transplantation is to allow the patient to achieve an independent and satisfying existence. However, the intensive follow-up program in the early months after surgery is both physically and psychologically demanding, and thus a life-style that approximates normal will not be immediate.

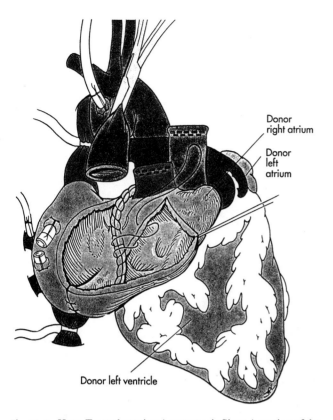

**Fig. 21-1.** Heart Transplantation Anastamosis Sites: A portion of the recipient's own right atrium, including the SA node, is preserved to provide the largest attachment site for the donor heart. Venous blood returns to the mixed recipient/donor right atrium via the recipient's vena cava inlet sites. The donor vena cava inlets are closed. (From Starzl TE, Shapiro R, and Simmons R: *Atlas of organ transplantation,* New York, 1992, Gower Medical Publishing.)

The patient usually has great hope of regaining and enjoying an improved level of activity in life; however, these expectations can also generate anxiety and apprehension. Posttransplant depression may be aggravated by unfulfilled expectations, rapid onset of postoperative complications, by sudden exposure to an unaccustomed life-style, other's expectations, or even unexpected abilities.

Exercise capacity is an acceptable measure of enhanced quality of life after transplantation. However, a good home rehabilitation program recognizes that exercise provides only one component of a patient's multifaceted needs when attempting to achieve satisfaction after organ transplantation.[40]

It must also be recognized that prolonged illness prior to transplantation may have caused considerable reduction in skeletal muscle performance, which may not recover spontaneously with the return to normal activity. Participation in a formal intensive rehabilitation program may result in a significantly improved exercise performance over time.[61]

**Heart transplant.** Following heart transplantation, individuals can expect to experience noticeably improved tolerance for activities of daily living because left ventricular systolic function is near normal both at rest and with exercise. However, altered hemodynamic performance, in part attributable to altered diastolic function, is present at rest and with exercise. Therefore, exercise capacity will not be as great as in the healthy population.[18]

According to Kavanagh, with the start of exercise in the person with a heart transplant, minute ventilation increases quickly, but heart rate does not increase, and stroke volume and cardiac output increase slower than usual. Therefore, oxygen consumption is inefficient and increases slowly. With continued exercise over time, oxygen consumption gradually becomes more efficient, and the person can achieve a true training effect.[23] Kavanagh further states that the threshold for this training effect occurs at approximately 60% of peak oxygen uptake, a level of effort usually attained even by those not adequately motivated to exert maximal efforts during exercise testing.[23]

Therefore, the person with a heart transplant *must* understand the benefits to be gained through regular participation in a well-designed training program. Once the individual with the transplant is hemodynamically stable, an invaluable portion of his or her education is provided by the physical therapist.

**Heart-lung transplant.** Persons with heart-lung transplants also have adequate capacity for activities of daily living with no serious limitations attributable to denervation of and disruptions in both the cardiac and pulmonary systems. Nonetheless, work capacity in these individuals is frequently limited and is related to freedom from serious complications in the heart or lung grafts.[40]

**Lung transplant.** Persons with either SLT or DLT have functional capacities and peak exercise levels,[61] that are substantially below the normal population. However, following transplantation and significantly restored lung function, a comfortable life-style and moderately higher amounts of work can be expected.[38]

Recipients of DLT have essentially normal pulmonary function; SLT recipients have a mild restrictive abnormality with varying degrees of airflow obstruction consistent with the disease in the native lung.[38,44] However, SLT and DLT recipients are not comparable for anthropometric data, so direct comparisons between the groups should be undertaken with caution.[61]

On a practical level, persons with SLT often have similar exercise capacity as those receiving the more extensive DLT and HLT procedures. Therefore, surgeons will look beyond the anticipated exercise capacity,[33] and often use the SLT for many different types of end-stage pulmonary disease. This practice should lead to optimal use of scarce donor lungs and may become the procedure of choice for most patients.[61]

## Mechanisms of rejection and immunosuppression medications

According to Mahon,[34] T-lymphocytes play a major role in recognizing the donor organ as being a foreign antigen. When the "antigen recognition structure" (CD-3 complex)

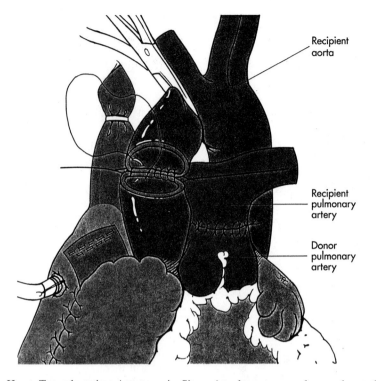

**Fig. 21-2.** Heart Transplantation Anastamosis Sites: Attachments are also made at the aorta, pulmonary artery trunk, and pulmonary veins (not shown). (From Starzl TE, Shapiro R, and Simmons R: *Atlas of organ transplantation,* New York, 1992, Gower Medical Publishing.)

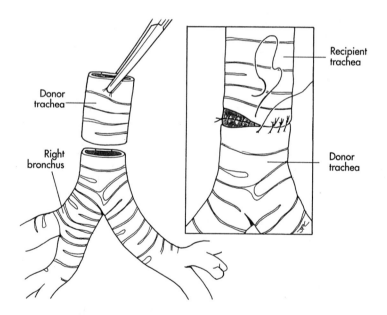

**Fig. 21-3.** Heart-Lung Transplantation Anastamosis Sites: The double lung attachment is located in the trachea just above the carina. The heart attachments are the same as Figs. 21-1 and 21-2. (From Starzl TE, Shapiro R, and Simmons R: *Atlas of organ transplantation,* New York, 1992, Gower Medical Publishing.)

on the T-cell surface engages an antigen, a signal is transduced to sensitize other T-cells to produce both cytotoxic T cells and lymphokines. Cytotoxic T cells then bind tightly with the donor organ and release cytotoxic substances into the organ's cells. Lymphokines are hormones that increase the activity of the cytotoxic T cells, increase accumulation of macrophages within the area of the donor organ, and enhance the efficiency of phagocytosis.

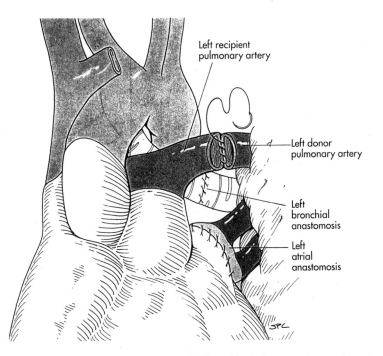

**Fig. 21-4.** Single Lung Transplantation Anastamosis Sites: Single lung attachment sites, shown here for the left lung, are at the left mainstem bronchus, left pulmonary artery, and left atrium. A portion of the recipient's right atrium is resected to accommodate a portion of donor atrium, which contains the inlets for the pulmonary veins. (From Starzl TE, Shapiro R, and Simmons R: *Atlas of organ transplantation,* New York, 1992, Gower Medical Publishing.)

B-lymphocytes also produce antibodies that attack the donor organ directly by weakening its cell membranes.

The presence of cytotoxic T cells, lymphokines, and antibodies weaken the donor organ's cells by making the cells more vulnerable to lysis or to acute allograft rejection.[34]

**Immunosuppression regimens.** Because the immune system of the organ recipient treats the donor tissue as foreign material, it is critically important to reduce the effects of the immune system, particularly the T-cell system that is responsible for rejection. Various medications are employed towards this end. Early after the transplant, the immunosuppression protocol, usually administered for the first few weeks, is called "triple drug therapy" and consists of cyclosporine, azathioprine, and corticosteroids (usually prednisone). If a specific anti-T-cell agent, such as antithymocyte globulin, is added, "quadruple drug therapy" is said to be used.

Long-term maintenance of immunosuppression is also commonly achieved with triple drug therapy. "Double drug therapy" includes only cyclosporine and prednisone, although some programs have used cyclosporine and azathioprine without corticosteroids.

Should acute allograft rejection occur, triple or quadruple drug therapy may be used, with variations in the doses depending on the histological grade and hemodynamic consequences of the rejection episode.[60,11]

Brief descriptions of commonly used drugs, their side effects, and consequences for physical therapy include:

Azathioprine: An immunosuppressant that can cause severe leukopenia, thrombocytopenia, macrocytic anemia, or bone marrow depression.[11]

Cyclosporine (Cyclosporin A, CyA): An immunosuppressant that with prolonged use can reduce aerobic capacity because of alterations in peripheral and renal blood flow, mitochondrial respiration, and multisystem toxicity.[40,47]

It can produce a wide range of vasoconstriction as a result of endocrine interactions.[47]

Exogenous Glucocorticoids (specifically prednisone): These synthetic steroid compounds have profound antiinflammatory effects:

Average and high doses can cause elevated blood pressure, salt and water retention, increased potassium and calcium excretion.[11]

Prednisone-induced diabetes mellitus is a common complication.[3]

They induce cardiac, skeletal, and respiratory muscle atrophy through protein catabolism with prolonged therapy.[11]

Muromonab CD-3 (OKT3): This drug is a monoclonal (i.e., each molecule is identical) antibody used in corticosteroid-resistant acute rejection.

Antilymphocyte globulin (ATG)/Antithymocyte globulin (ATM)

These immunoglobulins act mainly against circulating and lymph node T lymphocytes while sparing B cells and antibody production.

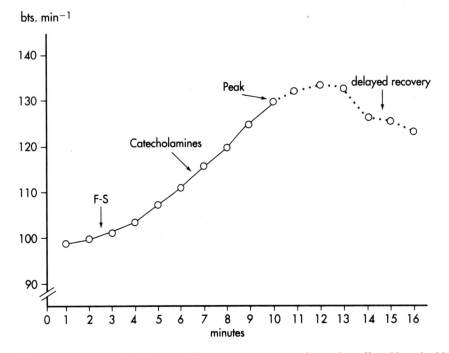

**Fig. 21-5.** Typical transplanted denervated heart rate response to increasing effort. Note the high resting rate, the delayed rate of acceleration during effort, the delayed deceleration during recovery, and the tendency for the rate to continue to rise after the termination of effort (peak exercise). (From Kavanagh T and Yacoub MH: Exercise training in patients after heart transplantation, *Ann Acad Med Singapore* 21:372, 1992.)

Gancyclovir sodium: This antiviral drug that is active against cytomegalovirus is used if either the donor or recipient is sero-positive.

**Physical therapy considerations related to immunosuppression.** In general, the patient should avoid situations of likely exposure to large numbers of endogenous or pathologic bacteria or viruses in closed spaces. Monitor immunosuppression-induced hypertension on a continual basis. Other things being equal, expect some decrease in aerobic capacity with continuing use of cyclosporine. Be aware of salt and water retention, unusual weight gain, lower extremity swelling, muscle weakness, osteoporosis, evidence of GI bleeding, and puffiness of the face with prolonged use of corticosteroids. New diabetes mellitus may occur with steroid use. Emphasize exercise in weight-bearing positions to decrease calcium loss from long bones attributable to prolonged steroid use. During initial treatment with Muronomab CD-3, avoid exercise until the risk of life-threatening reactions is past. Encourage liberal protein intake for muscle growth to offset steroid-induced catabolism.

### Exercise: expectations and limitations

**Heart transplant.** After cardiac transplantation, there are significant improvements in hemodynamic function and activity tolerance, although normalization does not occur.

*Heart rate.* Resting heart rates are higher than normal because of loss of parasympathetic innervation. Peak heart rates are below normal, but heart rates may continue to rise for minutes after the conclusion of exercise, then gradually decline to resting, at a slower pace than normal, thus prolonging recovery time (see Fig. 21-5).[24] The loss of sympathic innervation makes the patient dependent on return of boluses of blood from large exercising skeletal muscles at the start of exercise in order to increase stroke volume and cardiac output via the Frank-Starling mechanism. Shortly after surgery, cardiac output will increase only via changes in stroke volume during exercise because of the lack of any significant increase in heart rate. Later, heart rates will rise slowly, but significantly above resting, and further augment cardiac output during exercise.[18]

The recipient's own SA node may produce P waves that have a slower rate than the P wave rate of the donor's SA node because the former is still under parasympathetic control. However, the donor's SA node is unable to initiate a QRS complex in the donor heart.

*Blood pressure.* Resting diastolic hypertension is a common finding after heart transplantation and is related to stiffness of the left ventricular myocardium. Patients with the highest elevations in diastolic pressures during exercise compared to rest retain the greatest myocardial stiffness.[42] Although elevated diastolic pressure is to be expected when exercise begins, large increases place the myocardium at risk for loss of perfusion and ischemia. The therapist *must* monitor diastolic pressure with the patient at rest and during early exercise until a regular pattern of response is determined. Exercise while upright affords the heart improved compliance and better diastolic pressure than exercise while supine. Similarly, isometric exercise should be used cautiously, performed only after extensive warm-up, and should be interrupted regularly and frequently with aerobic exercise.

Systolic function and contractile reserve are in the high normal range early after transplantation but low normal later, probably because of undetected episodes of allograft rejection or coronary artery disease.[18] Peak systolic blood pressure, though, is reduced to approximately 80% of normal.[24]

*Other exercise hemodynamics.* With submaximal exercise, oxygen uptake following heart transplantation is normal, but perceived exertion, minute ventilation, and the ventilatory equivalent for oxygen (the ratio $\dot{V}E/\dot{V}o_2$) are elevated.[24] Stroke volume may be greater or less than normal,[8] and oxygen carrying capacity is normal,[22] but cardiac output is somewhat reduced, leading to higher extraction of oxygen by the tissues (e.g., widening of the arteriovenous oxygen difference).[48]

The switch to anaerobic metabolism occurs at lower levels, and peak work rates and cardiac output will not be as high as normal. Increased left ventricular filling pressures and volumes, decreased diastolic function, and impaired right ventricular function all contribute to a lower than normal exercise capacity.[18]

Peak power output and oxygen uptake are initially subnormal, attributable in part, to the surgical insults to the myocardium (i.e., temporary edema due to perioperative ischemia[20]). Transplant recipients have a 10% to 50% reduction in lean body mass, which can also decrease peak power output and oxygen uptake.[24] With an appropriately graded training regimen, power output and oxygen uptake have the potential for normalization.

Exercise capacity in the first 3 months is predictive of exercise capabilities during the year after transplant.[31]

*Ventilatory function.* The ventilatory response to exercise following cardiac transplantation is significantly improved to near normal after heart transplant, although conflicting results have been reported. Minute ventilation remains excessive, but this may reflect the blunted cardiac output response to exercise, abnormal intrapulmonary pressures, or persistent deconditioning.[36]

Forced vital capacity increases in proportion to the decrease in cardiac volume of the new organ. Patients without a smoking history have normal lung volumes in contrast to those with a smoking history.[36]

Perceived exertion and minute ventilation are elevated beyond normal with exercise. The switch to anaerobic metabolism occurs at lower levels, and peak cardiac output and work rates will not be as high as normal.

*Effectiveness of aerobic training.* Marked effects of aerobic training on hemodynamics have been demonstrated in persons with heart transplants under very differing circumstances. Examples include: supervised training periods ranging from 10 weeks to 2 years; supervised training beginning shortly after surgery to beginning many years posttransplant; and supervised training with persons who are highly motivated towards exercise versus those who have never trained.[5,23,25,27] A summary of the effects of aerobic training on the person with a heart transplant is shown in the box below.

**Heart-lung transplant.** Neurogenically, afferent and efferent nerves to both the heart and the lungs are lost in heart-lung transplantation, with the exception of postganglionic efferent nerves.[40] In the absence of normal innervation of heart and lung, there is dissociation of the ventilatory and circulatory responses to the onset of leg exercise.[4]

Loss of the pulmonary vagal afferents does not significantly influence resting breathing patterns,[40] and despite pulmonary denervation, the sensation of dyspnea is preserved after heart-lung transplant.[36]

**Lung transplant**

*Ventilatory factors.* The donor lung, regardless of size, will not fill the entire hemithorax vacated by a markedly overexpanded, emphysematous lung. Therefore, compensatory shifting of the mediastinum, in SLT, and elevation of the diaphragm are beneficial.[57] The donor lung, if larger in volume than the excised lung, may offer additional accommodation for the rise in pulmonary vascular pressures during exercise and in surface area for gas exchange, which may provide potential for earlier recovery of exercise capacity.[38] Ventilation/perfusion matching appears normal at rest or with exercise in the uncomplicated transplanted lung.[15]

---

**The effects of aerobic training on patients after a heart transplant**

*Conclusive evidence for:*

Normalization of heart rate response (lower resting heart rates; higher peak heart rates)[22]

Improved maximum oxygen uptake[27]

Significant decrease in diastolic blood pressure[23]

Doubling of MET levels[5]

Peak work output increases from 49% to 65%[23]

Increased body mass with a higher percentage of lean tissue[23]

*Inconclusive evidence that training has improved:*

Incidence of infection

Rejection rate

Longevity

Return to premorbid life style[46]

*Improvement in peak heart rate appears related to increased leg muscle strength, and is associated with:*

Improved power output

Later onset of anaerobic threshold

Lower perceived exertion

Lower minute ventilation[23]

Vital capacity, forced expiratory volume in one second, and diffusion capacity for carbon monoxide (DLCO) approach normal in DLT and HLT, but show moderate restriction and comparatively reduced DLCO in SLT, although the DLCO increases towards normal with exercise.

Gas exchange, measured by pulse oximetry and end-tidal $CO_2$ monitoring, during exercise appears well preserved. Exercise $SaO_2$ of 95% for DLT and 90% for SLT have been recorded and are more than adequate to meet oxygen delivery requirements during functional work levels for each group.[61]

Resting breathing patterns are essentially normal,[40] however increased respiratory rates occur and ventilation at any given workload is greater than normal. Thus, ventilatory factors do not seem to limit exercise, even in SLT recipients with an abnormal native lung.[33] In fact, breathing reserves and arterial blood gas values are adequate even at peak exercise levels.[61,13]

*Cardiovascular factors.* Exercise testing after lung transplantation has shown a persistent limitation in maximal exercise, without evidence for ventilatory limitation in either SLT or DLT groups.[38] Although $\dot{V}o_{2max}$ and exercise tolerance improve significantly following transplantation, continued deficits in these values occur and likely have multifactorial causes.[44]

Heart rate responses during submaximal exercise show appropriate exercise adaptation, but during maximal exercise, heart rates were only 70% and 74% of predicted values in DLT and SLT groups, respectively. This finding suggests that cardiac output is a limiting factor during exercise for persons with lung transplants.[61]

Although chronic anemia contributes to circulatory limitations,[38] reduced aerobic capacity and abnormal cardiovascular limitations are more likely to result from chronic deconditioning and peripheral muscle atrophy, or from myopathy secondary to steroid use.[33]

*Effectiveness of training.* DLT recipients often participate in more rigorous rehabilitation programs and show superior aerobic and peak exercise levels in comparison to HLT and SLT recipients.[33] Therefore, transplantation prior to severe deconditioning, or more aggressive postoperative training programs may be necessary for full exercise potential to be achieved.[61]

Superior aerobic and peak exercise levels and fullest potential functional results occur when patients with lung transplants undergo rigorous rehabilitation programs that attempt to reverse deconditioning and redevelop normal muscle mass and physiology.

## PHYSICAL THERAPY PROGRAM GUIDELINES FOR POST-TRANSPLANT CARE
### Immediate postoperative phase

During the immediate postoperative phase the patient is in the intensive care unit for hemodynamic stabilization, endotracheal extubation, and pulmonary care. For the uncomplicated case, this period usually lasts 2 to 5 days.

The heart and/or lung transplant patient may be encumbered by numerous internal and external restrictions such as:

- Sternotomy, unilateral or bilateral thoracotomy, or "clamshell" (sternotomy plus bilateral anterior subcostal) incisions and dressings
- Invasive monitoring of electrocardiogram, systemic, central venous and pulmonary blood pressures, cardiac output, and systemic venous oxygenation all inserted through the jugular vein and radial or femoral arteries
- External pacemaker inserted through the abdomen
- Noninvasive monitoring of arterial oxygen saturation and blood pressure
- Ventilator or supplemental oxygen tubing
- Mediastinal, pleural, and gastric drainage tubes
- Various peripheral venous lines
- Some degree of protective isolation, and limitation of family visitation

During this phase of care, common physical therapy goals should include:

1. Successful weaning from mechanical ventilation
2. Full aeration and secretion removal
3. Regaining preoperative range of motion
4. Achieving bed mobility and bed-to-chair transfers with minimal or no assistance
5. Active participation in light exercise for all extremities and trunk in reclining, sitting and standing positions within tolerance
6. Ambulation within tolerance
7. Preliminary awareness of the predischarge program of educational activities and exercise expectations

Physical therapy in the immediate postoperative period resembles that indicated for most thoracic surgery patients, and is likely to include any or all of the techniques described in Chapter 20.

Helpful education for thoracic surgery patients also includes alleviating the surgical pain-tension cycle and aiding lung recovery through frequent, slow, rhythmic reaching, turning, bending and stretching of the trunk and all extremities many times throughout the day, but especially after pain medication has taken effect.

**Heart transplant.** During this phase specific education for the patient with an uncomplicated heart transplant includes early instruction that the heart is denervated and is now dependent on the blood-pumping action of large muscles and on hormones (e.g., catecholamines) to stimulate the heart at the beginning of physical activity.

Introducing the concepts of warm-up, peak activity, and cool down, and their use in identifying parts of every treatment is helpful in fostering thorough understanding and follow-through when the patient is exercising independently.

During the intensive care period, it is often very encouraging for the patient to identify potential physical achievements to be gained by the time of discharge from the hospital. These achievements may include walking distance, time pedaling a stationary bike, stair climbing, and using small hand weights for upper body strengthening.

**Heart-lung and lung transplant.** Specific education of the patient with the heart-lung or lung transplant includes the information provided for the heart transplant patient. The following additional information applies to the patient with an uncomplicated heart-lung or lung transplant.

Because the lung is denervated surgically below the level of its anastamosis to the respiratory tree, reflex coughing in response to accumulation of secretions will not occur until the mucociliary elevator moves the secretions above the anastamosis site.

Also, because of postoperative extracellular edema, dependent portions of the lung can be boggy like a sponge. Frequent change of position will decrease the risk of localized prolonged overstretching of pulmonary and vascular tissue.

During the early postoperative period, the patient will need vigilant and regular changes of position, reminders to cough, manual chest wall stretching, and, possibly, active or resistive diaphragmatic exercise. The patient will become a more active participant, and must learn to accept responsibility for all aspects of care. These aspects include rolling, movement in and out of bed, trunk twisting and arm reaching, breathing exercises such as increased diaphragmatic excursion and use of an inspirometer, and frequent coughing to change the pressures in the lung, even if secretions are not raised with each cough.

Physical achievements used to encourage patients with lung transplants during the early acute, postoperative weeks are more difficult to anticipate in comparison to those with heart transplantation. In part, this difficulty is due to usually longer periods of chronic deconditioning, muscle atrophy, and malnutrition preceding the lung transplant. These changes, which are typically more peripheral, often do not recover spontaneously following surgery. For most patients, however, the renewed ability to perform simple bedside activities without the expected dyspnea is encouragement enough during this phase.

## Early conditioning phase

The early conditioning phase begins when the patient leaves the intensive care unit and continues through early recovery when effective organ functioning, incisional integrity, and basic functional activity in the community have been established. This period usually lasts 6 to 8 weeks in the uncomplicated heart or lung transplant, including 1 to 5 weeks of hospitalization.

At this time, the patient's restrictions are centered on limiting exposure to endemic or pathogenic bacteria and viruses that may compromise the newly immunosuppressed system.

During this early conditioning phase, common physical therapy goals include:

1. Achievement of uncompleted goals from initial postoperative phase
2. Independence in pulmonary hygiene
3. General strength of at least 3+/5
4. Return to normal or at least to preoperative posture and flexibility
5. Independence in functional mobility on flat surfaces and stairs in the home or community
6. Completion of a minimum of 20 minutes of aerobic exercise at the appropriate intensity indicated by patient tolerance
7. Understanding how the transplanted organ is different from normal while at rest and with exercise
8. Understanding the need for and means to protect and progress the transplanted organ's function via appropriate, effective, and safe exercise sessions

Physical therapy treatment at this time would include continuation of the treatment given in the immediate postoperative phase for as long as indicated. In addition, the following activities could be added during the early conditioning phase.

1. Bed mobility, transfers, and ambulation progressing to independence
2. Endurance walking or cycling
3. Stair climbing
4. Stretching and light resistive exercises
5. Posture awareness and correction
6. Extensive education

Common methods for easily quantifying exercise noninvasively in the clinic include the 6-minute walk test, in which the therapist records the distance traveled in 6 minutes at the fastest safe pace tolerated by the patient. The patient may rest, but the clock continues to run during rest periods, and the number and length of rests are documented. The MET × time product is used with the treadmill to measure endurance compared to time, although initially increases should be made in time rather than intensity. The product of Watts × Seconds, or Joules of energy, may be used with the cycle ergometer to measure endurance compared to time. As with the treadmill, early increases should emphasize time rather than intensity.[3,10]

*Patient education.* Several educational topics relate to the safe performance of exercise. It is particularly important for the patient to understand these topics because he or she may need to explain the correct way to take care of an individual with a transplanted organ to uninformed health care personnel and others.

The first topic regards how the patient can self-monitor to know when exercise intensity is appropriate. The following three monitoring parameters have been particularly useful, and their precautionary limits for peak activity are listed

## Descriptions of common self-monitoring parameters during exercise

### Dyspnea index

The patient inhales deeply then counts aloud slowly during exhalation from 1 to 15 over about 8 seconds time. If the patient runs out of breath, stop the count before the patient begins to strain. The patient inhales deeply again, begins the count where it was left off, and continues at the same slow pace. The patient notes the number of breaths needed to reach 15, including the initial breath. This index is an excellent indicator of workload because minute ventilation increases immediately and progressively with exercise.

### Perceived exertion

Either the Borg 15-grade Interval Scale or newer Category Scale with Ratio Properties can be used[6] (see Tables 21-1 and 21-2). The former scale is most common, but the latter scale may be more useful with a lung transplant, particularly if subjective symptoms of breathing difficulties persist. During exercise, the scales integrate information from peripheral working muscles and joints, from the cardiovascular and respiratory systems, and from the central nervous system by the patient's response to the question, "How much stress is this causing you?", using the descriptors listed in the scale. The scales correlate well with various physiological variables at different workloads.

### Symptoms

The patient should be aware of how the body responds to exercise. If light-headedness, dizziness, feeling cold or clammy, fatigue, tiredness in a certain body part, shortness of breath, discomfort, etc. occur, the intensity of the activity should be reduced. If the symptoms persist, the activity should be discontinued and the experience reported by the patient to the appropriate health care professional.

Also refer to the specific precautionary limits for each parameter, listed according to transplant, on p. 417.

**Table 21-1.** The 15-grade scale for ratings of perceived exertion, the RPE Scale

| 6 | |
|---|---|
| 7 | Very, very light |
| 8 | |
| 9 | Very light |
| 10 | |
| 11 | Fairly light |
| 12 | |
| 13 | Somewhat hard |
| 14 | |
| 15 | Hard |
| 16 | |
| 17 | Very hard |
| 18 | |
| 19 | Very, very hard |
| 20 | |

From Borg GAV: Psychophysical bases of perceived exertion, *Med Sci Sports Exer* 14:377, 1982.

**Table 21-2.** The new rating scale constructed as a category scale with ratio properties

| 0 | Nothing at all | |
|---|---|---|
| 0.5 | Very, very weak | (just noticeable) |
| 1 | Very weak | |
| 2 | Weak | (light) |
| 3 | Moderate | |
| 4 | Somewhat strong | |
| 5 | Strong | (heavy) |
| 6 | | |
| 7 | Very strong | |
| 8 | | |
| 9 | | |
| 10 | Very, very strong | (almost max) |
| • | Maximal | |

From Borg GAV: Psychophysical bases of perceived exertion, *Med Sci Sports Exer* 14:377, 1982.

below by transplant type. The parameters measured during warm-up will indicate intensity of exercise possible during peak activity, and during cool down from exercise, they will indicate the adequacy of recovery.

Other monitoring parameters the patient may be taught include heart rate and blood pressure. Skill with these parameters depends on the ability to palpate and count the pulse accurately or on the availability of easy-to-use equipment.

The second topic is understanding the concepts of warm-up, peak activity, and cool down, and how they fit together in an exercise session. The third educational topic includes understanding the benefits of aerobic exercise and identifying activities that provide aerobic benefit. Contrasting the characteristics of aerobic exercise to anaerobic, static, isometric, and other types of exercise, can help the

patient identify those exercises effective for maximum cardiac health, while complementing the individual's lifestyle preferences.

Topic four is understanding how to safely and independently progress the exercise program to achieve effective early aerobic conditioning. A daily exercise log, including vital signs, dyspnea index, perceived exertion spirometer data, monitoring parameters, exercise conditions, feelings and symptoms, may be motivating and will provide some data about trends.

**Heart transplant: specific guidelines.** Education specific for the uncomplicated heart transplant patient includes how the transplanted heart differs from the normal heart during rest and exercise. Heart rate responses, dependence on warm-up to increase stroke volume and catecholamine stimulation, and loss of sensory input on the ability to monitor symptoms of angina would be included in the education.

When monitoring parameters during *peak* activity after *heart* transplant, the following may be considered precautionary limits:

1. Dyspnea index
   a. Use two to three breaths to reach 15, which equals about 30 breaths per minute.
   b. If 4 breaths are needed—slow down; if only 1 breath is needed—increase intensity.
2. Perceived exertion
   a. 13 or "somewhat hard" on the interval scale
3. Heart rate
   a. greater than 120 bpm at rest
   b. increase of greater than 40 bpm above resting
4. Systolic blood pressure:
   a. greater than 170 mm Hg at rest
   b. with exercise—increase/decrease greater than 30 mm Hg
5. Diastolic blood pressure:
   a. greater than 120 mm Hg at rest
   b. with exercise—increase/decrease greater than 20 mm Hg

Reasonable activity goals by the end of this phase, if the patient is still hospitalized, include a one-half mile walk, 20-30 minutes work on a cycle ergometer, 2 flights of stairs, and 1- to 4-pound hand weights for upper body strengthening.

**Heart/lung and lung transplant: specific guidelines.** Education for the patient with a heart-lung transplant is similar to that for the heart transplant patient except for the following information for the uncomplicated lung transplant.

The patient has lost the protective mechanism of reflex coughing in response to airway stimulation distal to the anastamosis site. Therefore volitional coughing should be performed on a regular basis after surgery until the lung appears to be free of secretions, and volitional coughing should be performed whenever inhalation of anything but clean air is suspected.

After lung transplantation into a thorax with a chronic barrel-chest deformity, rib mobilization, chest wall stretching, strengthening of the external intercostal muscles, and lengthening with strengthening of the hemidiaphragm(s) should be employed. These exercises and techniques should help the hemithorax, which formerly held a markedly overexpanded emphysematous lung, return to normal shape, and the respiratory muscles to achieve more effective length-tension ratios.

When monitoring parameters during *peak* activity after *lung* transplant, the following may be considered precautionary limits:

1. Dyspnea index

a. assess dyspnea index at rest
   b. at peak exercise, 1-2 additional breaths to reach 15 with a maximum of 5, which equals about 38 breaths per minute
2. Perceived exertion
   a. 13 or "somewhat hard" on the interval scale
   b. 3 to 4 or "moderate" to "somewhat strong" on the category scale
3. Heart rate
   a. greater than 120 bpm at rest
   b. increase to greater than 50% of age-predicted target heart rate during unsupervised exercise
   c. increase to greater than 70% of age-predicted target heart rate during supervised exercise
4. Systolic blood pressure:
   a. greater than 170 mm Hg at rest
   b. with exercise—increase/decrease greater than 30 mm Hg
5. Diastolic blood pressure:
   a. greater than 120 mm Hg at rest
   b. with exercise a decrease greater than 20 mm Hg

Reasonable activity goals by the end of this period must be based upon a gradual progression to and beyond the highest activity level tolerated by the patient within 2 to 3 months prior to the transplantation. Emphasis of activity should be on endurance training of large muscle groups, particularly the lower extremities, to facilitate peripheral revascularization.

For those who have not walked farther than bed to chair without severe dyspnea for many months prior to surgery, a 6-minute walk of 150 feet with 1 to 2 brief standing rests, or pedaling at 45 rpm for 10 to 15 minutes may be major accomplishments. For others with fairly recent onset of disability and early organ transplantation, activity goals similar to those listed above for heart transplantation would be very achievable.

## Continuing conditioning phase

The continuing conditioning is the time period from the establishment of functional integrity of the grafted organ to death. The intensity of out-patient monitoring and follow-up gradually diminishes, and the patient returns to normal daily work, play, school, and avocational activities.

Physical therapy goals during this period may include:

1. Continue participation in a supervised rehabilitation program and an independent personalized exercise prescription.
2. Achieve all goals from the early conditioning phase not yet achieved.
3. Strengthen and increase bulk of large skeletal muscles towards normal and enhance their revascularization.
4. Progress aerobic conditioning towards cardiovascular fitness.

5. Increase understanding and monitoring for symptoms and side effects of immunosuppression and steroidal drugs, and taking appropriate action.

6. Develop a thorough awareness and skill in rating perceived exertion, interpreting symptoms of myocardial ischemia, and in knowing appropriate actions to take.

7. Develop increased understanding of cardiovascular and pulmonary risk factors and of life-style modifications that are needed to maximize the health and longevity of the donor organ and the individual.

Physical therapy treatment at this time would include dynamic activity, involving large muscle groups, to enhance cardiovascular fitness that can be accurately quantified and monitored. Pacing of the exercise prescription is based on 60% to 70% of peak oxygen uptake, coupled with the ventilatory threshold, and a perception of effort equivalent to 13 to 14 on the original Borg scale.

For years after a heart transplant, warm-up continues to be essential prior to exercise to allow contracting muscle masses to return large blood volumes to the heart to increase stroke volume and cardiac output, and to allow time for catecholamines to gradually increase HR before peak activity is begun. Cool down maintains a lighter activity level during the prolonged HR recovery time described on p. 412.

Highly individualized programs are indicated for patients with a history of severe deconditioning and muscle atrophy; however, many patients can be paced at walking 1 mile in 30 minutes, 5 times per week early in this phase. After the first four to six weeks, regardless of the pace, training sessions should last 30 to 60 minutes. Many individuals are able to progress to a walk-jog 4 to 5 miles 5 times per week.[24]

Education during this phase includes correct interpretation of symptoms of myocardial ischemia, such as excessive dyspnea, unusual fatigue, lightheadedness, and extrasystoles. In the case of denervation of the heart, atypical heart rate responses and the general absence of angina as a warning symptom make dependence on these signs and symptoms less useful than normal.

## COMPLICATIONS, HAZARDS, AND IMPLICATIONS OF ACUTE PATHOLOGY
### Infection

Bacterial infections are common during the first postoperative month. Later, viral infections are more common. Cytomegalovirus infections are very dangerous in CMV-seronegative recipients and mortality up to 90% has been reported.[19]

The incidence of extrapulmonary infections is low, thereby implicating the lungs as a primary focus of infection. The majority of bacterial infections involve the lower respiratory tract.[9] Therefore, vigilance in pulmonary hygiene and use of barriers to reduce incidence of opportunistic infections, particularly in the lungs, will reduce early postoperative morbidity.

### Rejection

**Heart transplant.** Acute rejection occurs at least once in over 95% of patients in the early phase after heart transplant, and in the vast majority of episodes, clinical symptoms are absent.[32] However, fatal ventricular dysrhythmias have occurred during severe acute rejection.[14] The damage resulting from early rejection is usually subclinical and may be apparent only by subtle change in tolerance for exercise or activity.[31] Interestingly though, compared to older infants, the neonatal immune system is remarkably receptive to foreign tissue, thereby reducing the chance of rejection.[39]

Classically, the "gold standard" for identification of cardiac cellular rejection has been the grading of endomyocardial biopsy specimens. However, immunofluorescent staining of coronary vascular endothelium more clearly identifies humoral or vascular rejection.[37] Chronic rejection is an important cause of late graft failures.[41] Heart grafts with chronic rejection most often show vaso-occlusive changes in the large and small vessels, along with varying degrees of interstitial fibrosis. Clinical manifestations of chronic rejection may include the sequelae of coronary artery occlusion and obstruction, dysrhythmias, mitral regurgitation, heart failure, and sudden death. A recent study reported chest pain as the presenting symptom of chronic rejection.[41]

Therefore, for the patient with a heart transplant, changes in exercise tolerance or symptoms of angina should be reported since they often indicate early rejection. A pattern of increased diastolic dysfunction with preserved systolic pressure would be expected in acute rejection. Chronic rejection is manifested by various cardiac symptoms.

**Heart-lung and lung transplant.** Lung rejection and opportunistic infections are the most common acute complications in heart-lung transplantation.[40] Lung allograft rejection has three distinct patterns:

1. *Classic rejection* always occurs in non-immunosuppressed transplant recipients and is associated with decreased ventilation and perfusion

2. *Atypical or alveolar rejection* is seen in patients receiving standard immunosuppression in whom fibrinous alveolar exudates and radiographic opacification are present. Atypical rejection is also associated with decreased ventilation but without a corresponding decrease in pulmonary perfusion.

3. *Vascular rejection* involves the small and medium vessels only in patients receiving cyclosporine. Vascular resistance is increased and blood flow to the transplanted lung is decreased, but alveoli and interstitial areas are normal.[9]

Bronchoscopy, bronchoalveolar lavage, transthoracic needle biopsy, and open lung biopsy have been used to detect pulmonary rejection, but none is universally accepted. Confirmation of acute rejection is assumed when rapid improvement of the chest radiograph occurs after high-dose cortiocosteroid administration.[9]

Effective interventions for rejection lead to decreasing pulmonary vascular resistance, which increases blood flow and normalizes the ventilation/perfusion ratio in the transplanted lung.[30]

Regarding heart-lung and lung transplantation, perception of increased dyspnea with exercise is the earliest feature of rejection.[40] In patients with heart-lung transplants, the lung allografts are susceptible to rejection earlier than the heart.

## Pulmonary disorders
### Heart-lung and lung transplants

*General problems.* Initially after surgery, the transplanted lung is at risk for compromise because of cough suppression due to denervation, perioperative ischemia, lymphatic interruption, injury from early rejection, transmission of infectious agents with the lung transplant, postoperative atelectasis, and a temporary restrictive ventilatory defect.[9]

Full recovery of lung volumes to pretransplant levels occurs about a year after transplantation when the chest wall and ribs have resumed their normal position.[40]

*Broncholitis obliterans (BO).* BO is a progressive, inflammatory, fibrotic reaction that obliterates the bronchioles with granulation and fibrous tissue. BO may be the end result of recurrent infections due to impaired defense mechanisms or a process of chronic rejection within the airways that produces diffuse intimal hyperplasia in the pulmonary vasculature. BO is the most serious long-term complication associated with lung transplantation.

Airflow obstruction usually does not become evident until several months after the transplant, but once present, the clinical course can progress in a rapid and irreversible manner. Clinically, the patient has bronchitic symptoms initially, followed by early development of dyspnea. Total lung capacity is decreased, and edema and hypoxemia occur. Bronchodilators are largely ineffective in reversing symptoms. Pulmonary function tests show both severe obstructive and restrictive lung disease, and chest radiographs show distinctive infiltrates.[9]

## Reimplantation response

The reimplantation response is that part of the postoperative pathological changes that could have resulted only from the surgical procedure itself. The symptoms and chest radiograph findings of the reimplantation response are consistent with pulmonary edema, but they are apparently independent of fluid overload, tissue rejection, or infection.

The reimplantation response can present as a transient and reversible defect in gas exchange, lung compliance, and vascular resistance, that usually occurs within 2 to 3 weeks of the transplant and resolves without specific therapy or with supplemental oxygen or ventilatory support.[9]

## Transplant coronary artery disease (TxCAD)

Endothelial activation in the donor organ caused by immune reactions seems to override the impact of conventional risk factors (i.e., smoking habits, hyperlipidemia) on coronary artery disease. These risk factors take several years to become clinically detectable.[41] However, acceleration of CAD in the heart-transplant population may be the single most important limitation to long-term survival.[23,49] TxCAD has *not* been identified as a complication of lung transplantation.

From 2% to 14% of persons with heart transplantation have significant TxCAD by one year after transplantation, 25% to 40% by year 3, and 42% to 60% by year 5. However, it has been difficult to assess the clinical relevance of these numbers because of a lack of posttransplant ventricular function studies.[41]

The lesions associated with TxCAD are different than those of naturally occurring CAD in that the former affect the whole length of the vessel and especially its small branches, including small intramyocardial tributaries, which may not be detectable on angiography.[10] Suggested causes include prolonged use of cyclosporine or steroids, postoperative infections with cytomegalovirus, or repeated bouts of rejection.[24]

## Hypertension (HTN)

During exercise, the systemic and pulmonary circulations normally can accommodate large increases in cardiac output. However, vasopressor effects, which can occur in the transplant population for various reasons, cause the circulation to behave in a noncompliant manner that, in this case, increases cardiac output leading to a rise in blood pressure.[47] Also, unopposed secretion of neuroendocrine hormones following denervation of the heart can alter control of fluid volume by the kidneys and contribute to hypertension.[7]

The high incidence of resistant hypertension increases progressively with time, if not treated pharmacologically. This increase can be further heightened by exercise with as little as 40% of peak power output.[7]

## Renal impairment

Azotemia, progressing to uremic syndrome, in which renal insufficiency causes retention of nitrogenous compounds and decreased preservation of the internal environment, as reflected in elevated plasma urea and creatinine, occurs in 45% to 100% of patients during the first 6 months of cyclosporine immunosuppression.[40]

## Anemia

Most drugs used for immunosuppression have the potential to cause anemia. With chronic or established anemia, maximal exercise capacity and $\dot{V}o_{2max}$ are decreased in proportion to the reduction in hemoglobin as a result of poorer oxygen delivery to peripheral muscles.[40] A gradual reduction in maximal exercise capacity and $\dot{V}o_{2max}$ secondary to anemia may be reversed quickly by infusion of appropriate blood products.

## SUMMARY OF ESSENTIAL POINTS FOR THE SUPERVISING CLINICIAN

General points for cardiac and/or lung transplantation:

- Ensure that barriers against opportunistic infection are respected in the first weeks after transplantation.
- The greater the pretransplant deconditioning and muscle atrophy, the poorer the initial postoperative physical capacity, and the longer the rehabilitation to regain potential exercise capacity.
- Persons with transplants should be aware that, barring complications, overall improvement in physical ability should occur with disciplined and extended rehabilitation.
- Patients must also have an understanding of the permanent physiological changes of the transplanted organ, and of acute changes that should be reported immediately to the appropriate health care professional.
- Offset the side effects of ongoing steroidal use by encouraging liberal protein intake for muscle growth, and by establishing a maximum of safely tolerated aerobic conditioning to diminish water and salt retention.
- A gradual decrease in peak exercise may indicate medication-induced anemia; a more acute decrease may indicate rejection.
- A gradual increase in hypertension with a decrease in peak power output may indicate need for pharmacologic change.
- Without effective pharmacologic treatment, hypertension would be expected to gradually increase over time at rest, and to increase further with as little as 40% of peak power output during exercise.[7]

When developing an exercise prescription therapists should:

- Monitor changes in blood pressures, perceived exertion, arterial oxygen saturation, heart rates and respiratory rates
- Note changes in diastolic blood pressure between rest, early, and continued exercise until a regular pattern of diastolic response is established
- Rely on measurements of oxygen uptake, not on target heart rates if the heart is denervated (note that accidental denervation of the heart can occur with lung transplantation, especially DLT[33])
- Use weight-bearing exercise for bone health when steroids are being used, and emphasize use of large muscle masses of the lower extremities for aerobic conditioning
- Note that a sudden increase in minute ventilation without a corresponding increase in workload may indicate crossing of the anaerobic threshold
- Be aware that cardiac output may be the limiting factor for peak exercise in either heart or lung transplantation because of structural changes in peripheral muscles secondary to deconditioning, atrophy, or steroid use

The following guidelines apply to heart transplants only:

- Expect hemodynamic responses similar to that of an older person, even though the donor usually is much younger.[63]
- Warm-up is *essential* before peak activity because it (1) increases the stroke volume via return of boluses of blood from large contracting muscles and (2) increases catecholamine release, which progressively increases heart rate.
- Whereas some change in diastolic blood pressure is to be expected at the start of exercise, large changes indicate ischemia or acute rejection.
- Chronic rejection may be manifest by various cardiac symptoms.
- Isometric exercise should be used cautiously and only in association with dynamic exercise.
- A true training effect can occur even at the modest level of effort of only 60% of peak oxygen uptake.[23]
- Only transplanted hearts in situ less than 3 to 4 months should be considered completely denervated.[62]
- Angina pectoris associated with myocardial ischemia or with chronic rejection, is absent initially, but may reappear years later.

The following guidelines apply to lung transplants only:

- Early attention to volitional coughing, frequent position change, regular pulmonary hygiene, and flexibility of the trunk and shoulder girdle areas assists in clearing lungs that are denervated distal to the anastamosis site.
- Volitional coughing, whenever inhalation of anything but clean air is suspected, will help protect denervated lung areas.
- Thoracic mobilization to reduce barrel-chest deformity, and diaphragmatic stretching and strengthening can improve efficiency of respiratory function.
- Satisfactory pulse oximetry values during work are 95% for DLT and 90% for SLT.
- Expect higher than normal respiration rates and minute ventilation at rest and with exercise.
- Sudden increase in dyspnea with exercise may indicate rejection in lung and heart-lung transplantation.
- During exercise, submaximal heart rates tend to be average or high, but at peak levels, maximal heart rates average only 72% of predicted values.

- Cardiac output may be a limiting factor during exercise in lung transplantation.

## SUMMARY

The entry-level physical therapist can play an invaluable role in educating and assisting the candidate for and recipient of a cardiac and/or lung transplant to achieve the greatest potential functional level possible during all phases of the transplant experience.

Before the surgery, progressive exercise below the thresholds for cardiac or pulmonary decompensation, and education about the active role the patient must play in the early postoperative phase aid in minimizing perioperative risk.

During the first few weeks after transplantation, prevention of postoperative pulmonary complications, minimization of donor heart deconditioning, early progression of endurance activities, basic education about the differences of the transplanted organ during rest and exercise, and self-monitoring of exercise are indicated.

In the period of return to normal life, the physical therapist motivates the individual into an aggressive training program over the long term to maximize exercise potential. Training programs may include endurance, strengthening, fitness, and flexibility components. Education at this stage includes more detailed understanding of and alertness to the signs of rejection, infection, or medication side effects, and of the actions to be taken.

Finally, when the individual with a heart or lung transplant consults a physical therapist in any practice setting, reinforcement of the activities and education of the above two phases, appropriate modification of the treatment recommendations, and alertness to long-term physiological changes associated with transplantation provide comprehensive direction not available through any other health care provider.

## REFERENCES

1. Appell HJ: Muscular atrophy following immobilisation: a review, *Sports Med* 10:42, 1990.
2. Arai Y and others: Modulation of cardiac autonomic activity during and immediately after exercise, *Am J Physiol* 256:H-132, 1989.
3. Arnold C: Physical therapy with the lung transplant patient, *Combined Sections Meeting of the American Physical Therapy Association,* San Francisco, 1992.
4. Banner N, and others: Ventilatory and circulatory responses at the onset of exercise in man following heart or heart-lung transplantation, *J Physiol* 399:437, 1988.
5. Block E and others: Influence of exercise on a heart transplant patient, *Arch Phys Med Rehabil* 71:153, 1990.
6. Borg GAV: Psychophysical bases of perceived exertion, *Med Sci Sports Exer* 14:377, 1982.
7. Braith RW and others: Abnormal neuroendocrine responses during exercise in heart transplant recipients, Circulation 86:1453, 1992.
8. Clough P: The denervated heart, *Clin Manage* 10:14, 1990.
9. Davis MJ and Parker JR: Postoperative pulmonary complications in heart-lung transplantation: a review of the literature, *Respir Care* 32:676, 1987.
10. Downs A: Aerobic exercise program for patients awaiting lung transplantation, *Combined Sections Meeting of the American Physical Therapy Association,* San Francisco, 1992.
11. *Drug Facts and Comparisons 1994 edition,* Olin RO and others, editors, Wolters Kluwer, St Louis, 1992.
12. Eschenbacher WL and Mannina A: An algorithm for the interpretation of cardiopulmonary exercise tests, *Chest* 97:263, 1990.
13. Estenne M, Primo G, and Yernault JC: Cardiorespiratory responses to dynamic exercise after human heart-lung transplantation, *Thorax* 42:629, 1987.
14. Gaer J: Physiological consequences of complete cardiac denervation, *Brit J Hospital Med* 48:220, 1992.
15. Gibbons WJ and others: Cardiopulmonary exercise responses after single lung transplantation for severe obstructive lung disease, *Chest* 100:106, 1991.
16. Glanville AR and others: Bronchial responsiveness to exercise after human cardiopulmonary transplantation, *Chest* 96:281, 1989.
17. Goldstein SA and others: Nitrogen and energy relationships in malnourished patients with emphysema, *Am Rev Respir Dis* 138:636, 1988.
18. Hartmann A and others: Serial evaluation of left ventricular function by radionuclide ventriculography at rest and during exercise after orthotopic heart transplantation, *Euro J Nucl Med* 20:146, 1993.
19. Holzinger C and others: (Infections in organ transplantation) Infektionen bei Organtransplantationen, *Zentralbl Chir* 115:1091, 1990 (published in German).
20. Hosenpud JD and others: Abnormal pulmonary function specifically related to congestive heart failure: comparison of patients before and after cardiac transplantation, *Amer J Med* 88:493, 1990.
21. Hosenpud JD and others: Lack of progressive "restrictive" physiology after heart transplantation despite intervening episodes of allograft rejection: comparison of serial rest and exercise hemodynamics one and two years after transplantation, *J Heart Transplant* 9:119, 1990.
21A. Hosenpud JD and others: The registry of the international society for heart and lung transplantation: eleventh official report—1994. *J Heart Lung Transplant* 13:561, 1994.
22. Jensen RL, Yanowitz FG, and Crapo RO: Brief reports: exercise hemodynamics and oxygen delivery measurements using rebreathing techniques in heart transplant patients, *Am J Cardiol* 68:129, 1991.
23. Kavanagh T: Exercise training in patients after heart transplantation, *Herz* 16:243, 1991.
24. Kavanagh T and Yacoub MH: Exercise training in patients after heart transplantation, *Ann Acad Med Singapore* 21:372, 1992.
25. Kavanagh T and others: Cardiorespiratory responses to exercise training after orthotopic cardiac transplantation, *Circulation* 77:162, 1988.
26. Kaye MP: The registry of the international society for heart and lung transplantation: tenth official report, *J Heart Lung Transplant* 12:541, 1993.
27. Keteyian S and others: Cardiovascular responses of heart transplant patients to exercise training, *J Appl Physio* 70:2627, 1991.
28. Kramer B, Massie B, and Topic N: Hemodynamic differences between supine and upright exercise in patients with congestive heart failure, *Circulation* 66:820, 1982.
29. Kriett JM and Kaye MP: The registry of the international society for heart and lung transplantation: eighth official report, *J Heart Lung Transplant* 10:491, 1991.
30. Krull K and Hatswell E: Single-lung allograft: a nursing perspective, *Crit Care Nurse* 8(6):35-56, 1988.
31. Labovitz AJ and others: Exercise capacity during the first year after cardiac transplantation, *Am J Cardio* 64:642, 1989.
32. Leonardi L (graft rejection reaction and immunosuppression following heart transplantation) Abstossungsreaktion and Immunosuppression nach Herztransplantation, *Ther Umsch* 47:147, 1990 (published in German).

33. Levy RD and others: Exercise performance after lung transplantation, *J Heart Lung Transplant* 12:27, 1993.

34. Mahon PM: Orthoclone OKT3 and cardiac transplantation: an overview, *Crit Care Nurse* 11:42, 1991.

35. Mancini DM and others: Value of peak exercise oxygen consumption for optimal timing of cardiac transplantation in ambulatory patients with heart failure, *Circulation* 83:778, 1991.

36. Marzo KP, Wilson JR, and Mancini DM: Effects of cardiac transplantation on ventilatory response to exercise, *Am J Cardiol* 69:547, 1992.

37. Miller LW and others: Vascular rejection in heart transplant recipients, *J Heart Lung Transplant* 12:S147, 1993.

38. Miyoshi S and others: Cardiopulmonary exercise testing after single and double lung transplantation. *Chest* 97:1130, 1990.

39. Nehlsen-Cannarella SL and Chang L: Immunology and organ transplantation in the neonate and young infant, *Crit Care Nurs Clin North Am* 4:179, 1992.

40. Otulana BA, Higenbottam TW, and Wallwork J: Causes of exercise limitation after heart-lung transplantation, *J Heart Lung Transplant* 11:S244, 1992.

41. Paul LC: Chronic rejection of organ allografts: magnitude of the problem, *Transplantation Proceedings* 25:2024, 1993.

42. Paulus WJ and others: Deficient acceleration of left ventricular relaxation during exercise after heart transplantation, *Circulation* 86:1175, 1992.

43. Ribeiro JP and others: Periodic breathing during exercise in severe heart failure: reversal with milrinone or cardiac transplantation, *Chest* 92:555, 1987.

44. Ross DJ and others: Hemodynamic responses to exercise after lung transplantation, *Chest* 103:46, 1993.

45. Rudas L, Pflugfelder PW, and Kostuk WJ: Comparison of hemodynamic responses during dynamic exercise in the upright and supine postures after orthotopic cardiac transplantation, *J Am Coll Cardiol* 16:1367, 1990.

46. Sciaky A: Mobilization of the intensive care unit patient: pathophysiology and treatment, *Physical Therapy Practice* 3(2):69, 1994.

47. Scott JP and others: Cyclosporine in heart transplant recipients: an exercise study of vasopressor effects, *Euro Heart J* 13:531, 1992.

48. Shephard RJ: Responses of the cardiac transplant patient to exercise and training, *Ex Sport Sci Rev* 20:297, 1992.

49. Smart FW and others: Detection of transplant arteriopathy: does exercise thallium scintigraphy improve noninvasive diagnostic capabilities? *Transplantation Proceedings* 23:1189, 1991.

50. Sobush DC: Work and rest: establishing ratios that are safe, tolerable, and productive, *University of Michigan Hospitals Physical Therapy Division Inservice,* March 20, 1991.

51. Squires RW: Exercise training after cardiac transplantation, *Medicine Science in Sports Exercise* 23:686, 1991.

52. Stevenson LW and others: Exercise capacity for survivors of cardiac transplantation or sustained medical therapy for stable heart failure, *Circulation* 81:78, 1990.

53. Sullivan MJ and others: Exercise training in patients with severe left ventricular dysfunction: hemodynamic and metabolic effects, *Circulation* 78:506, 1988.

54. Sullivan MJ and others: Increased exercise ventilation in patients with chronic heart failure: intact ventilatory control despite hemodynamic and pulmonary abnormalities, *Circulation* 77:552, 1988.

55. Theodore J and others: Augmented ventilatory response to exercise in pulmonary hypertension, *Chest* 89:39, 1986.

56. Theodore J and others: Cardiopulmonary function at maximum tolerable constant work rate exercise following human heart-lung transplantation, *Chest* 92:433, 1987.

57. Trulock EP and others: Single lung transplantation for severe chronic obstructive pulmonary disease, *Chest* 96:738, 1989.

58. Weber KT and others: Oxygen utilization and ventilation during exercise in patients with chronic cardiac failure, *Circulation* 65:1213, 1982.

59. Weisman IM and others: The role of cardiopulmonary exercise testing in the selection of patients for cardiac transplantation, *Chest* 102:1871, 1992.

60. Woodley SL and others: Immunosuppression following cardiac transplantation, *Cardiol Clin* 8:83, 1990.

61. Williams TJ and others: Maximal exercise testing in single and double lung transplant recipients, *Am Rev Respir Dis* 145:101, 1992.

62. Wilson RF and others: Evidence for structural sympathetic reinnervation after orthotopic cardiac transplantation in humans, *Circulation* 83:1210, 1991.

63. Younis LT and others: Left ventricular systolic function and diastolic filling at rest and during upright exercise after orthotopic heart transplantation: comparison with young and aged normal subjects, *J Heart Transplantation* 9:683, 1990.

# Physical Therapy for the Acutely Ill Patient in the Respiratory Intensive Care Unit

*Willy E. Hammon*

## OUTLINE

In many hospitals across the country, the physical therapist may be a relative newcomer to the critical care team. Unfortunately, student physical therapists receive minimal, if any, exposure to the intensive care unit (ICU). As a result, the request to provide care in the ICU may cause anxiety in many therapists. The area is viewed as forbidding and crisis oriented. The majority of patients are perceived to be medically unstable and perhaps close to death. The unit is full of unfamiliar equipment. The patients are frequently semiconscious, with multiple central and peripheral monitoring and therapeutic lines. The many monitors and their sensitive alarms can add to the therapist's uneasiness.

However, a more realistic viewpoint is important. The severity of illness in these patients spans the spectrum from medically stable, in good condition to the unstable whose survival is in question; however, the majority fall somewhere in between.

The numerous monitors should be viewed as friends, not foes, because they can provide rapid objective data on the patient's condition and tolerance to treatment. Like any area the physical therapist is unfamiliar with, the most effective way to gain confidence in the ICU is to spend time there learning about the various monitors and gaining experience treating those who are critically ill.

The purpose of this chapter is to describe the various physical therapy techniques that can be used effectively in treating the medical patient in the respiratory intensive care unit (RICU). Conditions requiring caution and special consideration are identified. Alterations of the normal respiratory defense mechanisms that predispose the critically ill to respiratory complications and frequently encountered pulmonary conditions are discussed. Also included is information regarding psychological disorders the critically ill occasionally suffer.

The physical therapist can make a valuable contribution in caring for the medical patient in the RICU. Our training in chest physical therapy and rehabilitative medicine adds an important dimension to the comprehensive treatment of the critically ill. To be excluded from this area is neither in our profession's nor in the patient's best interests, and such exclusion would certainly omit an important aspect of his or her care.

## RESPIRATORY DEFENSE MECHANISMS

The respiratory system can be divided into the upper and lower airways.[51] The upper airway consists of the nose, mouth, pharynx, and larynx. The lower airway consists of the tracheobronchial tree and lung parenchyma. The major upper and lower airway defense mechanisms and their alterations in critically ill patients are described below.

### Upper airway

The first respiratory defense mechanisms are encountered in the upper airway, particularly in the nose.[123] Inspiration draws air into the nostrils past the anterior nasal hairs and nasal turbinates with an airflow pattern that provides maximal exposure with the mucosa.[71] The nasal hairs and mucus covering the mucosa filter foreign particles from the inspired air. Ciliary action propels the particles posteriorly and eventually into the oropharynx, where they are swallowed. Large particles are expelled from the anterior nasal passages by sneezing or nose blowing.

Two other important functions of the upper airway are warming the air to body temperature and saturating it with water vapor.

### Larynx

The larynx connects the upper and lower airways. The glottis is located at the opening of the larynx and has an important function during the cough reflex (see section on cough). The mucosa of the larynx has receptors that are sensitive to mechanical or chemical irritation. Stimulation of these receptors will elicit the cough reflex to expel the irritant.[86] The cough reflex and the epiglottis (during swallowing) are the two major defense mechanisms that prevent aspiration and contamination of the lower respiratory tract.[86,123]

### Alterations by artificial airways

Critically ill patients commonly have artificial airways placed for adequate ventilation or effective removal of secretions. However, placement of an artificial airway bypasses the normal upper airway function and defense mechanisms, resulting in bacterial contamination of the tracheobronchial tree.[123] Air being delivered to the patient must be warmed and humidified to maintain adequate mucociliary function.[140] The presence of a foreign object (the artificial airway) in the trachea causes an increased production of secretions. Cuffed endotracheal tubes are known to reduce the clearance rate of tracheal mucus.[114] The effectiveness of the cough reflex is diminished because the glottis cannot close during the compressive phase of the cough. Also the potential for pulmonary aspiration is increased and has been reported in 15% to 20% of intubated critically ill patients.[17] For these reasons critically ill patients with artificial airways generally benefit from postural drainage, percussion, and vibration, all of which enhance the drainage of secretions.

### Mucociliary escalator

The mucociliary escalator is an important defense mechanism for clearing the airways of unwanted material.[62,104,129] The term "mucociliary escalator" describes the interrelationship between the mucous secretions and the cilia that propel the mucus. The airways are coated with a double (sol-gel) layer of mucus secreted by mucous glands and goblet cells. The outer layer is the viscous (gel) layer; the inner is the liquid (sol) layer in which the cilia beat. The cilia beat in unison, sweeping mucus and any material in the airways toward the the larynx at a rate of 1 to 2 cm per minute. Approximately 10 ml of mucus is cleared from the respiratory tract daily.[71]

The mucous blanket is composed of numerous substances that in combination probably have a role in the defense of the respiratory tract against infection.[50] These include secretory immunoglobulins (especially IgA), polymorphonuclear leukocytes, lysozymes, interferon, and others. For example, it is known that IgA antibodies have a viral neutralizing activity, and a deficiency of IgA is commonly associated with recurrent sinopulmonary infections. However, the precise activity of these substances in the defense of the respiratory system remains ill defined.

### Altered mucociliary transportation

The mucociliary transport rate can be affected by multiple factors.[140] Dehydration and the inhalation of dry gases cause the secretions to become more viscous and difficult to move.[30] Impaired cilia activity has been demonstrated in cystic fibrosis,[141,147] chronic bronchitis,[71] and asthma and in cigarette smokers.[139] Numerous drugs, including narcotics and acetylcysteine (Mucomyst),[140,141] breathing elevated concentrations of oxygen,[80,115] intubation with cuffed endotracheal tubes,[114] intermittent suctioning,[79] and bilateral diaphragmatic weakness slow mucociliary transportation. By contrast, hydration,[30] bronchial drainage,[30] and some drugs (e.g., aminophylline and acetylcholine)[140] can increase the rate at which secretions are cleared. An increased production of secretions can be caused by tracheobronchial inflammation from a variety of causes. The most common acute causes are infection and inhalation of noxious gases or materials. Many persons with chronic lung disease, especially chronic bronchitis or bronchiectasis, have long-standing hypersecretions of mucus.

These secretions can usually be removed adequately by the mucociliary escalator or by coughing, a second important clearance mechanism of the respiratory system. When performed properly, a cough propels secretions and foreign material through the airways toward the mouth. However, if respiratory clearance mechanisms become ineffective, the inability to remove secretions becomes clinically significant.[13]

## Cough

An effective cough is an important mechanism for clearing the airways of secretions or foreign material.[83,86] A cough has three distinct phases.[69] The first is a deep inspiration. The second, or compressive, phase begins with closure of the glottis. Both intrathoracic and intraabdominal pressure build with contraction of the expiratory respiratory muscles. The final, or expulsive, phase begins with opening of the glottis and expulsion of the trapped air. The diaphragm relaxes to provide for the transmission of the increased intraabdominal pressure into the lung. Usually airways above the fourth-generation bronchi are compressed by the high intrathoracic pressure.[91] The narrowed lumen of the airways is important for maintaining the high linear velocity of airflow required for an effective cough. The high lung volume, along with the increased static lung elastic recoil and the reduced airway frictional resistance, contributes to maximal expiratory flow rate during the final cough phase. The lung volume attained during inspiration also determines which airways are compressed during the expulsive phase.[98] Coughing at large lung volumes compresses large airways, but coughing at lower lung volumes compresses smaller airways. This observation has caused some to postulate that a series of coughs is more effective than a single cough.[98] After a deep breath, the initial cough would clear the secretions from the larger airways, and the following coughs, at successively lower lung volumes, would advance the secretions from smaller airways to larger ones. Another deep inspiration and series of coughs would begin clearing the most proximal secretions and continue advancing the secretions from smaller to larger airways.

The cough of the critically ill patient can be inadequate for a number of reasons.[69] Some chronic respiratory diseases such as advanced chronic obstructive pulmonary disease

(COPD)[87] and bronchiectasis[89] reduce cough effectiveness by limiting the maximal expiratory airflow rate. Pain,[26,40] depression of the central nervous system,[27] small tracheostomy tubes,[82] paralysis,[126] and weakness[82,134] have each been shown to alter one or more cough phases. This alteration can have especially serious implications in patients with an increased production of secretions. Therapists should analyze the quality of patients' coughs and try to improve their effectiveness. Some techniques we have found helpful for improving coughs are discussed on p. 429.

### Alveolar macrophage

The most important defense mechanism in the alveoli is the macrophage.[50,51] The alveolar macrophage is a large mononuclear ameboid cell that scavenges the surface of the alveolar epithelium.[123] Any foreign particles or organisms encountered by the macrophage are engulfed and digested. These cells are then removed from the alveoli either through the lymphatics or by migration to the terminal bronchioles, where they become attached to the mucus. The mucus transports the macrophages up the respiratory tract, and they are eventually expectorated or swallowed.

The rate of phagocytosis by the alveolar macrophage is reduced by multiple factors[50] including acute hypoxia, alcohol ingestion,[21] cigarette smoking, starvation, corticosteroids, air pollutants, and oxygen.

## COMPLICATIONS OF RETAINED SECRETIONS

Chest physical therapy is indicated in the removal of retained secretions and treatment of their complications. One of the most common complications is hypoxemia caused by secretions that partially occlude airways and cause ventilation-perfusion mismatching. We have found bronchial drainage and percussion effective in rapidly correcting this type of hypoxemia (Fig. 22-1).[31,55] In patients with copious secretions, improved oxygenation can result from treatment as frequent as every 2 hours (Fig. 22-2).

Atelectasis attributable to secretions completely occluding airways causes hypoxemia by shunting blood past nonventilated alveoli. This complication can also be reversed by bronchial drainage and percussion (Fig. 22-3).[40,52,55,94] Short-term results (after 1 treatment and after a 6-hour treatment period) using positioning with chest vibrations, hyperinflations, and suctioning are significantly better than hyperinflations and suctioning alone. At 24 and 48 hours both treatment regimens appear to be of comparable value.

On occasion, the inability to remove secretions effectively can present life-threatening problems. We have previously described, in a 21-year-old quadriplegic, a cardiopulmonary arrest attributable to complete occlusion of the trachea by a large volume of mucus.[55] One confirmed death has occurred at this medical center because of inspissated secretions. At the postmortem examination a

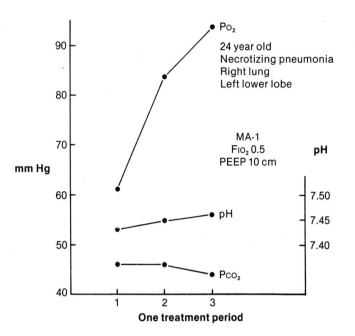

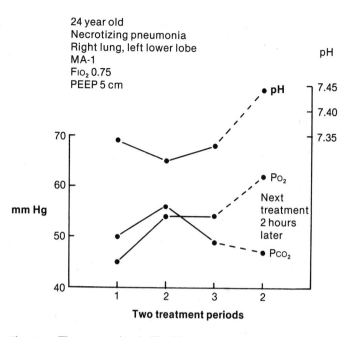

**Fig. 22-1.** This graph shows a dramatically improved $Po_2$ during and after a single 15-minute bronchial drainage, percussion, and vibration treatment in this critically ill patient. It was productive of copious amounts of sputum. *Point 1,* Reclining head up immediately before treatment; *point 2,* at the end of 15 minutes of treatment in the Trendelenburg position; *point 3,* reclining head up 30 minutes after treatment.

**Fig. 22-2.** The same patient in Fig. 22-1. *Point 1,* Reclining head up immediately before treatment; *point 2,* at the end of 15 minutes of treatment, in Trendelenburg position; *point 3,* reclining head up 30 minutes after treatment. The second point 2 was drawn at the end of a second 15-minute treatment, in Trendelenburg position, 2 hours after the first treatment. The further improvement in his $Po_2$ over the previous level *(point 3)* indicates some patients with copious secretions can benefit from treatments every 2 hours.

large mucous plug was found obstructing the trachea of a young asthmatic patient. Therapists should be aware of the importance of draining secretions from seriously ill patients, especially those with impaired respiratory clearance mechanisms.

## PATIENT ASSESSMENT

A complete review of the medical chart should precede the initial treatment. The therapist should briefly check the chart before each treatment to be certain the patient's status has not changed significantly. Ascertain the patient's state of health before he or she was admitted to the RICU. Chronic diseases should be noted, as well as acute episodes that caused the patient to be admitted to the critical care area. A history of acute and chronic cardiovascular disease should alert the therapist to the increased possibility of poor tolerance of bronchial drainage, percussion and vibration. The likelihood of any increased production of, or difficulty in, clearing secretions should be considered, as discussed in the previous sections of this chapter. Laboratory results should be reviewed to rule out coagulopathies that would contraindicate treatment. Any reference to thoracic or rib cage abnormalities should be noted. Therapists should be aware that long-term steroid use may contribute to osteopenia and may predispose to easily fractured ribs. The chest radiographs should be read. Is there any central nervous system or spinal cord disorder? If there is also an acute pulmonary problem, this patient will need aggressive chest

physical therapy. In short, therapists should carefully review the chart to glean as much information as possible about the patient.

The most recent chest radiograph should also be examined to visualize any infiltrates and determine if atelectasis is present.[55] Make a mental note taken of anatomic landmarks and their relation to the involved lobe to locate the precise area on which to concentrate percussion and vibration, should they be indicated. The film should be examined for signs of congestive heart failure (an enlarged heart, bilateral pleural effusions), rib lesions, or pneumothorax. The location of all lines and tubes should be noted.

Before treatment, the therapist should take a couple of minutes to study the patient's baseline heart rate and rhythm on the cardiac monitor. This is important, since cardiac dysrhythmias during treatment may occur in 36% of patients receiving bronchial drainage and percussion.[57]

The most recent arterial blood gas values must be identified as well. Is the patient hypoxemic? What is the acid-base status?

The nurse caring for the patient should be asked about the patient's current condition. The therapist should explain that he or she has come to do a bronchial drainage treatment. If this is the first time to see the patient, the nurse can provide important additional information. Is the patient alert and cooperative? How many people are needed to turn the patient? Most importantly, has he or she become unstable

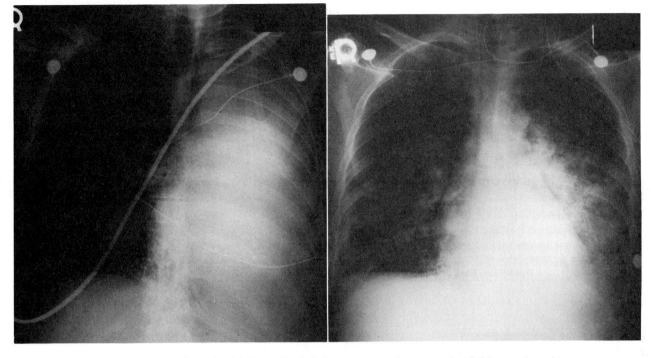

**Fig. 22-3. A,** A radiograph taken immediately before treatment shows complete left lung atelectasis in this 42-year-old man with dermatomyositis and left lower lobe pneumonia. **B,** A radiograph taken immediately after bronchial drainage, percussion, and vibration shows reexpansion of the left lung.

since the last note was written on the medical chart? For example, if the patient has developed significant dysrhythmias and is now receiving lidocaine, it probably would be best to allow him or her to become stabilized before the requested treatment is performed.

## PHYSICAL ASSESSMENT

The chest should be inspected before treatment. Are any chest deformities present? The lateral and anteroposterior dimensions of the chest should be noted. An increase in the anteroposterior diameter suggests underlying chronic obstructive pulmonary disease (COPD).[25] The patient's breathing should also be observed. Normally during quiet breathing, inspiration is active and expiration passive, each lasting approximately the same length of time. However, use of the sternocleidomastoids and other accessory muscles of inspiration indicates increased work of breathing. This increased inspiratory work and a prolonged forced expiration with contraction of the abdominal muscles are commonly seen during an exacerbation of COPD.[22] Next, the therapist should inspect the skin for abnormalities. Are there any scars from previous trauma or surgery? Are there needle marks or areas of ecchymosis present? These, or a Band-Aid on the back, may indicate that a thoracentesis has been performed recently. If this procedure has been done within the past few hours, the postthoracocentesis chest radiograph should be examined to rule out a residual pneumothorax before

proceeding. (See the discussions on precautions and special considerations, p. 432, and on thoracentesis, subclavian lines, and chest tubes, p. 435.)

With the hands, the therapist should palpate for symmetrical bilateral expansion of the chest. There is diminished chest movement over the area of lung disease.[29] The chest should then be auscultated, not only to locate the most congested segments,[103] but also to establish a base line for determining the effectiveness of treatment.[56] When breath sounds are diminished or absent, percussion is important to differentiate the conditions that may cause these findings, as Case 1 and Case 2 on p. 428 illustrate.

All acutely ill patients, whether in the ICU or not, should be examined for signs and symptoms of hypoxia and carbon dioxide retention (Table 22-1). These signs and symptoms should correspond with the previously reviewed arterial blood gas values. If they do not, the patient's condition may have deteriorated since the last sample was drawn. Before proceeding with treatment, the therapist should ask the nurse if the patient's physical condition has changed in the past few minutes.

The majority of health professionals are familiar with cyanosis as a sign of hypoxia and can recognize central cyanosis by looking at the color of the patient's lips and tongue. However, the signs and symptoms of carbon dioxide ($CO_2$) retention are often poorly recognized. The patient may be dozing and difficult to arouse. The redness of the skin

## CASE 1

A 19-year-old man with quadriplegia is noted to suddenly become diaphoretic and short of breath. Auscultation reveals absent breath sounds in the left lung, and there is dullness to percussion. A chest radiograph shows complete left lung atelectasis.[55] Bronchial drainage and percussion to the left lung are productive of several mucous plugs. Auscultation then indicates breath sounds in the previously silent lung and a normal resonance to percussion. The posttreatment chest radiograph shows resolution of the atelectasis. Dullness to percussion is most often found in pleural effusions, pneumonia, and atelectasis.[29]

## CASE 2

A 23-year-old man is evaluated for bronchial drainage 1 day after laparotomy for an abdominal gunshot wound. Auscultation reveals normal breath sounds in the left lung but absent breath sounds in the right. Percussion to the right lung was hyperresonate. A chest radiograph taken a few minutes earlier was read by the therapist and showed a large pneumothorax. The physician was notified, and he inserted a chest tube to treat the pneumothorax.

---

**Table 22-1.** Signs and symptoms of hypoxia and carbon dioxide ($CO_2$) narcosis

**Hypoxia**

*Symptoms*

Ethanol-like symptoms: confusion, loss of judgment, paranoia, restlessness, dizziness

*Signs*

Sympathetic response: tachycardia, mild hypertension, peripheral vasoconstriction
Nonsympathetic response: bradycardia, hypotension

**$CO_2$ narcosis**

*Symptoms*

Headache
Mild sedation→drowsiness→coma

*Signs*

Vasodilation: redness of skin, sclera, and conjunctiva caused by increased cutaneous blood flow; sweating
Sympathetic response: hypertension (systolic and diastolic); tachycardia

From Rogers RM: Acute respiratory failure, *Resident and Staff Physician* 25(5):39, 1979.

(especially the face), sclera, and conjunctiva caused by vasodilation is striking. Persons with these signs of $CO_2$ retention have reduced respiratory effort and usually have a greater need for ventilatory assistance than for drainage of secretions.

## TREATMENT PROCEDURES: BRONCHIAL DRAINAGE, PERCUSSION, VIBRATION

Most treatment regimens in the intensive care unit involve the application of multiple chest physical therapy techniques, depending on the physician's orders, patient's needs, etc. Although this section provides in-depth coverage of bronchial drainage, percussion, and vibration with the seriously-ill patient, it should not be interpreted as comprising the full scope of chest physical therapy.

If a patient has excessive secretions and an ineffective cough, treatments such as bronchial drainage, percussion, vibration, and hyperinflations, may be ordered by the primary physician or selected by the therapist.[13,44] Treatment begins with the therapist introducing himself or herself as a physical therapist and explaining that the physician has requested treatment to help the patient's breathing by clearing his or her lungs of secretions. The therapist will help the patient turn on his or her side and then percuss or clap the chest gently to help drain the secretions from the lungs. The head of the bed will be lowered to help the secretions drain toward the patient's mouth so that he or she can cough them out more easily.

If the patient, in particular the intubated patient, tries to communicate, the therapist should make a determined effort to understand.[6] This is an important aspect of developing rapport. Reading lips is the ideal way to communicate because many seriously ill patients find writing quite tedious.

There must be sufficient slack in all tubing and lines (heart monitor, central venous pressure [CVP], Swan-Ganz catheter, arterial lines) before the patient is turned onto the side. The ventilator tubing should be checked for accumulation of water. Sometimes when the patient is turned, several milliliters of water in the tubing can be "spilled" down the patient's airway, triggering paroxyms of coughing. Although probably not harmful, to the anxious, alert patient it is uncomfortable and frightening. Confidence in the therapist may be lost, and the patient may become uncooperative after such an episode.

One person can effectively turn most comatose patients onto the side. He or she should stand on the side toward which the patient is to be turned. The arm of the patient that will be uppermost when he or she is on the side should be adducted (with the elbow flexed) across the chest. With the patient supine, the therapist flexes the patient's farthest hip and knee. The hand is placed just above the knee, over the anterior lateral surface of the leg. Then the patient is pulled toward the therapist until the side-lying position is achieved. Pillows may be placed behind the patient's back to maintain the position better. The uppermost hip and knee should remain flexed to most effectively maintain this side-lying position. Pillows can also be used to support the uppermost arm and leg.

Patients can be turned to the prone position in a similar manner. The therapist stands on the side of the bed opposite the direction that the patient will be turned and slides the patient toward himself or herself. The therapist then takes the farther arm and adducts it against the patient's side, with the elbow extended and the hand pronated. The closer arm is adducted across the patient's chest with the elbow flexed. The closer hip and knee are flexed. The therapist then rolls the patient away, toward the prone position. Next the therapist pulls the dependent arm posteriorly, out from beneath the torso. One pillow can be placed under the uppermost shoulder, another under the flexed hip and knee.

The therapist should check to be sure that none of the attached lines are pulled taut in this position and the intravenous (IV) lines are running. The patient's heart rhythm and rate are then observed on the heart monitor and the patient is allowed a minute to stabilize before placing the bed in the head-down position (Trendelenburg) for treatment of the middle, lingula, or lower lobes.

Percussion over the involved lobe begins lightly and gradually increases to the patient's tolerance. Generally, heavier persons tolerate more vigorous percussion than thinner persons do.

If the cardiac electrodes are in proximity to the area being treated, the percussion may register on the cardiac monitor as tachycardia or artifacts. These artifacts can simulate serious dysrhythmias, such as ventricular tachycardia or flutter.[139] The brief conversation with the nursing staff before bronchial drainage can prevent an inappropriate emergency resuscitation being called. Observation of the heart rhythm as percussion is initiated is particularly helpful in distinguishing artifact from dysrhythmias. Briefly halting percussion is also useful in distinguishing artifact from dysrhythmias.

Percussion continues for 4 minutes. Then, after the patient has taken a deep breath, the therapist compresses and vibrates the thorax during expiration, repeating this for six consecutive breaths. Patients receiving mechanical ventilation can be given hyperinflations when the "sigh" button on the ventilator is pushed. Vibration can be performed during expiration and before the triggering of another breath.

The proper direction to compress and vibrate must be kept in mind. During inspiration the lateral chest wall rises as the ribs move upward and outward (bucket-handle effect). Hence, during expiration the ribs are moving downward and inward. To vibrate in the proper direction, many therapists stand near the head of the bed to compress and vibrate in the approximate direction of the patient's opposite hip. However, if vibration is done improperly (toward the patient's head), injuries can result, especially in persons with less mobile or osteoporotic ribs.

Vibration is an important part of the treatment. It is noteworthy that many persons expectorate secretions during this maneuver. Secretions have been observed (by bronchoscopy) moving into larger airways during vibration.[148] The precise manner by which this technique advances the sputum is unclear. In addition to the effect that a vibratory force might have on advancing secretions, I believe that there are other important reasons for vibration. The airways dilate and expand on inspiration. Conversely, during expiration the airways constrict. If there is a bolus of mucus in an airway, the deep inspiration moves an increased volume of air distal to the mucus. Expiration narrows the airway around this mucus. Compression and vibration of the lung tissue and the "confined" air may have an effect similar to a Heimlich maneuver by dislodgement of the bolus centrally. This would also explain, at least in part, the findings noticed during bronchoscopy.

Percussion is resumed for another 4 minutes before vibration is repeated. Length of treatment should be based, in part, on how productive bronchial drainage, percussion, and vibration have been on removing secretions. A patient should be treated as long as sputum is produced, provided that there are no signs of poor tolerance to treatment. Occasionally, patients with copious secretions may receive very lengthy treatments of 30 to 60 minutes. They may also benefit from frequent treatments done every 1 or 2 hours (see Fig. 22-2). The majority of patients receive treatments that range from 10 to 20 minutes. Patients should be suctioned as needed during and after treatment before the head of the bed is elevated. Some therapists prefer to use a 2-L anesthesia bag to give 6 to 8 hyperinflations, holding each hyperinflation at full inflation for up to 5 seconds, prior to suctioning. However, these procedures may also elicit dysrhythmias.

## IMPROVING COUGH

The therapist should listen to and analyze the quality of a cough. When a cough is abnormal, an attempt should be made to determine which phase or phases are reducing its effectiveness.[29,69] When inspiration is too shallow, a deeper breath may be attained if the person is taught diaphragmatic or lateral costal breathing. Another method to improve inspiration for spontaneously breathing patients is to deliver a deep inspiration using intermittent positive-pressure breathing. The patient then closes the glottis, removes the

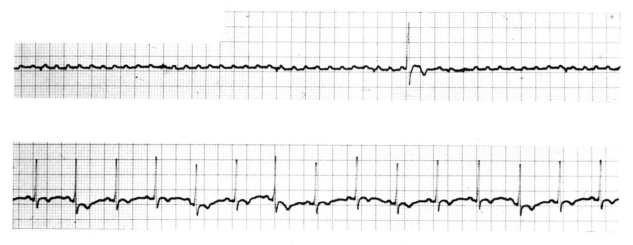

**Fig. 22-4.** The upper tracing shows a dysrhythmia (ventricular standstill) induced by suctioning of secretions of an intubated 42-year-old man receiving 40% oxygen. Preoxygenation with 100% oxygen results in no dysrhythmias during suctioning *(lower tracing)* of the same patient.

mouth-piece, and contracts the abdominal muscles to deliver a productive cough.

Glottic closure is not essential for an adequate cough.[69] However, if indicated in persons with artificial airways, an Ambu bag (breathing bag) can be compressed to resist expiration for a few seconds after the end of inspiration. This technique increases intrathoracic pressure for a more forceful expulsive phase. Assisted coughing is a useful technique for increasing the force of the expulsive phase, particularly in spontaneously breathing spinal cord-injured patients.[24,74] Assisted coughing is often helpful when used with postural drainage and percussion.[126] The therapist places one hand in the epigastric region of the patient's abdomen and the other hand on the lateral chest wall. At the end of inspiration, the therapist compresses the chest downward and the abdomen toward the diaphragm increasing the expiratory velocity of air. This procedure is effective for mobilizing secretions and reduces the need for frequent suctioning. Patients are also convinced of its benefit, since they frequently request abdominal compression when congested. Abdominal binders have also been used to increase the expiratory force of ventilator patients.[92]

## SUCTIONING

Suctioning is an important procedure for removing secretions from patients with artificial airways and from those who cannot cough well. However, suctioning must be done carefully to avoid the complications of hypotension, hypoxemia, and cardiac arrest.[3,70,123,125] Use of catheters with "ringed tips" is advocated to reduce tracheal mucosal trauma associated with suctioning.[72,113]

Hyperoxygenation to prevent arterial hypoxemia, which can lead to myocardial hypoxia and dysrhythmias, is very important. The effect of 100% oxygen on reducing dysrhythmias has been reported.[125] Fig. 22-4 also demonstrates this reduction.

The suction catheter in the trachea may cause dysrhythmias by vagal stimulation. To reduce this hazard, the catheter should not remain in the patient's trachea longer than 10 to 15 seconds.

The following procedure is recommended to suction patients:

1. Explain to the patient what you are going to do.
2. Set the wall-suction regulator at 100 to 120 mm Hg.
3. Using sterile technique, open the package containing the suction catheter and put the glove on. Then using the gloved hand, attach the catheter to the wall-suction tubing.
4. Hyperoxygenate the patient.
5. Pass the suction catheter through the airway, without vacuum, until resistance is met (usually the level of the carina).
6. Withdraw the tip of the catheter approximately 1 cm before applying intermittent suction.
7. The catheter should rotate between the thumb and forefinger as it is withdrawn, with intermittent suction being applied.
8. The catheter should not be in the airway longer than 10 to 15 seconds.
9. Hyperoxygenate the patient before reintroducing the suction catheter into the airway.
10. The tubing may be flushed with sterile water to clear it of secretions before reintroduction of the catheter into the airway.
11. The instillation into the airway of 5 to 10 ml of sterile water may be helpful in loosening especially tenacious secretions.
12. Reset the oxygen to the presuction value.
13. Wrap the suction catheter around the gloved fingers. Then, holding the catheter with the thumb, remove the glove over the suction catheter. The glove should

be inside out with the suction catheter in the center, ready to be discarded.

14. The suction may be shut off.
15. Wash your hands.

Closed system, in-line endotracheal suctioning is widely performed today, utilizing a suction catheter that remains enclosed in a clear plastic sleeve attached to the patient's ventilator tubing or T-piece, rather than opening and discarding a new package each time the patient is suctioned.[107] Otherwise, the procedure for suctioning is essentially the same as described above.

## TOLERANCE TO TREATMENT

Therapists should carefully monitor each ICU patient's response to all forms of physical therapy. The majority of patients manifest no ill effects from such intervention. However, therapists need to know the potential adverse effects of each treatment technique and recognize them if they occur. Especially when patients require a physical therapy regimen that includes bronchial drainage, percussion, and vibration, the therapist should be alert for signs of poor tolerance to treatment. These signs are most often associated with placing the patient in a head-down position to treat the lingula, right middle lobe, or lower lobe.[54,55,120]

## HEMODYNAMIC AND METABOLIC RESPONSES

Studies have examined the effects of routine daily activities on mechanically ventilated intensive care unit patients.[132] In one group of postoperative patients, chest physical therapy was associated with the greatest increases in metabolic rate, heart rate, and rate-pressure product.[143] This was probably caused by several factors, including pain, movement, and muscular tension in the chest and abdomen. Although chest physical therapy is generally well tolerated, it can cause significant hemodynamic and metabolic stress in some critically ill patients. These changes have been attenuated by the administration of a short-acting narcotic.[75] Therapists should carefully note all patients' tolerance to treatment, but especially those with underlying cardiac disease. Poorly tolerated treatments should be modified or discontinued.

## CARDIAC DYSRHYTHMIAS

Cardiac dysrhythmias may be one of the earliest manifestations of poor tolerance to treatment. At times dysrhythmias occur transiently when the patient is placed in the Trendelenburg position, and the rhythm returns to normal within 30 to 45 seconds. On other occasions dysrhythmias occur after percussion is begun. In a series of 72 initial treatments, coworkers and I found that major dysrhythmias occurred in 11.1%, minor dysrhythmias in 25% and no dysrhythmias in 63.9%.[57] Age >64 years and acute cardiac conditions were significant risk factors for dysrhythmias. Patients with major dysrhythmias also manifested a significantly lower blood pressure and respiratory rate, with an increased heart rate during treatment. Measuring these vital signs pretreatment and noting changes with treatment may alert therapists to impending dysrhythmias in high risk patients. Huseby and co-workers[67] observed dysrhythmias, including ventricular tachycardia, in the seriously ill during treatment. Laws and McIntyre[81] were prompted to study the cardiac output in a group of patients after two episodes of sudden death during bronchial drainage. The investigators apparently suspected that a cardiovascular mechanism was responsible. Hypoxemia during treatment may play a role in precipitating some dysrhythmias. However, co-workers and I have documented dysrhythmias in some critically ill persons with arterial blood gas values that showed $P_{O_2}$ well above 80 mm Hg.[57] An increase in sympathetic nervous system activity and elevated plasma catecholamine levels during bronchial drainage and percussion may contribute to dysrhythmias in critically ill patients.[2,57] It is possible that chest percussion itself to the left lung may stimulate dysrhythmias.[57] Rarely, chest percussion has been shown to interfere with pacemaker function.[78] Hence, an important part of any treatment is close observation of the cardiac monitor to recognize dysrhythmias that may occur.

## HYPOXEMIA

Hypoxemia is another indication of poor tolerance to treatment. Hypoxemia is more likely to occur in persons who do not expectorate sputum during treatment.[31] However, as Fig. 22-5 shows, hypoxemia can be seen in patients who

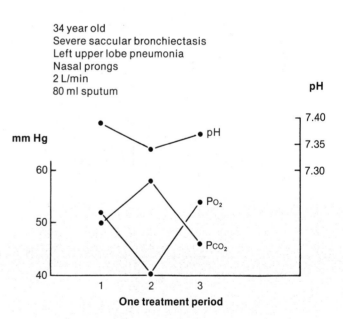

**Fig. 22-5.** Hypoxemia during a single bronchial drainage, percussion, and vibration treatment of a patient with severe bronchiectasis, which was productive of 80 ml of sputum. *Point 1,* Reclining head up immediately before treatment; *point 2,* at the end of 15 minutes of treatment, on his left side in Trendelenburg position; *point 3,* reclining head up 30 minutes after treatment. Note that the hypoxemia occurred at point 2 when the lobe involved with pneumonia was positioned dependent.

expectorate large volumes of sputum. Co-workers and I have found hypoxemia during treatment to be caused most often by ventilation-perfusion mismatching or shunting. A fall in cardiac output has been shown in some instances[12,81] and may also contribute to a fall in $Po_2$.

Huseby and co-workers[67] noticed that some of their patients who received bronchial drainage to multiple lung segments had a fall in mean $Po_2$ of 19 mm Hg. This fall was noticed most often when the involved lung was dependent (see Fig. 22-4). Remolina[108] and others[68] have also demonstrated a dramatically lower $Po_2$ when patients with unilateral acute lung disease were positioned with the involved lung dependent. Hence it is important to recognize that hypoxemia can occur or worsen during bronchial drainage. This is most likely when the involved lung segments are dependent. It is helpful to emphasize the involved lung by placing it uppermost during treatments and by draining it thoroughly so that the incidence of this complication is reduced.

If on physical examination the patient with unilateral radiographic involvement has developed bilateral congestion, both lungs must be treated. Certain modifications of treatment may be necessary to ensure adequate oxygenation. Some of these are described in the next section.

Many ICUs utilize transcutaneous pulse oximeters attached to patient's digits to monitor their arterial oxygen saturation, and to indicate when arterial blood gases should be obtained. However, often the arterial oxygen saturation provides only a relative measure of the patient's oxygenation and the numerical values can vary widely because of a loose or improper fit, positioning, motion, decreased peripheral perfusion, interference from ambient light sources and many other factors.[133] Low readings should also be correlated with other signs and symptoms of hypoxemia (Table 22-1). Also these oximeters do not provide monitoring of the patient's ventilatory status, $Paco_2$, or pH, which may reach dangerous levels in the presence of a normal arterial oxygen saturation.[34,133]

## SYMPTOMS ASSOCIATED WITH POOR TOLERANCE TO TREATMENT

Most patients who complain of difficulties during treatment have a demonstrable reason for their complaint. They may become agitated, orthopneic, dyspneic, weak, or diaphoretic with dysrhythmias. A change in blood pressure may also be noted. Agitation, shortness of breath, dyspnea, increased use of accessory muscles, and central cyanosis are often associated with hypoxemia. There are a few patients in whom dysrhythmias or hypoxemia can be demonstrated who do not become symptomatic. Therefore, whether or not the patient has monitors attached, the therapist should carefully consider all complaints of difficulty and watch for signs of poor tolerance to treatment. Often modifications can be made to allow the patients to receive effective bronchial drainage.

## MODIFICATIONS

If hypoxemia or dysrhythmias are a problem during bronchial drainage, certain adjustments can be made to permit a less physically demanding treatment. Secretions can be effectively drained with the patient in the horizontal rather than the head-down position, or some physicians may permit a temporary increase in the percentage of oxygen delivered during bronchial drainage to reduce the chances of hypoxemia and thereby ensure a safer treatment. If signs of poor tolerance are noted several minutes after initiation of bronchial drainage, it may be beneficial to shorten the length of treatment. Although treatments are shorter, the time interval between treatment sessions can be reduced and effective bronchial hygiene can still be provided.

Some patients with chronic obstructive pulmonary disease or neuromuscular or spinal cord dysfunction have great difficulty maintaining adequate ventilation in the head-down posture. In addition, an increased volume of secretions in the patient with a compromised cough can lead to atelectasis and life-threatening problems.[16,55] It is useful to coordinate treatment with a respiratory therapist who provides intermittent positive-pressure breathing (IPPB) as a means of assisted ventilation with the patient in the appropriate bronchial drainage position (Fig. 22-6). The patient is effectively ventilated with supplemental oxygen, and the necessary treatment can be performed with minimal distress.

## PRECAUTIONS AND SPECIAL CONSIDERATIONS
### Cardiac disease

Patients with coexistent pulmonary and cardiac conditions are frequently encountered in the ICU. Also, individuals with cardiomegaly have impaired ventilation of the left lower lobe.[4,5] Because acute cardiac conditions place individuals at increased risk for poor tolerance to treatment, especially when the lingula or left lower lobe is treated, these patients especially should be carefully evaluated and monitored.[57] Any signs of congestive heart failure—such as jugular vein distention, pulmonary edema, and pitting edema of the lower extremities—should be noted. The cardiac monitor should be observed for dysrhythmias. The therapist should also review the patient's electrocardiographic rhythm strips that have been recorded in the past 3 to 4 hours.

Not surprisingly, the author and coworkers noticed a significantly higher incidence of dysrhythmias in patients with underlying cardiac disease.[57] For example, patients with irregular rhythms before treatment had a tendency to deteriorate with bronchial drainage (i.e., they experienced an increased number of premature atrial contractions). Others who had received antidysrhythmia drugs within the past 48 hours developed a significant number of premature ventricular contractions that necessitated the early termination of treatment. Patients with cardiac disease have an increased tendency to tolerate treatment poorly and should be closely monitored.

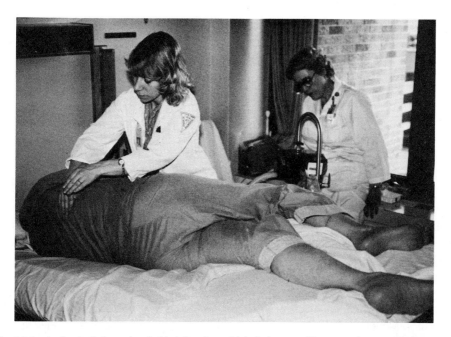

**Fig. 22-6.** A physical therapist *(left)* doing bronchial drainage with percussion to a patient who requires the assisted ventilation of an IPPB (intermittent positive-pressure breathing) machine operated by the respiratory therapist *(right)* to tolerate the head-down position.

### Congestive heart failure

Patients with significant congestive heart failure should not receive bronchial drainage in the Trendelenburg position. Experience has shown that these persons have increased respiratory distress and cardiac dysrhythmias while reclining head down.[57,58,96] Also this position increases venous return to the failing heart and can produce an increased amount of pulmonary edema. Posttreatment auscultation reflects this effect by a significant increase in rales throughout both lung fields. I prefer to treat patients with congestive heart failure in the horizontal (bed-flat) position rather than in the Trendelenburg position. Often after their cardiac status improves, they can tolerate the standard bronchial drainage positions.

### Carbon dioxide retention

Occasionally therapists are asked to treat nonventilated patients who are acidotic (pH < 7.30) with elevated carbon dioxide levels. These patients should also be treated cautiously. If the patient ventilates inadequately in a sitting position, being placed in the Trendelenburg position, with the diaphragm working against both gravity and the abdominal contents during inspiration, can further increase respiratory distress. It may be possible for the patient to tolerate the bed-flat position for short periods of time (5 to 10 minutes). Diaphragmatic and pursed-lips breathing may be helpful,[102,135] but these persons often require intubation and mechanical ventilation before effective bronchial drainage can be delivered.

### Adult respiratory distress syndrome (ARDS)

Some patients with the adult respiratory distress syndrome (ARDS) have an improved $Po_2$ after bronchial drainage, whereas others show a fall in both their $Po_2$ and their lung compliance. It appears that the fall in $Po_2$ may be related to an increased amount of fluid "leaking" into the extravascular spaces in the lung from the pulmonary vessels, perhaps caused by an increased venous return from being in the head-down position. Interestingly, similar findings have been noted in neonates with the respiratory distress syndrome.[122] The ARDS patient's response to treatment is individualized, and each should be assessed accordingly. If the cause of the ARDS is related to a pulmonary infection, these persons generally tolerate treatment better than those who develop the condition from pancreatitis, shock, or other extrathoracic insults.

### Pleural effusions

Questions often arise regarding the efficacy of treatment of persons with pleural effusions. Pleural effusions are not an indication for bronchial drainage but accompany many cardiac and pulmonary conditions seen in critically ill patients. Some may believe that the increased pleural fluid between the lung and chest wall would significantly reduce the effectiveness of percussion during bronchial drainage. However, if the fluid is not loculated, when the patient is positioned on his or her side (with the involved lobe uppermost) the fluid will track away from the lateral chest wall and accumulate medially. This will usually allow effective percussion of the lingula, middle lobe, and lower lobe. Auscultation can confirm this change in the location of the fluid. Breath sounds are distant with the patient sitting up (with dullness to percussion), but when the patient is positioned for bronchial drainage, breath sounds can almost always be heard (with resonant percussion). If these persons have an underlying pulmonary condition that necessitates chest physical therapy, pleural effusions usually do not present a problem.

### Pulmonary embolism

Pulmonary embolism is a common complication in critical illnesses.[22,23,105] On occasion therapists are asked to administer bronchial drainage to persons with increased secretions who also have a pulmonary embolism. Questions have arisen regarding the likelihood of bronchial drainage and percussion moving the embolus and causing further problems. It is important to remember that emboli lodge in the pulmonary artery system. These blood vessels become progressively smaller in diameter until they form the pulmonary capillary bed. Therefore the probability of advancing dislodged emboli along the narrowing pulmonary artery system is quite remote.

Most pulmonary thromboemboli originate from the deep veins of the legs or pelvis. One should weigh the possibility of causing additional emboli against the benefits of turning and positioning the patient for bronchial drainage. Three questions should be addressed before one proceeds. Is the patient anticoagulated? Has the nursing staff been turning the patient from side to side for nursing care? Does the patient have sufficient secretions to benefit significantly from bronchial drainage? If these questions can be answered affirmatively, the benefits generally outweigh the risks, and the treatment can proceed.

### Hemoptysis

Hemoptysis in all patients should be carefully evaluated. The cause must be known before initiation of bronchial drainage. Hemoptysis is a common finding after thoracic trauma with pulmonary contusion, and bronchial hygiene does not present any risk to the patient in this case.[88] Persons with bronchiectasis intermittently develop hemoptysis, but rarely is the bleeding of life-threatening proportions. I have seen patients with dysphagia develop hemoptysis from aspirating blood during nosebleeds resulting from trauma caused by nasotracheal suctioning. With the exception of not percussing the aforementioned bronchiectatics, therapists can treat patients in this group without creating an added risk. However, of major concern is hemoptysis in patients with coagulopathies caused by either anticoagulants or a very low platelet count (less than 20,000). Major bleeding from a lung abscess or a cavitating pulmonary carcinoma, especially after radiation therapy, has especially serious implications. At least two deaths have been reported during chest physical therapy in patients with pulmonary malig-nancies.[28,54] The therapist must be convinced that the benefits of treatment outweigh the risks before proceeding with the bronchial drainage.

### Osteopenia, osteoporosis, and rib fractures

Osteopenia, in particular when the ribs are involved, is another condition that necessitates precautions. On occasion patients with malignancies are admitted to the intensive care unit. Before chest percussion it is important to rule out, to the extent possible, metastasis to the ribs.

Osteoporosis, a condition that affects an estimated 15 million persons in this country, is most common in postmenopausal women. It is best to assume that elderly women, in particular those of slight body build, have some bone demineralization and to adjust treatment accordingly. Corticosteroids are used to treat asthma and many other nonthoracic conditions. Long-term steroid use may result in osteopenia and predispose the patient to rib fractures from mild stresses. One woman with lung disease treated for several years with steroids reported that she had fractured her ribs by pulling up a plant and trying to grab a gnat. Special caution must be used in treating these persons to determine an effective force that will not injure the ribs.

Rib fractures can be caused by trauma or metastatic disease or even be a complication of forceful coughing. Looking at the chest radiograph can be helpful in determining the location of the rib fractures. The majority occur either along the lateral or posterior chest wall. Because of the potential for a pneumothorax caused by the sharp edges of a fractured rib puncturing the lung, I prefer to slightly modify the treatment performed on these patients. If the fractures are along the posterior chest wall, the fracture site can be supported with one hand while percussion and vibration is done lateral to it. If the fracture is located on the lateral chest wall, it also is supported with one hand while the treatment is performed posteriorly. Experience at a number of trauma centers has shown that the majority of patients with rib fractures tolerate these treatments well.[88]

The sputum expectorated by patients with rib fractures and pulmonary contusions is frequently bloody. This is to be expected and should not be viewed with the same caution as the other causes of hemoptysis.

Conscious patients may have increased chest wall pain with treatment, and treatments should therefore be carefully coordinated with forms of pain management such as the administration of pain medications and intercostal nerve blocks or use of TENS units.

### Intracranial pressure

Questions have been raised concerning the effect of Trendelenburg positioning on intracranial pressure in patients with intracranial lesions. Although some have alluded to an increased intracranial pressure during an unspecified chest physiotherapy treatment,[101] we have rarely seen this. In an ongoing study, my co-workers and I have found that the greatest change in pressure occurs when the patient is repositioned from head up to supine.[56] The change from supine to Trendelenburg has been insignificant. Interestingly, as the intracranial pressure increases in the Trendelenburg position, so does the blood pressure. Hence cerebral perfusion pressure is not altered significantly.[97] However, if the patient has suffered a spontaneous cerebral hemorrhage, one must weigh the risk of additional bleeding against the benefit of treatment. It is often best to position the patient bed flat with the head supported for more conservative treatment.[45]

### Lung abscess

A lung abscess is a circumscribed, suppurative inflammation of the pulmonary parenchyma greater than 2 cm in diameter followed by central necrosis. It is usually caused by aspiration of oral anaerobic organisms and foreign material into the dependent segments of the lung. Approximately 75% are located in either the posterior segment of the right upper lobe or the superior segment of either lower lobe, because these segmental bronchi are most vertical when the patient is in the supine position.[18] Less commonly, lung abscess may be the result of hematogenous seeding from another infected site, bronchogenic carcinoma, bronchiectasis, or opportunistic organisms in immunocompromised patients.

Postural drainage, percussion, and vibration have been used for many years to drain the purulent material from these cavitary lesions. Because of the anaerobic infection, the sputum may be purulent, brown, and particularly foul smelling. Examining the radiograph before treatment can often help the therapist visualize the bronchi that lead to the lung abscess, especially when an air-fluid level is present within the cavity. In this way the postural drainage position can be modified to place the airway in the most vertical position.

Remembering airway dynamics is also helpful in promoting drainage of these abscesses. The airways dilate with inspiration and narrow with expiration. Therefore after placing the spontaneously breathing patient in the most appropriate postural drainage position, the therapist should have the patient take slow, deep inspirations, even holding the breath for 5 to 10 seconds to achieve a maximal dilation of the airway leading to the lung abscess. This often causes productive coughing within a few minutes of treatment.

### Human immunodeficiency virus (HIV) disease and acquired immunodeficiency syndrome (AIDS)

Patients with human immunodeficiency virus (HIV), HIV-related disease, and acquired immunodeficiency syndrome (AIDS) are being seen more frequently in many RICUs. In part, this is because more than one half of the patients with AIDS have involvement of the lungs. They are predisposed to a variety of opportunistic infections including *Pneumocystis carinii*, *Mycobacterium avium-intracellare*, and cytomegalovirus.[66,146] Because of respiratory distress

and increased pulmonary secretions, they are at times referred for chest physical therapy.

There is no reason to become unduly apprehensive about treating HIV infected or AIDS patients, because by using proper precautions the therapist can minimize his or her risk of being exposed to blood or body fluids. Even when exposure does occur, the risk of seroconversion remains quite small, with percutaneous exposure to blood as the most likely mechanism of transmission, rather than nonparenteral exposure to body fluids.[46,93,142] The possibility of such an exposure to therapists remains quite remote.

However, certain special considerations are in order. The universal precautions established by the Centers for Disease Control (CDC) do not generally apply to saliva or sputum.[138] But in the ICU many seriously ill patients have blood-streaked sputum as a result of such factors as intubation and suctioning. Hence it is prudent to take appropriate precautions to prevent being exposed to these fluids by wearing gloves and protective eyewear if one is going to be draining pulmonary secretions. When doing bronchial drainage, percussion, and vibration, some therapists prefer to stand behind the patient to further minimize the risk of being exposed to secretions during coughing or suctioning. In this way an effective treatment can still be administered.

## THORACENTESIS, SUBCLAVIAN LINES, AND CHEST TUBES

If the patient has had a thoracentesis, placement of subclavian lines, or placement of or removal of chest tubes, treatment should be withheld until the postprocedure chest radiograph rules out a pneumothorax. At times there will be a small residual pneumothorax, which the physicians elect to observe rather than reduce by inserting a chest tube. The therapist should view the untreated pneumothorax as a strict contraindication. Techniques that encourage the patient to cough will likely increase the size of a pneumothorax. One therapist treated a patient with an initially small pneumothorax. Thoracentesis had not been documented in the physician's or nurse's notes. The patient suffered a cardiopulmonary arrest. After successful resuscitation, the chest radiograph showed a much larger pneumothorax caused by the increased intrathoracic pressure during coughing.

## TUBE FEEDING

To reduce the potential for regurgitation, patients who receive tube feeding at regular intervals are best treated immediately before a feeding. Some therapists find it helpful to aspirate the stomach contents of these patients before placing the patient in the Trendelenburg position.

## CONDITIONS COMMONLY TREATED IN THE RICU
### Adult respiratory distress syndrome (ARDS)

The adult respiratory distress syndrome (ARDS) is a form of respiratory failure commonly encountered in the respiratory intensive care unit (RICU). It is characterized by respiratory distress (evidenced by severe dyspnea), hypoxemia that is unresponsive to high concentrations of oxygen (caused by intrapulmonary right-to-left shunting), decreased lung compliance, and a chest radiograph with diffuse bilateral pulmonary infiltrates (often sparing the costophrenic and cardiophrenic angles).[32] ARDS has been associated with a variety of conditions including the following:

1. Aspiration of gastric contents
2. Drug overdose
   a. Barbiturates
   b. Heroin
3. Infection
   a. Diffuse bacterial, fungal, or viral pneumonias
4. Inhalation of toxic gases
   a. Oxygen ($FIO_2 > 0.5$)
   b. Smoke
5. Near drowning
6. Shock
   a. Cardiogenic
   b. Hemorrhagic
   c. Septic (especially gram-negative)
7. Trauma
   a. Pulmonary contusion
   b. Head trauma

Regardless of the specific insult that precipitates ARDS, the resulting pulmonary pathological condition is similar—an alveolar-capillary membrane injury that increases the permeability of the pulmonary capillary bed.[32,65] An increased amount of fluid is allowed to flow into the interstitial and alveolar spaces, resulting in pulmonary edema and abnormalities of surfactant function. This abnormality causes a fall in lung compliance, and areas of atelectasis develop. The flow of blood past nonventilated alveoli (right-to-left shunt) results in hypoxemia. Severe hypoxemia is a leading cause of death in persons who do not respond to treatment.

**Medical treatment.** Treatment is directed primarily at maintaining adequate oxygenation and preventing additional complications.[32,65] All ARDS patients require supplemental oxygen. Many must be mechanically ventilated to maintain acceptable arterial oxygen levels. Large tidal volumes (15 ml/kg of body weight) and frequent hyperinflations may help prevent atelectasis. Positive end-expiratory pressure (PEEP) may be used to lower the inspired oxygen fraction below 50% to reduce the toxic effects of oxygen on the respiratory system, although PEEP must be used carefully to avoid compromising the patient's cardiac output. Frequent turning, suctioning, and bronchial drainage are often effective in draining secretions and preventing atelectasis. However, one must carefully monitor each patient's tolerance to bronchial drainage (see the discussion on precautions for ARDS, p. 435). Infections and sepsis are treated with appropriate

antibiotics. Corticosteroids may be administered, but their value remains controversial. The amount of fluid the patient receives is carefully regulated to prevent overhydration and worsening of the pulmonary problems. However, despite these aggressive measures the mortality remains high, between 20% and 75%.

## Chronic obstructive pulmonary disease (COPD)

Chronic obstructive pulmonary disease (COPD) is the most commonly encountered respiratory diagnosis in the RICU. It is characterized by increased airway resistance and prolonged forced expiration.[52] COPD is a general description that usually includes chronic bronchitis, emphysema, and asthma. Although these diseases are described separately, the majority of patients admitted to the RICU have some combination of all three. These persons typically have a long history of cigarette smoking and a chronic productive cough. They usually report intermittent episodes of wheezing. On physical examination one notes an increased anteroposterior diameter of the chest. There is moderate to pronounced contraction of the accessory muscles of inspiration, depending on the degree of respiratory distress. On auscultation one often notices bibasilar crackles, wide scattered to diffuse wheezes and rhonchi over both lung fields. With significant right-sided heart failure, neck-vein distention and pedal edema may be present. The chest radiograph shows hyperinflated lungs with flattened diaphragms. The other findings will vary according to each COPD patient's predominant disease process.

**Chronic bronchitis.** Chronic bronchitis is a disease characterized by a cough productive of sputum for at least 3 months and for 2 consecutive years.[60] The cause is prolonged exposure to nonspecific bronchial irritants, the most common of which is cigarette smoke.[123] The inhaled irritants cause hypersecretion of mucus and result in changes within the airways including tracheal mucous gland hypertrophy and goblet cell hyperplasia.[71,136] The abnormal ciliary function and a disrupted mucous blanket that accompanies this condition reduce the effective clearance of mucus. Hypersecretion of mucus combined with an impaired mucociliary transport system results in a chronic productive cough.

Because bronchitics often have a stocky body build and cyanosis (because of hypoxemia), they have been referred to as "blue bloaters."[123]

**Emphysema.** Emphysema is characterized by an irreversible destruction of interalveolar septal walls and of the connective tissue that provides much of the elastic recoil of the lung. This disease can be classified as centrilobular or panlobular. Centrilobular emphysema is characterized by destruction of the respiratory bronchiole and panlobular emphysema refers to a destructive enlargement of the alveoli.[136]

The cause of this disease remains obscure. Emphysema occurs more commonly in cigarette smokers than in nonsmokers, and its incidence increases with age. There are also hereditary predispositions, as evidenced by the severe panlobular emphysema that is found at a relatively early age in nonsmokers with an alpha$_1$-antitrypsin deficiency. Emphysema patients tend to be thin with an increased anteroposterior chest diameter. Because of the increased work of breathing they must do to maintain relatively normal arterial blood gas levels, they have been referred to as "pink puffers."[123]

**Asthma.** Asthma is a disease characterized by reversible intermittent attacks of airway obstruction because of an increased responsiveness of the smooth muscle of the trachea and bronchi to various stimuli. Asthma can generally be divided into two types: allergic or immunological (formerly called "extrinsic") and nonallergic or nonimmunological (sometimes called "intrinsic"), which is often associated with a history of recurrent respiratory tract infections.[60] Allergic asthma usually dates from early childhood, whereas the nonallergic type begins primarily in adulthood.[52]

During an acute attack, the lumen of the airways is narrowed by bronchial smooth muscle spasm, mucosal inflammation, and hypersecretions of mucus. This obstruction causes audible wheezing and rhonchi that persist despite frequent coughing.

**Medical treatment.** Most patients with COPD have elements of reversible airway obstruction. Therefore bronchodilators and corticosteroids are administered.[106] Antibiotics are given for respiratory infection.[23] Congestive heart failure is treated with diuretics. Arterial blood gas levels are closely monitored. Low-flow oxygen is given by nasal prongs or by Venturi mask to raise the $Po_2$ to approximately 60 mm Hg.[22,106,112] Carbon dioxide retention is initially treated with intermittent positive-pressure breathing (IPPB) for 15 minutes each hour.[20,60] Bronchial drainage, percussion, and vibration are given to aid in the expectoration of sputum, with the frequency varying according to the needs of the individual patient.[23,112] Diaphragmatic and pursed-lips breathing may also be useful to relieve dyspnea and improve arterial blood gas levels.[102,135] These measures are successful in 60% to 95% of patients with COPD in respiratory failure. If, however, the $Po_2$ falls below 40 mm Hg or the $Pco_2$ continues to climb with a corresponding deterioration in blood pH (<7.20), the patient is intubated and mechanically ventilated.[23,112]

### Disorders of the thoracic cage

Respiratory failure in patients with disorders of the thoracic cage is commonly seen in the RICU. The disorders can be divided into two major categories: a mechanical syndrome (scoliosis, obesity-hypoventilation, thoracoplasty) and a neuromuscular or paralytic syndrome (after poliomyelitis, spinal cord injury).[16] The common finding is alveolar hypoventilation at some time during the course of the disease.

**Mechanical syndrome.** The development of alveolar hypoventilation in patients with mechanical derangements differs from the neuromuscular category in that it is preceded by significant dyspnea on exertion.[16] Symptoms increase with advancing age. In particular, those with a scoliosis that approaches a 70-degree angle (at the intersection of upper and lower limbs of the thoracic curvature) during youth are much more likely to become symptomatic with age. Although respiratory failure is common, the incidence of secretions, atelectasis, and pneumonia is increased only in those with obesity-hypoventilation or thoracoplasty (Table 22-2). However, cor pulmonale, congestive heart failure, and pulmonary hypertension occur almost exclusively in this group rather than the neuromuscular group. Infection and congestive heart failure are the most common reasons they require admission to the RICU.

**Neuromuscular syndrome.** The onset of respiratory failure in the neuromuscular group can be abrupt (Guillain-Barré), episodic (myasthenia gravis), or chronic (muscular dystrophy, spinal cord injury). Acute respiratory failure develops in a relatively predictable manner.[16] All the diseases in this category affect both the inspiratory and expiratory muscles of respiration. Therefore the patient's ability to perform maximal inspiratory and expiratory maneuvers is impaired. The cough becomes progressively less effective.[127,134] The inspiratory capacity becomes progressively smaller, resulting in an inadequate sigh. As the inspiratory capacity falls to approximately one third the predicted value, alveolar hypoventilation becomes significant, causing hypoxemia and hypercapnia. The incidence of secretions, atelectasis, and pneumonia is increased within this entire group (Table 22-2) and, along with deteriorating arterial blood gases, frequently requires that the patient be admitted to the RICU.

**Medical treatment.** Treatment of disorders of the thoracic cage is similar to the treatment of chronic obstructive pulmonary disease.[16] It includes low-flow oxygen, intermittent positive-pressure breathing, antibiotics, bronchodilators, and diuretics. Bronchial drainage is indicated and effective for most patients in the neuromuscular category.[16,55,95,126] Special attention should be given to the left lung, particularly the left lower lobe, of patients with quadriplegia, multiple trauma, and neuromuscular conditions, since it is involved with pneumonia and atelectasis up to four times more often that the right.[9,43,55,117] It should also be performed on patients with scoliosis,[82] obesity-hypoventilation, and thoracoplasty.

In addition, efforts to strengthen and increase the endurance of the respiratory muscles are often begun in the RICU. This topic is more fully discussed elsewhere in this text.

Pharmacological ventilatory stimulants such as progesterone, caffeine, and theophylline may be administered, although their use remains controversial. Long-term ventilatory assistance at home may be necessary in the manage-

**Table 22-2.** Clinical description of respiratory failure in derangements of the thorax

| Category | Respiratory failure | | Clinical course | Secretions, atelectasis, pneumonia† |
| | Incidence | Severity* | | |
| --- | --- | --- | --- | --- |
| Mechanical | | | | |
| Scoliosis | Common | +++ | Slow | NL+ |
| Obesity-hypoventilation | Common | +++ | Periodic | NL or ↑ |
| Fibrothorax | Common | +++ | Slow | NL |
| Thoracoplasty | Common | +++ | Slow | NL or ↑ |
| Ankylosing spondylitis | Rare | + | Slow | NL |
| Neuromuscular | | | | |
| Postpoliomyelitis | Common | +++ | Slow | ↑ |
| Amyotrophic lateral sclerosis | Common | +++ | Fast | ↑ |
| Muscular dystrophies | Common | + | Slow | ↑ |
| Spinal cord injury | Common | ++ | Slow | ↑ |
| Multiple sclerosis | Uncommon | + | Slow | ↑ |
| Myasthenia gravis | Common | +++ | Periodic | ↑ |

From Bergofsky EH: *Am Rev Respir Dis* 119:694, 1979.
*+, Dyspnea on exertion; ++, dyspnea, mild hypoxemia, and hypercapnia only; +++, severe hypoventilation.
†*NL*, Normal lungs; ↑ = increased incidence.

ment of chronic or sleep-induced hypoventilation (see the discussion of discharge planning, pp. 441).[7,16,64] Also physical rehabilitation of the ventilator-dependent patient should be a major, ongoing effort, as described in a separate chapter.

## RESPIRATORY MUSCLE DYSFUNCTION

There has been increased interest in the role of the respiratory muscles in the precipitation and management of respiratory failure.[14,110,111,121] Persons predisposed to respiratory muscle weakness or fatigue include those with congestive heart failure, neuromuscular conditions, spinal cord injuries, and thoracic and pulmonary conditions associated with respiratory failure.* Unilateral or bilateral diaphragmatic paralysis may be caused or associated with spinal cord injuries, polyneuropathies, and cardiac surgery.[53] Unilateral diaphragmatic paralysis involves the left hemidiaphragm more often than the right, probably in part because of the close proximity of the left phrenic nerve to the pericardium.[1] It is more common in patients undergoing coronary artery bypass grafting with the internal mammary artery; perhaps this is related to surgical traction, electrocautery, hypothermia or a decrease in blood supply to the phrenic nerve.[1]

In addition, the respiratory muscles can atrophy in patients who require long-term mechanical ventilation. Inspiratory muscle fatigue in persons being weaned from mechanical ventilation is manifested by rapid, shallow breathing, paradoxical abdominal motion, and inspirations that alternate between predominant abdominal and rib cage movement.[90] Diaphragmatic flutter, a rare ventilatory pattern characterized by rapid, repetitive, involuntary diaphragmatic

contractions, can also result in a failure to wean from mechanical ventilation.[61]

Studies in normal subjects have shown that both inspiratory muscle strength and endurance can be increased by appropriate training.[14,73,83] Respiratory muscle training has also been demonstrated in persons with cystic fibrosis,[73] COPD,[8,128] and quadriplegia.[48] Such training has special significance in the latter two groups because the prevention of respiratory failure depends to a large extent on the strength and endurance of the inspiratory muscles.[35,36]

Physical therapists will have the opportunity to be more actively involved in designing and implementing exercise programs that strengthen weak respiratory muscles. Breathing against increased inspiratory resistance or progressively adding external resistance are the two methods most commonly used.* Placing the nonneuromuscular group patient in an upright sitting position with the arms supported enhances the use of accessory muscles and increases the length of time one can breathe at MVV.[11] Pressure support may be added through the ventilator to assist the muscles of inspiration and decrease the patient's work of breathing. Biofeedback is another technique that has been used successfully to wean paralyzed patients from ventilators.[33] This topic is discussed comprehensively in a separate chapter.

## PROGRESSIVE PHYSICAL ACTIVITY

The adverse effects of immobilization have been well documented. They include a decrease in circulating blood volume, which causes tachycardia and orthostatic hypotension when the patient is mobilized.[41] Immobilization also increases blood viscosity, which, along with venous stasis

* References 49, 58, 85, 90, 96, 110, 111.

* References 7, 8, 14, 37, 48, 53, 84.

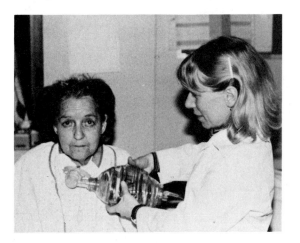

**Fig. 22-7.** This 62-year-old woman required mechanical ventilation for respiratory failure caused by an exacerbation of her chronic obstructive pulmonary disease (COPD). The physical therapist is bagging her in preparation for walking around the intensive care unit.

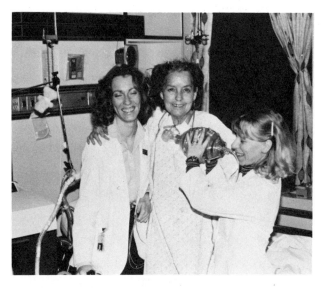

**Fig. 22-8.** Two physical therapists in the intensive care unit walking the patient shown in Fig. 22-7. The therapist on the left is supporting the patient and pulling the oxygen cylinder as the one on the right bags the patient.

from the reduced use of the leg muscles, predisposes to thromboembolism.[144] The first week of bed rest reduces skeletal muscle mass, contractive strength, and efficiency by 10% to 15%. By the end of 3 weeks of bed rest, physical work capacity may be reduced by 20% to 25%.[116,144] Hence, exercise can be important to minimize the adverse inactivity.

More unusual factors that contribute to weakness should be considered when the patient's exercise tolerance is disproportionately low compared to his length of immobilization. For example, electrolyte imbalances such as a low serum potassium (hypokalemia),[42] phosphate (hypophosphatemia),[10] or magnesium (hypomagnesemia)[100] can cause muscular weakness. Hypophosphatemia is common in alcoholism, with extended use of antacids, and following correction of diabetic ketoacidosis. Inadequate nutrition may also cause weakness.[39] The maintenance caloric requirement of the average adult is 20 to 25 Kcal/kg/day, but the average ICU patient may require 40 to 50 Kcal/kg/day. Inadequate nutrition is suggested by a serum albumin level below 3.0 mg/dL. Abnormal endocrine function, in particular hypothyroidism, can cause both respiratory and extremity muscle weakness.[109]

Moderate-to-severe weakness may be seen in patients that require high dose corticosteroids and/or neuromuscular blocking drugs (pancuronium, vecuronium) to treat status asthmaticus, COPD, ARDS, and other conditions.* Impaired renal or hepatic function contributes to the development of this type of weakness or paralysis.[119] Generalized severe weakness due to axonal neuropathy after sepsis and multiple organ failure has been classified as "critical illness neuropathy."[47,145,149] The recovery of strength and endurance loss because of these neuropathies or myopathies is more

* References 38, 47, 59, 76, 77, 124.

prolonged than for patients with weakness resulting from immobilization.

Another important aspect of exercise and ambulation of alert patients in the intensive care unit is the psychological benefit derived from these activities. Reaching the point of recovery from a catastrophic illness where physical rehabilitation is indicated gives the patient immense reassurance. Progressive exercise and ambulation of these persons is rewarding, even though they require mechanical ventilation.

While the ventilated patient is confined to bed, he or she should begin active exercises as soon as possible and progress to resistive exercises. When the patient is initially transferred to the bedside chair, I prefer to be present to observe the strength and coordination of the lower extremities. As soon as the patient is medically stable and can sit and be away from the life-support system for a few minutes, he or she can take short trips out of the ICU. If assisted ventilation is still necessary, an Ambu bag (breathing bag) with supplemental oxygen from a small oxygen cylinder can be used. After the patient gains confidence in a bed-to-chair transfer, he or she can prepare for ambulation by walking in place while still attached to the ventilator. If the patient does well for 20 to 30 seconds, arrangements can be made to ambulate around the ICU during the next treatment, maintaining ventilation with the Ambu bag and supplemental oxygen. The patient can try to increase the distance ambulated with each treatment session (Figs. 22-7 and 22-8).

If lack of motivation to walk is a problem,[137] the patient can be asked to walk to a wheelchair placed 20 to 30 feet away, before he or she takes the wheelchair ride out of the ICU. After returning to the ICU, the wheelchair is stopped approximately the same distance away from the bed and the

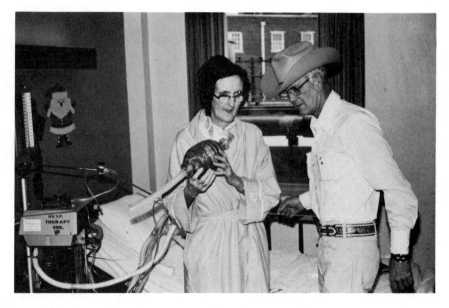

**Fig. 22-9.** This 55-year-old woman became ventilator dependent after an infarct to her brainstem, but she did not require oxygen. She was transferred to a general nursing floor and taught to bag herself for independence. The patient has just taken herself off the ventilator, has attached the Ambu bag (breathing bag) to her tracheostomy tube, and is going for a walk with her husband.

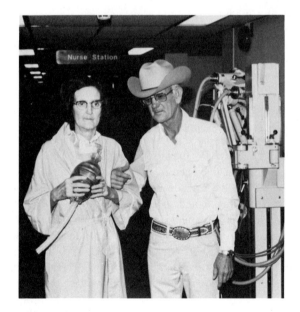

**Fig. 22-10.** The same patient as in Fig. 22-9, going down the hallway, past a nurse station, for a walk around the hospital.

patient walks back to bed. In this way the patient benefits physically from exercise as well as emotionally from brief trips out of the critical care area. This topic is more fully discussed in Chapter 18.

## PSYCHOLOGICAL ASPECTS OF CRITICAL ILLNESS

Patients with critical illnesses are anxious[6] and often terrified by their life-threatening conditions. The busy and crowded environment in the ICU has been implicated as

contributing to their anxiety. The frequent procedures and vital-sign measurements permit only minutes of uninterrupted sleep at one time. The rooms are usually plain and filled with unfamiliar machinery. The patient's personal items and clothing have been removed. Many lines, tubes, and needles are attached to or inserted into the patient's body. Continuously irritating sounds are heard from the ventilator, cardiac monitor, or some other type of life-support equipment. Impersonal communication and treatment of the patient as an inanimate object take their psychological toll as well. Psychologically, the patient may cope with these threats by temporarily retreating from reality (neurosis or psychosis) or humanity (psychoplegia).[118]

Professionals working in the ICU should be aware that temporary psychological disturbances have been reported in approximately 12.5% of critically ill patients.[63] Psychic disorders are commonly seen among those with respiratory failure or pulmonary insufficiency.[131] Alterations of memory, orientation, judgment, perception, concentration, or level of consciousness are common signs of psychological disturbance.

Those with a prolonged ICU stay may manifest a simple reactive apathetic depression when a significant improvement is made over their admission status.[137] They become apathetic and do not actively cooperate or participate in their own care. Although some have attributed this to sleep deprivation, there must be additional factors, because it occurs even when sleep is minimally disturbed.[118] Explaining to patients that the depression is normal and consistently reassuring them of recovery is helpful. Health professionals should be sympathetic but firm in dealing with persons with this type of disturbance.[137] Much less commonly, patients who have been weaned from ventilators may manifest great

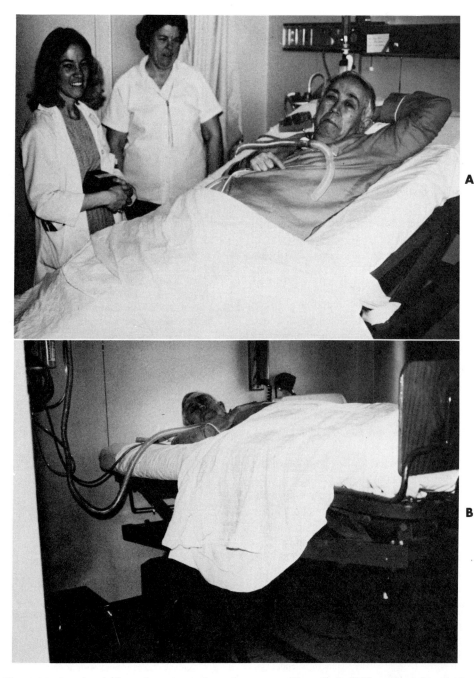

**Fig. 22-11.** A patient with respiratory muscle weakness caused by polio in 1950, on the rocking bed. The bed oscillates between, **A,** 30° head up and, **B,** 10° head down. He has been followed for over 1 year using this bed primarily to sleep on at home, without recurrent respiratory failure.

apprehension about going to sleep without ventilatory support. This is also transitory in most cases.

## DISCHARGE PLANNING

Occasionally patients cannot be weaned from the ventilator. This poses a serious dilemma and considerable controversy in patients with progressive systemic diseases. However, regardless of the cause, if the physician and patient are committed to long-term ventilator support, it is important that the patient be weaned from supplemental oxygen so that

he or she can eventually be transferred to a specialized facility, nursing home, or even to home, despite being ventilator dependent. The persons we have seen make the choice to go home have been most appreciative of the assistance and support received in this effort.

A measure of independence can be achieved by teaching the ambulatory patient self-ventilation with an Ambu bag while walking (Figs. 22-9 and 22-10). This is also a good safety measure, in case mechanical problems occur with the ventilator after the patient has been discharged.

Volume ventilators are often used for home ventilation. A chest cuirass, which looks like a turtle shell that covers the patient's abdomen and chest, may also be used. A suction tube protrudes from the center of the shell and creates a negative pressure at the desired inspiratory intervals. The diaphragm is pulled downward and the chest expands, drawing air into the lungs.

A pneumobelt can be used for assisted ventilation. It consists of an abdominal corset with an inflatable bladder anteriorly. When the bladder is inflated, it compresses the abdominal contents and moves the diaphragm upward, causing expiration. The bladder then deflates and allows the diaphragm to work more effectively during inspiration from this elevated position. It is especially useful in spinal cord-injured patients.[7]

The rocking bed is another means of assisted ventilation that was first used during the polio era. As it moves into the head-down position (about 10 degrees), the abdominal contents are pushed upward against the diaphragm, which moves upward and assists expiration.[1] Then, as the bed moves into the head-up position, the abdominal contents and diaphragm descend, assisting inspiration (Fig. 22-11). The number of respirations per minute is adjusted to the patient's needs. Interestingly, patients usually adjust quickly to the motion.

There are also portable ventilators available that can be mounted on wheelchairs to allow mobility of nonambulatory patients.[15]

The patient's family is instructed in the operation of the machines and how to trouble-shoot minor problems. They are also instructed in proper bagging and suctioning techniques. These duties are done by the family members many times in the hospital under the supervision of the health professionals. Training in exercises and ambulation is given to the family when appropriate. When the patient is discharged, the family members are competent in caring for him.

## REFERENCES

1. Abd AG and others: Diaphragmatic dysfunction after open heart surgery: treatment with a rocking bed, *Ann Intern Med* 111:881, 1989.
2. Aitkenhead AR and others: Effect of respiratory therapy on plasma catecholamines, *Anesthesiology* 61:44, 1984.
3. Albanese AJ and Toplitz AD: A hassle-free guide to suctioning a tracheostomy, *RN*, p 24, April 1982.
4. Alexander MS and others: Left lower lobe ventilation and its relation to cardiomegaly and posture, *Br Med J* 299:94, 1989.
5. Alexander MS and others: Impaired left lower lobe ventilation in patients with cardiomegaly, *Chest* 101:1189, 1992.
6. Allen CB: Just breathing, *Nursing '74*, p 22, Nov 1974.
7. Alvarez SE and others: Respiratory treatment of the adult patient with spinal cord injury, *Phys Ther* 61:1737, 1981.
8. Anderson JB and others: Resistive breathing training in severe chronic obstructive pulmonary disease: a pilot study, *Scand J Respir Dis* 60:151, 1979.
9. Appendix I: Chest physical therapy statistics showing the type and number of patients treated. In Mackenzie CF, editor: *Chest physiotherapy in the intensive care unit,* Baltimore, 1989, Williams & Wilkins.
10. Baker WL: Hypophosphatemia, *Am J N* 85:999, 1985.
11. Banzett RB and others: Bracing arms increases the capacity for hyperpnea, *Am Rev Respir Dis* 138:106, 1988.
12. Barrell SE and Abbas HM: Monitoring during physiotherapy after open heart surgery, *Physiotherapy* 64:272, 1978.
13. Bateman JR and others: Is cough as effective as chest physiotherapy in the removal of excessive tracheobronchial secretions? *Thorax* 36:683, 1981.
14. Belman MS and Sieck GC: The ventilatory muscles: fatigue, endurance and training, *Chest* 82:751, 1982.
15. Benvenuti CS: Independence for the quadriplegia: the Bantam respirator, *Am J Nurs* 79:918, 1979.
16. Bergofsky EH: Respiratory failure in disorders of the thoracic cage, *Am Rev Respir Dis* 119:643, 1979.
17. Bernhard WN and others: Adjustment of intracuff pressure to prevent aspiration, *Anesthesiology* 50:363, 1979.
18. Bernhardt WF and others: Lung abscess: a study of 148 cases due to aspiration, *Dis Chest* 43:620, 1963.
19. Bhaskar KR and others: Bronchial mucus hypersecretion in acute quadriplegia, *Am Rev Respir Dis* 143:640, 1991.
20. Birnbaum ML and others: Effects of interminent positive pressure breathing on emphysematous patients, *Am J Med* 41:552, 1966.
21. Bomalaski JS and Phair JP: Alcohol, immunosuppression, and the lung, *Arch Intern Med* 142:2073, 1982.
22. Bone RC: Acute respiratory failure and chronic obstructive lung disease: recent advances, *Med Clin North Am* 65:563, 1981.
23. Bone RC: Treatment of respiratory failure due to chronic obstructive lung disease, *Arch Intern Med* 140:1018, 1980.
24. Braun SR and others: Improving the cough in patients with spinal cord injury, *Am J Phys Med* 63:1, 1984.
25. Burnside J: *Physical diagnosis: an introduction to clinical medicine,* ed 16, Baltimore, 1981, Williams & Wilkins.
26. Byrd RB and Burns JR: Cough dynamics in the post-thoracotomy state, *Chest* 67:654, 1975.
27. Calvert JR and others: Halothane as a depressant of cough reflex, *Anesth Analg* 45:76, 1966.
28. Campbell CC: Appreciation for advice (letter), *Phys Ther* 60:809, 1980.
29. Cherniack RM and others: *Respiration in health and disease,* Philadelphia, 1972, WB Saunders Co.
30. Chopra SK and others: Effects of hydration and physical therapy on tracheal transport velocity, *Am Rev Respir Dis* 115:1000, 1977.
31. Connors AF and others: Chest physical therapy: the immediate effect on oxygenation in acutely ill patients, *Chest* 78:559, 1980.
32. Connors AF and others: The adult respiratory distress syndrome, *Disease-a-Month* 27(4): 10, 1981.
33. Corson JA: Use of biofeedback in weaning paralyzed patients from respirators, *Chest* 76:543, 1979.
34. Davidson JH and Hosie HE: Limitations of pulse oximetry: respiratory insufficiency—a failure of detection, *Br Med J* 307:372, 1993.
35. Derenne J: The respiratory muscles: mechanics, control and pathophysiology, Part 3, *Am Rev Respir Dis* 118:581, 1978.
36. Derenne J and others: The respiratory muscles: mechanics, control and pathophysiology, Part 1, *Am Rev Respir Dis* 118:119, 1978.
37. Derrickson J and others: A comparison of two breathing exercise programs for patients with quadriplegia, *Phys Ther* 72:763, 1992.
38. Douglas JA and others: Myopathy in severe asthma, *Am Rev Respir Dis* 146:517, 1991.
39. Driver AG and LeBran M: Iatrogenic malnutrition in patients receiving ventilatory support, *JAMA* 244:2195, 1980.
40. Egbert LD and others: The effect of site of operation and type of anesthesia upon the ability to cough in the postoperative period, *Surg Gynecol Obstet* 115:295, 1962.
41. Fareeduddin K and Abelmann WH: Impaired orthostatic tolerance after bed rest in patients with myocardial infarction, *N Engl J Med* 280:345, 1969.
42. Farley JC: Practical pointers, *Consultant* 25(4):154, 1985.

43. Fishburn MJ and others: Atelectasis and pneumonia in acute spinal cord injury, *Arch Phys Med Rehabil* 71:197, 1990.

44. Gallon Am: Evaluation of chest percussion in the treatment of patients with copious sputum production, *Respir Med* 85:45, 1991.

45. Garradd J and Bullock M: The effect of respiratory therapy on intracranial pressure in ventilated neurosurgical patients, *Austr J Physiotherapy* 32:107, 1986.

46. Gerberding JL and others: Risk of transmitting the human immuno-deficiency virus, cytomegalovirus and hepatitis B virus to health care workers exposed to patients with AIDS and AIDS-related conditions, *J Infec Dis* 156:1, 1987.

47. Gorson KC and Roper AH: Acute respiratory failure neuropathy: a variant of critical illness polyneuropathy, *Crit Care Med* 21:267, 1993.

48. Gross D and others: The effect of training on strength and endurance of the diaphragm in quadriplegia, *Am J Med* 68:27, 1980.

49. Guenter CA: The role of diaphragm function in disease, *Arch Intern Med* 139:806, 1979.

50. Guenter CA and Buchan KA: Acute infectious respiratory illnesses. In Guenter CA and Welch MH, editors: *Pulmonary medicine,* Philadelphia, 1977, JB Lippincott Co.

51. Hammon L: Review of respiratory anatomy. In Frownfelter D, editor: *Chest physical therapy and pulmonary rehabilitation: an interdisciplinary approach,* Chicago, 1978, Year Book Medical Publishers, Inc.

52. Hammon WE: Pathophysiology of chronic pulmonary disease. In Frownfelter D, editor: *Chest physical therapy and pulmonary rehabilitation: an interdisciplinary approach,* Chicago, 1978, Year Book Medical Publishers, Inc.

53. Hammon WE: Improving inspiratory muscle function in patients with bilateral diaphragmatic paralysis, *Cardiopulm Phys Ther J* 2(2): 10, 1991.

54. Hammon WE and Martin RJ: Fatal pulmonary hemorrhage associated with chest physical therapy, *Phys Ther* 59:1247, 1979.

55. Hammon WE and Martin RJ: Chest physical therapy for acute atelectasis, *Phys Ther* 61:217, 1981.

56. Hammon WE and others: Effect on bronchial drainage on intracranial pressure in acute neurological injuries (abstract), *Phys Ther* 61:735, 1981.

57. Hammon WE and others: Cardiac arrhythmias during postural drainage and chest percussion of critically-ill patients, *Chest* 102:1836, 1992.

58. Hammond MD and others: Respiratory muscle strength in congestive heart failure, *Chest* 98:1091, 1990.

59. Hirano M and others: Acute quadriplegic myopathy: a complication of treatment with steroids, nonpolarizing blocking agents or both, *Neurology* 42:2082, 1992.

60. Hodgkin JE: *Chronic obstructive pulmonary disease: current concepts in diagnosis and comprehensive care,* Park Ridge, Ill, 1979, American College of Chest Physicians.

61. Hoffman R and others: Diaphragmatic flutter resulting in failure to wean from mechanical ventilator support after coronary artery bypass surgery, *Crit Care Med* 18:499, 1990.

62. Hogg JC: The respiratory airways. In Guenter CA and Welch MH, editors: *Pulmonary medicine,* Philadelphia, 1977, JB Lippincott Co.

63. Holland JC and others: The ICU syndrome: fact or fancy, *Psychiatry Med* 4:241, 1973.

64. Holtackers TR and others: The use of the chest cuirass in respiratory failure of neurologic origin, *Respir Care* 27:271, 1982.

65. Hopewell PC: Adult respiratory distress syndrome, *Basics Respir Dis* 7:1, 1979.

66. Hopewell PC and Luce JM: Pulmonary involvement in the acquired immunodeficiency syndrome, *Chest* 87:104, 1985.

67. Huseby J and others: Oxygenation during chest physiotherapy (abstract), *Chest* 70:430, 1975.

68. Ibañez J and others: The effect of lateral positions on gas exchange in patients with unilateral lung disease during mechanical ventilation, *Intensive Care Med* 7:231, 1981.

69. Irwin RS and others: Cough: a comprehensive review, *Arch Intern Med* 137:1186, 1977.

70. Jacquette G: To reduce hazards of tracheal suctioning, *Am J Nurs* 71:2362, 1971.

71. Johanson WG Jr: Lung defense mechanisms, *Basics Respir Dis* 6:2, 1977.

72. Jung RC and Gottlieb LS: Comparison of tracheobronchial suction catheters in humans, *Chest* 69:179, 1976.

73. Keens TG and others: Ventilatory muscle endurance training in normal subjects and patients with cystic fibrosis, *Am Rev Respir Dis* 116:853, 1977.

74. Kirby NA and others: An evaluation of assisted cough in quadriparetic patients, *Arch Phys Med Rehabil* 47:705, 1966.

75. Klein P and others: Attenuation of the hemodynamic responses to chest physical therapy, *Chest* 93:38, 1988.

76. Kupfery and others: Prolonged weakness after long-term infusion of vencuronium bromide, *Ann Intern Med* 117:484, 1992.

77. Lacomis D and others: Acute myopathy and neuropathy in status asthmaticus: case report and a review of the literature, *Muscle Nerve* 16:84, 1993.

78. Lamb LS and Judson EB: Maximal rate response in a permanent pacemaker during chest physiotherapy, *Heart Lung* 21:390, 1992.

79. Landa JF and others: Effects of suctioning on mucociliary transport, *Chest* 77:202, 1980.

80. Laurenzi GA and others: *Mucus flow in the mammalian trachea,* Proceedings Tenth Aspen Ephysema Conference, US Public Health Service, publ 1787, p 27, 1967.

81. Laws AK and McIntyre RW: Chest physiotherapy: a physiological assessment during intermittent positive pressure ventilation in respiratory failure, *Can Anaesth Soc J* 16:487, 1969.

82. Leith DE: Cough, *Phys Ther* 48:439, 1968.

83. Leith DE and Bradley M: Ventilatory muscle strength and endurance training, *J Appl Physio* 41:508, 1976.

84. Lerman RM and Weiss MS: Progressive resistive exercise in weaning high quadriplegics from the ventilator, *Paraplegia* 25:130, 1987.

85. Libby DM and others: Acute respiratory failure in scoliosis or kyphosis: prolonged survival and treatment, *Am J Med* 73:532, 1982.

86. Loudon RG: Cough, a symptom and a sign, *Basics Respir Dis* 9:4, March 1981.

87. Loudon RG and Shaw GB: Mechanics of cough in normal subjects and in patients with obstructive respiratory disease, *Am Rev Respir Dis* 96:666, 1967.

88. Mackenzie CF and others: *Chest physiotherapy in the intensive care unit,* Baltimore, 1981, Williams & Wilkins.

89. Macklem PT: Physiology of cough, *Ann Otol* 83:761, 1974.

90. Macklem PT: Respiratory muscles: the vital pump, *Chest* 78:753, 1980.

91. Macklem PT and Wilson JJ: Measurement of intra-bronchial pressure in man, *J Appl Physiol* 20:653, 1965.

92. Maclean D and others: Maximum expiratory airflow during chest physiotherapy on ventilated patients before and after the application of an abdominal binder, *Intensive Care Med* 15:396, 1989.

93. Marcus R and others: Surveillance of health care workers exposed to blood from patients infected with the human immunodeficiency virus, *N Engl J Med* 319:1118, 1988.

94. Marini JJ and others: Acute lobar atelectasis: a prospective comparison of fiberoptic bronchoscopy and respiratory therapy, *Am Rev Respir Dis* 119:971, 1979.

95. McMichan JC and others: Pulmonary dysfunction following traumatic quadriplegia, *JAMA* 243:528, 1980.

96. McParland C and others: Inspiratory muscle weakness and dyspnea in chronic heart failure, *Am Rev Respir Dis* 146:467, 1992.

97. McQuillan KA: The effects of the trendelenburg position for postural drainage on cerebrovascular status in head-injured patients, *Heart Lung* 16:327, 1987.

98. Mead J and others: Significance of the relationship between lung recoil and maximum expiratory flow, *J Appl Physiol* 22:95, 1967.

99. Mier A and others: Tracheobronchial clearance in patients with bilateral diaphragmatic weakness, *Am Rev Respir Dis* 142:545, 1990.

100. Molloy DW and others: Hypomagnesemia and respiratory muscle power, *Am Rev Respir Dis* 129:497, 1984.

101. Moss E and others: The effects of nitrous oxide, Athesin, and thiopentone on intracranial pressure during chest physiotherapy in patients with severe head injuries. In Shulman K and others, editors: *Intracranial pressure,* IV, New York, 1980, Springer-Verlag.

102. Mueller RE and others: Ventilation and blood gas changes induced by pursed-lips breathing, *J Appl Physiol* 28:784, 1970.

103. Murphy R and Holford SK: Lung sounds, *Basic Respir Dis* 8:1, 1980.

104. Murray JF: *The normal lung,* Philadelphia, 1976, WB Saunders

105. Neuhaus A and others: Pulmonary embolism in respiratory failure, *Chest* 73:4, 1978.

106. Owens GR and Rogers RM: Managing respiratory failure in chronic airflow obstruction, *J Respir Dis* 3:24, 1982.

107. Redick EL: Closed system, in-line endotracheal suctioning, *Crit Care N P* 47, Aug 1993.

108. Remolina C and others: Positional hypoxemia in unilateral lung disease, *N Engl J Med* 304:523, 1981.

109. Riniker M and others: Prevalence of various degrees of hypothyroidism among patients of a general medical department, *Clin Endocrinol* 14:69, 1981.

110. Rochester DF: Respiratory disease: attention turns to the air pump, *Am J Med* 68:803, 1980.

111. Rochester DF and Braun MT: The respiratory muscles, *Basics Respir Dis* 6:4, 1981.

112. Rogers RM: *Respiratory intensive care,* Springfield, Ill, 1977, Charles C Thomas, Publisher.

113. Sackner MA and others: Pathogenesis and prevention of tracheobronchial damage with suction procedures, *Chest* 64:284, 1973.

114. Sackner MA and others: Effect of cuffed endotracheal tubes on tracheal mucous velocity, *Chest* 68:774, 1975.

115. Sackner MA and others: Effect of oxygen in graded concentrations upon tracheal mucous velocity, *Chest* 69:164, 1976.

116. Saltin B and others: Response to exercise after bed rest and training, *Circulation* 37-38(suppl 7):1, 1968.

117. Schmidt-Nowara WW and Altman AR: Atelectasis and neuromuscular respiratory failure, *Chest* 85:792, 1984.

118. Schoenfeld MR: Terror in the ICU, *Forum on Medicine,* p 14, Sept 1978.

119. Segredo V and others: Persistent paralysis in critically ill patients after long-term administration of vencuronium, *N Engl J Med* 327:524, 1992.

120. Selby DS: Chest physiotherapy may be harmful in some patients, *Br Med J* 298:541, 1989.

121. Shaffer TH and others: Respiratory muscle function, assessment, and training, *Phys Ther* 61:1711, 1981.

122. Shannon DC: Respiratory care in the newborn, *Crit Care Med* 5:10, 1977.

123. Shapiro BA and others: *Clinical application of respiratory care,* Chicago, 1975, Year Book Medical Publishers, Inc.

124. Shee CD: Risk factors for hydrocortisone myopathy in acute severe asthma, *Respir Med* 84:229, 1990.

125. Shim C and others: Cardiac arrhythmias resulting from tracheal suctioning, *Ann Intern Med* 71:1149, 1969.

126. Siebens AA and others: Cough following transection of spinal cord at C-6, *Arch Phys Med Rehabil* 45:1, 1964.

127. Smeltzer SC and others: Respiratory muscle function in multiple sclerosis, *Chest* 101:479, 1992.

128. Sonne LJ and Davis JA: Increased exercise performance in patients with severe COPD following inspiratory resistive training, *Chest* 81:436, 1982.

129. Staub NC: Lung structure and function, *Basics Respir Dis* 10(4):1, 1982.

130. Stiller K and others: Acute lobar atelectasis: a comparison of two chest physical therapy regimens, *Chest* 98:1336, 1990.

131. Strain JJ: Psychological reactions to acute medical illness and critical care, *Crit Care Med* 6:39, 1978.

132. Swinamer DL and others: Effect of routine administration of analgesia on energy expenditure in critically ill patients, *Chest* 92:4, 1988.

133. Szaflarski NL and Cohen NH: Use of pulse oximetry in critically ill adults, *Heart Lung* 18:444, 1989.

134. Szeinberg A and others: Cough capacity in patients with multiple dystrophy, *Chest* 94:1232, 1988.

135. Thoman RL and others: The efficacy of pursed-lips breathing in patients with chronic obstructive pulmonary disease, *Am Rev Despir Dis* 93:100, 1966.

136. Thurlbeck WM: Chronic bronchitis and emphysema: the pathophysiology of chronic obstructive lung disease, *Basics Respir Dis* 3:1, Sept 1974.

137. Tomlin PJ: Psychological problems in intensive care, *Br Med J* 2:441, 1977.

138. Update: universal precautions for prevention of transmission of human immunodeficiency virus, hepatitis B virus and other blood borne pathogens in health-care settings, *MMWR* 37:377, 1988.

139. Wang K and Berman DA: Artifacts simulating serious ventricular arrhythmia, *Postgrad Med* 69:98, 1981.

140. Wanner A: Clinical aspects of mucociliary transport, *Am Rev Respir Dis* 116:73, 1977.

141. Wanner A: Alteration of tracheal mucociliary transport in airway disease: effect of pharmacologic agents, *Chest* 80(suppl):867, 1981.

142. Weiss S and others: HTLV-III infection among health care workers: association with needle-stick injuries, *JAMA* 254:2089, 1985.

143. Weissman C and others: Effect of routine intensive care interactions on metabolic rate, *Chest* 86:815, 1984.

144. Wenger NK: Rehabilitation after myocardial infarction, *JAMA* 424:2879, 1979.

145. Witt NJ and others: Peripheral nerve function in sepsis and multiple organ failure, *Chest* 99:176, 1991.

146. Wollschlager CM and others: Pulmonary manifestations of the acquired immunodeficiency syndrome (AIDS), *Chest* 85:197, 1984.

147. Wong JW and others: Effects of gravity on tracheal mucus transport rates in normal subjects and in patients with cystic fibrosis, *Pediatrics* 60:146, 1977.

148. Zadai CC: Physical therapy for the acutely ill medical patient, *Phys Ther* 61:1746, 1981.

149. Zochodne DW and others: Critical illness polyneuropathy: a complication of critical illness and multiple organ failure, *Brain* 110:819, 1987.

## SUGGESTED READINGS

Frownfelter D, editor: *Chest physical therapy and pulmonary rehabilitation: an interdisciplinary approach,* Chicago, 1978, Year Book Medical Publishers, Inc.

Guenter CA and Welch MH, editors: *Pulmonary medicine,* Philadelphia, 1977, JB Lippincott Co.

Petty TL, editor: *Intensive and rehabilitative respiratory care,* ed 3, Philadelphia, 1982, Lea & Febiger.

Rogers RM: *Respiratory intensive care,* Springfield, Ill, 1977, Charles C Thomas, Publisher.

Tyler ML: Complications of positioning and chest physiotherapy, *Respir Care* 27:458, 1982.

Zadai CC, editor: *Pulmonary management in physical therapy,* Clinics in Physical Therapy, Churchill Livingstone, New York, 1992.

# CHAPTER 23

# Pulmonary Rehabilitation

*Lana Hilling and Jan Smith*

"Not everything faced can be changed, but nothing can be changed unless it's faced."—Motto of Mt. Diablo Medical Center's Pulmonary Rehabilitation Program.

## DEFINITION OF PULMONARY REHABILITATION

"I feel I've been able to pretty much return to the mainstream of life, both emotionally and physically."—Phil Peterson

"Pulmonary rehabilitation taught me how to live comfortably with my disease."—Beverly Striplin

"Pulmonary rehabilitation has made me feel I control my lung disease rather than letting it control me."—Marie Van Beveren*

To these patients, and others, pulmonary rehabilitation has been a life-saving pathway between inactivity and

*Pulmonary rehabilitation participants, Mt. Diablo Medical Center, Concord, Calif.

activity, isolation and socialization, depression and hope, and from being an observer of life to an active participant. These quotes and others like them truly give meaning to the definition of pulmonary rehabilitation as "the restoration of the individual to the fullest medical, mental, emotional, social, and vocational potential of which he or she is capable," as defined by the Council of Rehabilitation in 1942.

Although rehabilitation has been practiced for several decades by patients with musculoskeletal and neuromuscular disorders, 1970 marked the beginning of the modern era for rehabilitation of patients with chronic obstructive pulmonary disease.[120]

At its annual meeting in 1974, the American College of Chest Physicians' Committee on Pulmonary Rehabilitation adopted, the following definition: "Pulmonary rehabilitation may be defined as an art of medical practice wherein an individually tailored multidisciplinary program is formulated, which through accurate diagnosis, therapy, emotional support, and education, stabilizes or reverses both the physio- and psychopathology of pulmonary diseases, and attempts to return the patient to the highest possible functional capacity allowed by his pulmonary handicap and overall life situation."

In 1981 the American Thoracic Society published an official statement on pulmonary rehabilitation. The statement defines pulmonary rehabilitation, specifies objectives, lists the essential components, and recognizes the benefits and limitations of such programs.[13]

The American Association of Cardiovascular and Pulmonary Rehabilitation published the "Guidelines for Pulmonary Rehabilitation Programs" in 1993, to establish nationally recognized guidelines for program development, enhancement, and reimbursement.[3] Pulmonary rehabilitation programs have been inconsistent and varied in both setting and scope. The guidelines are flexible enough to allow for program and patient individualization, yet specific enough to promote improved patient health and program success. They include the essential components that a pulmonary rehabilitation program must provide, as listed in

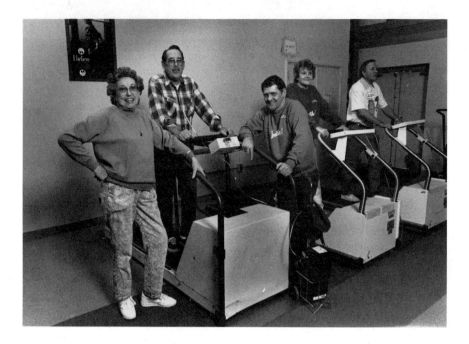

## Essential components of a pulmonary rehabilitation program

- Team Assessment
- Patient Training
- Exercise
- Psychosocial Intervention
- Follow up

the box above. These components will be expanded upon later in the chapter.

## Statistics

Statistics show that chronic obstructive pulmonary disease (COPD) and related conditions have advanced from the fifth to the fourth leading cause of age-adjusted death in the United States between 1990 and 1991, while heart disease, cerebrovascular diseases, and atherosclerosis are on the decline.[125] The prevalence of COPD, mostly chronic bronchitis and emphysema, was estimated to be 14 million persons in the United States in 1989. Of this total chronic bronchitis accounted for 12 million and emphysema for 2 million. These conditions have increased by 45.3% between 1979 and 1989. An estimated 11.6 million Americans suffer from asthma. Between 1980 and 1989 the prevalence of asthma increased 44% in males and 56% in females.[124] Morbidity related to COPD and asthma is significant. COPD and related conditions were considered to be the direct cause of death for 88,980 persons in the United States in 1990.[39]

Health care costs in the United States continue to escalate rapidly. Annually, more than $6.2 billion is spent on health care and indirect costs for people with asthma.[11] The estimated expenditure for COPD in 1988 was a total of $13.2 billion, which included the direct costs of treatment, morbidity, and mortality (The National Heart, Lung, and Blood Institute, unpublished data, 1991).[84] "These estimates do not take into account the costs in terms of human suffering."[84]

Life expectancy has increased rapidly for those over 65 years of age from 16.3 years in 1978 to 16.9 years more in 1987.[38] This increase in life expectancy is partly responsible for the trends of increased morbidity and mortality from COPD and allied conditions. Our patient population and its need for pulmonary rehabilitation (PR) will continue to grow.

## Patient interaction

Health care professionals often comment that they are frustrated and feel impatient when working with pulmonary patients, who can be very demanding, angry, anxious, hostile, depressed, stoic, etc. This type of response may demonstrate a lack of understanding of this type of patient by the health care professional. Perhaps the professional fears being inadequate, or not knowing how to help the chronically ill patient, especially when the patient is short of breath. We often want to cure, to help, to give someone the "quick fix", and to take care of patients who get well quickly. With chronic lung disease there is no such cure and no quick fix.

The first step in caring for pulmonary patients is to understand why they respond as they do. When the pulmonary patient is hurried or in distress and tries to save enough air to request something, the patient is seen as demanding. If patients are quiet, don't ask for anything, and try to deal individually with their problems, as they do every minute of their lives, they are labeled stoic. These patients are often apprehensive, tense, nervous, socially isolated, fatigued, and fearful that their next breath will not come. They live in an emotional straightjacket, as all expressions of emotion lead to distressing or disabling symptoms.[34,56,93,119,148] Theirs is a constant struggle to stay alive.

The day before he died, my father looked at me and said with calm reality, "Jan, the difference between breathing and not breathing is so small . . . there's so little difference and so much work. . . ." Later a wonderful patient was to liken the breathing of a pulmonary patient to stuffing a handkerchief in one's mouth and then placing a clothespin on one's nose and trying to breathe and walk and talk and just live. . . .

The satisfaction in working with pulmonary patients comes not with a quick fix, but with the knowledge that they can truly be helped through breathing retraining, relaxation, panic control, energy conservation techniques and exercise.

To instruct the patient in the skills needed to exercise and perform these techniques you must know your patient, be an empathetic listener, provide appropriate reassurance, positive reinforcement, realistic guidance, and have a calming touch. When working with this patient population never rush or communicate your own anxiety, and avoid making comments like "just relax."[34] Laughter is wonderful medicine.[178] "Try to tune into what the person's sense of humor is," as this will tell you "a lot about how their spirit is," as well as their outlook and motivation.[71]

Always remember: "COPD often makes a bad first impression, but you will find wonderful people underneath."[34]

## PULMONARY REHABILITATION TEAM

The value of a multidisciplinary team should not be underestimated. It is the collective knowledge, skill, and clinical experience of the professional staff that is essential to achieving desired comprehensive patient and program goals. The *patient* is always the central and most important member of the pulmonary rehabilitation team (Fig. 23-1).[170] Depending upon the resources of a facility, the team members' roles and composition may vary.[102,144] The following allied health professionals may be members of the PR team: medical director, physical therapist, respiratory care practitioner, dietitian, nurse, occupational therapist, pharmacist, social worker.[148] The minimum requirements of a PR team are the medical director and program director/coordinator. It is very helpful to have at least one full-time team member. The advantages of a multidisciplinary team are to allow each professional to assess the patient in his/her specialty area; to offer varied teaching tech-

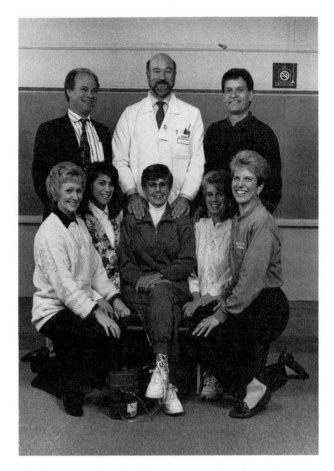

**Fig. 23-1.** The patient is always the central and most important member of the pulmonary rehabilitation team.

niques and good listening support; to reinforce information; and to collaborate toward the achievement of common goals.* Diversity does not detract from but rather contributes to excellence within the PR team.

## TEAM MEMBER ROLES/TEAM FUNCTION
### Medical director

The medical director should be a licensed physician who has training and/or special interest in PR and in the treatment of patients with pulmonary disease. The medical director's role and responsibilities will vary. He or she may function as an administrator, diagnostician, clinician, educator, and/or research coordinator. This individual should have knowledge of pulmonary function and exercise testing. The director is responsible for meeting with the team to discuss each patient's medical status and to reevaluate each patient's goals. To ensure an optimal treatment program for the patient and to obtain the support of the medical staff, the medical director should serve as a liaison between the team, patient, patient's primary care physician, and the medical staff.[3,27,41]

---

* References 13, 27, 71, 76, 93, 97.

## Program director/coordinator

According to the 1992-1993 National PR Survey, the program director's position is held by the following health care professionals: registered respiratory therapist (RRT), 33%, registered nurse (RN), 24%, exercise physiologist, 12%, certified respiratory therapy technician (CRTT), 11%, licensed physical therapist (PT), 3%, and others, 17%.[85]

Program directors/coordinators must be committed, good communicators, enthusiastic, and knowledgeable not only in the skills of their profession, but also in administration, program development, marketing, and education. A program director should be a health professional, with clinical experience in caring for pulmonary patients,[170] and must enjoy working with a diversified population from pediatrics to geriatrics. They must understand and believe in the philosophy and goals of PR, and be able to relate well to motivate patients with pulmonary disease.[114,144,148]

## Team conference

The purpose of the team conference is to address the patient's initial assessment, individualized goals and treatment modalities, progress, problems, and discharge plans. The conference provides the opportunity to enhance team communication, but may vary in structure and frequency from one program to another. The conference must be documented and signed by the medical director or program director/coordinator, and a report must be placed in the patient's medical chart (Fig. 23-2).[103,170]

## Goals

The primary goals of pulmonary rehabilitation programs (PRPs) are to improve the patient's quality of life, increase their strength and endurance, and to decrease their dyspnea. The overall goal is to positively alter the patient's life style or pattern of living.[3,13,27,65,111] The box on p. 449 lists these realistic goals.

PRPs *must* be individually tailored to meet the needs of the patient. The patient's goals need to be reviewed with him or her and their significant other prior to, or early in the program. Realistic short- and long-term goals need to be established. It is important to have the significant other, family member, or friend attend the program, whenever possible. This serves to encourage their support, increase patient motivation, improve their knowledge of lung disease, and provide them with the skills to cope with its debilitating symptoms.[103,144,151]

The most frequently expressed goals are to breathe better, be more active, stop using oxygen and decrease medications. The meaning of these goals to the individual patient should be carefully examined. Through experience we have learned that "to breathe better" or "be more active," may really mean returning to their predisease state. The patient may not be consciously aware that these are their expectations, but this needs to be clarified at the beginning of the program. PR cannot return patients to their predisease state, but it can improve the quality of their lives within the limits imposed by their lung disease.

If their goal is to stop using oxygen or to decrease their medication usage, they could be setting themselves up for failure during the program. It is important to address the reasons that these goals might not be realistic and to help them establish attainable goals.

## Outcomes

A comprehensive PRP can produce cost-effective outcomes. The box on p. 449 lists these beneficial outcomes.*

---

* References 4, 13, 32, 83, 87, 108, 110, 114, 121, 144, 164, 170.

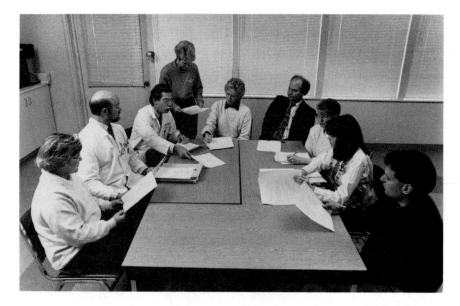

**Fig. 23-2** Team conference.

The Nation's health care delivery system is changing. We must learn to meet these changes and work within the new guidelines. It is imperative that we continue to show improvement in patient outcomes through objective documentation of decreased patient symptoms, increased functional status, continued cost-effectiveness, and prevention of future disease risks through earlier detection and education.

PR team members need to understand the complex concept of continuous quality improvement (CQI), and how it applies to pulmonary rehabilitation. Beginning in 1994, CQI will be a required mechanism of the accreditation process of the Joint Commission on Accreditation of Health Care Organizations (JCAHO).[1,79] CQI is replacing traditional quality assurance (QA). QA was based on the ability to provide high quality care, with the emphasis of monitoring and evaluation activities placed on individual performance; hence, traditional QA activities became synonymous with

reprimands. Because of this process, any good that could have come from the QA program was often lost.[57] The emphasis of CQI is on improving the process and desired outcomes. Patient care outcomes can be improved by assessing and improving the processes that most affect the outcome.[107] Most processes are carried out jointly by various clinical personnel, administration, and other managers. Integrated involvement of managerial and clinical leaders is required to improve these processes.

There are variations in PRPs both in scope and setting, but all programs must include the essential components discussed earlier. The outcome movement will help reduce these variations. The tools from which outcomes are determined are clinical indicators.[16,40,95,140,165] The American Association for Respiratory Care (AARC) has published a number of clinical practice guidelines and is currently working on many others for respiratory care practices including PR. These guidelines will facilitate the development of clinical indicators.[80,95] The American Association of Cardiovascular and Pulmonary Rehabilitation (AACVPR) is currently working on objective outcomes for PRPs. To have a successful program and achieve these outcomes, it is critical that the team members be enthusiastic, dedicated, able to motivate and relate well to the patient, and understand and apply the philosophy of PR. This philosophy includes striving, both individually and as a team, to maintain the highest standards of professionalism, knowledge, and confidentiality. Each team member must be a role model and must truly believe in the importance of prevention and early detection, not just treatment, of pulmonary disease.[3,97]

### Patient selection

Historically PRPs have provided care for patients with COPD and asthma. These programs are well established as a means of enhancing standard medical care, controlling and alleviating symptoms, and providing optimal functional capacity for these patients.[12,67,82,109,143] Too often the patient

---

### Pulmonary rehabilitation goals

**Patient-directed goals**

- Control and alleviate, as much as possible, the symptoms and pathophysiological complications (e.g., pulmonary hypertension) of respiratory impairment.
- Train the patient to achieve his or her optimal capacity to carry out activities of daily living.
- Decrease psychological symptoms such as anxiety or depression.
- Improve quality of life.
- Return the patient to gainful employment when possible.
- Promote independence and self-reliance.
- Increase exercise tolerance.
- Reduce exacerbations and hospitalizations.
- Encourage participation in recreational pursuits.

**Program goals**

- Design and implement a patient's individualized program under the medical direction of a physician with special knowledge or interest in pulmonary rehabilitation.
- Train, motivate, and rehabilitate the patient to his or her maximum potential in self-care through an organized team effort.
- Train, motivate, and involve the patient's significant others in the patient's treatment program.
- Reduce the economic burden of pulmonary disease on society through reduction of acute exacerbations, hospitalizations, emergency room visits, long-term duration of convalescence, and possible return of the patient to gainful employment or active retirement.
- Educate the general public and health care professionals about pulmonary health and rehabilitation.
- Increase awareness in the medical community regarding the importance of early detection of pulmonary disease through screening (e.g., spirometry).

From American Association of Cardiovascular and Pulmonary Rehabilitation: Selection and team assessment of the pulmonary rehabilitation candidate. In *Guidelines for pulmonary rehabilitation programs,* Champaign, Ill, 1993, Human Kinetics. Reprinted with permission.

---

### Demonstrated outcomes of pulmonary rehabilitation

Reduced hospitalizations and use of medical resources
Improved quality of life
Reduced respiratory symptoms (e.g., dyspnea)
Improved psychosocial symptoms (e.g., reversal of anxiety and depression and improved self-efficacy)
Increased exercise tolerance and performance
Enhanced ability to perform activities of daily living
Return to work for some patients
Increased knowledge about pulmonary disease and its management
Increased survival in some patients (i.e., use of continuous oxygen in patients with severe hypoxemia)

From Ries AL: Position paper of the American Association of Cardiovascular and Pulmonary Rehabilitation: Scientific basis of pulmonary rehabilitation, *J Cardiopul Rehab* 10:418, 1990. Reprinted with permission.

referred to PR is in end-stage disease. It must be remembered that PR is not just therapeutic, but preventive,[111,138] and the earlier the patient is referred into a program, the better the outcomes. Many patients ask why their physician did not refer them to the program earlier.

Pulmonary rehabilitation programs have also been shown to be beneficial for patients with other types of pulmonary diseases. Medical personnel need to be educated that any patient with physical limitations secondary to lung disease and who is motivated should be a candidate for PR.[13,68,103,128] These conditions may include restrictive pulmonary diseases and pulmonary vascular diseases, lung resection, lung transplantation, and neuromuscular disorders.[131,132,160,181] The box below lists the conditions that are appropriate for PR.

Significant or unstable medical or psychiatric conditions such as congestive heart failures, acute cor pulmonale, disabling stroke, metastatic cancer, significant liver dysfunction, substance abuse, dementia, or organic brain syndrome *may* be considered contraindications for PR. Once the unstable medical or psychiatric condition has been treated

and stabilized, the patient may be considered as a PR candidate.

In selecting patients for the PRP, it is important to assess whether the disease is causing any limitations for the patient, and if so what limitations the patient is experiencing.[46,74,144,148]

## COMPONENTS OF PULMONARY REHABILITATION
### Team assessment

The team assessment is individualized based upon the initial interview with the patient. A family member or significant other is encouraged to attend the interview and participate in the program.[103] This interview is an opportunity to:

- Meet the patient and family or significant other
- Discuss the program, goals, financial considerations, transportation, and time commitment
- Address any concerns that the patient may have
- Provide reassurance
- Work with the patient to prepare for the upcoming program
- Schedule necessary tests as listed in the box on p. 451
- Review the medical history
- Complete the questionnaire of symptoms, activities of daily living (ADLs), nutritional, social, and medication information

Keep in mind that the physician's list of prescribed medication and the patient's medication list may differ. Neither, in reality, may be accurate. This can occur because of multiple physicians, lack of patient understanding, poor compliance, and self-medicating. The patient's medication regimen needs to be reassessed throughout the program with careful attention to comments regarding vitamins, herbs, prescribed, and over-the-counter (OTC) medications.

The initial interview also provides the opportunity to identify which team member assessments may be beneficial. These could include assessments from the following: medical director, physical therapist (PT), occupational therapist (OT), respiratory care practitioner (RCP), pharmacist, social worker, or dietitian.[75,115]

A thorough initial assessment is an essential component of a comprehensive PRP. It provides the opportunity to evaluate other systems, including nasal/sinus, gastrointestinal, cardiovascular,[26] and musculoskeletal; detect exercise hypoxemia;[7] assess the need for supplemental oxygen; and determine the patient's initial strengths and weaknesses (Fig. 23-3).* For the purpose of this chapter, only the physical therapy assessment will be discussed thoroughly.

The physical therapy assessment serves to:

---

### Conditions appropriate for pulmonary rehabilitation

**Obstructive pulmonary disease**

Chronic obstructive pulmonary disease (COPD)
Asthma
Asthmatic bronchitis
Chronic bronchitis
Emphysema
Bronchiectasis
Cystic fibrosis

**Restrictive pulmonary disease**

Interstitial fibrosis
Rheumatoid pulmonary disease
Collagen vascular lung disorders
Pneumoconiosis
Sarcoidosis

**Restrictive chest wall disease**

Kyphoscoliosis
Severe obesity
Poliomyelitis

**Other conditions**

Pulmonary vascular diseases
Lung resection
Lung transplantation
Occupational/environmental lung diseases

From Beytas L and Connors GL: Organization and management of a pulmonary rehabilitation program. In Hodgkin JE, Connors GL, and Bell CW, editors: *Pulmonary rehabilitation: guidelines to success*, ed 2, Philadelphia, 1992, JB Lippincott. Reprinted with permission.

---

* References 12, 13, 46, 68, 74, 82.

1. Establish a baseline of strength, range of motion, posture, functional abilities, and activity
2. Determine any initial limitations or restrictions to activity that may require exercise or program modifications or special considerations, such as a patient with a hip or knee replacement or one with arthritis or scoliosis
3. Establish both patient and PT goals that will be worked on immediately and throughout the program
4. Determine any special needs that the patient may have, such as extra pillows when exercising on the floor, or perhaps a chair to facilitate getting up and down from the floor
5. Introduce the PR candidate to exercise in a friendly, individually-paced, calm, and confident manner

This evaluation is done individually just prior to the beginning of the program. At least 30 to 45 minutes should be allowed for each patient. See Fig. 23-4 for an example of an evaluation form. More important than the form that is

---

### Suggested tests during initial evaluation of a pulmonary rehabilitation candidate*

Spirometry pre/post bronchodilator
Lung volumes
Diffusing capacity
Resting arterial blood gas
Chest radiograph
Resting electrocardiogram
Complete blood count
Basic blood chemistry panel
Exercise test with cutaneous oximetry and/or arterial blood gas (simple or modified test such as 6- or 12-minute walk)
Master's step, calibrated cycle or ergometer, or motorized treadmill

*It is acceptable not to repeat these tests if done within the 3 months prior to entering the PRP or as determined by the PR medical director.

#### Other tests to consider for selected patients

Maximal voluntary ventilation
Maximal inspiratory and expiratory pressures
Theophylline level, when applicable
Pulmonary exercise stress test (metabolic study) with continuous ECG monitoring
Postexercise spirometry
Bronchial challenge
Cardiovascular tests (e.g., holter monitor, echocardiogram, thallium exercise stress test)
Polysomnography
Sinus radiographs
Upper gastrointestinal series
Skin tests

From American Association of Cardiovascular and Pulmonary Rehabilitation: Selection and team assessment of the pulmonary rehabilitation candidate. In *Guidelines for pulmonary rehabilitation* programs, Champaign, Ill, 1993, Human Kinetics. Reprinted with permission.

---

used is the very special interaction that occurs between the patient and the therapist throughout the evaluation. The following may serve as an example of how to use this form as a tool to facilitate the therapist's understanding of the total patient (Fig. 23-4).

The evaluation includes name, age, and date of the initial evaluation. The patient is asked to identify his or her diagnosis or chief physical complaint. This request is important because it gives the therapist a baseline of knowledge regarding the patient's understanding of the illness; whether the patient has been given a definitive diagnosis; and whether the patient (or family, in some cases,) acknowledges that he or she has a problem. Most of the time the patient will say, "My breathing of course," or "I can't breathe." Sometimes the patient will state in very definite terms the exact diagnosis and what it means. Other times patients will state that they have no physical problems at all, but that their doctor or some family member is making them participate. Sometimes they may give answers that reveal a sense of loss or frustration such as the statement, "I'm useless and I can't do anything." This answer gives the therapist a beginning background to know how to approach this patient.

The next question regards onset or "How long has this been a problem?" While it is important for billing purposes that all members of the rehabilitation team use the same date of onset, it is important to acknowledge that the onset of pulmonary problems may be difficult for patients to ascertain. They may associate onset with the date of a hospitalization or surgery, or they may believe that symptoms began only recently. You should acknowledge that this question may be difficult to answer, and they may not have thought about this issue before. This question often leads to a discussion and the realization of a gradual progression of shortness of breath and decrease in functional abilities. This realization is important since the therapist is establishing the need for a program of slow, consistent, progressive exercise beginning with the current level of function as a baseline. "COPD differs from other devastating illnesses in its *lack of a critical incident*. The disability is insidious yet invisible, and medical attention is sought late in its course."[33]

The patient may then give the therapist other information regarding general health or medical history that might be important, (e.g. surgeries). In most cases the therapist has already read a history form that the patient has completed, and sometimes the patient may feel that this written information is adequate. Occasionally, the patient may wish to relate specific parts of the medical history. This can be important information and may reveal the patient's perception of personal health and the relationship of other medical factors to current physical problems. Also, a surgical history is important because thoracic or abdominal surgery may result in pain and scar tissue development, causing restriction of thoracic movement (i.e., decreased ventilation). Scar tissue mobilization and massage may be introduced at an appropriate time during the program.

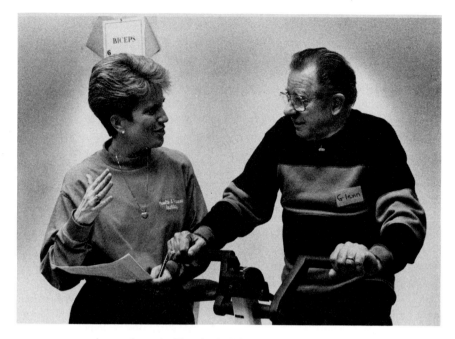

**Fig. 23-3.** The physical therapy assessment.

The patient is next asked about an orthopedic history to determine if modification of exercises might be necessary. It is important to ask specifically about a history of back, neck, shoulder, elbow, wrist, hand, hip, knee, ankle, or foot problems. The patient will often deny orthopedic problems but will comment "my right knee hurts." This also is a good place for general information regarding previous rehabilitation or physical therapy. Did they have an old injury, go to therapy, and "it really helped"? Did they go to therapy and it "didn't do a bit of good"? Have they never been sick or injured in their life until now, and thus have had no contact at all with rehabilitation personnel?

The next section, which may be checked off at any time during the evaluation, addresses body type. The patient may mention a significant loss of weight, poor appetite, or weight gain because of a decrease in activity or steroid use. This patient may benefit from a nutritional assessment to help with healthy caloric changes to begin while in the program.

The next question refers to the patient's usual daily activity. This is an important baseline in regard to the patient's quality of life. The answers may be: "I don't do anything..."; "I'm useless..." Sometimes the patient will reveal a sense of loss as in "I used to get up and go play golf..."; "I used to work in the garden..." It is important to ask when the activity was last done, i.e., "When was the last time that you played golf?" It has often been 2 to 3 years since the patient has actually participated in the activity. Make sure that you "give credit" for the activity such as, "That's great that you played golf 3 times a week since that lets me know that you like to exercise and that you were in good shape not long ago; but today tell me what you've done for activity on an average day for the last week."

The next part of the evaluation includes testing range of motion (Fig. 23-5) and strength. Testing may be modified as needed for the individual patient population and the therapist's own individual assessment styles.

Postural assessment is extremely important since the patient may be developing a forward head, elevated shoulders, and protracted scapular posture so commonly seen. Cervical and scapular motion may be restricted secondary to use of accessory muscles of respiration. Often the patient has noticed this change in posture and movement and has been concerned. It helps to reassure the patient that this change in posture is common and that many of the stretching and strengthening exercises included in the program are designed to improve both posture and motion.

Functional grading of dyspnea level is also very important initially, because patients will often forget at what level they began the program. Four weeks into the program, some may respond that they are "about the same." Referral back to this section may reveal that the individual had been extremely short of breath with any movement and could not tolerate getting up and down from the floor secondary to severe dyspnea. At the time of follow-up, he or she may be doing warm-up exercises, aerobic activity, and floor exercises before arriving at the "same" earlier level of dyspnea.

After evaluating the patient's functional dyspnea, the therapist must then determine whether or not to proceed with instruction in getting up and down from the floor. Some patients may tell you that they haven't been down on the floor in at least 30 years. (This may be the time for some humor—remind them that no one is still on the floor and that all who have entered your assessment area have left!) Emphasize that this activity does not have to

MT. DIABLO MEDICAL CENTER - PULMONARY REHABILITATION
PHYSICAL THERAPY EVALUATION

NAME: _____ AGE: _____ DATE: _____
(initial)

DIAGNOSIS: (CHIEF COMPLAINT): _____ DATE: _____
(final)

ONSET: _____ OTHER INFORMATION: _____
_____

MEDICAL HISTORY: _____
_____

ORTHOPEDIC HISTORY: _____
_____

BODY TYPE:        LITHE _____ MEDIUM _____ STOUT _____

AVERAGE DAILY ACTIVITY: _____

| RANGE OF MOTION | INITIAL | FOLLOW UP |
|---|---|---|
| CERVICAL | | |
| Forward flexion | | |
| Extension | | |
| Rotation R/L | | |
| Lateral flexion R/L | | |
| TRUNK MOBILITY | | |
| Forward flexion | | |
| Extension | | |
| Side-bending R/L | | |
| Rotation R/L | | |
| UPPER EXTREMITIES | | |
| Shoulders | | |
| Scapula | | |
| Elbows | | |
| Wrists and hands | | |
| LOWER EXTREMITIES | | |
| Hips | | |
| Knees | | |
| Ankles and feet | | |
| RIB MOBILITY | | |
| Opposite elbow to knee | | |
| HANDS BEHIND HEAD | | |
| HANDS BEHIND BACK | | |
| CHEST EXCURSION (INCH) | | |
| Inspiration-Exhalation | | |

**Fig. 23-4.** Physical Therapy Evaluation Form. (Reprinted courtesy of the PRP at Mt. Diablo Medical Center, Concord, Calif.)

| STRENGTH | INITIAL | FOLLOW UP |
|---|---|---|
| UPPER EXTREMITIES | | |
| Distal | | |
| Proximal | | |
| LOWER EXTREMITIES | | |
| Distal | | |
| Proximal | | |
| POSTURE | INITIAL | FOLLOW UP |
| A/P BALANCE | | |
| Head | | |
| Scapula | | |
| Thoracic Curve | | |
| Lumbar Curve | | |
| Abdomen | | |
| LATERAL BALANCE | | |
| Head Tilt | | |
| Shoulder Level | | |
| Chest (convex/concave) | | |
| Pelvic Level: | | |
| FUNCTIONAL GRADING | INITIAL | FINAL |
| DYSPNEA | | |
| At rest | | |
| With slight action | | |
| With level walking | | |
| With light activity | | |
| With unlimited walking | | |

FUNCTIONAL MOBILITY:
   Up and down from floor: _____

BREATHING PATTERN: _____

PATIENT'S GOALS: _____

PHYSICAL THERAPIST'S GOALS: _____

INITIAL ASSESSMENT: _____

FOLLOW-UP ASSESSMENT: _____

PHYSICAL THERAPIST: _____

**Fig. 23-4, cont'd.**

be pretty. Don't give them a lot of time to decide. Be positive, let them know you're there to help. Provide encouragement, lead them through each move, and do it with them! (Figs. 23-6 and 23-7.) This activity is important for several reasons:

1. Some patients have a terrible fear that if they fall they will never be able to get up. Because of their physical state, surgeries, breathing problems, barrel chest, etc.,

they have not been on the floor in years and may have determined that they could not get up if they got down. An immediate improvement in their self-confidence occurs when they are able to get up and down following instruction.

2. Doing this activity individually enables the therapist to watch the patient move and to work with the patient to develop the best way to get up and down (i.e., a person with a total knee or total hip replacement might

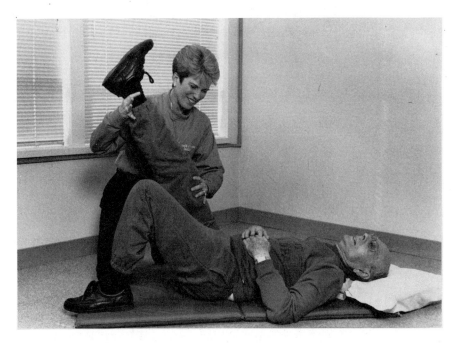

**Fig. 23-5.** Testing range of motion.

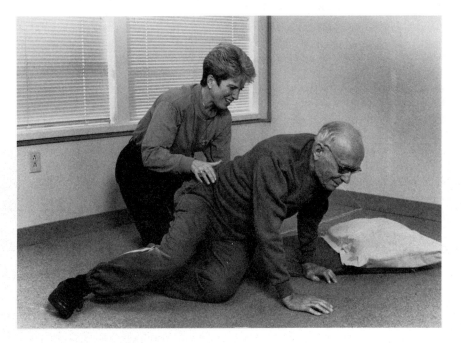

**Fig. 23-6.** Getting up and down from the floor.

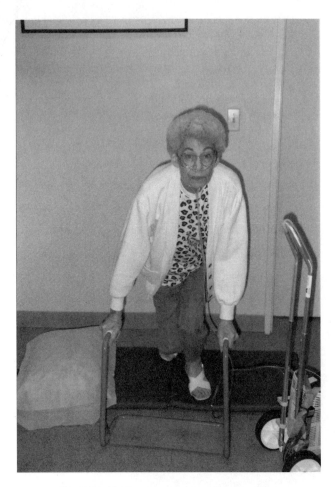

**Fig. 23-7.** Getting up and down from the floor.

need to modify his or her method when compared to a patient with arthritis in the hands and wrists). The patient can perform this movement at a comfortable pace and without fear of embarrassment.

3. The initial need for several pillows or wedge when lying supine can be identified. Improvement may be noted during follow-up regarding the patient's ability to relax now with fewer pillows or a decreased height of the wedge. The need for a chair next to the patient during floor exercises to help him or her get up and down can also be determined.

4. If the therapist determines that the patient is too short of breath or apprehensive to try this during the initial evaluation, instruction can be done the first day of floor exercise activity. This is another important aspect of progress to identify at a later time, i.e., initially the patient was unable to get up and down from the floor and now he or she is able. What an accomplishment!

The patient's breathing pattern may be noted throughout the evaluation along with the ability to perform pursed-lip breathing.

Next, the patient is asked about personal goals for the program. This point is extremely important. Answers to the question "If I treat you how will I make you better," may range from vague, "to breathe a little better," to very specific, "to be able to play 9 holes of golf using the cart twice a week."

The therapist may next discuss expected goals of treatment and rehabilitation. The assessment list may be used and discussed with the patient at this time (Fig. 23-8), with additional discussion of what will happen in the program and what to expect. The PR candidate can be told what to wear and what will happen during the class. Individual plans per the assessment can be discussed (Fig. 23-8).

Patients are reminded that if an exercise is uncomfortable or painful, they are NOT to do it but are to notify the therapist. This does not mean that patients can avoid an exercise, but rather that an exercise may be modified for their needs. The patients need to be reminded frequently that everyone is different and that exercise programs need to be individualized in order to be comfortable and most beneficial. Individual responsibility and control is emphasized.

The same form can be used at a follow-up evaluation in order to directly compare all components of the original assessment.

### Patient training

Patient training may include instruction and participation in correct inhaler technique, respiratory muscle training (RMT),* bronchial hygiene,[5,40,70] nutrition,[14,17,115] medications,† psychosocial interventions, exercise principles, activities of daily living (ADLs), smoking cessation,[6,53,54,127,175] oxygen rationale,[8,129] and self-assessment, and treatment. The various breathing, relaxation, and panic-control techniques are also included in this component. This information is delivered through a series of short, interactive lectures. The patient may feel overwhelmed by the amount of information presented. To minimize this feeling, it is important to provide each patient with a well-organized notebook, that he or she may refer to as needed.[72,171]

Learning is helped by:

- Providing adequate time for questions
- Keeping classes short
- Talking in lay terms (4th to 7th grade level)
- Alternating sitting classes with active classes
- Acknowledging the influence of physical and mental defects, i.e., hypoxia, hearing loss, visual problems, fluid and electrolyte imbalance, pain, memory loss, and low self-esteem
- Individualizing the program
- Providing support, praise, encouragement, and acceptance

The goal is to teach the patients to apply and coordinate their breathing techniques while performing activities of daily living.

---

* References 21, 25, 35, 135, 136, 159.
† References 58, 94, 96, 133, 169, 174.

# PHYSICAL THERAPY ASSESSMENT

P.T. Assessment #1: Inadequate strength of the upper extremities and/or lower extremities to perform functional activities.

Goal: Increase strength of the upper and/or lower extremities for functional activities.

Plan: Instruction and practice in upper/lower extremity exercises specific to difficult functional activities.

P.T. Assessment #2: Decreased range of motion of _____ resulting in inability or difficulty in performing functional tasks.

Goal: Increase the necessary range of motion to facilitate performing the functional activities.

Plan: Instruction and practice of stretching and flexibility exercises.

P.T. Assessment #3: Decreased joint protection techniques.

Goal: Increased knowledge of the principles of joint protection and the ability to relate it to ADL tasks.

Plan: Instruction and practice of joint protection techniques.

P.T. Assessment #4: Limited knowledge of exercise guidelines and dyspnea level.

Goal: Patient to know individual exercise guidelines and be able to use dyspnea level scale.

Plan: Teach and practice individual exercise guidelines and rating of dyspnea level.

P.T. Assessment #5: Poor posture or improper body alignment.

Goal: Patient to understand and work towards correct body alignment.

Plan: Teach correct posture and alignment and the stretching and strengthening exercises necessary to move towards this posture.

P.T. Assessment #6: Decreased strength of the _____.

Goal: Patient to increase strength of the _____.

Plan: Instruct in and practice strengthening exercises for the _____.

P.T. Assessment #7: Patient has pain located in the _____ with exercise.

Goal: Decrease the symptoms noted with exercise.

Plan: Instruct/use modalities and exercise modification as needed to decrease the symptoms and pain with exercise.

P.T. Assessment #8: _____ is the activity that causes the most dyspnea.

Goal: Patient to learn compensation measures that will assist in _____.

Plan: Instruct and allow the patient to practice the pacing and strengthening activities specific for the difficult activity. Establish a daily individual exercise program that will assist the patient in increasing his/her strength and endurance for the activity.

P.T. Assessment #9: Patient exhibits poor endurance for functional activities.

Goal: Increase endurance to allow the patient to perform functional activities.

Plan: Instruct patient in energy conservation and strengthening exercises to increase endurance.

P.T. Assessment #10: Patient exhibits muscle spasm/cramping when performing exercise or functional activities.

Goal: Decrease muscle spasm/cramping to allow the patient to exercise and/or perform functional activities.

Plan: Teach patient stretching, warm-up, and cool-down activities to minimize spasms. Instruct patient on what to do should cramping occur.

**Fig. 23-8.** Physical Therapy Assessment Form.

---

### Directions for proper use of a metered-dose inhaler

1. Remove dust cap.
2. Shake the inhaler.
3. Hold inhaler in the upright position.
4. Exhale normally.
5. Open mouth wide—hold mouthpiece approximately 2 inches from mouth.
6. Start to inhale slowly; depress the top of the canister.
7. Continue to inhale deeply and slowly, then hold the breath for 10 seconds, if possible.
8. Exhale slowly through pursed-lips.
9. Wait 1 to 10 minutes before repeating a dose (this is determined by a physician's directions and the type of medication).

---

Always keep in mind that patients can retain more when they not only hear the information, but also see it and demonstrate it as well. Repetition is essential to learning and each instructor should encourage the patient to practice the skills as much as possible.*

Only the following lectures will be individually discussed: metered-dose inhaler (MDI)/spacer, breathing retraining, i.e., pursed-lip breathing (PLB), diaphragmatic breathing, and (DB)/abdominal breathing, and exercise principles. For additional information regarding other training sessions, see references.[3,9,71]

**Metered-dose inhaler/spacer.** The metered-dose inhaler (MDI) is a simple, convenient, effective method used to deliver pharmacologic agents to the lower airways.[44,103,166]

The patient must be instructed in the correct technique for using the inhaler and supervised while demonstrating this technique.[2,15,96,133,154] The patient should be advised to use the bronchodilator inhaler within two hours prior to exercise and to carry it with him or her at all times.

Whenever the opportunity arises, the patient should be observed using the inhaler and reinstructed if necessary. The box above lists the directions for proper use of the MDI. If the patient is unable to use the MDI or is having difficulty using it properly, a spacer should be used. The purposes of the spacer are to avoid the need for coordinating inspiration and simultaneously activating the inhaler to remove the large droplets, which add toxicity; and to minimize the impact of the small droplets on the nasopharynx by slowing them down.[149,173] Currently, there are several brands of spacers on the market. Follow the manufacturer's directions for proper use and cleaning techniques.

The Rotahaler is another type of bronchodilator inhaler. This inhaler works by using the pressure of rapid inhalation and a mixing chamber to suspend an agent in powder form. Some patients report that the Rotahaler is easier and more convenient to use than the other inhalers.[133] As a P.T.

working with pulmonary patients, it is essential that you are familiar with the correct inhaler technique, frequency, and prescribed dosage.

**Breathing retraining.** Pursed-lip breathing (PLB) (Fig. 23-9) alleviates dyspnea by:

- Decreasing the respiratory rate with an accompanying increase in the tidal volume (TV) and oxygen saturation,[171] possibly altering the pattern of recruitment of the respiratory muscles[30]
- Enabling the patient to gain a feeling of control rather than panic when breathing discomfort occurs[30]

In chronic lung disease, airways collapse during exhalation, trapping air in the alveoli. PLB provides resistance to expiration, which increases airway pressure, and may prevent compression of airways.[40] In normal individuals, the diaphragm does approximately 80% of the work of breathing. In COPD the diaphragm is flattened because of air-trapping and is less effective as a result of the poor length-tension relationship of its fibers. The accessory muscles of respiration then assume the responsibility for breathing, requiring more oxygen to accomplish chest expansion and doing a less efficient job than the diaphragm. Diaphragmatic breathing (DB) will help strengthen the diaphragm and abdominal muscles, helping to decrease dyspnea. For patient instruction in PLB and DB see the box on p. 459. An improved ventilatory pattern (with increased tidal volume and a decrease in respiratory rate) has been demonstrated following breathing retraining.[122,123]

### Exercise principles

How much exercise should I do? How much should I push myself? How much is too much? If I can hardly get out of bed, there's no point in even considering an exercise program, right? Tell me, if I can only walk at a snail's pace, is there any point in doing it? Anyone who has ever worked in a PRP or with deconditioned patients has heard these questions. Even after the program has started, questions continue: "Why does the program start out slowly? Why is he/she doing more exercise than I am? Why do we do different exercises at the beginning of the exercise session than we do at the end? Why can't I just ride the bike? Why do you make me walk and work on my arm strength?" These and many other questions should be answered during the exercise lecture of the training component.

**The pulmonary athlete.** As a physical therapist guiding the exercise of an individual or a group of PR patients, where do you start? Perhaps first by truly looking at the audience. How would you describe them? They are individuals who are sharp, motivated, driven, hard-working, competitive, frightened, angry or depressed. Does this sound like a description of an injured athlete? Aren't we all athletes—industrial athletes, office athletes, professional athletes, pulmonary athletes? Whether performing our jobs, throwing a ball, making a bed, typing a report, building a fence, or walking to the kitchen with the greatest efficiency of

---

*References 18, 63, 89-91, 101, 105, 106, 117, 126, 137, 141, 158, 170.

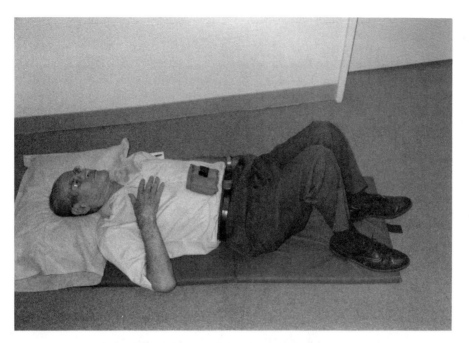

**Fig. 23-9.** PLB-DB with a weight on the diaphragm.

---

## Patient instructions for breathing techniques

**Pursed lip breathing**

1. Relax.
2. Inhale through your nose with your mouth closed. Take normal breaths, not a deep breath.
3. Exhale through your mouth with your lips pursed, as if you are going to whistle, kiss, or blow out a candle.
4. Exhale at least twice as long as you inhale. For example, inhale for 2 seconds; exhale for 4 seconds. When doing pursed-lip breathing, inhale through you nose for two counts—then purse your lips and exhale for four counts.

*Remember*

• Do not force the air out.
• Your breathing should be slow, easy, and relaxed.
• Practice this technique as often as possible. It will become a natural way of breathing when you are short of breath or doing any physical activity.
• It will help you relax.
• It gives you more control over your breathing.

**Diaphragmatic/abdominal breathing**

1. Place one hand on your stomach just at the base of your breastbone. This hand will tell you when your diaphragm presses down against your abdomen, pushing your stomach out.
2. Place your other hand on your upper chest. Use this hand to tell you how much movement is occurring in your chest muscles.

*Remember*

• Concentrate on exhaling at least twice as long as you inhale, just as you did with pursed-lip breathing.
• Keep your chest still so your diaphragm, and not your neck and chest muscles, does the work of breathing. Practice this exercise until you feel comfortable using diaphragmatic and pursed-lip breathing together.
• It will help you relax.
• It gives you more control over your breathing.

---

movement, strength, and energy, we are all developing a strategy, a game plan to do our best and meet the challenges that the game of life tosses to us. We are pacing ourselves, improving techniques, strengthening specific muscles and stretching others, setting goals along the way and striving to meet them.

Here in this classroom sit salesmen, construction workers, professionals, grandmas, grandpas, computer experts, engineers, nurses, doctors, and physical therapists separated from an active participation in their lives often only by shortness of breath. As one patient stated about the frustrating reality

of his life, "My mind makes promises that my body can't keep!" (Fig. 23-10) Here is the injured athlete in all of us. To rehabilitate any athlete we must address the whole person, including such aspects as strength, flexibility, psychology, stress, diet, self-esteem, and confidence. Life is indeed an individual sport—each person strives each day for a personal best. If one looks at those striving for the Olympic gold or on any sports field, he or she will see athletes striving, sacrificing, and giving their all. Nowhere will you see more effort, sacrifice, and determination than within this group of pulmonary patients who work harder than we can probably

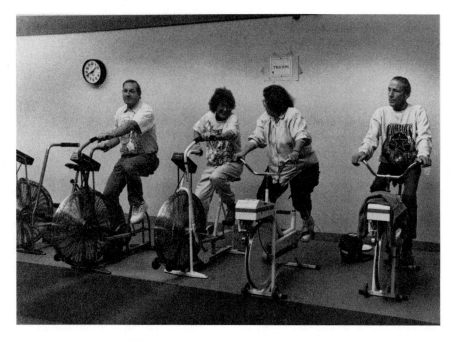

**Fig. 23-10.** "My mind makes promises that my body can't keep!"

ever imagine just to live, breathe, laugh, and do the things that just a short time ago they could do with ease.

You should recognize their loss, their anger, their frustration, their guilt ("I did this to myself"—cigarettes) and their shame, i.e., the patient who did not want to tell her church group that she was going to PR because she was so ashamed that she had done this to herself. You must also recognize and emphasize to the patients that for all athletes, rehabilitation is the only road back. You have the unique opportunity to introduce them to the creation of their exercise program, to help them rediscover the hidden athlete that might be camouflaged by oxygen tanks and barrel chests.

So how did they reach this point? For many the path has been downhill for sometime. Many have been making logical decisions daily that may be contributing to a decline in their health. Consider a patient with pulmonary disease who goes out for a walk, ascends some stairs, tries to make a bed, or unloads some groceries. Maybe they are having a bad day or trying to move too fast; regardless, the patient has a difficult time. The patient decides that it was wrong to have tried. Patients respond in what may seem a logical and certainly safer manner at the time by decreasing the distance or omitting the activity. Gradually, over time, the activities decrease, the distances walked decrease, and the muscle size and endurance decrease. Never is the adage, "If you do not use it—you will lose it," more true.

This is a good time to ask patients, "What is the most important muscle of the body?" They commonly respond, "The heart!" By looking down at their atrophied bicep or quadricep, they begin to visualize the deconditioning that may be occurring to their heart and respiratory musculature. This decline tends to increase their exertional dyspnea,

decreases functional capacity, and thereby reduces their quality of life.[148] See Fig. 23-11 for the dyspnea/deconditioning cycle. PR strives to break this cycle of dyspnea/deconditioning at the point of fear of exertion. Once the level of fear has decreased, the patient will be able to tolerate increased exercise[33] (Fig. 23-11).

The bad news is that a decline in quality of life is often the motivation to begin the PRP. The good news is that each patient has the power and control to strengthen muscles and improve their efficiency. Ask your audience, "What does a weight lifter do to strengthen his bicep?" They will quickly answer, "Lift weights—make it work!"

"So what do you need to do to your muscles, your heart, your respiratory system?" you ask. Again they reply, "Make them work!" They are now ready for a plan of action.

Any cardiopulmonary exercise program should include the following components: warm-up, aerobic/endurance, and cool-down (Fig. 23-12). Relaxation and breathing techniques may be practiced also.

Warm-up, the first phase of the exercise program, allows the heart rate to increase gradually to meet the demands of increased activity and signals the body that more work will follow. Warm-up begins to use the deconditioned muscles that have perhaps been in one position for a long time with the patient sitting or lying down. At this point the therapist can discuss the difference between static and dynamic stretching. Dynamic stretching allows a body part to move gently within the normal range of motion. The purpose of this type of stretch is to prepare muscle groups that are about to be used during the aerobic activity. These stretches are not fast, do not include bouncing, and are not forced to the end of the range of motion. Get the patients involved at this time. Tell them to "look up and look down," and proceed through

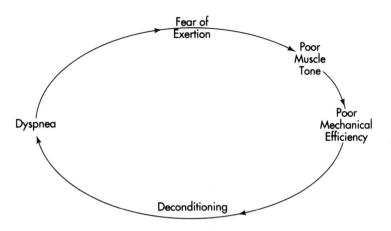

**Fig. 23-11.** Dyspnea/Deconditioning Cycle.

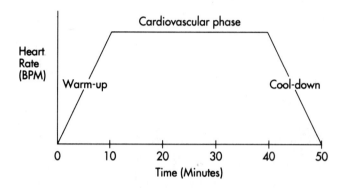

**Fig. 23-12.** Components of an exercise program.

a possible 5 to 10 minute warm-up. An example of an exercise routine, including warm-up, is presented later in the chapter.

During your lecture you have led the patients through an exercise warm-up and cool-down that can be done anytime and anyplace, even while sitting down. Patients realize that this activity does not require large amounts of time or energy. Most importantly, by having them do it initially with you, they can achieve their first success before ever going to the gym. Let them know, "You just did it!!! That was a warm-up. Great job!" The looks on the faces of these athletes says it all, "I'm exercising—I can do it!"

Emphasize at this point that each patient should pay attention to how their muscles feel and to evaluate their shortness of breath. This lays the ground work for their understanding of "perceived level of exertion/dyspnea." (See the box on p. 462.)

The next phase of the exercise program is the aerobic, cardiovascular, or endurance phase. This is the portion of the program that most patients will consider "exercise". Aerobic entails oxygen uptake and should be carried out for a long enough time to allow for the strengthening of the heart and improvement in the circulatory systems. The following elements of an exercise program should be considered during this phase.

**Frequency.** The frequency of a training program should be a minimum of 3 times per week for a training effect to be reached and maintained. Three to five times a week may be advisable,[10] although this is open to debate.[24,112] An alternate day schedule allows for a recovery period, if necessary. Individuals with COPD work at such a low intensity at first that a daily program can be employed without detrimental effects. Stopping exercise results in a loss of this training effect.[99,176] The stimulus must be maintained to prevent deconditioning. The ideal situation would include: exercise training, followed by an ongoing maintenance exercise program, and/or a home exercise program (HEP) for those who wish to continue independently.

**Intensity.** The importance of the intensity of training is often emphasized but is not clear.[81] It is most important to realize that exercise MUST be tolerable, enjoyable, and have realistic, attainable goals. In this training session, the patient is educated regarding the basis for the intensity of their program ("How hard do I exercise?"). Some programs use Karvonen's formula for determining target heart rate (THR) with 0.6 as the intensity factor:[86]

$$\text{Target HR} = [0.6 \times (\text{Peak HR-Resting})] + \text{Resting HR}$$

The advantage of this formula is that it takes into consideration both peak and resting heart rates, which is important because the formula for nonimpaired patients (e.g., 0.7 × peak HR) may calculate a target heart rate lower than the patient's resting heart rate.[81,82] Other methods to determine exercise intensity may be symptom-limited targets, such as perceived level of exertion[28] or perceived level of breathlessness scales.[22,64,179] With these limits some severe ventilatory-limited patients can reach levels during training that may approach 100% of their maximum exercise tolerance.[139,145,167]

Patients are told that they will be learning to monitor their heart rate and their dyspnea level (Fig. 23-13). They begin to attend to their bodies, so that they can exercise and recognize what responses are safe and acceptable and at what level they may continue. Patients also learn to exercise to

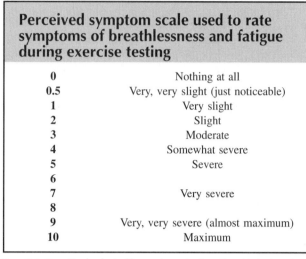

| Perceived symptom scale used to rate symptoms of breathlessness and fatigue during exercise testing | |
| --- | --- |
| 0 | Nothing at all |
| 0.5 | Very, very slight (just noticeable) |
| 1 | Very slight |
| 2 | Slight |
| 3 | Moderate |
| 4 | Somewhat severe |
| 5 | Severe |
| 6 | |
| 7 | Very severe |
| 8 | |
| 9 | Very, very severe (almost maximum) |
| 10 | Maximum |

From G.A. Borg: Psychophysical bases of perceived exertion, *Med sci sports exer* 14:377, 1982. Reprinted with permission.

"target" levels of heart rate or breathing comfort.[28] Many patients have a difficult time monitoring heart rate, and we have found dyspnea level to be the most valuable criterion for intensity. A good rule is that if a patient has enough air to say a word aloud, then it is okay to continue exercising. During exercise, heart rate and dyspnea level should always be monitored, and oxygen saturation and blood pressure may also be followed.

Regardless of studies and goals, the initial exercise program should focus on low-intensity training to maximize success and minimize the risk of injury. Initial emphasis should be on endurance rather than intensity of exercise.[130] Remember that exercise should be enjoyable as the patient moves from a sedentary life style to an active one. Compliance with an exercise program may decrease with high levels of exertion. Low-intensity, subanaerobic threshold training is adequate stimulus to produce modest gains in aerobic power in previously sedentary subjects.[23]

**Time.** The duration for which this aerobic exercise should be continued is set at approximately 12 to 30 minutes, plus a 5 to 10 minute warm-up, and an equally long cool down that includes stretching. Emphasize that this is a GOAL and that many may start at shorter training periods and progress as tolerated. The initial evaluation is important to help set a goal and then to aid the patient in determining his or her current status. For some, a walk from the bed to the kitchen may feel subjectively like the Boston Marathon. Perhaps by setting a progression of folding chairs along the way and beginning with 7 to 8 stops, the patient might complete this "marathon" successfully. During the next few days, weeks and months, the rest times may be shortened and the number of stops decreased by removing one chair, then two, then three, until the trip is done without a stop. This demonstrates progress and allows the patient to gain confidence and work toward the real goal of making it to meals with less exhaustion.

**Type.** The mode or type of exercise used for training the pulmonary patient can and should be varied, depending on the initial assessment. It is important to look at the specific activities with which the patient has difficulty and to work on those. Exercise and training are task and muscle specific. That is, patients tend to do best on activities and exercises for which they were trained.[33] Thus, if the evaluation shows limited endurance, training should include low-resistance and high-repetitions to increase endurance by increasing the vascularity of muscle fibers (number of capillaries and mitochondria in the muscle); to increase the myoglobin content and aerobic enzymes; and to develop muscle fibers that are fatigue-resistant.[21,25,99] If the patient lacks strength, some high-resistance and low-repetition activity (progressive overload) should be provided to increase strength by increasing the number of myofibrils in the white fibers (hypertrophy of the fibers as in weight lifting).

Resistive training has been recommended for healthy adults,[10] the elderly,[69,78] patients with cardiac[161] and neurological[118] disorders and COPD.[156] Studies have shown that inclusion of leg exercises is beneficial to patients with lung disease.[20,43,121,157,162] Clausen and others[41] found that when subjects' extremities were exercised, the decreased heart rate

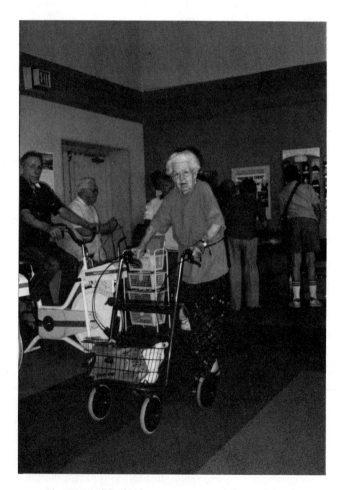

**Fig. 23-13.** Monitoring target rate and dyspnea level.

found with upper extremity trained subjects did not transfer to the lower extremity trained group or vice versa.

Many everyday tasks require unsupported upper extremity use. Patients with severe COPD often report a disproportionately high increase in dyspnea when performing tasks employing the upper extremities such as lifting, bathing, and grooming when compared to activities involving lower extremities.[37,51,111,144] For some of these tasks the actions of other muscle groups in the upper body are required (respiratory and postural). These include muscles with both thoracic and extrathoracic attachments such as: the upper and lower trapezius, latissimus dorsi, serratus anterior, subclavius, and pectoralis major and minor. These muscles can either help position the arms or shoulders, or if the arms are fixed, may exert a pulling force on the rib cage to enhance respiratory maneuvers. As the intensity of muscle function increases by exercise or by the increased impedance associated with respiratory disease, the accessory muscles of respiration are recruited. Expiration then is no longer passive and the accessory muscles of the rib cage, scapula, head and neck, shoulders, and pectoral region become active during inspiration.[159] When patients perform unsupported arm exercise, some shoulder girdle muscles must decrease their work in ventilation, thereby changing the pattern of ventilation which often increases dyspnea.[36,37,51] To avoid intolerable levels of dyspnea, patients often limit their upper extremity use.[144] This limitation of muscle function can result in muscle deconditioning, general disability, and emotional and social changes. Studies recommend unsupported upper extremity exercise to improve upper extremity performance,[62] using activities specific for the muscle groups and tasks involved in training.[50,55,116,162] Some researchers also believe in strengthening the muscles of respiration, as discussed fully in Chapter 17.[26,135,136,146]

It appears that varied modes of exercise should be performed,[179,180] based upon the initial and ongoing assessment of the pulmonary patient. This program should consist of a combination of specific exercises including: unsupported upper extremity exercises with or without weights,[60,155] leg exercises, aerobic conditioning, and respiratory muscle training.

Walking programs are especially good because everyone needs to walk. Emphasize the specificity of training. In order to increase one's ability to walk, a regular session of walking must be done.[138] Help the patient realize that many "tasks" or "jobs" can be incorporated into exercise training—these tasks "count!" Help them give themselves credit. In excessively hot or cold weather, patients can walk with the cart in the grocery store, mall, or large warehouse store, where they may "cruise" without stopping; after their exercise, they may stop and do the task (shop). Thus, walking enables them to enlarge social horizons, to get out and to be of help. ("I'll push the cart.") We have found that initially pushing a wheel chair or using a cart with a seat, enables the patient to go farther with more confidence and thus to progress faster.

Other aerobic activities include: treadmill, cycling, stationary bike, step exercise, rowing, water exercise, swimming, and modified aerobic dance. One of the values of an organized program is the use of varied aerobic equipment and socialization. The time seems to go faster when patients vary the activity and are having fun. The value of walking, stair climbing, etc., was well expressed by a patient who, returning from a rigorous trip to classical Greece, stated "I climbed hills, stairs, old ruins, and kept up with people younger and healthier than I. I couldn't have done that without attending the PRP."* Aerobic exercise has the added benefit of decreasing depression, fatigue, muscle stiffness, and enhancing subjective well being.[144]

Finally, once the patient has warmed-up and performed the aerobic activity, a 5 to 10 minute cool down should follow. This period allows the heart rate to decrease gradually and offers an opportunity for static stretching and floor exercise. *Static* means hold. This type of stretch involves holding a position for 10 to 30 seconds initially. These stretches should never be forced, painful, or done with a bounce. They are best done after the dynamic stretches in the cool down since a warmer muscle will relax and allow greater stretch to occur. Floor exercises include abdominal strengthening and stretching/strengthening of the postural and lower extremity musculature. Relaxation and breathing techniques may also be practiced at this time. Dyspnea is often accompanied by fear and anxiety. Some studies have reported significant improvement of symptoms with progressive relaxation techniques and yoga.[168]

**Exercise considerations.** Patients are encouraged to exercise 3 or more times per week. They may exercise at whatever time of day they prefer. The important thing is to find that time and make it a part of their life-style.

Clothing: Patients are encouraged to wear clothing that is loose and comfortable. Layers are often suggested so that the patient can remain comfortable as the activity level changes.

Shoes: Shoes are the most important article of clothing. There are all types of shoes and no one kind is right for everyone. Patients are encouraged to take in a pair of their favorite old, worn shoes and get expert advice on the best type for them. The goal is to provide good cushion, good shock absorption, and a neutral position of the foot. An appropriate shoe can prevent strains, sprains, and problems with back, hips, knees, and ankles.

Hats: If it is hot, patients are encouraged to wear a hat with a brim and a space between the top of their head and the hat to release heat. If it is cold, a stocking cap will help hold body heat in so that they will stay warm.

Scarf: A scarf is helpful in environments that are cold, humid, windy, or dusty. It may be worn around the neck and

* Pat Barrett, MDMC pulmonary rehabilitation participant.

then brought up around the mouth and nose when the patient goes out into adverse elements.

It is important to remind pulmonary patients to strive to be their own best friend, their own "favorite Aunt Matilda." We tend to be nicer and more supportive of our best friends and favorite aunts than to ourselves. Our best friend who begins an exercise program following an injury or illness, may be able to only sit up the first day and may be able to take a few steps by that afternoon. The next day "our friend" may be able to walk to the door and in a few days is walking in the hall. We would tend to think that "our friend" has made great progress. "Way to go!" we might say. When this happens to us and we walk out to the hall, we tend to say, "but I used to be able to walk 5 miles."

A previously very active person began PR when he had to drive to his mail box because he was too short of breath to walk. Starting at this baseline, he gradually increased his exercise tolerance until upon completion of the PRP, he was able to walk to the mailbox with less dyspnea, more confidence, and increased self-esteem. We must try to be supportive of ourselves, start at our baseline, and look at each step as progress and small successes on the way to improvement.

**Exercise component.** Much has been written regarding the value* and types† of exercises recommended for pulmonary patients. The clinical benefits of these exercises include: decreased fear of exercise, increased tolerance of dyspnea, better appetite, improved sleep, increased exercise tolerance, and an enhancement of the patient's ability to perform ADLs. We would like to present an example of a possible exercise program.

Before exercise you should remind the pulmonary patients to take the prescribed inhaler or aerosol treatment within two hours of beginning exercise, monitor the heart rate and level of dyspnea, and incorporate breathing techniques.

All exercise sessions must consist of a warm-up, aerobic/endurance phase, and a cool down.

## Sample exercise program
*Warm-up*
   Dynamic Stretching
      *Cervical*
      • Look up-down (nod "yes").*
      • Look left/right (shake "no").*
      • Left ear to left shoulder.*
      *Shoulder and Upper Extremity*
      • Shoulder circles forward.*
      • Shoulder shrugs* (up/relax).
      • Shoulders* (up-back-down).
      • Shoulder blade squeeze—With your hands resting on your shoulders, try to touch your elbows

together in front of your body. Pull them apart. Try to push them backward. Squeeze your shoulder blades together as you push. Breathe IN as you push elbows backward and breathe OUT as you bring elbows together in front.
      • Front arm raises (shoulder flexion)—Lift your arms overhead. Lower them in front of you slowly, as if pushing against resistance. Breathe IN when lifting and OUT when lowering.
      • Side-arm raises (abduction)—Lift your arms out to the side and up over head. Lower back to your sides slowly, as if pushing against resistance. Breathe IN as you lift and breathe OUT as you lower.
      • Arm circles forward*—With your arms fully extended and raised to shoulder level, slowly make small circles with your arms. Reverse. If the patient is extremely short of breath, he or she may lower the arms.
   *Trunk*
      • Trunk rotation* (side to side twists)—Start with your arms extended in front of you and slowly twist to the right and then to the left. Try not to move your hips.
      • Side-bending (right and left)—Reach one arm up over your head and lean to the opposite side. Reverse. Blow OUT as you bend and breathe IN as you straighten.
   *Lower Extremity*
      • Wall slide*—Stand with your hips and buttocks pressed as flat as you can against a wall. Shoulders should be relaxed. Slowly lower your body as if you were going to sit in a chair. Keep your hips above the level of your knees. Hold this position. Try to increase the holding time to at least two minutes.
      • Hip flexion*—Marching in place.
      • Toe tapping.*
   *Gastrocnemius/Soleus Stretch*
   Begin with 2 repetitions each and then increase slowly to 3 to 5 to 7 to 10. Once 10 repetitions of each can be done, a 1-pound weight may be added to the arm exercises. Remember to always breathe "IN" through your nose and "OUT" through pursed lips. Do pursed-lip breathing (PLB) throughout your activity. Do not hold your breath.
Aerobic/Endurance Phase (Fig. 23-14)
      • Walking
      • Stationary bike
      • Treadmill
      • Rowing machine
      • Stairstepper

---

* References 3, 12, 13, 19, 22, 26, 35, 42, 43, 81, 88, 92, 97, 120, 145, 153, 157, 164.
† References 10, 25, 60, 69, 99, 118, 136, 156, 161.

*In the (*) starred activities, the exact breathing pattern is not crucial as long as good PLB techniques are incorporated.

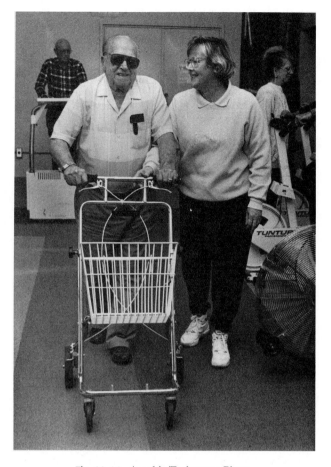

**Fig. 23-14.** Aerobic/Endurance Phase.

- Modified aerobic dance
- Cross-country ski
- Bicycle
- Swimming
- Water aerobics

*Frequency*
- Three or more times per week

*Intensity*
- Target heart rate and/or dyspnea level

*Time*
Individually determined depending on the preprogram test data. The goal is 12 to 30 minutes. Endurance is initially emphasized. Once the goal of 30 minutes has been attained, strengthening activities (i.e., bicycle tension, treadmill grade) may be added.

*Cool Down*
Any exercises from the warm-up phase plus static stretching and strengthening.

*Static Stretches*
Chest stretches (pectoral/corner stretch)—find a corner, bend your elbows and abduct your shoulders to 90°. Use your hands to support yourself as you slowly press your chest into the corner and then return to standing straight. Breathe IN as you lean into the corner and breathe OUT as you return to standing straight.

*Floor Exercises*
- Pelvic tilt.
  Bridges—With your knees bent, press the small of your back against the floor and slowly lift your hips up off the floor and slowly lower. Blow OUT as you lift your hips and breathe IN as you lower your hips.
- Partial sit-ups—keep knees bent, slowly reach for your knees, hold for two counts and slowly lower yourself back down. Only raise your upper back up to your shoulder blade level (curl halfway). Keep eyes and chin up toward the ceiling. Some patients may benefit from cradling their heads with their hands. Do not pull up on neck. Breathe OUT as you come up and breathe IN as you lower.
- Diagonal sit-ups—Same as partial sit-ups, *except,* slowly reach with your extended left hand toward the outside of your right knee, hold for two counts and slowly lower yourself back down. Repeat with your right hand and left knee.
- Leg lifts—Bend one knee and keep the other extended. Lift the extended leg up to the level of your bent knee and lower back down. Blow OUT as you lift your leg and breathe IN as you lower your leg.
- Side leg lifts (abduction).
- Hamstring stretches.
- Diaphragmatic/abdominal breathing—Add 1 to 5 pounds to abdomen for resistance.
- Relaxation exercises—If breathing allows, encourage the patients to lie prone and to remove one or more pillow to lie supine.

**Maintenance exercise program.** Studies have shown that when exercise stops, the effects gained by training are lost.[24,99,112] Thus, the optimal plan for a PRP is to provide a training phase and a maintenance phase. (Fig. 23-15) Various maintenance options should be provided including, an ongoing group program or an individual home program. The important things to consider when designing a maintenance program are to create a program that compliments the individual's personality, physical abilities, interests, opportunities, and environment. The activities should be as varied and easy to do as possible, both in simplicity and expense,[131,134] but should allow for attainment of small but realistic goals, improvement, and most of all some FUN!

Variety in the group program can mean the introduction of free weights, hydraulic weights, modified aerobic dance, use of Theraband/elastic tubing for strengthening, relays of lifting, stair climbing, etc.

### Psychosocial intervention

To optimize the patient's rehabilitation potential, the psychosocial component must be integrated into all aspects of the program.[61,93,98] Patients with pulmonary diseases are often depressed, anxious, angry, and feel a sense of loss,

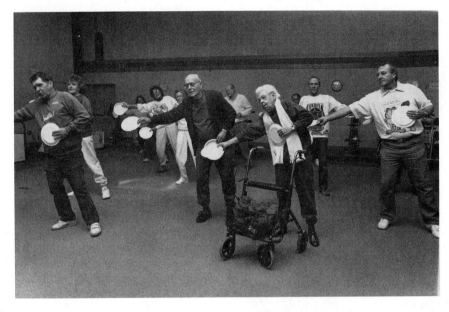

**Fig. 23-15.** Maintenance.

including their sexuality.* These feelings should be acknowledged as understandable. These individuals often look fine to others—no bandages, no swelling (unless you consider the bloat of prednisone or the barrel chest), no stitches, no bleeding, thus they often receive little, if any, acknowledgment for the amount of effort they expend throughout an average day. They may feel resentment when others state that they do not "look" sick, or when they are told "but you look great." One of our patients once stated boldly that she was going to have the statement, "But I Don't Feel Good," placed on her tombstone. When patients are unable to meet their social commitments, their friends may slowly drift away. Our patients have named this the "yo-yo" disease. One day they feel great and make plans and the next day they feel terrible and cancel them. For fear of disappointing themselves and others, they stop planning. Patients become socially isolated. Their lives may have taken a sharp turn from independent to dependent, fast to slow, working to nonworking, and healthy to disabled.

Patients face embarrassing moments such as coughing or having to use inhalers or oxygen in public. They may not be able to debate or argue because of the emotional energy that it involves. Their families have to adapt to their many limitations.[45,147,151,177]

As they share their feelings and experiences throughout the program, patients discover that others have felt the same isolation, experienced a lack of understanding, and felt the resentment and depression. They suddenly feel a sense of relief at learning that others share their problems and frustrations. Some of the structured ways the psychosocial issues can be addressed are through a support group, stress management, panic control, relaxation training[142,152] and individual/family counseling.

Because depression plays a major role in lung disease, it should be evaluated throughout the program. If a psychologist or psychiatrist is on the team, it might be necessary to refer the patient for further evaluation of his or her depression. Otherwise, the patient should be referred to his or her physician for this assessment. Oftentimes psychotropic medications and a referral to a mental health professional are helpful.[73,148] Remember, physical condition and response are directly influenced by these psychosocial impairments.[3,61] As one patient wrote: "Don't waste your breath. . . . A euphemism not perceived the same by all. How much for granted we take this bodily function that once for so many of us came as easy as the wink of an eye."*

### Follow-up

Follow-up activities have become an important component to help maintain the benefits accomplished during the program and to improve patient compliance. These activities often include: group outings (e.g., bowling, picnics, movies, day and overnight trips); newsletter; maintenance exercise; patient volunteers; phone follow-up by staff or volunteers; and monthly education/support groups. Some programs provide a support group for the spouses and significant others.[3,31,141]

### CONCLUSION

Dr. Hodgkin stated that an effective PRP is no longer a luxury but a necessity for lung patients.[4] It should be considered an essential part of the routine treatment of pulmonary disease. PR is not just for patients with COPD, but for others with any type of condition that has potential

---

* References 49, 52, 66, 100, 104, 150, 172.

* Phil Peterson, Mt. Diablo Medical Center pulmonary rehabilitation participant.

pulmonary involvement. It needs to be viewed as preventative care to educate potential smokers and other individuals at high occupational, environmental, or genetic risk. Early intervention helps to slow down the progression of the disease, to maximize the patient's quality of life before it is severely affected, and to reduce health care costs. The earlier PR is initiated, the greater the potential for individual success.

Remember that training or exercise alone does not constitute a PRP. Rather it is comprised of: team assessment, patient training, exercise, psychosocial intervention, and follow-up components. The success and longevity of any program depend on other important factors, which are documentation and reimbursement;[48,59,113] facilities (i.e., convenient parking and access for individuals with disabilities); location (i.e., inpatient, outpatient, and other settings);[47] marketing; group size; and program schedule. Emphasis is on giving the patient the training and information necessary to enable self-responsibility for improving their physical, mental, and spiritual quality of life.

Ideally, the physical therapist would serve as part of a multidisciplinary team. This role, however, could range from a single evaluation to the program director. More important than the role of the therapist is his or her understanding of the pulmonary patient and commitment to the philosophy of PR.

The rewards are immeasurable—team work, the determination, the laughter, the friendship—all evolving one breath at a time.

## DEDICATION

We would like to dedicate this chapter to Jan's dad, Jonald White, who died of lung disease; Lana's mom, Doris Larter, who died of lung cancer; Burton Culley, a PR patient who was special to everyone who came in contact with him; and to all of our patients in Pulmonary Rehabilitation whose determination, humor, and friendship continue to be a constant inspiration to all of us who are privileged to work with them.

## ACKNOWLEDGEMENTS

The following graduates and dedicated volunteers of the Mt. Diablo Medical Center Pulmonary Rehabilitation Program in Concord, Calif., assisted with the completion of this chapter. We wish to thank them for their generous support: Beverly Striplin, Volunteer Coordinator, who spent many hours typing the multiple drafts and references; Marie Van Beveren for her computer assistance; Dave Jenne for copying and collating the drafts; and Ruth Woods and our ROP student, Julius Nichols, for working on the references.

## REFERENCES

1. *Accreditation Manual for Hospitals:* Joint commission for accreditation of hospital organizations, Chicago, 1991.
2. Allen SC and Prior A: What determines whether an elderly patient can use a metered-dose inhaler correctly? *Br Jn Dis Chest* 80:45, 1986.
3. American Association of Cardiovascular and Pulmonary Rehabilitation: *Guidelines for pulmonary rehabilitation programs,* Champaign, Ill, 1993, Human Kinetics.
4. American Association for Respiratory Care: Pulmonary rehabilitation: the next ten years, *AARC Times* 12:54, 1988.
5. American Association for Respiratory Care: Postural drainage therapy. *Respir Care* 36(12):1418, 1991.
6. American Association for Respiratory Care: Smoking cessation resource list, *Respir Care* 1:19, 1991.
7. American Association for Respiratory Care: Exercise testing for evaluation of hypoxemia and/or desaturation, *Respir Care* 37(8):907, 1992.
8. American Association for Respiratory Care: Oxygen therapy in the home or extended care facility, *Respir Care* 37(8):918, 1992.
9. American Association for Respiratory Care: Selection of aerosol delivery device, *Respir Care* 37(8):891, 1992.
10. American College of Sports Medicine position stand: The recommended quantity and quality of exercise for developing and maintaining cardiorespiratory and muscular fitness in healthy adults, *Med Sci Sports Exer* 22:265, 1990.
11. American Lung Association: *Lung Disease Data* p. 7, 1993.
12. American Thoracic Society: Standards for the diagnosis and care of patients with chronic obstructive pulmonary disease (COPD) and asthma, *Am Rev Respir Dis* 136:225, 1987.
13. American Thoracic Society: Position statement on pulmonary rehabilitation, *Am Rev Respir Dis* 124:663, 1981.
14. Angelillo VA: Nutrition and the pulmonary patient. In Hodgkin JF, Connors GL, and Bell CW, editors: *Pulmonary rehabilitation: guidelines to success,* ed 2, Philadelphia, 1992, JB Lippincott.
15. Armitage JM and Williams SJ: Inhaler technique in the elderly, *Age Aging* 124:317, 1988.
16. Audet A, Greenfield S, and Field M: Medical practice guidelines: current activities and future directions, *Ann Intern Med* 113:709, 1990.
17. Axen KV: Nutrition in chronic obstructive pulmonary disease. In Haas F and Axen K, editors: *Pulmonary therapy and rehabilitation,* Baltimore, 1991, Williams & Wilkins.
18. Bartlett EE: Whither patient-centered care? *Pt Educ Counsel* 14:97, 1989.
19. Bass H, Whitcomb JF, and Forman R: Exercise training: therapy for patients with chronic obstructive pulmonary disease, *Chest* 57:116, 1970.
20. Beaumont A, Cockcroft A, and Guz A: A self-paced treadmill walking test for breathless patients, *Thorax* 40:459, 1985.
21. Belman MJ: Ventilatory muscle training in the pulmonary patient, *Respir Ther* p. 23, Sept/Oct 1983.
22. Belman MJ: Exercise in chronic obstructive pulmonary disease, *Clin Chest Med* 7:585, 1986.
23. Belman MJ and Gaesser GA: Exercise training below and above the lactate threshold in the elderly, *Med Sci Sports Exer* 23:562, 1991.
24. Belman MJ and Kendregan BA: Exercise training fails to increase skeletal muscle enzymes in patients with chronic obstructive pulmonary disease, *Am Rev Respir Dis* 123:256, 1981.
25. Belman MJ and Mittman C: Ventilatory muscle training improves exercise capacity in chronic obstructive pulmonary disease patients, *Am Rev Respir Dis* 121: 273, 1980.
26. Belman MJ and Wasserman K: Exercise training and testing in patients with chronic obstructive pulmonary disease. *Basics of Respir Dis* 10:1, 1981.
27. Blue Cross of California: Pulmonary rehabilitation guidelines, *Medicare Bulletin* 224:1, Sept 1987.
28. Borg GAV: Psychophysical bases of perceived exertion, *Med Sci Sports Exer* 14:377, 1982.
29. Breslin EH: Dyspnea-limited response in chronic obstructive pulmonary disease: reduced unsupported arm activities, *Rehab Nur* 17:676, 1992.
30. Breslin EH: The pattern of respiratory muscle recruitment during pursed-lip breathing, *Chest* 101:75, 1992.
31. Burns MR: Social and recreational support of the pulmonary patient. In Hodgkin JE, Connors GL, and Bell CW, editors: *Pulmonary*

*rehabilitation guidelines to success,* ed 2, Philadelphia, 1992, JB Lippincott.

32. Burns MR and others: Pulmonary rehabilitation outcomes, *J Respir Care Pract* 2:25, 1989.

33. Butts JR: Pulmonary rehabilitation through exercise and education, *Respir Ther* 37, Sept/Oct 1981.

34. Callahan M: C.O.P.D. makes a bad first impression, but you'll find wonderful people underneath, *Nurs* 12:67, 1982.

35. Carter R, Coast JR, and Idell S: Exercise training in patients with chronic obstructive pulmonary disease, *Med Sci Sports Exer* 24:281, 1992.

36. Celli BR, Criner GJ, and Rassulo J: Ventilatory muscle recruitment during unsupported arm exercise in normal subjects, *J Appl Physiol* 64:1936, 1988.

37. Celli BR, Rassulo J, and Make BJ: Dyssynchronous breathing during arm but not leg exercise in patients with chronic airflow obstruction, *N Engl J Med* 314:1485, 1986.

38. Center for Disease Control: United States health and prevention profile, National Center for Health Statistics, U.S. Department of Health and Human Services, DHHS Publication No. (PHS) 90-1232, Hyattsville, Md: 210, March, 1990.

39. Center for Disease Control: Monthly vital statistics report, National Center for Health Statistics, Bethesda Md: U.S. Dept of Health and Human Services, Public Health Service, August 28, 1991.

40. Certo C: Chest physical therapy. In Hodgkin JE, Connors GL, and Bell CW, editors: *Pulmonary Rehabilitation Guidelines to Success,* ed 2, Philadelphia, 1992, JB Lippincott.

41. Clausen JP and others: Central and peripheral circulatory changes after training of the arms or legs, *Am J Physiol* 225:675, 1973.

42. Cockcroft AE, Saunders MT, and Berry G: Randomized controlled trial of rehabilitation in chronic respiratory disability, *Thorax* 36:200, 1981.

43. Cockcroft A and others: Psychological changes during a controlled trial of rehabilitation in chronic respiratory disability, *Thorax* 37:413, 1982.

44. Cohen NH: Metered dose inhalers, National Board for Respiratory Care, Inc. *Horizons* 19:1, 1993.

45. Collins LL: COPD and family stress, *Advance* 4(47):14, 1991.

46. Connors GL, Hilling L, and Morris K: Assessment of the pulmonary rehabilitation candidate. In Hodgkin JE, Connors GL, and Bell CW, editors: *Pulmonary rehabilitation guidelines to success,* ed 2, Philadelphia, 1992, JB Lippincott.

47. Connors GL, Shnell-Hobbs S, and Syvertsen WA: Marketing the pulmonary rehabilitation program. In Hodgkin JE, Connors GL, and Bell CW, editors: *Pulmonary rehabilitation guidelines to success,* ed 2, Philadelphia, 1992, JB Lippincott.

48. Connors GL and others: Reimbursement: a determinant of program survival. In Hodgkin JE, Connors GL, and Bell CW, editors: *Pulmonary rehabilitation guidelines to success,* ed 2, Philadelphia, 1992, JB Lippincott.

49. Constain JS, Haas SS, and Salazar-Schicchi J: Sexual aspects of the pulmonary-impaired person. In Haas F and Axen K, editors: *Pulmonary therapy and rehabilitation,* Baltimore, 1991, Williams & Wilkins.

50. Couser JI, Martinez FJ, and Celli BR: Pulmonary rehabilitation that includes arm exercise reduces metabolic and ventilatory requirements for simple arm elevation, *Chest* 103:137, 1993.

51. Criner GJ and Celli BR: Effect of unsupported arm exercise on ventilatory muscle recruitment in patients with severe chronic airflow obstruction, *Am Rev Respir Dis* 138:856, 1988.

52. Curgian LM and Gronkiewicz CA: Enhancing sexual performance in COPD, *Nur Pract* 13:34, 1988.

53. Daughton D and Fix J: Smoking intervention techniques: historical and practical applications. In Hodgkin JE, Connors GL, and Bell CW, editors: *Pulmonary rehabilitation guidelines to success,* ed 2, Philadelphia, 1992, JB Lippincott.

54. Daughton DM and others: Effect of transdermal nicotine delivery as an adjunct to low-intervention smoking cessation therapy. A randomized, placebo-controlled, double-blind study, *Arch Intern Med* 151:749, 1991.

55. Davies CTM and Sargeant AJ: Effects of training on the physiological responses to one- and two-leg work, *Jn Appli Physiol* 38:377, 1975.

56. Dudley DL and others: Psychosocial concomitant to rehabilitation in chronic obstructive pulmonary disease, *Chest* 77:413, 1980.

57. Dunne P: Applying CQI in-home care, *AARC Times* 17:42, 1993.

58. Dwyer MS, Levy RA, and Mewawdes KB: Improving medication compliance through the use of modern dosage forms, *Jn Pharm Tech* p. 166, Jul/Aug 1986.

59. Elkousy NM and others: Outpatient pulmonary rehabilitation: a Medicare fiscal intermediary's viewpoint, *J Cardiopulm Rehab* 11:492, 1988.

60. Ellis B and Ries AL: Upper extremity exercise training in pulmonary rehabilitation, *J Cardiopulm Rehab* 11:227, 1991.

61. Emery CF: Psychosocial considerations among pulmonary patients. In Hodgkin JE, Connors GL, and Bell CW, editors: *Pulmonary rehabilitation guidelines to success,* ed 2, Philadelphia, 1992, JB Lippincott.

62. Epstein S and others: Impact of unsupported arm training (AT) and ventilatory muscle training (VMT) on the metabolic and ventilatory consequences of unsupported arm elevation (UAE) in patients with chronic airflow obstruction, *Am Rev Respir Dis* 143:81A, 1991.

63. Fahrenfort M: Patient emancipation by health education: an impossible goal? *Pt Educ Counsel* 10:25, 1987.

64. Fahyniaz K and Mahler DA: Writing an exercise prescription for patients with COPD, *J Respir Dis* 11:638, 1990.

65. Ferguson GT and Cherniack RM: Management of chronic obstructive pulmonary disease. *New Engl J Med* 328:1017, Apr 1993.

66. Fletcher EC and Martin RJ: Sexual dysfunction and erectile impotence in chronic obstructive pulmonary disease, *Chest* 81:413, 1982.

67. Foster S, Lopez D, and Thomas HM: Pulmonary rehabilitation in COPD patients with elevated $PCO_2$, *Am Rev Respir Dis* 138:1519, 1988.

68. Foster S and Thomas HM: Pulmonary rehabilitation in lung disease other than chronic obstructive pulmonary disease, *Am Rev Respir Dis* 141:601, 1990.

69. Frontera WR and others: Strength conditioning in older men: skeletal muscle hypertrophy and improved function, *J Appl Physiol* 64:1038,1988.

70. Garritan SL: Chest physical treatment of the patient with chronic obstructive pulmonary disease. In Haas F and Axen K, editors: *Pulmonary therapy and rehabilitation,* Baltimore, 1991, Williams & Wilkins.

71. Gibbons M: RRT uses lumberjack background in rehab program, *Advance for respiratory care practitioners,* p. 6, April 1991.

72. Gilmartin ME: Patient and family education, *Clin Chest Med* 7(4):619, 1986.

73. Glaser EM and Dudley DL: Psychosocial rehabilitation and psychopharmacology. In Hodgkin JE and Petty TL, editors: *Chronic obstructive pulmonary disease: Current Concepts,* Philadelphia, 1987, WB Saunders.

74. Goldstein RS and Avendano MA: Candidate evaluation. In Casaburi R and Petty TL, editors: *Principles and practice of pulmonary rehabilitation,* Philadelphia, 1993, WB Saunders.

75. Goldstein SA, Thomashow B, and Askonazi J: Functional changes during nutritional repletion in patients with lung disease, *Clin Chest Med* 7:141, 1986.

76. Green CA: What can patient-health education coordinators learn from their years of compliance research? *Pt Educ Counsel* 10:167, 1987.

77. Guidry GG and George RB: Pulmonary and critical care update. *American college of chest physician,* vol 6, 1990.

78. Hagberg JM and others: Cardiovascular responses of 70- to 79-year-old men and women to exercise training,*J Appl Physiol* 66:2589, 1989.

79. Hall LK: Quality assurance in cardiac and pulmonary rehabilitation, *J Cardiopul Rehab* (editorial), 10:117, 1990.

80. Hess, D: The AARC clinical practice guidelines, *Resp Care* 36:1398, 1991.

81. Hodgkin JE: Exercise testing and training. In Hodgkin JE and Petty TL (editors): *Chronic obstructive pulmonary disease: current concepts,* Philadelphia, 1987, WB Saunders.

82. Hodgkin JE: Pulmonary rehabilitation:structure, components and benefits, *J Cardiopul Rehab* 11:423, 1988.

83. Hodgkin JE: Pulmonary rehabilitation, *Clin Chest Med* 3:447, 1990.

84. Hodgkin JE: Pulmonary rehabilitation: definition and essential components, In Hodgkin JE, Connors GL, and Bell CW, editors: *Pulmonary rehabilitation guidelines to success,* ed 2, Philadelphia, 1992, JB Lippincott.

85. Hodgkin, JE: Pulmonary rehabilitation: Results of the 1993 National Survey, American Association for Respiratory Care 39th Annual Convention, unpublished data, presentation. Nashville, TN, Dec 12, 1993.

86. Hodgkin JE and Litzau KL: Exercise training target heart rates in chronic obstructive pulmonary disease, *Chest* 94:305, 1988.

87. Holden DA and others: The impact of a rehabilitation program on functional status of patients with chronic lung disease, *Respir Care* 35:322, 1990.

88. Holle RH and others: Increased muscle efficiency and sustained benefits in an outpatient community hospital-based pulmonary rehabilitation program, *Chest* 94:1161, 1988.

89. Hopp JW and Gerken CM: Making an educational diagnosis to improve patient education, *Resp Care* 28(11):1456, 1983.

90. Hopp JW, Lee JW, and Hills R: Development and validation of a pulmonary rehabilitation knowledge test, *J Cardiopul Rehab* 8:15, 1989.

91. Hopp JW and Neish CM: patient and family education. In Hodgkin JE, Connors GL, and Bell CW, editors: *Pulmonary rehabilitation guidelines to success,* ed 2, Philadelphia, 1992, JB Lippincott.

92. Hughes RL and Davidson R: Limitations of exercise reconditioning in COLD, *Chest* 83:241, 1983.

93. Inniss P: Psychosocial aspects of pulmonary rehabilitation. In Haas F and Axen K, editors: *Pulmonary therapy and rehabilitation,* Baltimore, 1991, Williams & Wilkins.

94. Jenne J: Pharmacology and use of respiratory medications in obstructive airway diseases. In Hodgkin JE, Connors GL, and Bell CW, editors: *Pulmonary rehabilitation guidelines to success,* ed 2, Philadelphia, 1992, JB Lippincott.

95. Joint Commissions Agenda for Change, characteristics of clinical indicators, *ORB* p. 330, Nov. 1989.

96. Kacmarek RM and VazFragoso CA: Aerosol therapy. In Hodgkin JE, Connors GL, and Bell DW, editors: *Pulmonary rehabilitation guidelines to success,* ed 2, Philadelphia, 1992, JB Lippincott.

97. Kane CS: An interdisciplinary approach to pulmonary rehabilitation, *J Respir Care* 2:16, 1993.

98. Kaplan RM, Eakin EG, and Ries AL: Psychosocial issues in the rehabilitation of patients with chronic obstructive pulmonary disease. In Casaburi R and Petty TL, editors: *Principles and practice of pulmonary rehabilitation,* Philadelphia, 1993, WB Saunders.

99. Keens TG and others: Ventilatory muscle endurance training in normal subjects and patients with cystic fibrosis, *Am Rev Respir Dis* 116:853, 1977.

100. Kieran J and Pjeatt N: No end to love, *American Lung Association Bulletin* December, 1981.

101. King JB: Illness attributes and the health belief model, *Health Educ Q* 3(4):287, 1984.

102. Kirilloff LH and others: Skills of the health team involved in out-of-hospital care of patients with COPD, *Am Rev Respir Dis.* 133:948, 1986.

103. Kochansky M: Pulmonary rehabilitation—more than the name implies, National Board for Respiratory Care, Inc. *Horizons* 18(2):1, 1992.

104. Kravetz HM and Pheatt N: Sexuality in the pulmonary patient. In Hodgkin JE, Connors GL, and Bell CW, editors: *Pulmonary rehabilitation guidelines to success,* ed 2, Philadelphia, 1992, JB Lippincott.

105. Lau RR and Hartman KA: Health as a value: methodological and theoretical considerations, *Health Psychol* 5:25, 1986.

106. Ley P: Cognitive variables in noncompliance, *J Compliance Health Care* 1:171, 1986.

107. Lynn ML and Osborn DP. Deming's quality principles: a health care application. *Hosp Health Serv Admin* 36:1, 1991.

108. Mahler DA: *Dyspnea*, Mt. Kisco, NY, 1990, Futura Publishing Co.

109. Make BJ: Pulmonary rehabilitation: myth or reality? *Clin Chest Med* 4:519, 1986.

110. Make BJ: Pulmonary rehabilitation—what are the outcomes? *Resp Care* 35(4):329, 1990, (editorial).

111. Make BJ: COPD: Management and rehabilitation, *Am Fam Phys* 43(4):1315, 1991.

112. Make BJ and Buckolz J: Exercise training in COPD patients improves cardiac function, *Am Rev Respir Dis* 143:80A, 1991.

113. Mall RW and Chaika-Medeiros M: Reimbursement for a community hospital-based program. In Casaburi R and Petty TL, editors: *Principles and practice of pulmonary rehabilitation,* Philadelphia, 1993:487, WB Saunders.

114. Mall RW and Medeiros M: Objective evaluation of results of a pulmonary rehabilitation program in a community hospital, *Chest* 94:1156, 1988.

115. Mancino JM, Donahoe M, and Rogers RM: Nutritional assessment and therapy. In Casaburi R and Petty TL, editors: *Principles and practice of pulmonary rehabilitation,* Philadelphia, 1993, WB Saunders.

116. Martinez FJ, Couser J, and Celli BR: Factors that determine ventilatory muscle recruitment in patients with chronic airflow obstruction, *Am Rev Respir Dis* 142:276, 1990.

117. Mast ME and VanAtta MJ: Applying adult learning principles in instructional module design, *Nur Educ* 11(1):35, 1986.

118. McCarthy N and others: The effects of strength training in patients with selected neuromuscular disorders, *Med Sci Sports Exer* 20:362, 1988.

119. McSweeny AJ and others: Life quality of patients with chronic obstructive pulmonary disease, *Arch Intern Med* 142:473, 1982.

120. Miller W: Historical perspective of pulmonary rehabilitation. In Hodgkin JE, Connors GL, and Bell CW, editors: *Pulmonary rehabilitation guidelines to success,* ed 2, Philadelphia, 1992, JB Lippincott.

121. Moser KM and others: Results of a comprehensive rehabilitation program: physiologic and functional effects on patients with chronic obstructive pulmonary disease, *Arch Intern Med* 140:1596, 1980.

122. Motley HL: The effects of slow deep breathing on the blood exchange in emphysema, *Am Rev Respir Dis* 88:484, 1963.

123. Mueller RE, Petty TL, and Filley GF: Ventilation and arterial blood gas changes induced by pursed-lip breathing, *J Appl Physiol* 28:784, 1970.

124. National Center for Health Statistics, U.S. Govt. Printing Office, 1990; DHHS Publication No. (PHS)90-1504 (Vital and Health Statistics: Series 10, No. 176).

125. National Center for Health Statistics: Advance report of final mortality statistics, 42(2):6, 1993.

126. Neish CM and Hopp JW: The role of education in pulmonary rehabilitation, *J Cardiopul Rehab* 8(11):439, 1988.

127. Nett LM: Nicotine addiction treatment. In Casaburi R and Petty TL, editors: *Principles and practice of pulmonary rehabilitation,* Philadelphia, 1993, WB Saunders.

128. Niederman MS and others: Benefits of a multidisciplinary pulmonary rehabilitation program, *Chest* 99:798, 1991.

129. Nocturnal Oxygen Therapy Trial Group: Continuous and nocturnal oxygen therapy in hypoxemic chronic obstructive lung disease: a clinical trial, *Am Inter Med* 93:391, 1980.

130. Olopade CO and others: Exercise limitation and pulmonary rehabilitation in chronic obstructive pulmonary disease, *Mayo Clin Proc* 67:144, 1992.

131. Orenstein DM: Cystic fibrosis, *Respir Care* 36(7):746, 1991.

132. Owen RR: Postpolio syndrome and cardiopulmonary conditioning. In Rehabilitation medicine: adding life to years (special issue), *West J Med* 154:557, 1991.

133. Owens MW, Anderson WM, and George RB: Pharmacologic therapy. In Casaburi R, Petty TL, (eds): *Principles and practice of pulmonary rehabilitation*, Philadelphia, 1993, WB Saunders.

134. Paine R and Make BJ: Pulmonary rehabilitation for the elderly, *Clin Geriatr Med* 2:313, 1986.

135. Pardy RL and Leith DE: Ventilatory muscle training, *Respir Care* 29:278, 1984.

136. Pardy RL and others: The effects of inspiratory muscle training on exercise performance in chronic airflow limitation, *Am Rev Respir Dis* 123:426, 1981.

137. Perry JA: Effectiveness of teaching in the rehabilitation of patients with chronic bronchitis and emphysema, *Nurs Res* 30:219, 1987.

138. Petty TL: Pulmonary rehabilitation: Why, who, when, what, and how? *J Respir Dis* 11(2):192, 1990.

139. Punzal PA and others: Maximum intensity exercise training in patients with chronic obstructive pulmonary disease, *Chest* 100:618, 1991.

140. Quality Review Bulletin: Characteristics of Clinical Indicators, *J Quality Assurance,* November 1989.

141. Reisman-Beytas LJ and Connors GL: Organization and management of a pulmonary rehabilitation program. In Hodgkin JE, Connors GL, and Bell CW, editors: *Pulmonary rehabilitation guidelines to success,* ed 2, Philadelphia, JB Lippincott.

142. Renfroe KL: Effect of progressive relaxation on dyspnea and anxiety state in patients with chronic obstructive pulmonary disease, *Heart Lung* 17:408, 1988.

143. Ries AL: Pulmonary Rehabilitation. In Fishman AP, editor: *Pulmonary diseases and disorders,* ed 2. New York, 1988, McGraw-Hill Book Co.

144. Ries AL: Position paper of the American Association of Cardiovascular and Pulmonary Rehabilitation: scientific basis of pulmonary rehabilitation, *J Cardiopulm Rehab* 10:418, 1990.

145. Ries AL and Archibald CJ: Endurance exercise training at maximal targets in patients with chronic obstructive pulmonary disease, *J Cardiopulm Rehab* 7:594, 1987.

146. Ries AL and Moser KM: Comparison of isocapnic hyperventilation and walking exercise training at home in pulmonary rehabilitation, *Chest* 90:285, 1986.

147. Rob C and Reynolds J: *The Caregivers Guide,* Boston 1991, Houghton Mifflin Company.

148. Rodriques JC and Ilowite JS: Pulmonary rehabilitation in the elderly patient, *Clinics in Chest Medicine* 14:429, 1993.

149. Sackner MA and Kim CS: Auxiliary MDI aerosol delivery systems, *Chest* 88(2):161, 1985.

150. Selecky PA: Sexuality and the patient with lung disease. In Casaburi R and Petty TL, editors: *Principles and practice of pulmonary rehabilitation,* Philadelphia 1993:382, WB Saunders.

151. Sexton DL: The supporting cast: wives of COPD patients. *J Geriatr Nurs* 10:82, 1984.

152. Sexton DL and Neureuter A: Relaxation Techniques and Biofeedback. In Haas F and Axen K, editors: *Pulmonary therapy and rehabilitation,* Baltimore, 1991, Williams & Wilkins.

153. Shephard RJ: On the design and effectiveness of training regimens in chronic obstructive lung disease, *Bull Eur Physiopathol Respir* 3:457, 1977.

154. Shim C and Williams, MH Jr.: The adequacy of inhalation of aerosol from canister nebulizer, *Am J Med* 69:891, 1980.

155. Silvestri GA and Mahler DA: Evaluation of dyspnea in the elderly patient, *Clin Chest Med* 14:393, 1993.

156. Simpson K and others: Randomised controlled trial of weight lifting exercise in patients with chronic airflow limitation, *Thorax* 47:70, 1992.

157. Sinclair DJ and Ingram CG: Controlled trial of supervised exercise training in chronic bronchitis, *Br Med J* 1:519, 1980.

158. Smith NA and others: Health beliefs, satisfaction, and compliance, *Pt Educ Counsel* 10:279, 1987.

159. Sobush D, Dunning, III M, and McDonald K: Exercise prescription components for respiratory muscle training: Past, present, and future. *Respir Care* 30:34, 1985.

160. Squires RW and others: Cardiopulmonary exercise testing after unilateral lung transplantation:a case report, *J Cardiopulm Rehab* 11:192, 1991.

161. Stewart K: Resistance training effects on strength and cariovascular endurance in cardiac and coronary prone patients, *Med Sci Sports Exer* 21:678, 1989.

162. Stramford BA and others: Task specific changes in maximal oxygen uptake resulting from arm versus leg training, *Ergonomics* 21:1, 1978.

163. Strijbos JH, Koeter GH, and Meinesz AF: Home care rehabilitation and perception of dyspnea in chronic obstructive pulmonary disease (COPD) patients. *Chest* 97:109s, 1990.

164. Strijbos JH and others: Objective and subjective performance indicators in COPD, *Eur Respir J* 2:666, 1989.

165. Summary second national invitational forum on clinical indicator development, Joint Commission on Accreditation of Health Care Organizations, 1989.

166. Summer W and others: Aerosol bronchodilation delivery methods: Relative impact on pulmonary function and cost of respiratory care, *Arch Intern Med* 149:618, 1989.

167. Swerts PMJ and others: Exercise training as a mediator of increased exercise performance in patients with chronic obstructive pulmonary disease, *J Cardiopulm Rehab* 12:188, 1992.

168. Tandon MK: Adjunct treatment with yoga in chronic severe airway obstruction, *Thorax* 33:514, 1978.

169. Theodore AC and Beer DJ: Pharmacotherapy of chronic obstructive pulmonary disease. In Make BJ, (guest editor): Pulmonary Rehabilitation, *Clin in Chest Med* (4)7 Philadelphia, 1986, WB Saunders.

170. Tiep BL: Pulmonary rehabilitation program organization. In Casaburi R and Petty TL, editors: *Principles and practice of pulmonary rehabilitation,* Philadelphia, 1993:302, WB Saunders.

171. Tiep BL and others: Pursed-lip breathing training using ear oximetry, *Chest* 90:218, 1986.

172. Timms RM: Sexual dysfunction and chronic obstructive pulmonary disease, *Chest* 81:398, 1982.

173. Tobin MJ and others: Response to bronchodilator drug administration by a new reservoir aerosol delivery system and a review of other auxiliary delivery systems, *Am Rev Respir Dis* 126:670, 1982.

174. Tresman K, Kamelhar D, and Meixler: Pharmocological therapy in chronic obstructive pulmonary disease. In Haas F and Axen K, editors: *Pulmonary therapy and rehabilitation.* Baltimore, 1991:144, Williams & Wilkins.

175. US Dept of Health and Human Services. The nicotine dependency program. NIH Pub #89.2961: Part 1, 2 and 3, Oct. 1989.

176. Vale F, Reardon JZ, and Zu Wallack RL: The long-term benefits of outpatient pulmonary rehabilitation on exercise endurance and quality of life, *Chest* 103:42, 1993.

177. Wasow M: Get out of my potato patch: A biased view of death and dying, *Natl Assoc of Soc Workers* 261, 1984.

178. Wooten P: Laughter as therapy for patient and caregiver. In Hodgkin JE, Connors GL, and Bell CW, editors: *Pulmonary rehabilitation guidelines to success,* ed 2, Philadelphia, 1992, JB Lippincott.

179. Zack MB and Palange AV: Oxygen supplemented exercise of ventilatory and nonventilatory muscles in pulmonary rehabilitation, *Chest* 88:669, Nov. 1985.

180. Zack MB and others: Ventilatory and nonventilatory muscle exercise in COPD rehabilitation. *Respir Ther* p. 41, Sept/Oct 1984.

181. Ziment I: Helping asthma patients help themselves, improving treatment compliance among your respiratory patients, *J Respir Dis* 2:1980.

# CHAPTER 24

# Physical Rehabilitation of the Ventilator-Dependent Patient

*Thomas R. Holtackers*

Ventilator dependency is a result of respiratory failure, which itself results from a patient's inability to maintain spontaneous ventilation for normal lung function. Primary causes of respiratory failure include complications of neuromuscular disease, trauma, and cardiopulmonary disease. Rehabilitation of ventilator-dependent patients is often tedious and limited, particularly during the acute stages of respiratory failure. However, rehabilitation programs should be based on the patient's condition, not determined by equipment he or she must use. Limited knowledge and understanding of the equipment may restrict the therapist's involvement with the patient receiving mechanical ventilation. This chapter provides the basis for developing a rehabilitation program for the ventilator-dependent patient.

Patients requiring mechanical ventilation because of respiratory failure are extremely vulnerable to complications. Mechanical ventilation itself may have serious side effects including an increased risk of pulmonary infection and tracheal damage. Positive-pressure ventilation may cause lung tissue damage (barotrauma) and, in the presence of hypovolemia, may decrease the blood pressure and cardiac output.[2] Additional potential problems associated with positive-pressure ventilation include an increase of intracranial pressure (ICP) with a concomitant decrease in cerebral profusion; a decrease of urinary output; changes in ventilation-profusion ratios ($\dot{V}/\dot{Q}$); oxygen toxicity, in the presence of high levels of oxygen; and absorption atelectasis. With chronic lung disease patients who breathe on a "hypoxic drive," bradypnea is also a potential hazard of positive-pressure ventilation. The use of a tracheostomy or endotracheal tube to access the lungs potentiates the increase of the work of breathing and trauma to the trachea. There is always the risk of mechanical and human error that places the patient at risk.[10] Other complications may result from multiple system failure, poor nutrition, psychological depression, poor patient motivation, lack of restful sleep, and lack of mobility.[1] These complications may further compromise the patient's already tenuous condition. A cyclic progression of respiratory failure, mechanical ventilation, complications, and further progression of respiratory failure may occur (Fig. 24-1). This cycle produces a frustrating, difficult situation for the patient and the health care practitioners.

Patients are often mechanically ventilated after trauma or surgery, but most are rapidly weaned from the ventilator and extubated. Although many of these patients require some degree of rehabilitation, the intent of this chapter is to focus on those who require prolonged ventilatory support.

It is often difficult to identify those ventilator patients who will benefit from aggressive rehabilitation. Delays in identification may contribute to the development of complications that inhibit effective rehabilitation.

## GOALS OF REHABILITATION

The ultimate goal of rehabilitation of ventilator-dependent patients is weaning from mechanical ventilation. Since this is not always possible, an alternative goal is to prepare the patient and family to live with ventilatory dependency. Patients who cannot be weaned may require long-term institutional care, though some can be managed

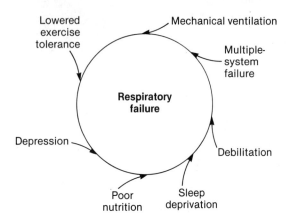

**Fig. 24-1.** A cyclic reaction of acute respiratory failure and mechanical ventilation.

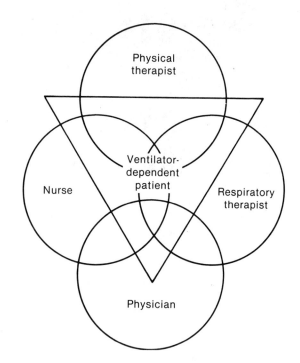

**Fig. 24-2.** Role overlap of health care team caring for the ventilator-dependent patient.

while on mechanical ventilators at home. Family and patient motivation, financial support, disease severity and complications, and the patient's level of physical function are variables that may determine long-term management and the ability to live a relatively independent life with ventilator support.

Some patients are not entirely dependent on mechanical ventilation. They breathe spontaneously during the day when awake but may require periodic or nocturnal mechanical ventilation and "freedom" from the ventilator. This capacity of occasional mechanical ventilation provides the long-term benefits of the maintenance of appropriate levels of arterial carbon dioxide ($Paco_2$), improved oxygenation, increased ability to perform activities of daily living, diminished hospitalization, decreased respiratory symptoms, increased respiratory muscle strength and decreased morbidity and mortality.[6]

## THE REHABILITATION TEAM

Rehabilitation is always a multidisciplinary endeavor. Rehabilitation of the ventilator-dependent patient is no exception. The team may be composed of physical therapists, nurses, occupational and recreational therapists, respiratory therapists, dietitians, social workers, and physicians. The physicians may include critical care specialists, pulmonologists, neurologists, and surgeons during the acute phases of care. Community medicine specialists, pediatricians, psychiatrists, and physiatrists may be involved during the chronic stages. Roles may be specific and structured in some institutions but quite flexible in others. In all cases, the roles should overlap to provide comprehensive teamwork for maximal patient care (Fig. 24-2).

## PATIENT EVALUATION

. The physical therapist's evaluation of the ventilator-dependent patient should include a thorough functional assessment of the patient's cardiac, pulmonary, neurological, and musculoskeletal systems. The therapist must also note

possible multiple system involvement. It is imperative to evaluate each system independently and all systems collectively before, during, and after each encounter with the patient.[5]

## Pulmonary assessment

Arterial blood gas analysis, respiratory muscle function testing, chest radiographs, and auscultation are the major tools for evaluating the respiratory system. Assessment of cough reflex, sputum culture and production, swallowing function, and shoulder girdle-chest wall mobility supplement the therapist's evaluation. The patient's respiratory rate and breathing pattern are also important but are dependent on the mode of mechanical ventilation.

**Arterial blood gases.** Analysis of the partial pressures of arterial oxygen ($Pao_2$) and carbon dioxide ($Paco_2$) provides an expression of the ability of the lung to deliver oxygen to and remove carbon dioxide from the blood. $Pao_2$ indicates oxygen dissolved in the blood plasma but reflects the potential for the amount of oxygen combined with hemoglobin, the main carrier of oxygen to the tissues. The percentage of hemoglobin saturated with oxygen ($Sao_2$) is directly proportional to $Pao_2$ and is described by the oxyhemoglobin dissociation curve. $Pao_2$ is dependent partially on the concentration of inspired oxygen ($Fio_2$), the $Paco_2$, and the barometric pressure (Pb). The partial pressure of carbon dioxide ($Paco_2$) is directly proportional to alveolar ventilation. An increase in $Paco_2$ represents hypoventilation, and a decrease in $Paco_2$ represents hyperventilation. Hypoventilation produces respiratory acidosis, and hyperven-

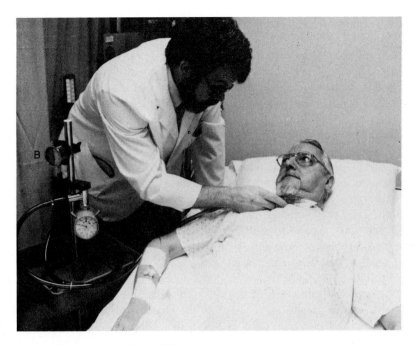

**Fig. 24-3.** Forced vital capacity (FVC) and maximum inspiratory and expiratory pressure measurements can be made with a portable spirometer, *A,* and manometer, *B.*

tilation produces alkalosis. Changes in pH can also be produced with fluctuations of bicarbonate ion ($HCO_3^-$) levels in the arterial blood.[3,11]

There are several methods by which the lungs' ability to add oxygen to arterial blood ($Pa_{O_2}$) can be compared to the $FI_{O_2}$. The alveolar-to-arterial (A-a) oxygen gradient reflects the difference in partial pressures of alveolar oxygen ($PA_{O_2}$) and arterial oxygen $Pa_{O_2}$). The normal A-a gradient when room air is breathed is less than 10 and less than 100 when 100% oxygen is breathed. The A-a oxygen ratio is another expression that compares the $PA_{O_2}$ to $Pa_{O_2}$. The $Pa_{O_2}/FI_{O_2}$ ratio, or P/F ratio, is also used as a comparison but is a less accurate value than the A-a gradient or ratio. The advantage of the P/F ratio is its simplicity of calculation. Increases in the A-a oxygen gradient and decreases in the A-a and P/F ratios indicate the lungs' inability to supply oxygen to the arterial blood.[3,11]

**Respiratory muscle function.** Respiratory muscle strength, endurance, and coordination are three elements of function. Evaluation of respiratory muscle function gives the therapist an indication of the patient's ability to breathe spontaneously.

The ability to produce maximum negative intrathoracic pressure ($PI_{max}$) and maximum positive intrathoracic pressure ($PE_{max}$) reflects inspiratory muscle and expiratory muscle strength, respectively. The $PI_{max}$ and $PE_{max}$ can be measured at the bedside with a portable static pressure manometer (Fig. 24-3). The manometer is easily attached to the endotracheal or tracheostomy tube. The patient is instructed to perform a maximal inspiratory effort from end expiration for $PI_{max}$ measurements, and to perform a

maximal expiratory effort at the end of full inspiratory volume for a $PE_{max}$ measurement. The maneuvers are repeated three or four times, and the best value is recorded. Both measurements are dependent on patient cooperation and effort.[2]

Forced vital capacity (FVC) measures the patient's ability to move the maximum amount of gas into or out of the lungs. Tidal volume ($V_T$) is the measurement of the patient's "normal" inspiratory or expiratory volume. FVC and $V_T$ can be measured at the patient's bedside with a portable spirometer (Fig. 24-3, *A*). The spirometer is attached to the endotracheal or tracheostomy tube, and the patient is instructed to breathe normally. After 10 breaths, the total expired volume is recorded and divided by 10 to establish the tidal volume. The patient is then instructed to breathe in as deeply as possible and to exhale as fully as possible to determine vital capacity. Because of the time and effort needed to measure FVC and $V_T$, the patient may need to be reconnected to the ventilator for short periods of time to prevent fatigue.

Graphs of the patient's $PI_{max}$, $PE_{max}$, FVC, and $V_T$ can indicate trends of improvement or deterioration of respiratory muscle function. When appropriate, these graphs can be an incentive to the patient.

One can evaluate respiratory muscle endurance by having the patient breathe spontaneously or with low ventilator settings that permit spontaneous breathing such as that occurring with intermittent mandatory ventilation (IMV). The length of time the patient can maintain spontaneous breathing without undue distress is one indication of respiratory muscle endurance. Respiratory rate, pulse rate,

ECG response, and arterial blood gases should be monitored during these trials.

Respiratory muscle coordination can be subjectively assessed during spontaneous breathing. Paradoxical chest and abdominal wall movements indicate respiratory muscle dyskinesis or, in the presence of normal accessory muscle function, diaphragm paralysis.

Respiratory muscle function is examined more fully elsewhere in this text.

**Chest radiographs.** Chest radiographs are an important clinical tool for the therapist. During the acute stages of respiratory failure, chest radiographs may be taken daily. Atelectasis, effusions, infiltrates, and pneumothorax can be identified from a radiograph and must be considered in the design and redesign of the physical therapy program.

**Chest assessment.** Auscultation, palpation, and inspection should be performed before each physical therapy session for assessment of the patient's pulmonary status. Changes in breath sounds, adventitious sounds, and chest-wall movement or configuration may indicate acute changes in the lung and may necessitate changes in the physical therapy program. Diminished or absent breath sounds may indicate atelectasis, but they should be corroborated with chest radiograph findings. Rales and rhonchi usually indicate retained secretions. Wheezes commonly indicate broncho-spasm of distal airways and may necessitate bronchodilators. Retention of secretions is often accompanied by decreases in $Pao_2$ and increases in $Paco_2$,[5] and postural drainage with manual techniques is indicated.

### Cardiovascular assessment

Assessment of the patient's cardiovascular status includes determination or estimation of heart rate, arterial blood pressure, electrocardiogram (ECG), pulmonary artery and pulmonary artery wedge pressures, cardiac output, and peripheral circulation. The patient's heart rate, blood pressure, and ECG status should be monitored before, during, and after physical therapy. Abnormalities during or after certain therapeutic procedures may preclude the use of those procedures. For example, a severe cardiac dysrhythmia may prevent the patient from assuming certain postural drainage positions, changes in blood pressure may occur during ambulation, and tachycardia may occur after vigorous exercises. Physiological responses to therapeutic exercise must be monitored and well documented. Pulmonary artery catheters, which measure pulmonary vascular dynamics and cardiac output, are used primarily during the acute stages of respiratory failure to monitor body fluid balance and peripheral vascular perfusion. Patients with poor peripheral circulation—for example, those with atherosclerosis obliterans or diabetes—may have difficulty with ambulatory activities.

### Neuromusculoskeletal evaluation

A thorough assessment of the patient's neurological status, muscular function and strength, and skeletal integrity is an important consideration when one is designing a rehabilitation program and should be included in the care of the ventilator-dependent patient. Emphasis is frequently placed on cardiopulmonary status, but because respiratory failure commonly results from neuromuscular disease, skeletal deformity, and trauma, the neuromusculoskeletal evaluation is imperative. Physical therapists' skills in evaluating and treating these systems should be utilized. The patient's sensory function, including proprioception, reflexes, coordination, and balance, should be assessed when one is developing a therapeutic regimen. Muscle strength and joint range of motion should also be assessed, though the patient's limited physical condition makes this task difficult and sometimes impossible to complete.

## PHYSICAL THERAPY TREATMENT PROGRAM

Weaning from mechanical ventilation and restoration to a maximal functional level of activity is the general goal of the physical therapy program for the ventilator-dependent patient. Specific objectives of the program include maintaining or improving muscle strength and endurance, joint range of motion, chest wall compliance, cardiovascular endurance, and secretion clearance. Other goals may include prevention and treatment of atelectasis and skin breakdown and maintenance of homeostasis. Psychological support and education of the patient and family in self-care and home activities are additional treatment considerations. The treatment program should be dynamic and flexible, responding to the patient's needs as ascertained through a thorough and continuing evaluation. Specific physical therapy procedures may include, but are not limited to, breathing-retraining exercises, postural drainage and manual techniques, range of motion and strengthening exercises, and ambulatory activities.

### Breathing-retraining exercises

The purpose of breathing-retraining exercises for the ventilator-dependent patient is to maintain or improve respiratory muscle endurance, strength, coordination, and rhythmicity. Although breathing-retraining exercises cannot be performed by all patients being mechanically ventilated, they are possible with many. The type and appropriateness of breathing exercise depends on the patient's degree of respiratory failure, associated complications, and the mode of mechanical ventilation.

**Coordination of breathing exercises and mechanical ventilation.** For a better understanding of how breathing-retraining exercises can be used during mechanical ventilation, the types or categories of ventilators, the modes of ventilation, and use of positive end-expiratory pressure (PEEP) should be explained.[4,8]

Following are several ways of categorizing ventilators:

1. Means of power
   a. Electrically driven
   b. Pneumatically driven

2. Mode of pressure delivered
   a. Negative
   b. Positive
3. Method of cycling or limiting breaths
   a. Pressure
   b. Volume
   c. Time
   d. Flow

The form of pressure delivered to the patient by the ventilator may be positive, as with most modern ventilators, or negative, as with earlier forms of ventilators such as iron lungs and cuirass ventilators. The method of powering the ventilator may be either electric or pneumatic. The means of cycling or limiting mechanical breaths may be with either time, pressure, flow, or volume.[8] For example, a ventilator may be categorized as an electrically powered, time-cycled, volume-limited, positive-pressure ventilator. Ventilators can almost be compared to automobiles: they can be powered by several means, they look different and have different features, but they have basically the same function.

Traditionally, there have been four modes of mechanical ventilation: control, assist, assist-control, and intermittent mandatory ventilation (IMV) (Table 24-1). The control mode simply does not "permit" the patient to initiate a ventilator breath, and all the breaths the patient receives are predetermined mechanical breaths. The type of ventilator used will determine the amount of tidal volume the patient receives during control ventilation. Volume-limited ventilators deliver a predetermined volume of gas. The volume of the pressure-limited ventilator's breath is established by a predetermined pressure limit. Basically, the ventilator "controls" the patient's ventilation. Patients requiring the control mode are often paralyzed or heavily sedated and are thus unable to breathe spontaneously.[4,8] Breathing-retraining exercises are usually not performed when this mode of ventilation is employed.

**Table 24-1.** Modes of mechanical ventilation

| | |
|---|---|
| Control | The patient is "guaranteed" a predetermined number of mechanical breaths but is unable or not permitted to initiate a mechanical breath or breathe spontaneously. |
| Assist | The patient is permitted to initiate a mechanical breath but is not guaranteed a predetermined number of mechanical breaths. |
| Assist-control | The patient is guaranteed a predetermined number of mechanical breaths and is permitted to initiate additional mechanical breaths. |
| Intermittent mandatory ventilation (IMV) | The patient is guaranteed a predetermined number of mechanical breaths and permitted to initiate spontaneous breaths through the ventilator. |

With the assist mode the patient "assists" the ventilator by inspiring to initiate a ventilator breath. Once the breath is initiated or "triggered," the ventilator will deliver a mechanical breath. This mode allows the patient to regulate his or her own respiratory rate. The volume of each breath is again determined by the type of ventilator being used.

The assist-control mode provides a preselected number of "control" breaths but permits the patient to "assist" the ventilator to receive additional mechanical breaths. The respiratory rate can vary with patient effort. Since the patient can trigger ventilator-supplied breaths, a lower limit of mechanical breaths is maintained with the control part of the mode.

Intermittent mandatory ventilation (IMV) is similar to the assist-control mode in that the ventilator provides a preselected number of breaths. Additional breaths that the patient initiates are spontaneous and not mechanical. The IMV mode provides an advantage over other modes by permitting the patient to breathe spontaneously during mechanical ventilation. The patient can thus maintain some degree of respiratory muscle endurance and coordination. When the IMV rate is lowered, the patient must initiate a greater number of spontaneous breaths to maintain minute ventilation.[4]

There are several other, less often encountered, mechanical ventilator modalities that have been introduced within the past decade. The newer vogue is referred to as "pressure support." It is used during the spontaneous breath part of an IMV mode of ventilation. During the breath the patient's inspiratory effort receives a little boost from a source of gas under a low pressure of, for instance, 10 cm $H_2O$. Patients may also receive support with continuous positive airway pressure, CPAP, which is basically the same as PEEP, except that the patient breathes spontaneously on a T-piece or through the ventilator on an IMV of 0. This provides support of the airways during exhalation in an attempt to improve oxygenation without higher levels of inspired oxygen. BiPAP is a relatively new mode of ventilation, a method of delivering CPAP during inspiration (IPAP) and during expiration (EPAP) via a nasal mask.[9]

**Diaphragmatic breathing.** Diaphragmatic breathing exercises can be utilized with patients receiving assist, assist-control, and IMV modes. These exercises help maintain proprioception and rhythmicity of the diaphragm and foster abdominal wall relaxation. When patients receive progressively lower IMV rates, diaphragmatic breathing exercises become increasingly more important because of the increased need for spontaneity of breathing. Diaphragmatic breathing exercises are performed by having the patient protrude the abdomen during inspiration as the diaphragm descends. Simultaneously, the abdominal wall must relax to prevent resistance to the excursion of the diaphragm. The patient is instructed to concentrate on diaphragm contractions without accessory respiratory muscle contraction. Placing the patient's hand on the abdomen provides information to the patient about the depth and rate of diaphragm contractions and the degree of abdominal wall tension. The patient should be in a position that promotes abdominal wall relaxation and unrestricted diaphragm excursion. The semisitting or side-lying positions with the hips flexed are optimal positions for encouraging diaphragm contraction in the ventilator-dependent patient. Coaching by the therapist during these exercises is very important. The therapist should initially instruct the patient in diaphragm breathing, but because the patient may require continued coaching while receiving mechanical ventilation, continued reminders from nurses and other health care personnel are imperative. Patients can be instructed in diaphragm breathing for short periods of time while detached from the ventilator; however, most instruction occurs with patients receiving mechanical breaths. Therefore the therapist must coordinate the instruction with the mode of ventilation. Attempts at diaphragmatic breathing with the patient on the assist mode will result in mechanical breaths, but during IMV the attempt at a diaphragmatic breath will result in spontaneous breaths.

**Deep breathing.** Deep-breathing exercises are an attempt to utilize all the inspiratory muscles to produce a maximum sustained breath.[5,7] This type of breathing exercise can be performed during mechanical ventilation, but again it is dependent on the mode of ventilation or the patient's ability to tolerate spontaneous ventilation for short periods of time. The type of ventilator may also determine the effectiveness of deep-breathing exercises. A pressure-limited ventilator will permit the patient to take a deep breath because the breath is limited by the preset pressure limit of the ventilator. With the volume- or time-limited ventilator, the breath is limited by the predetermined volume limit, inspiratory time, and flow rate. Patients receiving IMV can take deep breaths if the IMV rate is not too high. If the rate is high, the short time interval between mechanical breaths may not permit the patient to finish a deep breath before the next ventilator breath automatically occurs. However, some ventilators have synchronized IMV (SIMV), which may permit enough time for a deep breath. The therapist should again be instrumental in instructing and directing the deep-breathing exercises. Unlike diaphragm-breathing exercises, deep breathing need not be performed continuously. A program of 5 to 10 deep breaths, two to three times a day, can be utilized. Measurement of vital capacity with a spirometer at bedside provides a form of biofeedback for the patient and the therapist.

**Segmental breathing.** Segmental breathing emphasizes the expansion of a specific area of the chest wall during a deep breath.[5,7] The anterior-apical and lateral-basilar areas of the chest wall usually move freely with deep inspiratory efforts. The therapist's hands are placed over these areas, unilaterally or bilaterally, and the patient is instructed to inhale deeply, pushing the chest wall up against the pressure provided by the therapist's hands. This manual pressure is not sustained throughout the inspiratory effort but is released gradually as the patient continues with inspiration. A method of "quick release," however, utilizes constant pressure during inspiration with a rapid removal of the pressure at the end of the breath. This technique may facilitate a deeper breath and may locally alter the intrapleural pressure causing expansion of a lung segment. Another method of segmental breathing facilitation is the "quick stretch." A quick stretching of the chest wall at end expiration facilitates a stronger contraction of the accessory muscles in the area stretched, producing a deeper inspiratory effort. The effectiveness of these maneuvers requires excellent patient-therapist coordination. The mode of ventilation and the type of ventilator will also determine the efficacy of these techniques. A pressure-limited ventilator that cycles "off" when a predetermined pressure is reached is the most compatible with these facilitation techniques. The volume-limited or time-limited ventilator permits increased inspiratory efforts and chest wall excursion. However, the volume of each spontaneous breath is limited by the preset volume limit of the ventilator. Patients receiving the IMV mode of ventilation can achieve greater inspiratory volumes during the spontaneous phase of IMV. However, they can receive only the predetermined volume during the mechanical breaths, unless the ventilator is pressure limited. Whichever mode or type of ventilation the patient is receiving, segmental breathing should be attempted. Segmental breathing used with chest wall stretching and inspiratory muscle facilitation techniques will help maintain chest wall compliance and accessory respiratory muscle strength.

**Abdominal breathing.** Abdominal breathing emphasizes active expiration for patients who have paralyzed or extremely weak diaphragms, but with good accessory and abdominal muscle strength. Active expiration utilizes abdominal muscle contraction to increase intraabdominal pressure. This increased pressure "pushes" the diaphragm to an unusually high position in the thorax. When the intraabdominal pressure is reduced, the diaphragm passively "falls" to produce inspiration. The accessory muscles can assist with this inspiratory effort to produce a greater tidal volume. This type of breathing can be performed mechanically with a type of ventilator called a "pneumobelt." Two disadvantages of this type of breathing are that a conscious effort is necessary to breathe and the patient must be in an upright position to provide, using gravity, the maximum excursion of the diaphragm. Patients with paralyzed diaphragms who can effectively use abdominal breathing still require mechanical ventilation during recumbency and sleep.

Abdominal pursed-lip breathing is another form of abdominal breathing, more commonly used for patients with small airway disease, such as emphysema. This type of breathing permits the patient to maintain small airway patency during expiration by producing a controlled resistance at the lips. Pursed-lip breathing is not practical when the patient is intubated or tracheostomized but may be useful during weaning from the ventilator when the patient can breathe spontaneously through the mouth. Some ventilators can mimic pursed-lip breathing by retarding expiration. A valve to increase the resistance in the expiratory circuit of the ventilator can provide the pursed-lip effect.

## Breathing retraining and the "weaning" process

During long-term mechanical ventilation the patient's respiratory muscles lose endurance and strength. These functional losses are attributable, in part, to poor nutrition and weight loss. These respiratory muscle problems occur most commonly in patients ventilated with control, assist, or assist-control modes. Because intermittent mandatory ventilation (IMV) permits the patient to breathe spontaneously between ventilator breaths, loss of respiratory muscle strength and endurance is delayed. Weaning from mechanical ventilation requires that the patient breathe spontaneously with increased respiratory muscle strength and endurance. To increase endurance, the patient receives lower rates with IMV or is removed from mechanical ventilation completely to breathe spontaneously for short periods of time three or four times a day. One should monitor these weaning sessions by arterial blood gas analysis to determine if the patient can maintain adequate ventilation, as indicated by the $Paco_2$. Whichever method of weaning is used for breathing retraining, coaching and observation during weaning are important, both for breathing reeducation and psychological support. Breathing retraining and weaning must be coordinated with other rehabilitation activities. Suctioning and pulmonary hygiene should precede each breathing session to help reduce the amount of retained secretions and thereby reduce the work of breathing. Ambulation should be scheduled around the weaning sessions, but breathing retraining should be reinforced during both activities. Meals, nursing care, rest periods, and respiratory therapy have to be coordinated with weaning.

Weaning from mechanical ventilation can be tedious, time consuming, and frustrating for both the patient and the health care team. Weaning must be approached cautiously with a controlled and coordinated effort, particularly if the patient has been mechanically ventilated for a long time. Haphazard weaning with multiple, rapid attempts and failures produce patient anxiety, frustration, and discouragement.

## Pulmonary hygiene

Pulmonary or bronchial hygiene is the process of removing secretions from the tracheobronchial tree. Cough, mucociliary transport, physical activity, and deep breathing normally provide secretion removal. Impairment of these normal mechanisms promotes the retention of secretions. The predisposition to secretion retention is escalated in the presence of pulmonary disease that produce abnormally large amounts of mucus. Secretion retention impairs alveolar ventilation, promotes atelectasis, and results in reduced arterial oxygenation and increased arterial carbon dioxide. Secretion retention also increases the work of breathing and decreases airway compliance.[3]

Respiratory failure with mechanical ventilation potentiates secretion retention, making pulmonary hygiene an important treatment for ventilator-dependent patients. A comprehensive program of pulmonary hygiene for these patients may include suctioning, postural drainage, manual techniques, aerosolized bronchodilators and mucolytics, ambulation, and adequate hydration.

**Suctioning.** Suctioning for intubated and tracheostomized patients requires sterile technique to prevent contamination of the tracheobronchial tree. To prevent hypoxemia and atelectasis the patient must be well oxygenated and ventilated before and after each pass of the suction catheter. A self-inflating bag with an oxygen source is usually used to hyperventilate the patient, but the ventilator can be adjusted to provide the same results. After the patient is well oxygenated, the sterile catheter is passed through the endotracheal or tracheostomy tube until either a cough reflex is elicited or firm resistance is met. Suction is then applied by placement of the thumb over the suction port of the catheter, and the catheter is gradually withdrawn. The patient is then reoxygenated and hyperventilated. Passing and removing the catheter should take no more than 12 seconds from the time the oxygen is removed until it is reattached. Instillation of 3 to 5 ml of normal saline solution followed by hyperventilation may be necessary if the secretions are thick and tenacious. The suctioning procedure is repeated until the secretions removed by suction are minimal. The frequency of suction depends on the amount of secretions. Suctioning should follow postural drainage and manual techniques and should precede ambulation and breathing retraining.

**Postural (bronchial) drainage.** Postural drainage is positioning of the patient to permit gravity to drain secretions from lung segments.[2,5,7] A specific position is used to drain each lung segment. Because of specific surgery, trauma, or patient intolerance, modification of the suggested drainage position may be necessary. Nursing procedures that include turning and repositioning the patient may help prevent retention of secretions. However, when focal atelectasis or lobar consolidation occurs, a more specific program of postural drainage should be incorporated into the plan of care. Chest radiographs and auscultation are used to determine which lung segments have secretions. The appropriate drainage positions should then be used.

Postural drainage itself, in the absence of manual techniques, is a therapeutic entity. Although commonly accompanied by the manual techniques of chest percussion and vibration, postural drainage can be used alone to assist the drainage of pulmonary secretions. This fact is particularly important when patients cannot tolerate manual techniques or when there is limited access to persons who can provide manual techniques.

**Table 24-2.** A guide to the frequency of postural drainage treatments

| | |
|---|---|
| Daily or bid | General maintenance and prophylaxis |
| tid or qid | Moderate term care (i.e., postoperative linear atelectasis) |
| qid or q4h | Moderately severe retained secretion or lobar atelectasis |
| q2h | Copious amounts of secretion or total lung collapse (this frequency should only be maintained for a short duration [i.e., 12 to 18 hours]) |

The frequency and length of time for postural drainage depends on the amount of secretions, the number of segments to be drained, and the patient's tolerance. A guideline for the frequency of postural drainage is listed in Table 24-2.

The order of drainage for secretions in multiple segments is determined by procedural considerations and the patient's tolerance of certain positions. One suggestion is to drain the most involved segment last and maintain the patient in that drainage position after the treatment session. Another suggestion is to treat the most involved segment first, especially if the patient can tolerate the treatment for only short periods of time. This would ensure that the most involved segment would be effectively treated even though the other segments would receive only minimal drainage during that session.

Patients receiving postural drainage must be monitored during treatment for changes in cardiac rhythm, pulse rate, blood pressure, and respiratory rate. Additional caution must be used with patients who have preexisting cardiac dysrhythmias or vital sign instability. Because several postural drainage positions involve placing the patient in a head-down position, caution must be used with patients who have recent head injuries, life-threatening cardiac dysrhythmias, pulmonary hemorrhage, pulmonary edema, diaphragmatic and hiatal hernias, and gastrointestinal bleeding. When the patient is turned, care must also be taken not to dislodge or remove intravenous catheters, urinary catheters, or any other equipment or monitors attached to the patient.

**Manual techniques.** Chest percussion, vibration, and shaking are manual techniques applied to the chest wall during postural drainage to enhance the removal of pulmonary secretions.[2,5,7]

Chest percussion is performed by alternate striking of the thorax with cupped hands. This is done rapidly and as vigorously as the patient can tolerate to produce a mechanical force that is transmitted to the patient's airways. This force loosens mucus that has collected in the airways. The loosened mucus is drained proximally under the influence of gravity created by placement of the patient in a drainage position. Chest percussion is performed with caution over osteoporotic or fractured ribs, over hematomas, in the presence of bleeding disorders, and near incisions and chest tubes.

Vibration and shaking are performed on the thorax during expiration. Vibration is a finer, more rapid up-and-down motion, whereas shaking is coarser and slower. The same precautions are taken with vibration and shaking as with percussion, but vibration and shaking seem to be better tolerated. Vibration and shaking as facilitation techniques can supplement segmental breathing or can be used with other facilitation techniques such as "quick stretching" and "quick release." A quick stretch of the thorax at the end of expiration after vibration or shaking may facilitate both a stronger contraction of the intercostal muscles and relaxation of their antagonists. In patients with spasticity, a quick stretch will facilitate a reflex contraction of the intercostal and diaphragm muscles thereby producing a greater inspiratory effort. A quick release of manual pressure on the thorax at the end of inspiration "springs" the chest wall, facilitating a deeper breath before the next vibration or shaking cycle. These techniques can be used with patients on volume-limited ventilators, though quick stretch appears to be more effective for the patient on a pressure-limited ventilator.

The major indications for postural drainage and manual techniques are secretions and atelectasis. Patients with impaired mucociliary transport, such as smokers, patients with cystic fibrosis or chronic obstructive lung disease, and patients who have received a general anesthetic, are predisposed to retain secretions and develop atelectasis, particularly if their cough is impaired. Ineffective cough can result from inspiratory-expiratory muscle weakness, and pain can result from thoracic or abdominal surgery or trauma. Respiratory failure may result from any of these problems. Although intubated or tracheostomized and mechanically ventilated, the patient should be encouraged to cough to assist in the mobilization of secretions during suctioning and postural drainage.

**Joint range of motion exercise.** Maintaining joint range of motion (ROM) to prevent contractures is important for any immobilized or paralyzed patient, including those who are ventilator dependent. Joint and muscle contractures that develop could reduce functional activities and ambulation. Proper bed positioning, frequent turning and repositioning, use of splints and footboards, and encouragement of self-care activities supplement ROM exercises in preventing contractures. If contractures exist, it is imperative to stretch the involved joint or muscle.

One of the most difficult problems encountered with ROM exercises for ventilator-dependent patients, especially during the acute stages in intensive care, is the limitation of exercise on extremities with monitoring or life-support equipment attached. Restriction of specific joint movement occurs when intravenous or arterial lines, central venous pressure and pulmonary artery catheters, temporary cardiac pacemakers, traction devices, and renal dialysis cannulas are placed in arteries or veins close to or in a joint (Fig. 24-4).

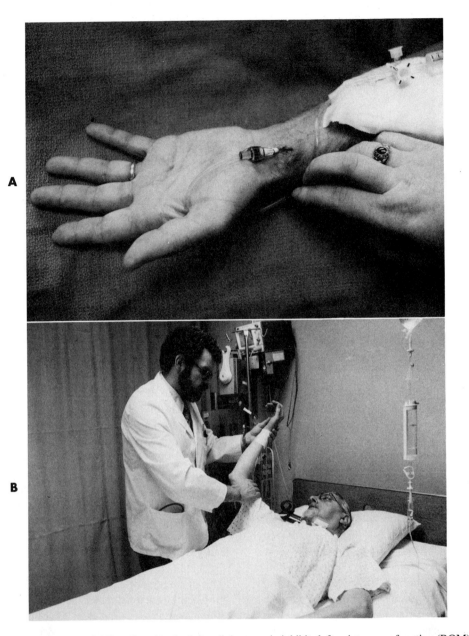

**Fig. 24-4.** An arterial line placed in the left radial artery, **A,** inhibits left wrist range of motion (ROM) but not ROM of other joints, **B.**

In most situations ROM exercises are not recommended for that joint. ROM exercises for other joints are not prohibited unless they change the position of another catheter or line. For example, shoulder elevation beyond 90 degrees may change the position of a transvenous pacemaker or pulmonary artery catheter placed in the basilic vein. Before initiation of ROM exercise, a careful inspection and assessment of the equipment attached to the patient is imperative.

Since active and active-assistive ROM exercises not only maintain or improve joint mobility but also help maintain or improve muscle strength, these exercises should be employed whenever possible.

**Strengthening exercises.** Maintaining or improving the strength of the ventilator-dependent patient is often a focal point of rehabilitation, particularly during the acute stages of respiratory failure. The effects of immobility are paramount and potentiate a multitude of complications, including muscle weakness. With immobility, loss of strength is rapid, but return of strength is slow. Prevention therefore is the best strategy for muscle weakness, and active exercises should be initiated as soon as possible. Manual resistance, isometric, and progressive resistance exercises (PRE) are three methods of maintaining and increasing strength.[7] These exercises are no different for the ventilator patient than they are for other patients, with one exception. Because most patients

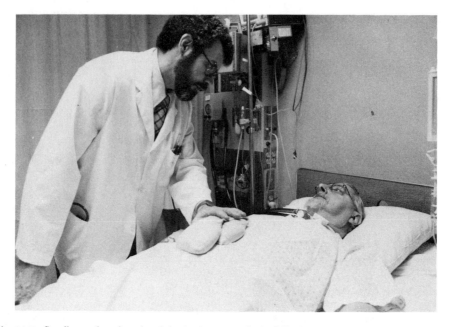

**Fig. 24-5.** Sandbags placed on the abdomen is one method of diaphragm-strengthening exercises for ventilator-dependent patients.

being mechanically ventilated are intubated or tracheostomized, they are unable to perform a Valsalva maneuver. The Valsalva maneuver—expiration against a closed glottis—increases intrathoracic pressure, which stabilizes the thorax during resistive exercise. Although not recommended for extended periods because it causes a decrease in blood pressure, the maneuver provides additional support during initiation of the resisted movement. The patent airway provided by the endotracheal or tracheostomy tube prevents the ventilator patient from closing the glottis, thereby preventing the increase in intrathoracic pressure. Patients may try to reproduce the effect by exhaling against the inspiratory cycle of the ventilator. However, this attempt interferes with the ventilator's normal inspiratory cycle by triggering the high-pressure alarm and "pop-off" valve of the ventilator. This sequence of events may limit the tidal volume delivered to the patient and may precipitously and dangerously increase intrathoracic pressure. This pressure increase is not recommended, and the physical therapist should encourage relaxation of abdominal and thoracic muscles during exercises and must provide longer rest periods between repetitions.

Strengthening the respiratory muscles, especially the diaphragm, may be of particular benefit for the ventilator-dependent patient. The ventilator provides much of the work of breathing previously provided by the respiratory muscles. Prolonged mechanical ventilation combined with weight loss will weaken and diminish the endurance of the diaphragm and other inspiratory muscles. Strengthening of the respiratory muscles must be incorporated into a rehabilitation program when the patient is capable of breathing spontaneously. The same principles of strengthening for skeletal muscles can be applied to respiratory muscles. This means that the respiratory muscles must be resisted during contraction. This has traditionally been accomplished with manual resistance to diaphragmatic excursion, placement of weights on the abdomen, or having the patient breathe with an inspiratory pressure restriction. The therapist can provide resistance by placing his or her hand on the patient's abdomen and manually resisting the excursion of the diaphragm during inspiration. The patient is asked to protrude the abdomen during inspiration, and the therapist can gradually increase the amount of resistance applied to the diaphragm as the patient begins to coordinate breathing with the ventilator's cycle. Abdominal weights can be used in place of manual resistance with increases in weight administered as the patient gains strength (Fig. 24-5). Resistance to inspiration provided by using the ventilator's inspiratory triggering sensitivity can also be effective but requires a thorough understanding of the ventilator. Each method requires much coaching by the therapist. The frequency, number of repetitions, and the amount of resistance must be carefully monitored by the physical therapist. A daily, or twice daily, inspiratory exercise session with three sets of 10 repetitions might be a starting or target regimen for manual resistance or abdominal weight training. Periodic testing of FVC, $V_T$, and $PI_{max}$ provides an objective assessment of the patient's progress (p. 473).

Using the ventilator's inspiratory resistance offers a different regimen of exercise. By decreasing the ventilator's "triggering" sensitivity to inspiration, the patient must create a greater negative pressure to initiate a ventilator breath during the assist or assist-control mode. This increased inspiratory effort can serve as a strengthening exercise. The number of repetitions is initially between 4 and 8, but may be increased as the patient progresses. The pressure needed to trigger the ventilator should also be kept low initially—between 3 and 10 cm $H_2O$ of negative pressure. With assist and assist-control modes of ventilation, this technique provides resistance to the initial excursion of the diaphragm. Once the ventilator is triggered, the remaining work of the breath is provided by the ventilator.

There is no evidence indicating which method of respiratory muscle strengthening is the most successful. Therefore the method of respiratory muscle strengthening used for the ventilator-dependent patient is determined largely by the clinical judgment of the physical therapist, with the condition of the patient and the mode of ventilation influencing the therapist's decision.

**Ambulatory activities.** The effects of immobilization on patients can be devastating. Pulmonary emboli, decubitus ulcers, orthostatic hypotension, and atelectasis are major complications of prolonged bed rest, which is often employed for treatment of acute respiratory failure. However, attempts to improve the patient's mobility should start early in the treatment program for acute respiratory failure. Frequent turning, ROM exercises, and progressive ambulation can help maintain or improve mobility.

The patient should not be permitted to remain in one position for more than 2 hours. Although turning patients is primarily a nursing responsibility, the physical therapist should provide recommendations about the positioning of patients, particularly those with paralysis. Proper positioning will prevent contractures and joint trauma. Proper placement of pillows to support flaccid extremities and to align the spine is a necessary part of the positioning procedure. For patients who are obtunded, paralyzed, or in traction, or are difficult to turn for other reasons, several types of turning beds may be utilized. The Stryker Frame, Foster Frame, and CircOlectric beds permit safe turning but limit the position of the patient to prone and supine. The RotoRest bed permits gradual turning from side to side in a continuous, slow motion.

Progression from sitting to standing to walking is an important aspect in mobilizing ventilator-dependent patients. Despite being mechanically ventilated, patients who are medically and physically able to increase their level of physical activity should have the opportunity to progress at their own rate during rehabilitative activities. The equipment used to support vital functions should not limit the patient's ambulation, but meticulous care is necessary to prevent dislodgement or accidental removal of therapeutic or monitoring machinery. In some cases it takes longer to arrange the equipment to permit ambulation than the time needed to actually have the patient ambulate! Assistance from nurses and respiratory therapists may be necessary to prepare the equipment. The therapist must remember that the equipment does not restrict mobility under most circumstances, but it is the patient's severely debilitated condition that becomes the inhibiting factor in rehabilitation.

The schedule for ambulation sessions must be coordinated with other activities or procedures the patient may need to receive. Generally, pulmonary hygiene, bronchodilator therapy, and endotracheal suction, if needed, should precede the ambulation session. Pulmonary hygiene, especially when provided before ambulation, helps remove secretions from the airways and reduces the work of breathing. Another consideration during ambulation sessions is allowing sitting time. The patient should have an opportunity to sit and rest after each attempt at ambulation. In addition, a "cooling-down" period after the physical therapy treatment may be necessary to permit the patient to recover from the fatigue caused by the physical demands of treatment.

Careful monitoring of the patient's pulse rate, respiratory rate, and blood pressure is imperative before, during, and after each ambulation session. The most likely time of critical changes in respiratory and hemodynamic status is when progressing from one stage of ambulation to another, such as walker to cane. Although there may be many pressures to have the patient walk, the therapist must control the progression of ambulation to ensure the tolerance of one stage before one advances to the next; for example, if the patient cannot tolerate sitting with good balance and stable vital signs, it is doubtful the patient will tolerate standing or walking.

When the patient begins to progress toward walking, a different method of mechanical ventilation must be provided. A portable, lightweight, pneumatically driven ventilator provides a degree of freedom for ambulation. A ventilator such as the Bird Mark VII can be attached to an E-sized cylinder of oxygen. The ventilator and attached oxygen source can be mounted on a walker with wheels (Fig. 24-6) or on a podium type of walker (Fig. 24-7). Intravenous lines and other equipment can be attached to the walker or placed on a portable intravenous-line pole. If the patient is receiving positive end-expiratory pressure (PEEP), portable PEEP valves can be attached to the walker and connected to the expiratory valve of the ventilator. If the patient has chronic obstructive pulmonary disease (COPD) and premature airway collapse, an expiratory retard cap can be added to the expiratory valve of the Bird ventilator. The expiratory retard cap acts similarly to pursed-lip breathing, which may enhance the patient's ability to tolerate the added physical stress of ambulation without becoming dyspneic. A self-inflating anesthesia or breathing bag is another method of ventilatory support while the patient is walking. These bags can also be attached to the E-sized oxygen cylinder on the walker, and the patient can be manually ventilated while walking. This can be a cumbersome task for the therapist, especially if the patient has difficulty ambulating because of weakness, instability, or the amount of equipment necessary.

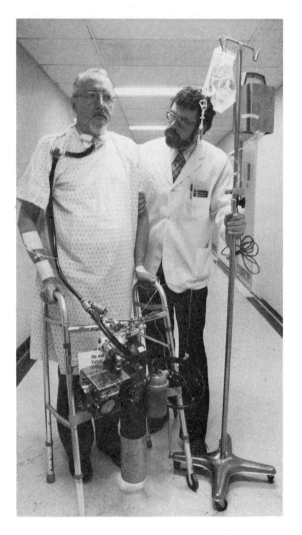

**Fig. 24-6.** Bird Mark VII ventilator attached to an orthopedic walker permits more mobility for the ventilator-dependent patient.

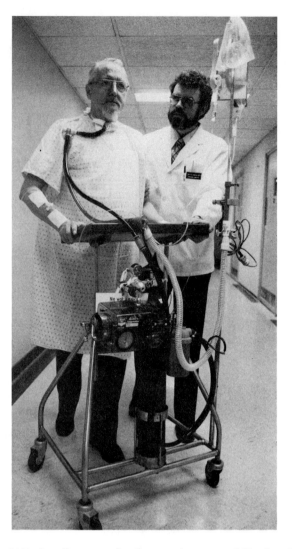

**Fig. 24-7.** A podium type of walker permits more mobility than the orthopedic walker, but it gives less support. Arterial line equipment and intravenous tubes are easily attached to the walker's intravenous tubing pole and, with modification of the ventilator positive end-expiratory pressure (PEEP), can also be used during ambulation.

However, it is an alternative method that can be used when portable ventilators are not available.

One can also increase exercise tolerance by having the patient work with a bicycle ergometer at the bedside. The ergometer enables the patient to exercise in the hospital room while attached to the ventilator. The patient may have some difficulty getting on and off the ergometer, which may necessitate the presence of a therapist to supervise the patient's safety.

Ambulation must be well controlled and coordinated with other patient-care activities to prevent conflicts. Careful interdisciplinary coordination and communication are vital for the patient's well-being, for professional rapport, and for prevention of one activity from interfering with another. The patient's schedule must be flexible to provide for special activities or procedures the patient may be involved in from time to time. One or two specific activities, such as renal dialysis, ambulation, or ventilator

weaning trials, should receive priority depending on the emphasis at that stage of rehabilitation. Some combination activities may be incongruous and injurious when attempted too soon. For instance, ambulation may be sufficiently fatiguing to interfere with subsequent trials of weaning from a ventilator. Decisions must be made to determine which activity should take priority. It may be necessary to temporarily inhibit one effort to permit the progression of another. It is my opinion that patients tolerate ventilator weaning better if they are able to tolerate walking. Hence ambulation should take priority over weaning if there is a conflict or intolerance between the two. However, if the patient is unable to walk but seems to be progressing well with ventilator weaning, the weaning should take priority over ambulation *if* there is a conflict between the two.

**Self-care activities.** Patients in intensive care units receive intensive nursing care that provides all aspects of body hygiene and nutrition. Those who are capable of providing some self-care are often not given the opportunity. These patients will become complacent and dependent on those who are providing their personal care. This dependency may be difficult to overcome despite an improvement in physical condition. Allowing patients to increase their self-care helps them develop a feeling of self-worth and provides some control over their personal environment. Undoubtedly some patients are physically unable to do anything for themselves. However, it is common to see patients being shaved or having their teeth brushed when they are capable of doing those tasks independently. Patients should be encouraged to perform independently, whenever possible, activities of daily living.

**Awareness of environment.** An intensive care unit (ICU) can be an overwhelming and threatening environment for the patient and family. The patient, in a situation of extraordinary need, is removed from the normal home environment, separated from family, and placed in the care of strangers using strange equipment. Intensive care emphasizes a multidisciplinary approach that inundates the patient with different medical and paramedical services. Patients may become confused regarding who is responsible for different phases of their care. To reduce their confusion, one must keep the patient and family informed of the reasons for and goals of the various therapies and equipment being used.

As procedures and equipment are changed, the reasons for the change must be explained. Open and frank communication helps develop a trusting, honest relationship with the patient. Without good communication the patient and family may develop resentment and mistrust, which can undermine the therapeutic effect.

## DISCHARGE PLANNING

Continued mechanical ventilation is occasionally required for the patient after discharge from the hospital. With the increase in technological support available to treat patients with respiratory failure and the increase in caregiver support outside of the hospital, along with the increase in awareness of the independent living needs of the disabled, home care for the ventilator-dependent patient has become feasible for an increasingly large number of patients. In addition, there is an increase in the number of skilled nursing facilities that are more likely to accept ventilator-supported patients. At some institutions, long-term chronic care facilities have been established to meet the demands of ventilator-dependent patients. The dramatic rise in the availability of durable medical equipment (DME) dealers and home-care companies that provide nurses and respiratory therapists specifically trained in ventilator home-care management, along with the increased availability of home-care rehabilitation services, has added to the competent support of the patients at home or in skilled nursing facilities.

Discharge planning, like the rehabilitation process, is always a multidisciplinary effort. The discharge team is usually comprised of the same disciplines involved with the patient's rehabilitation. Discharge planners, social workers, DME vendors, and home-health agency personnel are added to the team as the needs arise. The members of the team must be prepared to work cooperatively and communicate effectively to provide an efficient mechanism to prepare the patient for discharge. This cooperative communication is vital to the development of a secure, emotionally "safe" environment for the patient and his or her significant others.

The discharge planning process could be thought of as beginning when the patient is placed on the ventilator for the first time. Therefore every patient who is mechanically ventilated for any length of time should be considered as being potentially ventilator dependent. When the patient is identified as being appropriate for initiation of the discharge process, preliminary screening may be started by the physician, primary nurse practitioner, or any member of the health care team involved with the patient. A patient may be deemed appropriate if weaning failure has occurred after several attempts and if the patient is medically stable. Emphasis during this early stage is on assessment, goal setting, and continuation of the weaning and rehabilitation process. The patient must be given optimal opportunities to succeed at being weaned during the discharge planning phase. In other words, the rehabilitation process should continue through the discharge process with weaning always the ultimate goal. In many situations the various team members have already been involved to some degree with the long-term care of the patient and need only be advised that discharge planning has begun. A discharge-planning coordinator is made aware of the patient's status and begins the assessment. The patient and family members may also be advised of the return home or discharge to another institution. This "first alert" will permit the various team members to make necessary assessments and inquiries, develop goals, develop a discharge plan based on the patient's needs, and facilitate dialogue with other team members.

Once the initial screening and assessment has occurred, a team conference should be initiated without the patient and family in attendance. During this conference each team member outlines his or her assessment and goals for the patient and then discusses responsibilities, roles, and tasks for each of the team members. In addition, the possible role of the patient and significant others can be determined at that time. With the conclusion of the initial patient care-discharge conference, a well-planned outline of the discharge process, team member responsibility, and projected length of time before discharge should be agreed upon. Additional conferences are scheduled as necessary; the next conference should include the patient and his or her available significant other. These additional conferences should focus on the progress of the patient and possible revisions of the preliminary goals of each of the team members. As future conferences are discussed and planned, other providers, such as DME vendors and home health agency personnel, are introduced at the appropriate times. The roles of the hospital-based care providers and home health providers should be determined before these external agencies are added to the discharge process. Without clear-cut delineation of roles of all care providers, the efficiency of the discharge program can be compromised. The patient's room is not the appropriate place for turf battles and differences of opinion on the ideologies of patient instruction. These "battles" need to take place without the patient getting caught in between the warring factions. Without role delineation and compromise, the patient and others may well become confused as to which way to perform certain tasks and disillusioned with the whole discharge process.

The development of a comprehensive discharge plan is an important part of the discharge process. Each discharge plan has to be individualized to meet the individual patient needs. Each member of the patient care team needs to have his or her own goals that are incorporated into the whole scheme. The discharge plan should include, but not be limited to: patient/significant other involvement; assessment of resources such as emotional and physical environment, financial support, and medical care; support services; a plan of instruction; equipment and supplies; identified goals; and projected schedule of events toward discharge. The plan needs to be comprehensive enough to include an assessment of the patient's physical, emotional, and financial resources, identification of support services and medical care available in the community, long- and short-term goals from all disciplines involved with the discharge, an instructional plan from each of the members of the team, an estimated time of discharge, and documentation of the equipment and supplies needed for the patient.

As the projected time of discharge becomes closer, it is wise to provide home-care equipment while the patient is still in the hospital. For instance, if the patient is going to be ventilated with a ventilator model different from the one being used in the hospital, providing the patient with the home-care model for a period of time before discharge would permit the patient to acclimate to the different ventilator. Discharge from the ICU to a "step-down unit" or a ward in the hospital where patients with ventilators are fairly common can also ease the process and permit acclimation to a more self-reliant environment. It may be a rude awakening to be transferred directly from an ICU environment to a home environment. If an apartment-type setting is available, a predischarge stay gives the patient and his or her caregivers a chance to experience a home-care environment without leaving the hospital.

An important part of discharge planning includes instructing the patient, significant others, and support personnel in the various components of the patient's care. This is a time-consuming process and should be well planned to avoid last-minute rushes that are educationally counterproductive. Each member of the health care team has some instructional function that should be syncronized with the other team members' instructional goals. The efficiency of this process depends on communication through verbal and written documentation. The preinstructional agreement discussed in the nonparticipating patient care conference becomes an important phase in the global process of discharge. Follow-up conferences are needed to keep the process fluid and to directly discuss the patient's progression with the patient and his or her significant others.

The responsibilities of the physical therapist vary, depending on the needs of the patient and the physical therapy goals. The primary responsibility of the physical therapist is the physical and functional assessment of the patient's upper- and lower-extremity strength, coordination, and endurance, the patient's sitting, standing, and walking balance, and the patient's mobility needs, such as wheelchairs or walkers. However, physical therapists may also have input into the pulmonary hygiene procedures, such as postural drainage and manual techniques, that the patient may require at time of discharge. Unfortunately, at many institutions those responsibilities have been "taken over" by nurses and respiratory therapists. It is for that reason that communication among disciplines and delineation of roles are important before the patient is instructed in these techniques and is discharged.

It is imperative that the patient and significant others thoroughly understand and demonstrate proficiency in all techniques and skills necessary for safe and effective living with mechanical ventilation at home. The preparation includes teaching the patient and significant others to maintain and clean the ventilator, tracheostomy tubes, and suctioning equipment. Instruction must also include an explanation of the many different kinds of therapy the patient may require. If patients and significant others are motivated and reasonably skillful and have good financial support, it may be feasible for the patient to be maintained at home. The needs of the patient are many, and if they cannot be adequately met at home, arrangements should be made for discharge to a skilled nursing facility.

The amount of care involved with the activities of daily living and recreation of the discharged ventilator-dependent patient can be extreme. Reinforcement of and instruction in activities demonstrated and explained while the patient is in the ICU become less threatening as the patient and significant others become more proficient at engaging those activities. Usually, significant others must provide pulmonary hygiene (including postural drainage and manual or mechanical techniques and suctioning), care for the patient's ventilator and other equipment, and assistance with ROM exercises, personal hygiene, and ambulatory activities, depending on the patient's status.

The equipment involved with support of the mechanically ventilated patient can be almost overwhelming. The equipment may include, but is not limited to, mechanical ventilator, oxygen source, suction equipment, tracheostomy tubes, cleaning equipment, distilled water, electric wheelchair, hospital bed, urinary catheter supplies, feeding gastrostomy equipment, and various adaptive equipment for activities of daily living. The expense of acquiring equipment is burdensome and the maintenance time-consuming. Social-service agencies can work closely with DME vendors to dispel some the frustration by arranging to have the equipment in the home by the time of the patient's discharge from the hospital. The family can purchase or rent the equipment needed; however, medical equipment companies usually provide for repair of rented equipment more readily than for purchased equipment. Many rental agencies strongly recommend the use of back-up equipment in the home, which increases the expense of renting.

After discharge from the hospital, recheck to visit and follow-up communications maintain a vital link between the discharging institution, the patient, and the support systems providing patient care in the home or the skilled nursing care facility.

## REFERENCES

1. Burton G and others: *Respiratory care,* Philadelphia, 1977, JB Lippincott Co.
2. Bushnell SS: *Respiratory intensive care nursing,* Boston, 1973, Little, Brown & Co. (Morrison ML, editor: ed 2, 1979.)
3. Cherniack R and others: *Respiration in health and disease,* Philadelphia, 1972, WB Saunders Co.
4. Egan D: *Fundamentals of respiratory therapy,* ed 4, St Louis, 1982, Mosby.
5. Frownfelter D: Chest physical therapy and pulmonary rehabilitation, Chicago, 1978, Year Book Medical Publishers, Inc.
6. Hodgkin J and others: *Pulmonary rehabilitation,* Philadelphia, 1993, J.P. Lippincott Co.
7. Kottke F and others: *Krusen's handbook of physical medicine and rehabilitation,* Philadelphia, 1982, WB Saunders Co.
8. McPherson S: *Respiratory therapy equipment,* ed. 4, St Louis, 1989, Mosby.
9. Pierson D and Kacmarek R: *Foundations of respiratory care,* New York, 1992, Churchill Livingstone.
10. Pilbeam S: *Mechanical ventilation,* St Louis, 1992, Mosby.
11. West J: *Respiratory physiology,* Baltimore, 1979, The Williams & Wilkins Co.

# CHAPTER 25

# Physical Therapy for the Neonate With Respiratory Disease

*Linda D. Crane*

It is not uncommon for physical therapists to assess and treat pediatric patients or patients with cardiopulmonary dysfunction. However, when the patient is less than 16 inches long, weighs under 1200 g, is receiving mechanical ventilation, and is attached to an ECG monitor (among other things), many physical therapists suddenly become uncomfortable and unwilling to be involved. The neonatal intensive care unit (NICU) seems to be one step beyond adult and pediatric intensive care units, and when it is first encountered, this setting often strikes fear in the hearts of health care workers. In reality, however, the technology, care delivered, and patient problems typical of a neonatal ICU are not very different from those of other ICUs, except for the size of the average patient (Figs. 25-1 and 25-2). Therapists should also be encouraged by the fact that treating any patient (including neonates) in an ICU setting is likely to be safer than treating patients in most other settings because of the availability of monitoring, emergency equipment, and personnel.

Physical therapists have a role in the NICU. We have a responsibility to recognize both the neonate's physical and developmental problems and the potential contribution of physical therapy to this continuously evolving and very exciting area of health care. Infants have special problems related to their age, stage of development, and size. Even though neonates represent a unique population, many of the same principles of physical therapy management employed for children and adults can be applied safely to this patient group if done with skill and full consideration of their special needs.

This chapter discusses physical therapy management of the neonate with cardiopulmonary dysfunction. Pulmonary problems related to immaturity, neonatal distress and asphyxia, infection, gastroesophageal reflux and medical and surgical procedures are described. The chapter then presents guidelines for assessment and treatment of infants with cardiopulmonary dysfunction with special emphasis on a specific rationale for treatment procedures as they relate to

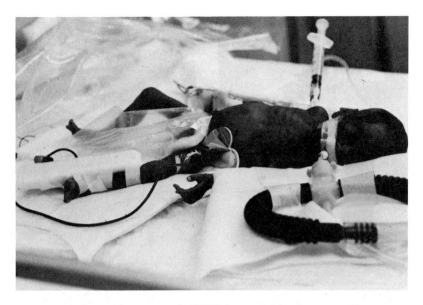

**Fig. 25-1.** Tiny neonate in NICU (neonatal intensive care unit).

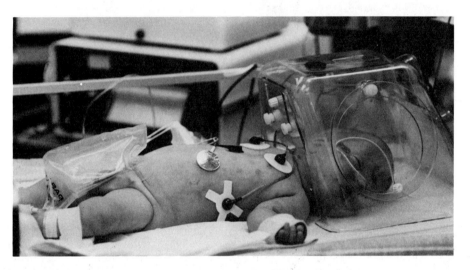

**Fig. 25-2.** Infant in NICU.

physiology and pathophysiology. Finally, this chapter provides guidelines for discharge planning and home programs with emphasis on parent education.

Consider the following examples of "typical" patients in the NICU who may be referred to a physical therapist (p. 488). (The case studies presented in this chapter are hypothetical and are intended to represent infants with problems commonly encountered in the NICU setting.)

## ANATOMICAL AND PHYSIOLOGICAL DIFFERENCES OF NEONATES

Many anatomical and physiological differences exist between infants and older children and adults. These differences increase the infant's vulnerability to respiratory distress, airway obstruction, and respiratory failure.[15,46,62] Furthermore, the structural and functional differences of

premature infants exaggerate their susceptibility to cardiopulmonary problems and medical complications.[46] Some differences are protective and functional in a normal healthy baby but may contribute to problems in a sick or compromised infant.[15,42,50]

*Anatomical differences* that affect cardiopulmonary function in neonates include the following:

1. A *high larynx,* which enables the newborn to breathe and swallow simultaneously up to approximately 3 to 4 months of age.[50] The high laryngeal position and the relatively low resistance of the nasal air passage contribute to the possibility that a neonate could be an obligate nose breather. Any compromise of the dimension of the nasal airway will significantly increase the work of breathing in an obligate nose breather.

---

**CASE 1 ▼ B. L.**

B.L. is a 2-day-old male, admitted to the regional neonatal ICU 30 minutes after birth. B.L. is approximately 30 weeks of gestation by dates and 28 weeks by Dubowitz.[28] B.L.'s mother is 28 years old and has miscarried twice (2 and 5 years ago). Labor was precipitated by premature rupture of the membranes (PROM) 20 hours before B.L.'s birth. Apgar scores were reported as 5 at 1 minute and 8 at 5 minutes. B.L. breathed spontaneously once his mouth and nose were suctioned and almost immediately showed signs of respiratory distress manifested by subcostal retractions, expiratory grunts, and nasal flaring.

B.L.'s condition deteriorated rapidly, and when his arterial blood gases indicated a $Pao_2$ of 30 and $Paco_2$ of 70, he was intubated and placed on continuous positive airway pressure (CPAP) with an $Fio_2$ of 0.4. At 48 hours a ductal murmur, secondary to patent ductus arteriosus (PDA), was detected on auscultation.

---

**CASE 2 ▼ A. C.**

A.C. is a 4200 g female, 24 hours old. She is 43 weeks of gestation, and her Apgar scores were 3 at 1 minute and 9 at 5 minutes. A.C. was meconium stained at birth but gasped before her airways could be suctioned. Several milliliters of meconium-stained fluid were eventually suctioned from the nose, mouth, pharynx, and trachea. A.C. demonstrated severe substernal and intercostal retractions within 12 hours of birth. Her $Pao_2$ was 28 mm Hg, $Paco_2$ 22 mm Hg, and respiratory rate 72. A.C. was placed under an oxygen hood and received 50% oxygen. A.C.'s chest radiograph at 24 hours showed hyperinflation and streaky atelectasis. A.C. developed hypercapnia and required intubation and mechanical ventilation with high positive pressures (30 cm $H_2O$). At 36 hours A.C. developed a left pneumothorax requiring surgical insertion of a chest tube.

---

2. Lymphatic tissue may be enlarged in the small infant and may contribute to upper airway obstruction.[42]

3. The full-term infant has approximately one twentieth the alveolar surface area of an adult.[42] Alveolar multiplication is rapid during the first year of life and continues to approximately 8 years of age.[78] The capacity of infants to increase alveoli is *protective*. In contrast to this postnatal alveolar growth, the formation of conducting airways is complete by 16 weeks of gestation.[63] Airway diameter and structural support are reduced in infants and children, and so the chances of airway obstruction and collapse are increased.

4. Channels for collateral ventilation in the lungs (pores of Kohn and Lambert's canals) are found in small numbers in the lungs of newborns.[63] Although little is known about these structures, an observation that the right middle and right upper lobes (RML and RUL) have fewer collateral channels may be associated with the increased incidence of RML and RUL atelectasis in neonates.

5. Rib cage configuration is circular in the horizontal plane in the infant. The diaphragm's angle of insertion is horizontal so that when it is combined with the horizontal and more cartilaginous rib cage, there is less efficiency of ventilation and more distortion in the chest wall shape.[21,49,62]

*Physiological differences* affecting cardiopulmonary function include the following:

1. Decreased compliance (or distensibility) of the neonate's lungs. Normal full-term infants demonstrate increases in lung compliance in the first week of life.[73] Low compliance means that greater inflation pressures must be generated to maintain lung volume and infants must work harder to ventilate their lungs. This problem is exacerbated when surfactant is deficient and alveoli are maintained at lower volumes (decreased functional residual capacity, FRC), as commonly occurs in several neonatal diseases.

2. Neonates normally exhibit irregular respiratory patterns (the more immature the infant, the more irregular the breathing pattern).[73] Apnea, occurring for long enough periods of time to produce bradycardia (probably secondary to hypoxemia), is considered serious.[74] Apnea is commonly seen in infants distressed by intraventricular cerebral hemorrhage and sepsis. Reduced apnea in the *prone* position in premature infants may result from greater ventilation and improved oxygenation.[22,56,84]

3. Neonates compensate for respiratory difficulties by increasing the rate rather than the depth of ventilation.[24]

**Table 25-1.** Factors contributing to pulmonary dysfunction in the premature infant

| Anatomical | Physiological |
|---|---|
| Capillary beds not well developed before 26 weeks gestation | Increased pulmonary vascular resistance leading to right-to-left shunting |
| Type II alveolar cells and surfactant production not mature until 35 weeks of gestation | |
| Elastic properties of lung not well developed | Decreased lung compliance |
| Lung "space" decreased by relative size of the heart and abdominal distention | |
| Type I, high-oxidative fibers compose only 10% to 20% of diaphragm muscle | Diaphragmatic fatigue; respiratory failure |
| Highly vascular subependymal germinal matrix not resorbed until 35 weeks of gestation increasing the vulnerability of the infant to hemorrhage | Decreased or absent cough and gag reflexes; apnea |
| Lack of fatty insulation and high surface area to body-weight ratio | Hypothermia and increased oxygen consumption |

4. Newborns sleep up to 20 hours per day and may spend up to 80% of sleep in rapid eye movement (REM) sleep (as compared with 20% REM sleep in adults).[62] There is greatly increased work of breathing during REM sleep secondary to decreased postural muscle (and therefore intercostal muscle) tone, which causes the upper rib cage to move inward as the diaphragm contracts.[62] Work of breathing is further increased because of a 30% reduction in FRC during REM sleep.[41]

5. The diaphragm of the neonate has a reduced percentage (approximately 25% as compared with 50% in an adult) of type I, red, slow-twitch, fatigue-resistant, and high-oxidative muscle fibers.[62] The diaphragm of a premature infant may have as little as 10% type I muscle fibers. The lack of oxidative fibers in the diaphragm increases the susceptibility of infants to respiratory muscle fatigue.[21]

## PATIENT PROBLEMS

Newborns in a neonatal intensive care unit present with and develop a myriad of problems related to immaturity, postmaturity, adverse prenatal or postnatal events, congenital defects, and iatrogenic complications. Although many problems of the neonate are interrelated, this section briefly addresses only those problems that primarily or secondarily affect the cardiopulmonary systems. Medical complications of cardiopulmonary problems and their management, which are important for the physical therapist to recognize and incorporate in a problem-solving approach to managing sick neonates, are also discussed.

### Pulmonary problems secondary to immaturity

The premature infant and small-for-gestational-age (SGA) baby often develop pulmonary problems. Factors contributing to the normal newborn's susceptibility to airway obstruction and respiratory failure have been dis-

cussed. The tiny premature baby's vulnerability is compounded by the addition of several anatomic and physiological factors (Table 25-1).

The most common pulmonary disorder of the newborn is called the "idiopathic respiratory distress syndrome" (IRDS). IRDS, also called "hyaline membrane disease" (HMD), is characterized by alveolar collapse because of a deficiency of surfactant. Surfactant, composed of phospholipids and protein, is produced by type II alveolar epithelial cells and reduces surface tension of the fluid lining of alveoli.[31,42,85] Maturity of the surfactant system occurs at about 35 weeks of gestation. Therefore the risk of IRDS increases as the gestational age of the premature baby decreases. IRDS is also associated with several other factors that decrease surfactant production including (1) cesarean section, (2) maternal diabetes, (3) perinatal asphyxia, and (4) being the second born of twins.[28,74] Although the mechanisms are not completely understood, hypoxia and acidosis also contribute to surfactant deficiency.

Clinical signs and symptoms—including tachypnea, intercostal and sternal retractions, flaring of nasal alae, and expiratory grunting—usually appear within 2 to 3 hours after birth.[31] Pulmonary status deteriorates within 24 to 48 hours. Mortality usually occurs within, and recovery occurs after, 72 hours from birth.[28] If mechanical ventilation is required, the course of the disease is often prolonged and the incidence of complications is increased because of both the severity of the disease and the consequences of intubation and assisted ventilation.[65]

Treatment of infants with IRDS is supportive and generally includes adequate oxygenation, (to maintain cell metabolism), nutrition, thermal regulation, and often some type of continuous positive airway pressure.[28,74,85] Intratracheal administration of surfactant has been under clinical trials for the last decade. Intratracheal administration of surfactant (bovine, porcine, human amniotic, and artificial) in premature infants with HMD indicates favorable outcomes. The reported effects of surfactant therapy include improved oxygenation, decreased requirements for ventilatory support, decreased incidence of pulmonary airleaks and decreased mortality.[16,35,37,67,91]

Bronchial drainage techniques are advocated in the literature for infants with IRDS.[18,24,29,58] Bronchial drainage is appropriate for treatment of airway clearance problems and prevention of pneumonia, atelectasis, and other complications of IRDS and its management.[18,71] The application of these techniques, as well as developmental therapeutic interventions, must be done judiciously after carefully weighing the risk-benefit considerations so as not to compromise oxygenation unnecessarily.

## Pulmonary problems secondary to neonatal distress and asphyxia

The *meconium-aspiration syndrome* (MAS) occurs in approximately 5%[89,90] of infants who are meconium stained at birth. Meconium, the dark, "sticky," fecal material that accumulates in utero, is passed in approximately 10% to 20% of all deliveries,[52] especially when the fetus is at term or past term.[4,89] SGA infants and infants who are in breech position are also at risk for MAS.[2] Once meconium is passed, the neonate is at risk for aspirating this substance, which can cause symptoms of chemical pneumonitis and airway obstruction within 12 to 24 hours after birth.[74] Passage of meconium and its aspiration are almost invariably associated with fetal hypoxia and often fetal distress and intrapartum asphyxia.[4,36,52,74] Gregory and coworkers[36] found that the presence of meconium in the trachea does not necessarily result in MAS. The incidence of MAS has decreased since intrapartum oropharyngeal suctioning and immediate postnatal intubation and direct tracheal suctioning of meconium-stained neonates has been performed routinely.[4,77,89,90] The prevention of MAS by early suctioning has been controversial,[27,89] but the current literature supports this practice in all meconium-stained neonates.[89,90]

MAS characteristically causes partial airway obstruction with a "ball-valve" effect that causes hyperaeration of the lungs. Hyperaeration may result in pneumothorax or pneumomediastinum. Airway obstruction also contributes to right to left cardiopulmonary shunting, with resultant hypoxemia and hypercapnia (increased $Paco_2$). Persistance of fetal circulation (PFC), or persistent pulmonary hypertension, is also occasionally associated with MAS.[74]

Once respiratory distress is manifested secondary to MAS, the treatment is supportive. In severe MAS that doesn't respond to conventional oxygenation and mechanical ventilation, extracorporeal membrane oxygenation (ECMO) is being used effectively as a lifesaving therapy.[3] Gregory and coworkers[36] advocated postural drainage and "thoracic physical therapy" for the first 8 hours of life if the infant was born through particulate, "pea-soup" meconium and meconium was suctioned from the trachea, or if the chest radiograph was consistent with meconium aspiration.

*Central nervous system damage* secondary to perinatal asphyxia can result in severe pulmonary problems often characterized by hypoventilation and poor airway clearance. Perinatal asphyxia may be caused by a variety of circumstances and events including, but not limited to, umbilical cord compression, maternal placenta previa and abruptio placentae, placental insufficiency, excessive maternal anesthesia and analgesia, bilateral choanal atresia (imperforate nares), tracheal web, and diaphragmatic hernia. The infant's failure to breathe at birth is attributable to suppression of intrinsic central nervous system mechanisms secondary to acidemia, hypoxemia, and drugs.[74]

Indicators of fetal status (fetal heart rate and scalp blood gases) may be monitored during labor and delivery. Approximately 1% to 2% of all deliveries result in an infant with severe resuscitation problems. Low Apgar scores are useful in documenting a problem at 1 minute and are predictive of possible neurological damage at 5 minutes. The kidneys and brain may be damaged as a result of shock and hypoxemia secondary to asphyxia. Severe hypoglycemia and hypocalcemia are frequently associated with perinatal asphyxia. Initial muscular flaccidity with subsequent seizures and respiratory depression are most likely the result of significant central nervous system damage.[74] IRDS and aspiration syndromes are common complications in asphyxiated newborns. Other common complications of neonatal asphyxia include depressed cough, gag, and sneeze reflexes and defective swallowing mechanisms. These deficits, along with frequent episodes of hypoventilation, put the infant at great risk of developing pulmonary infection, atelectasis, airway obstruction, and respiratory failure.

## Respiratory complications of gastroesophageal reflux

Gastroesophageal reflux (GER) is the retrograde entry of acidic gastric contents into the esophagus most likely related to an incompetent sphincter and delayed gastric emptying.[44] GER is very common with the highest incidence in premature infants and within the first year of life.[43,44,81] GER in neonates and children has been associated with a number of respiratory problems including apnea, asthma, recurrent pneumonia, near-miss sudden infant death syndrome, bronchopulmonary dysplasia and chronic pulmonary disease (including cystic fibrosis).[38,43,44,81]

Not all GER results in respiratory symptoms, and reflux-related symptoms are less common in premature infants less than 39 weeks gestation. The duration of reflux during sleep appears to be associated with worsening of respiratory symptoms. Esophageal pH monitoring helps with the diagnosis of GER.[38,43]

The relationship of GER and respiratory symptoms is still unclear, especially since many infants and children have GER but do not have the symptoms. Three theories of the mechanism of how GER may precipitate respiratory symptoms include: (1) reflex constriction of the airways and larynx secondary to acidic stimulation of esophageal receptors; (2) direct stimulation of bronchospasm due to aspiration of reflux material and (3) GER may increase vagal tone. The good news is that GER is treatable by dietary, pharmacological and surgical means.[44,80]

The incidence of GER has been shown to be increased in three groups of infants who were treated with bronchial drainage (postural drainage, percussion, vibration, and cough stimulation by abdominal compression or manual tracheal pressure) treatments three hours after feeding. The three groups represented normal controls, infants with emesis, and infants with acute pulmonary disease. The increased incidence of GER was not associated with the cough stimulation phase of the treatment.[80]

### Pulmonary problems secondary to surgery

Respiratory complications of general anesthesia and incisions in the thorax or upper abdomen are well documented.[6,9,79] Infants are believed to have decreased sensitivity to pain or decreased nervous system irritability.[75] This postulated imperception of pain may help prevent postoperative pulmonary complications in infants if there are no other complicating factors. A literature search revealed no studies that measured the incidence of postoperative pulmonary complications in this age group. My clinical experience is that if the infant requires prolonged intubation and mechanical ventilation (greater than 24 hours) and is compromised by either preexisting lung lesions, central nervous system depression, general immobility, or other factors, the infant is very susceptible to pulmonary complications after surgery. The addition of chest physical therapy to the care of these infants may reduce the incidence of postoperative pulmonary complications.[34]

The mechanisms of postoperative pulmonary complications are described in detail in Chapter 20. Some common congenital abnormalities requiring surgical repair are discussed below:

*Diaphragmatic hernia* is a defect of the posterior diaphragm where abdominal contents may herniate into the chest cavity.[48,74] The result is a hypoplastic lung on the affected side (usually the left).[48] A neonate with this defect exhibits respiratory distress at birth and requires immediate surgical intervention, usually by an abdominal approach.[48] Because the abdomen may be too small to contain the gut, closure of the abdominal wall may be delayed to avoid tension on the diaphragm.[74]

*Esophageal atresia and tracheoesophageal (TE) fistulas* are suspected in infants whose feeding results in excessive saliva, respiratory distress, and choking.[48,74] There are several variations in these anomalies, with the most common being esophageal atresia and a fistula between the distal esophagus and the trachea at a point above the carina. Surgical repair of these anomalies is commonly accomplished retropleurally through a right thoracotomy incision.[74] Aspiration pneumonia is common in infants with esophageal atresia and TE fistula. The survival rate in

uncomplicated cases is 90%. Surgical repair in infants at risk may proceed in stages, starting with a gastrostomy to provide for adequate nutrition.[74] Swallowing may be impaired in infants who have had these surgical procedures. Dyskinesia of the distal esophagus, uncoordinated peristalsis, and gastroesophageal reflux may also occur.[74]

Many other surgical procedures involving the thorax and abdomen may be necessary in neonates with specific abnormalities. Some of the more common abnormalities are congenital lobar emphysema, necrotizing enterocolitis, Hirschsprung's enterocolitis, meconium ileus, and congenital heart defects.

### Respiratory problems consequent to neonatal ICU management

*Bronchopulmonary dysplasia* (BPD) is commonly associated with the use of mechanical ventilation with positive pressure and oxygen therapy in premature infants with IRDS.[47,65,74,88] Bronchopulmonary dysplasia is a form of chronic obstructive lung disease and was first described by Northway and others[65] in 1967. There is controversy regarding the exact cause of BPD[47]; however, all descriptions indicate that this syndrome is iatrogenic. Improved care in the neonatal intensive care nursery has been associated with decreased severity of BPD.[5,11]

The disease progresses from an acute stage, in which the pathological condition is indistinguishable from IRDS, through three additional stages, to a chronic stage with atelectasis, emphysema, and cystic changes.[65] Onset of bronchopulmonary dysplasia often occurs within the first few days of life with symptomatic and pathological progression continuing until approximately 1 month. Survivors of this disease usually require long-term follow-up care because of both the slow process of weaning from supplemental oxygen and the high incidence of recurrent pulmonary infection.[34,47,83] Lengthy hospitalizations during the critical first months of life and complex programs of home care are often necessary for infants with BPD (Fig. 25-3). Studies that are just recently becoming available on the long-term "outcome" for children with BPD show variable results. Infants with mild to intermediate chronic lung disease appear to have pulmonary function that approaches normal by 3 years of age.[32] Conversely, infants with severe BPD have more variable and generally abnormal pulmonary function into childhood and adulthood.[10,11] Surfactant-treated infants appear to have less severe and prolonged abnormal pulmonary function.[11]

Some common complications and consequences of BPD include pulmonary hypertension and right-sided heart failure, frequent lower respiratory tract infections, poor growth, increased oxygen consumption, and complex emotional and behavioral problems.[82,83,87]

*Mikity-Wilson syndrome* (MW), or pulmonary dysmaturity, is often confused with BPD because its radiographic and clinical course is comparable.[47] The Mikity-Wilson syn-

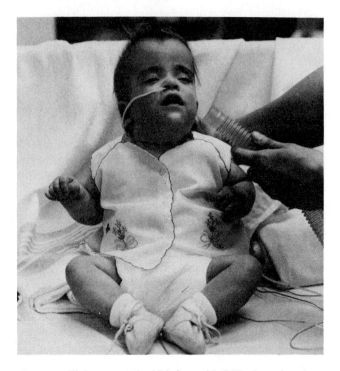

**Fig. 25-3.** Eighteen-month-old infant with BPD (bronchopulmonary dysplasia).

drome is a separate entity of unknown cause that occurs in very premature infants and has not been directly associated with oxygen or ventilator therapy.[47,88] The pathogenesis of the Mikity-Wilson syndrome is now believed to be associated with unequal distribution of ventilation in the immature lung.[47,88] The problem with this hypothesis is that not every premature neonate develops this syndrome.

*Subglottic and bronchial stenosis* is associated with prolonged intubation and frequent endotracheal suctioning in some infants.[64,74] Subglottic narrowing can result in mild or pronounced upper airway obstruction. This problem often results in inspiratory stridor and may require tracheostomy until the infant grows. Once the diameter of the upper airway increases sufficiently to allow for adequate ventilation, the tracheostomy will be removed.

*Iatrogenic infection* is not uncommon in any area of a hospital. A newborn's deficient immune system usually means that most infections in a newborn are systemic. Signs and symptoms of systemic infection are varied and often nonspecific and can include apnea, cyanosis, bradycardia, retractions, vomiting, difficulty feeding, and unstable temperature. Prevention is best accomplished by frequent and effective handwashing and isolation of infants with identified pathogens (especially gram-negative organisms).

### Problems secondary to maternal substance abuse

The problem of substance abuse in the United States continues to grow and has severe implications if the user is pregnant. Approximately 400,000 infants are born each year to drug-using women who have been exposed to heroin, methadone, cocaine, amphetamines, PCP, and marijuana.[45] The incidence of infants born to mothers who abuse alcohol, the most abused drug in the United States, is approximately 3 in 1000 births.[68]

Some of the effects of fetal exposure to drugs and alcohol, which potentially could lead to cardiorespiratory problems, include neurological abnormalities (including hypotonia) with fetal alcohol syndrome (FAS); vasoconstriction (leading to fetal hypoxia and prematurity) with exposure to cocaine; and respiratory distress and CNS disturbances with neonatal abstinence syndrome (NAS) with exposure to opiates. In general, infants born to drug-abusing mothers are at risk for infections (e.g., AIDS) and developmental delay.[45]

### Patient problems that complicate management

Neonates and premature infants are prone to develop respiratory distress and pulmonary dysfunction. These infants are also susceptible to other complications of immaturity and neonatal ICU management. Many of these complications affect the subsequent management of the infant, especially chest physical therapy.

The most common of these problematic complications are described briefly below. How these problems affect physical therapy assessment and treatment is discussed later in this chapter.

*Pneumothorax, pneumomediastinum,* and *pneumopericardium* occur frequently in tiny infants with poorly compliant lungs, who require positive-pressure ventilation. Pneumomediastinum is often inconsequential and requires no specific therapy.[74] Pneumopericardium often occurs in association with pneumothorax and pneumomediastinum and can be serious if sufficient air collects in the pericardial sac to cause cardiac tamponade (pressure on the major vessels entering and leaving the heart). Tension pneumothoraces increase pressure in the intrapleural space resulting in decreased cardiac output, mediastinal shift to the contralateral hemithorax, and rapid clinical deterioration of the infant. Emergency treatment usually consists of insertion of a sterile needle into the pleural space to remove air. When the infant's condition improves, one or more chest tubes are surgically inserted to remove the pleural air.[47]

*Hypothermia* is a common problem of premature and sick neonates. Thermal regulation of the infant is extremely important because infants have a high surface area-to-body weight ratio, poor vasomotor control, and poor fat insulation to help protect them against hypothermia.[74] The neutral thermal temperature zone (NTTZ) is the environmental temperature at which oxygen consumption is minimized. Temperatures above and below the neutral thermal temperature zone increase oxygen consumption.[74] Hypothermia is associated with apnea, hypoxemia, metabolic acidosis, and, if it continues over time, poor weight gain and hypoglyce-

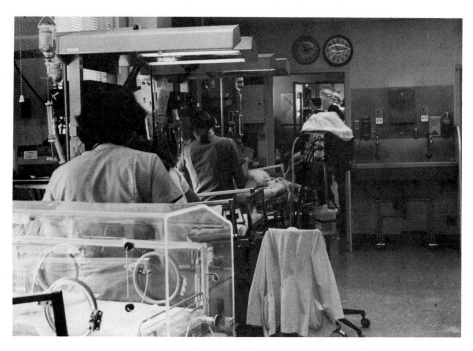

**Fig. 25-4.** Typical scene in NICU.

mia.[2] Incubators and radiant warmers with servoregulation are used to help maintain a constant thermal environment. Radiant warmers tend to produce more evaporative water loss and slightly higher basal metabolic rate compared to incubators.[51] Insensible water loss and convective heat loss can be reduced by use of a head shield[74] (inside an incubator) or transparent plastic wrap.[34,51] Large decreases in body temperature, which occur with approximately 20 minutes of routine nursing care and/or bronchial drainage treatments, in premature infants take up to two hours to return to the NTTZ.[60]

*Congestive heart failure* (CHF) and cor pulmonale (right-sided heart failure) may occur in neonates secondary to patent ductus arteriosus (PDA), increased pulmonary vascular resistance, right-to-left shunting, and other associated problems and congenital anomalies. Diuretics and digitalis are used to treat the peripheral and pulmonary edema that may result from heart failure.

*Persistent fetal circulation* (PFC) is characterized by pulmonary hypertension, probably caused by pulmonary vasoconstriction (vasospasm), increased pulmonary vascular smooth muscle, and decreased pulmonary vascular bed cross-sectional area.[47,72] A persistent fetal circulation results in increased hypoxemia and hypoxia because of right-to-left shunting of blood flow (usually through the foramen ovale or ductus arteriosus). Infants with persistent fetal circulation usually require high concentrations of oxygen and minimal handling.

*Intraventricular hemorrhage* (IVH)—or, more appropriately, subependymal hemorrhage/intraventricular hemor-

rhage (SEH/IVH) is the most common neuropathological finding in premature infants.[34] SEH/IVH is most closely correlated with vaginal delivery (versus cesarean), gender (males more than females), and hypoxemia ($Pao_2$ less than 45 mm Hg).[8] Other associations have been made between SEH/IVH and gestational age, positive-pressure ventilation, idiopathic respiratory distress syndrome, continuous positive airway pressure (CPAP), pulmonary air leaks, patent ductus arteriosus, administration of bicarbonate, and others.[8] The incidence of SEH/IVH is not clear. Because intraventricular hemorrhage is asymptomatic in most cases, noninvasive diagnostic tests such as computed tomography (CT) and high-frequency real-time ultrasound (RTU) scanning are invaluable. Intraventricular hemorrhage is graded I to IV according to the extent of bleeding.[34] Mortality with intraventricular hemorrhage is higher with grade IV lesions. Little is known about SEH/IVH. Important questions include the predictive morbidity according to the grade of the lesion and the relationship between common treatment techniques (e.g., endotracheal suctioning[66]) and the incidence of IVH. Bejar and associates[8] state that hemorrhage does not continue beyond the first week of life, and Ahmann and coworkers[1] found progressive hydrocephalus in only 23% of survivors of SEH/IVH.

## ASSESSMENT AND PREPARATION

As mentioned earlier, entering a NICU can be an overwhelming experience for a therapist until the patients and the equipment become more familiar (Fig. 25-4). Table 25-2 describes some of the common equipment found in the

**Table 25-2.** Equipment commonly encountered in the neonatal intensive care unit

| Equipment | Description |
|---|---|
| Radiant warmer (Fig. 25-5) | Unit composed of mattress on an adjustable table top covered by a radiant heat source controlled manually and by servo-control mode. Unit has adjustable side panels. *Advantage:* provides open space for tubes and equipment and easier access to the infant. *Disadvantage:* open bed may lead to convective heat loss and insensible fluid loss; increased metabolic rate. |
| Self-contained incubator (Isolette) (Fig. 25-7) | Enclosed unit of transparent material providing a heated and humidified environment with a servo system of temperature monitoring. Access to infant through side portholes or opening side of unit. *Advantage:* less convective heat and insensible water loss. *Disadvantage:* infection control; more difficult to get to baby; not practical for a very acutely ill neonate. |
| Thermal shield | Plexiglass dome placed over the trunk and legs of an infant in an Isolette to reduce radiant heat loss. |
| Oxygen hood (Fig. 25-12) | Plexiglass hood that fits over the infant's head; provides environment for controlled oxygen and humidification delivery. |
| Mechanical ventilator Pressure ventilator (Fig. 25-6) | Delivers positive-pressure ventilation; pressure-limited with volume delivered dependent on the stiffness of the lung. |
| Volume ventilator | Delivers positive-pressure ventilation; volume-limited delivering same tidal volume with each breath. |
| Negative-pressure ventilator | Ventilator that creates a relative negative pressure around the thorax and abdomen thereby assisting ventilation without endotracheal tube. NOTE: Difficult to use in infants weighing less than 1500 grams.[20] |
| High frequency ventilator | Ventilator that creates adequate alveolar ventilation and oxygenation at low tidal volumes and supraphysiologic ventilatory frequencies. The main advantage is decreased barotrauma.[33] |
| Nasal and nasopharyngeal prongs | Simple system for providing continuous positive airway pressure (CPAP) consisting of nasal prongs of varying lengths and adaptor to pressure-source tubing. |
| Resuscitation bag | Usually a self-inflating bag with a reservoir (so high concentrations of oxygen may be delivered at a rapid rate) attached to an oxygen flowmeter and a pressure manometer. |
| ECG, heart rate, respiratory rate, and blood pressure monitor (Fig. 25-8) | Usually one unit will display one or more vital signs on oscilloscope and digital display. High and low limits may be set, and alarm sounds when limits exceeded. |
| Transcutaneous oxygen monitor (Fig. 25-9 to 25-11) | Noninvasive method of monitoring partial pressure of oxygen from arterialized capillaries through the skin. The electrode is heated, placed on an area of thin epidermis (usually abdomen or thorax). The monitor has capability of providing both a digital display and a continuous recording of $TcPo_2$ values. |
| Pulse oximeter | Noninvasive method of continuously monitoring oxygen saturation with a real-time, beat-to-beat calculation of arterial oxygen saturation. Sensors are not heated so no possibility of skin burns exists and rotation of sensor placement is not necessary. Sensor placement is commonly on a digit (finger or toe).[40] |
| Intravenous infusion pump (Fig. 25-12) | Used to pump intravenous fluids, intralipids, and transpyloric feedings at a specified rate. Pump has alarm system and capacity to monitor volume delivered, obstruction of flow, and other parameters. |

NICU (also Figs. 25-5 to 25-11). One of the first tasks of a therapist when assessing an infant in a NICU is to become familiar with the monitors, equipment, and supplies on and around the baby (Fig. 25-12). This should be done even before looking at the baby.

Preliminary activities of the therapist, before assessing the infant, include reviewing the medical record and chest radiographs (when available) and discussing the infant with the nurse and physician. In *reviewing the chart,* the therapist should be sure to review:

1. Complete history of labor and delivery
2. Assessment of infant including:
   a. Apgar scores
   b. Dubowitz gestational age scores[23]
3. Clinical course of infant from birth to present
4. History of respiratory distress and oxygen and ventilation assistance provided since birth
5. Arterial blood gas history
6. Report on previous chest radiographs (CXR)
7. Mode and frequency of nutrition and feedings
8. Physician orders (e.g., run special tests) doublecheck the order for physical therapy)

The chest radiographs can be very helpful in identifying or locating a pulmonary pathological condition, indicating specific areas of the lung that may be involved, and assisting the therapist to identify anatomical landmarks on a very tiny baby. In many NICUs the chest radiographs are readily available in the unit. The therapist will most likely need assistance interpreting these films.

Talking with the physician and the nurse taking care of the infant can provide the therapist with invaluable current information, some of which may not yet have been placed in the chart. Some common questions the physical therapist may ask include the following:

1. What kind of day (or afternoon, evening, night depending on when assessment is done) has the baby had?
2. Has the baby had any evaluation or treatment procedures performed within the last hour or two?
3. Is the baby being fed orally or orogastrically, and when was the last feeding?
4. How does the baby respond to handling: i.e., does transcutaneous oxygen ($TcPo_2$) drop, or does the baby have apnea and bradycardia?

## CHEST EVALUATION

Once this preliminary information is gathered, the therapist assesses the infant. The evaluation of an infant's

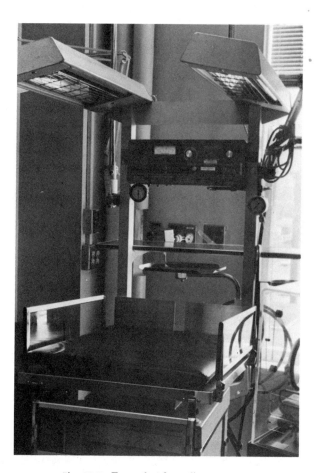

**Fig. 25-5.** Example of a radiant warmer.

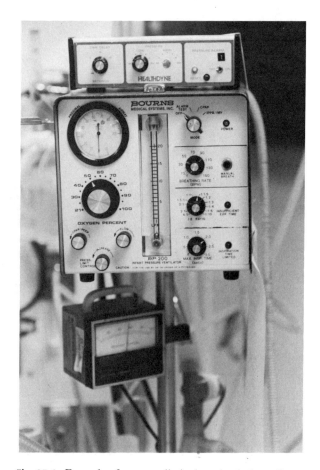

**Fig. 25-6.** Example of pressure-limited mechanical ventilator.

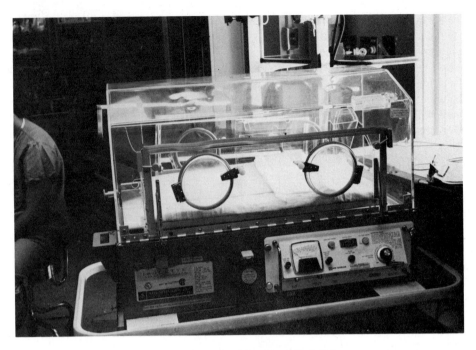

**Fig. 25-7.** Example of incubator (Isolette).

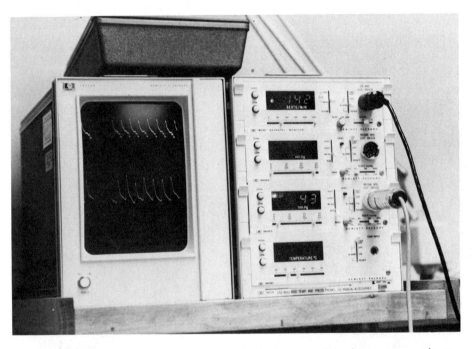

**Fig. 25-8.** Example of electrocardiographic, blood pressure, and respiratory rate monitor.

chest incorporates the four major skills used to assess any patient with pulmonary disease: observation and inspection, auscultation, palpation, and, rarely, mediate (i.e., indirect) percussion. *Observation* and *inspection* of a neonate include:

1. Signs of respiratory distress (these may not be evident in infants who are intubated and receiving mechanical ventilation).

   a. *Retractions* can be suprasternal, subcostal, substernal, or intercostal. Retractions occur because of the

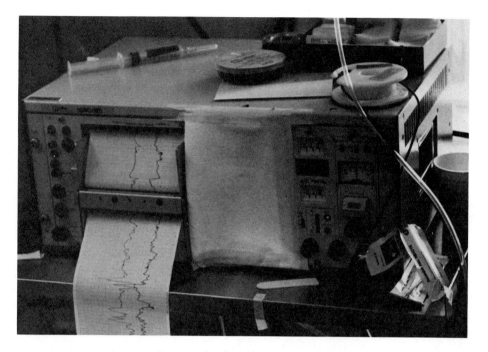

**Fig. 25-9.** An example of transcutaneous oxygen monitor.

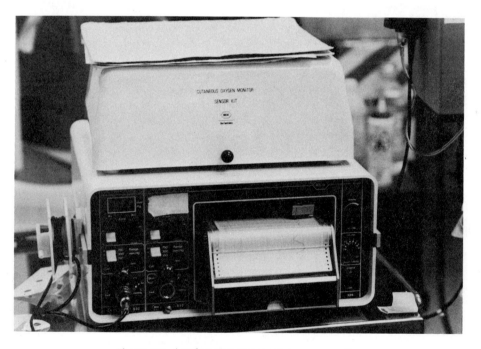

**Fig. 25-10.** Another transcutaneous oxygen monitor.

infant's very compliant chest wall, which is pulled inward by the high negative pressures generated in making greater than normal respiratory efforts. Severe retraction limits anteroposterior expansion of the chest and limits effective ventilation.[15,69] Mild retractions may be normal.

b. *Nasal flaring* is a reflex dilatation of the dilatores naris muscles. The resulting widening of the nares is believed to decrease airway resistance in the nasal passages and is most likely a primitive response.[15]

c. *Expiratory grunting* is an effort to increase functional residual capacity and improve both the distribution of ventilation and the ventilation-to-

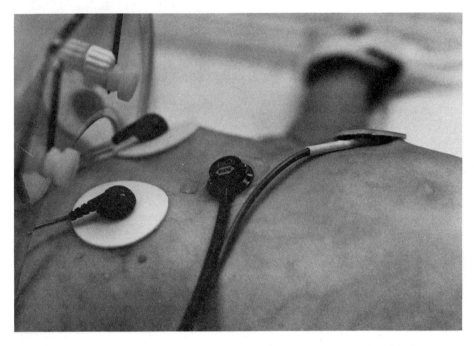

**Fig. 25-11.** Transcutaneous oxygen electrode *(center of photograph in black).*

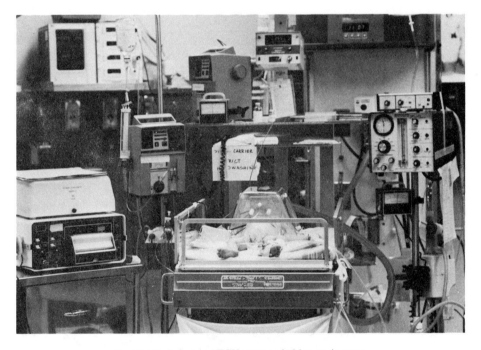

**Fig. 25-12.** Infant in NICU surrounded by equipment.

perfusion relationships by retarding expiration. The sound is produced by either expiration against a partially closed glottis or reflectory approximation of the vocal cords.[15,69]

d. *Stridor* on inspiration occurs with obstruction or collapse of the upper airway (upper two thirds of the trachea and larynx). The intensity of stridor

may change with the position of the infant, especially the degree of neck extension (NOTE: extending the neck of an infant tends to collapse the trachea).

e. *Head bobbing* occurs in infants who are attempting to use accessory respiratory muscles (sternocleidomastoid, scaleni) to assist in ventilation. Because neck extensor muscles of infants are not strong enough to stabilize the head, accessory muscle use often produces head bobbing.

    f. *Bulging* of the intercostal muscles occurs when obstruction to expiration creates high pleural pressures during expiration.[74]

2. Chest configuration: some abnormal findings in sick neonates include *barrel-shaped chest* (indicating overinflation or air trapping within the lungs) and *pectus excavatum* (funnel chest), a depression of the sternum that may be acquired secondary to prolonged periods of sternal retractions in the first months of life.

3. Skin color:

    a. *Cyanosis,* if apparent in the mucous membranes and around the lips and mouth, is a significant sign of hypoxemia. Cyanosis is a *very unreliable* clinical sign because it depends on both the relative amount of hemoglobin in the blood and the adequacy of peripheral circulation. When cyanosis is present it is *very* significant clinically.

    b. *Plethora,* or redness that may be noticed in a newborn with polycythemia.

    c. *Pallor, mottling,* or *webbing* of the skin is commonly seen in distressed infants and may be associated with hypoxemia, sepsis, intraventricular hemorrhage, and other problems. Pallor in an infant is also considered a sign of respiratory distress and of anemia.

4. Breathing pattern:

    a. *Tachypnea* is considered a sign of respiratory distress in infants. A normal newborn breathes most efficiently at approximately 40 breaths per minute.[69,73]

    b. *Irregularity* of respiration is *normal* in a newborn. Therefore one must count respiratory rates over a long period of time (i.e., 60 seconds) to account for the irregularity. Premature infants often have a breathing pattern called *"periodic breathing."* Periodic breathing is characterized by respirations of irregular rate and depth interrupted by apneic pauses of 5 to 10 seconds not associated with cyanosis or bradycardia.[73]

    c. *Apnea* is also considered a clinical sign of respiratory distress, sepsis, intraventricular hemorrhage, and other stresses of the premature baby. Apnea is commonly differentiated from periodic breathing by the length of the nonbreathing episode. Most sources consider an apneic pause of 20 seconds or longer to be true apnea. Apnea is also commonly associated with bradycardia. Increasing environmental oxygen may be helpful in decreasing apneic episodes. Other techniques used to decrease apnea and bradycardia in neonates include cutaneous stimulation, nasal continuous positive airway pressure, administration of theophylline (a central nervous system stimulant), and placement of an alternating pressure cushion (sometimes referred to as a "whoopee cushion") under the infant.

5. Coughing and sneezing: sneezing occurs more frequently in neonates than coughing does probably because of a better developed neural pathway.[69] The gag reflex and sneeze seem to be more important protective mechanisms for the infant's airways than coughing is. It will be helpful for the physical therapist to determine if a cough can be stimulated or if the infant coughs or sneezes spontaneously.

## AUSCULTATION

Auscultation of an infant or child is a gross assessment, at best, because of the thin chest wall, proximity of structures, and easy transmission of sounds. These problems are even more confounding when one is auscultating the chest of a premature infant or an infant who is being mechanically ventilated.

The *stethoscope* used may vary according to the size of the infant or the personal preference of the therapist. Fig. 25-13 shows two sizes of stethoscopes commonly used for auscultation. The stethoscope should have both a bell and a diaphragm because it is often helpful to use both portions when listening to a neonate's chest.

Before attempting to auscultate an infant who is intubated or has a tracheostomy, the therapist should be sure to empty the corrugated ventilator tubing of all water. Water will precipitate in the tubing from the humid water vapor delivered with inspired gases. Water bubbling in ventilator tubing can mask breath sounds and mimic adventitious sounds. A baby who is receiving intermittent mandatory ventilation (IMV) may be receiving as little as two breaths per minute from the ventilator. It may be very difficult to hear breath sounds when the infant is breathing spontaneously. However, the mechanical breath will often enhance breath sounds.

The therapist listens for normal and abnormal breath sounds as well as for adventitious sounds (Figs. 25-14 and 25-15). Abnormal sounds can be distinguished from normal sounds by thorough and careful auscultation.

Whenever possible, the therapist should auscultate with the infant's head in the midline position, since turning the head to the side may cause decreased breath sounds in the opposite side.[15] In infants the specific location of the sound does not necessarily correspond with the underlying lung segment. It is extremely important to correlate physical signs, such as auscultation, with radiographic evidence of a pathological condition. The anteroposterior (AP) and lateral chest radiographs help to localize areas of atelectasis, infiltrate, and pneumothorax, but these abnormalities are not always present. The therapist must often rely on auscultatory findings to indicate areas for treatment emphasis and to

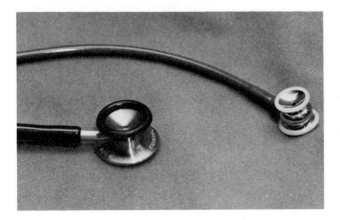

**Fig. 25-13.** Two sizes of pediatric stethoscopes.

describe the results of bronchial drainage techniques. Auscultation is therefore an *essential* component of the chest evaluation of neonates.

## PALPATION

Chest palpation of a neonate is limited to palpating for the position of the mediastinum (position of trachea in suprasternal notch) for subcutaneous emphysema, edema, or rib fracture (Fig. 25-16). Symmetry of chest wall motion is generally not palpable because the chest wall in a tiny baby moves very little. Paradoxical motion of the chest can be palpated in a neonate.

## MEDIATE PERCUSSION

Mediate (or indirect) percussion is seldom appropriate for a small infant. Exceptions may include percussing for the presence of pneumothoraces, diaphragmatic hernia, enlarged liver, and masses. Percussion in an infant's chest is performed by one finger directly on the chest (direct percussion).

## OTHER SYSTEMS

Assessment of systems other than the pulmonary system, particularly as they relate to physical therapy intervention, is extremely important in sick neonates.

The *cardiovascular system* is interrelated with the pulmonary system both anatomically and physiologically. Many patient problems affecting one system eventually affect the other. An example of this interrelationship would be the pulmonary vascular constriction caused by hypoxia and hypercapnia in neonates secondary to pulmonary dysfunction. Pulmonary hypertension, or increased pulmonary vascular resistance, increases the pressure in the right ventricle, which may lead to shunting of blood through the ductus arteriosus or foramen ovale and possibly right-sided heart failure (cor pulmonale).

Vital signs, such as heart rate (HR) and blood pressure (BP), must be monitored carefully in the infant. These signs indicate cardiovascular status and reflect the infant's response to assessment and treatment techniques. The autonomic nervous system is well developed in the neonate, and vasomotor regulatory mechanisms are present in the premature and term infant.[61] The sympathetic tone of the myocardium is incompletely developed in the premature and newborn infant, who may therefore not respond to stress, postural changes, or other situations in the same way as the adult.[47,95]

Detection of murmurs by auscultation of the heart may be important to the physical therapist. The murmur of a patent ductus arteriosus is usually characterized by a short ejection murmur with maximal impact along the left sternal border.[74]

Signs of poor peripheral circulation include pallor, cyanosis, weblike markings of the extremities, cool extremities, and poor correlation of transcutaneous oxygen ($TcPo_2$) values with arterial oxygen ($Pao_2$) values.

Arterial blood gas (ABG) values are extremely important indicators of adequacy of ventilation and oxygenation. So called normal ABG values for preterm and term infants vary greatly according to age, size, and pathological condition. Noninvasive and continuous monitoring of $O_2$, $CO_2$, and $O_2$ saturation are now available in most NICUs. Transcutaneous monitoring of $O_2$ and $CO_2$ and pulse oximetry, which monitors $O_2$ saturation, are invaluable to physical therapists evaluating and treating these sick and physiologically labile infants.

$TcPo_2$ and $TcPco_2$ values obtained are generally 5 to 10 mm Hg below $Pao_2$ and $Paco_2$ values because of some absorption by the skin. It is also important to realize that the validity and reliability of transcutaneous monitoring depends on periodic comparisons with ABG values. One complication of transcutaneous monitoring is possible skin burns caused by the heated electrode. Pulse oximetry measurement of $O_2$ saturation is a real-time beat-by-beat measurement. Motion artifact is a potential problem with this type of monitoring. It is also important that the therapist interpret $O_2$ saturation readings in the context of the infant's respiratory and metabolic state as shifts in the oxyhemoglobin-dissociation curve could result in inappropriate interpretations of an infant's oxygen "state" (e.g., if curve is shifted to the left, $O_2$ saturation will appear to be high, even at relatively low $Pao_2$ levels, but the infant could be very hypoxic because of the increased affinity of hemoglobin and oxygen).[14,94]

In a physical therapy assessment of the *skeletal* status of the infant, the therapist uses radiographic and blood chemistry data. Hypocalcemia, hypophosphatemia, and vitamin-deficiency syndromes can result in acquired rickets or osteoporosis.

The *skin* should be assessed for signs of breakdown and bruising. Recent incisions should also be noted.

The therapist should be aware of the mode of *nutritional support* for the infant. Infants with respiratory distress are

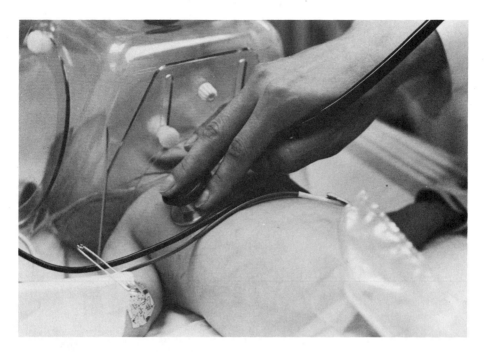

**Fig. 25-14.** Auscultation of the infant's lungs with larger stethoscope.

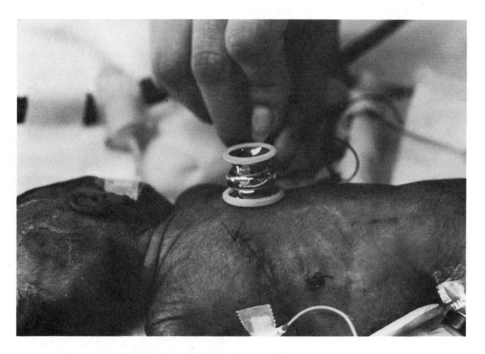

**Fig. 25-15.** Auscultation of infant's lungs with small, neonatal stethoscope.

seldom fed orally. Gavage or orogastric (OG) feeding is as common as transpyloric nutrition (TPN) or nasojejunal feeding. With transpyloric feeding, vomiting and aspiration is not common. Infants fed orally or orogastrally are often placed on their right sides for 20 to 30 minutes to assist with gastric emptying.[34] Abdominal distention should be noted

because it may interfere with ventilation, especially with the baby in a head-down position.

The *neuromuscular* system is often affected by prematurity, hypoxia, and various prenatal, intranatal, and postnatal problems. The most common causes of central nervous system abnormalities in neonates are hypoxia and hemor-

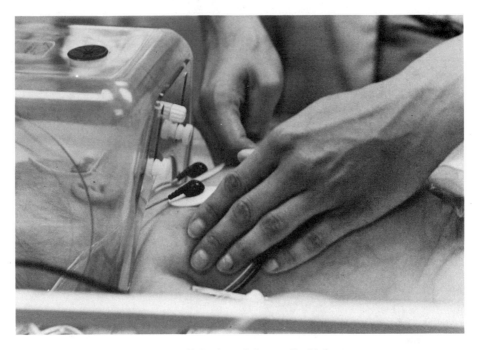

**Fig. 25-16.** Palpation of chest wall of infant.

rhage. Physical therapists are more often encountering infants in NICU nurseries who have CNS abnormalities due to fetal exposure to drugs and alcohol. Physical therapy assessment of the neurological and neuromuscular status of a neonate includes, but is not limited to, the following:

1. Primitive reflexes
2. Muscle tone
3. Limb movements and postures
4. Sucking and swallowing
5. Deep tendon reflexes
6. Behavioral assessment
7. State of quiet alertness
8. Joint range of motion

## CASE STUDIES: ASSESSMENT

Consider the two cases presented earlier in this chapter with physical therapy assessment information included. (See Case 1 assessment and Case 2 assessment on p. 503.)

## CHEST PHYSICAL THERAPY

Chest physical therapy (CPT) appropriate for an infant is limited to the bronchial drainage techniques of positioning for gravity-assisted drainage, chest percussion, vibration, and airway suctioning. The techniques listed above are few, and therefore one might assume CPT for the neonate is relatively simple and straightforward. Unfortunately, the application of CPT techniques to tiny infants is more involved than it sounds.

The first complicating factor involves careful and appropriate determination of *need*. Sick neonates, especially prematures, often do not tolerate handling well, even with routine procedures.[76] Investigators have found that many procedures (e.g., heel sticks, intravenous insertion, position changes, feedings, diaper changes, chest percussion, and suctioning) result in hypoxemia and increased oxygen consumption.[54,76,92,93] It is therefore very important that CPT procedures be performed only when clearly indicated for an existing problem or when a potential problem in an infant at risk is to be prevented.

Another complicating factor involves selection of the safest and most appropriate combination of CPT procedures for this population. There are many precautions and contraindications for various positions, chest percussion, vibration, and suctioning. The most appropriate and safest treatment program must be individually designed for each infant. Unfortunately, much confusion and inconsistency exist in the literature regarding the safety and efficacy of various CPT procedures. Many of the studies lump all of the procedures together and report that "CPT" may be dangerous. Therapists must be particularly careful in evaluating the methods and conclusions of reports in the literature regarding CPT for neonates.[70]

The third complicating factor is related to the size of the baby. The infant who weighs less than 1000 g is extremely tiny, and manual techniques (chest percussion and vibration) are therefore more difficult to administer and can be injurious.

## POSITIONING

Positioning for postural drainage (PD) traditionally employs 12 classic positions to drain the bronchopulmonary

## CASE 1 ▼ Assessment of B. L.

B.L. was evaluated on his third day of life by the physical therapist. B.L. had a patent ductus arteriosus ligated 24 hours before the assessment and was being weaned from the mechanical ventilator and supplemental oxygenation. B.L.'s pulmonary diagnosis is idiopathic respiratory distress syndrome (IRDS).

Before assessment of the infant's physical signs and symptoms, the following data were collected:

B.L. is intubated with an orotracheal tube and is receiving 28% oxygen at an intermittent mandatory ventilation (IMV) of 12 breaths per minute. Positive and expiratory pressure (PEEP) is +2 cm $H_2O$.

Arterial blood gases: pH 7.41; $Paco_2$ 36; $Pao_2$ 68; $TcPo_2$ reading in the low 60s; chest radiograph (today) shows reticulogranular pattern infiltrate and air bronchograms consistent with IRDS. Right lower lobe and left lower lobe atelectasis are apparent.

B.L. had a transpyloric tube in place and was receiving continuous infusion of formula.

An umbilical arterial catheter (UAC) was inserted.

B.L. is on a radiant warmer and has ECG leads, temperature servocontrol probe, and $TcPo_2$ electrode attached to his chest, back, and abdomen, respectively.

B.L. had a real-time ultrasound scan, which revealed a grade II SEH/IVH (subependymal hemorrhage/intraventricular hemorrhage).

The nurse caring for B.L. reports only one episode of apnea and bradycardia since surgery. Once his endotracheal tube was suctioned, he had no further problem. She reports having suctioned B.L. 3 hours ago with the return of a moderate amount of yellow secretions. She reports B.L. does not exhibit a cough reflex when suctioned.

Chest evaluation revealed the following:

A tiny infant with a left thoracotomy incision (after patent ductus arteriosus ligation).

B.L.'s respiratory rate was 52 with mild retractions during his spontaneous ventilatory efforts.

On auscultation B.L. had harsh vesicular breath sounds, slightly decreased on the left. Crackles were noticed over the left anterior chest, and occasional rhonchi were heard bilaterally on expiration.

B.L.'s trachea was palpated in the midline and mild rhonchal fremitus was felt over the anterior chest wall.

Heart rate was 160 bpm.

Blood pressure was 82/39 mm Hg.

B.L.'s skin was fragile and bruised. Blood studies demonstrated normal values for coagulation.

B.L. exhibited general hypotonia but could weakly suck a small nipple when stimulated.

B.L. was easily irritated with quick and noxious tactile stimuli. There was a decrease in his $TcPo_2$ during suctioning, during drawing of blood samples, and with turning, though the $TcPo_2$ returned to baseline value within 2 to 3 minutes after he was turned with no additional oxygen required.

## CASE 2 ▼ Assessment of A. C.

A.C. was 36 hours old when a physical therapy consultation was requested. Her pulmonary diagnosis was MAS (meconium-aspiration syndrome). She was extubated and was receiving 50% $O_2$ by oxygen hood when evaluated.

The following data were collected before the chest evaluation:

Arterial blood gases: $Fio_2$ 50%; pH 7.29; $Paco_2$ 51; $Pao_2$ 70; base excess (BE) +4.

Chest radiograph: hyperinflated lungs with patchy atelectasis bilaterally; infiltrate noted in right middle lobe; no sign of pneumothorax; right chest tube in place.

A.C. has ECG leads, temperature probe, and urine collection bag attached to her; an intravenous line was inserted into the left wrist.

A.C. has a transpyloric tube for nutritional support.

The nurse reported A.C. has been somewhat agitated. She reported suctioning meconium-stained secretions from A.C.'s mouth and nose every 3 to 4 hours. A.C. coughs when stimulated with a catheter. There was some concern about A.C. developing persistent fetal circulation (PFC), but so far this has not occurred.

Chest evaluation revealed the following:

A large infant; very pale; head under an oxygen hood.

A chest tube was sutured in place on the right anterior hemithorax and connected to suction by an underwater seal.

A.C. exhibited the following signs of respiratory distress; mild substernal retractions, nasal flaring, and tachypnea (respiratory rate is 60).

On auscultation A.C. had decreased breath sounds in the right lung fields and coarse crackles were heard diffusely throughout the chest.

Heart rate was 152 bpm.

Blood pressure was 98/56 mm Hg.

segments. The 12 postural drainage positions vary from 45° sitting to 45° head down and prone to sidelying to supine. A neonate's conducting airways are completely developed, and therefore the classical positions are appropriately applied for postural drainage. Fig. 25-17 demonstrates the 12 positions for a neonate.

Many precautions and a few contraindications (Table 25-3) for some of the positions in some infants may necessitate modification. As a general rule, a modified postural drainage position should be as close as possible to the classical position. In many cases a position within one-fourth turn and 10° to 20° from the classic position is well tolerated, safe, and effective. The intensive care setting and special problems of neonates often dictates some form of modified postural drainage, especially for head-down positions. Crane and associates[19] found significant increases in heart rate and blood pressure in a group of neonates with hyaline membrane disease in response to a 20-degree head-down position for chest physical therapy. These

changes, however, were all well within normal ranges for those vital signs, and they returned to pretreatment levels within 30 minutes.

Positioning may also be helpful to infants with pulmonary dysfunction because of the effects of some positions on ventilation-perfusion relationships and lung volumes and capacities.[59] The *prone position,* in particular, has been shown to affect oxygenation, lung compliance, state of alertness, vital signs, and other factors[56,84] (Table 25-4 and Fig. 25-18). Semierect positions as described by Ennis and Harris[25] may also improve oxygenation as compared to flat positions.

## MANUAL PERCUSSION AND VIBRATION

Percussion and vibration are techniques used to accelerate the loosening and movement of secretions and mucous plugs in the conducting airways. Either or both techniques, when combined with postural drainage, have been shown to improve oxygenation, decrease the incidence of postextu-

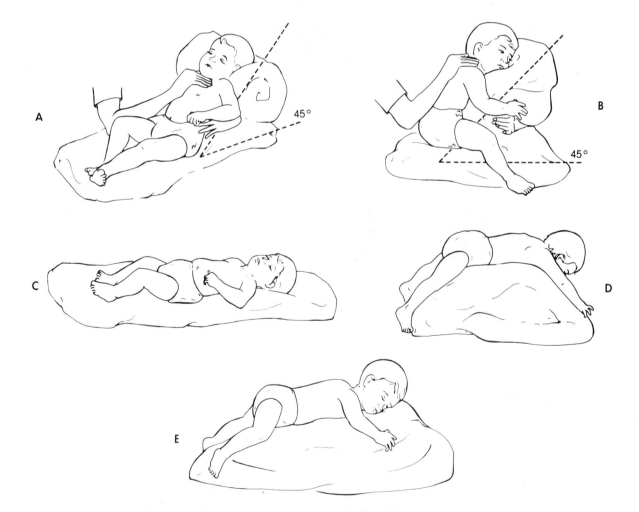

**Fig. 25-17.** Twelve positions for postural drainage (with **H** and **I** lying on right and left sides).

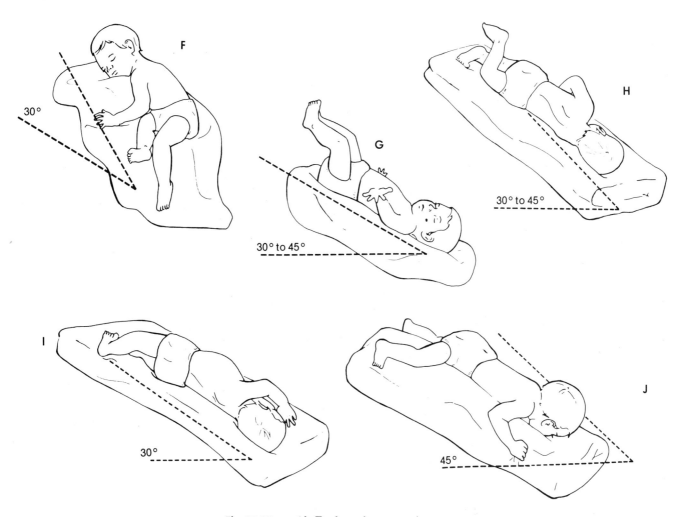

**Fig. 25-17, cont'd.** For legend see opposite page.

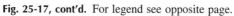

| Table 25-3. Precautions and contraindications for postural drainage in a neonate | | |
| --- | --- | --- |
| **Position** | **Precaution** | **Contraindication** |
| Prone | Umbilical arterial catheter<br>Continuous positive airway pressure in nose<br>Excessive abdominal distention<br>Abdominal incision<br>Anterior chest tube | Untreated tension pneumothorax |
| Trendelenburg position (head down) | Distended abdomen<br>SEH/IVH* (grades I and II)<br>Chronic congestive heart failure or cor pulmonale<br>Persistent fetal circulation<br>Cardiac dysrhythmias<br>Apnea and bradycardia<br>Infant exhibiting signs of acute respiratory distress<br>Hydrocephalus<br>Less than 28 weeks gestational age | Untreated tension pneumothorax<br>Recent tracheoesophageal fistula repair<br>Recent eye or intracranial surgery<br>Intraventricular hemorrhage (grades III and IV)<br>Acute congestive heart failure or cor pulmonale |

*Subependymal hemorrhage/intraventricular hemorrhage.

**Table 25-4.** Effects of the prone versus supine position on the neonate

| Effect when prone | Reference | Significance |
|---|---|---|
| More quiet sleep | Brackbill, Douhitt, and West[12] (30 full-term neonates) | <0.05 |
| More active sleep | | <0.05 |
| Less crying | | <0.01 |
| Less motor activity | | <0.01 |
| More regular respirations | | NS |
| Slower heart rates | | NS |
| Increased arterial oxygen tension | Martin and co-workers[56] (16 premature infants) | <0.001 |
| Decreased chest wall asynchrony | | <0.001 |
| Increased arterial oxygen tension | Wagaman and co-workers[84] (14 neonates; mean gestational age, 34.5 weeks) | <0.05 |
| Increased lung compliance | | <0.05 |
| Increased tidal volume | | <0.05 |
| Decreased number of apnea episodes | Dhande, Kattwinkel, and Darnall[22] (5 premature infants) | <0.001 |
| Higher $TcPo_2$ values | | <0.005 |
| $TcPo_2$ values higher postextubation | Lioy and Manginello[53] (18 premature infants) | 0.00001 |
| Lower respiratory rates | | NS |
| Lower retraction scores | | NS |
| $\dot{V}_T$ (mil) and $\dot{V}_E$ (mil) slightly higher in prone | Warren and Alderson[86] (49 neonates; mean gestational age, 36 weeks) | NS |

*NS*, Not significant.

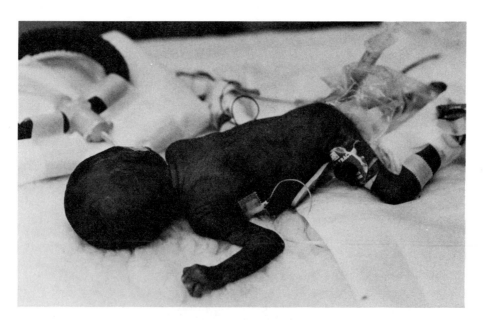

**Fig. 25-18.** Infant placed in prone position despite mechanical ventilation and artificial airway.

**Table 25-5.** Precautions and contraindications for chest percussion of a neonate

| Precautions | Contraindications |
|---|---|
| Poor condition of skin | Intolerance to treatment as |
| Coagulopathy | indicated by low TcPo$_2$ |
| Presence of a chest tube | values |
| Healing thoracic incision | Rib fracture |
| Osteoporosis and rickets | Hemoptysis |
| Persistent fetal circulation | |
| Cardiac dysrythmias | |
| Apnea and bradycardia | |
| Signs of acute respiratory | |
| distress | |
| Increased irritability during | |
| treatment | |
| Subcutaneous emphysema | |
| Bronchospasm, wheezing, | |
| rhonchi | |
| Subependymal hemorrhage/ | |
| intraventricular hemorrhage | |
| (SEH/IVH) | |
| Prematurity (less than 28 | |
| weeks gestational age) | |

**Table 25-6.** Precautions and contraindications for vibration of a neonate

| Precautions | Contraindications |
|---|---|
| Increased irritability/ | Untreated tension pneumothorax |
| crying during | |
| treatment | |
| Persistent fetal | Intolerance to treatment as |
| circulation | indicated by low TcPo$_2$ |
| | values |
| Apnea and bradycardia | Hemoptysis |

bation atelectasis, and increase the volume of secretions removed in newborn infants with pulmonary disease.[26,29,30]

There are many precautions and contraindications for using these techniques (Tables 25-5 and 25-6) with neonates (especially percussion). It is therefore very important to consider percussion and vibration *separately* and use them individually or together as appropriate for each infant.

*Percussion* for a small infant can be administered manually or with one of a variety of percussion "devices" (Fig. 25-19). Manual percussion may be performed with the fully cupped hand, four fingers cupped, three fingers with the middle finger "tented," or the thenar and hypothenar surfaces of the hand (Figs. 25-20 to 25-24). The therapist's choice of hand position is personal and depends on the size of the hand, the baby, and the shape of the area to be percussed. Most percussion techniques include a larger area of the chest wall than the surface adjacent to the affected lung area segment. The therapist should avoid percussing over the liver, spleen, kidneys, or other structures by paying close attention to the borders of the lungs and surface anatomy.

Percussion is often well tolerated by infants and its rhythmic, nonpainful stimulus seems to soothe some babies to sleep. Regardless of the method used for percussion, a cupping effect should be maintained. When percussion is administered manually, the motion should come primarily from the therapist's wrist with firm support applied to the opposite side of the chest wall (Figs. 25-25 and 25-26). In most cases a thin blanket, sheet, or article of clothing should cover the area being treated (Fig. 25-27). In some premature infants, it is important to continually observe the chest wall

for anatomical landmarks and to watch for signs of respiratory distress; therefore percussion is administered directly over the skin.

*Vibration* can be administered manually or with a mechanical vibrator. There are fewer precautions and contraindications for vibration (Table 25-6), and so vibration can often be used in place of manual percussion in a chest physical therapy treatment (Fig. 25-28). Curran and Kacho-yeanos[20] advocate the use of a padded electric toothbrush for vibration. The mechanical vibrator (of which the electric toothbrush is one form) has not been conclusively demonstrated to be more effective or safer than other manual chest physical therapy techniques in infants. The therapist should be cautious that no electric motor capable of producing a spark is used around high concentrations of oxygen in which a spark could trigger an explosion.

One performs manual vibration by placing the palmar surface of the fingers over the chest wall surface to be vibrated and isometrically contracting the muscles of the hand and arm to create a fine, tremulous vibration. Very little pressure should be applied when one is vibrating the chest wall of a neonate. Vibration is traditionally done during the expiratory phase of breathing. That coordination may be impossible when an infant is breathing above 40 to 50 breaths per minute. If the baby is receiving mechanical ventilation with intermittent mandatory ventilation (IMV), vibration can easily be coordinated with the expiratory phases of the ventilator-assisted breaths.

Postural drainage, percussion, and vibration should be administered for at least 3 to 5 minutes per position to be effective. If postural drainage is used alone, the time for drainage in each position must be longer, at least 20 to 30 minutes. I strongly recommend that the therapist not attempt to employ all the positions necessary for a baby during one treatment session if it means significantly decreasing the time in each position. Rather, the therapist should first treat the areas showing signs of the most severe pathological condition and then treat the less-involved segments using short, frequent treatments. In this manner all areas of the lung requiring drainage will be adequately treated.

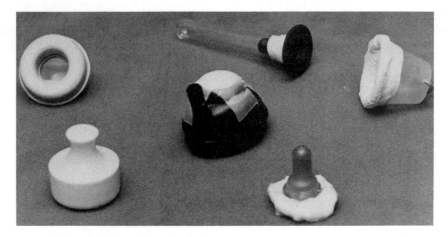

Fig. 25-19. Commercially available and adapted devices for percussion.

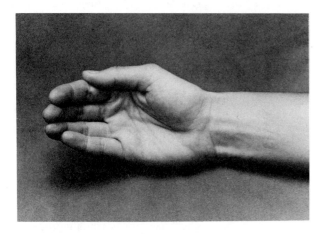

Fig. 25-20. Fully cupped hand for percussion.

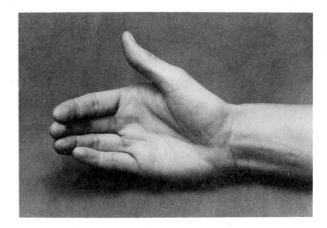

Fig. 25-21. Four fingers cupped for percussion.

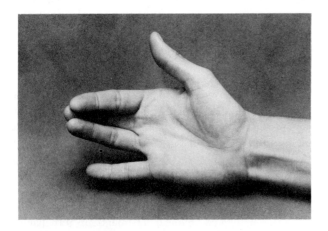

Fig. 25-22. Three fingers cupped for percussion with middle finger "tented"—palmar view.

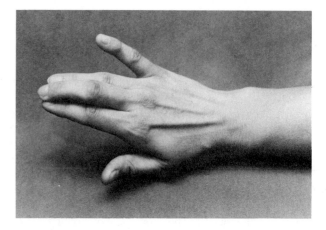

Fig. 25-23. Three fingers cupped for percussion with middle finger "tented"—dorsal view.

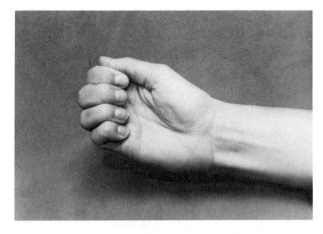

**Fig. 25-24.** Thenar and hypothenar surfaces for percussion.

## AIRWAY SUCTIONING

*Airway suctioning* is usually required to help the infant clear the secretions loosened by the bronchial drainage treatment. Suctioning may also be considered an emergency procedure if a large airway or tube becomes obstructed by secretions. Physical therapists working with infants with pulmonary dysfunction should know how to suction endotracheally with an airway present (endotracheal or tracheostomy tube). Suctioning is always potentially dangerous for the infant.[13,17,54] The risks can be reduced if suggested procedures are carefully followed and precautions are taken.

As a general rule, unless the situation is an emergency, nasotracheal suctioning should not be attempted without an endotracheal (ET) or tracheostomy tube. Deep tracheal suctioning is most effectively and more safely performed through an artificial airway. The therapist can suction the nasal and oral pharynges and try to stimulate a cough in an infant without an ET tube or tracheostomy. If the infant has an adequate cough and suctioning can be deferred, it is better not to perform the procedures.

When suctioning is necessary, the following procedure is suggested:[18,57]

1. *Preparation:* Place the infant supine, preferably with the head positioned in the midline. Be sure the suction apparatus is working properly and is connected, the suction is turned on, and the vacuum level is set between 60 and 80 cm $H_2O$. Make sure the oxygen flow is turned on and attached to the self-inflating breathing bag and the pressure manometer is connected. Check to see what pressures the ventilator is delivering to the baby or what pressure is required to properly ventilate the infant.

2. *Hyperventilation:* With a self-inflating bag and artificial airway connector, hyperventilate the infant at approximately 20 breaths per minute above the rate delivered by the ventilator up to a maximum of 60

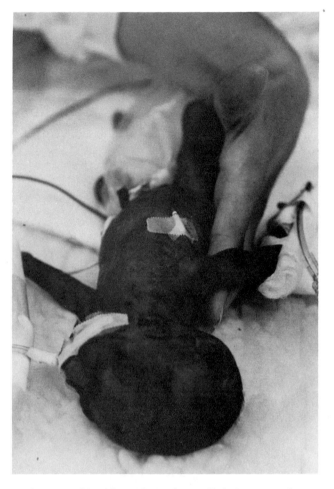

**Fig. 25-25.** Manual support to chest wall during percussion.

breaths per minute at the pressure noted in step 1. Hyperoxygenate the infant by delivering an oxygen concentration 10% to 20% higher than the inspired concentration ($FIO_2$) the infant was receiving. The bag should be attached to a manometer so ventilating pressures can be maintained (e.g. not too high or too low).

If the $FIO_2$ is 0.5 or higher, deliver 100% oxygen. Hyperventilation and hyperoxygenation should precede and follow each pass of the suction catheter.

3. *Lavage* (OPTIONAL): Instill 0.5 to 1 ml, or 2 or 3 drops, of sterile normal saline solution (NaCl) directly into the endotracheal or tracheostomy tube. Instillation of saline can be done safely before bagging as well.[7]

4. *Suction:* Using sterile procedure:
   a. Wet the catheter in sterile saline.
   b. Insert the catheter (with *no* suction applied) into the airway until resistance is met. Pull the catheter back slightly and then withdraw the catheter while applying intermittent suction and turning the catheter. Suction should not last longer than 10 seconds.

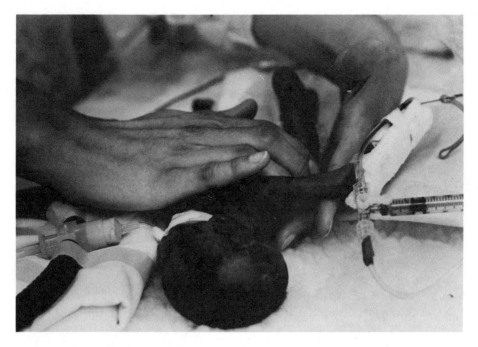

**Fig. 25-26.** Manual chest percussion using three fingers with middle finger tented.

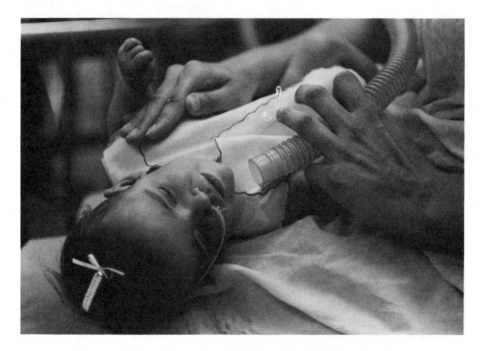

**Fig. 25-27.** Manual percussion with light article of clothing over chest.

c. Repeat if necessary.
d. Suction the nasal and oral pharynges.

Hypoxemia and hyperoxemia can be *minimized* during chest physical therapy if the infant is monitored with a transcutaneous oxygen (TcPo$_2$) monitor.[54]

## CASE STUDIES: TREATMENT

The cases presented earlier in the chapter provide examples of chest physical therapy treatment of infants with pulmonary dysfunction. Notice the careful consideration of precautions and contraindications and individualized treatment plans. (See Case 1 treatment on p. 511 and Case 2 treatment on p. 512.)

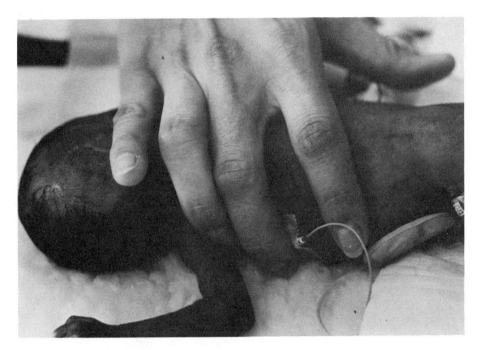

**Fig. 25-28.** Manual chest vibration on an infant with a thoracotomy incision.

---

**CASE 1 ▼ Treatment of B. L.**

B.L. is almost ready to be extubated and the following treatment is planned:

Short, frequent (approximately every 2 or 3 hours) bronchial drainage treatments to begin at least 1 hour before extubation and to continue for at least 48 hours. As a result of the chest radiograph and auscultation, treatment emphasis is placed upon the left lower lobe. Also emphasized are the right upper lobe and right middle lobe, which are susceptible to postextubation atelectasis. A maximum of four positions will be used for each treatment with a maximum of 15 minutes of treatment time. Vibration will be used in lieu of percussion because of a thoracotomy, coagulopathy, bruised skin, and intraventricular hemorrhage. Modified postural drainage positions will be used because of the intraventricular hemorrhage to avoid greater than 15° with the head down. Postural drainage and vibration will be followed by suctioning through the endotracheal tube. Once the extubation is done, suctioning will be limited to stimulation of a cough reflex with the catheter and suctioning of the mouth and nose.

Nursing personnel will perform the chest physical therapy treatments at night to provide for 24-hour continuity of treatment. Between chest physical therapy treatments, B.L.

will be positioned for modified postural drainage of lung segments not treated during the formal treatment session. If B.L.'s $TcPo_2$ drops during treatment, the $Fio_2$ will be increased slightly to keep the $TcPo_2$ between 40 and 70 mm Hg.

B.L. was able to breathe without the mechanical ventilator for 72 hours, but the left lower lobe infiltrate did not respond to antibiotic therapy and the infant became progressively more hypoxemic and hypercapnic with increased episodes of apnea and bradycardia. B.L. was reintubated to receive mechanical ventilation for 1 week. He was 13 days old. His chest radiograph then began to exhibit signs of early bronchopulmonary dysplasia (BPD), and copious amounts of secretion were suctioned from his endotracheal tube.

**PLAN:** Continue bronchial drainage treatments for all lung segments as tolerated. As B.L.'s infiltrate improves, his condition will still have changes consistent with bronchopulmonary dysplasia, and he will therefore be extremely susceptible to respiratory infection, airway obstruction, and respiratory failure. Chest physical therapy should continue routinely for prophylaxis until discharge, and B.L.'s parents should be instructed in chest physical therapy techniques for use at home.

---

## DISCHARGE PLANNING

Preparing the parents of an infant in the NICU for their baby's discharge is almost as important as preparing the baby. Discharge planning and teaching must begin early. Parents of infants requiring long hospitalizations should become involved in the care of their baby long before discharge.

The transition from hospital to home can be a crisis for the parents of a baby who has spent a long time in a NICU.[39,55] The stresses of discharge are, however, over-

---

**CASE 2** ▼ **Treatment of A. C.**

The following treatment plan was recommended for A.C.:

**BRONCHIAL DRAINAGE:**

1. Position to drain the right middle lobe (one-fourth turn from supine, right side up) and the right lower lobe (15° to 20° head down, modified because of respiratory distress) with percussion and vibration performed for 3 to 5 minutes every 4 hours.
2. Treat the remaining lung segments as tolerated with modified head-down positions for lower lobe segments.
3. Follow chest physical therapy with cough stimulation and suctioning. NOTE: If a good cough is not evident and lower airways remain obstructed, temporary intubation for direct suctioning may be considered by the neonatologist.

If A.C. is agitated by vibration, percussion alone should be performed except where the chest tube exits the chest.

Agitation may be secondary to hypercapnia: $Paco_2$. One performs vibration around the chest tube site by slipping the index and middle fingers on either side of the tube and vibrating at regular intervals. As respiratory distress abates, postural drainage should be performed in the classical positions.

The therapist must observe for signs of increasing hypoxemia—increased respiratory distress, cyanosis, tachycardia, or bradycardia—and must observe for spontaneous pneumothorax—sudden clinical deterioration with bradycardia or tachycardia, cyanosis or pallor, increased respiratory distress, shift of the mediastinum away from the side of the pneumothorax, and decreased or absent breath sounds on the side of the pneumothorax.

---

shadowed by the benefits, which include decreasing the fatigue of travel, decreasing the financial burdens of prolonged hospitalization, and ending the separation of the parents from the child.

If the NICU is a regional newborn intensive care nursery, the parents may live a long distance from the hospital. This distance can present a problem when it becomes necessary for the parents to visit the hospital frequently to learn the infant's home care. It is imperative that planning for parent involvement with the infant's care and teaching in preparation for discharge be started early, as soon as it is evident that the baby will eventually go home.

In most NICU settings someone is designated as the discharge planner. Often it is a nurse who coordinates the efforts of the team to assure that the plans are carried out.

### Team assessment of needs

In most cases several disciplines will be involved in the care of the baby. As the infant progresses and the time for discharge approaches, the team members must communicate their assessments and plans to each other. This process is extremely important for consolidation of plans and avoidance of inconsistencies and duplication of effort in dealing with the parents.

The *physical therapist* has much to contribute to the parents' knowledge and skills. The physical therapist can assist parents regarding an infant's pulmonary, neurological, or orthopaedic problems. This section discusses only the discharge planning for an infant with chronic pulmonary problems.

### Bronchial drainage at home

If the infant has an airway clearance problem secondary to some form of chronic lung disease, central nervous system dysfunction, or infectious process, bronchial drainage should be continued at home. Requiring parents to perform these treatments may present some inconvenience and interruption of the normal family routine. One advantage, however, is that treatments provide a period of time for the infant and parent to interact and be in close physical contact. When viewed in this way, bronchial drainage may be considered mutually beneficial.

### What to include in the home program

*Positioning* can often be limited to six or less modified postural drainage positions for prophylaxis or emphasis on problem areas. The positions chosen depend on many factors, including the following:

1. Location of the pathological condition in the lung
2. Condition or conditions requiring modification of positions
3. What positions the infant is likely to be in most of the time

When teaching parents bronchial drainage for an infant with diffuse chronic lung disease, the author recommends the following six positions:

1. Sitting, leaning back 45° from vertical
2. Sitting, leaning forward 45° from vertical
3. Lying one-fourth turn from supine with the right side up and head and thorax tilted 30° down from the horizontal
4. Lying on left side with the head and thorax tilted 45° down from the horizontal
5. Lying on right side with the head and thorax tilted 45° down from the horizontal
6. Lying prone with the head and thorax tilted 45° down from the horizontal

The *manual technique* usually taught to parents is chest percussion. Vibration may also be taught if, in the opinion of the therapist, the baby will benefit *and* the parents can learn the technique. The therapist should urge and observe for adequate force of percussion. Parents are reluctant to use sufficient percussion force, believing they might harm the baby. Percussion and vibration should be practiced several times by the parent with the therapist present to assure that good technique is used.

Parents may need to be taught how to stimulate a cough. They also need to know that infants commonly swallow cleared secretions and may vomit if a large amount of mucus accumulates in the stomach. This vomiting is usually *normal.*

### Suctioning at home

If an infant has a tracheostomy, airway suctioning may be necessary. Parents must learn sterile, or "clean," techniques of airway suctioning and should practice this procedure with supervision. It is helpful for parents and baby to "room in" in a regular hospital room to practice routine care with assistance and encouragement close at hand. The therapist should caution parents to avoid bronchial drainage for at least 1 hour after feeding. Preferably, the treatment should be just before feedings. The frequency of treatment is variable and depends on the infant's needs. The therapist and physician should consider the emotional effects frequent chest physical therapy treatments may have on the family.

Parents must also recognize signs and symptoms of respiratory infection. Early intervention with antibiotics, more frequent bronchial drainage treatments, and other measures may help avoid rehospitalization when an infection occurs at home.

## SUMMARY

As NICU technology improves and more neonates of lower gestational ages survive the perinatal period, the role of the physical therapist in the NICU increases in importance. Tiny babies are very susceptible to cardiopulmonary, neurological, and orthopedic problems. The physical therapist assesses and treats a neonate to prevent and remediate physiological and functional problems. Chest physical therapy is often indicated for neonates with pulmonary dysfunction to improve airway clearance, enhance ventilation, and decrease the work of breathing. Determining the need for physical therapy and designing appropriate treatment programs is especially important for this patient population. A physical therapist in a NICU must be familiar with the unique problems of small, sick neonates. When applied conscientiously, chest physical therapy can be safely and effectively administered to the tiniest babies.

### REFERENCES

1. Ahmann P and others: Intraventricular hemorrhage in the high risk preterm infant, *Ann Neurol* 7:118, 1980.

2. Aloan CA: *Respiratory care of the newborn: a clinical manual,* Philadelphia, 1987, JB Lippincott Co.

3. Anastassios C and others: Lung mechanics during and after extracorporeal membrane oxygenation for meconium aspiration syndrome, *Crit Care Med* 20:751, 1992.

4. Bacsik RD: Meconium aspiration syndrome, *Pediatr Clin North Am* 24:463, 1977.

5. Bancalari E and Sosenko I: Pathogenesis and prevention of neonatal chronic lung disease: Recent developments, *Pediatr Pulmonol* 8:109, 1990.

6. Bartlett RH and others: Studies on the pathogenesis and prevention of postoperative pulmonary complications, *Surg Gynecol Obstet* 137:925, 1973.

7. Beeram MR and Dhanireddy R: Effects of saline instillation during tracheal suction on lung mechanics in newborn infants, *J Perinatol* 12(2):120, 1992.

8. Bejar R, Coen RW, and Glock L: Hypoxic-ischemic and hemorrhagic brain injury in the newborn, *Perinatol Neonatol* 6:69, 1982.

9. Bendixen HH and others: Atelectasis and shunting during spontaneous ventilation in anesthetized patients, *Anesthesiology* 25:297, 1964.

10. Berman W and others: Long-term follow-up of bronchopulmonary dysplasia, *J Pediatr* 109:45, 1986.

11. Bhutani VK and Abbasi S: Long-term pulmonary consequences in survivors with bronchopulmonary dysplasia, *Clin Perinatol* 19(3):649, 1992.

12. Brackbill Y, Douthitt TC, and West H: Psychophysiologic effects in the neonate of prone versus supine placement, *J Pediatr* 82:82, 1973.

13. Brandstater B and Muallem M: Atelectasis following tracheal suction in infants, *Anesthesiology* 31:468, 1969.

14. Cassady G: Transcutaneous monitoring in the newborn infant, *J Pediatr* 103:837, 1983.

15. Chrisman MK: *Respiratory nursing: continuing education review,* Flushing, NY, 1975, Medical Examination Publishing Co, Inc.

16. Collaborative European Multicenter Group: Surfactant replacement therapy for severe neonatal respiratory distress syndrome: an international randomized clinical trial, *Pediatrics* 82:683, 1988.

17. Cordero L and Hon EH: Neonatal bradycardia following nasopharyngeal stimulation, *J Pediatr* 78:441, 1971.

18. Crane L: Physical therapy for neonates with respiratory dysfunction, *Phys Ther* 61:1764, 1981.

19. Crane LD and others: Comparison of chest physiotherapy techniques in infants with HMD (abstract), *Pediatr Res* 12:559, 1978.

20. Curran CL and Kachoyeanos MK: The effects on neonates of two methods of chest physical therapy, *Matern Child Nurs J* 4:309, 1979.

21. Davis GM and Bureau MA: Pulmonary and chestwall mechanics in the control of respiration in the newborn, *Clin Perinatol* 14:551, 1987.

22. Dhande VG and others: Prone position reduces apnea in preterm infants (abstract), *Pediatr Res* 16:285A, 1982, part 2 of 2 parts.

23. Dubowitz L, Dubowitz V, and Goldberg C: Clinical assessment of gestational age in the newborn infant, *J Pediatr* 77:1, 1970.

24. Dunn D and Lewis AT: Some important aspects of neonatal nursing related to pulmonary disease and family involvement, *Pediatr Clin North Am* 20:481, 1973.

25. Ennis S and Harris TR: Positioning infants with hyaline membrane disease, *Am J Nurs* 78:398, 1978.

26. Etches PC and Scott B: Chest physiotherapy in the newborn: effect on secretions removed, *Pediatrics* 62:713, 1978.

27. Falciglia HS and others: Does DeLee suction at the perineum prevent meconium aspiration syndrome? *Am J Obstet Gynecol* 167:1243, 1992.

28. Farrell PM and Avery ME: State of the art: hyaline membrane disease, *Am Rev Respir Dis* 111:657, 1975.

29. Finer NN and Boyd J: Chest physiotherapy in the neonate: a controlled study, *Pediatrics* 61:282, 1978.

30. Finer NN and others: Postextubation atelectasis: a retrospective review and a prospective controlled study, *J Pediatr* 94:110, 1979.

31. Frownfelter DL, editor: *Chest physical therapy and pulmonary rehabilitation,* Chicago, 1978, Year Book Medical Publishers, Inc.

32. Gerhardt T and others: Serial determination of pulmonary function in infants with chronic lung disease, *J Pediatr* 110:448, 1987.

33. Gerstmann DR, deLemos RA, and Clark RH: High-frequency ventilation: issues of strategy, *Clin Perinatol* 18(3):563, 1991.

34. Goldsmith JP and Karotkin EH: *Assisted ventilation of the newborn,* Philadelphia, 1981, WB Saunders Co.

35. Goldsmith LS and others: Immediate improvement in lung volume after exogenous surfactant: Alveolar recruitment versus increased distension, *J Pediatr* 119:424, 1991.

36. Gregory GA and others: Meconium aspiration in infants: a prospective study, *J Pediatr* 85:848, 1974.

37. Hallman M and others: Exogenous human surfactant for treatment of severe respiratory distress syndrome: a randomized prospective clinical trial, *J Pediatr* 106:963, 1985.

38. Halpern LM and others: The mean duration of gastroesophageal reflux during sleep as an indicator of respiratory symptoms from gastroesophageal reflux in children, *J Pediatr Surg* 26(6):686, 1991.

39. Harrison A: *The premature baby book: a parent's guide to coping and caring in the first years,* New York, 1983, St Martin's Press.

40. Hartsell MB: Noninvasive oxygen monitoring, *J Pediat Nurs* 2:64, 1987.

41. Henderson-Smart DJ and Read DJ: Depression of respiratory muscles and defective responses to nasal obstruction during active sleep in the newborn, *Aust Paediatr J* 21:261, 1976.

42. Johnson TR, Moore WM, and Jeffries JE, editors: *Children are different: developmental physiology,* ed 2, Columbus, Ohio, 1978, Ross Laboratories.

43. Jolley SG and others: The relationship of respiratory complications from gastroesophageal reflux to prematurity in infants, *J Pediatr Surg* 25(7):755, 1990.

44. Jones SP: Relationship between apnea and GER: What nurses need to know, *Pediatr Nurs* 18(4):413, 1992.

45. Jorgensen KM: The drug-exposed infant, *Crit Care Nurs Clin N A* 4(3):481, 1992.

46. Kattan M: Long-term sequelae of respiratory illness in infancy and childhood, *Pediatr Clin North Am* 26(3):525, 1979.

47. Klaus MH and Fanaroff AA: *Care of the high-risk neonate,* ed 2, Philadelphia, 1979, WB Saunders Co.

48. Kottmeier PK and Klotz D: Surgical problems in the newborn, *Pediatr Ann* 8:60, 1979.

49. Krumpke PE and others: The aging respiratory system, *Clin Geriatr Med* 1:143, 1985.

50. Laitman JT and Crelin ES: Developmental change in the upper respiratory system of human infants, *Perinatol Neonatol* 4:15, 1980.

51. LeBlanc MH: Thermoregulation: Incubators, radiant warmers, artificial skins, and body hoods, *Clin Perinatol* 18(3):403, 1991.

52. Levine MI and Mascia AV: *Pulmonary diseases and anomalies of infancy and childhood,* New York, 1966, Hoeber Medical Division, Harper & Row, Publishers.

53. Lioy J and Manginello FP: A comparison of prone and supine positioning in the immediate postextubation period of neonates, *J Pediatr* 112:982, 1988.

54. Long JG, Philip AG, and Lucey JF: Excessive handling as a cause of hypoxemia, *Pediatrics* 65:203, 1980.

55. Lund C and Lefrak L: Discharge planning for infants in the intensive care nursery, *Perinatol Neonatol* 6:49, 1982.

56. Martin RJ and others: Effect of supine and prone positions on arterial oxygen tension in the preterm infant, *Pediatrics* 63:528, 1979

57. McFadden R: Decreasing respiratory compromise during infant suctioning, *Am J Nurs* 81:2158, 1981.

58. Mellins RB: Pulmonary physiotherapy in the pediatric age group, *Am Rev Respir Dis* 110 (6 part 2):137, 1974.

59. Menkes H and Britt J: Physical therapy: rationale for physical therapy, *Am Rev Respir Dis* 122:127, 1980.

60. Mok Q and others: Temperature instability during nursing procedures in preterm neonates, *Arch Dis Child* 66:783, 1991.

61. Moss AJ, Duffie EF, and Emmanouilides G: Blood pressure and vasomotor reflexes in the newborn infant, *Pediatrics* 32:175, 1963.

62. Muller NL and Bryan AC: Chest wall mechanics and respiratory muscles in infants, *Pediatr Clin North Am* 26:503, 1979.

63. Murray JF: *The normal lung,* Philadelphia, 1976, WB Saunders Co.

64. Nagaraj HS and others: Recurrent lobar atelectasis due to acquired bronchial stenosis in neonates, *J Pediatr Surg* 15:411, 1980.

65. Northway WH and others: Pulmonary disease following respirator therapy of hyaline membrane disease: bronchopulmonary dysplasia, *N Engl J Med* 275:357, 1967.

66. Perlman JM and Volpe JJ: The effects of oral suctioning and endotracheal suctioning on cerebral blood flow velocity and intracranial pressure in the preterm infant (abstract), *Pediatr Res* 16:303A, 1982.

67. Pfenninger J and others: Lung mechanics and gas exchange in ventilated preterm infants during treatment of hyaline membrane disease with multiple doses of artificial surfactant (Exosurf), *Pediatr Pulmonol* 14:10, 1992.

68. Pietrantoni M and Knuppel R: Alcohol use in pregnancy, *Clin Perinatol* 18:93, 1991.

69. Polgar G: Practical pulmonary physiology, *Pediatr Clin North Am* 20:303, 1973.

70. Raval D and others: Chest physiotherapy in preterm infants with RDS in the first 24 hours of life, *J Perinatology* 7:301, 1987.

71. Remondiere R and others: Interet de la kinesitherapie respiratoire dans le traitement de la maladie des membranes hyalines du nouveau-né, *Ann Pediat* 23:617, 1976.

72. Rudolph AM: High pulmonary vascular resistance after birth, *Clin Pediatr* 19:585, 1980.

73. Scarpelli EM, editor: *Pulmonary physiology of the fetus, newborn and child,* Philadelphia, 1975, Lea & Febiger.

74. Scarpelli EM, Auld PAM, and Goldman HS, editors: *Pulmonary disease of the fetus, newborn and child,* Philadelphia, 1978, Lea & Febiger.

75. Smith RM: *Anesthesia for infants and children,* ed 3, St Louis, 1968, Mosby.

76. Speidel BD: Adverse effects of routine procedures on preterm infants, *Lancet* 1:864, 1978.

77. Sun SC and others: Meconium aspiration and tracheal suction, *J Med Soc NJ* 74:542, 1977.

78. Thurlbeck WM: Postnatal growth and development of the lung, *Am Rev Respir Dis* 111:803, 1975.

79. Tisi GM: State of the art: pre-operative evaluation of pulmonary function, *Am Rev Respir Dis* 119:293, 1979.

80. Vandenplas Y and others: Esophageal pH monitoring data during chest physiotherapy, *J Pediatr Gastroenterol Nutr* 13:23, 1991.

81. Veereman-Wauters G, Bochner A, and Van Caillie-Bertrand M: Gastroesophageal reflux in infants with a history of near-miss sudden infant death, *J Pediatr Gastroenterol Nutr* 12(3):319, 1991.

82. Vohr BR, Bell EF, and Oh W: Infants with bronchopulmonary dysplasia, *Am J Dis Child* 136:443, 1982.

83. Voyles JB: Pulmonary problems in infants and children: bronchopulmonary dysplasia, *Am J Nurs* 81:510, 1981.

84. Wagaman MJ and others: Improved oxygenation and long compliance with prone positioning of neonates, *J Pediatr* 94:787, 1979.

85. Wallis S and Harvey D: Respiratory distress: its cause and management, *Nurs Times* 75:1264, 1979.

86. Warren RH and Alderson SH: Breathing patterns in infants utilizing respiratory inductive plethysmography, *Chest* 89:717, 1986.

87. Weinstein MR and Oh W: Oxygen consumption in infants with bronchopulmonary dysplasia, *J Pediatr* 99:958, 1981.

88. Wesenberg RL: *The newborn chest,* New York, 1973, Harper & Row, Publishers, Inc.

89. Wiswell TE and Henley MA: Intratracheal suctioning, systemic infection and the meconium aspiration syndrome, *Pediatrics* 89(2):203, 1992.

90. Wiswell TE, Tuggle JM, and Turner BS: Meconium aspiration syndrome: Have we made a difference? *Pediatrics* 85(5):715, 1990.

91. Yee WFH and Scarpelli EM: Surfactant replacement therapy, *Pediatr Pulmonol* 11:65, 1991.

92. Yeh TF and others: Changes of $O_2$ consumption ($VO_2$) in response to NICU care procedures in premature infants (abstract), *Pediatr Res* 16:315A, 1982.

93. Yeh TF and others: Increased $O_2$ consumption and energy loss in premature infants following medical care procedures, *Biol Neonate* 46:157, 1984.

94. Yelderman M and New W: Evaluation of pulse oximetry, *Anesthesiology* 59:349, 1983.

95. Young IM and Holland WW: Some physiological responses of neonatal arterial blood pressure and pulse rate, *Br Med J* 2:276, 1958.

# CHAPTER 26

# Physical Therapy for the Child With Respiratory Dysfunction

*Jeanne A. DeCesare, Carole A. Graybill-Tucker, and Anne L. Gould*

## FRAME OF REFERENCE

Improved diagnostic, surgical, and medical techniques have had an impact on pediatric care. In 1967, at the

☐ We would like to thank biomedical photographer, James Koepfler, Department of Orthopedic Surgery, Children's Hospital, Boston, for his outstanding contribution to this chapter; Claire McCarthy, Michelina Cassella, and the Physical Therapy staff at Children's Hospital, Boston; and the patients and parents who so willingly agreed to pose for photographs. ☐ This chapter is dedicated to the memory of Jeffrey S. O'Connell, who lived his life so well, with enviable strength and spirit.

Children's Hospital in Boston, the average length of stay for a patient was 14.0 days. By 1978 that number had been reduced to 8.3 days; by 1988 it was further reduced to 6.7 days; and in 1992 the average length of stay was 5.8 days. The number of days in the hospital for patients over 21 years of age almost doubled from 1967 to 1981, with an additional 7.1% increase from 1981 to 1988.[11] These statistics probably reflect changes in medical care, causing increased life expectancy of patients with chronic life-limiting diseases. For example, the patients with cystic fibrosis born today have a much better chance of living into their twenties than those of previous years.[150] On the other end of the spectrum, premature infants who would have died in past years are now surviving the newborn period because of improved, intensive neonatal care. Chemotherapy and aggressive surgical intervention have helped improve the life expectancy for many pediatric patients with neoplasms. Some patients with bone marrow dysfunction, such as acute leukemia and aplastic anemia, can undergo bone marrow transplantation, which may cure their otherwise fatal disease. Pediatric patients with congenital malformations or end-stage disease of various solid organs—such as kidney, heart, liver, or lung—can now receive transplants for their failing organ that offer them an increased chance of survival and increased well-being.

Cardiac and thoracic surgical advances also account for earlier correction of abnormalities in newborns and infants and survival of those with previously uncorrectable anomalies.

A wider range of care for every age group from the premature infant to the young adult has evolved with medical advances and has redirected the pediatric clinician's focus. Physical therapy evaluation and treatment must therefore reflect this diversification in pediatric care.

### The developing lung

It is an accepted fact that children are different from adults. Not only do their emotional responses and small stature set them apart, but anatomical and physiological differences are apparent. Total care of the pediatric patient means consideration of growing systems—cardiopulmonary, skeletal, neurological, and so on.

Lung growth is not complete at birth. Normal growth and remodeling of the lung continues until adulthood.[108] The bronchial tree is fully formed by approximately 16 weeks of gestation. After birth the conducting airways continue to increase in diameter and length but not in number. Primitive alveoli are present at birth, but mature alveolar growth and development take place after birth. There is some controversy as to when the development of new alveoli stops. It has been suggested that by 8 years of age the number of alveoli is the same as that in the adult.[108] However, there is some evidence that the number of alveoli increases until 12 years of age.[33] The alveoli are developing throughout most of childhood. Alveolar diameter also changes with age. The diameter of alveoli at 2 months is approximately 60 to 130 microns. This diameter increases to a range of 100 to 200 microns in older children, whereas the adult has alveoli of 200 to 300 microns in diameter.[33] Changes in morphology and size of the alveoli appear to parallel increases in the lateral chest wall dimension.[21] The contour of an infant's chest is more rounded than that of an adult's, which has an elliptical shape. A rounded chest with ribs positioned horizontally, as seen in an infant, places the intercostals and accessory muscles of respiration at a mechanical disadvantage. An elliptical-shaped chest, as seen in the adult, provides a mechanical advantage for the intercostal and accessory muscles.[44]

Branching of the pulmonary artery at 19 weeks of fetal life is the same as the adult pattern. Alveolar capillaries multiply as rapidly after birth as the alveoli do.

There appears to be greater density of mucous glands in relationship to the size of the bronchial surface in the young child. Nearly twice the density of glands per unit surface is present in children less than 4 years old compared with the adult.[33] Goblet cells, which generally do not extend beyond the cartilaginous portion of the tracheobronchial tree, often migrate rapidly into the bronchioles and replace ciliated cells in disease. These findings may explain why the severity of obstructive pulmonary disease is more striking in infants and young children with small airways than in older patients.

Because of the lack of smooth muscle development, which occurs by about 3 to 4 years of age, there is weakness in the bronchioles of infants and young children. This weakness may contribute to airway collapse and air trapping. It has also been found that peripheral airway conductance, or the freedom with which air flows through an airway, increases substantially at about 5 years of age.[33] Children up to 5 years of age have a greater proportion of narrow airways as compared with adults. Fifty per cent of peripheral airways are less than 2 mm in diameter in infants as opposed to only 20% in adults. In addition, the lung volume at which airway closure occurs is higher in children under 7 years of age. This

may be the result of decreased elastic recoil. This, combined with narrower airways, predisposes young children to airway obstruction and collapse and increases their susceptibility to complications from small airway diseases such as bronchiolitis.

In addition to the lack of structural support in the small airways in the early years, collateral ventilation offered by the pores of Kohn and Lambert's canals is limited. Development of the pores of Kohn may not occur until 12 to 13 years of age[33] Lambert's canals may not exist until 6 to 8 years of age.[21] The young child is therefore at higher risk for development of atelectasis and infection.

Lung volume and surface area increase steadily through adolescence and most likely relate to an increase in alveolar size and number. When ill, the infant and young child have less pulmonary reserve to depend on than the adult does. This poor reserve is probably attributable to a child's increased resting oxygen consumption demand in relationship to the lung surface area.[33]

Some investigators have noticed that lung compliance and distensibility may be low in young children. Elastic tissue may not develop in the walls of the alveoli until after adolescence.[141] In addition to lung compliance being decreased in children, chest wall compliance is increased. This disparity can lead to severe chest retractions and loss of mechanical advantage to the inspiratory musculature during respiratory distress. Prior to 8 months of age, type 1, fatigue resistant muscle fibers are not present in adult proportions. This along with a small glycogen supply in the muscle contributes to respiratory fatigue for the infant.[132]

It is apparent from what we know about lung growth and development that the infant and young child represent a high-risk population for pulmonary dysfunction. Improved pulmonary reserve, greater airway support and patency, and collateral ventilation occur with growth. Chest physical therapy for the pediatric patient is therefore a challenge in both the treatment and prevention of pulmonary complications.

## Importance of the family

Years ago family participation was not encouraged in pediatric care; today, however, it is enthusiastically welcomed. The family, primarily parents, is an excellent resource to health professionals. Parents are needed to construct a comprehensive medical history of their child. They can offer vital information regarding their child's personality and usual responses to the environment. It is essential to establish a good relationship with both family and patient.

Family participation and cooperation during the care of a hospitalized child can mean better understanding and compliance with a home care program. Poor communication and exclusion of parents from their child's care can result in noncompliance with a treatment regimen. Comprehensive parental education is crucial to ensure continued care for the

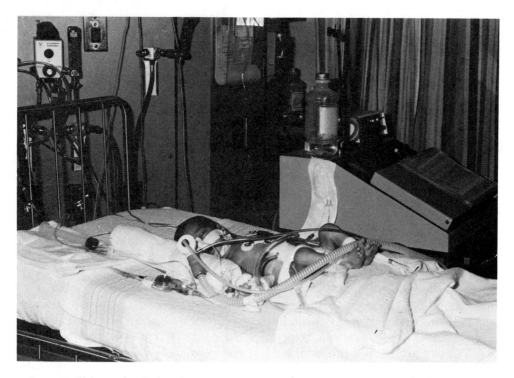

**Fig. 26-1.** Elaborate medical equipment becomes part of the environment of an acutely ill child.

pediatric patient at home. If the parents are unavailable or uninvolved, then whoever will be the primary caretaker must be included in home treatment planning.

## PATIENT PROBLEMS
### Physical considerations

**Easy fatigue, disturbed schedules.** The infant and child are experiencing growth and physiological changes that must be considered by the physical therapist when planning treatment. As has been discussed, lung growth and remodeling are taking place throughout childhood and possibly adolescence. The previous discussion of the anatomical and physiological immaturity of the growing lung shows that such immaturity contributes to airway collapse and increased airway resistance, atelectasis, and lack of pulmonary reserve during stress. This decreased reserve leads to easy fatigability. As a result, the length of chest physical therapy treatment sessions may have to be reduced for an acutely ill infant or child. Shorter, more frequent treatments may be indicated. Use of frequent position changes is essential and should be a part of a bronchial hygiene program.

When caring for an acutely ill child, one must carry out many medical interventions throughout the day and night. Sleep cycles and schedules can be disturbed easily. Chest physical therapy may be needed every 2 to 3 hours. One approach to this rigorous routine of medical care is to place a child on "stress precautions." This is an attempt to protect the child from unnecessary disturbances by using a strict intervention schedule, with structured periods of rest and minimal contact. Physical therapy should be coordinated with this synchronized approach to help reduce patient stress.

Fig. 26-1 shows the medical equipment needed for the care of an acutely ill infant. This elaborate technological armamentarium becomes part of the infant's environment.

**Small chests.** The size of an infant's or child's chest will alter treatment technique. Hand positioning for bronchial drainage and the force of percussion techniques will have to be modified. The use of one hand or three fingers in a tented position may be sufficient to cover the indicated area of the chest for percussion techniques (Fig. 26-2).

**Gastroesophageal reflux.** An incompetent lower esophageal sphincter mechanism causing repeated return of stomach contents into the esophagus is known as "gastroesophageal reflux" (GER). If the stomach contents reach the pharynx, partially digested food may be aspirated into the lungs causing respiratory problems. Interest in gastroesophageal reflux helped to identify it as a possible cause of recurrent pneumonias and pulmonary problems in children who repeatedly experienced aspiration of refluxed gastric contents.[55] In the absence of vomiting, diagnosis of this problem becomes more difficult. It may be overlooked or misdiagnosed as bronchopulmonary dysplasia in the premature infant or allergic bronchitis or asthma in the older child. Many infants have mild gastroesophageal reflux that resolves when they begin to sit upright. The majority of cases (60%) will resolve by 18 months of age. However, about 30% will continue to have significant reflux until at least 4

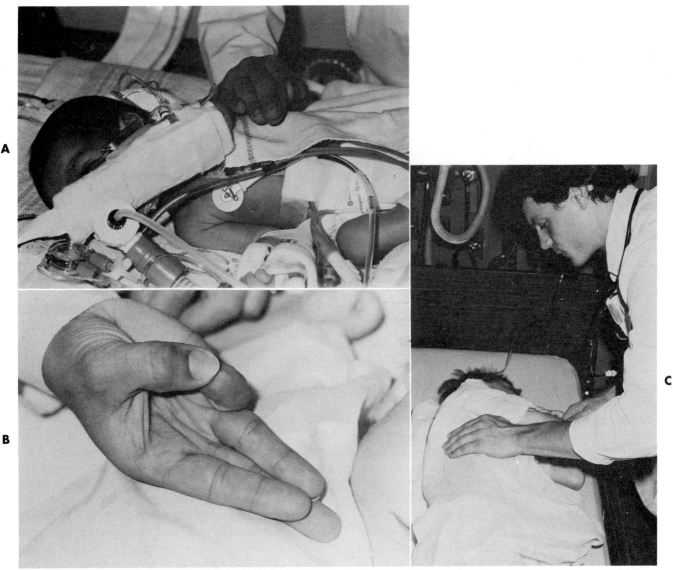

**Fig. 26-2. A,** "Tented" position of hand for percussion of small infant's chest. **B,** Underside view. **C,** Use of one hand for percussion on chest of small child.

years of age and sometimes longer.[55] Gastroesophageal reflux also appears to be common in children with severe neurological impairment, although the reason for this has not been identified.[54] Hendren and Lillehei[54] recommended that if a feeding gastrostomy is being considered for a neurologically impaired patient, then gastroesophageal reflux should be evaluated and the need for an antireflux surgical procedure be examined. It has been determined that a feeding gastrostomy can actually create reflux.[64] The physical therapist should be aware of these possibilities when working with any patient with neurological dysfunction or a feeding gastrostomy tube.

Conservative medical treatment may require that the child maintain an upright position after feedings or constantly when gastroesophageal reflux is severe. An upright prone position appears less favorable to reflux because the esophagogastric junction is located at the uppermost part of the stomach and the contents are less likely to be regurgitated[55] (Fig. 26-3). Prone positioning also encourages extensor muscle activity and strengthening, which is a fringe benefit to the motor development of an infant. However, if bronchial drainage is necessary, the physician should be consulted regarding positioning—especially if lower lobe secretions are present. The benefits of head-down positioning for bronchial drainage must be considered. Bronchial drainage is always recommended before a meal or no earlier than 1 hour after meals. Treatment before a meal is preferred for any child suspected of having gastroesophageal reflux. If strict positional therapy must be maintained, bronchial drainage may have to be done in a modified position.

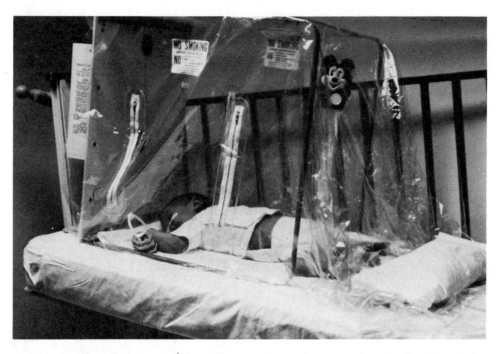

**Fig. 26-3.** Infant upright prone position to decrease chance of gastroesophageal reflux. The plastic oxygen tent is supplying necessary oxygen to the infant, but it provides a limited environment.

Percussion and vibration techniques can be used without any precautionary measures.

Strict adherence to a premeal schedule for bronchial drainage is also recommended for the infant with feeding problems and the child with cystic fibrosis who has difficulty maintaining adequate nutritional intake and is likely to vomit when coughing. The therapist should always inquire if bronchial drainage has a tendency to cause vomiting.

**Developmental delay.** Developmental delay is another significant problem for a sick infant or child. Prolonged or frequent hospitalizations of a child or dependency on oxygen can create a limited environment (Fig. 26-3). There may be a lack of sensorimotor stimulation no matter how sensitive a hospital staff may be to this issue. Psychobiological deprivation studies clearly point out that a growing neurological system needs appropriate stimulation to develop.[103]

The physical therapist working in pediatric chest care must realize that many patients requiring prolonged hospitalizations can experience secondary lung problems. These children will experience decreased environmental stimulation and be at risk for delays in sensorimotor development. The child with primary lung problems may also require extended hospitalizations and may be oxygen dependent. Increased secretions may interfere with feeding and normal oral motor development. Children with bronchopulmonary dysplasia may have constant oxygen requirements that, even when delivered at home, can restrict their ability to explore their environment. Physical therapists must be acutely aware of the developmental needs of their maturing patients regardless of the primary diagnosis.

### Psychological considerations

It is essential when working in pediatrics to be aware of the emotional impact an illness has on a child. A large part of the problem is a child's inability to verbalize fears and concerns. Interpreting the cries of an infant is not an easy task.

Illness can disrupt family security and unity. Anxiety regarding separation from parents and siblings may be acute for the hospitalized child. Welcoming parents to stay during treatment may help alleviate some of this anxiety. The fear of pain and invasive medical procedures can be overwhelming. Reassurance that chest physical therapy will not require use of a "needle" may help. Recognizing the fear and responding with concern and sensitivity can be the key to successful treatment. For example, the fear of dislodging a small intravenous needle in the arm or hand can prevent a child from moving or sleeping well. A therapist must respect these fears and assure the child that the intravenous line will be carefully watched and supported during treatment. A child's unwillingness to move may be caused by this anxiety and not by uncooperative behavior.

Making treatment as comfortable and pleasant an experience as possible is also very important. Using games or songs to obtain therapeutic results will help capture the child's attention and cooperation.

Frequent or prolonged illness may interfere with normal social development. The hospitalized infant or child may receive too much attention from many different caretakers. Hospitalization may also reduce peer contact, which is important for the self-image of older children and adolescents. Respiratory illnesses especially may prevent participation in normal play and sports because of shortness of breath and fatigue.

Dealing with an illness can bring about stresses such as anger, guilt, and resentment in a child or adolescent who is often not emotionally mature. Acting out and inappropriate behavior may result. Feelings may be manifested through noncompliance with the medical regimen, as is often seen in the adolescent.

Young patients grappling with a chronic disease may find that life-style changes, such as entry into college, require much planning and often compromise future goals and dreams.

### Death and dying

Working with a dying patient is never easy and can be particularly difficult when the patient is a child. Several texts have been written about the topic.[74,116] Death brings to light our own personal death awareness and the fears we harbor regarding the loss of life. The physical therapist who works with children with respiratory illnesses cannot escape facing a dying child. Schowalter,[120] who has written about the reactions of caregivers dealing with fatal illnesses in children, makes special mention of the physical therapist. He believes that physical therapists may experience specialized stresses when working with patients who do not improve but are maintained or deteriorate despite a rehabilitative approach. In the pediatric setting, therapists may personalize the loss of patients. Younger patients may be close in age to a therapist's own children or siblings. For older patients, the age difference between patient and therapist may be small and may create in the therapist a heightened sense of personal vulnerability. In view of this, an emotional bond may be established between patient and therapist. Facing the death of such a patient can have a significant impact upon the therapist.

We recommend that regular sessions with a staff psychologist, psychiatrist, or other trained professional be arranged for physical therapists who are faced with the stress of working with dying patients. It is not unusual for a therapist working in a major center for patients with cystic fibrosis to face several deaths in a short period of time.

An understanding of our own feelings and reactions toward loss of life can often help when working with someone who is facing a terminal illness. In pediatrics, one deals with dying patients who have widely different conceptions of death, depending on their age and maturity. It is probably easiest to respond as naturally as possible and to continue to foster a therapeutic and personal relationship despite the grave prognosis. Finding the right words to say to a patient facing the end of life is the most difficult. The therapist should depend on the relationship he or she has already developed to ease the difficulty.

It is important that a therapist continue treatment for a dying patient with whom he or she has developed a relationship. The treatment components may change because of a lack of patient tolerance, but continued contact is essential. A child who expects daily physical therapy should believe it is being continued, even though modified, despite his or her deterioration. We are fortunate as therapists to have our manual skills to offer comfort and express our closeness and concern for the dying patient. Massage can be a soothing experience for a distressed, breathless patient. Parents or family members can be taught simple massage strokes to use in the therapist's absence. This technique may give parents an opportunity to offer comfort and remain physically close to their child. The therapist may discover that opportunities to offer comfort through massage or other manual techniques can replace the need to "find the right words."

### Diseases

**Chronic obstructive lung diseases.**  Chronic obstruction of the airways can be caused by increased secretions, bronchospasm, inflammation or destruction of the bronchial walls, or a combination of the above. There is an interference of the normal flow of air within the lung. Some reversibility of the obstructive components can be achieved through the use of bronchodilator or antiinflammatory drugs (steroids) and chest physical therapy. For example, the airway obstruction in asthma is often reversible.

Lung changes attributable to structural damage as seen in cystic fibrosis are irreversible, but chest physical therapy continues to be extremely important in clearing airways of excessive secretions.

*Asthma.*  Asthma is a condition characterized by intermittent airway obstruction, airway inflammation, and increased irritability or hyperactivity of the tracheobronchial tree caused by an assortment of stimulants. Recurrent episodes of wheezing or dyspnea that are reversed or spontaneously with medication constitute the clinical picture of asthma. Asthma has been classified into two types. Extrinsic asthma is caused by allergens or environmental factors, whereas intrinsic asthma is caused by nonallergic factors including psychosomatic components. Childhood asthma is primarily of the extrinsic type, though a mixture of the two types may occur.

The primary clinical signs of an asthma "attack" include an increased respiratory rate, spasmodic cough, prolonged expiration with wheezing, and pulmonary hyperinflation. Initially the cough may be dry, but as secretions increase, the cough may become productive. If symptoms progress, severe bronchial obstruction may occur in part because of bronchospasm and secretions. The patient becomes so "tight" that little air is moving in the lungs and the patient becomes fatigued. Respiratory failure can ensue with the need for oxygen therapy and possible mechanical ventilation.

The medical management of an acute asthma episode relies on inhaled bronchodilators, oral or inhaled corticosteroids, and intravenous sympathetic nervous stimulants such as epinephrine or aminophylline (See pp. 310-311, 313). If the child's bronchospasm is not improved by this medical therapy, the child is considered to be in status asthmaticus.[132] Standard long-term outpatient medical treatment consists of drug therapy, primarily with oral or inhaled bronchodilators and, in severe cases, corticosteroids. Environmental controls can minimize dust and other offending allergens, and reduction of emotional stress can help. Hyposensitization through injection of gradually increasing doses of the offending allergens may offer some relief. Exercise induced asthma is common in children, and strenuous exercise or sudden cold may precipitate an exacerbation.[132]

The physical therapist has much to offer the child with asthma. Outpatient treatment programs should include relaxation and controlled breathing techniques, exercises for thoracic mobility, and general conditioning exercises. Included also is parental and patient education with an emphasis on how to minimize attacks.[121] Treatment during an acute attack should focus on relaxation and controlled diaphragmatic breathing. A child in status asthmaticus initially may be unable to cooperate with physical therapy intervention secondary to their severe respiratory distress.[132] Once bronchodilation has taken place, bronchial drainage with percussion and vibration may help clear secretions. If the patient has difficulty with excessive secretions, instruction of parents or patient in bronchial drainage techniques for home care may be indicated. Bronchial drainage may be of benefit to the child with asthma on an intermittent basis when the child is developing or has a respiratory infection.

***Cystic fibrosis.*** Cystic fibrosis is the most common life-limiting genetic disease among white children.[150] It is characterized by generalized exocrine gland dysfunction. It affects many organ systems, but an elevated salt content in the sweat, chronic pulmonary disease, and pancreatic insufficiency resulting in nutritional compromise are the primary manifestations. Increased awareness of the disease and a valid diagnostic test (the sweat test) have aided in earlier recognition of symptoms and diagnosis. The cloning of the cystic fibrosis gene and the identification of many mutations of the gene have led to the use of direct DNA analysis for diagnostic testing.[6] The clinical course of the disease is variable. However, with medical advances, including appropriate antibiotic therapy and chest physical therapy to control lung infection, the life expectancy with cystic fibrosis has improved significantly, with many patients living into adulthood.[93,123] In recent years lung transplantation has become a treatment option for some children and adults with advanced lung disease.

Cystic fibrosis accounts for much of the chronic lung disease seen in children. Possible impairment of mucociliary transport, production of copious mucous secretions, mucous plugging of peripheral airways, recurrent infections, and eventual bronchial wall destruction all contribute to the obstructive lung disease. As the pulmonary involvement progresses, habitual coughing, abnormal distribution of

ventilation, decreased pulmonary function, and weight loss compromise exercise tolerance. Airway instability also appears to be a contributing factor.[76,151]

Complications of cystic fibrosis include atelectasis, recurrent infection, pneumothorax, hemoptysis, and cor pulmonale.[57,93,119] Hospitalization and intensive therapy are generally indicated for control of exacerbations of pulmonary infections or other complications such as pneumothorax or massive hemoptysis. However, recent studies[34,75] indicate that patients previously hospitalized for pulmonary exacerbations can be treated as effectively at home. These home treatment regimens are substantially less costly and allow patients to remain in a comfortable and familiar setting. Home treatment regimens do require that the patient or patient's family help provide the additional care and time needed to carry out the expanded medical regime during this time. Home care professionals may be available to help with intravenous management and chest physical therapy.

Nutritional, pulmonary, and psychosocial needs of patients with cystic fibrosis are met through care at nationally recognized and supported cystic fibrosis centers. The physical therapist is an integral part of the medical team caring for the patient with cystic fibrosis.[133] Bronchial drainage (with percussion, rib shaking, and vibration to all bronchopulmonary segments), breathing exercises and retraining, and postural and general conditioning exercise are the primary techniques incorporated into a person's treatment program. Family instruction regarding the various chest physical therapy techniques is essential for care at home. Normal physical activity and play should also be encouraged to promote mobilization and expectoration of secretions. Techniques for secretion removal—such as the forced expiration technique (FET),[105,106,132,137] self-applied positive expiratory airway pressure with a mask (PEP),* and autogenic drainage[28,29,31,132]—have been used in Great Britain and Europe with cystic fibrosis patients. These techniques are beginning to be included in treatment programs here in the United States. New aerosolized medications that reduce the viscosity of the purulent sputum have promising results for the treatment of lung disease.[58] As improvements in medical management in cystic fibrosis occur, many people with cystic fibrosis are surviving into adulthood. Recent medical literature is focusing on management and complications of cystic fibrosis in adults.[93] The physical therapist must help educate and encourage adolescents to take an active role in decision making with regards to their pulmonary hygiene program. This will help facilitate the adolescent's transition into adulthood, which brings added responsibilities to provide his or her own health care.

The psychosocial support needed by patient and families facing a genetically inherited and lethal disease cannot be overestimated.[100] The autosomal recessive pattern of inheritance in cystic fibrosis results in a one-in-four chance of two

---

* References 31, 37, 47, 56, 97, 125, 132, 140, 142.

carriers producing a child with the disease and dictates the need for genetic counseling. With an increased number of patients living into adulthood, career and marital counseling should also be available. Finally, and most importantly, a hospital staff should be trained and prepared to offer support, care, and concern when a patient is facing deteriorating pulmonary status and terminal hospital admission or death at home.

**Restrictive lung diseases.** Restrictive lung disease is characterized by a reduction of lung volume caused by extrapulmonary or pulmonary factors.[43] Chest wall stiffness and deformity and respiratory muscle weakness can cause decreased thoracic excursion resulting in decreased lung volumes including vital capacity and total lung capacity. Loss of lung tissue caused by tumor or surgical removal, atelectasis, and pneumonia are also causes of restrictive pulmonary problems.

Primary causes of extrapulmonary restrictive lung disease in the pediatric population include the following particular disease entities.

*Muscular weakness.* Respiratory muscle weakness can lead to respiratory insufficiency with subsequent respiratory failure, which can be fatal—especially in patients with progressive muscular diseases such as muscular dystrophy. Inability to take deep breaths because of weak respiratory muscles can result in patchy areas of atelectasis.[94] The cough musculature may be weak and effective removal of secretions thereby reduced. Patients with muscular weakness are at risk for aspiration pneumonia because of poor coordination of the muscles involved in swallowing. A hyperactive gag reflex, as seen in cerebral palsy, may cause frequent choking and aspiration.

Even when a neuromuscular disease is not progressive, skeletal and soft-tissue deformities resulting from inactivity and poor positioning can be progressive and can alter respiratory function. Decreased pulmonary reserve and the likelihood of confinement to bed or wheelchair add to the risk of pulmonary infection for children with neuromuscular disease.

Intercostal and diaphragmatic muscle weakness, ventilatory insufficiency, chronic alveolar hypoventilation, and ventilatory failure are potential complications of muscular and neurological diseases.[94]

Many muscle diseases involve the diaphragm and the intercostals. Diaphragmatic weakness is much more disabling than intercostal weakness because of the primary inspiratory function of the diaphragm. Fortunately, in Duchenne muscular dystrophy, weakness of the diaphragm is not apparent until the end stage of the illness. In cerebral palsy, lack of neuromotor control and coordination and weakness of respiratory muscles may both be a factor in respiratory dysfunction.[112] Increasing intolerance of the supine posture is an indication of progressive diaphragmatic weakness. With a weakened diaphragm, the vital capacity will decrease in the supine position and improve in the upright position.[94] These clinical signs may aid the therapist when assessing diaphragmatic function.

The volume of a voluntary deep breath and the force of a cough will be diminished with ventilatory insufficiency caused by muscular weakness. This may result in small atelectatic areas, which may reduce lung compliance.[41] Dyspnea upon exertion and accessory muscle use during inspiration are likely clinical signs.

Hypoventilation during sleep, in addition to diaphragmatic muscle weakness, can result in chronic alveolar hypoventilation. Increased $Paco_2$ and decreased $Pao_2$ with evidence of cyanosis occur during sleep, with some correction obtained through conscious hyperventilation. A decrease in nocturnal hypoventilation can result in elevation of daytime arterial oxygenation and improved function.[94]

Ventilatory failure marks a serious decline in the patient's respiratory status and usually occurs in the end stage of progressive muscular diseases. The patient may be restless and confused with noticeable cyanosis and respiratory distress. Prolonged carbon dioxide retention may lead to coma and death.

Patients with muscular weakness have many physical therapy needs. Emphasis in the early stages of treatment is on improving muscle tone, maintaining strength and range of motion (including thoracic and spinal flexibility), and promoting physical function at an optimal level.

Emphasis on proper body alignment, especially in sitting and recumbent positions, is essential. Proper alignment may prevent deformities of the extremities, thorax, and vertebral column, which can alter respiratory function. Effective coughing and breathing exercises facilitate and maintain ventilation, chest mobility, and intercostal and diaphragmatic function. As physical function declines or confinement to a wheelchair occurs, close observation of respiratory status is important. As abdominal strength decreases, an abdominal binder or corset may help maintain a normal resting position of the diaphragm through external support.[1] The corset may also be helpful during coughing. A treatment priority is the maintenance of effective coughing through emphasis on abdominal muscle use and support and manually assisted coughing techniques. Manually assisted coughing is described in detail in Chapter 28. Parents should be taught this technique for use at home. If acute infection or chronic mucous retention occurs, a regimen of bronchial drainage with percussion and vibration must be incorporated into the treatment program.

*Skeletal abnormalities*

*Scoliosis.* Chest deformities may compromise lung function by restricting the space in which the lung must grow and function. Scoliosis can cause thoracic deformity and respirator dysfunction in varying degrees depending on the severity of the malalignment. The size and shape of the lungs may be abnormal. Some lobes of the lung are involved more than others and the actual number of alveoli is reduced.[108]

The lung in the convex hemithorax is generally the larger and more important to respiratory function.

Pulmonary function can range from normal for a patient with mild scoliosis to severely reduced in a patient with a severe rotational curve. In more advanced curves lung volume can be affected with reductions in total lung, functional, residual, and vital capacities. In addition to reduced lung volume, decreased compliance of the lung and chest wall may occur. Bjure and others[8] believe that in patients of all ages with severe curves, premature airway closure may be a leading cause of respiratory problems.

The most common blood gas abnormality is a reduced $Pao_2$. Carbon dioxide tension is often normal, but it increases in older patients with scoliosis and in those with obstructive pulmonary disease.[68]

Scoliosis may be congenital, idiopathic, or associated with muscular weakness or spasticity. The patient with neuromuscular disease experiences the double insult of respiratory muscle weakness and the thoracic restriction from a scoliotic deformity.

Physical therapy in the nonsurgical management of scoliosis should always include exercises to improve deep breathing and thoracic mobility in the effort to improve ventilation and prevent atelectasis.

Operative correction of scoliosis is generally indicated for curves of 40° or more in the growing child, and for those curves that are greater then 50° after the end of growth.[17] Surgical access to the spine may be through a posterior vertebral approach or an anterior thoracotomy. Patients who undergo an anterior approach may be at higher risk for postoperative pulmonary complications because of the thoracotomy, diaphragm detachment, and lung manipulation necessary to gain access to the spine. Patients with neuromuscular disease or severe congenital curves are also at higher risk postoperatively than those with idiopathic curves.

Patients without specific pulmonary problems postoperatively benefit from deep-breathing exercises and coughing to prevent atelectasis.[72] If secretion retention, atelectasis, or infection occurs, bronchial drainage with percussion and vibration may be indicated. Precautions should be taken when using Trendelenburg positioning. Depending on the operative procedure performed, stress on the spine must be avoided. The bottom of the bed may have to be raised on blocks to maintain straight spinal alignment. Incisional discomfort may necessitate modification of percussion or vibration.

*Pectus excavatum.* Pectus excavatum, or "funnel chest," consists of an obvious depression of the sternum. The deformity has been thought to be a cosmetic problem that generally does not alter cardiac or pulmonary function.[95] However, patients have reported that symptoms improve following surgical correction, and recent studies have provided physiological data to support these reports. The salient points of these studies were recently highlighted by Hendren and Lillehei.[54] Improvements have been noted in maximal voluntary ventilation and exercise tolerance as measured by total exercise time and maximal oxygen uptake.[15] In 13 patients impressive increases were observed in both right and left ventricular volume postoperatively pointing to possible relief of cardiac compression.[101] In some patients regional ventilatory deficits and regional perfusion abnormalities, especially of the left lower lobe, became normal after surgery.[9] Postoperatively, the patient with a repaired pectus excavatum may need deep breathing exercises and effective coughing to prevent atelectasis. If there is secretion retention, bronchial drainage techniques may be indicated. Patients may have an external metal strut in place to hold the sternum in the corrected position. Discussion should be held with the surgeon regarding precautions that should be observed around the operative site.

### The immunosuppressed patient

*Immunological deficiencies.* There are several syndromes classified as immunological deficiencies. Hypogammaglobulinemia and agammaglobulinemia are two such deficiencies that the pediatric physical therapist may encounter. Patients with these disorders have increased susceptibility to infections, especially bacterial. This susceptibility is caused by a generalized or specific lack of immunoglobulins, which are important for immune function. Hypogammaglobulinemia can be transient when a young infant fails to synthesize his or her own immunoglobulins and is subject to recurrent infections in which the lungs are a common locus. Infants with this syndrome usually recover between 9 and 15 months of age.[5] However, recovery may not occur. In agammaglobulinemia, where there is a lack of all immunoglobulins, infections continue into childhood, resulting in chronic otitis media, sinusitis, and bronchiectasis.

Treatment of these patients is focused primarily on prevention of infection. Physical therapy is directed toward bronchial hygiene for prophylaxis of lung infection. The resulting effects of chronic obstructive pulmonary problems, such as dyspnea, decreased exercise tolerance, and postural abnormalities, must also be considered.

*Bone marrow transplantation.* Human bone marrow transplantation was first attempted in the late 1950s on radiation accident victims.[134] Discovery of histocompatibility typing in the 1960s made it possible to match a recipient's (patient's) tissue with that of a donor's marrow, the treatment rationale being that engraftment of healthy marrow from a donor would provide normal marrow function to the patient and eradication of the disease process. Transplantation is now considered when the patient's disease does not respond to conventional therapy and transplantation is the only hope for a cure.[96]

The most common diseases treated with bone marrow transplantation are leukemia and aplastic anemia. Other diseases that have been successfully treated with bone marrow transplantation include neuroblastomas, lymphomas, Fanconi's anemia, thalassemia, Wiskott-Aldrich syndrome, and severe combined immune disease.[67]

For the patient's body to accept the donor's marrow and allow it to be engrafted, total suppression of the patient's own immune system is required before the transplantation of marrow from the donor. This suppression is accomplished by toxic doses of chemotherapy and possible total body irradiation. Common side effects of these treatments are nausea, vomiting, diarrhea, and alopecia.

After the immunosuppression is accomplished, the immune system is nonfunctional, and the patient has increased susceptibility to infection until successful engraftment occurs. To reduce, and hopefully eliminate, the risk of infection during this time, the patient is placed in a sterile environment such as a laminar airflow room (LAFR) until his or her new immune system is functioning. The patient also undergoes daily baths and bowel preparations to ensure skin and gut sterilization. Everyone entering the LAFR, including family, must scrub hands and forearms with antibacterial soap and wear a gown

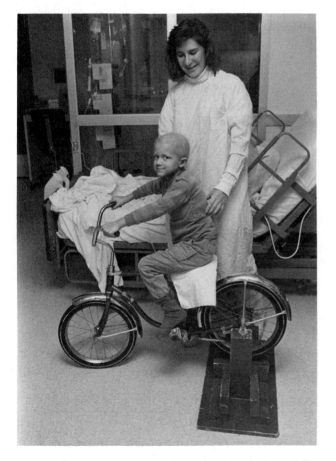

**Fig. 26-4.** Physical therapist with a patient in a laminar airflow room. The stationary bicycle is being used as part of the therapeutic exercise program for this patient who has undergone bone marrow transplantation.

(Fig. 26-4). Engraftment can occur as early as eighteen to thirty days, but may take as long as six to eight weeks.

After the patient is in the LAFR and immunosuppressed, the bone marrow transplant is performed. The usual route for administration of the donor marrow is intravenous. Rejection of the bone marrow transplant and complications such as infection and graft-versus-host disease are the major problems of bone marrow transplantation and can result in death.[135]

The physical therapist is part of the team of medical professionals who address the complex needs of these patients and their families. The relationship between therapist and patient entails weeks or months of hard work and understanding. A complete physical therapy evaluation should be done before the initiation of chemotherapy and the onset of its side effects.[63] The evaluation should include assessments of range of motion, muscle strength, functional, developmental, and respiratory status. The respiratory evaluation should be thorough since patients with marrow diseases and a suppressed immunological system may have a history of recurrent pulmonary infections with possible chronic obstructive changes.

The patient is at risk for infection from the point of total suppression of bone marrow in preparation for the transplant until total engraftment of donor marrow. Patients are particularly susceptible to viral illness. The most common infectious complication is interstitial pneumonia, which usually occurs after the marrow graft shows some function.[135] Cytomegalovirus and the effects of irradiation are possible causes of this type of pneumonia. Chest physical therapy, including bronchial hygiene and instruction in relaxed breathing patterns and effective coughing, are indicated. General mobility, maintenance of strength and range of motion, and encouragement of developmental milestones in the younger patient are all necessary in the rehabilitation of the restricted bone marrow transplant patient (Fig. 26-4). Platelet counts will be compromised while the patient is immunosuppressed and should be considered before one institutes daily treatment (see p. 547).

***Pediatric acquired immunodeficiency syndrome.*** By September of 1992, a total of 4051 cases of acquired immunodeficiency syndrome (AIDS) in children less than 13 years of age had been reported to the Centers for Disease Control (CDC). An estimated 10,000 to 20,000 children are currently infected with the human immunodeficiency virus type 1 (HIV-1), and AIDS was the ninth leading cause of death in children aged 1 to 4 years in the United States.[4]

*Diagnosis.* It is important to make a distinction between AIDS in adults and that seen in children. Criteria for the diagnosis of AIDS in adults and children established by the CDC are available and worth reviewing.[19,20,107] The term "pediatric AIDS" is used to refer to children under the age of 13 years who are afflicted with the disease. When diagnosing pediatric AIDS, all primary and secondary causes for immunodeficiencies must be excluded. Individuals are generally tested for the presence of the antibody for HIV. The HIV antibody test should be positive for the diagnosis of HIV infection, and recurrent or serious bacterial infections should also be present. The CDC has recently added histologically documented lymphoid interstitial pneumonitis (LIP) in children under 13 years of age (with a positive HIV test) as an acceptable criterion for the diagnosis of pediatric AIDS.[19] Not all individuals infected with HIV automatically develop AIDS. Approximately 50% infected with HIV are presently asymptomatic.[10] Others develop AIDS-related complex (ARC), which describes the condition of those who have some of the symptoms of AIDS—such as prolonged fevers, weight loss, swollen lymph glands, and fungal infection of the mouth—but lack the tumors and opportunistic infections present with AIDS. The final stage of infection with HIV is fully expressed AIDS.

*Transmission.* The majority of pediatric AIDS cases (75% to 80%) in the United States are a result of transmission of the HIV from infected mothers to infants during the perinatal period.[4,10,25,79] An infected mother will transmit the virus to her baby an estimated 20% of the time.[4] It is important to note that infants who are seropositive for the antibody to HIV but without clinical symptoms are not automatically considered to be infected with the virus before the age of 14 to 15 months. This is because passively transmitted maternal antibodies can cause an infant to test positive for the HIV antibody test even when the actual virus has not been transmitted.

HIV transmission beyond the neonatal period may occur by infusion of infected blood products, or high risk behaviors, such as sharing intravenous needles or sexual contact with an infected person. Most children with transfusion-related HIV disease were infected prior to 1985, and hemophiliacs make up a large portion of this group.[4,10,79] A growing percentage of HIV infected adolescents is noted due to increased practice of high risk behaviors.

*Symptoms.* If acquired perinatally, symptoms of AIDS are usually manifested during the first 6 months of age.[2,25] Infected infants are usually small for gestational age. Other symptoms and clinical findings in pediatric AIDS include failure to thrive, present in all children at some time during their disease course, recurrent pneumonias, upper respiratory infections, otitis media, persistent or recurrent oral candidiasis, chronic diarrhea, parotitis, hepatosplenomegaly, and lymphadenopathy.[2,4,10,25,113] More rapid disease progression is associated with the presence of opportunistic infections such as pneumocystis carinii pneumonia (PCP) or progressive neurological disease.[4] Hepatomegaly, splenomegaly, parotitis, and lymphocytic interstitial pneumonitis (LIP) are symptoms associated with longer survival.[4] As the disease progresses, children develop the same opportunistic infections as adults with AIDS. The following is a list of clinical findings that are unique to the pediatric age group:

1. Kaposi's sarcoma is very rare
2. Presence of parotitis or chronic parotid swelling
3. Presence of lymphoid interstitial pneumonitis (LIP)
4. Neurological sequelae that are different from those seen in adults

*Pulmonary sequelae.* The two major pulmonary diseases affecting patients with pediatric AIDS are lymphoid interstitial pneumonitis (LIP) and infections. PCP is the leading infectious cause of pulmonary disease. The lung disease seen in pediatric AIDS is most responsible for the morbidity and mortality of affected children.[107]

Lymphoid interstitial pneumonitis is seen only in pediatric AIDS patients and not in adults with AIDS. LIP is characterized by diffuse infiltration of the interstitial spaces and peribronchiolar areas by lymphocytes, plasma cells, and immunoblasts.[2,22] Significant and widespread lymphadenopathy, cough, digital clubbing, salivary gland enlargement, and a nodular pattern on chest radiography are also present.[25,113] The pulmonary disease is characterized by an insidious onset of respiratory distress with mild to moderate hypoxemia. The etiology of LIP and why some children develop LIP and others do not have not been determined. Symptoms may come and go, or continue unchanged for months or years. Children with LIP do not have as many opportunistic infections, although they may have persistent Epstein-Barr virus infection.[113] Despite the possibility of severe pulmonary sequelae, AIDS patients with LIP have a lower mortality rate than those with many opportunistic infections.[10] Also, infants with LIP present at the age of approximately 14 months, as opposed to approximately 6 months of age for those with opportunistic infections.

The two most common life-threatening opportunistic infections affecting the lungs in pediatric AIDS are pneumocystis carinii pneumonia (PCP), and cytomegalovirus (CMV). High fever, dry cough, hypoxemia, abnormal auscultatory findings, and tachypnea when at rest are presenting clinical signs of PCP. Onset of PCP is generally acute, with rapid progression of respiratory distress, as opposed to LIP, with its more insidious onset with milder symptoms. Early in the disease, chest radiographs may appear normal; later in the disease, however, bilateral alveolar and interstitial infiltrates can be seen.[2] CMV pneumonia is characterized by interstitial inflammation and edema, alveolar cell hyperplasia, and occasional hyaline membranes.[2] The onset of CMV can be rapid or slow. Radiographic changes consist of either a diffuse interstitial pattern or a more alveolar pattern.

Other opportunistic pulmonary infections seen are mycobacterium avium-intracellular (MAI), mycobacterium tuberculosis, Epstein-Barr virus (EBV), and adenoviruses.[2,66] In addition, reactive airways disease is also common.[22]

The correct diagnosis of the pulmonary disease is important and will directly affect the patient's treatment. LIP and PCP frequently can be distinguished by clinical signs and laboratory data;[25,113] however, it can be extremely difficult to distinguish different infectious agents without a more invasive procedure. The procedure of choice for diagnosis of the infectious agent in adults with AIDS is fiberoptic bronchoscopy.[90] However, the diagnosis of PCP, CMV, or other infectious agents in children generally requires an open lung biopsy.[2] There is some evidence in the literature of success with bronchoscopy and bronchoalveolar lavage for diagnosis of PCP and other organisms in children with AIDS though research has been limited.[14]

*Cardiac sequelae.* Recent literature indicates that children with congenital AIDS, as well as adults with AIDS, are at risk for developing cardiac complications. The primary cardiac complication is dilated cardiomyopathy, with resultant electrocardiograph abnormalities, pericardial effusions, and congestive heart failure with right ventricular hypertrophy.[127] The exact etiology of the cardiac involvement is unknown, however the virus itself seems to be able to initiate the process.[22]

*Neurological sequelae.* Neurological complications exist in children with HIV disease.[7,51] It is estimated that 50% of HIV-infected children and 90% of children with AIDS have some type of neurological involvement.[25] Central nervous system effects may include static or progressive encephalopathy, acquired microcephaly, developmental delay, cognitive deficits, bilateral pyramidal tract signs, and basal ganglion calcifications. Motor dysfunction is often a combination of weakness, flaccidity, hyperreflexia, and spasticity.[22] Central nervous system opportunistic infections are not as common in pediatric patients as they are in adult patients with AIDS.[7] Rather, evidence suggests that AIDS encephalopathy in children results from direct HIV infection of the central nervous system.

*Treatment.* There is no known cure for AIDS, however HIV disease can no longer be considered untreatable.[27] Many medications are being used with some success,[113,114,124] however only two drugs, zidovudine and didanosine, are approved by the Food and Drug Administration for use in children.[27]

The physical therapist is a vital member of the medical team treating patients with AIDS. The physical therapist working with AIDS patients must address the multiple disease processes and problems that result from this illness, including the complications created by immunosuppression, neurological disorders, and general debilitation.

For patients with pulmonary infections chest physical therapy can help remove secretions and thus improve ventilation and breathing control. With PCP, CMV, and LIP pneumonitis, a nonproductive cough is typical. Bronchial drainage would not be indicated in these cases, but often there are concomitant infections causing production of thick secretions and therefore warranting intervention. In older pediatric patients functional levels can be improved through paced breathing exercises. General conditioning exercises can help endurance. Range of motion exercises, developmental stimulation, gait assessment, and use of assistive devices may be indicated if neurological sequelae exist.

Home programs with appropriate instruction to the parents or guardians should be designed. A thorough assessment of each patient and his or her individual problems must be outlined and a program planned accordingly.

AIDS is not easily transmitted, but it is very important for physical therapists to be aware of infection control when treating any patient. Both the Centers for Disease Control (CDC) and the American Academy of Pediatrics (AAP) have published valuable guidelines regarding infection control in health care settings.[18,131] Essentially all patients should be considered to be potential HIV carriers. "Universal Precautions" are presently being put into effect in most health care settings. Handwashing with some type of skin detergent before and after contact with a patient should be carried out. If there is a possibility of contact with blood or body fluids, gloves should be worn. Gowns should be worn if clothing could be soiled. A gown is also recommended when working with children who are not toilet trained. Masks and goggles should be worn if there is a possibility of splashing of body fluids such as during tracheal suctioning (Fig. 26-5).

At the same time, patients with AIDS or HIV disease are immunosuppressed and must be protected from outside contaminants. If a therapist has a sore throat, cold, cough, or any airborne contagion, a mask is recommended. Gloves should be worn if there is a chance of spreading a contagion

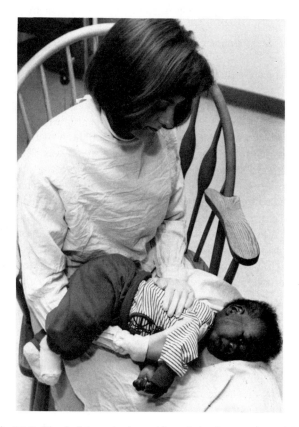

**Fig. 26-5.** Physical therapist dressed for universal precautions while performing a lap drainage on an infant. Gowns are recommended when treating children who are not toilet trained, and gloves should be worn if there is a possibility of contact with body secretions.

through contact. A mild infection for a healthy person could be devastating to an immunosuppressed patient.

In summary, treating a pediatric patient with AIDS requires the physical therapist to consider many issues. The therapist must be aware of the effect of the underlying disease as well as of the secondary infections and sequelae. Evaluating each individual's clinical picture in light of the broad spectrum of the disease's symptoms and complications is essential. The therapist should consider the impact of a fatal disease on a child's comprehension and also maintain close communications with the parents or primary caretakers. The emphasis of treatment must be on physical potential and quality of life.

### Acute problems

*Bronchiolitis.* Bronchiolitis, which is commonly caused by the respiratory syncytial virus (RSV), is a leading cause of respiratory distress with wheezing in the young infant. The RSV infection usually occurs during November to March in infants under 2 years of age, with the majority being under 6 months.[109] The clinical picture is one of a preceding upper respiratory infection followed by an abrupt onset of dyspnea, retractions, tachypnea, and wheezing. A chest radiograph can show air trapping, peribronchiolar thickening, consolidation (which is usually segmental), and collapse. Histologically, there may be necrosis of bronchiolar epithelium with concurrent cilia destruction. Infiltration of lymphocytes into the peribronchial tissue, edema, and mucous plugging of the airways add to the problems.[149] The poor development of collateral ventilation in the lungs of infants enhances the chance of atelectasis and decreased arterial oxygenation.

Treatment includes administration of oxygen and fluids, as well as vigorous chest physical therapy. Bronchodilators are usually not effective.[109] The antiviral drug ribavirin has recently been used in infants and children with RSV infection. Initial research had shown ribavirin was effective in reducing the severity of illness and improving arterial oxygen tension.[46,49] Ribavirin is generally administered via nebulization for up to 20 hours a day.[62] More recently, concern has been raised over whether ribavirin's long-term side effects outweigh the degree of actual clinical improvement observed.[145] More research is needed, and presently ribavirin is recommended primarily for RSV-infected patients who are considered at very high risk, such as infants younger than 12 months of age with cyanotic congenital heart lesions and those with severe bronchopulmonary dysplasia or severe pulmonary anomalies. Infants with cystic fibrosis with significant pulmonary involvement may also be considered at high risk. Diminished cilia function compounded by increased necrotic tissue and mucus in the small airways dictate the need for frequent bronchial drainage with percussion and vibration as tolerated. If spontaneous coughing does not occur, nasotracheal suctioning is necessary. Wheezing should be evaluated before and after percussion techniques. If percussion causes an increase in wheezing or

respiratory distress, positioning with only vibration may be effective. It is recommended that caretakers who are treating patients undergoing ribavirin therapy follow stringent precautions to minimize their exposure to the aerosolized drug.[36,89]

There is increasing evidence that respiratory sequelae may continue through adulthood in children who have had bronchiolitis. Many of these children develop asthma, increased airway resistance, and abnormal arterial oxygen levels.[13,69,111,149]

*Pertussis.* Pertussis is an acute, contagious bacterial infection of the respiratory tract caused by *Bordetella pertussis.* The more serious respiratory manifestations are seen in children under 2 years of age.[35] It is also known as "whooping cough" because of the characteristic spasmodic cough followed by a high-pitched inspiratory "whoop." Cell infiltration and edema are present in the entire mucosal lining of the respiratory tract. Secondary pneumonia can occur causing an accumulation of pus and mucus within the alveoli. Obstruction of the airways caused by mucus, bronchospasm, and edema can cause paroxysmal coughing spells and cyanosis. The symptoms of pertussis last about 8 weeks. The paroxysmal stage, lasting 2 to 4 weeks, is the most severe. Fortunately, immunization against pertussis is available to infants and has greatly reduced the incidence of the infection.

Bronchial drainage with percussion and vibration is indicated to aid the removal of tenacious sputum and prevention of bronchial obstruction.

*Aspiration.* Aspiration involves inhalation of foreign matter into the lungs. The foreign material may cause local irritation and inflammation with the possibility of eventual infection. The right lower lobe is most prone to gastric aspiration, but in severe cases both lungs can be affected.[24] Neurological immaturity or insult may cause swallowing dysfunction, which can result in choking and aspiration of food or liquid. Aspiration can also accompany gastroesophageal reflux. It has also been our clinical observation that in children with gastroesophageal reflux or recurrent aspiration, the right upper lobe is also a common locus for aspiration.

Mouthing objects is a means of exploration for the infant and young child, and these objects can be aspirated into the lungs. Improperly chewed food can result in choking and subsequent aspiration. Peanuts or other nuts are among the most common types of food that are aspirated.[26] The phenomenon of foreign-body aspiration and treatment has been examined over the years in many pediatric institutions.[12,26,77] The clinical manifestations are cough, wheezing, and cyanosis. Radiographic examination may show evidence of airway obstruction represented as air trapping or localized atelectasis. The small airways of children are easily blocked by foreign objects.

In the early 1970s, the usual treatment of immediate bronchoscopic removal of a foreign body was challenged by

Cotton and Burrington.[12,26] They reported an 80% success rate of foreign-body removal using a combination of inhaled bronchodilator and bronchial drainage with chest percussion over a 24-hour period. In 1976, Law and Kosloske[77] reported a study of 76 patients treated for foreign-body aspiration. This later study did not confirm the high success rate of the bronchodilator inhalation and bronchial drainage regimen. Law and Kosloske suggested that a limited trial of 24 hours of bronchodilation and bronchial drainage was of value only in the early management of foreign-body aspiration. If this early trial failed, they recommended bronchoscopy. In addition, they stated that long-standing aspiration of a month or more duration should be treated initially with bronchoscopy.

Bronchodilatation and bronchial drainage performed in the initial stage should be frequent, with vigorous percussion, vibration, and specific positioning for the affected lobe. Because of the anatomical configuration of the major airways, the foreign bodies lodge most often in the right main bronchus and are found less frequently in the left main bronchus and trachea.

We strongly recommend bronchial drainage with percussion and vibration after bronchoscopic removal of a foreign body to clear any retained secretions or resultant acute pulmonary process.

Cotton and associates[26] recorded cases of cardiorespiratory arrest during the therapy treatment. Law and Kosloske[77] postulated that a mobilized foreign body, especially in a main bronchus, could migrate. This migration could obstruct another bronchus or the glottis and might be accompanied by reflex bronchospasm. We strongly recommend that the physical therapist carry out treatment where cardiac monitoring, oxygen, and resuscitation equipment are available.

## Indications for surgery

The benefits of chest physical therapy for the surgical patient have been well documented.[72] Surgical intention in the pediatric population may result in postoperative pulmonary complications. The following section describes conditions in which thoracic or abdominal surgery is indicated for the pediatric patient.

***Cardiac anomalies.*** The physical therapist is an important part of the medical team caring for the infant or child who undergoes open-heart surgery for correction of cardiac anomalies. The types of anomalies and the corrective procedures are many and varied.[115]

Preoperative and postoperative physical therapy evaluations are essential.[110] Postoperative treatment should place emphasis on improving ventilation and mobilizing secretions if present. However, in some cardiac conditions, especially those involving pulmonary venous obstruction and hypertension, pulmonary congestion may be present preoperatively. These preoperative factors place the patient at a higher risk for postoperative pulmonary complications. In infants and children pulmonary congestion may arise from valvular regurgitation, left ventricular outflow, pulmonary venous obstruction, or from any primary myocardial disease.[129] Pulmonary venous hypertension can lead to engorgement of the pulmonary vessels with blood. Alveolar and airway mucosal edema can develop, resulting in bronchial compression and obstruction of airflow, which leads to atelectasis and pulmonary infection. In addition to airway obstruction, pulmonary edema can lead to changes in lung surfactant and decreased lung compliance.[129] These alterations, when added to the risk of pulmonary infection and decreased lung volume because of an enlarged heart, can severely reduce pulmonary reserve. The result may be an increased work of breathing. The problems of pulmonary vascular overload can be surgically corrected. However, patients undergoing surgery may already have chronic lung problems and should be identified for vigorous treatment by the physical therapist.

Postoperative chest physical therapy for the pediatric cardiac patient should include frequent position change, breathing exercises, and instruction in effective coughing with incisional splinting or airway aspiration as necessary. Modified bronchial drainage techniques with consideration of the necessary postoperative precautions are performed only if there is secretion retention. Mobility exercises including range of motion, bed mobility, and progressive ambulation should also be part of the postoperative program.

***Tracheoesophageal malformations.*** Malformations of the trachea or esophagus can cause respiratory distress in infancy. Tracheomalacia is a condition in which the tracheal lumen is reduced because of absence or malformation of the cartilaginous rings of the trachea. Narrowing of the tracheal lumen becomes exaggerated during expiration because of this lack of structural support. Clinically, the infant may have an increased respiratory rate, stridor, wheezing, cough, and possibly cyanosis. Increased pulmonary secretions may cause further distress and may interfere with feeding. Symptoms become exaggerated with crying. Conservative treatment is directed toward prevention of infection and management of secretions. If an infection occurs, bronchial hygiene is indicated to mobilize excessive secretions, especially before feeding. Recovery is promising as the infant grows and cartilaginous development occurs. Most clinical symptoms resolve by 6 months of age.[117]

Tracheoesophageal fistula (TEF) is a more difficult problem characterized by one or several interconnections between the trachea and esophagus. Overflow of food or liquids into the lung through these anatomical interconnections causes continued pulmonary injury and is a source of infection. This malformation comes in a variety of types and is often coincident with atresia, or absence, of part of the esophagus.

Presenting signs include significant coughing, choking, and cyanosis with the ingestion of fluids, or a history of recurrent pneumonia or upper lobe collapse. If the malformation is not diagnosed quickly, chronic pulmonary disease may occur because of continued irritation of the lungs by aspirated material.

Before and after surgical corrections through a lateral thoracotomy, many infants with tracheoesophageal fistula have lengthy hospitalizations. Upright positioning is necessary if gastroesophageal reflux is also present. After surgery oral feeding is postponed, and deep endotracheal suctioning is contraindicated until suture healing occurs.

The physical therapist is often involved before diagnosis and after surgical correction. Pulmonary care is directed toward maintaining bronchial hygiene and resolving pulmonary infection. Developmental stimulation for gross motor and oral function also becomes a necessary part of the treatment.

*Solid organ transplantation.* The first solid organ transplantations were performed in the 1950s, but high mortality rates and poor graft survival limited their use as a routine treatment option.[52] Over the years solid organ transplantation has become more feasible as a result of improvements in surgical techniques, in organ procurement methods, and in the controlling of graft rejection.

Improvements in surgical techniques and donor organ procurement have advanced steadily, and graft failures related to the surgery or injury to the donor organ during transport have decreased. Currently the most difficult aspect of care of the transplant recipient is related to the management of graft rejection.

All solid organ transplant recipients require chronic suppression of their immune system to prevent graft rejection and commonly have complications related to increased incidence of infections or to the side effects of the immunosuppressive drugs. Most transplant recipients receive a combination of corticosteroids, azathioprine (Imuran), and cyclosporine on a constant basis to prevent rejection. Cyclosporine, discovered in the late 1970s, is the most effective drug to date in controlling the body's immune system to prevent tissue rejection while leaving the recipient sufficient immune activity to control infection.[148] With the introduction of cyclosporine, lower doses of corticosteroids could be used and a decrease in the frequency of bacterial and fungal infections, frequently found in patients on chronic corticosteroid regimens, was seen.[60] Viral infections, particularly herpes simplex and cytomegalovirus (CMV), continue to be common in transplant recipients. When episodes of graft rejection occur, the patient's immunosuppressive regimen is increased and may include a 3 to 5 day pulse of corticosteroids, or a 1 to 2 week course of a different immunosuppressive drug such as antithymocyte globulin (ATG) or Orthoclone OKT3 (OKT3).

There are many other side effects of chronic immunosuppressive therapy in addition to increasing susceptibility to infections. Corticosteroids can cause osteoporosis and avascular necrosis of weight-bearing bones. However, the steroid-related side effects can be reduced with alternate-day dosage.[92] Cyclosporine can be toxic to the liver and kidneys,

may cause neurological complications and induce seizures, and may increase the recipient's risk of developing lymphoproliferative disorders.[52,60,148] The potential side effects of long-term immunosuppressive therapy, especially in the pediatric population, and the side effects of the newer immunosuppressive drugs such as OKT3 are not well known.

Currently renal, heart, and liver transplants are the most commonly performed solid organ transplants in the pediatric population. The use of lung and heart-lung transplants to treat the pediatric patient with end-stage disease has increased during the past few years. Physical therapy evaluation and treatment is an important component both preoperatively and postoperatively for all children undergoing a solid organ transplantation.[45] More specific aspects of renal, heart, liver, and lung transplants are presented below.

*Renal transplantation.* Renal transplants are frequently performed in children for treatment of various forms of congenital nephrotic syndrome. Uncontrolled rejection is still the major cause of graft failure in renal transplants.[98] Unlike other solid organ transplants, many of the side effects of immunosuppressive therapy can be reduced by sacrificing the grafted kidney, halting the immunosuppression, and resuming hemodialysis or retransplanting in the future.

The majority of the patients who require a renal transplant have been maintained on chronic hemodialysis before their transplant and may be deconditioned or developmentally delayed secondary to their chronic illness. Those patients who have received peritoneal dialysis frequently have weakened abdominal muscles secondary to overstretching of their abdominal wall during the dialysis procedure. A pretransplant physical therapy evaluation is important to assess the patient's base-line status and to instruct the patient in pulmonary care techniques.[45]

At the time of transplantation the patient is started on an immunosuppressive regimen, and good handwashing and gowns are required for people coming into contact with the transplant recipient. During the perioperative period, infections from the environment or any that were harbored within the donated kidney are most common. During the first 6 months after transplantation, the recipient is prone to viral infections.

During the first 1 to 2 weeks, the patient's mobility and positioning may be restricted to prevent increased abdominal pressure while the surgical anastomoses are healing. A regular program of pulmonary care with emphasis on deep-breathing exercises and effective coughing is especially important during this period of mobility restriction. Gentle percussion over the lower lobes and more vigorous percussion over the upper lobes can be done, although positioning may have to be modified. Active trunk flexion and the prone position are generally avoided for 2 to 4 weeks after transplantation, although modifications may be made after consultation with the renal transplant surgical team. The patient is allowed to sit but must attain sitting from a side-lying position, decreasing the use of his abdominal muscles during this time period. The patient should be progressed as allowed to a program consisting of mobility, ambulation, and developmental stimulation as indicated.

*Heart transplantation.* Heart transplants in infants and children are generally performed on patients with either congenital heart disease resulting in poor cardiac function despite maximal surgical and medical intervention, or those with end-stage cardiomyopathy. There are two classifications of heart transplants: orthotopic, in which the recipient's heart is removed and the donor's placed; and heterotopic, in which the recipient's heart is left in place and the donor's is "piggybacked" onto it. Orthotopic is the more common form. Heterotopic heart transplants are performed when there is increased pulmonary vascular resistance, which would overload the donor heart's right ventricle and lead to its failure. It is more difficult to assess for rejection after a heterotopic transplant, since catheterization is technically more difficult. Another problem associated with heterotopic transplants is that the recipient's diseased heart may throw clots, necessitating chronic anticoagulant therapy for prevention.

The majority of children who require heart transplants are deconditioned and have a significantly decreased activity tolerance. A preoperative physical therapy evaluation should include an assessment of the patient's endurance, a muscle examination (to evaluate for a generalized myopathy), and respiratory evaluation.[45] Preoperative teaching emphasizing the immediate posttransplant physical therapy program is especially important, since the unfamiliar intensive care unit environment can be frightening to a child.

The transplant recipient starts the immunosuppressive regimen within the perioperative period and is placed on protective precautions on return from surgery. People having contact with the patient need to wear gowns and gloves. Masks may be required during seasons with increased frequency of viral respiratory infections.

In heart transplantation the immunosuppressive regimen is designed to prevent rejection, since repeated or chronic rejection can interfere with cardiac function. Chronic rejection has been shown to increase graft atherosclerosis and cause myocardial fibrosis. Therefore rejection—detected by clinical signs or by tissue changes on cardiac endometrial biopsy obtained via cardiac catheterization—is vigorously treated.

Transplant recipients who have an uncomplicated perioperative course can generally be extubated within the first 48 hours. There are no general restrictions on range of motion or mobility although this might vary in individual cases. The physical therapist needs to be aware of the various monitoring lines and equipment, such as intracardiac lines, mediastinal drainage tubes, and pacer wires, commonly seen immediately after the operation. In general, no special treatment modifications are required with regard to the above, except to avoid placing the hands or exerting pressure

directly over them. Percussion over the upper anterior chest is avoided while the sternum is healing from the midsternal incision. If the patient requires postural drainage to maintain pulmonary hygiene, the head-down position is allowed once the patient is hemodynamically stable.

In addition to pulmonary hygiene, the physical therapy program should stress early mobility by initiating an exercise or developmental stimulation program and ambulation as indicated. The majority of children undergoing heart transplants have been sedentary; they may prefer low-energy-expending activities, and may even be fearful of or dislike exercise. In addition, the implanted donor heart is denervated, and longer transition periods before and after exercise are therefore needed to allow for changes in cardiac output. The physical therapist must take this into account as the program is developed and develop a program as enjoyable as possible to promote long-term compliance. The transplant recipient, as well as his or her primary caretakers, will benefit from the guidance provided by physical therapy in helping to develop an increased tolerance for activity and exercise.

*Liver transplantation.* Liver transplantation in the pediatric population was pioneered by Starzl[126] in the late 1960s. However, it was not until the 1980s, with the advent of improved immunosuppressive regimens, that survival rates improved. Biliary atresia occurs in about 1 of 15,000 births and is the reason for about 75% of the pediatric liver transplantations.[54] Atresia of the bile duct causes an inability to excrete bile because of obstruction, distraction, absence, or reduction in the number of bile ducts. Biliary atresia was almost always a fatal disease, but the advent of liver transplantation has now increased survival rate to 80% within the first year of surgery.[54] Indications for liver replacement in parenchymal and metabolic diseases have also been described.[91] The Boston Center for Liver Transplantation (BCLT) group stated that over half of the children receiving transplants during a 30 month period were less than 2.5 years old.[143]

Like all solid organ transplantation patients, those undergoing liver transplants are maintained on immunosuppressive drug therapy with drugs such as cyclosporine and steroids. The group studied by the BCLT experienced hypertension and bacterial infections as the two most common postoperative complications.[143]

The following are several common postoperative respiratory complications:[73,136]

1. Pulmonary edema, caused in large part by transfusion of large amounts of blood products intraoperatively. This usually resolves early in the postoperative period.
2. Lobar atelectasis, especially on the right, as a result of peribronchial edema and upward displacement and decreased excursion of the diaphragm caused by abdominal distention and right hemidiaphragmatic dysfunction resulting from right phrenic nerve damage (Fig. 26-6). These problems may also predispose the

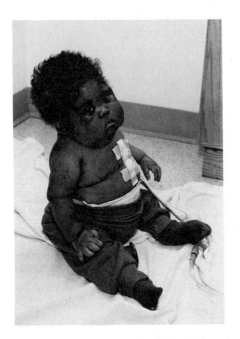

**Fig. 26-6.** The enlarged abdomen of this child with liver disease can cause decreased excursion of the diaphragm and tachypnea in a sitting position.

patient to persistent hypoventilation, which is compounded by incisional pain and splinting and general muscle weakness if a patient is severely malnourished.

3. Right pleural effusions of a transient nature during the first few days posttransplantation. If they do not resolve spontaneously, a thoracentesis may be indicated.

4. A depressed central respiratory drive resulting from a metabolic alkalosis caused by fluid retention, nasogastric drainage, and diuretic therapy.

Pulmonary infections are uncommon in the early postoperative period. Pneumonias usually do not occur until 1 to 2 months after transplantation. Fungal infections and viral infections, such as cytomegalovirus and respiratory syncytial virus, are seen. *Pneumocystis carinii* pneumonia can also occur.

A significant postoperative cardiovascular complication is that of severe systemic hypertension. This hypertension may persist for months, becoming less severe with time; it is most severe in the first postoperative week.[136]

Postoperatively, the patient spends some time in the intensive care unit until medically stable. During this period protective precautions or reverse precautions are used to prevent the recipient from infection. The physical therapist also generally follows a platelet protocol for treatment (see p. 547) because of the occurrence of thrombocytopenia. When treating a liver transplant patient one should also consider the possibility of decreased reserve secondary to a poor premorbid condition of general health, a long operative period with increased blood loss, and the presence of a high

transverse abdominal incision making coughing more difficult. Length of intubation and mechanical ventilatory support should be noted.

Recent research of liver transplants in adults has shown an increased frequency in neurological complications, including seizure disorders, cerebellar toxicity, and paresis following transplantation.[102,144] The etiology of these complications is unclear. However, the monitoring of a patient's neurological status should be included in the therapeutic program.

During the early postoperative period, patient needs vary, but generally there is an indication for chest physical therapy. Bronchial drainage with percussion and vibration may be very helpful in clearing secretions and resolving atelectasis.[73] If bronchial drainage is indicated, besides considering platelet counts, the physical therapist should also observe vital signs—in particular, respiratory rate. An enlarged abdomen can further compromise respiratory status when pushed against the diaphragm in a Trendelenburg position. Range of motion, bed mobility, and proper positioning are emphasized to prevent contractures and/or decubiti. In addition, parents are introduced to and educated about physical therapy techniques (if this was not done preoperatively), developmental stimulation, and plans for discharge.

As a patient's status improves, developmental issues are emphasized. Frequently, children who have undergone transplants experience developmental delays resulting from their disease.[128] Stewart and others[128] found that, among infants with liver disease, both mental and motor development were significantly related to growth. In children, development was related more to measures of liver function than to growth. However, physical complications from liver disease can alter a child's experiences and interactions with his or her environment. Because they have an enlarged abdomen, children with liver disease often are tachypneic when sitting and are not comfortable when prone (Fig. 26-6). Abdominal musculature is often weak and lack of experience in sitting and the prone position compound to cause decreased extensor tone, which in turn creates diminished trunk support and delays in standing and walking. These factors should be considered when planning a developmental program. It should also be noted that prone positioning is often limited until about 2 weeks to a month postoperatively because of the excessive abdominal distention and concern for graft integrity. However, if prone positioning is necessary for pulmonary hygiene, discussion with the surgeon should take place. Despite developmental deficits, with intensive intervention most children exhibit catch-up growth or maintain normal growth velocity postoperatively. Moreover, liver transplantation does not appear to have any effect on cognitive ability.[154] Progress is associated with graft function and general well-being.

*Lung and heart-lung transplantation.* During the 1980s lung and heart-lung transplantation became an accepted therapeutic option for adults with end-stage lung disease.

Since 1990 several pediatric lung transplant programs have been developed. Between 1991 and 1993, 27 patients were evaluated by the Lung Transplant Program at The Children's Hospital, Boston. Eight of these children have undergone lung transplants; two have undergone heart-lung transplants.

Appropriate candidates for lung transplants are children with end-stage lung disease who have adequate nutritional status and psychosocial supports. The child should not be dependent on steroids or have any other systemic disease. In the pediatric population single-lung transplant is indicated for patients with pulmonary hypertension and pulmonary fibrosis. Children with septic lung disease, such as cystic fibrosis, require double-lung transplants. A single-lung transplant would be at risk for developing infection from the native, septic lung. Patients with congenital heart disease, pulmonary vascular disease, or parencymal lung disease with cardiac dysfunction may be candidates for heart-lung transplants.

Prior to being listed with the regional organ bank, patients are evaluated by a multidisciplinary team including: cardiology, infectious disease, nutrition, psychology, anesthesia, otolaryngology, dentistry, social work, and physical therapy. The evaluation determines if the child is an appropriate candidate, which type of transplant is appropriate, and if there are any problems which should be addressed prior to surgery.

The physical therapy evaluation includes assessment of muscle strength, flexibility, posture, gait, respiratory status, and activity or developmental level. Older children perform a six-minute walk test and a modified exercise test to assess their exercise tolerance. Most children with end-stage lung disease have sedentary life styles due to limitations of their pulmonary disease. Patients and parents are educated about the importance of maximizing/maintaining the child's strength and exercise tolerance pretransplant, as well as the role of physical therapy posttransplant. An exercise program is initiated to improve or maintain the child's strength and endurance while waiting for the transplant. Infants and toddlers may be involved in a developmental stimulation program. The patients are followed closely by the physical therapist during this period for reassessment and progression or modification of the program.

Single-lung transplant is performed through a posterolateral thoracotomy. Double-lung transplant is performed through bilateral anterior thoracotomies connected by a transverse sternal incision. This approach allows for exploration of the pleural space for division of adhesions which are common in patients with cystic fibrosis. Double-lung transplant may be performed as sequential single-lung transplants. This procedure may avoid the need for cardiopulmonary bypass and anticoagulation.[99] Heart-lung transplant is performed through a midline sternotomy.

The transplanted lung is denervated; therefore, there is loss of the cough reflex below the level of the anastomosis. Injury to the airway mucosa results in slowing of mucociliary clearance and interruption of the lymphatic drainage which affects the response of the immune system. In addition, a small number of bacteria aspirated in the donor lung may produce clinically significant bacteria in the immunocompromised patient.[30] Chest physical therapy to promote mobilization and clearance of secretions is an important component of the postoperative treatment of the lung-transplant patient. Treatments of postural drainage, percussion, and vibration/shaking should be done frequently. During the first few postoperative days the patient may be hypoxemic because of pulmonary edema that results from capillary injury due to ischemia, reperfusion, and fluid overload. There is usually a good response to vigorous diuresis and many patients are extubated during the first 72 hours following surgery.[138] The lung transplant patient will continue to benefit from treatment techniques to facilitate airway clearance, as well as encouragement to do deep breathing and coughing exercises. A weak ineffective cough may be due to incisional pain. Most patients receive epidural infusions of morphine for pain control; additional medication may be necessary prior to chest physical therapy treatments.

Range of motion and strengthening exercises are usually initiated during the first 48 hours postsurgery. The exercise program is progressed to include standing activities and ambulation. The rate of progression of the exercise program is dependent on the patient's pretransplant strength and exercise tolerance, the postoperative course, and the motivation and cooperation of the patient. Choosing exercises and activities that the child enjoys is beneficial to a successful program. The use of stickers and charts to reinforce good effort and document progress are often helpful. Some patients develop diffuse chest wall pain, which may be due to changes of the thoracic musculoskeletal configuration or excessive coughing.[84] Flexibility exercises and massage may be used to alleviate this discomfort.

The lung-transplant patient is closely monitored for signs and symptoms of rejection and infection. Lung and airway infections are a common problem because of the continual exposure to the air in the environment. Following heart-lung transplant, lung rejection is more common than cardiac rejection and can occur independently.[78] Medical management of these patients involves determining adequate immunosuppression to prevent rejection without leaving the patient defenseless against infection. Bronchoscopies are done periodically to monitor for signs of rejection and for clinical signs of an infection. Pulmonary infection may present with fever, cough, shortness of breath, and a decrease in spirometry and oxygen saturation in the blood. During the early postoperative period, bacterial infections are more common; later, opportunistic infections, such as cytomegalovirus, are more likely to occur.[30]

The signs and symptoms of lung rejection are similar to those of infection. The patient may have symptoms of decreased exercise tolerance, a decrease in spirometry and oxygen saturations, fever, loss of appetite, and fatigue. The classical pattern of acute rejection is infiltration of lymphocytes in the perivascular and peribronchiolar region.[78] It is essential that the rejection be detected and treated before the graft is irreparably damaged. Chronic rejection may present as a progressive obstructive disease due to peribronchiolar infiltration of lymphocytes and obliteration of bronchioles.[78] Some infections, such as cytomegalovirus, appear to predispose the graft to chronic rejection.[78,84] Patients with severe chronic rejection usually develop a productive cough and dyspnea on exertion. Pulmonary function tests are usually compatible with both an obstructive and restrictive impairment. Airway clearance techniques are beneficial for these patients. Early detection of both infection and rejection are essential. It is important that the physical therapist is aware of a decline in oxygen saturations or any signs of dyspnea or fatigue during the exercise program. Patients and parents are instructed to be aware of the signs and symptoms of rejection and infection. Patients are given a spirometer and oximeter and instructed to record daily measurements at home.

The physical therapy program for the lung-transplant patient is individualized to address the specific needs of each child. Older children may exercise on a treadmill or cycle; younger children may do more "play" activities with balls or jump ropes. The physical therapist continues to work closely with the child and family throughout the hospitalization and later discharge as the patient's strength and endurance improves and he or she assumes normal age-appropriate activities. Lung transplantation has enabled many patients with end-stage lung disease to return to school or work, keep up with their peers, and participate in sports.

The goal of all solid organ transplants is to provide the transplant recipient with an increased quality of life. The physical therapist is an integral member of any transplant team, working together with other team members to return the transplant recipient to a functional life-style.

***Congenital lobar emphysema.*** Although uncommon, congenital lobar emphysema is one of the few reasons for a lobectomy in an infant.[130] The cause is unclear, and it appears that some infants are born with a larger than normal lobe of the lung. The lower lobes are rarely involved. The syndrome may represent a developmental abnormality of the alveoli or a multialveolar lobe where the number of alveoli is up to five times that of normal.[108] The emphysematous lobe will usually compress and displace the remaining lung, causing varying degrees of atelectasis and diaphragmatic compression on the ipsilateral side. Mediastinal shift may also be present with atelectasis and compromise of the contralateral lung. The degree of respiratory distress will vary depending on the severity of the emphysema.

Immediate surgical correction is recommended. This involves thoracotomy and removal of the emphysematous lobe. The prognosis for these children is very good, and many are free of serious pulmonary problems or infections

with recovery of normal lung volume and size postoperatively.[88] Chest physical therapy may be indicated postoperatively if there are any problems with secretion retention or atelectasis.

## PATIENT EVALUATION
### Considerations

Approaching a sick infant or child is often a difficult task. As has been mentioned, children are often fearful of any procedures and may be overstimulated and stressed by the hospital environment. Evaluation and treatment of an infant or child must always include a thorough explanation to the family and patient of the physical therapy procedures. This explanation should be in clear, simple language. Capturing the cooperation and understanding of the family members and patient is important.

### Techniques

The evaluation techniques of observation, inspection, palpation, auscultation, measurement, and interview are not only used for the adult respiratory patient, but are also applicable to the pediatric patient. However, depending on the age of the child, the therapist may have to rely more on acute observational skills to gather necessary information. Actual handling of an infant or child may increase anxiety and alter evaluative findings. The therapist should always be cognizant of the temperature of his or her hands and stethoscope. Cold hands on a warmly swaddled infant can begin a stress reaction of crying and increased respiratory rate. A pediatric patient may not be able to verbalize about the level of comfort or anxiety. Noting general posture and whether speech is even or gasping can help determine the level of comfort during an evaluation of respiratory status. A physical therapist can gather much information regarding the infant or child by observation without any manual contact.

Interviewing techniques also take on added importance during an evaluation of a pediatric patient. If the child is young, a therapist must depend on information from parents, based on their understanding and perception of their child's pulmonary problems. Questions should be asked that require several-word answers, not just "yes" or "no." The therapist should phrase questions to avoid suggesting signs or symptoms. For example, do not say, "Do you think your child experiences shortness of breath or tires easily with active play?" but rather, "What are your child's favorite activities?" A response of "watching television" or "reading books" may indicate a limited activity level. More additional information, of course, would be necessary to confirm this suspicion. Good interviewing technique can be extremely beneficial in constructing a detailed patient profile.

### A comprehensive evaluation

Before any chest physical therapy evaluation, it is important to obtain a complete medical and surgical history through chart review, interview, and physician communication. Emphasis should be placed on the history of the respiratory illness, arterial blood gases, chest radiograph findings, and pulmonary function tests. Pulmonary function tests are generally not done with a child under 6 years of age because of lack of cooperation and understanding of the procedures.[87]

If the patient is hospitalized, nursing progress notes and discussion with the patient's nurse provide current information about the child's status and vital signs over the previous 24 hours. Proper identification of all equipment, lines and tubes attached to and around the patient is important. If the patient has undergone surgery, it is essential to make note of the incisional areas. If the patient is acutely ill, mechanical ventilator settings, electrocardiograph, and vital sign recordings must be noted. Saturation of hemoglobin in arterial blood, as well as pulse rate, can be continually monitored or checked periodically through the use of a pulse oximeter.

**Respiratory evaluation.** Observing the patient without laying on hands provides information regarding skin color, respiratory rate, nasal flaring, breathing pattern, chest symmetry, posture, and general comfort. Listening carefully for evidence of stridor, audible wheezing, and grunting can also be done before touching the patient. Any peripheral edema, wounds, or scars should be noted. Skin color can be observed with attention to the eyes, mucous membranes, and nailbeds. If cyanosis is present in these areas, then the patient most likely is hypoxemic. Lack of oxygenated hemoglobin in the capillaries will create a bluish cast to the areas mentioned above. Cyanosis in a dark-skinned child can be noted at the tongue. An infant can easily be observed from the bedside. However, a toddler or older child may become anxious just by seeing someone approach the bed. Therefore comfort and posture, color, and breathing pattern and rate may be observed from a distance before one approaches the child.

Once contact is made with the patient, there should be a simple explanation of what is to be done. Initially, efforts to reduce fear and anxiety take precedence over therapeutic tasks.

The following summary of evaluative findings are specific to the pediatric patient and will aid the clinician.

*Respiratory rate.* The pulmonary mechanics of the infant and child are such that the resting respiratory rate is higher than that in the adult. Respiratory rate is generally slower during sleep. This difference is more pronounced in the younger child.[118] The average respiratory rate for an awake, normal infant in the first year of life ranges between 30 and 40 breaths per minute. There will be a sharp decline in the rate during the second year to about 25 to 30 breaths per minute. A slow, steady fall in rate continues through childhood (20 to 25 per minute) and adolescence (15 to 20 per minute), when the rate approaches the adult level.[146] In other words, the younger a child, the higher the normal resting respiratory rate.

Respiratory rate should be determined with the child relaxed and unaware that his or her rate is being recorded. Respiratory rate can be observed at a distance from a child or while one is presumably taking a pulse. Observation of thoracic excursions is usually sufficient to obtain a respiratory rate, though the stethoscope may be used on the chest of a sleeping child. The rate should be taken for a full minute for accurate measurement.

If a child has an underlying chronic pulmonary condition, it is important to assess breathing rate in relationship to the child's base-line respiratory rate, as well as to the normal rate for that child's age.[44] It is also important to remember that respiratory rate may be altered due to factors unrelated to the pulmonary condition. Stress, pain, presence of fever, or crying can increase the respiratory rate. Central nervous system depression caused by drug effects or intracranial pressure can abnormally decrease the respiratory rate.[44]

*Pulse rate.* Pulse rate can vary among children and can be altered by activity level or stress. A newborn's heart rate is between 100 and 160 bpm. From 1 to 4 years of age, the rate can range from 80 to 120 bpm. As the child approaches adolescence, the pulse rate becomes comparable to the adult range of 60 to 80 bpm.[118] It is most important to monitor any sudden change or irregularity in heart rate. If the heart rate rises or drops significantly in response to treatment, this change should be noted and reported. Modifying or discontinuing the treatment session may be appropriate. An infant's pulse is best palpated at the brachial or femoral artery. The pulse of an older child can be monitored at the radial artery.

*Breathing pattern.* Retractions are a sign of increased inspiratory effort. A common occurrence in infants, whose chests are more compliant than those of older children, is depression of the lower sternum accompanying a labored inspiration. Intercostal retractions, if present, may indicate decreased compliance or airway obstruction. Suprasternal retractions may indicate an upper airway obstruction such as croup. Subcostal retractions may indicate flattening of the diaphragm and diffuse lower airway obstruction.[48]

Intercostal bulging during expiration may be present when air trapping occurs because of airway narrowing as seen in asthma, cystic fibrosis, or bronchiolitis. This bulging represents increased expiratory effort.

During respiration the synchronization between the upper chest and abdomen should be observed. Normally, both areas should expand on inspiration. When an infant is distressed and respiratory muscles are fatigued, a "seesaw" phenomenon occurs in which the upper chest expands during inspiration while the abdomen is pulled inward and the reverse occurs during expiration. Accessory muscles are recruited for use during a labored inspiration. The neck flexors, particularly the sternocleidomastoid, are commonly used to augment inspiration. That these muscles are being used by an infant can be inferred from head bobbing. The child's head will bob forward during inspiration as the neck flexors contract against neck extensor muscles that cannot stabilize the head. This action is particularly apparent when the child is held with the neck flexors placed in a shortened position. Nasal flaring is another indicator of increased work of breathing and is often present during accessory muscle use. It is believed that widening of the nares during respiratory distress may aid in diminishing airway resistance. Grunting during exhalation may also be audible in an infant who is experiencing respiratory distress.

Disruption of normal breathing patterns, grunting, postural splinting, or agitation upon movement may accompany chest pain or discomfort in an infant or child.

*Auscultation.* Interpretation of breath sounds is the same for children as for adults. However, the ease with which auscultation can be accomplished may be altered by the child's respiratory rate or cooperation. Breath sounds often appear louder in an infant or child when compared to an adult's because of the proximity of the child's airways to the skin surface. The breath sounds of a child are often audible during both inspiration and expiration. Crying can alter the sound, allowing clearly heard inspiratory sounds but muffled expiratory sounds. Wheezing in an infant often originates in the major airways because of their small diameter compared with adult airways. Secretions in any part of the respiratory tree may be audible throughout the chest. The examiner must rule out upper airway sounds, which may be transmitted to other parts of the chest. Comparing auscultative findings to chest radiograph findings is very desirable in the younger age group secondary to the difficulties that may occur in interpretation of breath sounds. Expiratory grunting can be heard either through the stethoscope or with the unaided ear. Auscultation is an excellent tool for evaluating the benefits of a chest physical therapy treatment. Improvements or changes in breath sounds can be ascertained by comparing pretreatment with posttreatment findings.

The technique of auscultation of an infant's or child's lungs is similar to that used on an adult. The following suggestions should be kept in mind. Before placing the diaphragm or bell of the stethoscope on the child's chest, always make sure it is warm. Give the child the opportunity to see and feel the stethoscope (Fig. 26-7). Explain simply what you are going to do and that it will not hurt. Demonstrating auscultation on a doll or favorite toy may ease the child's fears. Stethoscopes designed specifically for pediatric patients are commercially available. Some believe that although small stethoscopes offer no acoustic superiority, they accommodate a small chest better.[118]

*Palpation.* Before palpating a child's chest you should explain what you are going to do. Locating the position of the trachea at the suprasternal notch can give information regarding equality of pressure and volume between the two sides of the chest. A shift to one side or the other may indicate an abnormality such as atelectasis or pneumothorax. A complete atelectasis in one lung with loss of volume would cause a shifting of the trachea and mediastinum toward the

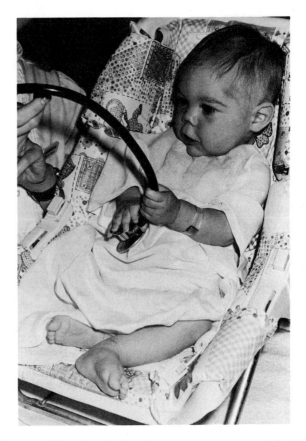

**Fig. 26-7.** This infant is given the opportunity to see and feel the stethoscope before it is used for auscultation.

atelectatic side. A tension pneumothorax in one lung would create a shift of the trachea and mediastinum toward the unaffected lung. The presence of subcutaneous emphysema, edema, or asymmetry of the chest can also be noted through palpation.

**Functional and developmental assessment.** Developmental assessments should always be part of the physical therapy evaluation of an infant or young child. Evaluation should be postponed until the child is free from stressful respiratory symptoms. Respiratory distress can alter muscle tone and the patient's normal activity level. Premature infants are often at risk for developmental delay and other subtle neurological manifestations. Consider the weeks of prematurity when determining the developmental age. Parents can provide helpful information about their child's developmental level before the illness.

A gross- and fine-motor assessment with evaluation of cognitive and social skills is important. Feeding and oral motor evaluations should also be performed on infants with respiratory problems. Respiratory illness and excessive secretions can make breathing while sucking or eating very difficult and may diminish nutritional intake. The child may appear to suck weakly or swallow poorly. Weak or spastic oral musculature and abnormal sucking, swallowing, or gag reflexes must be ruled out.

A functional assessment including an activities of daily

A        B        C

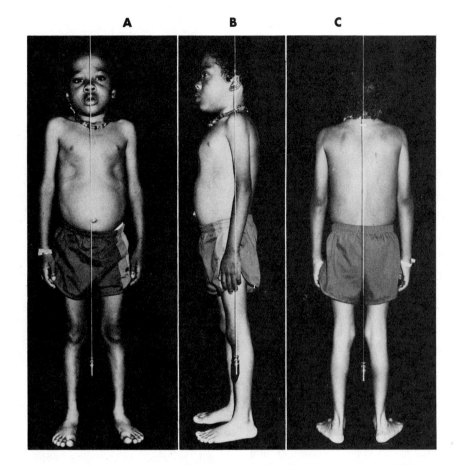

**Fig. 26-8.** Postural abnormalities in child with cystic fibrosis. **A,** *Anterior view.* Notice that the shoulders are held high especially on the right, a posture that appears to allow better mechanical advantage to the accessory muscles for breathing. The lower ribs are flared, and the thorax appears barreled and elongated because of the hyperinflation of the lungs. A full postural evaluation might reveal other less obvious abnormalities. **B,** *Lateral view.* The thoracic kyphosis and barreled chest seen here are common findings in children with obstructive pulmonary disease and hyperinflation of the lungs. **C,** *Posterior view.* The shoulders appear high with protraction of the scapulas. Notice the enlargement of the thorax in relation to the rest of this patient's body. Pronated feet are also noticeable.

living (ADL) survey is important when one is evaluating an older child or adolescent. These ADL surveys offer much insight into the extent the respiratory problem limits function. Specific questions regarding favorite play, sports activities, and hobbies can indicate a child's exercise tolerance. Children often lack the fear of becoming overfatigued that adult respiratory patients may harbor. A child with a respiratory problem will often function within his or her physical capability, being limited only by overprotective parents.

**Postural assessment.** Postural alignment is often altered by an underlying respiratory disease. A postural evaluation should be carried out with any respiratory patient, especially a growing child. Muscle groups that are often tight or weak are the pectorals, scapular, neck, low back, anterior hip, and the hamstring tendons. Hyperinflation of the lungs, often seen in the obstructive lung diseases such as cystic fibrosis, can result in an increased anteroposterior thorax diameter and rigid barrel chest. The tight musculature in combination

with a rigid, enlarged chest can greatly reduce thoracic excursion and spinal flexibility. Rigid deformities can result in thoracic spine kyphosis and functional or rotational scoliosis (Fig. 26-8). Postural abnormalities can further compromise pulmonary function. Discovering and treating these abnormalities before growth has ceased can possibly modify their progression.

**Strength and range of motion assessment.** Alterations in gross muscle strength and joint range of motion are seen in patients with chronic lung disease. Emphasis on evaluation of trunk musculature, especially the abdominal, back extensor, and scapular musculature, is indicated. Good abdominal strength is important for effective coughing. Back extensor and scapular musculature may be weak because of a kyphotic posture. Decreased range of motion from tight musculature may be evident in the neck and shoulders, especially in children with chronic pulmonary problems.

**Home program assessment.** Evaluation of patient and family compliance with treatment is an important part of the home program assessment. Answers to specific questions regarding frequency and length of treatments provide insight into compliance and involvement of the family.

The following are examples of questions that should be asked:

1. Is any chest physical therapy done at home?
2. Can you describe the type of treatment?
3. How often is the treatment carried out? If it is daily, what time or times of the day?
4. How long does it take to do a treatment?
5. Does anyone help the patient with treatment, or does the patient do the treatment alone?
6. Is any special equipment used to aid in treatment? Describe the equipment.
7. Are any aerosol medications taken before or after treatment?
8. When was the last time a physical therapist reviewed the home program or therapy techniques?
9. Are there any specific problems with the home treatment program—e.g., with scheduling, performing treatment techniques, or compliance?

**Evaluation of the surgical patient.** A preoperative physical therapy evaluation may be requested for a patient who is scheduled for major abdominal or thoracic surgery. Postoperative pulmonary complications are common, and the benefits of postoperative chest physical therapy are well documented.[72,110] A full respiratory, functional, and postural evaluation should be done. The therapist should understand the type of surgery to be performed, the surgical approach, the anticipated muscle or bone resections, and the respiratory and musculoskeletal limitations expected after surgical intervention. The evaluation session should also include an explanation to the parents and patient of the rationale for and demonstration of postoperative chest physical therapy. Preoperative explanation of postoperative procedures is extraordinarily important in pediatric care to help allay fears of the child or parents. A child, regardless of age, is entitled to explanations of the surgical experience. Fig. 26-9 is an example of a coloring book designed by Sylvia Dick, P.T., for preoperative instruction in chest physical therapy for the cardiac patients at Children's Hospital, Boston. This type of resource gives the child an opportunity to understand, in a very nonthreatening way, the procedures he or she will experience.

## PATIENT TREATMENT
### Considerations

One of the challenges of chest physical therapy is capturing the cooperation of the pediatric patient. Imagination and patience are the keys to holding the attention of a child and obtaining the desired results. Once rapport is established, treating a child is both enjoyable and rewarding. When one is treating children, many modifications and alternative treatment approaches have to be employed to

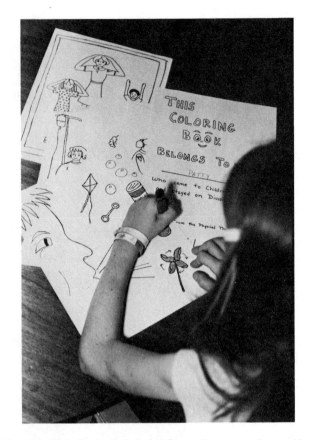

**Fig. 26-9.** Coloring book designed for use in preoperative teaching of the pediatric cardiac surgical patient.

accommodate small chests and bodies, alter behavior, allay fears, and respond to unpredictable changes in status. Treatment of the pediatric patient also presumes the importance of parents and family in the care of their child.

### Techniques

**Positions for breathlessness.** Positions for the breathless patient should promote comfort and increase relaxation. The positioning should encourage mobility of the thorax and support of the spinal column. Hip flexion should be incorporated to relax the abdominal area and aid in increasing intraabdominal pressure for coughing. Data suggest that postural relief for dyspnea may be related to an improved length-tension state of the diaphragm, which may increase its efficiency.[122] Some suggested positions for children who experience dyspnea are shown in Fig. 26-10. Diaphragmatic breathing with pursed-lips expiration combined with these illustrated positions should be taught to all patients who experience shortness of breath. Asthmatics, especially, can utilize these techniques during wheezing episodes to possibly avoid stressful attacks.

**Deep-breathing exercises and retraining.** The cognitive level of a patient will dictate the ability to execute deep-breathing exercises. With infants, a therapist must rely on neurophysiological facilitation techniques such as quick

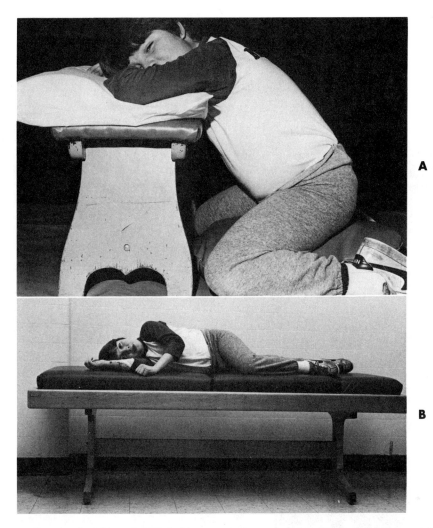

**Fig. 26-10.** Suggested positions for relief of dyspnea. *At home:* **A,** Relaxed foward kneeling or sitting position with the upper chest supported on a pillow and the spine straight, allowing free excursion of the abdominal area for diaphragmatic breathing. **B,** Lying on one side either flat or propped up on three or four pillows. Hips and knees should be flexed with the top leg in front of the one underneath. Shoulders should be relaxed and spine straight. *During play or sports activities:* **C,** Leaning back against telephone pole or wall, spine straight and supported with relaxed neck and shoulder muscles and slight hip flexion. **D,** Forward sitting position with a straight spine and relaxed neck and shoulder muscles, the wrists or forearms resting on the thighs. *In the hospital:* **E,** High side-lying position with head elevated 45°, hips and knees flexed with pillow between the knees, relaxed neck and shoulder muscles, small pillow under waist to straighten spine. **F,** Forward leaning over bed tray, upper chest supported on a pillow, neck and shoulders relaxed, hips flexed.

stretching of the diaphragm and intercostals to obtain an increased contractile response of these muscles for inspiration.

Toddlers and young children may begin to participate in blowing games when they can imitate and voluntarily take a deep breath. This ability usually begins around 2 years of age. Some suggested blowing games are shown in Fig. 26-11.

Older children, like adults, can be taught deep-breathing exercises by using manual contact and verbal reinforcement. Before children are engaged in deep-breathing exercises, it is useful to establish an understanding of their thoracic anatomy. Ask them to locate their lungs, ribs, and abdomen. If they are unsure, a simple explanation will enhance their understanding of deep breathing and augment their physical response to the exercises. Placing a small toy on the upper abdomen and asking the child to gently raise the toy up toward the ceiling on inspiration may promote use of the diaphragm. The therapist should be aware of any muscle substitutions for diaphragmatic contraction on inspiration. The child may attempt to raise the abdomen by thrusting the abdominal muscles outward by arching the lower back.

Breathing retraining with use of paced breathing techniques should not be overlooked for the pediatric population.

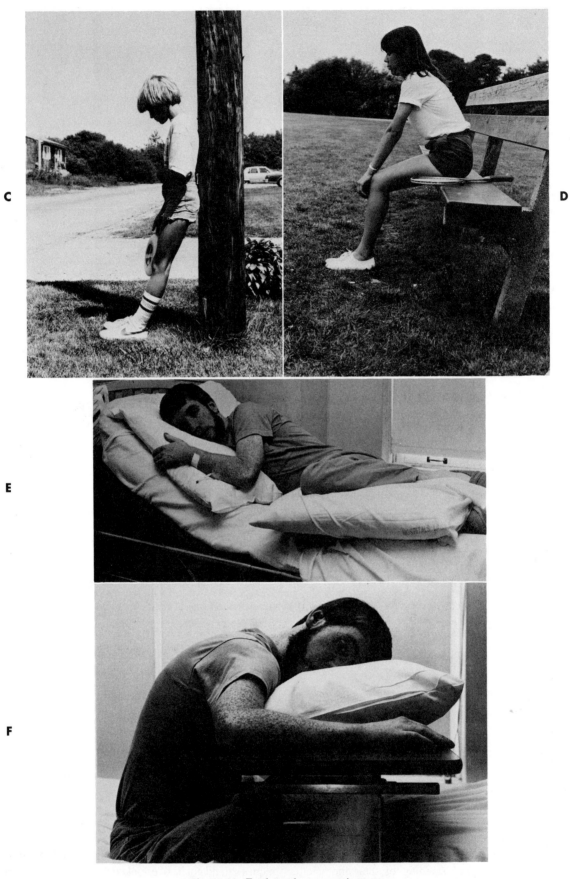

**Fig. 26-10.** For legend see opposite page.

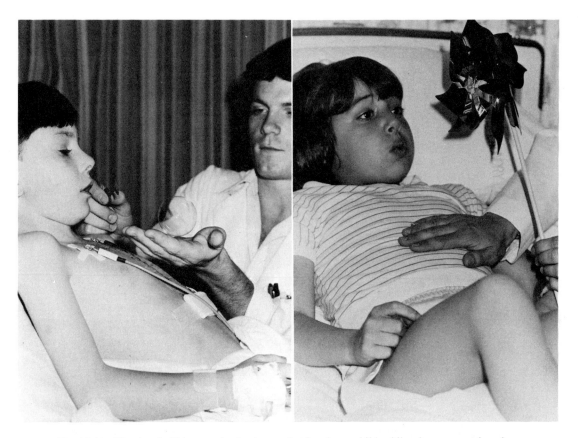

**Fig. 26-11.** Blowing bubbles or pinwheels can be fun for a child while also encouraging deep breathing.

Patients with cystic fibrosis, especially those with advanced disease and dyspnea during functional activities, can benefit from breathing control techniques. The therapist should first carefully assess particular activities that cause breathlessness. The patient should be instructed in controlled and paced diaphragmatic breathing while lying, sitting, standing, walking, and stair climbing. Once this sequence is mastered, the patient can practice combining paced breathing with simulated activities such as carrying a weighted load to imitate handling schoolbooks. Breathing control should be taught to the younger patient who complains of dyspnea during bicycle riding, play, or sports activities. Paced breathing techniques can be used with any patient old enough to understand the concept of regulating breathing rate and pattern with physical activity.

**Bronchial drainage, percussion, vibration, and shaking.** Modifications of these techniques will vary, depending on the age and condition of the patient. Regardless of the size of the patient, adaptation of the therapist's hand position can accommodate any size of chest. A tented position of the fingers is recommended for small infants. One hand can accommodate a toddler and young child's chest (Fig. 26-2, *C*). The force of the percussion, vibration, and shaking will also vary with the age and condition of the patient. Since an infant's chest is more compliant than an adult's, the force of manual techniques should be of less magnitude. Our opinion

is that manual techniques, rather than adapted or mechanical equipment, are highly recommended with infants and young children. Use of the hands allows easier monitoring of the force of the technique. Rib shaking is generally reserved for an older child or patient with a rigid chest as is often seen with advanced cystic fibrosis. Coordinating manual vibration with the expiratory cycle of an infant who breathes at a rapid respiratory rate is difficult. Therefore short, rapid bursts of vibration coordinated as well as possible with expiration are recommended.

Bronchial drainage positioning for the infant and toddler is often performed on the therapist's lap. Transition from the lap to a drainage table or bed is recommended when the child is approximately 2 years old or too large to handle comfortably and safely on the lap. Suggested positioning for lap drainage for the different lung segments is shown on infants in Chapter 25. Care should be taken when handling infants or children with decreased head and neck control to avoid excessive neck flexion and neck rotation. Excessive neck flexion can predispose the infant to obstruction of the upper airway, while excessive neck rotation can decrease breath sounds or air entry on the side opposite of that toward which the head is turned.

Frequent position changes (approximately every 2 hours) are recommended for the child or infant who is unable to move independently or is being mechanically ventilated.

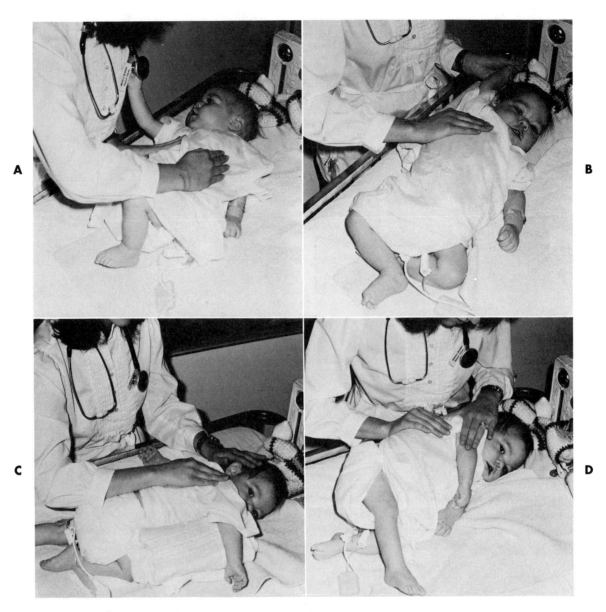

**Fig. 26-12.** Modified bronchial drainage positions. **A,** Anterior segments of the upper and lower lobes can be drained in a supine position. **B,** Right middle lobe or the lingula segment can be drained by positioning in a one-fourth turn from supine. **C,** The posterior segments of the upper and lower lobes can be drained in a three-fourth prone position. **D,** The lateral segments of the lower lobes can be drained in a side-lying position.

Changing position not only promotes pulmonary drainage but also alleviates skin pressure to prevent decubiti. The benefits of position changes for the bedridden patient have been reviewed by Kigin,[72] Zadai,[153] and Hyland.[61] Position changes that promote bronchial hygiene are shown in Fig. 26-12. These positions are used in combination with percussion and vibration when modified bronchial drainage positioning is necessary.

A good understanding of regional ventilation and how it is affected by postural changes is essential for therapists. Studies by Heaf and others[53] and Davies and others[32] begin to explain the differences seen in infants and young children as compared with adults. Heaf and co-workers discovered

that in infants (ages 2 days to 8 months old) with unilateral lung disease, transcutaneous oxygen pressure was greater with the good lung uppermost than with the good lung dependent or in the supine position. There were no changes in carbon dioxide pressure. The reverse is true for adults: pulmonary gas exchange is better when the patient with unilateral disease is positioned with the good lung dependent.[152] Davies went on to study 18 infants and young children (ages 11 days to 27 months old) with and without abnormal chest radiographs. Regardless of chest radiographic findings, it was found that ventilation is preferentially distributed to the uppermost lung. This again demonstrated the reversal of the adult pattern. Davies proposes

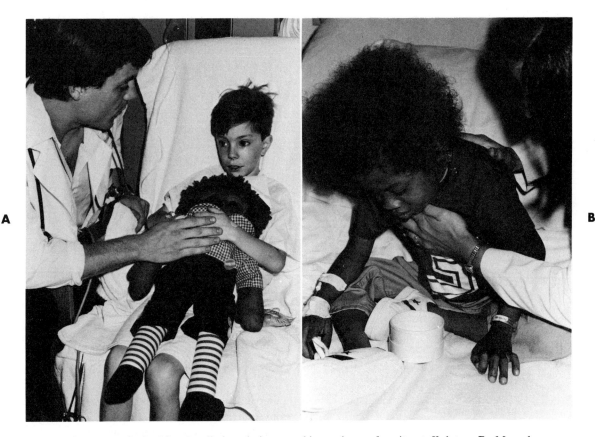

**Fig. 26-13. A,** Incisional splinting during coughing using a favorite stuffed toy. **B,** Manual compression over the midsternum to facilitate sputum expectoration.

reasons for this phenomenon.[32] Further research is needed to determine the age at which the adult pattern is seen. This information is important to the therapist. Care should be taken when positioning a child to do bronchial drainage on the involved side or in supine. Careful monitoring of oxygen saturation level and other vital signs should take place.

**Coughing techniques.** Eliciting a voluntary cough from a pediatric patient can be a challenge. Refusal to cough may stem from fear, pain, or just not being in the mood. Much time may be spent trying to convince a strong-willed child that it is important to cough. Instead, success may come by making coughing a game. For example, a child can be motivated to cough by earning a colorful star on a "cough score sheet" for each good cough. The child can then proudly display these efforts to parents, doctors, and nurses. Children who enjoy drawing are told that each time they cough, they may draw part of a face or object. The therapist then guesses who or what has been drawn! Huffing techniques to promote coughing can be performed during the story of the big bad wolf who "huffed and puffed and blew the house down." Imaginative approaches often work when a more straightforward approach has failed.

To ease the discomfort or fear of coughing for surgical patients, the therapist can have them splint their incision with a favorite stuffed animal or teach the parents to give a gentle hug with incisional support. Children will usually not welcome manual incisional support from the therapist (Fig. 26-13, A). Patients who have spasmodic coughing episodes or thickened secretions may benefit from manual compression or vibration over the midsternal area to facilitate sputum expectoration (Fig. 26-13, B).

The technique of tracheal stimulation or tickling can be used for young patients who do not understand the concept of coughing. It is recommended only if the therapist is trained in the technique and the child is not unduly distressed by the maneuver. The stimulation is performed by placing the index finger or thumb on the anterior side of the neck against the trachea, just above the sternal notch. A gentle but firm inward pressure in a circular pattern as the patient begins to exhale may elicit a reflex cough. Fig. 26-14 shows finger placement for tracheal tickling.

Endotracheal suctioning is often needed to stimulate coughing and raise secretions in the intubated and acutely ill infant or child. When large amounts of secretions are present, suctioning may be needed both during and after therapy.

**FET, PEP, and autogenic drainage techniques.** As was mentioned, techniques such as forced expiration technique (FET), self-applied positive expiratory airway pressure with a mask (PEP), and autogenic drainage (AD) are being used overseas. Therapists here in the United States are beginning to review and evaluate these techniques.[29a]

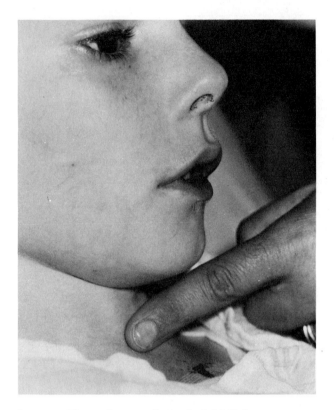

**Fig. 26-14.** Finger placement for tracheal "tickle" maneuver.

***Forced expiration technique.*** Bernice Thompson has taught the technique of forced expirations (huffing) for many years in New Zealand.[137] Therapists at the Brompton Hospital in London have used this technique extensively and researched its effectiveness with cystic fibrosis patients.[105,106] The FET employs a forced expiration or huff following a medium-sized breath. The patient should tighten the abdominal muscles firmly while huffing, without contracting the throat muscles. The "huff" should be maintained long enough to attempt removing distal bronchial secretions without going into a spasmodic cough. The important part of FET is the periods (15 to 30 seconds) of relaxation with gentle diaphragmatic breathing following 1 or 2 huffs. This helps relax the airways. Once secretions are felt in the larger, uppermost airways, a huff or double cough should remove them. This technique is especially helpful to those patients who experience bronchospasms or premature airway closure and have problems with exhaustive, spasmodic coughing. FET is often used in coordination with bronchial drainage. It was found that bronchial drainage using the FET with a physical therapist performing percussion and vibration was as effective as the cystic fibrosis patient treating him- or herself with the FET in terms of length of treatment and secretion production.[105] It is a treatment technique that may allow a patient to be more independent in carrying out a pulmonary hygiene program. However, this technique is generally too strenuous for a patient to carry out effectively when he or she is very fatigued or acutely ill.

***Positive expiratory pressure (PEP) mask therapy.*** In 1983 Stafanger and co-workers[125] described a technique of pulmonary hygiene for cystic fibrosis patients. It consisted of self-applied PEP produced by breathing through a specifically designed mask that created expiratory resistance. The principle behind PEP mask therapy is that the technique allows more air during inspiration to enter peripheral airways via collateral channels. This air then escapes during expiration, following pressure to build up behind sputum plugs moving secretions centrally toward larger airways. A patient can then more easily cough and clear sputum. This technique is generally taught with the patient sitting up and leaning forward with both elbows on a table. The PEP mask is placed over the mouth and nose, and a resistor is attached to the mask. The patient breathes abdominally against a resistance of 10 to 15 cm $H_2O$, which is measured by a manometer. A slightly active expiration is encouraged. After a number of breathing cycles, the mask is removed and secretions are raised by using the FET or by coughing. This continues for 15 to 20 minutes or until as much sputum is raised as possible. Research has indicated such benefits as improvement in transcutaneous tension of oxygen and sputum production with single treatments and significant falls in residual volumes over prolonged treatment periods. Comparisons have been made between PEP therapy and conventional postural drainage treatments.*

The PEP masks necessary to carry out this type of therapy have not been approved as yet by the Food and Drug Administration in this country. It is hoped controlled studies evaluating the PEP mask therapy here in the United States will begin soon.[31]

***Autogenic drainage.*** A less well-known technique of chest physical therapy for pulmonary hygiene in this country is that of autogenic drainage (AD).[132] The technique, done in a sitting position, teaches patients the ability to determine (through proprioceptive, sensory, and auditory signals) at which generation of bronchi secretions exist. The patient then learns: (1) to "unstick" mucus in the peripheral portions of the lungs by very low lung-volume breathing, (2) proceeding then to "collect" mucus in the middle to large airways by low lung-volume breathing, and (3) finally to evacuate the mucus in the central airways by normal to high lung-volume breathing. Minimal research exists regarding the effectiveness of AD.[28,29,31] However, proponents believe it can be applied in all types of obstructive lung disease and postoperative treatments, and can be taught to children as young as 5 to 6 years of age. Intensive training in the technique is necessary before it can be used effectively.

In conclusion, all three techniques discussed above (FET, PEP, AD) are specialized chest physical therapy techniques that require skill to be effective. Though these approaches are new in the United States, it is important for practicing therapists to become acquainted with them and pursue the

---

* References 31, 37, 47, 56, 97, 125, 140, 142.

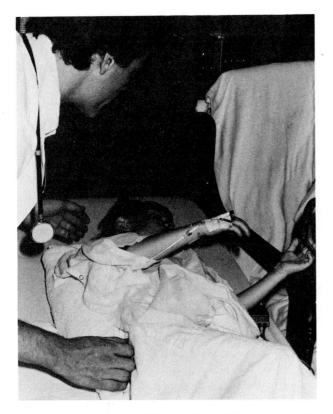

**Fig. 26-15.** Independent mobility in bed should be emphasized for the postoperative patient.

necessary training in these techniques if they are to be practiced. The principles of the above techniques are based on much of Macklem's work, and it is worthwhile to review these articles.[80-83]

**General mobility.** Whenever an ill infant's or toddler's status allows, bronchial drainage using the therapist's lap is preferable to treatment in bed. Regardless of lines or tubes attached to the child, holding a sick infant during therapy is encouraged. The tactile stimulation may be quite comforting.

Range of motion exercises to maintain joint mobility should always be part of chest physical therapy when the patient is unconscious or bedridden.

Early mobility should be stressed for the postoperative patient. Emphasis is placed on mobility in bed immediately after surgery with ambulation when indicated (Fig. 26-15). Specific range of motion exercises of a joint near an incisional site are often necessary. Thoracic surgical patients especially need help with motion of the upper extremity on the side of the thoracotomy. Thoracic mobility exercises to prevent muscular tightness and enhance thoracic excursion for deep breathing are also a necessary part of the postoperative program. Children who are aware that they have had surgery often assume a rigid posture. During gait there is a lack of proper spinal alignment, hip and knee flexion, and arm swing. Infants and toddlers without postoperative anxieties often move more freely than older children.

Musculoskeletal mobility, particularly of the thorax and shoulder girdle, is important to the patient with respiratory dysfunction. Decreased range of motion and tight muscles in the shoulder and thorax can create ineffective patterns of ventilation and increased work of breathing. Exercises should emphasize mobility of the spine, thorax, and shoulder girdle in coordination with deep breathing. Making the exercising fun is very important in pediatrics. Games like "Simon Says" or songs like "The Itsy-Bitsy Spider" or "Bend and Stretch" can be quite appealing. Ball games can promote both upper extremity and thoracic mobility. Exercising to music geared toward the age level of the child or adolescent can also be quite successful.

**Physical exercise and conditioning.** The importance of physical exercise and conditioning for the pediatric pulmonary patient is being recognized. Chapter 27 discusses this topic in detail. This information is essential for therapists working with children and young adults with compromised pulmonary function.

**Postural exercises.** As discussed on p. 323 skeletal abnormalities are often present in patients with chronic respiratory disease. Thoracic surgical patients are also at risk for developing postural problems because of large thoracic incisions, muscle resections, and incisional splinting from pain. Postural exercises for the respiratory patient should emphasize stretching for the pectorals and anterior hip muscles and strengthening for the scapular, upper back extensor, and abdominal muscles. One can perform thoracic spine flexibility exercises sitting in front of a mirror to provide visual feedback and promotion of pelvic stability.

If scoliosis is suspected, an orthopedic surgeon should be consulted to assess the severity of the curve and presence of a rotational component. An exercise program should be based on the surgeon's findings. Deep breathing is always coordinated with any exercises performed by a respiratory patient.

### Treatment precautions

There are few absolute contraindications or reasons to discontinue chest physical therapy. The risks and benefits of modifying or discontinuing a treatment because of a precarious situation should be carefully weighed and discussed with the patient's physician. Certain modifications of treatment techniques and precautionary measures should be considered when the therapist encounters the following 9 situations. These guidelines will be helpful in making sound decisions.

**Respiratory or cardiac instability.** Respiratory or cardiac instability may require modification of treatment techniques. Positioning to tolerance in an attempt to achieve at least a level horizontal position is recommended. Careful monitoring of skin color, respiratory rate, heart rate, and oxygen saturation levels is essential. It is important to work with respiratory therapists and nursing personnel to achieve the most stable condition possible for a patient in which to carry out safe and effective treatment.

**Severe gastroesophageal reflux.** Supine and Trendelenburg positioning may enhance gastroesophageal reflux (GER) (p. 518). The severity of a child's GER and the need for flat or Trendelenburg positioning for therapeutic bronchial drainage must be carefully considered with the physician. Modified bronchial drainage in an upright position may be necessary for children with severe GER with treatments scheduled before feedings. Following surgical correction of GER, positioning restrictions are generally not necessary. Discussion with the surgeon should take place to clarify any concerns regarding positioning.

**Hemoptysis.** Hemoptysis, or coughing up blood, is one of the complications of chronic lung disease. It is often seen in older patients with advanced cystic fibrosis.[57,93] Fresh blood streaking of sputum is common in patients with cystic fibrosis because of inflammation of the bronchial mucosa with resultant venous bleeding with no further consequence. However, there is great concern when the patient coughs up larger volumes of blood with evidence of little or no sputum. The amount of hemoptysis can range from a teaspoonful to several cupsful, the latter being a medical emergency. Patients will often describe a feeling of "warmth" or "gurgling" in one area of the chest before the hemoptysis. Hemoptysis can occur anytime and is not always related to strenuous activity or vigorous coughing. Some patients complain that they bleed when in a head-flat position, but they are fine when upright.

Most modifications of treatment involve bronchial drainage techniques and vary with each patient based upon the amount of bleeding and precipitating factors. A patient who raises only 5 to 10 ml of blood but whose sputum is clear of blood with subsequent coughing may not need the treatment altered. However, if the bleeding continues, vigorous percussion and positions that appear to induce bleeding should be avoided. Depending on the amount of hemoptysis, breathing exercises, modified positions, vibration, and instruction in controlled, effective coughing may continue. A patient who is not receiving some form of chest physical therapy may find that coughing becomes difficult and strained, thereby imposing added intrapulmonary pressures on inflamed and bleeding bronchial walls. Therapy will aid in mobilizing blood and secretions from the airways so that the effort of coughing is reduced. Full treatment may be resumed once the active bleeding has stopped and should emphasize clearance of retained secretions and blood from the airways. It is crucial for the therapist to reassure the patient that continued, careful reevaluation of the patient's status will occur during treatment, with necessary modifications made as indicated. Discussion and education of the physician regarding the chest physical therapy management of a patient who has experienced hemoptysis are important. Decisions should be based on individual situations, and the importance of modified, but continued, physical therapy should be stressed to the physician.

If a patient experiences a significant episode of hemoptysis during treatment, the therapist should help the patient into an upright position. A basin into which the patient can expectorate should be quickly provided. Above all, the patient should be encouraged to relax as much as possible with slow, controlled breathing to avoid a rise in blood pressure. The therapist should never leave the patient, but notify the nurse and physician as soon as possible.

**Pneumothorax.** Pneumothorax can occur as a complication of cystic fibrosis, severe asthma, or any pulmonary problem necessitating mechanical ventilation with high inspiratory pressure. Chest physical therapy is contraindicated in the presence of an untreated, progressing, or tension pneumothorax. Treatment can continue with a small, stable pneumothorax and with a pneumothorax that has resolved through treatment with a thoracostomy and insertion of a chest tube for vacuum drainage of air.

A patient with a chest tube in place has some discomfort. Scheduling of treatment after pain medication is recommended. If bronchial hygiene is needed, percussion should not be performed directly over the chest tube site, but percussion to tolerance is acceptable elsewhere on the thorax. If subcutaneous emphysema is present, percussion is often uncomfortable and vibration is recommended. Depending on the site of chest tube placement, modification of some bronchial drainage positions may be necessary to ensure chest tube patency at all times. Pressure on or kinking of the tube must be avoided (Fig. 26-16). An understanding of the negative-pressure treatment apparatus is important for recognition of the presence of air leaks.

Although dislodging a chest tube from the chest is a rare circumstance, if it should happen, the therapist should immediately apply pressure to the thorax at the chest tube site. If the tubing ever becomes disconnected from the negative-pressure apparatus, the therapist should immediately clamp the portion of tubing inserted into the chest. All these measures will prevent the reaccumulation of air in the pleural space. A case study describing the physical therapy program for a patient with cystic fibrosis and a pneumothorax can be found on p. 554.

**Bronchoconstriction.** There has been some concern that manual chest techniques, particularly percussion, can increase bronchoconstriction during treatment.[16] However, Huber and associates[59] studied 21 asthmatic children, 11 of whom received bronchial drainage including percussion and vibration. The treated group demonstrated a 40% increase in forced expiratory volume in 1 second at 30 minutes after treatment. The control group showed no improvement. Huber and associates concluded that bronchial drainage techniques were not detrimental for mildly to moderately obstructed asthmatic patients. However, the use of percussion should be carefully considered during treatment of patients with asthma or others who have a bronchospastic component to their disease. These patients may benefit from an aerosol bronchodilator before and possibly during treatment to reduce the risk of increased bronchoconstric-

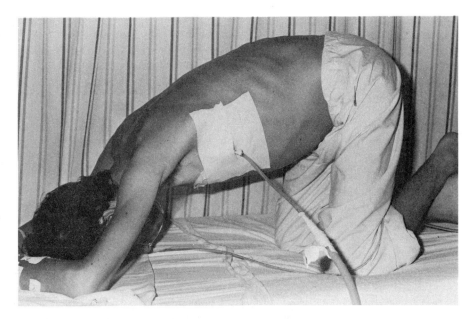

**Fig. 26-16.** Alternative position for the posterior segments of the lower lobes in a patient with a chest tube. This position would be particularly recommended for a patient who has anterior placement of a chest tube.

tion. Auscultation of the chest before and immediately after percussion can be used to monitor increased wheezing. The patient may also complain of feeling "tighter." With evidence of increased bronchoconstriction, bronchial drainage and only vibration with controlled coughing may allow the safe continuation of treatment. Sound judgment in choosing the appropriate techniques and the use of a bronchodilator may help reduce the risk of increased bronchospasm.

Exercise-induced bronchospasm (EIB) is a recognized and common complication of asthma in childhood.[39,70] Khan and Olson[71] reviewed the subject in relationship to physical therapy in 1975. Several studies have indicated that certain types of exercises are more likely to cause bronchospasm. The consensus is that activities involving running are more likely to cause EIB than cycling.[3] Swimming may be the least likely cause of EIB.[42,65] The severity of EIB also appears to relate to the rate of work and duration of exercise.[39,42] Jones and co-workers[65] found that short-term exercises of 1 to 2 minutes in duration caused bronchodilatation, but longer exercise of 4 to 12 minutes resulted in bronchoconstriction. These factors should be considered when one is planning an exercise program for children who have asthma or other bronchospastic problems. Exercises of short duration interspersed with periods of relaxation should be planned for the asthmatic child.

**Decreased platelet counts.** Children who have decreased production of platelets (thrombocytopenia) are predisposed to bruising. Platelets are essential for the maintenance of the integrity of the capillary walls. Platelets also donate substances that aid in coagulation or clotting. The normal platelet count is approximately 259,000 platelets

per cubic millimeter of blood. Patients with acute leukemia may have platelet counts of less than 50,000. A severely traumatized or ill patient may experience disseminated intravascular coagulation with a resultant drop in platelets. Vigorous techniques, such as chest percussion or resistive exercises, can cause bruising in a pediatric patient with a low platelet count. Guidelines for appropriate bronchial drainage techniques or exercises for such patients should be established. A guideline proposed at The Children's Hospital, Boston, is as follows: if the platelet count is greater than 50,000, percussion and vibration and resistive exercise is acceptable with caution; counts between 20,000 and 50,000 dictate the use of vibration and positioning only for bronchial drainage, as well as active-assistive and active exercise; below 20,000 only bronchial drainage positioning and active exercises are used. Breathing exercises and coughing may continue regardless of the platelet count. As with any general guidelines, exceptions may occur in specific cases, and discussion with the physician should be carried out to clarify which techniques are appropriate.

**Increased intracranial pressure.** Position changes, especially during turning or when placing one's head downward, cause an increase in intracranial pressure (ICP). Suctioning may also have the same effect on the ICP. Tomney and Finer[139] found that in infants with severe head injury, spontaneous movements were related to the greatest increases in ICP. In other conditions, such as surgery to the head and Reye's syndrome, control of ICP is essential in preventing brain damage.

Ciesla's work[23] with patients with space-occupying lesions revealed that percussion and vibration did not cause any untoward effects on ICP. More care should be taken when making position changes with patients with increased ICP. Ciesla recommends the use of a tilt test as a practical assessment of cerebral compliance, which can be defined as the body's ability to return ICP to base line following an elevation. Review of this information is recommended.

Intracranial pressure can be recorded constantly through the placement of cranial monitoring bolts. If the ICP becomes significantly elevated and does not return to base line within a very short period of time, limitations on positioning changes may have to be used. In cases where an intracranial monitoring bolt is not in place, blood pressure and central venous pressure readings may be of value in the assessment of ICP changes. Discussion with the physician should take place and appropriate guidelines for maximum allowable values of ICP or other vital signs during physical therapy treatments should be determined.

**Surgical precautions.** Because of the size of pediatric patients, some postoperative precautions may be necessary. Percussion techniques used over thoracic incisions will cause the patient great discomfort. Because of the highly compliant developing thorax, percussion is also avoided over the anterior chest of a child having had a recent midsternal incision. This precaution is not only to reduce discomfort but also to prevent the seesaw effect of percussion on the incisional area. Vibration within the child's tolerance is acceptable if indicated. Percussion is also avoided on the anterior chest of any patient with an unstable open sternum caused by a wound infection. The sternal area, in this case, should be supported manually during treatment.

Chest physical therapy can be initiated in postoperative pediatric cardiac patients while intracardiac lines are in place. However, because of the small size of a child's heart and the importance of monitoring lines, excessive pressure on the chest should be avoided while the lines are in place. These delicately placed lines are inserted intraoperatively in the patient's atria, ventricles, or pulmonary artery to monitor hemodynamic values postoperatively. Extra care should be taken with ventricular lines, as moving them could cause ventricular irritation, which could lead to dysrythmias.

**Osteoporosis.** Children with advanced or severe paralytic conditions may develop thin, osteoporotic bones. A lack of the normal muscular forces exerted on the bones can compromise the integrity and strength of the bony matrix. Osteoporosis or fragility of the ribs may occur in children with paralysis. With evidence of thoracic osteoporosis, caution should be employed with percussion or vigorous shaking techniques. A recent study by Gibbens and co-workers[40] has pointed to a prevalence of osteoporosis among patients with cystic fibrosis. It was found that osteoporosis is a complication of cystic fibrosis and is not related to the patient's age. It is, however, more predominant in patients with more severe disease. This may be the result of a malabsorption of fat and fat-soluble vitamins such as vitamin D. Calcium malabsorption is also commonly found in patients with cystic fibrosis. Gibbens determined that decreased bone density was more prevalent in the more undernourished. Therapists should be aware of this complication when performing vigorous manual techniques on patients with advanced disease.

## DISCHARGE AND HOME CARE
### Discharge planning

In an acute care setting, a pediatric patient's status can change quickly, and many can substantially improve in a few days. Therapists working in an acute care facility know only too well that a decision for discharge can be made quickly and with little time for preparation and planning. Although this may sound premature, discharge planning should begin the first day of treatment, especially if a need for home care or follow-up physical therapy is anticipated. A specific plan of treatment cannot always be determined early in the hospitalization, but the process must begin so that with a quick decision for discharge, home treatment planning and family instruction are possible. Therapists should always schedule a return appointment in 1 to 2 weeks for review of the home instructions.

Early contact between the therapist and family or other primary caretaker is ideal. Several sessions, if possible, should be scheduled for parental and patient instruction. Discharge planning and home instructions carried out under severe time constraints will be frustrating for both the therapist and family. Early planning is particularly important when the patient has been diagnosed to have a chronic illness such as cystic fibrosis. It is important to allow time for careful assessment of the family's abilities to carry out the necessary treatment. This assessment will help in determining a family's need for community support. Community physical therapists can help monitor a family's or patient's performance of the treatment at home and can provide direct care if necessary.

Part of discharge planning also involves good communication with other medical team members for the patient. Taking part in and offering necessary input at discharge planning meetings is essential.

### Home care

A physical therapist's primary responsibilities regarding home care are to plan a comprehensive and realistic program and to instruct and educate those involved.

When planning a home program of chest physical therapy for an infant or child, the therapist must remember that the treatment regimen will be in addition to daily routine child care. Parenting is a difficult task, and appreciation of the daily stresses experienced by a family with a child with respiratory dysfunction provides an essential framework in which to plan appropriate treatment.

Practical suggestions regarding scheduling and duration of treatment are always greatly appreciated by the family. Involvement of both parents, responsible siblings, and relatives may help ease the treatment burden. If the patient is older, encouraging responsibility for self-care will diminish the dependency on parents.

A family may have the added burden of caring for more than one child with a respiratory dysfunction. Cystic fibrosis is an inherited disease, and often more than one child in a family is afflicted. Reviewing family histories of patients with asthma may also reveal other siblings who have the disease.

Although the ultimate responsibility of home respiratory care rests with the family, community support may help ease the stress on the family. Qualified physical therapists working for either a home health agency or privately can help evaluate a family's or patient's performance of the treatment or can offer direct care as necessary. Private insurance policies or state aid through children's programs may pay for, or supplement, the cost of these treatments.

For patients with cystic fibrosis or other chronic lung diseases, daily chest physical therapy may be indicated from the time of diagnosis throughout the patient's life. As children grow, they face many critical stages of emotional development and life-style changes. It is no surprise, then, that a constant routine in one's life, such as chest physical therapy, must also "weather the storm" of emotional crises. The physical therapist must be aware of these critical periods during which treatment schedules and components may have to be modified. Additional guidelines and support may be needed to promote family or patient compliance with treatment. The following discussion presents critical stages during which families or patients may need review of chest physical therapy skills, as well as reevaluation and revision of treatment plans.

**The resistant toddler.** It is a difficult time for parents who are earnestly attempting to comply with treatment but are meeting great resistance from their small, but rebellious toddler. This is the appropriate time to make the transition from bronchial drainage on the lap to a bed or drainage table. This change will ease management of the child in different positions, and should add to the child's feelings of independence. The idea of having a special place to do therapy might be quite appealing. Treatment time may have to be altered to accommodate shorter attention spans. It is better to do a shorter, effective treatment than a lengthy, emotionally exhausting treatment on a crying, squirming child. The therapist should suggest dividing the bronchial drainage treatment into two or three shorter sessions rather than one long session. Simple effective methods to increase the attention span of the child during treatment may include reading or telling the child a favorite story, watching an appealing television show, or listening to a musical recording. A sibling can often be recruited to keep a brother or sister entertained during treatment.

The concept of coughing should be introduced early, between 2 and 3 years of age, or before if possible, and encouraged as a vital part of treatment. Blowing games can be used effectively in early childhood to aid in improving ventilation (Fig. 26-11).

The most important thing for young children with respiratory problems to learn is that therapy is a regular event in their lives. Consistency is important. As soon as the regularity or routine of the therapy is disturbed, cooperation of the child may be lost.

**Issues regarding the school-aged child.** When a child is ready for school, treatment schedules must be arranged accordingly. If treatment is needed before school, additional time for this must be provided. A therapist may be helpful in organizing a treatment session for the early morning that is more directed and focused upon problem areas of the lungs.

School absenteeism, which is often high in children with respiratory diseases, is another concern. The child may struggle to keep up with the class, adding to feelings of alienation. Children who fatigue easily or need chest physical therapy at midday may not be able to complete a full day of school and must attend part time. Efforts to teach a school nurse or other responsible adult bronchial drainage techniques could be useful in providing a midday treatment that might allow full attendance.

A child will often work hard to suppress coughing to avoid embarrassment and may return from school very congested and fatigued. Therapists should reinforce the importance of coughing when necessary. If a child is adamantly against coughing in the classroom, suggesting the lavatory as a private place for coughing may be helpful.

Activity and sports, within tolerance, should be encouraged. Parents can be reassured that physical exercise is good and aids in mobilizing secretions. Guidelines for the child with exercise-induced bronchospasm can be suggested.

**The rebellious adolescent.** Coping with a respiratory illness during the adolescent years can become challenging for all concerned. The emphasis on physical appearances in adolescence can create much stress for the teenager with lung problems. Adolescents with cystic fibrosis often experience weight loss from nutritional problems. Barrel chests and digital clubbing may be obvious in patients with more advanced chronic lung disease. These physical changes are hard to hide. A chronic cough and frequent illnesses can further alienate the adolescent from peers whose acceptance is so important.

It is no surprise that teenagers frequently express anger about their disease. This anger may take the form of rebellion and noncompliance with the treatment regimen. Medications may not be taken. This noncompliance can be detrimental for the asthmatic who must maintain a therapeutic level of medication to control wheezing and a severe bronchospastic attack may result. Chest physical therapy is the treatment against which the child most often rebels. Treatments are time consuming and often require the participation of a parent or other authority figure. This reliance on others becomes a threat to independence.

The physical therapist must be acutely aware of how these issues affect compliance with therapy. Instruction in self-care techniques should begin when the patient is both interested in and responsible for carrying out self-care. When the child reaches 12 or 13 years of age, it is often appropriate to begin teaching bronchial self-drainage techniques with either manual or mechanical percussion, the forced expiratory technique, PEP mask therapy, or autogenic drainage. The technique(s) chosen will depend on the patient's readiness and level of understanding as well as the availability of necessary equipment and qualified instructors. Self-drainage with percussion can be easily attained for all anterior and lateral bronchopulmonary segments. Percussion for posterior segments often requires the aid of another person. However, some mechanical percussors are designed to allow access to areas of the upper back. Parents must be reassured that instructing adolescents in self-care may help sustain compliance without compromising the effectiveness of treatment. Even though the adolescent may assume some responsibility for care, he or she may still need and seek out the encouragement that only a parent can offer. On the other hand, parental advice and support may be the last thing an adolescent would want. An outside professional may have more success in getting an adolescent to comply with treatment. Adolescent patients need both support and independence.

Emphasis should also be placed on designing an acceptable treatment program that encourages compliance and independence without compromising therapeutic goals. When discussing therapy with a teenager, the therapist should not lecture about the necessity of pulmonary care, but should allow some compromise and decision making on the part of the patient. For example, an agreement may be reached whereby a trial period of 3 months of routine therapy is tried by the patient. If there is benefit noted from the regimen, the patient may take it upon himself or herself to continue on a regular basis. It should be suggested that therapy can be done while the patient is watching television or listening to music. Headphones can allow appreciation of music while diminishing the sounds of chest percussion.

A regular program of exercise should always be encouraged and outlined for an adolescent patient. A program of physical exercise can aid sputum removal and improve conditioning (see Chapter 27). An exercise program may also be more socially acceptable to the adolescent. A firm commitment on the part of the therapist to therapeutic goals with sensitive consideration of the needs of the adolescent may spell success.

**The college-bound or working young adult.** As a teenager matures and grows toward college age and young adulthood, other issues surface. The patient faces a decision to leave the security of family life to begin living independently. The young adult living independently has the total responsibility of care. The demands of a college program can mean physically and mentally rigorous sched-

ules. Patients with more advanced lung disease often experience a decline in their health because of the stress of school. Hospitalizations may interfere with classes and exams. Keeping up with academic and social schedules of classmates can be difficult and can lead to dropping out of school temporarily or permanently.

The therapist may help by organizing a realistic treatment schedule and suggesting and demonstrating the use of a mechanical percussor to ease the stress of self-drainage. Arranging treatments through a hospital near campus, home health agency, or student health facility on campus may be helpful. An understanding roommate or college friend can be taught the skills of percussion and vibration. Many patients, however, do not want to burden friends or reveal the needs imposed upon them by their illness, and the latter suggestion may be rejected.

The young adult with lung disease often finds job hunting difficult. Describing a chronic illness to a prospective employer may be difficult, and many questions may be asked. Once a job is begun, the patient is faced with the stress of staying well to meet the responsibilities of the job. Therapy, which becomes even more important, may be more difficult to schedule into a busy day. Careful scheduling, organization of treatment time, and planning more directed treatment for involved areas of the lung may become necessary.

**Friendship, dating, and marriage.** Friendship, dating, and marriage bring another significant person into the life of a patient. This important person can offer much support and help and should be encouraged to take part in the care of the patient. A close friend may be willing to learn various chest physical therapy techniques to help a patient who is living independently or who refuses family support. A dating partner may also be willing to assist and encourage chest physical therapy. Instructing a prospective spouse in therapy techniques is important to the future marital relationship when a patient needs pulmonary care at home. It is healthy for prospective spouses to understand and accept the daily demands of their partner's illness before the marriage. Spouses are often more enthusiastic about regular treatments than patients themselves and can make significant contributions to the maintenance of optimal health of their partners. Often it is the patient's reluctance to accept assistance rather than the partner's lack of enthusiasm to help that stands in the way of effective care.

### Equipment suggestions

**Mechanical percussors and vibrators.** Mechanical devices that approximate chest percussion and vibration are available for home use. The most commonly used are mechanical percussors. These are designed with a small motor that drives a shaft onto which attaches a padded, cup-shaped head. Most percussors of this type weigh approximately 3 pounds. The padded head is placed on a designated area of the chest, and the motor will drive the

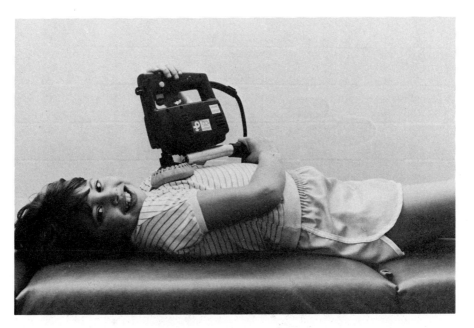

**Fig. 26-17.** Patient using mechanical percussor over anterior segment of right upper lobe.

shaft up and down. The head will then rhythmically strike the chest to provide percussion (Fig. 26-17). The speed of the shaft is variable, creating diversified amounts of force on the chest. There are many types of percussors including smaller models that accommodate a child's chest.

There are some questions concerning the effectiveness of mechanical percussion versus manual percussion. Study results have been limited and variable.[38,86,104] We believe that manual techniques are preferable over mechanical means for providing chest percussion, especially for the younger child. Manual percussion allows more sensitivity for the therapist regarding forces on the chest. Monitoring the force of percussion is very important when one is working with small, compliant chests. However, the mechanical percussor has its place in the care of patients requiring bronchial drainage. The percussor offers independence to some patients who, because of choice or circumstances, cannot employ manual percussion. Percussors are portable and can be taken on trips or to college. Parents may elect to use mechanical means to administer percussion and vibration because they lack the ability or physical dexterity to perform manual skills.

Mechanical vibrators are also commercially available. However, they can create sliding of the skin over the rib cage rather than the quick up and down force of manual vibration.

Before deciding to purchase a mechanical percussor or vibrator, the patient and parents should both see and try the machine to be sure it is sufficient. The device should be easy to use and should offer the desired results. Careful evaluation of the mechanics, effectiveness, and comfort of the apparatus during use is necessary before a machine is purchased.

**High Frequency Chest Compression (HFCC).** High frequency chest compression (HFCC) system is a relatively new concept that offers assistance to patients who require pulmonary hygiene. The system includes a custom fitted, inflatable vest. The vest is worn snugly over the patient's entire torso. Attached to the vest are flexible hoses that deliver pulsating air at different frequencies. The system is based on the theory that the gentle and rhythmic pulses of air that are delivered via the vest will force mucus towards the larger airways (Fig. 26-18).

Patients generally perform 30-minute therapy sessions. Each session is organized into 5-minute intervals at each of 6 frequencies (6,8,14,18, and 20 Hz). At the end of each interval, deep breathing exercises using the HFCC at 25 Hz during exhalation followed by effective coughing are done. Some patients require a weaning-in process to adjust to the system. Performing HFCC 1 to 2 minutes at each frequency and increasing accordingly, or doing only a few intervals at either the high or low frequencies may be desirable.

Contraindications to the use of HFCC include chest tubes, untreated pneumothorax, or hemoptysis. Precautions for the use of HFCC include low platelets (<60,000), hepatosplenomegaly, mild hemoptysis (streaking in the sputum), or rib fractures. Discussion with the physician should take place before initiation of HFCC treatment with patients with these conditions.

Warwick and Hansen described the HFCC system and later performed a study with 16 patients with cystic fibrosis to assess the effectiveness of HFCC on clearance of mucous secretions from the airways.[50,147] They concluded that HFCC could replace manual postural drainage techniques, thus offering more independence to adolescents and young adults with cystic fibrosis. There was evidence of a decrease in progression of lung disease during the HFCC therapy trial period.

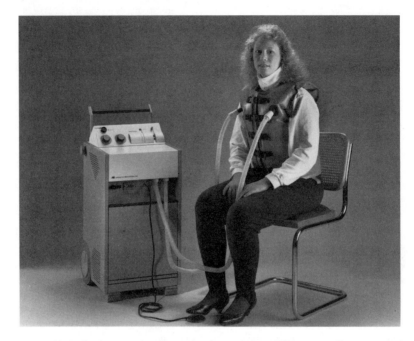

**Fig. 26-18.** A high frequency chest compression system. Photo compliments of American Biosystems, Inc., Stillwater, Mn.

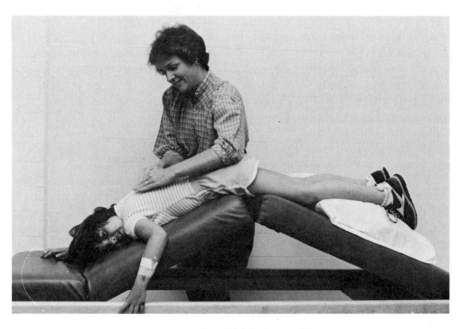

**Fig. 26-19.** Bronchial drainage table.

**Drainage tables.** Bronchial drainage tables are commercially available and are designed to offer comfortable positioning for both the patient and the parent administering treatment. Various degrees of head-down positioning can be obtained with most tables. An example of a type of table made expressly for the purpose of bronchial drainage is shown in Fig. 26-19. Several tables are also available that are small, light-weight, and easily transportable, making them ideal for people who travel or attend college. Many talented parents have been able to design and construct their own table once they understand the principles of bronchial drainage.

Money spent buying equipment such as mechanical percussors and bronchial drainage tables is often reimbursed, at least in part, by third-party payers. Justification by the physician for the equipment may be required before payment is approved.

**Home positioning methods.** Therapists must be prepared to offer suggestions on ways to accommodate

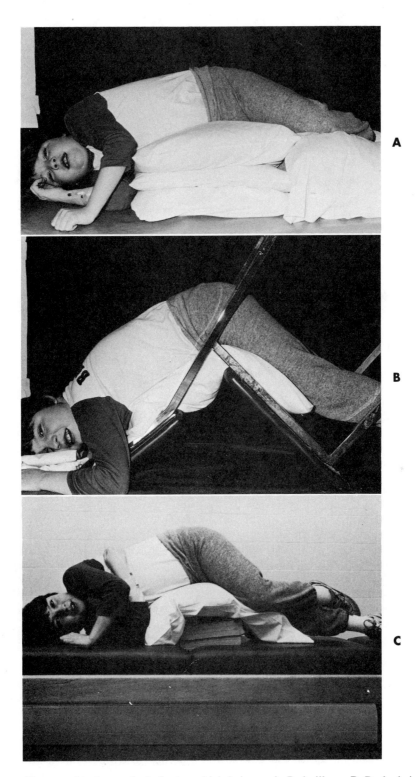

**Fig. 26-20.** Home positioning methods for bronchial drainage. **A,** Bed pillows. **B,** Desk chair. **C,** Stack of magazines with bed pillow.

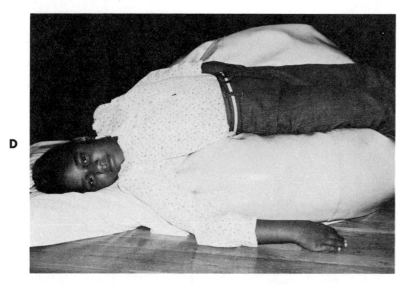

**Fig. 26-20, cont'd. D,** Bean-bag chair.

## CASE 1    A Teenager with Cystic Fibrosis

The patient is a 15-year-old female with cystic fibrosis. She was diagnosed by sweat test at age 3, following a history of recurrent pneumonia. Her course, until recently, has been characterized by moderate respiratory and minimal gastrointestinal symptoms. Her first hospitalization for pulmonary cleanout, consisting of intravenous antibiotics and intensive chest physical therapy, was at age 10. She has had 5 hospitalizations since then, all for pulmonary cleanouts. Although she has no evidence of cor pulmonale, she has experienced a decrease in exercise tolerance limiting her activities to attending school and climbing one flight of stairs. This patient had been active in extracurricular activities and lives at home with her parents. Her most recent pulmonary function tests in July 1986 were as follows: vital capacity = 41% predicted; forced expiratory volume in 1 second = 21% predicted; maximal mid-expiratory flow rate = 5% predicted. Arterial blood gases: $Pa_{O_2}$ – 60; $Pa_{CO_2}$ – 48; pH 7.38.

Five days before her most recent admission to The Children's Hospital in Boston, on July 19, 1986, the patient experienced a gradual onset of left posterior chest pain. This pain, which increased over the next few days, was especially evident on inspiration. She took no pain medication. The patient was taken to her local physician, who ordered a chest radiograph, which showed a small left apical pneumothorax. In view of this finding, arrangements were made for her admission to The Children's Hospital in Boston. A repeat chest radiograph on admission showed a 20% left pneumothorax, and a chest tube was placed anterolaterally in the left third intercostal space. The chest radiograph following tube insertion showed that the left lung was essentially reexpanded except for a 5% residual pneumothorax. There was also the presence of pleural fluid at the left base and dense opacification (infiltrate versus atelectasis) and bronchiectasis in the left upper lobe. Chronic changes on the right side were stable. On July 21, 1986, a physical therapy referral was written as follows: "Chest physical therapy as indicated to right lung, vibration as tolerated to left lung." Arrangements were made to see the patient when she was medicated for pain caused by insertion of the chest tube. Tables 26-1 to 26-3 describe the initial evaluation and treatment plan, and the long-range treatment plan developed for this patient.

Trendelenburg positioning for home drainage if a family is unable or chooses not to purchase a drainage table. Fig. 26-20 shows a few ideas that can be adapted for home use. In addition, tiltboards available in sporting goods stores for situps and other exercises may provide another low-cost method for bronchial drainage positioning.

### Follow-up

It is important to schedule a follow-up visit with patients and parents who have been instructed in a chest physical therapy home program. Reevaluation of the patient's status, compliance, and ability to carry out a home treatment program can take place at the follow-up visit.

Components of the treatment program can be reviewed as needed. The follow-up visit also helps promote communication between the therapist, patient, and family. Additional outpatient appointments at established intervals may be indicated as the therapist deems necessary. The first follow-up appointment after discharge or initial instruction

*Text continued on p. 559.*

**Table 26-1.** Initial evaluation

| Information needed | Therapist's method | Results |
|---|---|---|
| Medical history (past and present) Complications/ contraindications | Medical records Review chart | As noted in summary. Chest tube inserted 7-19-86 by surgeon into left third intercostal space, anterolateral position. |
| | Discussion with physician regarding the status of the chest tube and chest radiograph findings Subjective data from patient | As stated in summary, chest radiograph showed good placement of chest tube and reexpansion of lung, except for small residual (5%) pneumothorax. Physician stated that chest tube was functioning well but requested vibration only to left chest. Patient complaining of left chest pain, especially around chest tube site; was very anxious about moving and coughing. |
| Respiratory status | Check vital signs Check degree of respiratory distress | RR = 2, HR = 100 + regular, temperature = 98.6° F. Patient sitting in a semi-Fowler's position, evidence of mild supraclavicular and intercostal retractions. No nasal flaring. There was minimal digital clubbing and nailbed cyanosis. No obvious perioral cyanosis. |
| | Evaluate breathing pattern/ chest mobility | Breathing with use of accessory musculature, obvious splinting of chest, causing pain, resulting in decreased chest mobility (left greater than right). Poor diaphragmatic breathing pattern. |
| | Assess anteroposterior diameter of chest | A slight increase in anteroposterior diameter, without sternal bowing. |
| | Auscultation | Auscultation revealed breath sounds generally decreased and coarse (left greater than right); crackling (rales) evident in left apices. |
| | Assess presence of subcutaneous emphysema | Minimal subcutaneous emphysema palpable near chest tube insertion. |
| Postural alignment | Observation | Patient sitting with lateral C curve to left in a protective posture in response to pain from increased weight shift onto left buttocks. Further posture evaluation waived until after chest tube removal. |
| Range of motion of left shoulder | Gross assessment of range of left shoulder motion  Active assistive  Passive  Scapular motion | Patient limited in active-assistive flexion (approximately 110°) and abduction (approximately 95°) resulting from pain and restriction from extensive taping around chest tube. Rotation and extension within normal limits. Passively, patient able to reach almost full flexion but could not move beyond 95° abduction because of pain and taping and not joint restriction. Scapula appeared to be moving and free, but taping of chest made this difficult to evaluate. |
| Exercise tolerance/functional status | Assess dyspnea on exercise and/or fatigue upon position change and coughing Assess functional status through patient interview | Patient experienced a slight increase in respiratory rate when asked to move and cough, triggered primarily by discomfort from chest tube and anxiety.  Patient stated she had been experiencing increasing shortness of breath with activities over the last few months. She found it difficult to keep up with her extracurricular activities, with most difficulty occurring when climbing stairs, riding her bike, and during running activities. She complained of one flight and one block dyspnea. Plans made to further assess exercise tolerance once the chest tube was removed. |
| Patient's social/emotional status with regard to adjustment to disease, home pulmonary care | Patient interview and discussion with cystic fibrosis clinic psychologist who follows patient | Patient expressed concern over onset of pneumothorax, but felt secure with being in the hospital. She was most concerned with managing school activities in view of her progressing pulmonary problems. She also expressed frustration with home program of bronchial drainage, finding it difficult to do on a daily basis and questioning its necessity and importance. Her family is very supportive and wants to be involved in her care. They encourage and help her with bronchial drainage at home. |

**Table 26-2.** Initial treatment plan

| Goals | Treatment methods | Results |
|---|---|---|
| Improve bronchial drainage | Postural drainage to all lobes including: Positioning to tolerance with progression to tipped positions Percussion and vibration to right side Vibration only on left side with progression to percussion as tolerated | Initially, patient tolerated only modified drainage with head elevated 45°. Arrangements were made so that patient was medicated for pain before treatment. Percussion and vibration were tolerated well on the right side; vibration only was tolerated on the left side with special care regarding the chest tube and other apparatus. NOTE: Treatment progression was discussed with physician—a new order was written for "CPT as indicated." Within 24 hours after initial treatment, patient was progressed to bronchial drainage with a modified tip (20°) for lower lobe drainage and tolerated light to moderate percussion on the left. Within 48 hours patient was tolerating a full bronchial drainage treatment, but was unable to lie completely on left side or prone because of chest tube. Before treatment breath sounds were decreased (L > R) and coarse throughout. Following treatment, breath sounds increased minimally with less coarseness, but were still quite diminished in left upper lobe. |
| Promote effective coughing | Instruct in controlled coughing Forward sitting position Precede cough with maximal inspiratory effort Maximum of three coughs to one breath Instruct in splinting chest with manual self-support over tube site | Initially, her cough was weak and painful with little sputum production. Efficiency of coughing was enhanced when performed in a forward sitting position preceded by 2-3 maximal inspirations and manual support over chest tube area. As pain decreased and cough improved, sputum production increased to ±10-15 ml of green purulent secretions per treatment. |
| Maximize ventilation and chest mobility | Breathing exercises Diaphragmatic Lateral costal expansion with pursed lips expansion Relaxed in supported semi-Fowler's position Reinforce with verbal cuing | With verbal reinforcement and manual contact during exercises, chest mobility was increased on left side. Deeper inspirations and less accessory muscle activity resulted in improved diaphragmatic breathing and decrease in respiratory rate. |
| Improve left shoulder/scapular range of motion | Range of motion exercises to left shoulder Progress from active-assistive to active PNF diagonals: flex/add/ext.rot.-ext/abd/int.rot. flex/abd/ext.rot.-ext/add/int.rot. Encourage use of left upper extremity in functional activities | Patient was initially apprehensive about moving left upper extremity because of discomfort. She did participate in shoulder exercises with therapist and in a self-program using assistance from right upper extremity. As patient's pain and anxiety decreased, range of motion of left shoulder girdle was improved to within normal limits. Patient gradually began participating in self-care activities (e.g., bathing), using left upper extremity. |
| Achieve good postural alignment while in bed | Development of postural awareness Instruction in importance of good alignment to prevent deformity | Patient made aware of correct postural alignment with emphasis on symmetrical shoulder height and even weight distribution on buttocks. Initially, patient assumed a position of left lateral C-curve posture, but with verbal reinforcement was able to correct to good alignment in approximately 2 days. |

**Table 26-3.** Long-range treatment plan

| Goals | Method | Results |
|---|---|---|
| **Patient/family education** | | |
| Improve bronchial drainage | Review postural drainage positions and techniques with patient and family | Self-drainage techniques were reviewed with patient. Arrangements were made for her parents to come to hospital for observation of their percussion and vibration techniques and for review of bronchial drainage positioning. Patient and family demonstrated good bronchial drainage techniques. Several suggestions were made for tipping for lower lobe drainage because of dissatisfaction with methods presently being used at home. |
| | Emphasize necessity and rationale for home care | |
| | Suggest home tipping methods | |
| | Discuss treatment frequency | In view of patient's frustration and complaints regarding the need for daily bronchial drainage, much time was spent emphasizing the rationale and importance of such drainage. It was suggested that bronchial drainage be done while she watched her favorite television program or listened to her favorite music. The patient and her family were to make a strong effort to be faithful with this until her next clinic appointment, at which time we would review and evaluate benefits of daily bronchial drainage program. |
| Improve functional status/ breathing retraining | Instruct in paced diaphragmatic breathing techniques | *Level surfaces:* patient complained of mild dyspnea when walking on level surfaces greater than 1 block and when carrying weighted objects (e.g., schoolbooks, shoulderbag). Following instruction in paced diaphragmatic breathing (inspiratory cycle : expiratory cycle = 2 : 5) and assimilating the activity of ambulating while carrying a weighted object, patient was able to walk the equivalent of 1 block with less dyspnea and fatigue than when paced breathing not used. |
| | Instruct in coordination of paced breathing with functional activities/energy conservation | |
| | Review positions for dyspnea coordinated with diaphragmatic breathing | *Stair climbing:* patient instructed in paced breathing coordinated with stair climbing (inspiratory cycle: expiratory cycle = 1 : 2). Patient able to climb two flights of stairs with less dyspnea than previously exhibited. |
| | High side-lying | |
| | Forward sitting | *Daily activities:* suggestions were made regarding organization of work areas so as to conserve on energy expenditure. Emphasized importance of pacing breathing in with all strenuous activities. Patient stated she had found relief from breathlessness by assuming forward sitting position. |
| | Standing, with forward trunk flexion | |
| Increase exercise tolerance/ maintain general strength and range of motion | Low-level general conditioning exercises coordinated with diaphragmatic breathing | Once chest tube removed and physician approval obtained, patient began low-level group exercise program once daily with two other cystic fibrosis patients. Over three sessions patient progressed from (1) 10 repetitions to 20 repetitions of contralateral arm and leg lifts, (2) 3 minutes to 5 minutes on stationary bicycle with minimal resistance, (3) 1 minute to 2 minutes of jogging in place. |
| | Contralateral arm and leg lifts | |
| | Stationary bicycle | |
| | Jogging in place | NOTE: General muscle strength and range of motion were in good range. |
| | | All were performed with good pulse and respiratory rate response and near return to resting level following 3-minute rest. A home program was suggested, but patient felt she could not be faithful to it in view of demands of school and extracurricular activities. It was suggested that the matter be discussed further at her next clinic appointment when patient was more settled at home but emphasized the importance of improving her general condition so as to increase her exercise tolerance. |

*Continued.*

**Table 26-3.** Long-range treatment plan—cont'd.

| Goals | Method | Results |
|---|---|---|
| Maintain postural and trunk flexibility | Pectoral stretching exercise, standing and facing corner of room<br>Trunk flexibility exercises in sitting, hands behind neck | Patient's posture evaluation (following chest tube removal) was relatively unremarkable except for forward rounding of shoulders, protracted scapulae, and tight pectoral muscles. Scapular and abdominal muscle strength was in good range. Trunk flexibility was generally within normal limits.<br>a. Patient instructed in pectoral stretching exercise. She was able to maintain good stretch through range.<br>b. Trunk lateral flexion and rotation performed well with normal flexibility attained.<br>Both exercises performed coordinated with diaphragmatic breathing and patient given home program to be done once daily. |
| Psychological support | Team support from social worker, nurses, physician, psychologist, and physical therapist in coping with chronic decline and terminal aspects of disease | Patient received much support from medical team members during hospitalization and after discharge. The psychological support from physical therapy centered around emphasizing the positive—*abilities* rather than limitations. Patient's biggest concern was her difficulty in continuing with her previous life-style. Teaching patient to function within her capabilities with less distress through improved breathing patterns was emphasized.<br>Follow-up after discharge with reevaluation of status and home program. |

in the home program should be scheduled for 1 to 2 weeks later. If distance or transportation prevents a return outpatient visit, follow-up can be arranged through a local facility or home health agency.

## Role of physical therapist in the pediatric outpatient clinic

The role of the physical therapist in a cystic fibrosis or pulmonary specialties outpatient clinic is usually consultative. The physical therapist is part of the team made up of physicians, nurses, social workers, nutritionists, and psychologists.

Therapists who act as consultants to outpatient clinics should have specialized knowledge of the physical therapy management of pediatric patients with pulmonary disorders. They should demonstrate the ability to assist physicians in determining when chest physical therapy is indicated and then suggest appropriate referrals.

They should carry out interviews with patients and parents and introduce them to the role of chest physical therapy in the management of their child's specific lung problem. Therapists should be prepared to answer any questions regarding chest physical therapy.

The physical therapy consultant may be responsible for arranging physical therapy appointments for instruction or review of home programs. They should also have a comprehensive knowledge of chest physical therapy resources available in surrounding communities and coordinate follow-up or home care with outside agencies as necessary.

It is recommended that the physical therapist attend team conferences, offer input on total patient management, and teach the other medical professions about chest physical therapy.

## REFERENCES

1. Alvarez SE, Peterson M, and Lunsford BR: Respiratory treatment of the adult patient with spinal cord injury, *Phys Ther* 61:1737, 1981.
2. Amodio JB and others: Pediatric AIDS, *Semin Roentgenol* 22:66, 1987.
3. Anderson S and others: Comparison of bronchoconstriction induced by cycling and running, *Thorax* 26:396, 1971.
4. Annunziato PW and Frenkel LM: The epidemiology of pediatric HIV-1 infection, *Pediatr Ann* 22(7):401, 1993.
5. August S and Ellis EF: Disorders of immune mechanisms. In Kempe CH, Silver HK, and O'Brien D, editors: *Current pediatric diagnosis and treatment,* ed 3, Los Altos, Calif, 1974, Lange Medical Publications.
6. Beaudet AL: Genetic testing for cystic fibrosis, *Pediatr Clin North Am* 39:213, 1992.
7. Belman AL and others: Pediatric acquired immunodeficiency syndrome—neurological syndromes, *Am J Dis Child* 142:29, 1988.
8. Bjure J and others: Respiratory impairment and airway closure in patients with untreated idiopathic scoliosis, *Thorax* 25:451, 1970.
9. Blickman JG and others: Pectus excavatum in children: pulmonary scintigraphy before and after corrective surgery, *Radiology* 156:781, 1985.
10. Boudin K: Respiratory implications of AIDS, *Cardiopulm Rec* 3:12, 1988.
11. Brown J: Personal communication, Boston, 1993.
12. Burrington JD and Cotton EK; Removal of foreign bodies from the tracheobronchial tree, *J Pediatr Surg* 7:119, 1972.
13. Burrows B, Knudson RJ, and Lebowitz MD: The relationship of childhood respiratory illness to adult obtructive airway disease, *Am Rev Respir Dis* 115:751, 1977.
14. Bye MR and others: Diagnostic bronchoalveolar lavage in children with AIDS, *Pediatr Pulmonol* 3:425, 1987.
15. Cahill JL, Lees GM, and Robertson HT: A summary of preoperative and postoperative cardiorespiratory performance in patients undergoing pectus excavatum and carinatum repair, *J Pediatr Surg* 19:430, 1984.
16. Campbell AH, O'Connell JM, and Wilson F: The effect of chest physiotherapy upon the $FEV_1$ in chronic bronchitis, *Med J Aust* 1:33, 1975.
17. Cassella MC and Hall JE: Current treatment approaches in the nonoperative and operative management of adolescent idiopathic scoliosis, *Phys Ther* 71:897, 1991.
18. Centers for Disease Control: Recommendations for prevention of HIV transmission in health care settings, MMWR 36:25, 1987.
19. Centers for Disease Control: Revision of the CDC surveillance case definition for acquired immunodeficiency syndrome, MMWR 36 (suppl 15):35, 1987.
20. Centers for Disease Control and Prevention: *HIV/AIDS surveillance report,* Atlanta, Ga, Oct 1992, Centers for Disease Control and Prevention.
21. Charnock EL, Fischer BJ, and Doershuk CF: Development of the respiratory system. In Lough MD, Doershuk CF, and Stern RC, editors: *Pediatric respiratory therapy,* ed 2, Chicago, 1979, Year Book Medical Publishers, Inc.
22. Church JA: Clinical aspects of HIV infection in children, *Pediatr Ann* 22(7):417, 1993.
23. Ciesla N: Chest physiotherapy for special patients. In Mackenzie, CF, editor: *Chest physiotherapy in the intensive care unit,* Baltimore, 1981, Williams & Wilkins.
24. Clutario BC and Holzman BH: Uncommon diseases, extrapulmonary diseases, system diseases, and toxins. In Scarpelli EM, Auld PAM, and Goldman HS, editors: *Pulmonary disease of the fetus, newborn and child,* Philadelphia, 1978, Lea & Febiger.
25. Cooper EP, Pelton SI, and LeMay M: Acquired Immunodeficiency Syndrome: a new population of children at risk, *Pediatr Clin North Am* 35:1365, 1988.
26. Cotton EK and others: Removal of aspired foreign bodies by inhalation and postural drainage, *Clin Pediatr* 12:271, 1973.
27. Cvetkovich TA and Frenkel LM: Current management of HIV infection in children, *Pediatr Ann* 22(7):428, 1993.
28. Dab I and Alexander F: Evaluation of the effectiveness of a particular bronchial drainage procedure called autogenic drainage. In Baran D and Van Bogaert E, editors: *Cystic fibrosis,* Ghent, Belgium, 1977, European Press.
29. Dab I and Alexander F: The mechanism of autogenic drainage studied with flow-volume curves, *Monogr Paed* 10:50, 1979.
29a. Darbee J: Personal communication, Philadelphia, 1988.
30. Dauber JH, Paradis IL, and Dummer JS: Infectious complications in pulmonary allograft patients, *Clin Chest Med* 11:291, 1990.
31. Davidson AGF and others: Physiotherapy in cystic fibrosis: a comparative trial of positive expiratory pressure, autogenic drainage, and conventional percussion and drainage techniques, *Pediatr Pulmonol* 4(suppl 2):132, 1988.
32. Davies H and others: Regional ventilation in infancy—reversal of adult pattern, *N Engl J Med* 313:1626, 1985.
33. Doershuk CF, Fischer BJ, and Matthews LW: Pulmonary physiology of the young child. In Scarpelli EM, editor: *Pulmonary physiology of the fetus, newborn, and child,* Philadelphia, 1975, Lea & Febiger.
34. Donati MA and others: Prospective controlled study of home and hospitalized therapy of cystic fibrosis pulmonary disease, *J Pediatr* 111:28, 1987.

35. Eller JJ: Infections: bacterial and spirochetal. In Kempe CH, Silver HK, and O'Brien D, editors: *Current pediatric diagnosis and treatment,* ed 3, Los Altos, Calif, 1974, Lange Medical Publications.

36. Fackler FC and others: Precautions in the use of ribaviron at the Children's Hospital, *New Engl J Med* 322:634, 1990.

37. Falk M and others: Improving the ketchup bottle method with positive expiratory pressure, PEP, in cystic fibrosis, *Eur J Respir Dis* 65:423, 1984.

38. Flowers KA and others: New mechanical aid to physiotherapy in cystic fibrosis, *Br Med J* 2:630, 1979.

39. Ghory JE: Exercise and asthma: overview and clinical impact, *Pediatrics* 56(suppl):844, 1975.

40. Gibbens DT and others: Osteoporosis in cystic fibrosis, *J Pediatr* 113:295, 1988.

41. Gibson GJ and others: Pulmonary mechanics in patients with respiratory muscle weakness, *Am Rev Respir Dis* 115(3):389, 1977.

42. Godfrey S, Silverman M, and Anderson S: The use of treadmill for assessing exercise induced asthma and the effect of varying severity and duration of exercise, *Pediatrics* 56(suppl):893, 1975.

43. Gold M: Restrictive lung disease, *Phys Ther* 48:455, 1968.

44. Gould AL: *Cardiopulmonary evaluation of the infant, toddler, child, and adolescent, pediatric physical therapy,* Baltimore, 1991, Williams & Wilkins Co.

45. Graybill CA: Cardiopulmonary physical therapy in pediatric solid organ transplantation, *Cardiopulm Phys Ther J* 1(3) 1990.

46. Groothius JR and others: Early ribaviron treatment of respiratory syncytial virus infection in high risk children, *J Pediatr* 117:792, 1990.

47. Groth S and others: Pattern of ventilation in cystic fibrosis during positive expiratory pressure (PEP) and deep inspirations, *Pediatr Pulmonol* (suppl 1)133, 1987.

48. Gundy JH: Physical examination. In Gundy JH: *Assessment of the child in primary health care,* New York, 1981, McGraw-Hill Book Co, Inc.

49. Hall CB and others: Aerosolized ribavarin treatment of infants with respiratory syncytial virus infection, *N Engl J Med* 308:1443, 1983.

50. Hansen LG and Warwick WJ: High frequency chest compression system to aid in clearance of mucus from the lung, *Biomed Instrument Tech* 24:289, 1990.

51. Harris-Copp M: The HIV infected child: a critical need for physical therapy, *Clin Man Phys Ther* 8:16, 1988.

52. Harwood CH and Cook CV: Cyclosporine in transplantation, *Heart Lung* 14:6, 1985.

53. Heaf DP, and others: Postural effects of gas exchange in infants, *N Engl J Med* 308:1505, 1983.

54. Hendren WH and Lillehei CW: Pediatric surgery, *N Engl J Med* 319:86, 1988.

55. Herbst JJ: Gastroesophageal reflux, *J Pediatr* 98:859, 1981.

56. Hofmeyer JL and others: Evaluation of positive expiratory pressure as an adjunct to chest physiotherapy in the treatment of cystic fibrosis, *Thorax* 41:951, 1986.

57. Holsclaw DS: Common pulmonary complications of cystic fibrosis, *Clin Pediatr* 9:346, 1970.

58. Hubbard RC and others: A preliminary study of aerosolized recombinant deoxyribonuclease in the treatment of cystic fibrosis, *New Engl J Med* 326:812, 1992.

59. Huber AL, Eggleston PA, and Morgan J: Effect of physiotherapy on asthmatic children (abstract), *J Allergy Clin Immunol* 53:109, 1974.

60. Hunt SA: Complications of heart transplant, *Heart Transplantation* 3:70, 1983.

61. Hyland J: Neonatal and pediatric therapy. In Frownfelter D, editor: *Chest physical therapy and pulmonary rehabilitation,* Chicago, 1978, Year Book Medical Publishers, Inc.

62. Isaacs D: Ribavarin, *Pediatrics* 79:289, 1987.

63. James M: Physical therapy for patients after bone marrow transplantation, *Phys Ther* 67:6, 1987.

64. Jolley SG and others: Lower esophageal pressure changes with tube gastrostomy: a causative factor of gastroesophageal reflux in children? *J Pediatr Surg* 21:624, 1986.

65. Jones RS, Wharton JJ, and Bustong OH: The effect of exercise on ventilatory function in the child with asthma, *Br J Dis Chest* 56:78, 1962.

66. Josephs S and others: Parainfluenza 3 virus and other common respiratory pathogens in children with human immunodeficiency virus infection, *Pediatr Infect Dis J* 7:207, 1988.

67. Kadota RP: Bone marrow transplantation for diseases of childhood, *Mayo Clin Proc* 59:171, 1984.

68. Kafer ER: Respiratory and cardiovascular functions in scoliosis and the principles of anesthetic management, *Anesthesiology* 52:339, 1980.

69. Kattan M and others: Pulmonary function abnormalities in symptom free children after bronchiolitis, *Pediatrics* 59:683, 1977.

70. Kattan M and others: The response to exercise in normal and asthmatic children, *J Pediatr* 92:718, 1978.

71. Khan AU and Olson DL: Physical therapy and exercise induced bronchospasm, *Phys Ther* 55:878, 1975.

72. Kigin CM: Chest physical therapy for the postoperative or traumatic injury patient, *Phys Ther* 61:1724, 1981.

73. Krowka MJ and Cortese DA: Pulmonary aspects of chronic liver disease and liver transplantation, *Mayo Clin Proc* 60:407, 1985.

74. Kübler-Ross E: *On death and dying,* New York, 1969, The Macmillan Publishing Co, Inc.

75. Kuzemko JA: Home treatment of pulmonary infections in cystic fibrosis, *Chest* 94(suppl 2):1635, 1988.

76. Landau LJ and others: Contribution of inhomogenity of lung units to the maximal expiratory flow-volume curve in children with asthma and cystic fibrosis, *Am Rev Resp Dis* 111:725, 1975.

77. Law D and Kosloske AM: Management of tracheobronchial foreign bodies in children: a reevaluation of postural drainage and bronchoscopy, *Pediatrics* 58:362, 1976.

78. Lawrence EL: Diagnosis and management of lung allograft rejection, *Clin Chest Med* 11:269, 1990.

79. Leads from the MMWR: Update: Acquired Immunodeficiency Syndrome (AIDS)—Worldwide, *JAMA* 259:3104, 1988.

80. Macklem PT: Airway obstruction and collateral ventilation, *Physiol Rev* 51:368, 1971.

81. Macklem PT: Physiology of cough, *Ann Otol* 83:761, 1974.

82. Macklem PT and Mead J: Factors determining maximum expiratory flow in dogs, *J Appl Physiol* 25:159, 1968.

83. Macklem PT and Wilson NJ: Measurement of intrabronchial pressure in man, *J Appl Physiol* 20:653, 1965.

84. Malen JF and Boychuk JE: Nursing perspectives on lung transplantation, *Crit Care Nurs Clin North Am* 1:202, 1989.

85. Martin L: Pulmonary physiology in clinical practice: The essentials for patient care and practice, St Louis, 1987, Mosby.

86. Maxwell M and Redmond A: Comparative trial of manual and mechanical percussion technique with gravity-assisted bronchial drainage in patients with cystic fibrosis, *Arch Dis Child* 54:542, 1979.

87. McBride JT and Wohl MEB: Pulmonary function tests, *Pediatr Clin North Am* 26:537, 1979.

88. McBride JT and others: Lung growth and airway function after lobectomy in infancy for congenital lobar emphysema, *J Clin Invest* 66:962, 1980.

89. McIntosh K: Respiratory syncitial virus infections in infants and children: diagnosis and treatment, *Pediatr Rev* 9:191, 1987.

90. Meredith T and Acierno LJ: Pulmonary complications of acquired immunodeficiency syndrome, *Heart Lung* 17:173, 1988.

91. Mowat AP: Liver disorders in children: the indications for liver replacement in parenchymal and metabolic diseases, *Transplant Proc* 19:3236, 1987.

92. Mukwaya G: Immunosuppressive effects and infections associated with corticosteroid therapy, *Pediatr Infec Dis J* 17:499, 1988.

93. Murphy S: Cystic fibrosis in adults: diagnosis and management, *Clin Chest Med* 8:695, 1987.

94. Newsom-Davis J: The respiratory system in muscular dystrophy, *Br Med J* 36:135, 1980.

95. Nolan SP and others: Letter: Does pectus excavatum cause functional disability? *J Thorac Cardiovasc Surg* 71:148, 1976.

96. Nuscher R and others: Bone marrow transplantation—a lifesaving option, *Am J Nurs* 84:764, 1984.

97. Oberwaldner B and others: Forced expirations against a variable resistance: a new chest physiotherapy method in cystic fibrosis, *Pediatr Pulmonol* 2:358, 1986.

98. Oh CS and others: Increased infections associated with the use of OKT3 for the treatment of steroid resistant rejection in renal transplantation, *Transplantation* 45:68, 1988.

99. Patterson GA and others: Experimental and clinical double lung transplantation, *J Thorac Cardiovasc Surg* 95:70, 1988.

100. Patterson PR, DeMing C, and Kutscher A: Psychological aspects of cystic fibrosis: a model for chronic lung disease, New York, 1973, Columbia University Press.

101. Peterson RJ and others: Noninvasive assessment of exercise cardiac function before and after pectus excavatum repair, *J Thorac Cardiovasc Surg* 90:251, 1985.

102. Pier C and others: Central nervous system toxicity after liver transplantation, *N Engl J Med* 317:861, 1987.

103. Proceedings of the special session of the fourth meeting of the PAHO Advisory Committee on Medical Research, 1965: *Deprivation in psychobiological development,* Pub No 134, Washington, DC, 1966, Pan American Health Organization–World Health Organization.

104. Pryor JA, Parker RA, and Webber BA: A comparison of mechanical and manual percussion as adjuncts to postural drainage in treatment of cystic fibrosis in adolescents and adults, *Physiotherapy* 67:140, 1981.

105. Pryor JA and Webber BA: An evaluation of the forced expiratory technique as an adjunct to postural drainage, *Physiotherapy* 65:304, 1979.

106. Pryor JA and others: Evaluation of the forced expiration technique as an adjunct to postural drainage in the treatment of cystic fibrosis, *Br Med J* 2:417, 1979.

107. Reichert C, Kelly V, and Macher A: Pathologic features of AIDS. In Devita V, Hellman S, and Rosenberg SA, editors: AIDS, Philadelphia, 1985, JB Lippincott Co.

108. Reid L: The lung: its growth and remodeling in health and disease, *Am J Roentgenol* 129:777, 1977.

109. Reynolds EOR: Bronchiolitis. In Kendig EL, editor: *Pulmonary disorders,* vol 1, Philadelphia, 1972, WB Saunders Co.

110. Rockwell GM and Campbell SK: Physical therapy program for the pediatric cardiac surgical patient, *Phys Ther* 56:670, 1976.

111. Rooney JC and Williams HE: The relationship between proved viral bronchiolitis and subsequent wheezing, *J Pediatr* 79:744, 1971.

112. Rothman JG: Effects of respiratory exercises on the vital capacity and forced expiratory volume in children with cerebral palsy, *Phys Ther* 58:421, 1978.

113. Rubenstein A and others: Pulmonary disease in children with acquired immunodeficiency syndrome and AIDS-related complex, *J Pediatr* 108:498, 1986.

114. Rubenstein A and others: Corticosteroid treatment for pulmonary lymphoid hyperplasia in children with acquired immunodeficiency syndrome, *Pediatr Pulmonol* 4:13, 1988.

115. Sade RM, Cosgrove DM, and Casteneda AR: *Infant and child care in heart surgery,* Chicago, 1977, Year Book Medical Publishers.

116. Sahler OJZ, editor: *The child and death,* St Louis, 1978, Mosby.

117. Salzberg AM: Congenital malformations of the lower respiratory tract. In Kendig EL, editor: *Pulmonary disorders,* vol 1, Philadelphia, 1972, WB Saunders Co.

118. Scarpelli EM: Examination of the lung. In Scarpelli EM, Auld PAM, and Goldman H, editors: *Pulmonary diseases of the fetus, newborn, and child,* Philadelphia, 1978, Lea & Febiger.

119. Schidlow DV, Taussig L, and Knowles, MR: Cystic Fibrosis Foundation consensus conference report on pulmonary complications of cystic fibrosis, *Pediatr Pulmonol* 15:187, 1993.

120. Schowalter JE: The reaction of caregivers dealing with fatally ill children and their families. In Sahler OJZ, editor: *The child and death,* St Louis, 1978, Mosby.

121. Seligman T, Randel HO, and Stevens JJ: Conditioning program for children with asthma, *Phys Ther* 50:641, 1970.

122. Sharp JT and others: Postural relief of dyspnea in severe chronic obstructive pulmonary disease, *Am Rev Respir Dis* 122:201, 1980.

123. Shwachman H, Kowalski M, and Khaw KT: Cystic fibrosis: a new outlook, *Medicine* 56:129, 1977.

124. Slim J: Highlights of the third international conference on AIDS, *Med Aspects Human Sex* 21:13, 1987.

125. Stafanger G and others: Long-term study of effect of PEP-mask in cystic fibrosis patients. In Adam G and Valassi-Adam H, editors: Proceedings of the twelfth annual meeting of the European working group cystic fibrosis, *Am J Dis Child* 96:6, 1983.

126. Starzl TE and others: Pediatric liver transplantation, *Transplant Proc* 19:3230, 1987.

127. Steinherz LJ, Brochstein JA, and Robins J: Cardiac involvement in congenital acquired immunodeficiency syndrome, *Am J Dis Child* 14:1241, 1986.

128. Stewart SM and others: Mental and motor development correlates in patients with end-stage biliary atresia awaiting liver transplantation, *Pediatrics* 79:882, 1987.

129. Talner NS: Congestive heart failure. In Moss AJ, editor: *Heart disease in infants, children, and adolescents,* Baltimore, 1968, Williams & Wilkins Co.

130. Tapper D and others: Polyalveolar lobe: anatomic and physiologic parameters and their relationship to congenital lobar emphysema, *Pediatr Surg* 15:931, 1980.

131. Task Force on Podiatric AIDS: Pediatric guidelines for infection control of human immunodeficiency virus (Acquired Immunodeficiency Virus) in hospitals, medical offices, schools and other settings, *Pediatrics* 82:801, 1988.

132. Tecklin JS: Pulmonary disorders in infants and children and their physical therapy management. In Tecklin JS, editor: *Pediatric physical therapy,* ed 2, Philadelphia, 1994, JB Lippincott.

133. Tecklin JS and Holsclaw DS: Cystic fibrosis and the role of the physical therapist in its management, *Phys Ther* 53:386, 1973.

134. Thomas ED and others: Bone marrow transplantation (part 1), *N Engl J Med* 292:832, 1975.

135. Thomas ED and others: Bone marrow transplantation (part 2), *N Engl J Med* 292:895, 1975.

136. Thompson AE: Aspects of pediatric intensive care after liver transplantation, *Transplant Proc* 19(suppl 13):34, 1987.

137. Thompson BJ: The physiotherapist's role in rehabilitation of the asthmatic, *N Z J Physiother* 4:11, 1973.

138. Todd TRJ: Early post-operative management following lung transplantation, *Clin Chest Med* 11:259, 1990.

139. Tomney PM and Finer NN: A controlled evaluation of muscle relaxation in ventilated neonates (abstract), *Crit Care Med* 8:228, 1980.

140. Tonnesen P and Stovring S: Positive expiratory pressure (PEP) as lung physiotherapy in cystic fibrosis: a pilot study, *Eur J Resp Dis* 65:419, 1984.

141. Turner JM and others: Elasticity of human lungs in relation to age, *J Appl Physiol* 25:664, 1968.

142. Tyrrell JC and others: Face mask physiotherapy in cystic fibrosis, *Arch Dis Child* 61:598, 1986.

143. Vacanti JP and others: Liver transplantation in children: the Boston Center experience in the first 30 months, *Transplant Proc* 19:3261, 1987.

144. Vogt D and others: Neurological complications of liver transplantation, *Transplantation* 45:1057, 1988.

145. Wald ER, Dashefsky B, and Green M: In re ribavirin: a case of premature adjudication? *J Pediatr* 112:154, 1988.

146. Waring W: The history and physical examination. In Kendig EL, editor: *Pulmonary disorders*, vol 1, Philadelphia, 1972, WB Saunders Co.

147. Warwick WJ and Hansen LG: The long term effects of high frequency chest compression therapy on pulmonary complications of cystic fibrosis, *Pediatr Pulmonol* 11:265, 1991.

148. White DJG: Cyclosporin A—clinical pharmacology and therapeutic potential, *Drugs* 24:322, 1982.

149. Wohl ME and Chernick V: State of the art: bronchiolitis, *Am Rev Resp Dis* 118:759, 1978.

150. Wood RE, Boat TF, and Doershuk CF: State of the art: cystic fibrosis, *Am Rev Respir Dis* 113:833, 1976.

151. Zach MS and others: Bronchodilators increase airway instability in cystic fibrosis, *Am Rev Resp Dis* 131:537, 1985.

152. Zack MB and others: The effect of lateral positions on gas exchange in pulmonary disease: a prospective evaluation, *Am Rev Resp Dis* 110:49, 1974.

153. Zadai CC: Physical therapy for the acutely ill medical patient, *Phys Ther* 61:1746, 1981.

154. Zitelli BJ and others: Pediatric liver transplantation: evaluation and selection, infectious complications, and life-style after transplantation, *Transplant Proc* 19:3309, 1987.

# Exercise Testing and Exercise Conditioning for Children With Lung Dysfunction

*Joan Darbee and Frank Cerny*

The positive beneficial effects that therapeutic exercise conditioning has on children with lung disease have been well documented.* The exercise intolerance and lack of physical fitness generally observed in children with chronic lung disease can be improved through regular exercise.[62,63] Children who experience exercise-induced bronchospasm (EIB) can safely improve their exercise tolerance and cardiorespiratory fitness with appropriate preexercise medication. Similarly, most individuals with cystic fibrosis (CF) can participate in an exercise program to improve their level of physical fitness and possibly slow the progressive deterioration of lung function.

---

* References 3, 17, 18, 28, 44, 59, 62, 63, 76, 84, 85.

The psychological complications associated with chronic lung disease[12,48,74,79] also may be affected positively by an appropriately prescribed exercise program.[28] Physical and social restrictions accompanying a chronic lung disease and its vigorous therapeutic regimen can be minimized through organized therapeutic exercise. Several studies have shown improvements in self-concept for physically, mentally, and emotionally handicapped groups following physical conditioning.[13,22,30,32,41]

Although most children will not become elite athletes, all can benefit physically and psychologically from regular physical activity and should not be excluded from physical activity by physical educators, parents, physicians, physical therapists, or themselves because of lung disease. Virtually all children with chronic lung disease can safely participate in physical rehabilitation programs as long as those programs are specifically tailored to meet the individual needs of the child. The goals of any exercise conditioning program include improving the level of physical fitness and psychological wellness of the individual, thereby permitting the young person to function independently at the highest possible potential. The first step in the development of the individual exercise prescription is the comprehensive exercise evaluation.

## EXERCISE EVALUATION

The evaluation of a child during dynamic exercise testing provides the physical therapist with a great amount of information that cannot be obtained from the resting physical examination (see box on p. 564). Patients and parents will often deny or have difficulty recognizing and accurately describing physical limitations or symptoms such as shortness of breath. Often, those with chronic lung disease have a reduced exercise capacity but are not aware of their physical limitations because of the slow, insidious onset of

### Indications for performing an exercise test

1. Determine functional exercise capacity
2. Evaluate cardiorespiratory response to exercise
3. Identify reduction in cardiopulmonary reserves
4. Determine presence of or threshold for onset of exertional dyspnea
5. Document known or suspected cardiac or pulmonary disease
6. Provide a basis for safe exercise prescription
7. Document effects of treatment or therapy

the disease and the slow adaptation of their life-style to these limitations. In addition, less than 80% of the pulmonary capacity of the healthy child is used even during maximal exercise. This 20% reserve provides a buffer against the effects of deterioration of lung function on the exercise response. Severe lung dysfunction must be present before the effects of the disease will become evident at rest, but an exercise test, which may stress the lung capacity sufficiently to encroach on the reserves, may allow detection of even mild to moderate pulmonary deterioration.

### Exercise tests

The correct exercise test protocol (Fig. 27-1) can be selected and safely executed when the individuals administering the test have appropriate background information about the patient to be tested. Additionally, the test results can be interpreted within the context of the patient's history and can provide more useful information from a functional standpoint.

Before an exercise test the child should undergo a complete clinical evaluation including a thorough review of the medical history, a chest physical examination, and musculoskeletal screening. The therapist also should review chest radiographs, pulmonary function test results, and blood gas analyses. Children with known or suspected pulmonary disease should undergo pulmonary function testing and a chest radiograph before testing. Specific pulmonary function testing guidelines for the known or suspected young asthmatic patient should be followed and are described at length elsewhere.[23,24,29] In spite of suggestions that the exercise response can be predicted from resting pulmonary function tests,[26,49] it must be stressed that it is difficult to accurately predict decreases in arterial oxygenation during exercise based on either a resting pulmonary function test or resting oxygen saturation values because there are so many individual exceptions.[40]

Infants and small children under the age of 3 years generally are not able to participate in formal exercise testing performed in a laboratory setting because of their young age and their inability to cooperate. Infants can be evaluated during the resting state and under stressful conditions such

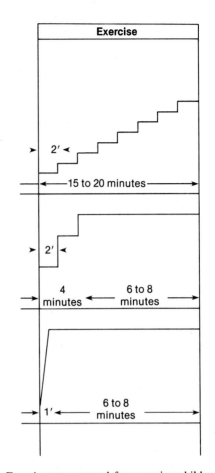

**Fig. 27-1.** Exercise test protocol for assessing children with lung disease. *Top,* A progressive, incremental test with workload increasing every 2 minutes; used for determining peak work capacity and/or the response to several work levels. *Middle,* A protocol used to measure the response to a submaximal work level where a steady state is necessary; the initial stages are used as an accommodation period. *Bottom,* The suggested protocol to be used identifying exercise-induced bronchospasm; a single load, sufficient to increase ventilation to high levels and sustainable for 7 to 8 minutes, is necessary for this test.

as during feeding, crying, hospital procedures, and handling (Table 27-1). Quantitative and qualitative measurements that can be made during exercise in this age group are shown in Table 27-1. Heart rate (HR) and arterial oxygen saturation ($Sao_2$) monitoring are necessary for safety and the interpretation of the exercise response.

Exercise performance can be quantified in children 3 to 6 years old using a motor driven treadmill (Fig. 27-2). It is recommended that a trained member of the evaluating team straddle the treadmill belt standing behind the child to offer support. Difficulties with the treadmill test in this age group are that most small children will want to hold on to guardrails for additional support, making it difficult to quantitate workloads accurately and that it is difficult to elicit heart rates in excess of 160 beats per minute (BPM). Treadmill testing for this age group, however, does provide valuable information since most children normally do not perform

**Table 27-1.** Recommended observations and measurements during exercise testing

| Age | Exercise | Observations and measurements |
|---|---|---|
| <3 years | Crying, feeding, crawling, walking | Heart rate by telemetry Arterial hemoglobin oxygen saturation by ear oximetry Respiratory rate Cyanosis Breathing pattern as indicator of increased shortness of breath |
| 3 to 6 years | Treadmill, stairs | All of the above plus blood pressure monitoring |
| >6 years | Treadmill, stairs, cycle ergometer | All of the above plus exhaled gas monitoring, end-tidal $CO_2$, mixed expired $O_2$ and $CO_2$, minute ventilation, $O_2$ consumption, respiratory exchange ratio |

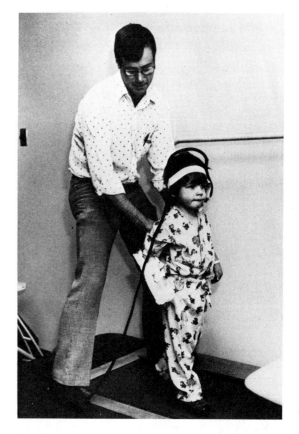

**Fig. 27-2** Ear oximetry monitoring during treadmill submaximal exercise testing.

levels of sustained exercise at heart rates above 160 BPM. As in younger children, the same parameters can be monitored as mentioned above (Table 27-1).

For children exceeding 6 or 7 years of age, a more formal exercise test can be performed using a variety of ergometers (Table 27-1). These tests include monitoring of ventilatory and metabolic variables during exercise (Table 27-1). It is imperative that the proper protocol be selected based on the child's age, disease severity, level of physical activity, and purpose for performing the test (see Fig. 27-1). Children with severe lung disease will need to start the exercise test at relatively low workloads, and incremental increases in work levels need to be small.

It is extremely important that all involved in the administration of the exercise test for children with cardiopulmonary disease be properly trained before initiating an exercise testing program. Physical therapists should have a sound working knowledge of the normal and abnormal physiological responses to exercise[6,14,82] to safely conduct testing and to be able to interpret test results, therefore making the effort expended meaningful to the young patient. The physical therapist should be competent in measuring and interpreting blood pressure (BP) and electrocardiogram (ECG) readings to provide a safe testing environment. Specialized training is usually necessary to learn expired gas collection and analysis techniques. The authors encourage newcomers to visit exercise laboratories in which children

are routinely tested to better understand the special needs of children.

**Exercise test protocols**

The purpose of the exercise test must be defined clearly to provide insight regarding the type of exercise test protocol to choose (see box, p. 564). There are several protocols for assessing the cardiopulmonary response to exercise in the child with lung disease.[20,26,33,42] (Fig. 27-1).

A progressive, incremental test (Fig. 27-1, top) is used when the patient's maximum oxygen consumption ($\dot{V}_{O_{2}max}$) or peak work capacity is to be determined. Workloads are progressively increased each minute until the subject can no longer continue exercising because of exhaustion or because the test is terminated for safety reasons[29] (see box on p. 566).

A progressive test in which the workload is increased every 2 minutes is used to document the cardiopulmonary response to increasing exercise levels. The patient may exercise to "peak" capacity and not $\dot{V}_{O_{2}max}$. The 2-minute exercise stage is long enough for the steady state to be attained and recorded before moving to the next level. Measurements are made and recorded during the last 30 seconds of each stage, before increasing the workload.

| **Criteria for termination of the exercise test** |
| --- |
| Patient request |
| Clinical observation of pallor or extreme dyspnea |
| $Sao_2$ decreases by >10% or below 80% $Sao_2$ |
| ECG dysrhythmias |
| A decrease in systolic or pulse pressure with increasing effort |
| Systolic pressure >250 mm Hg |
| Diastolic pressure >100 to 110 mm Hg |

These protocols can be performed on a variety of ergometers (see Table 27-1) using several methods of determining the workload or power output increments.

Godfrey's protocol[33] consists of a progressive maximal exercise test in which the resistance on the cycle ergometer is based on the subject's height and is increased in 1-minute intervals. The increments of resistance are 10, 15, and 20 watts for children shorter than 125 cm, those 125 to 150 cm, and those taller than 150 cm, respectively.

Cerny and associates[20] and Cropp and others[26] describe a protocol that starts subjects pedaling at 0.3 watts per kilogram of body weight (W/kg) for weaker and small individuals and at 0.6 W/kg for stronger and larger subjects. The workload is progressively increased every 2 minutes by 0.3 W/kg until peak exercise capacity is reached.

An incremental exercise test described by Jones and Campbell[42] is often encountered in the pediatric pulmonary literature. Workloads are increased every minute on the cycle ergometer by 100 kilogram meters per minute $(kg \cdot m \cdot min^{-1})$ or 17 watts.

If a treadmill is being used, speed should be adjusted in accordance with the size and skill of the patient. The speed and elevation should be selected to allow even the patient with severe dysfunction to exercise at two to three levels. A speed of 2 to 3 km/hr, 4 to 5 km/hr, and 6 to 8 km/hr is comfortable for small children, adolescents, and adults, respectively. Grade increases of about 2% will elicit 10 BPM increases in HR with each increment.

A standardized exercise bronchoconstriction provocation test[23] is selected when a patient is being evaluated for known or suspected exercise-induced bronchospasm (EIB), as is commonly done for the young person with asthma. Since EIB is related to the heat lost from the airways at high levels of minute ventilation, the exercise test need consist of only one work level of high intensity.[56] The patient exercises at approximately 85% of age-predicted maximum HR for a steady-state period of 6 to 8 minutes. Subjects need to be exercising at a HR of at least 170 BPM. The test can be optimized by having the patient inspire dry air (bottled gas) or cold, dry air.

A progressive exercise test to a single[5] or several submaximal[6,35] levels is useful to assess the effects of therapy or of a physical conditioning program over a period of time. Children serve as their own control, and the same test is administered whenever the exercise response is assessed. Heart rate, dyspnea scores, and $Sao_2$ are measured at each work level, and improvement or deterioration in the exercise response is monitored. For example, if HR has decreased at a given level of work during retesting, a conditioning effect has occurred, or an improvement in exercise $Sao_2$ may indicate improved arterial oxygenation as a result of a hospitalization or treatment. Heart rates obtained at a point of desaturation can serve as a guideline within which to prescribe exercise, and changes in this point may indicate the positive effects of treatment or the negative effects of a disease process.

Field tests also can provide valuable information on a patient's exercise capacity. A 3-, 6-, 9-, or 12-minute sustained walking endurance test can be performed over a premeasured distance, such as in a hallway, according to the procedures outlined by McGavin.[57] This easy-to-conduct field test has functional value and serves as a frequent test of choice, particularly for individuals with severe to very severe lung disease, since it is safe and does not require using equipment. The distance covered in a specified time period is measured and can be used to monitor changes in exercise capacity.

## Monitoring during an exercise test

Patients should be closely observed at all times before, during, and following the exercise test. Of those variables that can be monitored during an exercise test HR, ECG, and $Sao_2$ are the most critical (Table 27-1).

Percent arterial oxygen saturation should be measured and recorded for all patients undergoing testing as a gauge of levels of arterial hypoxemia and to ensure that the exercise prescription does not induce severe desaturation. Resting arterial blood oxygen levels are closely related to exercise tolerance.\* Measurement of $Sao_2$ should be mandatory for all individuals with a forced expiratory volume in 1 second $(FEV_1)$ of less than 50% of predicted, since reports indicate that individuals with an $FEV_1$ less than 50% of predicted may desaturate during exercise testing.[20,26,29] Noninvasive oximetry in which a probe is applied to either the ear or finger is easily used to measure $Sao_2$. Ear probes are preferable since reduced accuracy and delayed desaturation response time can pose problems for finger probes.[69] There are a number of stationary, as well as battery-operated, portable oximeters marketed that are extremely convenient to use. The tester should be familiar with the relationship between $Sao_2$ and $Pao_2$ as described by the oxyhemoglobin dissociation curve (Fig. 27-3). It is important to note that small changes in $Sao_2$ from 96% to 90% are associated with large decreases in $Pao_2$ and should not be treated lightly. As $Sao_2$ falls below 90%, the curve is steeper, so that for larger decreases in $Pao_2$, the $Sao_2$ decreases at an increasing rate. The table showing the relationship between $Sao_2$ and $Pao_2$

_____
\* References 17, 18, 20, 26, 27, 40, 49, 53, 81.

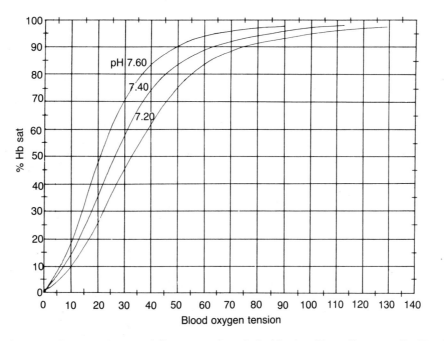

**Fig. 27-3.** Oxyhemoglobin dissociation curve for whole blood. (From Spearman R: *Egan's fundamentals of respiratory therapy,* ed 4, St Louis, 1982, Mosby.)

should be available in the exercise laboratory using oximeters.

Electrocardiogram, HR, and BP should be monitored throughout the exercise test to evaluate the cardiovascular responses. The ECG should be monitored for exercise-induced dysrhythmias. The linear relationship between $\dot{V}o_2$ and HR makes the HR a useful tool for the prescription and monitoring of therapeutic exercise programs (see section on exercise prescription later in this chapter).

The pulmonary responses to exercise can be documented in terms of gas exchange and respiratory mechanics. Percent arterial oxygen saturation is a simple, noninvasive method of monitoring $O_2$ exchange. The adequacy of carbon dioxide ($CO_2$) elimination can be determined by measuring end-tidal $CO_2$. End-tidal $CO_2$ is measured by sampling the inhaled and exhaled gases at the mouth using a one-way breathing valve and one of many $CO_2$ analyzers available. Total minute ventilation ($\dot{V}_E$) and its components, breathing frequency and tidal volume, can be used to monitor the mechanical adjustment to exercise. Abnormal changes in breathing frequency or tidal volume are indicative of abnormal pulmonary mechanics. These variables are measured using a gasometer, dry gas meter, or a flow meter attached to the expiratory side of the one-way breathing valve.

Mixed expired gas can be collected in a gasometer or an expiratory mixing chamber[42] and analyzed using $O_2$ and $CO_2$ gas analyzers. With $\dot{V}_e$ these values are used to calculate oxygen consumption ($\dot{V}o_2$) for each submaximal workload and peak or $\dot{V}o_{2max}$ during the final workload.[42]

Energy expenditure or $\dot{V}o_2$ can be determined and then expressed as metabolic equivalents (METS) using the following equation.[1]

$$\dot{V}o_2 = \dot{V}_I \, (F_Io_2) - \dot{V}_E(F_Eo_2) \tag{1}$$

where $\dot{V}_I$ and $\dot{V}_E$ are inspired and expired volumes per unit time; $F_Io_2$ and $F_Eo_2$ are inspired and expired fractions of $O_2$ in dry air, respectively; $F_Io_2$ is a constant value 20.93% or 0.2093; $F_Eo_2$ is measured by a gas analyzer.

To obtain $\dot{V}_I$ use a second equation:

$$\dot{V}_I(F_IN_2) = V_E(F_EN_2) \tag{2}$$
$$\dot{V}_I = \frac{\dot{V}_E(F_EN_2)}{F_IN_2}$$

where $F_IN_2$ is a constant value 79% or 0.789; $F_EN_2 = 1.0 - (F_Eco_2 + F_Eo_2)$; therefore,

$$V_I = V_E \, \frac{1 - (F_Eo_2 + F_Eco_2)}{79.0} \tag{3}$$

Energy expenditure expressed in METS:

$$E = \dot{V}o_2 \cdot \frac{1 \text{ MET}}{3.5 \text{ ml } O_2 \cdot kg^{-1} \cdot min^{-1}} \tag{4}$$

Subjects should be closely observed for signs of increased work of breathing disproportionate to what is expected. These signs include increased accessory neck muscle pulling, nasal flaring, dyspnea, and cyanosis. Dyspnea scales,[11,75] which quantify the patient's subjective sensation of respiratory work, can be used before, during, and following the exercise test.

The Borg Scale of Ratings of Perceived Exertion (RPE)[11] and the Visual Analogue Scale (VAS)[75] have been adapted

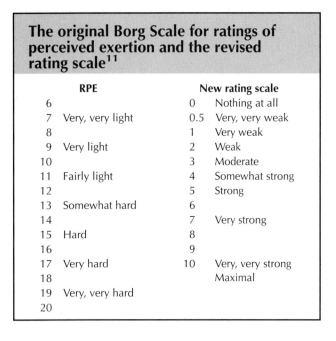

**The original Borg Scale for ratings of perceived exertion and the revised rating scale[11]**

| | RPE | | New rating scale |
|---|---|---|---|
| 6 | | 0 | Nothing at all |
| 7 | Very, very light | 0.5 | Very, very weak |
| 8 | | 1 | Very weak |
| 9 | Very light | 2 | Weak |
| 10 | | 3 | Moderate |
| 11 | Fairly light | 4 | Somewhat strong |
| 12 | | 5 | Strong |
| 13 | Somewhat hard | 6 | |
| 14 | | 7 | Very strong |
| 15 | Hard | 8 | |
| 16 | | 9 | |
| 17 | Very hard | 10 | Very, very strong |
| 18 | | | Maximal |
| 19 | Very, very hard | | |
| 20 | | | |

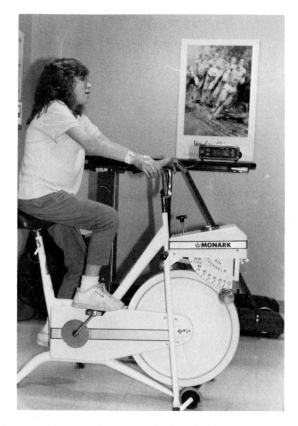

**Fig. 27-4.** Finger oximetry monitoring during cycle ergometry submaximal exercise.

for use by pulmonary patients.[1,10,75] Patients are asked to select a number between 6 and 20 that best quantifies the subjective impression of their dyspnea at rest and during exercise and recovery (see box above). The VAS consists of a 10 cm line that is anchored at each end by the phrases "no difficulty breathing" at the left and "unable to breathe" at the right. Subjects are asked to place an "X" on the line to best describe their breathing effort. Chest auscultation is also performed to assess for wheezing and any other adventitious changes in breath sounds. Measurements are usually recorded before testing, during the last 30 seconds of each exercise stage, and for 7 to 10 minutes after the exercise test or until the HR and BP have approached pretesting baseline values.

To safely conduct any exercise test, exercise and monitoring equipment must be well maintained and periodically calibrated. Professionals performing the physiological monitoring of the exercise test should be trained and certified in cardiopulmonary resuscitation. A fully equipped resuscitation cart, including up-to-date drugs and supplies, and a physician should always be available.

### Equipment considerations

A cycle ergometer is often the preferred mode for testing exercise in children with lung disease* (Fig. 27-4). $\dot{V}o_2$ can be predicted accurately since the mechanical efficiency for pedaling a cycle is independent of body weight and is nearly the same for everyone. This predictability is important when it is not feasible to perform expired gas collection and analyses.[6] Cycle ergometers are relatively light, can be relocated readily, and are much less costly than treadmills. Children easily adapt to pedaling and are generally less intimidated by the cycle than the treadmill. Electrocardio-

gram, BP monitoring, and expired gas collection are easily obtained from stationary individuals on the cycle. A disadvantage of the cycle ergometer is that peak or maximum $\dot{V}o_2$ values can be spuriously low because of local leg fatigue during cycle pedaling.

If children are too small to be fitted to a cycle, free-walking or walking on the treadmill are the preferred testing modes. Treadmills tend to be expensive, noisy, and poorly mobile. Young children require orientation to treadmill walking before the actual exercise test. Since there are individual and age-related variations in the mechanical efficiency associated with treadmill walking[6,70] and since the work performed depends on body weight, energy expenditure varies greatly and is difficult to predict. Higher $\dot{V}o_2$ values are obtained during treadmill work since greater muscle mass is exercising. Free-walking in a corridor or around a large room also can provide an opportunity to observe exercise response in small children, but quantitative measurements are difficult.

### Ventilatory limitations during exercise

The cardiovascular system normally limits the maximal work capacity during exercise.[82] In children with pulmonary disease, however, the ventilatory system limits the exercise capacity, and the maximal work capacity is thus said to be ventilatory-limited.

---

* References 20, 26, 33, 34, 62, 63.

EIB limits the exercise capability of children and adolescents with asthma.[33,43] A reduced physical fitness, as evidenced by a lower peak work capacity and a lower peak $\dot{V}O_2$, has been documented in children with EIB compared with nonasthmatic control subjects.[63] Dyspnea, high dyspnea scores, oxygen desaturation, decreased flow rates, and wheezing are signs of EIB. A respiratory function scoring system also has been developed for the interpretation of exercise-induced bronchospasm.[23] A documented postexercise drop of 10% to 15% or greater in peak expiratory flow rate, measured by a Wright Peak Flow Meter, provides a simple, rapid, quantitative evaluation of EIB.[33]

Children with chronic obstructive pulmonary disease (COPD) usually experience exercise intolerance as a result of deficiencies in exercise capacity,[20,26,53,62] gas exchange,* and poor pulmonary mechanics.[16,20,21,34] Patients develop progressively increased exercise limitation as lung disease worsens. Peak exercise capacity and peak $\dot{V}O_2$ are decreased in those with moderate to severe pulmonary dysfunction.[20,26,62] Some children with CF will experience oxygen desaturation during exercise.[20,26,40] Hypoxemia in this group of patients has been attributed to a low ventilation-perfusion ratio caused by lung tissue and pulmonary capillary bed destruction resulting from recurrent infection and scarring.[27] $CO_2$ retention, as evidenced by elevated end-tidal $CO_2$ values, has been observed in patients with severe lung dysfunction. The inability to appropriately eliminate $CO_2$ has been ascribed to alveolar hypoventilation and abnormal lung mechanics.[20]

In children with mild lung dysfunction, exercise $\dot{V}_E$ is the same as that of healthy children. The increased $\dot{V}_E$ response to exercise becomes more exaggerated as lung dysfunction worsens and is an attempt by the respiratory system to maintain normal alveolar ventilation in the presence of increased dead space ($\dot{V}_D$). Normally $\dot{V}_E$ encompasses about two thirds of the maximum voluntary ventilation (MVV) during maximal exercise. However, at high exercise levels, these young patients breathe at a very high $\dot{V}_E$, closely approximating their own MVV, indicating that the upper limits of ventilation are being reached. The high $\dot{V}_E$ in patients with severe lung dysfunction is accomplished by higher than expected breathing frequency and little or no change in tidal volume.[16] These altered respiratory mechanics during exercise are the result of disease-related resting hyperinflation. A recurrent cycle of secretion retention, airways obstruction, and pulmonary infection leads to lung tissue damage as demonstrated by decreased expiratory flow rates and increased hyperaeration. Increases in functional residual capacity and chest wall anteroposterior diameter result from hyperaeration. This cycle of complications leads to impaired pulmonary mechanics and an inability to further increase inspiratory capacity and exercise tidal volume.[16] Changes in

length-tension relationships of the respiratory muscles may occur because of increased functional residual capacity, placing the respiratory musculature at mechanical disadvantage and thus reducing respiratory muscle force generation.[52,67] These mechanical alterations result in a higher than expected work of breathing such that the respiratory muscles consume a large percentage of the total body $\dot{V}O_2$, and muscle fatigue may contribute further to exercise intolerance.[51]

That the exercise limitation in children with COPD is ventilation limited is supported by the HR response. Resting heart rates tend to be higher in individuals with obstructive lung disease than in normal subjects.[20,26] In children with CF, the HR response is heightened for each submaximal work load, although the rate of increase is normal. However, at maximal exercise capacity, maximum age-predicted heart rates are usually not attained in children with CF, reflecting the ventilatory limitation.

Recent work suggests that, in some patients, the lung disease and concomitant hypoxemia may limit cardiac function by increasing pulmonary vascular resistance.[53] Alternatively, the nutritional status of the patient appears to be critical[21] and may result in a reduction in muscle mass, which in turn could limit performance.[45] Nutritional state may also result in altered cardiac function by a reduced stroke volume and increased heart rate response due to a smaller exercising muscle mass.[83]

## CHEST WALL DEFORMITIES

Under normal conditions the chest wall of the healthy child is very compliant, requiring only small changes in transthoracic pressures to obtain large changes in intrathoracic volume. Compliance is decreased when congenital deformities, such as pectus excavatum or scoliosis, or acquired thoracic cage deformities, such as kyphoscoliosis caused by neuromuscular disease, exist. In children with thoracic cage deformities, a large inspiratory effort is required to expand a rib cage that is poorly compliant, stiff, rigid, and somewhat fixed. The increased work of breathing associated with the inspiratory effort of a child with a stiff rib cage can be identified by observation as exertional dyspnea. Dyspnea on exertion may be an indication for exercise testing to determine if the exercise capacity is limited because of cardiac or ventilatory dysfunction. When severe, chest wall deformities such as pectus excavatum and kyphoscoliosis are often thought to impose a circulatory limitation on exercise capacity, although it has been shown that the limitation is usually ventilatory.[15] $\dot{V}_E$ was inordinately high and the HR response was higher than expected for each workload in a group of adults with chest wall deformities.[68] Because of the difficulty in expanding the thoracic cage, $\dot{V}_E$ for increased workloads is achieved primarily through large increases in respiratory rate and a less than normal increase in tidal volume. A typical breathing pattern during exercise in children with a restrictive chest

---

* References 20, 21, 26, 27, 34, 40, 53.

wall deformity is characterized by a rapid respiratory rate and shallow breathing. As a result of the inability to appropriately increase $\dot{V}_E$ exercise capacities have been shown to be lower for children with restrictive chest wall deformities than for age-matched controls.

## EXERCISE PRESCRIPTION

Nearly all children with lung disease can participate in some type of therapeutic exercise program. Activity programs must be highly individualized and be based on a thorough history, evaluation, and exercise test. When prescribing an exercise program, the therapist should consider exercise mode, intensity, frequency, and duration.

### Exercise mode

Exercise programs should include endurance or cardiovascular activities, as well as strengthening and flexibility or stretching exercises. The purpose of the endurance component is to improve cardiorespiratory and musculoskeletal function, which will be reflected in increased exercise capacity and $Vo_{2max}$. The recommended exercises should be enjoyable and varied to avoid boredom and attrition from the program. Activities should be chosen to provide opportunities for lifelong enjoyment. Compliance to a prescribed program improves when exercises are performed with a family member or friend. Parents of young children are encouraged to be physically active regularly with their entire family so that an active life-style pattern is developed early for the youngster growing up with lung disease. Some children adhere better to exercise when they participate in organized sports activities. Others may do less well in public or group settings because of a reduced body image or physical self-image.

Popular endurance activities include brisk walking, jogging, bicycling, swimming, rowing, and cross-country skiing. Although several of these activities are seasonal, equipment is available so that one may exercise year-round indoors. Children with lung disease who engage in physical activities and sports can promote camaraderie and socializing with their peers.

Strength training will typically consist of isotonic resistive exercises involving the use of hand-held pulleys or free weights. Two important principles should be observed during isotonic strengthening.[66] First, the muscle groups being trained need to be stressed beyond their normal load (overload); second, additional load or resistance must be added progressively over time for strengthening to occur. Through trial and error the correct amount of weight is determined so that 10 to 12 repetitions can be performed before fatigue occurs and a rest is necessary. A minimum of two sets of these 10 to 12 repetitions should be done for each exercise in a session.

Strengthening exercises, especially for the upper body, have potential advantages for the respiratory muscle pump.[76] These exercises should emphasize shoulder girdle muscu-lature, and muscles of the chest wall (i.e., pectoralis major and minor, intercostal, serratus anterior, trapezius, erector spinae, rhomboid, latissimus dorsi, and abdominal muscles). The benefits of upper body strengthening exercises are not well known, although patients report subjectively that they generally feel better about their bodies. Breath holding, which often accompanies lifting "too much weight," should be avoided by teaching participants to exhale during the contraction. Strengthening of quadriceps and hamstring muscle groups can help prevent knee pain and injuries often incurred by less fit individuals engaged in running sports. Resistance training should focus on building strength instead of muscle bulk by emphasizing higher repetitions rather than high weight with few repetitions.

Stretching exercises are performed to promote musculoskeletal flexibility and to prevent potential deformities and contractures, especially of the thorax. Areas to be emphasized include the muscles of the chest wall and the hamstring muscles.

### Exercise intensity

The prescribed level of exercise intensity will depend on the child's physical fitness as determined by the exercise test. The better a child performs on a test, or the more fit the individual, the greater the intensity of exercise needed to further improve or maintain the fitness level. Conversely, the less fit an individual, the lower the intensity required to improve the fitness level. The linear relationship between HR and $\dot{V}o_2$ allows the use of HR to prescribe exercise intensity and to monitor progress. Exercise intensity is prescribed as a percentage of the heart rate reserve (HRR = Peak HR − Rest HR) based on the exercise test (Exercise heart rate = [HRR · %] + Rest HR). The initial exercise prescription for a child with a below normal fitness level, or one who has been inactive for an extended period, should be 40% to 50% of HRR and can be increased progressively to 60% to 80% of HRR. Children with obstructive lung disease can eventually exercise between 50% and 70% of the HRR; those individuals with normal lung function and mild lung dysfunction may be able to exercise between 70% and 80% of HRR. Regular endurance exercise at a given workload stimulates a cardiovascular adaptation such that the exercise HR is lower for that workload. The HR-based exercise prescription takes advantage of this conditioning-induced decrease in HR; to maintain the prescribed exercise HR, exercise intensity must be increased periodically to ensure a continued training effect. It is important to note that there will be individual exceptions.

For individuals who significantly desaturated during the exercise test, the exercise HR should be below the rate at which desaturation occurred, or $O_2$ supplementation should be used to keep $Sao_2$ above 90%. Supplemental oxygen should be provided at 0.5 liter increments to maintain $Sao_2$ above 90%. However, the lowest acceptable $Sao_2$ will vary among institutions, and the criteria for supplemental oxygen administration in such cases should be determined in conjunction with the attending physician. Patients with severe to very severe reduction in lung function will not be able to exercise at a specified intensity. At best, they will usually choose to walk, since walking is most functional and the intensity will be self-determined by their ability to coordinate walking speed with their breathing pattern.

Most children with asthma will be able to exercise at a heart rate between 70% and 85% of the peak HR achieved on a progressive maximal exercise test. These children should take their bronchodilator inhalants before exercising. In most children, EIB can be managed successfully pharmacologically with either cromolyn or beta-adrenergic aerosol administration 20 to 30 minutes before exercise.[63]

### Exercise duration

The benefits of cardiovascular conditioning cannot be attained with exercise lasting less than 15 minutes, and they typically require exercise for 20 to 30 minutes. Endurance exercise is usually preceded and followed by a 5 to 10 minute warm-up and cool-down period, respectively. Duration and intensity of exercise are related. High-intensity exercise is usually performed for a shorter duration, and low-intensity exercise is usually of longer duration. However, some individuals with a low exercise tolerance are able to sustain only low-intensity exercise for short periods of time as compared with more fit individuals who may sustain higher-intensity exercise for long periods. The intensity and duration are highly individualized and require frequent adjusting to ensure a conditioning response. For individuals with severe to very severe pulmonary disease and for unfit individuals, the duration of exercise may be only 3 to 5 minutes initially. These patients do well with intermittent exercise, in which short bouts (30 seconds to 3 minutes) of exercise are alternated with equal or longer duration rest periods. The total exercise time may be as much as 15 minutes, but it is interspersed with a rest period every 3 or 5 minutes. Over time, the exercise periods are lengthened, and rest periods are shortened or eliminated entirely. The goal should be to increase the duration of the exercise session to between 15 and 20 minutes of continuous exercise. Individuals with cor pulmonale are the exception to these guidelines because these patients are hypoxemic and in right-sided heart failure. They should walk frequent, short distances at a slower pace.

### Exercise frequency

Endurance exercise should be performed three to four times weekly on alternate days to optimize the conditioning effect. Children with advanced lung disease who are exercising at low intensities for 5 to 10 minutes can exercise two to four times daily. Exercise for these patients may consist of only a brief walk several times daily.

Strengthening exercise also can be performed every other day. To avoid boredom, two or more strengthening routines can be developed and alternated.

Stretching is an important part of any exercise program and plays a significant role in reducing injuries. Stretching should be done slowly. The muscle should be stretched until tension is evident and held for about 30 seconds. After 30 seconds the tension will decrease, at which point it should be increased again. This cycle is repeated for a total of 2 minutes. Ideally, all parts of the body should be stretched before and after the exercise session. In practice, some stretches are done before and some after as part of the warm-up and cool-down period.

## RESPIRATORY MUSCLE TRAINING

Respiratory muscle function is considered the principal factor in limiting exercise tolerance in adult patients with COPD.[37,73] The reduced respiratory muscle strength and endurance in COPD have been attributed to hypoxemia, respiratory muscle length/tension changes caused by hyperinflation, malnutrition, and increased work of breathing. Respiratory muscle strength and endurance can also be compromised in individuals who develop respiratory problems caused by neuromuscular disorders in which there is respiratory muscle weakness, such as quadriplegia, muscular dystrophy, or poliomyelitis, and disorders of the chest wall, such as kyphoscoliosis.

### Inspiratory muscles

Patients should begin a program of respiratory muscle training (RMT) only if respiratory muscle function is, in fact, the limiting factor to exercise tolerance. The goal of RMT is to delay the onset of inspiratory muscle fatigue and to improve ventilatory performance during exercise.

Inspiratory muscles have been trained using voluntary normocapneic hyperpnea,[9,44,50] resistive breathing exercise,[2,64,65,72] and threshold load training[36,47] in adults with COPD,* patients with quadriplegia,[36] and patients being weaned from mechanical ventilators.[8]

Voluntary normocapneic hyperpnea or respiratory muscle endurance training requires that subjects train by breathing through an elaborate rebreathing circuit that permits rapid breathing at a sustained increase in $V_i$ to a targeted level while maintaining normal $O_2$ and $CO_2$ levels. Subjects are required to train in a laboratory setting. Resistive strength training is much simpler and is easily performed at home. Inspiratory muscle training devices are readily available and require individuals to breathe in against resistance for 15 minutes twice daily (Fig. 27-5). Once a certain resistance is easily tolerated for 30 minutes daily, a higher resistance is imposed. Training should be carried out for a minimum of 6 to 8 weeks.

---

* References 2, 36, 47, 64, 65, 72.

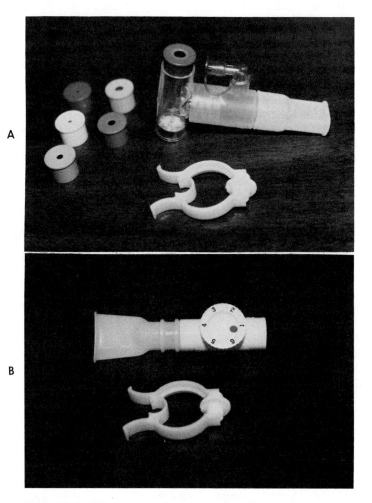

**Fig. 27-5. A,** DHD Medical Products inspiratory muscle trainer device and resistors. Note the pressure monitoring/supplemental oxygen port with port cap in place. **B,** PFLEX inspiratory muscle trainer with a dial selector to control resistance.

Resistive devices should have a means by which to measure mouth pressures to set training intensity. A pressure transducer is used to measure maximum static inspiratory mouth pressure (MSIP) from functional residual capacity. Resistive training should occur daily, 5 to 7 days per week, at an intensity between 30% and 40% of MSIP.[50] Training intensity should be based on periodic measurements of MSIP.

Through altering breathing strategy during resistive training, a slower breathing rate will reduce inspiratory flow rate and inspiratory load, making the training stimulus variable. More recent studies[36,47] have employed a loaded breathing device in which a threshold valve opens only once a predetermined threshold pressure is achieved. In contrast to the resistive devices, the inspiratory pressure load remains constant and is independent of inspiratory flow rate. While two studies[36,47] have evaluated this technique and agree that ventilatory muscle function can be improved, they disagree on the effect of threshold loading on exercise performance.

Inspiratory muscle training has resulted in improvements in maximum sustained ventilatory capacity (MSVC),[9,44,50]

maximum voluntary ventilation (MVV),[50,72] maximum critical mouth pressures $(Pm_{crit})$[38] maximum inspiratory mouth pressures $(Pm_{max})$,[36,38] inspiratory muscle endurance,* maximum resistive load,[2] $Vo_{2max}$,[9,72] $V_{Emax}$,[9,72] and exercise tolerance[2,9,44,47,64] without alterations in pulmonary function. It must be pointed out that these results are not consistent across the literature, suggesting that the use of inspiratory muscle training should be evaluated on an individual basis.

Early studies show that untrained individuals with CF have greater ventilatory muscle endurance[44] and strength[4] than do non-CF control subjects. This has been attributed to constant breathing against an elevated airway resistance in CF patients. Recent work shows that CF individuals can have ventilatory muscle strength similiar to that of controls.[46] Inspiratory muscle function appears to be unaffected by changes in lean body mass suggesting a selective training effect secondary to chronic lung disease. Specific ventilatory muscle endurance training, as well as nonspecific upper

* References 2, 9, 36, 47, 50, 65.

body exercise (e.g., swimming and canoeing), were shown to improve the endurance of the respiratory muscles in individuals with CF to a greater extent than in normal subjects.[44] Inspiratory resistance in CF patients will also increase inspiratory muscle strength but does not result in improved exercise performance.[4]

### Expiratory muscles

Expiratory muscle function in children with lung disease has not been well documented. Patients with asthma have a higher than normal expiratory muscle strength and endurance.[58] Abdominal muscle exercises have been shown to improve exercise performance in adult patients with COPD,[80] suggesting that part of the exercise limitation in these patients is a result of expiratory muscle dysfunction. On the other hand, in healthy adults, abdominal muscle conditioning had no effect on expiratory muscle strength and endurance, whereas expiratory resistive breathing exercises did improve both strength and endurance.[19] This topic requires further study.

The optimal method by which to train the respiratory muscles and the benefits of respiratory muscle training remain unclear. Further research investigating RMT in various patient populations needs to be done, and, most important, it needs to be determined if the effects of RMT are long lasting and whether they translate into improved exercise performance and function.

## SUPPLEMENTAL OXYGEN DURING EXERCISE

Hypoxemia leads to dyspnea, increased work of breathing, increased HR, and, at times, tachycardia, general fatigue, poor appetite, exercise intolerance, and reduced mental alertness. Chronic hypoxemia plays a major role in the development of pulmonary hypertension and cor pulmonale. The proper administration of supplemental $O_2$ can help alleviate or minimize these symptoms. Oxygen administration can improve exercise capacity in an otherwise medically stable child with advancing pulmonary disease, thereby permitting the child to be more functional at a reduced ventilatory and cardiovascular cost with less chance of experiencing exercise-induced desaturation.[21,25,54,60]

The need for $O_2$ supplementation is determined by arterial blood gas analyses or noninvasive oximetry. In our pediatric pulmonary clinic, oximetry is routinely performed on the ear or finger during outpatient clinic visits, with the child at rest and during walking. For inpatients, oximetry is performed during rest, sleep, chest physical therapy, activities of daily living, and exercise. Evaluation of $O_2$ requirements with oximetry should be approached in a deliberate and methodical manner. The decision to use $O_2$ must be assessed carefully before supplemental $O_2$ use is begun, because the need for $O_2$ indicates a deterioration in pulmonary status. The initial use of supplemental $O_2$ should be handled with sensitivity because of the emotional impact that often accompanies its first introduction.

Our goal is to maintain resting and exercising $Sao_2$, with exception of exercise testing, at a minimum of 90%, which correlates with a $Pao_2$ of 58 mm Hg, assuming the arterial pH is 7.4. Before engaging in physical activity, a resting $Sao_2$ above 90% is desirable because this provides a margin for exercise-induced desaturation to occur while still maintaining $Sao_2$ at or above 90% during activity. Periodic reassessment of $O_2$ requirements during various activities should be done. Simultaneously, dyspnea scales, respiratory rate, HR, and signs of increased work of breathing should be recorded.

During in-hospital activity, portable E cylinder $O_2$ tanks can be wheeled by most patients. A walker with an attached E cylinder $O_2$ tank enables ambulation with support for the more debilitated patient. Typically, portable liquid $O_2$ systems are used during ambulation outside the home and are refilled via a stationary home liquid $O_2$ system. The development of $O_2$-saving delivery systems has helped reduce financial costs and increase duration time of portable liquid $O_2$ systems, therefore enabling individuals to be away from home for extended periods.[77] These $O_2$ conservation systems include demand delivery systems,[7,55,77,78] $O_2$-conserving nasal reservoir cannulae,[71,78] transtracheal $O_2$ delivery,[31,39] and electronic demand solenoid valve systems.[61] These systems deliver $O_2$ flow only during the inspiratory phase of the respiratory cycle. Older children prefer to carry portable liquid $O_2$ systems in backpacks centered high up on their backs. Backpacks most favored are those with padded straps since some tanks weigh nearly 10 pounds. This preferred method is cosmetically acceptable, mechanically efficient, and permits free use of both arms and hands.

## SUMMARY

Children with chronic lung disease commonly experience a reduced exercise capacity and are usually less fit than their healthy peers. Through monitored exercise testing, individual exercise prescriptions can be designed. Children with asthma who experience EIB can safely engage in physical activity by using medication before exercise. Most individuals with CE are able to maintain a normal exercise response because they have a normal pulmonary reserve in gas exchange. Those with advanced lung disease require closer monitoring, specially tailored exercise regimens, and, when indicated, $O_2$ supplementation. Children with lung disease can improve their cardiovascular fitness and achieve the same benefits as their healthy peers through regular physical activity. Improved muscle endurance and increased resistance to fatigue specific to ventilatory muscles is achieved by respiratory muscle training, as well as general conditioning. Pulmonary function remains unchanged by endurance training programs; however, specific respiratory muscle training improves respiratory muscle strength and endurance. Studies assessing the long-term effects of exercise on longevity and lung disease progression need to be performed for children.

## CASE 1    14-Year-Old Patient with Cystic Fibrosis

S.R. is a 14-year-old girl with cystic fibrosis. She was admitted to the hospital with complaints of increased fatigue, decreased exercise tolerance, increased cough with increased mucous production, a 5-pound weight loss over the past 2 months, a temperature of 101° F, and periodic hemoptysis. The patient has a history of repeated hospital admissions and was last hospitalized 2 months ago. Her home treatment consisted of supplemental pancreatic enzymes, oral antibiotics, a high-calorie diet, postural drainage with percussion and vibration three times daily, and an exercise program. Hospital admission physical examination sitting at rest:

RHR = 120 bpm
BP = 100/64 mm Hg
RRR = 32 breaths/min
2+ clubbing

Mild to moderate cyanosis at lips and nailbeds. Breathing pattern: mild respiratory distress, increased accessory muscle activity with 2+ hypertrophy, and retractions. Breath sounds: decreased at bases bilaterally; inspiratory crackles throughout right chest. Cough: weak, productive of dark green sputum.

|  | Admission | | Discharge | |
|---|---|---|---|---|
| Height (cm) | 149 | | 149 | |
| Weight (kg) | 31 | | 35 | |

| Lung function | Actual | % Predicted | Actual | % Predicted |
|---|---|---|---|---|
| FVC(L) | 1.13 | 39 | 1.64 | 57 |
| FEV$_1$(L) | 0.63 | 25 | 0.95 | 37 |
| FEF$_{25\%-75\%}$(L/sec) | 0.24 | 8 | 0.42 | 14 |
| RV | 3.32 | 437 | 2.65 | 349 |
| Sao$_2$% | 88.6 | | 94 | |

S.R. was hospitalized for 21 days. In-hospital treatment consisted of intravenous antibiotic therapy, 3 liters of supplemental O$_2$, postural drainage with percussion and vibration four times a day, and a high-calorie diet.

At the time of hospital discharge, physical examination sitting at rest:

RHR = 96 bpm
BP = 90/60 mm Hg
RRR = 22 breaths/min
2+ clubbing

No cyanosis was present. Breathing pattern was improved with minimal accessory muscle activity. Breath sounds: chest markedly clearer; increased air entry to bases; fewer inspiratory crackles throughout right chest. Cough: stronger, less productive of lighter green sputum.

Over the course of the hospitalization, S.R. was weaned

from supplemental O$_2$. Before hospital discharge S.R. performed a submaximal exercise test on a Monarck cycle ergometer. Initial resistance was set at 0.25 kp while pedaling at 50 rpm (75 · kpm min$^{-1}$). Workload was increased every 2 minutes in 2-minute increments. HR, Sao$_2$, and Borg scale ratings of perceived exertion were recorded during the last 30 seconds of each workload.

S.R. was able to perform three stages of the exercise test before the test was terminated at S.R.'s request because of shortness of breath. The highest submaximal workload achieved was 225 kpm · min$^{-1}$. Peak heart rate was 150 bpm, and the final RPE was 17. Saturation dropped to 88% from a resting level of 94%. HR was 135 bpm when Sao$_2$ was 90%. One year previously, S.R. was able to perform five stages of the exercise test with minimal desaturation. The test at that time was terminated because of shortness of breath. Peak heart rate was 160 bpm, and the final RPE was 15.

*INTERPRETATION*

*Pulmonary function.* S.R. has moderate to severe lung dysfunction. Discharge values indicate severe airflow obstruction of the large airways (37%) and very severe airflow obstruction of the small airways (14%). An FVC of 57% indicates a moderate restrictive component. The increased RV indicates severe hyperinflation.

*Submaximal exercise test.* The patient has a reduced exercise capacity. One year ago peak submaximal work load was 375 kpm · min$^{-1}$ as compared with 225 · kpm min$^{-1}$ now. Peak submaximal heart rate is lower than previously, yet heart rates during the first three stages are higher than previously, indicating a deterioration in the level of fitness.

Desaturation is more apparent than before and indicates that S.R. should exercise at heart rates below 135 bpm to avoid desaturation below 90%.

*Exercise prescription.* As an outpatient, S.R. can perform a brisk walk coordinated with a diaphramatic breathing pattern or exercise on a stationary bicycle. S.R. was shown how to monitor her pulse rate and was instructed to exercise at a HR below 135 bpm. S.R. was able to walk briskly for 20 to 30 continuous minutes at a HR below 135 bpm without desaturating significantly.

On the stationary bicycle initially, S.R. tolerated pedaling for 10 continuous minutes against resistance alternated with several minutes of pedaling without resistance because of local leg fatigue. Over the next several days, longer periods of pedaling against resistance were alternated with shorter periods without resistance until S.R. could eventually pedal for 20 to 30 minutes with resistance to elicit a HR of 135 bpm. Sao$_2$ monitoring during cycle exercise is performed every 2 months during outpatient clinic visits to see if exercise intensity needs to be readjusted based on Sao$_2$ and HR response.

S.R. also performs three sets of 10 to 12 repetitions of strengthening exercises for the upper body, specifically the shoulder girdle, the back musculature, and the biceps and triceps. Stretching was performed for the upper anterior chest, the lateral thoracic region, and hamstring muscle group.

## CASE 2 ▼ 18-Year-Old Patient with Cystic Fibrosis

(Illustrates the use of exercise test to determine functional capacity and exercise prescription, as well as to track changes over time.)

This patient is an 18-year-old man with cystic fibrosis. Diagnosis was made at age 10 months through duplicate positive sweat tests. Normal home treatment consists of daily enzyme replacement therapy, oral antibiotics, and chest physical therapy, consisting primarily of postural drainage and percussion in several positions. The patient has had a history of repeated admissions to the hospital for acute exacerbations of the lung disease associated with cystic fibrosis.

The following tests were done when the patient was clinically stable as an outpatient (A), on admission to the hospital for treatment of an acute exacerbation (B), and at the time of discharge 13 days later (C).

Pulmonary Function Tests: forced vital capacity (FVC), forced expired volume in 1 second ($FEV_1$), and forced expired flow between 25% and 75% of FVC ($FEF_{25\%-75\%}$) were measured with standard spirometry; functional residual capacity (FRC) with body plethysmography. Arterial $O_2$ saturation ($SaO_2$) was estimated using an ear oximeter (see table at right).

*EXERCISE TEST*

*Electronic cycle ergometer.* Initial power output set at 0.3 W/kg; subsequent power output established as 0.3 W/kg increments every 2 minutes. ECG/heart rate (HR), minute ventilation ($V_E$), $SaO_2$, blood pressure, and end-tidal $CO_2$ were measured during the last 30 seconds of each load.

|  | A | B | C |
|---|---|---|---|
| Height (cm) | 172 | 174 | 174 |
| Weight (kg) | 52 | 53.2 | 55.3 |

| Test | Actual A | Actual B | Actual C | % Predicted A | % Predicted B | % Predicted C |
|---|---|---|---|---|---|---|
| FVC(L) | 3.4 | 3.3 | 3.4 | 82 | 78 | 81 |
| $FEV_1$(L) | 2.6 | 2.2 | 2.8 | 68 | 56 | 71 |
| $FEF_{25\%-75\%}$(L/sec) | 1.8 | 1.1 | 1.5 | 40 | 24 | 33 |
| FRC | 2.8 | 3.3 | 3.1 | 111 | 128 | 119 |
| $SaO_2$ | 94 | 89 | 92 | | | |

Peak workload when clinically stable was 2.7 W/kg; on admission to the hospital it was reduced to 1.5 W/kg, and had increased to 1.8 W/kg at the time of discharge. End-exercise $SaO_2$ had decreased to 90, 81, and 89 for test periods A, B, and C respectively. Peak exercise $V_E$ was 98 1/min$^{-1}$, 107 1/min, and 92 1/min at the three time periods respectively. End-tidal $CO^2$ at peak exercise was 29 mm Hg, 49 mm Hg and 36 mm HG for the outpatient, admission, and discharge tests respectively.

## Raw data for patient with cystic fibrosis

| Power output (W/kg) | HR (bpm) A | HR (bpm) B | HR (bpm) C | $SaO_2$ (%) A | $SaO_2$ (%) B | $SaO_2$ (%) C | $\dot{V}_E$ (L/min) A | $\dot{V}_E$ (L/min) B | $\dot{V}_E$ (L/min) C | End-tidal $CO_2$ (mm Hg) A | End-tidal $CO_2$ (mm Hg) B | End-tidal $CO_2$ (mm Hg) C |
|---|---|---|---|---|---|---|---|---|---|---|---|---|
| Rest | 78 | 83 | 84 | 94 | 89 | 92 | 12 | 13 | 14 | 38 | 40 | 39 |
| 0.3 | 85 | 94 | 94 | 94 | 88 | 92 | 18 | 19 | 20 | 38 | 41 | 39 |
| 0.6 | 96 | 107 | 109 | 95 | 88 | 92 | 25 | 29 | 30 | 39 | 43 | 40 |
| 0.9 | 105 | 119 | 118 | 94 | 87 | 92 | 33 | 58 | 43 | 38 | 44 | 38 |
| 1.2 | 118 | 132 | 138 | 94 | 84 | 92 | 41 | 79 | 56 | 37 | 46 | 37 |
| 1.5 | 129 | 145 | 151 | 93 | 81 | 91 | 50 | 107 | 70 | 35 | 49 | 36 |
| 1.8 | 140 | | 167 | 92 | | 89 | 62 | | 92 | 33 | | 36 |
| 2.1 | 151 | | | 92 | | | 74 | | | 33 | | |
| 2.4 | 160 | | | 90 | | | 86 | | | 31 | | |
| 2.7 | 165 | | | 90 | | | 98 | | | 29 | | |

| | Preexercise Actual | Preexercise % Predicted | Postexercise Actual | Postexercise % Predicted | Postbronchodilator Actual | Postbronchodilator % Predicted |
|---|---|---|---|---|---|---|
| FVC (L) | 2.07 | 77 | 1.41 | 52 | 2.22 | 82 |
| $FEV_1$ (L) | 1.5 | 62 | 0.92 | 36 | 1.45 | 57 |
| $FEF_{25\%-75\%}$ (L/sec) | 1.51 | 46 | 0.50 | 15 | 1.05 | 32 |
| $FEV_1$/FVC (%) | 78% | >72% | 65% | >78% | 65% | >78% |
| Peak flow (L/min) | 273 | 77 | 135 | 38 | 174 | 48 |

## CASE 2 ▾ 18-Year-Old Patient with Cystic Fibrosis—cont'd

*INTERPRETATION*

*Pulmonary function.* This patient has moderate to severe lung dysfunction. The reduced flow rates (68% and 40% of expected values) under condition A indicate severe obstructive disease. The slightly increased FRC shows that this patient has minimal hyperinflation. On admission to the hospital, the lung volume is reduced, the flow rates have deteriorated further, and moderate hyperinflation is present.

*Exercise test.* This patient had a moderately reduced peak *work capacity* of 2.7 W/kg while clinically stable. This was reduced further (1.5 W/kg) at the time of admission and had increased over the period of admission to 1.8 W/kg. The *HR response* to exercise was normal (i.e., the slope of the heart rate/power output relationship was normal). Peak heart rates were reduced at all test intervals indicating that exercise capacity was reduced as a result of pulmonary limitations. *Minute ventilation* was higher than expected during all tests. The increase was further exaggerated at the time of admission and was reduced over the period of hospital treatment. $SaO_2$ *desaturation* was evident at the end of all tests, but was most severe at admission. Hospitalization reduced the degree of desaturation, but there was still an abnormal decrease in $SaO_2$ at the time of discharge. $CO_2$ *retention,* a sign of alveolar hypoventilation, was seen only during the test administered at admission to the hospital.

*Exercise prescription.* As an outpatient this individual had no activity restrictions. His exercise prescription was based on a target heart rate of between 60% and 75% of the heart rate reserve. Target = (Peak HR − RHR) · % + (RHR).

During the first 3 days of the hospitalization, supplemental $O_2$ was required to keep the $SaO_2$ above 90%; exercise sessions lasted from 5 to 10 minutes two times per day and consisted of a light load (1 W/kg) sufficient to increase the HR to about 120 bpm. Over the next 10 days power output was increased gradually to increase HR to 130 to 140 bpm for a duration of 15 to 20 minutes twice per day.

At the time of discharge, the patient did not desaturate significantly until the peak load. Exercise prescription was again based on the heart rate reserve.

## CASE 3 ▾ Patient with Asthma

K.M. is an 11-year-old girl with asthma. The patient has been under treatment since wheezing was noticed at age 2. Intermittent medication with theophylline has been necessary. The child has inhaled isoproterenol to use as needed and has received training in the indications for use of the inhaler.

Exercise, or the hyperpnea of exercise, has been identified as a trigger of this patient's asthma. This was confirmed with a previous exercise test where the patient exercised while breathing dry air. Significant decreases in postexercise pulmonary function tests confirmed the presence of exercise-induced asthma.

The patient's physician suspected that the child's parents were so concerned about the asthma that they were not allowing the child to participate in regular activities. An exercise evaluation was ordered so that appropriate exercise could be prescribed.

Height (cm): 148.5
Weight (kg): 30.1

Pulmonary function tests: Lung volumes and flows were measured using standard spirometry; peak flow was measured with a peak flow meter. The tests were done before exercise, 5 to 10 minutes after exercise, and after inhaling the bronchodilator, isoproterenol, and 20 minutes postexercise.

*Exercise test*

Initial power output was 0.6 W/kg and was increased by 0.3 W/kg every 2 minutes. The test was terminated when the patient could no longer continue. Heart rate, blood pressure, end-tidal $CO_2$, and minute ventilation were measured during the last 30 seconds of each workload.

Peak power output was 1.8 W/kg, peak HR was 191 bpm, peak $CO_2$ was 34 mm Hg, and peak $V_E$ was 33 L/min.

### Raw data for exercise test done on patient with asthma

| Power output (W/kg) | HR (bpm) | End-tidal $CO_2$ (mm Hg) | $\dot{V}_E$ (L/min) |
|---|---|---|---|
| Rest | 85 | 39 | 6 |
| 0.6 | 110 | 40 | 15 |
| 0.9 | 130 | 41 | 17 |
| 1.2 | 153 | 41 | 20 |
| 1.5 | 174 | 37 | 26 |
| 1.8 | 191 | 34 | 33 |

*Interpretation.* Mild to moderate airway obstruction. Moderately severe exercise-induced bronchospasm, which was partially reversible with a bronchodilator aerosol.

Low-normal degree of *physical fitness* as indicated by the peak work capacity of 1.8 W/kg. The peak HR of 191 indicates normal cardiovascular reserves. The exercise test showed that there was no cardiopulmonary reason to limit activity in this patient.

*Exercise prescription.* An activity program was prescribed for this patient. The program was based on a point system whereby the patient received points for doing various types of activities for periods of time. She was given point goals to attain on a weekly basis, and incentives were offered if she attained these goals. On follow-up, this patient had increased her participation in physical education and daily activities, although her asthma did at times prevent full participation.

## REFERENCES

1. American College of Sports Medicine: *Guidelines for graded exercise testing and exercise prescription.* Philadelphia, 1986, Lea & Febiger.
2. Andersen JB and others: Resistive breathing training in severe chronic obstructive pulmonary disease, *Scand J Respir Dis* 60:151, 1979.
3. Andreasson BB and others: Long-term effects of physical exercise on working capacity and pulmonary function in cystic fibrosis, *Acta Paediatr Scand* 76:70, 1987.
4. Asher MI and others: The effects of inspiratory muscle training in patients with cystic fibrosis, *Am Rev Respir Dis* 126:855, 1982.
5. Astrand PO: *Experimental studies of physical working capacity in relationship to sex and age,* Munksgaard, Copenhagen, 1952.
6. Astrand PO and Rodahl K: *Textbook of work physiology,* New York, 1977, McGraw-Hill, Inc.
7. Auerbach D, Flick MR, and Block AJ: A new oxygen cannula system using intermittent-demand nasal flow, *Chest* 74:39, 1978.
8. Belman MJ: Respiratory failure treated by ventilatory muscle training (VMT), *Eur J Respir Dis* 62:391, 1981.
9. Belman MJ and Mittman C: Ventilatory muscle training improves exercise capacity in chronic obstructive pulmonary disease patients, *Am Rev Respir Dis* 121:273, 1980.
10. Belman MJ and others: Breathlessness index, a simple and repeatable exercise test for patients with chronic obstructive pulmonary disease (abstract), *Am Rev Respir Dis* 127 (suppl): 109, 1983.
11. Borg GV: Psychophysical bases of perceived exertion, *Med Sci Sports Exercise* 14(5):377, 1982.
12. Boyle IR and others: Emotional adjustment of adolescents and young adults with cystic fibrosis, *J Pediatr* 88(2):318, 1976.
13. Brinkman JR and Hoskins TA: Physical conditioning and altered self-concept in rehabilitated hemiplegic patients, *Phys Ther* 59:859, 1979.
14. Brooks GA and Fahey TD: *Exercise physiology,* New York, 1985, Macmillan Publishing Co.
15. Casey LC and Weber KT: Chronic lung disease and chest wall deformities. In Weber KT and Janicki JS, editors: *Cardiopulmonary exercise testing-physiologic principles and clinical applications,* Philadelphia, 1986, WB Saunders Co.
16. Cerny FJ: Ventilatory control during exercise in children with cystic fibrosis (abstract), *Am Rev Respir Dis* 123:195, 1981.
17. Cerny FJ: Relative effects of chest physiotherapy and exercise for in-hospital care of cystic fibrosis, *Phys Ther* 69:633, 1989.
18. Cerny FJ, Cropp GJA, and Bye MR: Hospital therapy improves exercise tolerance and lung function in cystic fibrosis, *Am J Dis Child* 138:261, 1984.
19. Cerny FJ, Loeffler R, and Stull A: Does abdominal muscle training improve expiratory muscle strength or endurance? *Med Sci Sports Exer* 22:S53, 1990.
20. Cerny FJ, Pullano TP, and Cropp GJ: Cardiorespiratory adaptations to exercise in cystic fibrosis, *Am Rev Respir Dis* 126:217, 1982.
21. Coates AL and others: The role of nutritional status, airway obstruction, hypoxia, and abnormalities in serum lipid composition in limiting exercise tolerance in children with cystic fibrosis, *Acta Paediatr Scand* 69:353, 1980.
22. Collingwood T and Willet L: The effects of physical training upon self-concept and body attitudes, *J Clin Psychol* 27:411, 1971.
23. Cropp GJ: The exercise bronchoprovocation test: standardization of procedures and evaluation of response, *J Allergy Clin Immunol* 64(6):627, 1979.
24. Cropp GJA: Pulmonary function and bronchial challenge testing in office and hospital practice, *Annals Allerg* 51:13, 1983.
25. Cropp GJA and others: Effects of oxygen breathing on exercise tolerance in cystic fibrosis (abstract), *Am Rev Respir Dis* 135:286, 1987.
26. Cropp GJ and others: Exercise tolerance and cardiorespiratory adjustments at peak work capacity in cystic fibrosis, *Am Rev Respir Dis* 126:211, 1982.
27. Dantzker DR, Patten GA, and Bower JS: Gas exchange at rest and during exercise in adults with cystic fibrosis, *Am Rev Respir Dis* 125:400, 1982.
28. Edlund LD and others: Effects of a swimming program on children with cystic fibrosis, *Am J Dis Child* 140:80, 1986.
29. Eggleston PA and others: Guidelines for the methodology of exercise challenge testing of asthmatics, *J Allergy Clin Immunol* 64(6):642, 1979.
30. Folkins C: The effects of physical training on mood, *J Clin Psychol* 32:583, 1972.
31. Frye K, Shukla L, and Selecky P: A new device for transtracheal oxygen therapy in patients with cuffless tracheostomy tubes (abstract), *Chest* (suppl) 94:32S, 1988.
32. Gary V and Guthrie D: The effect of jogging on physical fitness and self-concept in hospitalized alcoholics, *OJ Studies Alcohol* 33:1073, 1972.
33. Godfrey S: *Exercise testing in children,* Philadelphia, 1974, WB Saunders Co.
34. Godfrey S and Mearns M: Pulmonary function and response to exercise in cystic fibrosis, *Arch Dis Child* 46:144, 1971.
35. Golding LA and others: YMCA bicycle test. In *The Y's way to physical fitness,* YMCA of the USA, Chicago, 1982.
36. Goldstein R and others: Applicability of a threshold loading device for inspiratory muscle testing and training in patients with COPD, *Chest* 96:564, 1989.
37. Grassino A and others: Inspiratory muscle fatigue as a factor limiting exercise, *Bull Eur Physiopathol Respir* 15:105, 1979.
38. Gross D and others: The effect of training on strength and endurance of the diaphragm in quadriplegia, *Am J Med* 68:27, 1980.
39. Hansen LA and others: Transtracheal oxygen therapy: long term follow-up (abstract), *Chest* 94(suppl):32S, 1988.
40. Henke KG and Orenstein DM: Oxygen saturation during exercise in cystic fibrosis, *Am Rev Respir Dis* 129:708, 1984.
41. Johnson WR, Fretz SR, and Johnson JA: Changes in self-concept during a physical development program, *Res O* 39:560, 1968.
42. Jones NL and Campbell EJM: *Clinical exercise testing,* Philadelphia, 1975, WB Saunders Co.
43. Kattan M and others: The response to exercise in normal and asthmatic children, *J Pediatr* 92(5):718, 1978.
44. Keens TG and others: Ventilatory muscle endurance training in normal subjects and patients with cystic fibrosis, *Am Rev Respir Dis* 116:853, 1977.
45. Lands LC, Heigenhauser GJF, and Jones NL: Analysis of factors limiting maximal exercise performance in cystic fibrosis, *Clin Science* 83:391, 1992.
46. Lands LC, Heigenhauser GJF, and Jones NL: Respiratory and peripheral muscle function in cystic fibrosis, *Am Rev Respir Dis* 147:865, 1993.
47. Larson JL and others: Inspiratory muscle training with a pressure threshold breathing device in patients with chronic obstructive pulmonary disease, *Am Rev Respir Dis* 138:689, 1988.
48. Lawler RH, Nakielny W, and Wright N: Psychological implications of cystic fibrosis, *Canad Med Ass J* 94:1043, 1966.
49. Lebecque P and others: Diffusion capacity and oxygen desaturation effects on exercise in patients with cystic fibrosis, *Chest* 91(5):693, 1987.
50. Leith DE and Bradley M: Ventilatory muscle strength and endurance training, *J Appl Physiol* 41:508, 1976.
51. Levison H and Cherniack RM: Ventilatory cost of exercise in chronic obstructive pulmonary disease, *J Appl Physiol* 25:21, 1968.
52. Loke J, editor: Exercise: physiology and clinical applications, *Clin Chest Med* 5:35, 1984.
53. Marcotte JE and others: Multiple factors limit exercise capacity in cystic fibrosis, *Pediatr Pulmonol* 2:274, 1986.
54. Marcus CL and others: Supplemental oxygen and exercise performance in patients with cystic fibrosis with severe pulmonary disease, *Chest* 101:52, 1992.

55. McDonnell TJ and others: Efficacy of pulsed oxygen delivery during exercise, *Respiratory Care* 31:883, 1986.

56. McFadden ER: Respiratory heat and water exchange: physiological and clinical implications, *J Appl Physiol* 54:331, 1983.

57. McGavin CR, Gupta SP, and McHardy GJB: Twelve-minute walking test for assessing disability in chronic bronchitis, *Br Med J* 1:822, 1976.

58. McKenzie DK and Gandevia SC: Strength and endurance in inspiratory, expiratory, and limb muscles in asthma, *Am Rev Respir Dis* 134:999, 1986.

59. Nickerson BG and others: Distance running improves fitness in asthmatic children without pulmonary complications or changes in exercise-induced bronchospasm, *Pediatrics* 71:147, 1983.

60. Nixon PA and others: Oxygen supplementation during exercise in cystic fibrosis, *Am Rev Respir Dis* 142:807, 1990.

61. O'Donohue WJ: Oxygen conserving devices, *Respiratory Care* 32:37, 1987.

62. Orenstein DM and others: Exercise conditioning and cardiopulmonary fitness in cystic fibrosis, *Chest* 80:392, 1981.

63. Orenstein DM and others: Exercise conditioning in children with asthma, *J Pediatr* 106:556, 1985.

64. Pardy RL and others: Inspiratory muscle training compared with physiotherapy in patients with chronic airflow limitation, *Am Rev Respir Dis* 123:421, 1981.

65. Pardy RL and others: The effects of inspiratory muscle training on exercise performance in chronic airflow limitation, *Am Rev Respir Dis* 123:426, 1981.

66. Pollock ML, Wilmore JH, and Fox SM: *Exercise in health and disease,* Philadelphia, 1984, WB Saunders Co.

67. Rochester D and Arora N: Respiratory muscle failure, *Med Clin North Am* 67:573, 1983.

68. Schneerson JM: The cardiorespiratory response to exercise in thoracic scoliosis, *Thorax* 33:457, 1978.

69. Severinghaus JW and Naifeh KH: Accuracy of response of six pulse oximeters to profound hypoxia, *Anesthesiology* 67:551, 1987.

70. Skinner JS and others: Comparison of continuous and intermittent tests for determining maximal oxygen intake in children, *Acta Paediat Scand* 217(suppl):24, 1971.

71. Soffer M and others: Conservation of oxygen supply using a reservoir nasal cannula in hypoxemic patients at rest and during exercise, *Chest* 88:663, 1985.

72. Sonne LJ and Davis JA: Increased exercise performance in patients with severe COPD following inspiratory resistive training, *Chest* 83:436, 1982.

73. Spiro SG and others: An analysis of the physiologic strain of submaximal exercise in patients with chronic obstructive bronchitis, *Thorax* 30:415, 1975.

74. Spock A and Stedman DJ: Psychological characteristics of children with cystic fibrosis, *NC Med J* 27:426, 1966.

75. Stark RD, Gambles SA, and Chatterjee SS: An exercise test to assess clinical dyspnoea: estimation of reproducibility and sensitivity, *Br J Chest* 76:269, 1982.

76. Strauss GD and others: Variable weight training in cystic fibrosis, *Chest* 92:273, 1987.

77. Tiep BL: New portable oxygen devices, *Respiratory Care* 32:106, 1987.

78. Tiep BL and others: A new pendant storage conserving nasal cannula, *Chest* 87:381, 1985.

79. Tropauer A, Franz MN, and Dilgard VW: Psychological aspects of the care of children with cystic fibrosis, *Am J Dis Child* 119:424, 1970.

80. Vergeret J and others: Expiratory muscles and exercise limitation in patients with chronic obstructive pulmonary disease, *Respiration* 52:181, 1987.

81. Versteegh FGA and others: Relationship between pulmonary function, $O_2$ saturation during sleep and exercise, and exercise responses in children with cystic fibrosis, *Adv Cardiol* 35:151, 1986.

82. Wasserman K and Whipp BJ: Exercise physiology in health and disease, *Am Rev Respir Dis* 112:219, 1975.

83. Webb JG, Kiess MC, and CC Chan-Yan: Malnutrition and the heart, *Can Med Assoc J* 135:753, 1986.

84. Zach MS, Oberwaldner B, and Hausler F: Cystic fibrosis: physical exercise versus chest physiotherapy, *Arch Dis Child* 57:587, 1982.

85. Zach MS, Purrer B, and Oberwaldner B: Effect of swimming on forced expiration and sputum clearance in cystic fibrosis, *Lancet* 2:1201, 1981.

# CHAPTER 28

# Respiratory Rehabilitation of the Patient with a Spinal Cord Injury

*Jane L. Wetzel, Brenda Rae Lunsford, Margery J. Peterson, and Susan Enriquez Alvarez*

## CLASSIFICATION OF PATIENTS AND THEIR PROBLEMS

Patients with an injury to the spinal cord vary in levels of breathing function as a result of the degree of neurological deficit. For patients with significant impairment, respiratory rehabilitation is an important determinant in achieving their maximal functional level. The problem of decreased ventilation occurs as a result of (1) decreased strength, (2) decreased thoracic mobility, and (3) inadequate bronchial hygiene.

Ventilation, or the ability to circulate new air, is a result of inspiration and expiration.[15] In normal persons the muscles of inspiration are the diaphragm, neck accessory muscles, and external intercostals.[1,8,22] Expiration is passive.

Forced expiration or coughing is produced primarily by contraction of the abdominal muscles.[19]

### Mechanics of breathing

The diaphragm is a dome-shaped muscle, innervated by nerve roots C3 to C5, that originates from the dorsal aspect of the xiphoid process, the last six ribs, and the bodies and transverse processes of the upper thoracic vertebrae. The fibers insert onto a central tendon.[13] When the diaphragm contracts, it descends on the abdominal contents increasing intraabdominal pressure. The descending action of the diaphragm and the contraction of external intercostal muscles cause an increase in vertical and horizontal dimensions of the thoracic cavity, thereby decreasing intrathoracic pressure. This change creates a pressure gradient and air moves into the lungs.[2,5,17] Although the diaphragm and external intercostals are responsible for this inspiratory action during normal quiet breathing, neck accessory muscles assist in elevation and stabilization of the ribs during stressful inspiration.[17]

To produce adequate ventilation the muscles of breathing must overcome the elasticity of the soft tissues of the thorax. According to Hooke's law, the property of a substance that deforms as a force is applied to it and returns to zero when the force is removed is that of elasticity. At the point of relaxed expiration, the soft tissues are in a resting position. When the muscles of inspiration contract, they produce a force that causes the thorax to change shape primarily by elevating the ribs. The force that allows the thorax to return to its original shape is the elasticity of the tissues. The change in inspiratory volume relative to the quantity of force generated by the inspiratory muscles describes the phenomenon of compliance.

The function of abdominal muscles in the upright position is to counter the increase in abdominal pressure created during the descent of the diaphragm.[8] Normal tone in the abdominal muscles maintains the intraabdominal pressure necessary to allow the diaphragm to return to its elevated resting position. This elevated position is necessary to provide for full excursion of the diaphragm during inspiration. Forced expiration is produced by active contraction of abdominal muscles during high levels of activity. The active contraction forces the diaphragm further up into the thoracic cavity and thus increases the intrathoracic pressure, forcing air out of the lungs. A cough is produced as a result of a deep inspiration and a quick, forceful contraction of the abdominal muscles.[9]

## Ventilatory reserve

There are two basic questions that need to be answered regarding the breathing ability of a patient with a spinal cord injury. First, is there adequate muscle strength for the patient to breathe without assistance from a mechanical ventilator? If the answer is yes, then what amount of ventilatory reserve does the patient have for activity? Ventilatory reserve is defined as the amount of vital capacity greater than the resting tidal volume. It is logical that the lower the level of spinal injury, that more muscles will be active and therefore the greater will be the ventilatory reserve.

Given the segmental innervation to the muscles of breathing, patients can be grouped or classified according to the muscles that are preserved. For example, the patient who is neurologically intact at the level of C6 will have normal innervation and function of both the sternocleidomastoid and the diaphragm.[11,13,16] Patients in this group will have minimal ventilatory reserve for high levels of physical activity (Fig. 28-1). The concept of ventilatory reserve has become especially important today when many spinal cord–injured patients have a diagnosis of an incomplete injury. For example, the patient with a complete lesion at C6 will not have obvious ventilatory restrictions to activity because he or she has so little innervated skeletal muscle with which to challenge his respiratory system. On the other hand, the patient with an incomplete lesion at C6 who has skeletal muscles preserved that allow him or her to walk will have severe restrictions because of the ability to challenge a limited ventilatory reserve.

The muscles of ventilation work together to produce the most efficient method for moving air through the lungs. Each of the muscles in normal breathing is responsible for producing specific motions that contribute to the whole respiratory process. The paralysis of selected muscles causes deficiencies in ventilation, thoracic mobility, and cough function. The severity of these problems is best seen after a detailed evaluation is completed.

## EVALUATION

The respiratory evaluation is an important phase of assessing the functional potential of the spinal cord–injured patient. The evaluation allows the physical therapist to

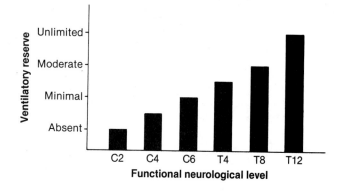

**Fig. 28-1.** Patient classification.

determine any problems with ventilation, thoracic mobility, or cough. In addition to a thorough review of a patient's medical history, the following must be included in a clinical examination to assure a complete assessment:

Respiratory rate
Breathing pattern
Chest mobility
Vital capacity
Muscle strength
Cough effectiveness

## Medical information

All available information regarding each patient's respiratory function must be thoroughly reviewed before the therapist begins any physical evaluation. The therapist should interview the patient and consult with appropriate personnel to be sure facts are complete and sensible. A record of past medical history and a recent report of the physician's physical exam are primary sources of information. Information concerning diagnosis, present symptoms, problems, and physical findings are assessed. The following areas are important:

1. Past history of lung disease (obstructive, restrictive?)
2. Present history of pulmonary complications
    a. Chest radiographs
    b. Thoracic surgeries
3. Laboratory findings
    a. Arterial blood gas values
    b. Pulmonary function tests
4. Respiratory equipment
    a. Type of respirator
    b. Tracheostomy equipment
    c. Suctioning equipment
    d. Intermittent positive-pressure unit
5. Chest trauma
    a. Rib fractures
    b. Pleural effusion
    c. Pneumothorax-hemopneumothorax
    d. Contusions to lung or heart
    e. Trauma to diaphragm

6. Prior treatment for complications
    a. Medical
    b. Other (e.g., respiratory therapy, postural drainage)

Once a thorough review of the patient's medical history has been completed, a detailed evaluation can begin.

## Respiratory rate

The function of evaluating rate is to determine the efficiency of respiratory muscles to ventilate the patient.[2] The respiratory rate for normal adults is 12 to 16 cycles per minute.[22] One cycle is measured from the beginning of inspiration through the end of expiration. When assessing the respiratory rate, the therapist counts the number of cycles completed in 1 minute with the patient at rest, breathing quietly. The therapist begins counting when it is evident that the patient is not aware of any evaluation. Results are accurate only when the patient does not know his or her breathing frequency is being monitored. Anxiety and attempts by the patient to "make an effort" will alter the rate.

If the diaphragm in the spinal cord–injured patient is normal and there are no other complications, there should be no change in respiratory rate related to muscle paralysis, since the diaphragm alone can maintain normal tidal volume. However, the patient with a high cervical lesion may have a diaphragm that functions less than normally. Here, an increase in respiratory rate may be substituted to maintain adequate ventilation and prevent hypoventilation, which may occur because of inadequate respiratory muscle strength. Hypoventilation must be identified as soon as possible so that the patient can be properly managed. If muscle weakness is the problem, ventilatory assistance may be needed, as discussed in the next section.

## Breathing pattern

Muscle groups in the neck, chest, abdomen, and diaphragm contribute to normal breathing.[1,8] When the breathing pattern is assessed, four points are used to describe the degree to which each muscle group is responsible for displacement of thoracic and epigastric regions during full inspiration. The normal breathing pattern consists of thoracic expansion and epigastric rise. Thoracic expansion results from the contraction of the external intercostal muscles, and the epigastric rise is the result of diaphragm contraction. With normal breathing the patient would have a "2-diaphragm, 2-chest" pattern, since both thoracic and epigastric regions are moving equally.

Evaluation of the breathing pattern is an observational assessment of how the patient gets air into the lungs. When the therapist inspects the breathing pattern, the patient should be in the supine position, breathing quietly. The displacement of thoracic and epigastric areas at full inspiration should be compared with their position at the end of expiration (Fig. 28-2). Palpation is then used to complement the findings of observation. One hand is placed on the midthoracic region while the other hand rests on the epigastric region (Fig. 28-3). The dominance of one area or another may be palpated to confirm observational assessment.

When chest movement is questionable, the hands can determine the amount of thoracic excursion. The therapist places the hands, with the fingers spread and the thumbs together, over the middle of the sternum, 1 inch below the top of the rib cage. At full inspiration the therapist observes the amount of separation between the thumbs. The greater the distance between the thumbs, the more the chest muscles are acting to expand the chest.

The patient with a low cervical spinal cord lesion will have chest muscle paralysis and isolated diaphragm movement. The epigastric rise is dominant, and there is no chest expansion. Since the diaphragm is the only active muscle, the patient is considered a diaphragmatic breather. This pattern should be recorded as "4-diaphragm" to indicate the dominance of the diaphragm (Fig. 28-4).

Patients with a high cervical spinal cord lesion will have chest muscle paralysis and diaphragmatic weakness. When the breathing pattern is observed, there will be an epigastric rise (diaphragm contraction) with no chest expansion. However, contraction of the neck muscles will be evident by their prominence. This breathing pattern is variable. It may be "1-neck, 3-diaphragm," or "2-neck, 2-diaphragm," or even "3-neck, 1-diaphragm" depending on the degree of displacement in the upper chest and epigastric region.

Patients with midthoracic lesions may show signs of active contraction of some intercostal muscles. The chest rises slightly along with the epigastric rise, which is still dominant. These patients are primarily diaphragmatic breathers but are assisting inspiration with chest muscles. Therefore the pattern is "3-diaphragm, 1-chest." Patients with lower thoracic injuries approach the normal breathing pattern because the intercostal muscles are working more effectively to raise the chest.

## Chest mobility

During maximum inhalation, the thorax is enlarged in three diameters—transverse, anteroposterior, and vertical.[21] The movements of the thorax in the anteroposterior and transverse diameters are inseparable. The intercostal muscles lie between the ribs and consist of short, parallel fibers that run oblique to the ribs. The external intercostals lift the ribs to increase the size of the thoracic cavity. The internal intercostals depress the ribs and decrease the size of the thoracic cavity. There are changes in both the transverse and anteroposterior diameters.[11,16,17] The vertical thoracic dimension is enlarged through diaphragm contraction. Chest expansion refers to the change in the transverse and anteroposterior dimensions and therefore relates to intercostal function.[21]

Chest expansion is defined as the circumferential change

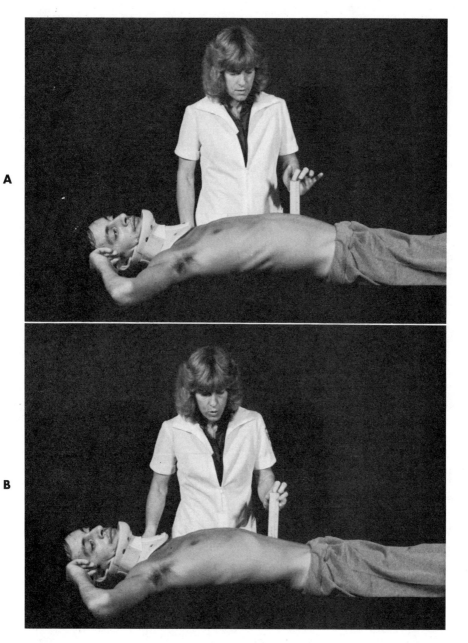

**Fig. 28-2. A,** Patient shown at maximum inspiratory effort. **B,** Same patient at his maximal expiration. Notice ruler, which shows 1½-inch change.

from full forced expiration to maximum inspiration.[6] With the patient supine, measurement of circumferences are taken with a soft, flexible tape measure at both the xiphoid process and the axilla. The xiphoid process is easy to palpate and thus assures that measurements can be accurately reproduced (Fig. 28-5). A reading is also taken at the axilla to monitor the expansion of the upper thorax.

Normal chest expansion when measured at the axilla in 20- to 30-year-old women is 3¼ inches ± ¼ inch.[6] The chest and the epigastric region rise simultaneously. The diaphragm and the intercostals work together to expand the chest by increasing the volume of air brought into the lungs.

Patients with low thoracic spinal cord lesions have initially decreased chest expansion. All muscles of respiration are fully innervated, but clinically the expansion measurements at the xiphoid level average 2 or 2½ inches. This decrease in inspiratory muscle activity shortly after the injury is transient, and normal values for chest expansion recur by the end of an intensive rehabilitation program.

Midthoracic injuries result in weakness of intercostal and abdominal muscles. This weakness contributes to a decrease in chest expansion. Since the abdominal muscles are weak or absent, forced expiration may not be complete. With

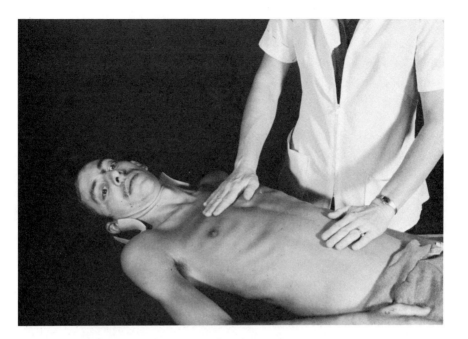

**Fig. 28-3.** Hand placement during resting-breathing evaluation.

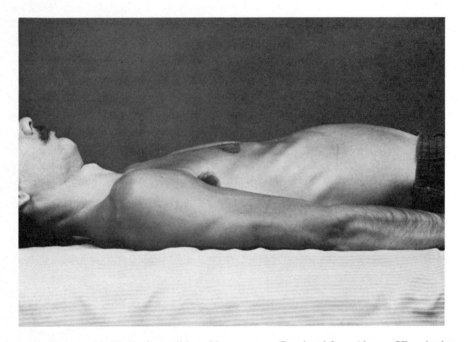

**Fig. 28-4.** Patient with "4-diaphragm" breathing pattern. (Reprinted from Alvarez SE and others: *Phys Ther* 61:1737, 1980, with the permission of the American Physical Therapy Association.)

intercostal muscle weakness, chest expansion is diminished.

The degree of epigastric rise increases as the diaphragm dominates inspiration. A patient with an upper thoracic spinal injury may have larger chest-expansion measurements at the axilla than at the xiphoid process because only the upper intercostal muscles are working. Patients with cervical spine injury breathe without the assistance of intercostal muscles and rely totally on the diaphragm. Their

chest-expansion measurements are between ½ inch and −½ inch.

The negative values for chest expansion are attributable to contraction of the diaphragm without intercostal muscle opposition. The rib cage is retracted as the diaphragm descends during inspiration.[2,4,17] This is called "paradoxical movement," since the action works to decrease chest expansion. Anatomically, lung size increases, but only in the

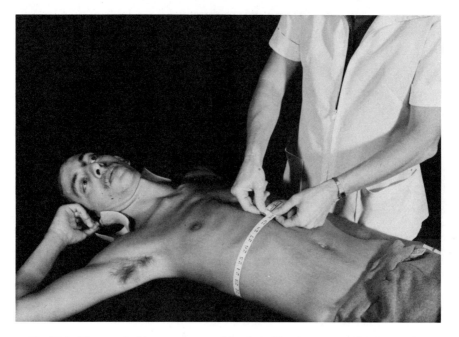

**Fig. 28-5.** Placement of tape measure and hand position to measure chest expansion.

vertical dimension. The transverse and anteroposterior dimensions are not increased, and chest expansion values of $-\frac{1}{4}$ inch to $-\frac{1}{2}$ inch are common.

Chest expansion should be measured throughout the respiratory program. Increases occur as intercostal muscle strength or chest mobility improve.

### Vital capacity

Vital capacity is the total of the inspiratory reserve volume, the tidal volume, and the expiratory reserve volume.[9] Vital capacity is defined as the maximum amount of air that can be expelled from the lungs after peak inspiration.[5,9] The vital capacity is an objective and reproducible measurement that is used to monitor changes in respiratory muscle strength and chest mobility. Because of its ease of use and portability, a hand-held spirometer is a convenient instrument for measuring vital capacity within the clinical setting. The volume on most spirometers is recorded in cubic centimeters or milliliters. Each set of patient values is matched to predicted normal values in regard to sex and height.[5,8,18] The patient's volume is compared with the normal to establish a percentage. Shortly after the injury vital capacity measurements are commonly less than 25% of normal in high cervical injuries and as high as 80% for low thoracic injuries.[2]

Frequent vital capacity determinations throughout the treatment program are important to document progress. As strengthening and chest stretching techniques are employed, the ventilatory ability improves. Because the vital capacity is tested repeatedly, a standard method for its measurement is necessary. Testing should be done with the patient supine. The patient inhales maximally, places the lips fully around the mouthpiece, and then exhales maximally. On exhalation

there must be no leakage around the mouth or through the nose. The patient must leave the lips around the mouthpiece until having completely and forcefully exhaled one full breath (Fig. 28-6). This sequence is repeated three times, and the best value is recorded.

Caution must be taken when measuring vital capacity. Trunk spasticity, which does not reflect the volitional and functional ability of the respiratory muscles, may invalidate the testing procedure. Rib fractures, chest trauma, and other medical complications will also alter values.

The patient with an injury at the C3 to C5 levels may have a vital capacity equal to the tidal volume.[9] The patient tested in the supine position should be retested in the sitting position. The effects of gravity in the upright posture act to decrease vital capacity in the absence of abdominal support. The sternocleidomastoid muscles assist strongly with inspiration in patients who have no reserve volume (i.e., vital capacity equals tidal volume). Although these patients have adequate vital capacity for ventilation, the lack of reserve volume does not permit adequate ventilation during activity. Although vital capacity is an important measure of breathing ability, the muscles that contribute to the breathing pattern and their strength ultimately determine a patient's breathing efficiency. For example, two patients with equal vital capacities may be using different muscles for ventilation. A patient who uses neck muscles will have less endurance than a patient using the diaphragm because ventilation with the diaphragm uses less metabolic energy than ventilation with the neck muscles.[1]

### Muscle evaluation

The purpose of evaluating the muscles of respiration is to identify specific areas of muscle weakness and to be aware

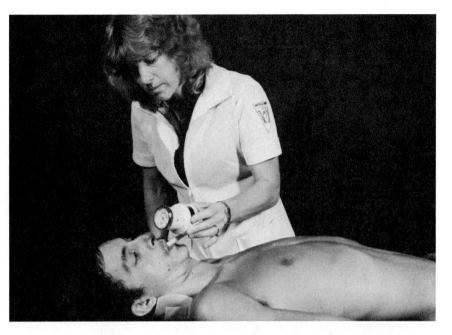

**Fig. 28-6.** Recording vital capacity using hand-held spirometer.

of potential restriction of activity because of ventilation problems. This evaluation is best accomplished by specific muscle testing of the diaphragm, sternocleidomastoid, intercostal, and abdominal muscles. A grade should be separately designated for each group. The neck and truck muscles can be evaluated with standard muscle-testing procedures.[11,16] The strength evaluation of the diaphragm and intercostals involves interpretation of the total neurological picture, component respiratory evaluations, and observational techniques. These evaluations provide a measure of the contributions of each muscle to the total ventilatory effort.

**Diaphragm.** The strength of the diaphragm is best evaluated with the patient in the supine position. The epigastric rise should be examined first for visible action resulting from diaphragm movement. The patient is observed by placing one's eyes level with his or her trunk, which is then viewed from the side. Recall that the patient with normal chest and diaphragm movement has a 2-chest, 2-diaphragm breathing pattern. If the patient has no assistance from the intercostal muscles and has a 4-diaphragm breathing pattern, the epigastric rise should have full excursion with maximum inspiration (Fig. 28-4). This response indicates at least a "fair" muscle grade for the diaphragm. Since the diaphragm is innervated by roots C3 to C5, a patient with an injury at the C6 level and lower is expected to have normal innervation to the diaphragm. The diaphragm in Fig. 28-7 is less than "fair," since it does not complete normal excursion. The sensory dermatomes and muscles in the C3 to C5 nerve distribution must be evaluated to assist in the interpretation of diaphragm strength. For example, the patient with C5 quadriplegia or higher may not have a full epigastric rise.

Once diaphragm strength is graded at least "fair," resistance is applied. This is done with the patient in the supine position. The therapist's hands are placed over the epigastric area with fingers spread. The patient is asked to inhale while maximal manual resistance is applied. If the patient has complete epigastric rise and holds the contraction firmly against this resistance, the diaphragm is "good" in grade. It is important to remember that the presence of spasticity or volitional control of the abdominal muscles may invalidate this test.

Diaphragmatic weakness designated as "less than fair" must be studied critically because its contraction may be difficult to palpate. To help confirm an independent finding of a weak diaphragm, the therapist should test the upper extremity muscles and the sensory dermatomes that are supplied by the same nerve roots as the diaphragm (sternocleidomastoid, C3; upper trapezius, C4; deltoid, C5). If weakness or sensory impairment is found, the suspicion of diaphragm weakness is reinforced. The patient with C4 quadriplegia who is able to breathe without continuous mechanical ventilation may be using the sternocleidomastoid muscles to assist with breathing. The therapist should observe the patient breathing quietly in the supine position. Active contraction of sternocleidomastoid will indicate a weak diaphragm. The patient should be reevaluated for the use of the sternocleidomastoid muscles for ventilation in the sitting position and again during activity. Active contraction of the sternocleidomastoid in C4 or C5 quadriplegics indicates that diaphragm function alone is too weak to maintain tidal volume. When the patient demonstrates neck breathing, the tidal volume and vital capacity are often found to be equal. Therefore the diaphragm is "poor."

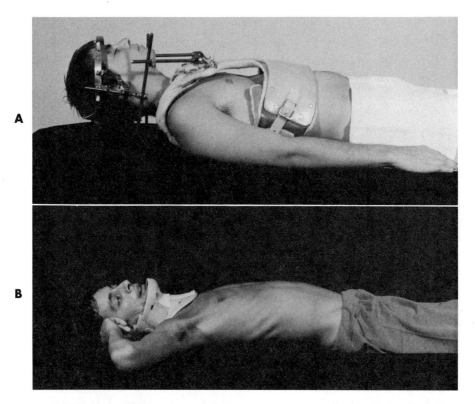

**Fig. 28-7. A,** Patient with fully innervated diaphragm showing normal epigastric rise. **B,** Patient with C5 level of injury showing less than full epigastric rise.

The patient with a "poor" diaphragm may have additional diagnostic evaluations to document its excursion. Fluoroscopy or radiographs are used to provide an objective record of diaphragm excursion.[7,8,20]

Fluoroscopy is a cineradiograph of the patient's breathing. As the patient breathes quietly, the excursion of the diaphragm is recorded on film. During quiet breathing the normal excursion should be at least one intercostal space (1.5 cm). During deep inspiration the diaphragm will descend at least three to four intercostal spaces (7 to 13 cm).[20,21] The diaphragm is dome-shaped on observation but is always higher on the right side because of displacement by the liver[7] (Fig. 28-8). A poor or worse diaphragm is evident when the movement is the same for deep breathing and quiet breathing.

When no contraction of the diaphragm during quiet breathing is observed with fluoroscopy, the therapist should ask the patient to sniff. This action will cause a contraction if the diaphragm is innervated. Fluoroscopy will also help determine an imbalance in diaphragm strength when right and left excursion is unequal.[7] Radiographs, used as an alternative to fluoroscopy, are less expensive and do not expose the patient to as much radiation. One radiograph is taken at full inhalation, and one is taken at full exhalation. One picture is superimposed on the other, the anatomical landmarks are matched, and the excursion of the diaphragm is determined by a count of the intercostal spaces as is done with fluoroscopy.

Patients with a high quadriplegia will have weak or paralyzed diaphragms and require ventilators. It is important to learn about the ventilator and emergency care procedures before evaluation of the condition of the diaphragm. The therapist must establish good rapport with the patient and become familiar with the hospital's philosophy and protocol for phasing quadriplegic patients from the ventilator. The therapist should consult with the appropriate personnel and together determine the patient's tolerance to being detached from the ventilator. Initially the patient can usually tolerate 10 seconds comfortably. Tolerance is increased gradually to approximately 1 minute without ventilatory assistance.

Once the patient is comfortably detached from the respirator, diaphragm strength can be assessed. Litten's sign is useful when one is confirming the presence of an extremely weak diaphragm. Litten's sign, which is more easily observed on thin patients, is a rippling action that may be seen between the intercostal spaces of the eighth, ninth, and tenth ribs.[2,8] Litten's sign can be seen only when there is total paralysis of the intercostal muscles. As the diaphragm contracts and pulls from its costal origins, there is a decrease in intrathoracic pressure causing the intercostal spaces to move inward so that this rippling action results (Fig. 28-9).

**Sternocleidomastoid muscles.** The sternocleidomastoid muscle is the primary muscle of substitution in patients with diaphragm weakness. This muscle assists with inspiration during quiet breathing when the tidal volume is inadequate. With the head fixed, either by its own weight or if the patient

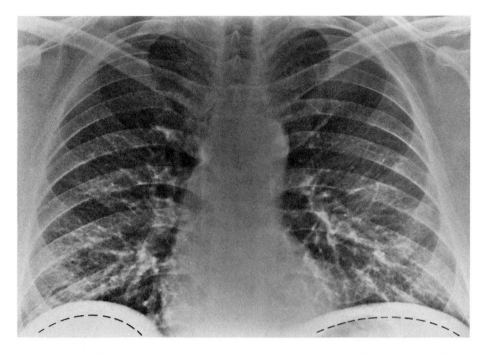

**Fig. 28-8.** Cineradiograph showing patient with a "poor" diaphragm. *Dotted line,* Position of diaphragm at maximal inspiratory effort. Excursion is less than one full intercostal space.

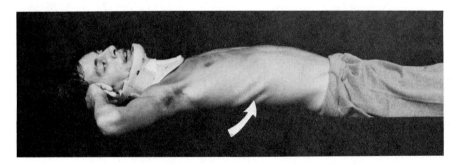

**Fig. 28-9.** Litten's sign demonstrated as patient initiates inspiratory effort.

is in a halo vest, the bilateral action of the sternocleidomastoids is to pull the chest toward the head. It is important to have complete knowledge of the condition of the spine before muscle testing of the sternocleidomastoids. The therapist should consult the physician regarding the stability of the spine and any contraindications to positioning or moving the head and neck for testing.

Initially the patient may be positioned supine in traction or in a halo vest, each of which restricts movement of the head and neck. In this case palpation of the sternocleidomastoid should be done. The patient should be asked to perform an isometric contraction to determine the presence or absence of contraction of the muscle (Fig. 28-10).

After the patient has received medical clearance for active motion, muscle strength up to "fair" can be tested. It is not uncommon to find limitation in neck range of motion because of bony block, fusion, or wiring. After the flexion range has been identified passively, the therapist asks the patient to produce the same movement actively. If pain at the fracture site occurs during motion, the physician should be consulted. Once the patient is cleared for resistive testing, the strength of the sternocleidomastoid can be determined by standard muscle-testing procedures.

**Abdominal and intercostal muscles.** Standard muscle-testing techniques are used when one is evaluating trunk musculature.[11,16] Precautions should be discussed with the physician before testing. Because motion of the spine is often contraindicated, the evaluation of abdominal muscle strength may be limited to palpation. When no palpable contraction is obtained, one way to verify that the abdominal muscles are absent (0) is to ask the patient to cough.

Intercostal strength is evaluated indirectly by measurement of chest expansion. Taking measurements at both the axillary and xiphoid landmarks provides a comparison of upper and lower intercostal function. Again, external intercostals lift the rib cage up and out during inspiration, whereas the internal intercostals depress the ribs pulling down and in during forced expiration. Observation

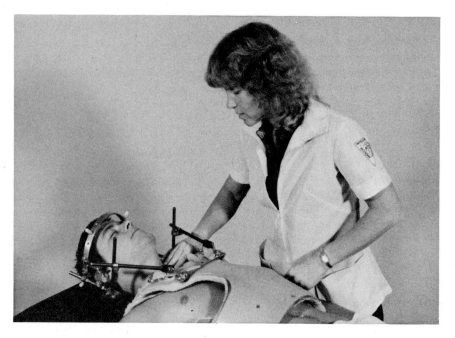

**Fig. 28-10.** Muscle testing can be done even when patient is in a halo vest. An isometric contraction gives information about presence and quality of muscle belly.

of these actions is important to confirm intercostal contraction.

### Cough evaluation

In the normal person, forced expiration is accomplished primarily by the abdominal muscles, which are assisted by the internal intercostals.[19] These muscles function to clear secretions or foreign material adequately from the lungs. Initially, when one is evaluating a cough, it is best to have the patient in the supine position. Both hands of the evaluator are placed on the patient's abdominal muscles to palpate for their contraction. The patient is asked to cough.

The cough is graded as "functional," "weak-functional," or "nonfunctional." The degree of expulsive force is determined by sound and the ability to cough twice within one exhalation. A functional cough will be loud and vigorous. The patient will be able to repeat at least two vigorous expulsive forces in one exhalation. Such a patient can adequately clear secretions. A weak-functional cough is less vigorous, and the sound is soft. The patient is not able to repeat the cough effort more than once during exhalation. The weak-functional cough is adequate only for clearing the throat. A nonfunctional cough has no expulsive force and sounds like a sigh or clearing the throat.

Clinically, patients can change cough function by altering volume or by eliciting abdominal spasticity. Patients without abdominal muscles and vital capacities over 2000 cc generally have a weak-functional cough. These patients are able to compensate for the lack of abdominal muscles by using a quick volume release to generate force.

## OBJECTIVES AND TREATMENT METHODS

The appropriate treatment plan is designed to increase ventilation by improving any or all of these three parameters:

Strength
Chest mobility
Bronchial hygiene

Attention to all of these parameters is critical. However, the interpretation of the respiratory evaluation may indicate that one parameter contributes more significantly to the problem of decreased ventilation. The respiratory evaluation is integrated with the complete physical therapy evaluation and pertinent evaluations noted by other members of the medical team.

Once treatment priorities have been established, the therapist must select the best mode to improve strength, chest mobility, and bronchial hygiene. As various treatment programs are employed, the patient should be periodically reevaluated for changes in ventilation. As medical conditions change, the treatment program must also be altered to meet the patient's needs. This section on treatment method will provide guidelines for planning and progressing a patient through respiratory rehabilitation.

### Diaphragm strengthening

Diaphragm strengthening can be beneficial to any patient with a less than normal vital capacity. Thus all patients with cervical and high thoracic injuries are candidates for intensive diaphragm strengthening. Patients with lower thoracic or lumbar injuries will have decreased vital capacity caused by limited activity. These patients, until they are

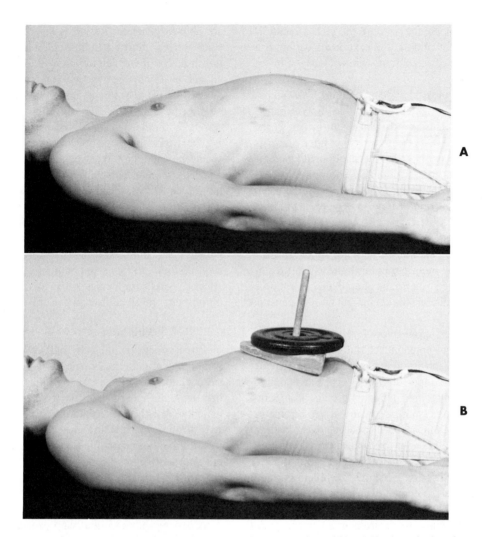

**Fig. 28-11. A,** Patient shown with full epigastric rise. **B,** Same patient still has full epigastric rise after diaphragm weights are added.

again fully active, will benefit from a daily routine of coughing, deep-breathing, and abdominal exercises. The strength of the diaphragm is used to determine which treatment technique to employ. Patients with fair+ strength of the diaphragm are candidates for progressive resistive exercise, whereas patients who have less strength must use active or active-assistive exercise techniques.

When beginning a strengthening program, the therapist should examine the methods of resisting the movement of the diaphragm. The resistance should allow the diaphragm to contract through its full range so that ventilation in the normal breathing pattern for the patient is not altered. Some methods of progressive resistive exercise are (1) weights, (2) manual, (3) positioning, and (4) incentive inspiratory spirometry.

Progressive resistive exercise by use of weights is one method for diaphragm strengthening. To begin, the patient is placed in the supine position. The diaphragm weight pan is placed over the epigastric region.[1,12] To allow full excursion

of the diaphragm, the weight pan should not rest on the ribs. The degree of epigastric rise should remain the same after weight is added (Fig. 28-11). The patient with a neurologically intact diaphragm can usually start comfortably with 5 pounds. The amount of weight used as resistance is appropriate when the patient can maintain a coordinated, unaltered breathing pattern for 15 minutes. The therapist should observe the degree of epigastric rise and the sternocleidomastoid muscles as well. If the patient begins to use the sternocleidomastoid muscles or noticeably alters his or her breathing pattern, the weight should be decreased.[1]

The benefits of progressive resistive exercise for strengthening the diaphragm are documented by increased weight and increased vital capacity. Progressive resistive exercise should continue with weights added* until the patient's

---

* As weights are added, there is an increased tendency for the weights to topple off the patient at full inspiration. Precaution should be taken to protect the patient's arms.

strength reaches a plateau: that is, until the vital capacity is the same from one evaluation to the next or the patient can tolerate the challenge of full activity without early signs of fatigue.

When the diaphragm is "fair," caution must be taken not to overchallenge and fatigue a muscle that must function throughout the day. Unlike other skeletal muscles, the diaphragm has no total rest period to recover after exercise. It is important to recognize that the abdominal contents provide resistance to the diaphragm. The force of the abdominal contents acting against the diaphragm increases in the head-down position. At a 15-degree head-down incline, this force is equivalent to 10 pounds.[12] Resistive strengthening by altering patient position or by diaphragm weights must be done carefully so as not to fatigue the diaphragm. Inspiratory muscle training by resistive breathing is being investigated as a means of applying appropriate workloads that will challenge the diaphragm without causing fatigue.[14]

Incentive spirometers provide low-level resistive training while minimizing the potential of fatigue to the diaphragm.[3,14] Incentive spirometers are designed to provide the patient with visual input during a sustained maximal inspiration. These devices are commonly used in postoperative conditions. The major purpose of incentive spirometry is to prevent alveolar collapse. Its secondary goals of cough stimulation and strengthening of weakened respiratory muscles are important benefits to spinal cord–injured patients. The visual input of balls rising in chambers, colored lights, or dials reflects the degree of inspiratory effort.

The supine position for the patient is preferred when the patient is instructed in incentive spirometry. A patient with a fair+ diaphragm will tolerate a level position, whereas one with only a fair diaphragm will do better in a 10- to 15-degree head-up incline. This incline will be adequate to relieve the resistance applied by the abdominal contents. Once positioned correctly, the patient should take four slow, easy breaths, letting the air out normally between the first three. After the fourth breath the air should flow out slowly until the patient cannot exhale any more. The patient should place the spirometer mouthpiece in the mouth and form a tight seal. The patient then takes a slow, deep breath in through the mouthpiece to elicit the visual input, that is, balls rising, lights, and so on. The visual cue should be maintained as long as possible. The patient should then remove the mouthpiece and relax. The procedure should be repeated eight to ten times and three or four sessions per day.

Presently, commercially available incentive spirometers are used to increase inspiratory effort by increasing the volume of inspired air. As more volume is inspired, resistance is increased only minimally as a result of increased flow through the spirometer. Primarily this is an active inspiratory exercise. New incentive spirometers that measure mouth pressure are under development. Mouth pressure reflects the amount of force the respiratory muscles

are able to generate. Resistive inspiratory muscle training studies have shown that muscular force passes a certain threshold beyond which fatigue will eventually result.[14] The advent of clinically practical mouth pressure–measuring devices should provide therapists with an objective means of monitoring appropriate low-level resistive training to inspiratory muscles.

The patient with "poor" diaphragm strength requires special consideration with regard to position and fatigue. As with any skeletal muscle when strength is poor, the arc of motion is decreased and fatigue occurs rapidly. The patient with a poor diaphragm may breathe comfortably when resting supine. There is no epigastric rise, since the diaphragm cannot displace the abdominal contents. This patient rests comfortably when supine because the ventilatory requirement for resting supine is less than for upright. An active-assistive device, such as the pneumobelt (exhalation belt), must be used when this patient begins to sit.

### Abdominal supports

**Pneumobelt (exhalation belt).** When a patient has a weak diaphragm, he or she will automatically use the sternocleidomastoid to assist in the breathing effort when breathing difficulty or distress is encountered. Since the patient with a high cervical injury (C3 and C4) gains function only through use of head and neck motions that are required to use a mouthstick or chin-controlled electric wheelchair, it is important to preserve use of the neck muscles for these activities. Therefore the following sequence and technique are recommended for the patient with a weak diaphragm that fatigues rapidly.

A patient with an initial vital capacity between 500 and 1000 cc, when upright, is a candidate for a pneumobelt. A pneumobelt is a corset with an inflatable bladder (Fig. 28-12). The pneumobelt corsets come in small, medium, and large sizes with an inserted inflatable bladder placed over the abdominal area. It is easy to modify most custom corsets to accommodate both the inflatable bladder and varying sizes of patients. The bladder is connected to a respirator by a hose. The respirator must be able to deliver positive pressure with an easily adjustable respiratory rate. The rate and pressure should be set according to the person's comfort. It may be necessary to increase the pressure setting when the activity level increases.

The mechanics of the pneumobelt depends on the passive descent of the abdominal contents; thus it must be used when the patient is sitting. Inflation of the bladder causes exhalation by pushing the abdominal contents in and up and thereby pushing the diaphragm into optimal ascended position within the thoracic cavity. Inspiration becomes active assistive, since the abdominal contents will passively descend as pressure is decreased in the bladder.

Fatigue of the diaphragm can occur even when a patient uses the pneumobelt. Monitoring the patient for fatigue is done by observation for contraction of the sternocleidomas-

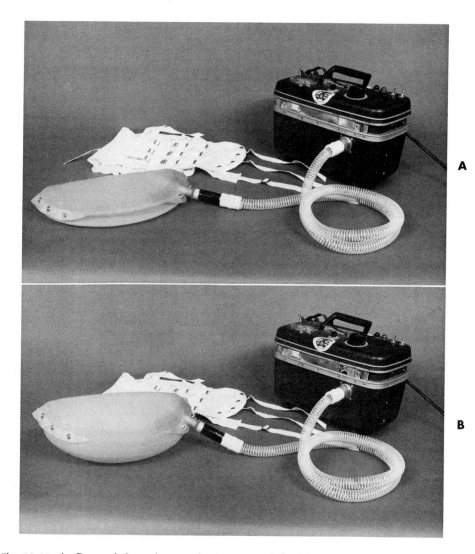

**Fig. 28-12. A,** Pneumobelt equipment shown: corset, inflatable bladder, and positive-pressure respirator. **B,** Pneumobelt equipment with bladder inflated. (Reprinted from Alvarez SE and others: *Phys Ther* 61:1737, 1980, with the permission of the American Physical Therapy Association.)

toid muscles during inspiration. When these contractions occur, the therapist should increase the pressure delivered to the bladder to see if the additional assistance to the diaphragm will decrease the patient's need for the sternocleidomastoids. If these neck muscles are still being used, the patient should be put back to bed. It is important to continue daily attempts to increase tolerance of the upright posture with the pneumobelt.

When the patient has been upright on an active program for 8 hours without signs of fatigue, the therapist should begin phasing the patient off the pneumobelt. First, the pressure in the bladder is decreased with the patient sitting but not active. If the sternocleidomastoid muscles are used, the therapist increases the pressure to the lowest level that will prevent their use. Once the patient can tolerate decreased pressure during inactive periods, the therapist can begin decreasing pressure when the patient is active, that is, while

using chin control or during mouthstick training. The therapist continues to watch for signs of fatigue. Eventually, the patient will tolerate less pressure assistance from the bladder and should begin to wear the pneumobelt only for activity sessions but should wear a corset during quiet periods. The ability of the patient to breathe without a pneumobelt will always depend on fatigue. Some patients develop adequate combined strength of their diaphragm and neck muscles to permit using the neck to assist breathing, without equipment, in addition to functional activities. However, caution is encouraged to not "phase" from equipment too early, or potential muscle strength may be lost.

**Corsets.** If the abdominal muscles are weak, that is, "less than fair," a patient will have a diaphragm that rests in the descended position because of the gravitational pull of the abdominal contents. The excursion of the diaphragm during contraction is therefore decreased (Fig. 28-13, *B*). A decrease in inspiratory reserve volume is the result of this decreased mechanical advantage of the diaphragm. A corset helps compensate for weak or absent abdominal muscles by supporting the abdominal contents and displaces the diaphragm to a higher resting position in the thoracic cavity.[2,17] The range of diaphragm descent during contraction is therefore increased and inspiratory reserve volume also increases (Fig. 28-13, *C*).

The corset should lie just over the last two floating ribs and cover the iliac crest over the anterior superior iliac spines (ASIS) bilaterally. If the corset is applied too high, it will restrict chest mobility and will not support the abdomen. The lower buckles should be tighter than the upper ones. The appropriate fit is firm yet allows a hand to be slipped between the abdomen and the corset on the upper border with the patient supine (Fig. 28-14).

Corsets may be custom fit or stock sized. Patients with partial innervation to abdominal muscles may get sufficient support with a stock elastic binder. The elastic component must be evaluated for effective support of the abdominal contents. Corsets with metal stays should be used with caution because skin pressure problems can result from them.

Another indication for using a corset is the patient who becomes hypotensive when sitting. When this happens, the therapist should be sure to check the corset for snug fitting. Well-fitting elastic stockings are also necessary to prevent blood pooling.

Careful monitoring of blood pressure and heart rate will provide information to evaluate the effectiveness of the corset in prevention of blood pooling caused by splanchnic nerve dysfunction.

The patient may discontinue use of the corset if the diaphragm strength improves or abdominal tone increases to adequately support the abdominal contents. Before discontinuing the use of the corset, the patient should be tested in bed with and without the corset while positioned with the head up and the body inclined 45°. The therapist evaluates vital capacity and breathing pattern and checks the vital signs. When there is no difference without the corset in ease of breathing and vital signs, the patient may be progressed to more upright postures. Eventually the patient will tolerate the sitting position without a corset with legs down.

It is especially important to test the patient in the upright position without a corset before he or she bathes. Bathing any spinal cord–injured patient will alter his or her blood pressure through changes in body temperature, which increase circulation to the periphery and increase splanchnic blood pooling. If the patient cannot tolerate 8 hours upright without a corset, an extra corset should be available to wear while bathing. The patient will ventilate better, and the body can more effectively adapt to temperature changes when the corset is worn.

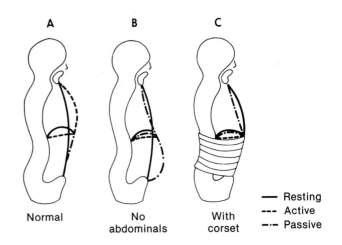

Fig. 28-13. A, Normal diaphragm positioning. B, Weak abdominal muscles allow diaphragm to rest in descended position because of gravitational pull. C, Corset application allows optimal positioning of the diaphragm. (Reprinted from Alvarez SE and others: *Phys Ther* 61:1737, 1980, with the permission of the American Physical Therapy Association.)

### Chest mobility

A strengthening program means little if joint mobility is not maintained. Just as a knee-flexion contracture can impair walking, so can chest wall tightness prevent strong respiratory muscles from effectively ventilating the patient. The treatment technique selected will depend on the muscles the patient has functioning and any contraindications. Deep breathing, positive pressure, manual chest stretching, airshift manuever, and glossopharyngeal breathing are methods for improving chest mobility. Specific chest mobilization treatment is indicated in patients whose chest-expansion range with deep breathing is less than 2 inches.

**Deep breathing.** Patients who have a voluntary chest-expansion range of greater than 2 inches should be encouraged to take a few deep breaths followed by a cough every day they are confined to bed. Even though they may have no specific neurological deficit that affects their breathing, the effects of long-term bed rest are generally debilitating. Deep breathing is a good way to avoid possible complications later.

**Air shifts.** For the patient with good chest wall range of motion and intercostal weakness, chest mobility may be maintained by doing an air shift. Technically, an air shift is a maneuver in which a person inhales maximally, closes the glottis, and relaxes the diaphragm to allow the air to shift from the lower to upper part of the thorax. Once successfully mastered, air shifts can potentially expand the chest from ½ inch to 2 inches. To maintain chest mobility, patients are instructed to do air shifts every day.

To teach the patient an air shift, the therapist should place one hand on the patient's epigastric area and one hand on the upper part of the chest. The therapist next asks the patient to

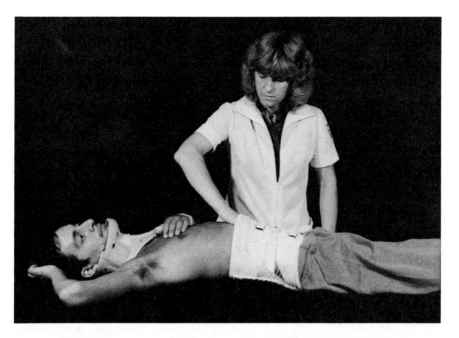

**Fig. 28-14.** A proper fitting corset will not restrict chest expansion.

take a deep breath and hold it and then tells the patient to suck the stomach in and move the air to the upper part of the chest (Fig. 28-15). If the technique is done correctly, the therapist's top hand should rise. The therapist should be aware that the patient may hyperventilate and become dizzy.

Not only is an air-shift maneuver beneficial to the range of motion to the rib cage, it is also a method of learning laryngeal control as a precursor to glossopharyngeal breathing. To be sure that the patient is closing the glottis and not holding air in the lips or cheeks, the therapist can have the patient hold his or her breath with the mouth open. An air shift should be reproducible when the mouth is open.

**Positive pressure.** Routine intermittent positive pressure (RIPP) is a method of mobilizing the chest.[9] The patient with poor chest wall range of motion and intercostal weakness may benefit from this method of chest mobilization. However, for the patient with a complete cervical injury and no potential intercostal muscle activity, use of this technique is not warranted. Unlike intermittent positive-pressure breathing (IPPB), there are no medications administered. For RIPP to be administered, the patient should wear a corset or cloth binder. The abdominal restriction will ensure that the volume of air expands the chest in the transverse plane. The rate and pressure of air delivered to the patient are controlled by the therapist. Initial treatment begins at 5 cm $H_2O$ and progresses to a maximum of 40 cm $H_2O$ pressure.

A positive-pressure respirator can be adapted to provide passive chest stretching. The respirator hose is attached to a tubular Y fitting. A sterilized mouthpiece tubing is inserted over one end of the Y. The therapist controls the air entering the lungs by moving a thumb over the air-relief valve. When the air-relief valve is completely closed off, the pressure, as set on the machine, is delivered to the patient (Fig. 28-16).

When beginning RIPP treatment, the therapist explains the purpose of the treatment to the patient. As the patient breathes normally, the therapist observes the respiratory rate and begins to move air into the lungs slowly at the same rate that the patient is breathing (Fig. 28-17). The treatment consists of three sets of five breaths, with an increase of the pressure, if tolerated, at each set. After each set, the therapist asks the patient if the pressure and rate are comfortable. Pressure is increased in 5 cm increments. The pressure reading at the end of inspiration is observed. If it does not reach the pressure dialed, there is a leak in the system. Either the patient is leaking air through the mouth or nose, the hoses are not connected completely, or the therapist does not have the thumb completely over the air-relief valve.

The RIPP treatment progresses from 1 week to 6 weeks depending on the patient. The patient is progressed to 40 cm $H_2O$, which has been found to be a safe limit for chest expansion.[9] The treatment is discontinued once the patient is active and has learned an air-shift maneuver to maintain chest mobility. If for some reason the patient is placed on bed rest, positive pressure would be reinitiated.

RIPP is contraindicated in patients with chronic obstructive airway disease, since fragile airways may rupture under high pressure. RIPP is also contraindicated in patients who have respiratory infections producing secretions. Positive pressure delays healing in patients who have an unhealed tracheostoma. Patients with rib fractures may not tolerate RIPP, although they may tolerate careful manual stretching to the opposite side.

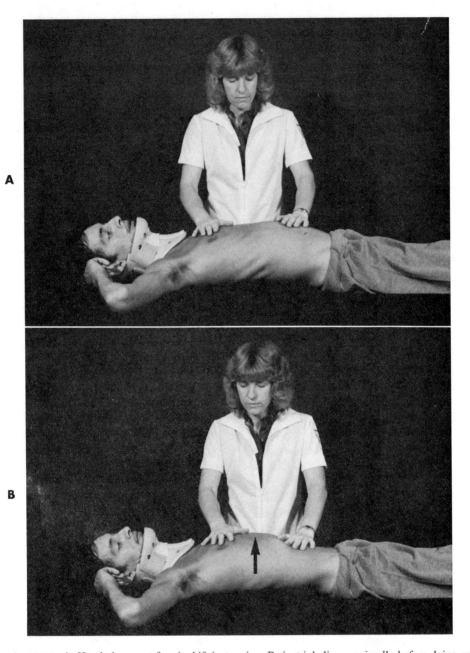

**Fig. 28-15. A,** Hand placement for air-shift instruction. Patient inhaling maximally before doing an air shift. **B,** Same patient having completed the air-shift maneuver. Notice increase in chest expansion.

**Manual chest stretching.** Manual chest stretching is done segmentally to lower, middle, and upper thoracic areas. This technique is often used in conjunction with the air-shift maneuver to maintain chest wall mobility for the patient with poor intercostal strength. The patient is supine while the therapist applies the treatment technique illustrated in Fig. 28-18.

The therapist can employ any technique that is safe and creates movement at the costal articulation. Stretching once a day maintains the range of motion; stretching more often helps increase the range.

**Glossopharyngeal breathing (GPB).** Glossopharyngeal breathing (GPB) is a substitute method of increasing the volume of air that is brought into the lungs.[10] Glossopharyngeal breathing is a specialized technique that is difficult to teach and learn. However, an individual with respiratory muscle paralysis may be well served to learn this method since it can be lifesaving. It is indicated to increase chest expansion for any patient with intercostal muscle paralysis or weakness. Glossopharyngeal breathing is an alternate method of breathing for respirator-dependent patients. Also any patient with loss of abdominal muscles can use

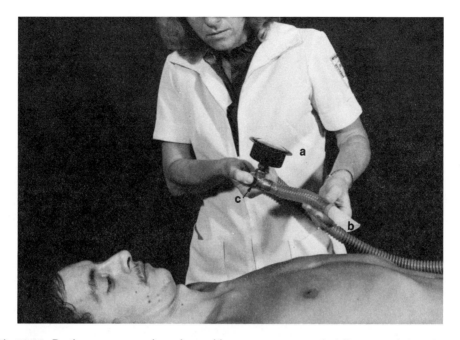

**Fig. 28-16.** Postive-pressure respirator hose with pressure gauge, *a;* air-delivery mouthpiece, *b;* and air-relief valve, *c.*

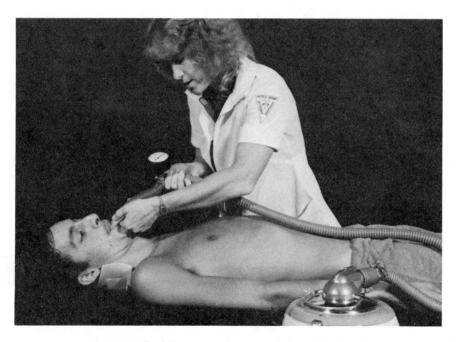

**Fig. 28-17.** Positive-pressure treatment being administered.

## Bronchial hygiene

glossopharyngeal breathing to improve the force of coughing. The patient learns to force air into the lungs by using the mouth, tongue, and pharyngeal and laryngeal structures (Fig. 28-19). The use of glossopharyngeal breathing can increase lung volumes by as much as 1000 cc. The details of this technique are beyond the scope of this chapter.[10]

Clear airways must be maintained in all spinal cord–injured patients. Patients with cervical or high thoracic injuries can develop respiratory infections rapidly if bronchial hygiene is not adequate. Once respiratory complications develop they are difficult to clear. Thus these patients are

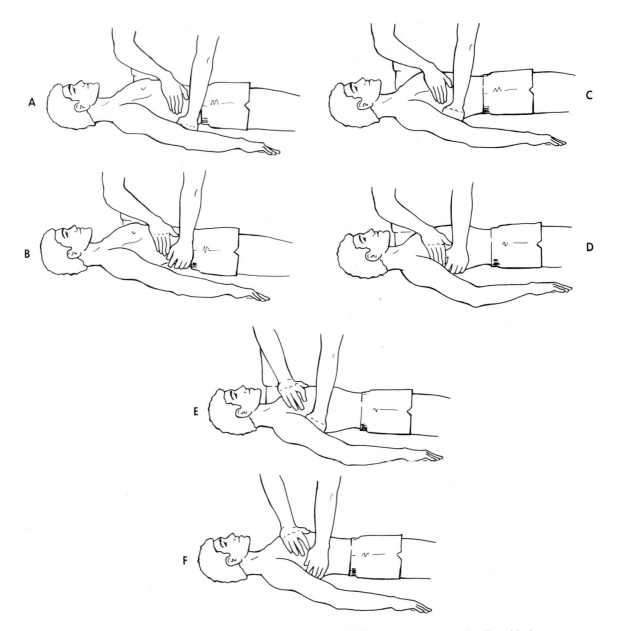

**Fig. 28-18. A,** Beginning position for manual chest stretch: One hand is placed under ribs with tips of fingers on transverse processes. Place other hand on top of chest with heel of lateral palmar area to the sternum. **B,** Stretching motion: Bring hands together in wringing motion. Do not force on edge of ribs or sternum. Distribute pressure over entire surface of your hands. Progress up the chest, alternating hands. **C,** Beginning position. **D,** Stretching motion. To effectively range the upper chest (**E** and **F**), top hand should be just inferior to the clavicle in the last position. **E,** Beginning position. **F,** Stretching motion.

taught bronchial hygiene as a preventive measure and as necessary to treat pulmonary infections. The patient depends on help from the family or attendant to provide manual cough assistance, postural drainage, and suctioning. A good preventive program will reduce the likelihood of respiratory complications, decrease the need for IPPB treatments, and diminish the need for mechanical ventilation.

**Coughing.** A patient with absent or weak abdominal muscles can attain adequate coughing power for clearing secretions. The following techniques may be employed—manual cough, self-manual cough, glossopharyngeal breathing, or, for patients with very low vital capacities, alternating use of the manual ventilation bag with abdominal compression.

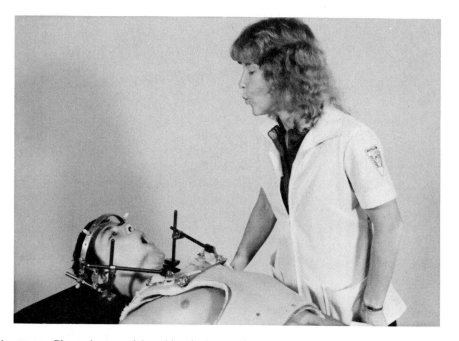

**Fig. 28-19.** Glossopharyngeal breathing is learned by imitation. Therapist is demonstrating this breathing technique for patient.

**Manual cough.** The manual cough is an excellent method for clearing secretions and maintaining good bronchial hygiene. It is appropriate for any patient with weak cough force as a result of abdominal muscle weakness or paralysis.

The technique is a maneuver similar to the Heimlich maneuver taught in cardiopulmonary resuscitation classes. The patient is in the supine position while the assister places his or her hands over the patient's epigastric area. The heel of one hand is placed over the abdomen, between the umbilicus and 2 inches below the xiphoid process. The other hand is placed on top of the first with the fingers spread apart so that both hands can interlock. The patient is instructed to take as deep a breath as possible and then attempt to cough. The assister pushes down and inward toward the head, compressing the abdomen quickly but with caution to avoid pressure against the xiphoid process. The force of the push should be timed carefully with the patient's attempt to cough (Fig. 28-20).

Manual coughing technique may be done with the patient prone, sitting, or standing; however, in other than the supine position, it is hard to get the mechanical advantage to correctly compress the abdomen. Any means of cautious but quick abdominal compressions is acceptable during emergency situations when the patient's airway is blocked.

Patients with high cervical injuries find it difficult to achieve sufficient lung volume to produce a forceful manual cough. The vital capacities in these patients are below 1000 cc. To assist the coughing maneuver, one must increase the inspiratory volume either with effective glossopharyngeal breathing (GPB) or with positive-pressure apparatus. For patients who have not been taught GPB, the manual ventilation bag is used for lung inflation just before a manual cough. These patients will have a tracheostomy and may be able to spend some time detached from the respirator. The ventilation bag is attached with a tracheostomy adapter. The therapist should be sure the adapter fits the tracheostomy tube. As the patient inhales, the bag is compressed manually to provide additional inspiratory volume. The bag is then removed. The patient should try to hold the air briefly by closing the glottis so that the therapist can effectively assist. Quickly the therapist places the hands on the abdomen and signals the patient to cough as the abdomen is compressed. This technique may be repeated until secretions are adequately cleared.

**Self-manual cough.** Self-manual cough can be taught with the patient in the supine or sitting position. A patient with full upper extremity function can lock the hands together across the epigastric region and push in diagonally toward the head while attempting to cough. Patients with injuries as high as C6 can learn self-manual cough in the sitting position by throwing their arms across the epigastric area and falling forward in time with the cough attempt. Coughing force can be improved in the patient with quadriplegia by placement of a pillow on the lap to increase abdominal compression. GPB will also improve cough force.

**Postural drainage.** For most patients with paraplegia standard postural drainage positions may be used. Patients with higher injuries may have difficulty breathing in positions that restrict the movement of the diaphragm. All

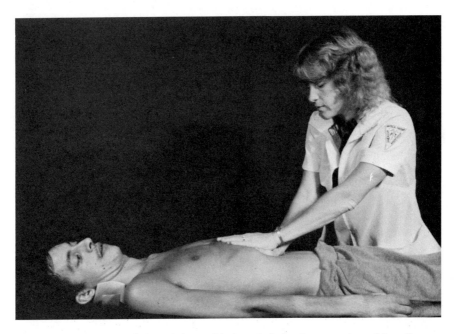

Fig. 28-20. Manual cough technique with therapist's hands one on top of the other.

patients must be positioned carefully when there is spinal instability. Auscultation of the chest for adventitious breath sounds should be done to determine the particular lobes of the lungs that require drainage. The appropriate positions for postural drainage should be selected based on the lobes that require drainage.

Patients with diaphragmatic weakness may not tolerate the Trendelenburg position, since this places the weight of the abdominal contents on the diaphragm. Even patients with a "good" diaphragm may have difficulty tolerating this position, which increases the burden of moving air through the resistance of secretion-filled airways. Upright positions of angles greater than 30 degrees will also increase the demand on the diaphragm. A corset may be necessary in this position. Side-lying positions for posterior segments of the upper lobes require a one-fourth turn onto the chest with the arm over a pillow. This semiprone position should be modified to keep pillows from restricting diaphragm movement.

**Suctioning.** Suctioning is indicated along with postural drainage when there is excessive mucous accumulation in the lungs. The patient with quadriplegia commonly needs to be suctioned because of poor cough function. The therapist should suction these patients before breathing reeducation or GPB lessons to assure clear airways. The therapist should also be aware of emergency procedures for patients in respiratory distress.

The condition of the tracheostomy may be acute or chronic. The acute form of a tracheostomy condition is most vulnerable to infection for the first 8 weeks. Therefore sterile techniques for suctioning are mandatory. Any patient with known bradycardia should be carefully monitored during suctioning. Suctioning may stimulate the vagus nerve and will further decrease the heart rate. The patient with the chronic form of a tracheostomy condition may be suctioned by use of clean techniques. Portable suction units may accompany the patient to the physical therapy department. Everyone working with the patient should be instructed in suctioning procedures. Patients with paraplegia can learn to suction themselves; however, patients with high spinal cord injuries will usually depend on family or attendant for suctioning at home.

### Emergency considerations for respirator-dependent patients

It is important to know adequate emergency procedures in the event of power failure or respirator equipment malfunction. Essential information to gather before treatment of any respirator-dependent patient includes knowing the patient's abilities, the equipment, and the secondary systems available. The therapist should be skilled in artificial respiration techniques. The patient's ability to breathe without the respirator can be lifesaving in an emergency. Patients who have sustained a C1 or C2 quadriplegia have no diaphragm function but may be able to use glossopharyngeal breathing if the tracheostomy is plugged. The therapist should know the endurance of the patient for glossopharyngeal breathing. Patients with weak inspiratory musculature may be able to continue breathing for extended periods of time when detached from the respirator. In the event of a power failure, it is important to identify those patients who require immediate attention.

Familiarity with the equipment can also be lifesaving. The therapist should know the type of respirator—that is,

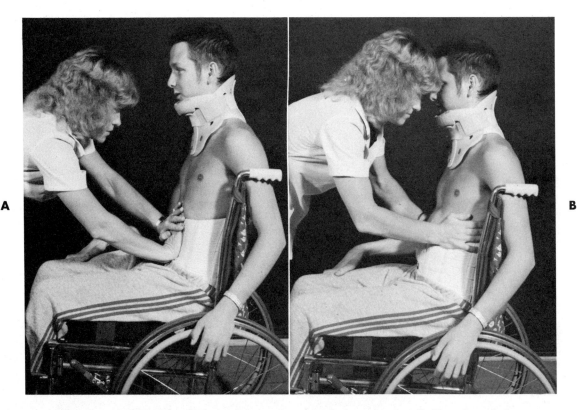

**Fig. 28-21. A,** Manual ventilation technique using abdominal compression. **B,** Manual ventilation using hands on either side of ribs.

positive or negative pressure, volume or pressure ventilator and learn how to ventilate the patient manually. Some respirators will have a hand pump. The pump attachment should be readily available, and the therapist should know how to assemble it quickly. If there is no manual pump mechanism for the respirator, alternative methods for manual ventilation can be sought. The manual ventilation bag is primarily used. This bag should go with the patient to all appointments and always be kept within reach of the patient. The therapist should know the size of the tracheostomy tube and have the tracheostomy adapters within easy reach.

Each facility should have a preestablished procedure for power failure emergencies. It is advisable to know the philosophy of the facility in the event of life-threatening emergencies. Many facilities will have secondary systems for electrical power operated by an alternate generator. Electrical outlets powered by this generator should be easily recognizable. When there are no alternatives—that is, electrical back-up, manual pump, or manual ventilation bag—and the patient has no time off the respirator, the therapist must use artificial ventilation.

Artificial ventilation is done by mouth or manually. Therefore when using mouth-to-nose, the therapist closes off both the tracheostomy and the mouth. If mouth-to-mouth is used, the nose and tracheostomy are closed off. When doing mouth-to-tracheostomy, the therapist closes off the mouth and nose. Manual ventilation is less efficient, is extremely

fatiguing for the person delivering the care, and is used only when mouth breathing is not practical. There are many techniques for manual ventilation; however, abdominal compressions, similar to manual cough, are most readily applied with the patient in any position (Fig. 28-21). An alternative technique is to place the hands laterally on the rib cage with one hand on either side of the lower half of the chest. The ribs are pushed down and released suddenly, using a normal breathing rate with the patient assisting inspiration if possible.

## DISCHARGE PLANNING

Preparation for discharge includes a good bronchial hygiene program that will prevent pulmonary complications. The patient should be performing deep breathing with airshifts or glossopharyngeal breathing, or both, daily. If chest expansion is less than 2 inches, the family should be instructed in manual chest-stretching techniques. Daily coughing to prevent an accumulation of secretions in the lungs is necessary at home. The patient and the family should demonstrate the ability to make the cough functionally productive, either with manual assistance or by compensation with increased volume.

The family should be taught how to do postural drainage and manual coughing and be able to recognize the indications for both. Increase in mucus, respiratory infection, and history of pulmonary complications are indications for cough assistance or postural drainage, or both. The therapist should emphasize the importance of immediate action by the family whenever the patient has even the slightest increase in respiratory symptoms. If the patient has a history of chronic respiratory infections, IPPB equipment should be provided in the home. The therapist should instruct the family in the use of IPPB equipment. IPPB treatments should be administered 30 minutes before postural drainage.

Family members can be taught how to auscultate for significant breath sounds. The family should be instructed about drainage positions that have been most productive and advised about the frequency of the treatment (three or four times a day as necessary when the patient is productive). Once in the morning to clear nightly mucous accumulation and once at night are good frequencies to suggest when planning a preventive program.

A patient using a ventilator can go home if the family environment is supportive. Full evaluation of the home setting should be done to aid the patient and family in planning adaptations that will be necessary for the respirator-dependent patient to return home. Any ventilator-dependent patient should have either a gasoline-powered emergency generator or a backup system with batteries at home. The family will have to become competent in the operation and maintenance of the equipment and all emergency procedures. Important to successful discharge with this type of patient is family experience with the patient and equipment at home.

---

## CASE 1 ▾ Young Man with C5 Fracture

Bill is a 20-year-old man who was injured April 9, 1977, while diving into a river. He sustained a C5 vertebral teardrop fracture with slight posterior displacement. He was placed in Crutchfield tongs with reduction of the fracture. The third day of his admission to the acute care facility he contracted pneumonia and was placed on a volume-limited respirator. Within 3 weeks the tongs were removed, and he was placed in a halo vest so that he could be mobilized to a rehabilitation center.

The initial physical therapy evaluation (see chart on p. 602) showed a functional neurological level of C4 quadriplegia. Clinically the patient had a nonfunctional cough and a breathing pattern of 1-neck, 3-diaphragm. The strength of the diaphragm was considered "poor" as demonstrated by an incomplete epigastric rise. The strength of the deltoids bilaterally was consistent with the finding of a weak diaphragm.

Because of recurrent episodes of pneumonia, the first treatment ordered by the physician was postural drainage with sterile suctioning procedures. On fluoroscopy examination the patient was observed to have slight movement of the diaphragm on the right with an excursion of one intercostal space for the diaphragm on the left. His vital capacity was 500 cc. When Bill could tolerate 20 minutes off the ventilator, special attention was paid to his diaphragm function.

Once Bill had confidence in the physical therapist, the therapist began treatment by inclining the bed to 15° before removing Bill from the ventilator. This slightly upright position decreased the force required to move the abdominal contents when the patient inhaled. A large mirror was attached over Bill's bed to allow him to view both the neck muscles and epigastric area. The therapist verified the diaphragm contraction by placing the fingers slightly under the edge of the sixth, seventh, and eighth ribs. Bill was instructed to take a deep breath in an attempt to increase the epigastric rise. While he viewed this movement in the mirror, he could also see if he was using any neck muscles. The therapist could palpate to evaluate the patient's attempt to use the diaphragm. Bill gradually increased his epigastric rise and ceased using his sternocleidomastoid muscles. The treatment time was kept to 5-minute sessions three times a day to avoid fatigue to the diaphragm. Bill felt comfortable off the ventilator for 5 minutes and could concentrate on diaphragmatic breathing.

Diaphragm strength was improving; however, Bill was also instructed in isometric neck strengthening to prevent disuse atrophy while in the halo vest. The sigh mechanism on the respirator was used to maintain chest mobility, since routine intermittent positive pressure could not be done with pneumonia present, and manual chest stretching was limited by the halo vest.

One month after admission Bill was able to tolerate being without the respirator for several hours during the day. In preparation for early wheelchair activities, thigh-high compression stockings and a corset with a bladder for a pneumobelt were ordered. The purpose of stockings was to aid venous return, and the purpose of the corset was to both reduce splanchnic blood pooling and improve the mechanics of the diaphragm. Once sitting, he was trained in the use of the pneumobelt to prevent diaphragm fatigue.

Two weeks later Bill's vital capacity had increased from 500 to 600 cc. The lung congestion had subsided, and he was able

**CASE 1        Young Man with C5 Fracture—cont'd**

to give full attention to learning glossopharyngeal breathing (GPB). Bill's vital capacity with GPB was 700 cc, which increased the force of his cough. Inspiratory incentive spirometry was added to the diaphragm-strengthening program, since the epigastric rise was still incomplete. Postural drainage, IPPB, and manual cough were decreased in frequency. Eight weeks after admission his epigastric rise reached full excursion. Vital capacity was now 900 cc without GPB and 1100 cc with GPB.

Two months after the injury the halo vest was removed and a cervical orthosis was placed on the patient. Manual resistive exercise was initiated to provide a mild challenge to the diaphragm. Diaphragm weights could not be used, since epigastric rise against external resistance was not full. Bill continued with incentive inspiratory spirometry and learned to do air shifts while the tracheostomy was plugged. Because he was no longer congested, the therapists could initiate routine intermittent positive-pressure breathing through the tracheostomy with a tracheostomy adapter. The RIPP treatments were started at a pressure of 20 cm $H_2O$. Bill initially tolerated three sets of five breaths each. Meanwhile, he was improving his upright time to 3 hours and tolerating brief periods of mouthstick training from the occupational therapy staff while respiration was assisted by the pneumobelt.

Three months after admission Bill was tolerating a plugged tracheostomy through the night as well as during the day. The tracheostomy sizes were gradually decreased, and finally he was decannulated. Routine intermittent positive pressure and daily use of air-shift maneuvers were discontinued to allow healing of the open tracheostomy site. Manual chest stretching was substituted for continued chest mobilization. The patient continued to have difficulty increasing upright and activity tolerance even when using the pneumobelt. His upright tolerance increased from 3 to 4 hours. Strengthening techniques for the diaphragm were limited to incentive spirometry and gentle manual resistance. By the end of the fourth month, the tracheostoma had healed, and so routine intermittent positive-pressure and air-shift maneuvers were reinitiated. At that point the vital capacity was 1200 cc, or 23% of normal. Chest-expansion measurements were taken: without an air-shift maneuver expansion was zero; with an air-shift expansion was 1/4 inch. He continued short periods of mouthstick training and an active-assistive upper extremity exercise program with occupational therapy. His upper extremities had now improved enough to allow him to use hand controls to operate the electric wheelchair.

In September, 5 months after his admission and a plateau period of 6 weeks, Bill began to again improve his respiratory function. His vital capacity was 1300 cc, or 29% of normal. The patient had full epigastric rise without fatigue. The strengthening program for the diaphragm was altered to begin

lifting the weight of the weight pan (1/4 lb). Upright activity tolerance increased to 6 hours, and Bill was able to decrease use of the pneumobelt gradually. He controlled his electric wheelchair well and began feeding and personal hygiene training. Even though the diaphragm strength improved to "fair," as evidenced by a full epigastric rise, Bill still required the pneumobelt, since his tolerance for being upright decreased during activity and his diaphragm would fatigue. His active chest expansion began to show negative values as the diaphragm strength increased. However, with an air shift he improved from $-1/2$-inch chest expansion to $+3/4$ inch (xiphoid).

By mid-October, 6 months after his admission, Bill's vital capacity was 41% of normal (1800 cc) and 45% of normal (2000 cc) with GPB. He was completely phased out from the pneumobelt. Routine intermittent positive pressure progressed to higher pressures (30-35-40 cm $H_2O$). The patient progressed over the next 2 weeks from 1/4 to 2 1/2-pound weights to the diaphragm. He plateaued at this point, since his vital capacity was 2700 cc and the same from one evaluation to the next. Bill was now close to discharge. He was using the electric wheelchair with a left-hand control and had tried manual propulsion of a wheelchair with hand rim projections. He was independent with feeding and personal hygiene after being set up. The family was instructed in postural drainage and manual cough. They were instructed to do preventive postural drainage to the left lower lobe because Bill's pneumonia history had primarily involved that segment of the lung.

On discharge evaluation, Bill had the following:

**RESPIRATORY EVALUATION**

| BREATHING PATTERN | | DIAPHRAGM FUNCTION |
|---|---|---|
| Neck | 0 | |
| Diaphragm | 4 | |
| Chest | 0 | *Fair +* |
| Abdomen | 0 | |

| COUGH | | VC | VC GPB |
|---|---|---|---|
| Functional | | | |
| Weak funct. | **X** | cc *2700* | cc *3500* |
| Nonfunct. | | % *66* | % *85* |

| CHEST EXPANSION (Xiphoid) | |
|---|---|
| Active | *– 1/2 inch* |
| With airshift | *2 inches* |

The strength of the diaphragm improved to fair +. Chest expansion was $-1/2$ inch because of the paradoxical movement of the strong diaphragm but was +2 inches with an air shift. Bill could produce a weak functional cough by compensating with increased volume produced by glossopharyngeal breathing.

## Physical therapy evaluation done on 4/21/89

### SENSATION EVALUATION:

Key: N = NORMAL
− = IMPAIRED
O = ABSENT

| | SUPERFICIAL PAIN | | LIGHT TOUCH | |
|---|---|---|---|---|
| | R | L | R | L |
| C2 | N | N | N | N |
| 3 | N | N | | |
| 4 | N | N | | |
| 5 | N | − | ↓ | |
| 6 | O | O | O | ↓ |
| 7 | | | | O |
| 8 | | | | |
| T1 | | | | |
| 2 | | | | |
| 4 | | | | |
| 5 | | | | |
| 8 | | | | |
| 10 | | | | |
| 12 | | | | |
| L1 | | | | |
| 2 | | | | |
| 3 | | | | |
| 4 | | | | |
| 5 | | | | |
| S1 | | | | |
| 2 | | | | |
| 3 | | | | |
| 4 | ↓ | ↓ | ↓ | ↓ |

### PROPRIOCEPTION

| | R | L |
|---|---|---|
| SHOULDER | N | N |
| ELBOW | − | O |
| WRIST | − | O |
| THUMB | − | O |
| HIP | O | O |
| KNEE | ↓ | ↓ |
| ANKLE | | |
| GREAT TOE | ↓ | ↓ |

76S611 RD241 (R4-79)

### RESPIRATORY EVALUATION:

BREATHING PATTERN
Neck — 1
Diaph. — 3
Chest — 0
Abdom. — 0

DIAPHRAGM FUNCTION

*Poor*

Volume ventilator setting
Tidal volume—650 cc

| COUGH | Functional | | VC | VC GPB |
|---|---|---|---|---|
| | Weak funct. | | cc *(MA-1)* | cc |
| | Nonfunct. | | % | % |

CHEST EXP. Active
(Xiphoid) c̄ Air shift — *NT 2° to halo*

### NECK STRENGTH

Sternocleidomastoids—present*
Extensors—present*

### TRUNK MUSCLES

Abdominals—0
Back extensors—0

### UPPER EXTREMITY STRENGTH

| | R | L |
|---|---|---|
| Upper trapezius | P ↑ | P ↑ |
| Middeltoid | P ↑ | P ↑ |
| Anterior deltoid | P ↑ | P ↑ |
| Pectoralis (clavicular and sternal) | 0/0 | 0/0 |
| Biceps | P | P |
| Triceps | 0 | 0 |
| Wrist extensors (radial and ulnar) | T/0 | 0/0 |
| Wrist flexors (radial and ulnar) | 0/0 | 0/0 |
| Intrinsics | 0 | 0 |

### LOWER EXTREMITIES—0

*Isometric contraction is the only allowable motion.
*GPB,* Glossopharyngeal breathing.
*MA-1,* Trade name for a volume respirator.
*NT 2° to halo,* Not tested; secondary to the patient being in a halo vest.
P ↑ , Method of indicating minimal muscle grade when resistance is not allowed; arrow indicates that strength may be greater than given grade.
*VC,* Vital capacity.

## REFERENCES

1. Adkins HV: Improvement of breathing ability in children with respiratory muscle paralysis, *Phys Ther* 48:577, 1968.
2. Alvarez SE and others: Respiratory management of the adult patient with spinal cord injury, *Phys Ther* 61:1737, 1980.
3. Bartlett RH and others: Respiratory maneuvers to prevent postoperative pulmonary complications, *JAMA* 224:1017, 1973.
4. Bergofsky EH: Mechanisms for respiratory insufficiency after cervical cord injury: a source of alveolar hypoventilation, *Ann Intern Med* 61:435, 1964.
5. Canter HG: Practical pulmonary physiology, *GP* 35:104, 1967.
6. Carlson B: Normal chest excursion, *Phys Ther* 53:10, 1973.
7. Carter RE: Medical management of pulmonary complications of spinal cord injury, *Adv Neurol* 22:261, 1979.
8. Dail CW: Muscle breathing patterns, *Med Arts and Sci* 10:64, second quarter, 1956.
9. Dail CW: Respiratory aspects of rehabilitation in neuromuscular conditions, *Arch Phys Med Rehabil* 46:655, 1965.
10. Dail CW and others: *Glossopharyngeal breathing,* Downey, Calif, 1979, Professional Staff Association of the Rancho Los Amigos Hospital, Inc.
11. Daniels L and Worthingham C: *Muscle testing,* ed 4, Philadelphia, 1980, WB Saunders Co.
12. Gayrard P and others: The effects of abdominal weights on diaphragmatic position and excursion in man, *Clin Sci* 35:589, 1968.
13. Gray H: *Anatomy of the human body,* ed 29, Philadelphia, 1973, Lea & Febiger.
14. Gross D and others: The effect of training on strength and endurance of the diaphragm in quadriplegia, *Am J Med* 68:27, 1980.
15. Guralnik DB and Friend JA: *Webster's new world dictionary of the American language,* Cleveland, 1968, The World Publishing Co.
16. Kendall HO, Kendall FS, and Wadsworth GE: *Muscles,* ed 2, Baltimore, 1971, Williams & Wilkins.
17. Luce C: Respiratory muscle function in health and disease, *Chest* 81:82, 1982.
18. McMichan JC and others: Pulmonary dysfunction following traumatic quadriplegia—recognition, prevention, and treatment, *JAMA* 243:528, 1980.
19. Siebens AA and others: Cough following transection of spinal cord at C-6, *Arch Phys Med* 45:1, 1964.
20. Stone DJ and Keltz H: The effect of respiratory muscle dysfunction on pulmonary function, *Amer Rev Respir Dis* 88:621, 1964.
21. Wade OL: Movements of the thoracic cage and diaphragm in respiration, *J Appl Physiol* 124:193, 1954.
22. West JB: *Respiratory physiology,* Baltimore, 1974, Williams & Wilkins.

# Glossary

*abruptio placentae* Premature separation of the placenta from the uterus, which often leads to hemorrhage.

*adrenergic* Type of medication or receptor site that stimulates the sympathetic nervous system.

*adventitious sounds* Breath sounds not normally heard that can be superimposed over normal breath sounds, such as crackles and rhonchi.

*aerobic* Type of energy produced using oxygen.

*afterload* The workload applied to the heart during systole by the resistance of the systemic vasculature.

*allograft (homograft)* A tissue transplant between two humans who are not identical twins.

*alveolar macrophages* Defense cells within the lungs that engulf and digest foreign particles within the alveoli.

*alveolar proteinosis* A disorder in which plasma proteins, lipo-proteins, and other blood components accumulate in the pulmonary alveoli.

*alveolar ventilation* Amount of air that actually enters the alveolar region of the lungs to take part in gas exchange.

*alveolus* Smallest distal air sac involved in gas exchange.

*anaerobic* Type of energy produced without using oxygen.

*anastomosis* Surgical joining of two tubular structures, such as arteries.

*aneurysm* A large area of akinetic myocardium that bulges or balloons out when the heart contracts.

*angina pectoris* Severe chest pain caused by insufficient myocardial oxygen supply.

*angiography* Examination of the coronary arteries or other blood vessels by use of contrast medium and recording of flow on film.

*antibodies* A protective substance that plays a role in the immune response to foreign substances including microorganisms.

*antidysrhythmics* Medications that reduce the incidence and frequency of cardiac dysrhythmias, such as quinidine, procaineamide (Procan-SR), disopyramide phosphate (Norpace), and beta blockers.

*aortic stenosis* Abnormally constricted opening of the aortic valve.

*Apgar scores* 10-point scoring system to assess newborn status, usually performed at 1 and 5 minutes of life.

*apical* Referring to the apex or upper portions of the lung.

*aplastic anemia* Blood disorder characterized by lack of production of blood cells by the bone marrow.

*apnea* Lack of breathing.

*arteriovenous oxygen (a-$\bar{v}o_2$) difference* Arterial oxygen content minus central venous oxygen content.

*atelectasis* Alveolar collapse because of poor lung expansion or complete obstruction of an airway.

*atrial fibrillation or flutter* High-rate atrial dysrhythmias. Atrial fibrillation is characterized by the absence of clearly distinguishable P waves and an irregular ventricular response. Atrial flutter is characterized by a pattern of saw-toothed P waves with an atrial rate of 300 and a variable P wave to the ventricular response rate.

*auscultation* Listening with a stethoscope.

*azotemia* Retention of excessive amounts of nitrogenous materials in the blood commonly associated with renal failure.

*barotrauma* Pulmonary trauma associated with high levels of inspiratory pressure from a mechanical ventilator.

*basilar* Referring to the bases or lower portions of the lung.

*beta-adrenergic receptor–blocking medications (beta blockers)* Medications that inhibit the beta-adrenergic receptor–blocking activity of the autonomic nervous system, such as atenolol, nadolol (Corgard), propranolol hydrochloride (Inderal), and timolol hydrogen maleate (Blocadren).

*bronchiole* Small, distal airway.

   *respiratory bronchiole* Small, distal airway characterized by the appearance of alveoli within the airway wall.

   *terminal bronchiole* Smallest, most distal bronchiole with no obvious alveoli.

*bronchodilator* Medication that reduces bronchial smooth muscle spasm and thereby increases the size of the bronchial lumen.

*bronchopleural fistula* An abnormal connection between a bronchus and the pleural space.

*bronchoscopy* Inspection of a bronchus after passage of a rigid or flexible tube into the airway for either diagnostic or therapeutic procedures.

*bronchus* Larger, more central airways below the trachea characterized by cartilage plates, respiratory epithelium, and glandular elements.

*calcium antagonist medications* Medications used to control dysrhythmias, hypertension, and vasospasm, such as diltiazem (Cardiem, Cardizem, Dilzem), nifedipine (Procardia), and verapamil hydrochloride (Isoptin).

*cardiac catheterization* Specialized procedure using catheters and opaque dye to analyze heart function and coronary blood flow.

*cardiac tamponade* Compression of the heart due to the accumulation of blood in the pericardial sac following rupture of the wall of the heart.

*cardiogenic shock* A situation in which the heart cannot maintain an adequate cardiac output.

*catecholamines* A group of sympathomimetic compounds that have significant cardiopulmonary effects.

*central training effects* Training effects that can be measured by changes in cardiac function.

*cholinergic* Type of medications or receptor sites that stimulate the parasympathetic nervous system.

*chronotropic* Affecting the rate of the heart beat.

*cilia* Hairlike projections from respiratory epithelial cells that propel mucus and debris toward the pharynx.

*coagulopathy* Disorder of clotting.

*commissurotomy* A surgical procedure to separate adherent leaves of a stenosed mitral valve.

*compliance* (1) The ability of tissue (lung or chest wall) to expand. High compliance means easy expandibility; low compliance means poor expandibility. Measured as ratio of volume change to pressure change. (2) A patient's adherence to program instructions and to suggestions for risk-factor reduction.

*congestive heart failure* Inability of the left side of the heart to maintain cardiac output at rest, which results in pulmonary congestion.

*cor pulmonale* Right-sided heart failure because of pulmonary hypertension caused by pulmonary disease.

*coronary collateralization* Development of blood vessels in or around areas of poor blood flow.

*coronary insufficiency* Inadequate blood flow through the coronary arteries to meet myocardial oxygen demands.

*CPK isoenzyme fraction* Blood-borne isoenzyme that is released after myocardial necrosis. The isoenzyme of creatine phosphokinase (CPK) is MB.

*decubitus posture* Side-lying position.

*defibrillation* Electrical shock of sufficient power to cause a fibrillating heart to resume normal electrical activity.

*dehiscence* Splitting open of a surgical wound.

*diaphoresis* Sweating.

*diffusion* Random movement of gas molecules along a gradient based on differences in partial pressure of gas. Accounts for the movement of oxygen into and carbon dioxide out of the blood in the pulmonary capillaries.

*dimer* A compound formed by the union of two radicals or two molecules of a simpler compound.

*distribution* Dispersion of gas throughout the lung fields.

*diuretic* Type of medication used to decrease body fluid and thereby decrease blood volume. Often used to control congestive heart failure and hypertension. Examples include furosemide (Lasix), Dyazide (triamterene and hydrochlorothiazide), and the thiazide diuretics.

*driving force* Force generated by respiratory muscles to move air through the airways.

*dysphagia* Pain and difficulty during swallowing.

*dyspnea* Inability to take a normal breath because of labored breathing. The sensation of not being able to catch your breath.

*echocardiography* Ultrasonic waves directed through the heart and reflected back towards the source to study the structure and motion of the heart.

*effusion* Abnormal collection of fluid (commonly seen in the pleura).

*egophony (tragophony)* The change in a voice sound from *a* to *e*, somewhat like the bleating of a goat (from Greek *aix, aig-,* 'goat,' and *phōnē,* 'voice').

*ejection fraction* A hemodynamic measurement of the stroke volume divided by end-diastolic volume. Ejection fraction indicates resting heart function, with normal being 55 to 65 m².

*empyema* The accumulation of pus in a body cavity, such as the pleural space, especially with bacterial infection.

*endotracheal tube* A plastic tube that is inserted orally or nasally to provide direct access into the trachea. These tubes are commonly attached to mechanical ventilators.

*eosinophil* White blood cell associated with asthma and allergy.

*epiglottis* Cartilage that protects the trachea from aspirated foodstuff during the normal swallowing process.

*esophageal atresia* Incomplete development of the esophagus.

*extracorporeal oxygenation* Use of an artificial membrane outside the body to provide for oxygenation in a patient with severe lung disease.

*fibrillae* The many tiny threads that a striated muscle fiber can be split into.

*fibrinolysis* Destruction of fibrin by fibrinolysin.

*fissure* Clearly discernible divisions in lung tissue that separate the lobes of the lungs.

*Frank-Starling mechanism* The force exerted with a heart beat is directly proportional to the degree of stretch or lengthening of the myocardial fibers.

*fremitus* Vibrations within the thorax that can be palpated.

*gastroepiploic foramen* A passage between the peritoneal cavity and the monetal bursa.

*glycogenolysis* Change of glycogen into glucose for use by body tissues.

*goblet cells* Mucus-producing cells found in the respiratory epithelium.

*hemopneumothorax* An accumulation of air and blood in the pleural cavity.

*hemoptysis* Pulmonary hemorrhage.

*huffing* Forced expiration with an open glottis to replace coughing when pain is a major factor that limits coughing.

*hydrostatic densitometry* Underwater weighing to determine a person's lean to fat body weight.

*hypercapnia (hypercarbia)* Increased arterial carbon dioxide level.

*hyperlipidemia* Excessive fat content in the blood, specifically elevated cholesterols and triglycerides.

*hyperoxygenation* The use of high concentrations of inspired oxygen before and after endotracheal aspiration.

*hypertrophic cardiomyopathy* Abnormal cardiac hypertrophy, having numerous causes, that results in poor cardiac function.

*hyperventilation* Increase in alveolar ventilation resulting in decreased arterial carbon dioxide level.

*hypoadaptive blood pressure* (see also **hypotension**) Abnormally low blood pressure at rest.

*hypocapnia (hypocarbia)* Decreased arterial carbon dioxide level.

*hypotension* (see also **hypoadaptive blood pressure**) A fall in systolic blood pressure with an increase in exertion or heart rate, or both.

*hypoventilation* Decrease in alveolar ventilation resulting in increased arterial carbon dioxide level.

*hypoxemia* Low arterial oxygen tension.

*immunofluorescent staining* A technique for identifying an antigen by exposing it to known antibodies tagged with fluorescent dyes that cause an antigen-antibody reaction that appears luminous under fluorescent light.

*immunoglobulins* Circulating antibodies that protect against foreign substances, including microorganisms.

*insufflation* To blow gas or powder into a tube, cavity, or organ to permit visual inspection, to remove an obstruction, or to apply medication.

*intermittent mandatory ventilation* A mode of mechanical ventilation that guarantees a specific minute volume to the patient but simultaneously permits the patient to breathe spontaneously.

*intraventricular conduction defects* Loss of the normal electrical conduction system in the ventricles.

*ischemia* Inadequate blood flow to meet the metabolic demands of tissue.

*isocapnic* Condition in which the carbon dioxide level remains unchanged despite changing levels of ventilation.

*Lambert's canals* Channels connecting alveoli with respiratory bronchioles.

*laparotomy* Surgical incision into the peritoneal cavity.

*lavage* The process of washing out an organ for therapeutic purposes.

*ligand* An organic molecule attached to a specific site on a surface or to a tracer element.

*lipolysis* Destruction of lipids or fats.

*lithotripsy* A procedure for eliminating a kidney stone by crushing or dissolving it in situ.

*lymphokines* Chemical products of T lymphocytes that attract macrophages to a site of infection or inflammation and prepare them for attack.

*meconium* The first stool passed by a newborn.

*metabolic acidosis* Decreased arterial pH caused by a nonrespiratory disorder.

*metabolic alkalosis* Increased arterial pH caused by a nonrespiratory disorder.

*minute ventilation* The volume of air inspired or expired in 1 minute.

*moeity* Part of a molecule that exhibits a particular set of chemical and pharmacologic characteristics.

*mouthstick* Mouth-operated control stick for a power wheelchair.

*mucociliary transport* The process of removal of mucus and debris within the mucus by means of the wavelike motion of cilia lining the respiratory epithelium.

*muscle bridging* Myocardium bridges over one or more of the large epicardial coronary vessels causing constriction during systole.

*MV̇o₂* Myocardial oxygen consumption.

*myocardial infarction* Death of heart muscle tissue.

*obstructive disease* Disorders characterized by obstruction of airways.

*orthotopic* In the normal or usual position.

*osteoarthropathy* Swelling and pain within the joints caused by numerous chronic pulmonary infections and other disorders. Can mimic early rheumatoid arthritis.

*osteopenia (osteoporosis)* Reduction in the amount of bone substance per unit volume of bone tissue.

*oximeter* Device used to measure oxygen level.

*oxygen toxicity* An inflammatory response of the lung tissue to exceedingly high concentrations of inspired oxygen over long periods.

*parietal pleura* The layer of the pleural sac adjacent to the chest wall.

*pathophysiology* The science of pathological processes and their effects on normal tissue.

*pectoriloquy* Transmission to the chest of a whispered sound.

*pectus carinatum* "Pigeon breast" deformity, a protrusion of the sternum and costal cartilages.

*pectus excavatum* "Funnel chest" deformity, a sunken sternum and costal cartilages.

*perfusion* Flow of pulmonary blood or other fluid through the vessels.

*pericarditis* Inflammation of the pericardium (sac that encloses the heart).

*phenotype* Inherited blood type. Referred to here in relation to cholesterol levels in the blood.

*physiologic dead space* Areas of the lung that are well ventilated but poorly perfused with blood.

*placenta previa* Development of the placenta low in the uterus that may cause the uterus to rupture and hemorrhage.

*plethysmograph* Airtight "body box" that is used to measure various pulmonary function values.

*pleura* Two-layered sac that encases the lungs.

*plexus* Group of nerves.

*pneumomediastinum* Leakage of free air into the mediastinum.

*pores of Kohn* Channels connecting adjacent alveoli.

*positive inotropic* Pertaining to any phenomenon that increases cardiac contractility; most commonly a glycoside medication like digoxin or digitalis.

*preload* The volume of blood in the left ventricle just before systole, the end-diastolic volume.

*progression of coronary artery disease* Worsening of the obstructive processes of coronary atherosclerosis.

*R-on-T phenomenon* A dysrhythmia characterized by premature ventricular contraction that occurs on or before the completion of the T wave of the previous beat. Associated with acute ventricular fibrillation and sudden death.

*radiolucent* Radiographic density that appears very dark, indicating material through which the x-ray beam passes easily, such as air.

*radionuclide ventriculography* Use of a radiopaque contrast medium by which to examine a heart ventricle.

*radiopaque* Radiographic density that appears white, indicating material through which the x-ray beam does not pass well, such as bone or metal.

*rate-pressure product* Heart rate multiplied by systolic blood pressure. A clinical indicator of myocardial oxygen demand.

*regression of coronary artery disease* Decrease in the obstructive processes of coronary atherosclerosis.

*respiratory acidosis* Decreased arterial pH caused by respiratory disorder.

*restrictive disease* Disorders characterized by restriction of expansion by the lungs or chest wall.

*revascularization* Ischemic or potentially ischemic areas that are provided, either surgically or naturally, with an alternative blood supply.

*splenorrhaphy* Suturing a ruptured spleen.

*stenosis* Narrowing of a tube, such as tracheal stenosis.

*stroke volume* Volume of blood, in millimeters, ejected from the heart with each beat.

*subcutaneous emphysema* Leakage of free air into the subcutaneous tissue.

*subendocardial* Pertaining to a nontransmural infarction. Myocardial necrosis is limited to the subendocardium.

*surfactant* Material produced by type II alveolar cells that serves to reduce surface tension in the alveoli.

*sympathomimetic bronchodilators* Medications that are useful in reducing bronchial muscle spasm because of their action that mimics the sympathetic nervous system response, resulting in reduced smooth muscle spasm.

*sympathomimetics* Group of pharmacologic agents that mimic activity of the sympathetic nervous system to achieve a response by various organs and structures.

*syncope* Sudden, but transient, unconsciousness. (Pronounced sing'ko-pee)

*thoracentesis (thoracocentesis)* Removal of fluid from the thorax, usually through a wide-lumen syringe.

*torr* Unit name for mm Hg (millimeters of mercury).

*tracheoesophageal fistula* Abnormal communication between the esophagus and trachea.

*tracheomalacia* Eroding of the trachea because of excessive pressure from a cuffed endotracheal tube.

*transmural infarction* Necrosis that extends across the full thickness of the myocardium from the endocardium to the epicardium.

*unstable angina pectoris* Preinfarction chest pain characterized by discomfort occurring at rest and low levels of activity.

*uremic syndrome* Toxic amounts of urea and other nitrogenous waste materials accumulating in the blood, as occurs in renal failure.

*ventilation* The process in which air moves into the lungs in preparation for gas exchange.

*ventricular dysfunction* Myocardial dysfunction within the ventricles that exhibits abnormalities in contraction and wall motion.

*ventricular tachycardia* Life-threatening dysrhythmia usually associated with a high rate and a series of ventricular ectopic beats (three in a row).

*ventriculotomy* Incision into a ventricle.

*visceral pleura* The inner layer of pleura that is adjacent to the external lung tissue.

*weaning* Coordinated effort to remove the patient from dependency on mechanical ventilation.

# Index

Page numbers in *italics* indicate illustrations. Page numbers followed by a *t* indicate tables.